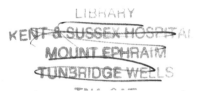

TRAUMA NURSING

From Resuscitation Through Rehabilitation

KAREN A. MCQUILLAN, RN, MS, CCRN, CNRN
Clinical Nurse Specialist, R Adams Cowley Shock Trauma Center
University of Maryland Medical Center
Baltimore, Maryland

KATHRYN TRUTER VON RUEDEN, RN, MS, FCCM
Senior Clinical Consultant
APACHE Medical Systems, Inc.
McLean, Virginia

ROBBI LYNN HARTSOCK, RN, MSN, CRNP
Trauma Nurse Coordinator, R Adams Cowley Shock Trauma Center
University of Maryland Medical Center
Baltimore, Maryland

MARY BETH FLYNN, RN, MS, CNS, CCRN
Clinical Nurse Specialist/Educator and Senior Instructor
University of Colorado Health Science Center
School of Nursing
Denver, Colorado

EILEEN WHALEN, RN, BSN, MHA
Director, Critical Care and Emergency Services
Saint Mary's Regional Medical Center
Reno, Nevada
(Past president of the Society of Trauma Nurses)

TRAUMA NURSING

From Resuscitation Through Rehabilitation

3rd Edition

W.B. SAUNDERS COMPANY

A Harcourt Health Sciences Company

Philadelphia   London   New York   St. Louis   Sydney   Toronto

W.B. SAUNDERS COMPANY
A Harcourt Health Sciences Company

The Curtis Center
Independence Square West
Philadelphia, Pennsylvania 19106-3399

Vice President and Publishing Director, Nursing: Sally Schrefer
Executive Editor: Susan Epstein
Senior Developmental Editor: Sharon Malchow
Project Manager: John Rogers
Project Specialist: Cheryl Abbott
Designer: Kathi Gosche

Library of Congress Cataloging-in-Publication Data

Trauma nursing : from resuscitation through rehabilitation.—3rd ed. / Karen A.
McQuillan ... [et al.].
    p. ; cm.
    Includes bibliographical references and index.
    ISBN 0-7216-8441-6
    1. Wounds and injuries—Nursing.   I. McQuillan, Karen A.
    [DNLM: 1. Emergencies—nursing.   2. Wounds and Injuries—nursing. WY 154 T777 2002]
RD93.95 .T73 2002
617.1′026′024613—dc21

                                                                    2001042916

Trauma Nursing: From Resuscitation Through Rehabilitation, 3rd Edition   ISBN 0-7216-8441-6

Printed in the United States of America

Last digit is the print number: 02   03   04   05   GW/MV   9   8   7   6   5   4   3   2   1

To my family:
My mom and dad,
who taught me life's most important lessons
that proved so valuable in persevering to complete
this project;
my husband, who taught me to believe in myself; and
my children, who taught me what is most important in life.

Karen A. McQuillan

To my parents,
Genevieve and Edmund Truter,
and to my sister,
Carolyn Truter Johnson,
for their encouragement, counsel, and unmitigated love.

Kathryn Truter Von Rueden

To my parents,
Lewis and Mildred,
whose unconditional love and support has
been ever-present throughout my life.

Robbi Lynn Hartsock

To my parents,
husband, and children,
who believed in me and supported me
through this endeavor and
throughout my career.

Mary Beth Flynn

I want to thank my husband
Bob
and my son
Alex Heilig
for their encouragement, love, and support.
Our life is never without adventure!
Special thanks to the members
of the Society of Trauma Nurses
because your vision is key
to the advancement of trauma nursing.

Eileen Whalen

CONTRIBUTORS

SHARON L. ATWELL, RN, PhD(c), CFRN
Flight Nurse
Critical Air Medicine
Galveston, Texas
Trauma in the Elderly

MARY BEACHLEY, MS, RN, CEN
Director, Office of Hospital Programs
Maryland Institute for Emergency Medical Services Systems
Baltimore, Maryland
Evolution of the Trauma Cycle

JANET M. BEEBE, MS, CRNP-A, CCRN
Nurse Practitioner
Bowie Internal Medicine
Bowie, Maryland
Substance Abuse and Trauma Care

SHARON A. BOSWELL, RN, BSN
Full Partner and Research Nurse
R Adams Cowley Shock Trauma Center
University of Maryland Medical Center
Baltimore, Maryland
Initial Management of Traumatic Shock

T. CATHERINE BOWER, RN, BSN, CPAN
Senior Partner, Nursing PCA Service
University of Maryland Medical Center
BelAir, Maryland
Analgesia, Sedation, and Neuromuscular Blockade in the Trauma Patient

PATRICIA B. CASPER, RN, CRNP
Nurse Practitioner
R Adams Cowley Shock Trauma Center
University of Maryland Medical System
Baltimore, Maryland
Infection and Infection Control

FRANKI CHABALEWSKI, RN, MS
Professional Services Coordinator
United Network for Organ Sharing (UNOS)
Richmond, Virginia
The Organ and Tissue Donor

DONNA YORK CLARK, RN, MS
Program Director
Dartmouth–Hitchcock Advanced Response Team
Lebanon, New Hampshire
Prehospital Care of the Trauma Patient

CHERYL EDWARDS, RN, MS, CS
Organ Transplant Coordinator
Yale New Haven Hospital
Waterbury, Connecticut
The Organ and Tissue Donor

JOCELYN A. FARRAR, RN, MS, CCRN, ACNP
Instructor
Villa Julie College, School of Nursing
Mount Airy, Maryland
Psychosocial Impact of Trauma Care

MARY KATE FITZPATRICK, RN, MSN
Trauma Program Manager
Division of Traumatology and Surgical Critical Care
University of Pennsylvania Medical Center
Philadelphia, Pennsylvania
Performance Improvement in Trauma Care

MARY BETH FLYNN, RN, MS, CNS, CCRN
Clinical Nurse Specialist/Educator
University of Colorado Hospital
and
Senior Instructor
University of Colorado Health Science Center,
    School of Nursing
Denver, Colorado
Burn Injuries • Wound Healing

CAROLYN J. FOWLER, PhD, MPH
Director, Injury Prevention Program
Baltimore County Department of Health
and
Assistant Public Health Professor
Center for Injury Research and Policy
The Johns Hopkins Bloomberg School of Public Health
Towson, Maryland
Injury Prevention

ROBBI LYNN HARTSOCK, RN, MSN, CRNP
Trauma Nurse Coordinator
R Adams Cowley Shock Trauma Center
University of Maryland Medical System
Baltimore, Maryland
Nursing Practice Through the Cycle of Trauma • Thoracic Injuries

ROBERT W. HEILIG, JD, MPH, RN
Principal
Robert W. Heilig & Associates
Incline Village, Nevada
Legal Concerns in Trauma Nursing

KAREN KLENDER HEIST, RN, MS
Management Consultant
Ellicott City, Maryland
Trauma Rehabilitation

CONNIE A. JASTREMSKI, MS, MBA, RN, ANP-CS, FCCM
Assistant Vice President, Nursing
Rome Memorial Hospital
Cazenovia, New York
Economic Issues in Trauma Care

MANJARI JOSHI, MD
Associate Professor of Medicine
R Adams Cowley Shock Trauma Center
University of Maryland Medical System
Baltimore, Maryland
Infection and Infection Control

CATHERINE J. KLEIN, PhD, RD
Clinical Coordinator in Research
Division of Critical Care Medicine
R Adams Crowley Shock Trauma Center
University of Maryland Medical System
Baltimore, Maryland
*Metabolic and Nutritional Management
  of the Trauma Patient*

JORIE D. KLEIN, RN
Director, Trauma Services
Parkland Health and Hospital System
Dallas, Texas
Mechanism of Injury

BARBARA MCLEAN, MN, RN, CCRN, CCNS-NP, FCCM
Critical Care Consultant
Grady Memorial Hospital
Atlanta, Georgia
Shock and Multiple Organ Dysfunction Syndrome

JANET MCMASTER, RN, MS
Trauma Performance Improvement Coordinator
Division of Traumatology and Surgical Critical Care
University of Pennsylvania Medical Center
Philadelphia, Pennsylvania
Performance Improvement in Trauma Care

KAREN A. MCQUILLAN, RN, MS, CCRN, CNRN
Clinical Nurse Specialist
R Adams Cowley Shock Trauma Center,
University of Maryland Medical System
Baltimore, Maryland
*Traumatic Brain Injuries • Maxillofacial Injuries • Soft Tissue
  Injuries*

PAMELA H. MITCHELL, PhD, RN, CNRN, FAAN
Associate Dean for Research, Elizabeth S. Soule Professor
  of Nursing and Adjunct Professor
School of Public Health and Community Medicine
University of Washington
Seattle, Washington
Traumatic Brain Injuries

**PATRICIA A. MOLONEY-HARMON,
  RN, MS, CCNS, CCRN**
Advanced Practice Nurse/Clinical Nurse Specialist,
  Children's Services
The Children's Hospital at Sinai
Baltimore, Maryland
Pediatric Trauma

JEAN M. MONTONYE, RN, MS
Clinical Therapy Specialist
Hill-Rom Company, Inc.
Golden, Colorado
Abdominal Injuries

DONNA A. NAYDUCH, RN-CS, MSN, ACNP
Regional Trauma Director
Banner Health System
Evans, Colorado
Genitourinary Injuries and Renal Management

JOAN M. PRYOR-MCCANN, PhD, RN, CNS
Associate Professor of Nursing
Otterbein College
Westerville, Ohio
Ethics in Trauma Nursing

BRADLEY C. ROBERTSON, MD, DDS
Associate Professor and Chief,
Plastic, Reconstructive, and Maxillofacial Surgery
R Adams Cowley Shock Trauma Center
University of Maryland Medical System
Baltimore, Maryland
Maxillofacial Injuries

TAMMY A. RUSSO-MCCOURT, RN, BSN, CCRN
Full Partner, Neurotrauma Critical Care Unit
R Adams Cowley Shock Trauma Center
University of Maryland Medical System
Baltimore, Maryland
Spinal Cord Injuries

THOMAS M. SCALEA, MD, FACS, FCCM
Physician-in-Chief
R Adams Cowley Shock Trauma Center
University of Maryland Medical System
Baltimore, Maryland
Initial Management of Traumatic Shock

SUZANNE FREY SHERWOOD, RN, MS
Full Partner, Trauma Resuscitation Unit
R Adams Cowley Shock Trauma Center
University of Maryland Medical System
and
Clinical Instructor
University of Maryland at Baltimore, School of Nursing
Baltimore, Maryland
Thoracic Injuries

NAVIN SINGH, MD
Assistant Professor,
Plastic, Reconstructive, and Maxillofacial Surgery
R Adams Cowley Shock Trauma Center
University of Maryland Medical Systems
Baltimore, Maryland
Soft Tissue Injuries

LYNN GERBER SMITH, MS, RN
Clinical Education Coordinator
R Adams Cowley Shock Trauma Center
University of Maryland Medical Systems
Baltimore, Maryland
The Pregnant Trauma Patient

SARAH C. SMITH, RN, MA, CRNO
Advanced Practice Nurse
Department of Ophthalmology
The University of Iowa Hospitals & Clinics
Oxford, Iowa
Ocular Injuries

GENA STIVER STANEK, RN, MS
Clinical Nurse Specialist
R Adams Cowley Shock Trauma Center
University of Maryland Medical System
Baltimore, Maryland
*Metabolic and Nutritional Management
of the Trauma Patient*

BETH A. VANDERHEYDEN, PharmD, BCPS, FASHP
Critical Care Specialist
University of Maryland Medical System
Belcamp, Maryland
*Analgesia, Sedation, and Neuromuscular Blockade in the
Trauma Patient*

THOMAS C. VARY, PhD
Professor, Department of Cellular and Molecular
Physiology
Pennsylvania State University College of Medicine
Hershey, Pennsylvania
Shock and Multiple Organ Dysfunction Syndrome

KATHRYN TRUTER VON RUEDEN, RN, MS, FCCM
Senior Clinical Consultant
APACHE Medical Systems, Inc.
McLean, Virginia
*Nursing Practice through the Cycle of Trauma • Shock
and Multiple Organ Dysfunction Syndrome*

COLLEEN R. WALSH, RN, MSN, ONC, CS, ACNP
Faculty, Graduate Nursing
University of Southern Indiana
Evansville, Indiana
and
Adjunct Assistant Professor
University of South Alabama
Mobile, Alabama
Musculoskeletal Injuries

JOHN A. WEIGELT, DVM, MD
Professor and Vice Chairman, Department of Surgery
Medical College of Wisconsin
and
Medical Director, Trauma Program
Froedtert Memorial Lutheran Hospital
Milwaukee, Wisconsin
Mechanism of Injury

EILEEN WHALEN, MHA, BSN, RN
Director, Critical Care/Emergency Services
Saint Mary's Regional Medical Center
Reno, Nevada
Administrative Issues in Trauma Care

REVIEWERS

ANDREW R. BURGESS, MD
Professor and Interim Chair
Department of Orthopedic Surgery
University of Maryland School of Medicine
Baltimore, Maryland

EDWARD E. CORNWELL III, MD, FACS, FCCM
Chief, Adult Trauma Services
The Johns Hopkins University
Baltimore, Maryland

C. MICHAEL DUNHAM, MD, FACS, FCCM
St. Elizabeth Health Care Center
and Northeastern Ohio Universities College of Medicine
Youngstown, Ohio

MARY KATE FITZPATRICK, RN, MSN
Trauma Program Manager
University of Pennsylvania Medical Center
Philadelphia, Pennsylvania

PAMELA FRANKEL, RN, MS, ACNP-CS
Portland, Oregon

ERKAN HASSAN, PharmD, FCCM
Director of Pharmacotherapy
VISICU
Baltimore, Maryland

PEGGY HOLLINGSWORTH-FRIDLUND, RN
Trauma Nurse Coordinator
University of California—San Diego
San Diego, California

ANNE GRAFTON HOPKINS, RN, MS, CCRN
Full Partner
R Adams Cowley Shock Trauma Center
University of Maryland Medical System
Baltimore, Maryland

NICHOLAS T. ILIFF, MD
Director of Oculoplastic and Reconstructive Surgery
Associate Professor of Ophthalmology
The Johns Hopkins University
Baltimore, Maryland

ELENA KELLER, RN, CRNP
Nurse Practitioner
Soft Tissue Service
R Adams Cowley Shock Trauma Center
University of Maryland Medical System
Baltimore, Maryland

MAJOR GRETA L. KRAPOHL, RN, MSN
Fort Bragg, North Carolina

ANN BUTLER MAHER, MS, RN, FNPC, ONC
Family Nurse Practitioner
Jersey Battered Women's Service
Morris Plains, New Jersey

ROBERT C. MCINTYRE, JR., MD
Associate Professor of Surgery
University of Colorado Health Sciences Center
Denver, Colorado

DAVID A. NAGEY, MD, PhD
Director, Perinatal Outreach Program
Associate Professor
Department of OB/GYN, Population and Family Health
    Sciences
The Johns Hopkins University
Baltimore, Maryland

CAROL A. RAUEN, RN, MS, CCRN
Georgetown University School of Nursing
Washington, District of Columbia

H. NEAL REYNOLDS, MD
Associate Professor of Medicine
University of Maryland School of Medicine
R Adams Cowley Shock Trauma Center
Baltimore, Maryland

MICHAEL RHODES, MD, FACS
Chairman
Department of Surgery
Christiana Care Health Services
Wilmington, Deleware
and
Professor of Surgery
Thomas Jefferson University
Philadelphia, Pennsylvania

RALPH N. ROGERS, MD, MBA, FACEP
Associate Clinical Professor of Medicine
Michigan State University
and
Medical Director and COO
Aero Med at Spectrum Health
Grand Rapids, Michigan

Bonnie Sakallaris, RN, MSN, CCRN
Director of Cardiology/Cardiac Services
Washington Hospital Center
Washington, District of Columbia

Carl A. Soderstrom, MD
Director of Physician Education
R Adams Cowley Shock Trauma Center
University of Maryland Medical System
and
Professor of Surgery
University of Maryland School of Medicine
Baltimore, Maryland

Laura A. Stephens, RN, BSN
Hospital Development Coordinator
Donor Alliance
Denver, Colorado

Lance R. Stone, DO
Medical Director, Rehabilitation Services
University of California—San Diego Medical Center
San Diego, California

David P. Tarantino, MD, MBA
Director of Pain Management Services
R Adams Cowley Shock Trauma Center
University of Maryland Medical System
and
Assistant Professor of Anesthesiology
University of Maryland School of Medicine
Baltimore, Maryland

Deborah Tribett, RN, MS, CS, CRNP
Adult and Acute Care Nurse Practitioner
Chesapeake Cardiology
Easton, Maryland

Linda Vader, RN, CRNO
Head Nurse
W.K. Kellogg Eye Center
University of Michigan
Ann Arbor, Michigan

Charisse Wasem, RPh, BCNSP
Clinical Pharmacist
University of Colorado Hospital
Denver, Colorado

FOREWORD

In 1985, I was fortunate to be one of a group of clinical specialists working at the R Adams Cowley Shock Trauma Center in Baltimore, Maryland. Our Director of Nursing at the time was Elizabeth Scanlon, RN, MS, a visionary in the field of trauma nursing. She believed that what had been learned up to that time about the care of trauma patients from a nursing perspective should be integrated into a textbook and that her clinical specialists should be the authors and editors for this project. For the next three years, we assembled expert practitioners in the field of trauma to make this venture become a reality, and in 1988 the first edition of *Trauma Nursing: From Resuscitation Through Rehabilitation* was published.

I had been dedicated to trauma nursing since 1967, when I spent a year in Vietnam caring for the wounded in an evacuation hospital. I was inspired by how soldiers with devastating injuries could survive without the technology and medications that are standard in trauma centers today. It was there that I learned the "art" of trauma nursing. There were no cardiac monitors, sophisticated ventilators, or even enough medical supplies. But as we watched our patients, we came to recognize that physical changes were imminent and thus were able to institute treatments that were effective. After Vietnam I continued my career in trauma care, now working with traumatically injured patients as a case manager for the military.

Trauma nurses are exposed to great sadness and heartache when patients do not survive or are permanently disabled. They share the shock and devastation of families as they guide them through the most difficult time of their lives. When a brain-injured patient follows commands for the first time, they also rejoice with the patient and family. Likewise, when a patient who survives devastating injury leaves the trauma center, they rejoice in the miracle of God's work, sometimes not recognizing or understanding how their own valiant efforts and dedication to established trauma protocols played a hand in the patient's survival. When patients are lost, trauma practitioners ask, "What more could I have done?" We must never stop asking that question, because it allows the continued development of protocols and research to verify medical and nursing treatments. The need for this development will always be there.

During the past 30 years, gigantic steps in trauma management have revolutionized this multidisciplinary field of care. While technology has assisted in this advancement, intuition and development of evidenced-based protocols that have been tested time after time guide the care of the traumatically injured. Centers of excellence for trauma care have multiplied, but there is still work to be done to improve outcomes for injured patients.

Trauma nursing also continues to expand into new territory. Trauma nurses play a vital role in trauma prevention initiatives such as being active in legislative efforts to enact laws that protect the public from traumatic injury. They also work collaboratively with physicians and industries to design safer consumer products and to develop innovative devices and techniques that improve the care of injured patients. Expert trauma nurses also speak in forums throughout the world on trauma and nursing care.

Advances in trauma care are so rapid and ever changing that one can hardly publish them before they are outdated. The second edition of *Trauma Nursing* carried on the task of offering the trauma practitioner the latest in trauma care. And now a third edition has evolved. I am confident this edition will be the best yet. The editors of this edition are dedicated practitioners who understand the "disease" of trauma. They have invited new authors to share their knowledge and expertise and have expanded the topics to create the most comprehensive text on trauma nursing yet. I hope that many more editions will follow, for they will always be necessary to keep practitioners abreast of the latest in trauma care.

I am proud to have been one of the original authors of this textbook, and I am honored to contribute to this third edition. I am even more proud to watch new authors and editors put into writing the expertise they have achieved in the field of trauma nursing. This edition will not disappoint you. Just as the previous editions have been instrumental in the training and education of today's trauma nurses, this collaborative effort will make the third edition a classic in the training and education of future trauma nurses.

My respect for trauma nurses never wanes. They are dedicated, energetic individuals who strive to keep learning so that the best care can be provided. Godspeed to the authors, editors, and readers of this textbook, as well as to those who will come in the future.

Virginia D. Cardona, MS, RN
Case Manager
Sierra Military Health Services
Baltimore, Maryland

PREFACE

Research developments and practice changes in the dynamic field of trauma care necessitate a third edition of the highly acclaimed text, *Trauma Nursing: From Resuscitation Through Rehabilitation*. Like the first two editions of this text, the third edition provides a comprehensive description of the art and science of trauma nursing. It builds on the strengths of the previous editions while updating content, expanding on specific topics, and introducing relevant new material.

The third edition of *Trauma Nursing: From Resuscitation Through Rehabilitation* employs the unique cycle of trauma framework that was used in previous editions. This format provides the reader with an easy-to-follow organization of material describing evaluation and management of the trauma patient through the continuum of trauma care, including prevention and prehospital considerations; resuscitation; and the operative, critical, intermediate, and rehabilitation phases of care. Evidence-based information about issues that effect trauma care systems, injury pathophysiology, and currently recommended assessment and care of the trauma patient are described for each phase of the trauma cycle.

This edition of *Trauma Nursing: From Resuscitation Through Rehabilitation* has added new chapters focusing on performance improvement, trauma prevention, and prehospital care reflecting the greater emphasis on these areas in the current health care environment. These chapters highlight the essential roles that nurses have in these areas of trauma care. Clinical decisions regarding the use of sedation, analgesia, and neuromuscular blockade often occur in tandem, and therefore an expanded discussion about sedation strategies and neuromuscular blocking agents has been added to the chapter on pain management. Soft tissue injuries and maxillofacial trauma have been separated into two distinct chapters to provide a more thorough discussion of each type of injury.

The four major parts of the text include:

Part I, "General Concepts in Trauma Nursing," covers healthcare concerns that affect trauma care facilities and trauma systems, ultimately affecting the care of trauma patients. These concerns include economic, administrative, quality improvement, ethical, and legal issues related to trauma care. Injury prevention, prehospital care, and rehabilitation of trauma patients are also discussed in this section.

Part II, "Clinical Management Concepts," addresses specific issues that affect all trauma patients regardless of their injury. These topics include mechanism of injury; pathophysiology and management of traumatic shock; psychosocial adaptations of the patient and family; infection; wound healing; metabolic and nutrition management; and management of pain, sedation, and neuromuscular blockade.

Part III, "Single System Injuries," describes the pathophysiology, assessment, and state-of-the-art treatment of specific types of systemic injuries throughout each of the phases of trauma care.

Part IV, "Unique Patient Populations," reviews the special trauma care considerations and needs of unique patient groups such as pregnant women, children, the elderly, burned patients, those with a history of substance abuse, and organ donors.

This text, authored by content experts from around the country, will serve as an excellent research-based reference for the novice and the experienced nurse caring for trauma patients in a variety of settings. Clinicians, advanced practitioners, researchers, administrators, managers, educators, and students will find this text a useful and comprehensive reference for trauma-related issues. It is our hope that knowledge gained using this resource will enhance your ability to achieve optimal outcomes for your patients as they progress through the cycle of trauma care.

Karen A. McQuillan, RN, MS, CCRN, CNRN
Kathryn Truter Von Rueden, RN, MS, FCCM
Robbi Lynn Hartsock RN, MSN, CRNP
Mary Beth Flynn, RN, MS, CNS, CCRN
Eileen Whalen, RN, BSN, MHA

ACKNOWLEDGMENTS

We wish to thank the following authors, whose contributions to the first and second editions made this textbook such a successful endeavor:

Judith K. Bobb
Virginia D. Cardona
Howard R. Champion
Warren T. Chave
Linda S. Cook
Christine Cottingham
Margareta K. Cuccia
Sandra L. Deli
Patricia C. Epifanio
Pamela Phillips Gaul
Erkan Hassan
Benny Hooper
Nancy J. Hoyt
Patricia D. Hurn
Connie Joy
James W. Karesh
Marguerite T. Littleton Kearney
Paula M. Kelly
Barbara J. Keyes
Karen M. Kleeman
Melva Kravitz
Steven Linberg
Susan M. Luff
Marcia S. Mabee

Mary E. Mancini
Janet A. Marvin
Paula J. Bastnagel Mason
Roy L. Mason
Patricia E. McCabe
Paul McClelland
Anne F. McCormack
Gerri Spielman McGinnis
Carolyn Milligan
Mary Murphy-Rutter
Lisa Robinson
Elizabeth Scanlan
Ann M. Scanlon
Barbara E. Schott
Ellen K. Shair
Julie Mull Strange
Peggy Trimble
Susan W. Veise-Berry
Constance A. Walleck
Neil Warres
JoAnne D. Whitney
Margaret Widner-Kolberg
Charles E. Wiles III
Joyce S. Willens

We would also like to thank Linda J. Kesselring, MS, ELS, who did a spectacular job providing us with feedback that enhanced the quality of our written message, and Carolyn G. Schmitt, who unselfishly gave of her time and talents to provide secretarial support for this project.

CONTENTS

PART IV   UNIQUE PATIENT POPULATIONS 717

29   Pediatric Trauma

30   Trauma in the Elderly   *Sharon L. Atwell* 772

31   Burn Injuries   *Mary Beth Flynn* 788

32   Substance Abuse and Trauma Care

33   The Organ and Tissue Donor

GENERAL CONCEPTS IN TRAUMA NURSING

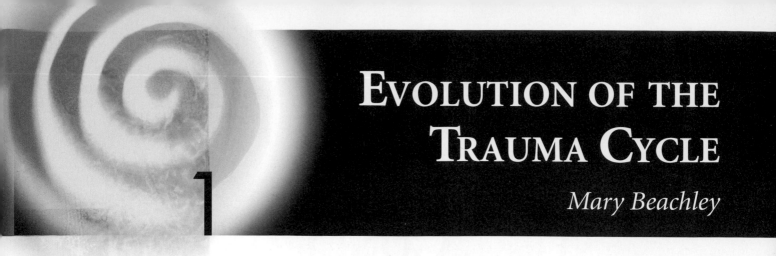

EVOLUTION OF THE TRAUMA CYCLE

Mary Beachley

For everything there is a season, and a time for every matter under heaven:
a time to be born, and a time to die;
a time to plant and a time to pluck up what is planted;
a time to kill, and a time to heal;
a time to break down and a time to build up;
a time to weep, and a time to laugh;
a time to mourn, and a time to dance;
a time to cast away stones, and a time to gather stones together;
a time to embrace, and a time to refrain from embracing;
a time to seek, and a time to lose;
a time to keep, and a time to cast away;
a time to rend, and a time to sew;
a time to keep silence, and a time to speak;
a time to love, and a time to hate;
a time for war, and a time for peace.

Ecclesiastes 3:1-9 (RSV)

Trauma continues to occur in epidemic proportions in our society today; however, this is not a new phenomenon. Traumatic injury has been recognized as a part of the human experience since early civilization. Anthropologic studies of the bony remains of Neanderthal humans have shown that this group sustained a great deal of trauma during their lifetime.[1] Disfigured skeletal structures and long-term bony calcification are evidence that the trauma that they experienced was a result of their relatively dangerous lifestyle. Many injuries were sustained secondary to constant exposure to the raw elements of nature, including frequent encounters with wild animals.

Although the concept of traumatic injury as a recognized societal affliction has remained unchanged since the time of the Neanderthals, the incidence, magnitude, cause, mechanism, and treatment of traumatic injury *have* changed. Human interaction with the environment at given points throughout our life span and the effects of a variety of forces—industrialization, societal influences (including belief systems), and educational orientation and level—have influenced the ways in which injury occurs in our society today. Currently, traumatic injury is a major public health problem in the United States and the world, and the incidence of traumatic injury is predicted to increase worldwide in the twenty-first century.

TRAUMA SYSTEMS DEVELOPMENT

Trauma is one of the major challenges in emergency, critical care, medical, surgical, and rehabilitation nursing practices today. To recognize and develop a keen appreciation for trauma nursing as a specialty field, one must not only examine state-of-the-art practices but also review the historical events that led to the creation of a systems approach to care and to the development of the clinical knowledge base that has formed the foundation for this distinct area of clinical nursing practice.

The term *trauma* is used to describe a variety of injuries, and the concept of trauma embodies several associated terms—*shock, injury, accident, accidental injury, fatality,* and *casualty.* These terms are sometimes used synonymously and may be used interchangeably in this book, although use of the term *accidental* is avoided when possible because it implies that an event is unexpected or unavoidable. Over the years a deeper understanding of the underlying causes of traumatic injury has led to the belief that most unintentional events are predictable and therefore preventable.

MAGNITUDE OF THE PROBLEM

In the United States, unintentional injury is the most common cause of death for individuals age 1 to 34 years. In 1997 injury became the third leading cause of death in the 34 to 44 age group. Acquired immunodeficiency syndrome (AIDS) replaced injury as the most common cause of death, and cancer was the second most frequent cause of death in this age group. Injury is the fifth leading cause of death of individuals of all age groups, exceeded only by deaths occurring from cardiovascular disease, cancer, cerebrovascular disease, and chronic obstructive pulmonary disease.[2] It is estimated that more than 60 million injuries occur annually in this country. In 1997, of the total number of injuries that occurred, 93,800 resulted in death.[2] This was only a

0.5% decrease from the fatality rate of the previous year, still representing an exorbitant figure. Although ranked fifth as the cause of death for all age groups, injury is the leading killer of one of our nation's most valued resources—young people. Children and youths between 15 and 24 years of age have a greater chance of dying from unintentional injury than from any other cause. More than three of four individuals in this age group who die from injury are male.[2]

The National Safety Council's 1999 report on injuries showed the incidence of unintentional injury deaths was unchanged compared with the 1997 report. The report estimated these deaths to total 92,200 in both 1997 and 1998, down 3% from the final 1996 count of 94,948. The 1998 number is 6% greater than the 1992 total of 86,777 (the lowest annual total since 1924). However, this report concluded that the steady death toll combined with the continuing population growth meant that the death rate in 1998 was the second lowest on record: 34.1 unintentional injury deaths per 100,000 population. The lowest death rate was 34.0 in 1992.[3]

Motor vehicle crashes, falls, ingestion, drowning, and burns represent the primary causes of unintentional injury.[2] Motor vehicle crashes caused 46,200 deaths in 1997 (16.1 per 100,000 population). The motor vehicle death rate per 100,000,000 vehicle miles was 1.71 in 1997, which was a 2% decrease from the 1996 rate of 1.74. A further reduction in motor vehicle deaths was reported in 1998. There were 41,000 reported motor vehicle deaths, with a rate of 15.2 per 100,000 persons (a 3% decrease from 1997).[2]

The 1999 National Safety Council Report cites falls as the second most common cause of unintentional injury type for ages 55 through 79. Falls become the primary cause of unintentional injury deaths for people age 80 and older, accounting for half that type of death in this age group.[2] Although the number of deaths caused by motor vehicle crashes is on the decline, the number of deaths from falls increased from 15,300 in 1997 to 16,600 in 1998, an 8% increase in one year.[2]

Deaths from fires, burns, and injuries in conflagrations totaled 4000 in 1997 (1.4 per 100,000), representing a 12% increase from the 1996 figures. However, in 1998 there was an 8% decline in the number of deaths caused by this injury type, to 3700. The most frequent victims are children up to 4 years of age and the elderly (65 years and older).[2]

Injury continues to be a major health care problem affecting millions of U.S. citizens and creates a significant resource demand for health care services. Nonfatal injuries cause approximately 2.6 million people to be hospitalized for treatment each year; approximately 34.9 million people are treated in emergency departments and 87.6 million go to physicians' offices for treatment of injuries. In addition, one in four people, or 61.3 million, seek medical attention or suffer at least one day of activity restriction as a result of an injury.[2]

Between 1912 and 1998 the unintentional injury death rate declined gradually. Since 1912 unintentional deaths decreased 77%, from 30 to 7 per 100,000. During this same period, motor vehicle deaths decreased 94% per 10,000 registered vehicles. There were 3100 motor vehicle deaths in 1912, when the number of registered vehicles totaled only 950,000. In 1998 there were 215.4 million vehicles registered, with 41,200 reported fatalities.[2] The decrease in motor vehicle deaths during the past 86 years is in part due to the development of emergency medical systems and trauma care systems, as well as improvements in road design, enhanced vehicle safety design, and increased use of passenger restraints.

Injury is a significant public health problem that affects all ages and all levels of society. The number of people injured from all causes annually is astounding. The National Safety Council reported that 60,452,000 people were injured in 1997; of this number, 3,198,000 were injured in a moving vehicle.[2] As a result of these injuries, there were 37,222 visits to emergency departments in 1997, with an annual rate of 36.9 emergency department visits per 100 persons.[2] Therefore, approximately 14.2 visits per 100 persons were necessitated by injury, increasing the demand on emergency department services, as well as on other hospital acute care and rehabilitation services.[2]

In addition to the human loss and disability resulting from trauma, the economic cost also must be considered. The National Safety Council defines a disabling injury as one that results in some degree of permanent impairment. This includes injuries that render the injured person unable to effectively perform regular duties or activities for a full day beyond the day of the injury. Cost estimates therefore include wage losses, medical expenses, insurance administration costs, property damages in motor vehicle crashes, fire losses, and indirect work loss from accidents. (Indirect loss from work injuries is the money value of time lost by noninjured workers and includes time spent filling out accident reports or giving first aid to injured workers and time lost as a result of production slowdowns.) The cost for unintentional injuries, including those in which deaths or disabling injuries occurred together with motor vehicle crashes and fires in which no injury took place, was estimated at $478.3 billion in 1997.[2] The portion of the total cost estimate for motor vehicle crashes was $200.3 billion.[2]

Despite an alarmingly high incidence of unintentional injury over the years, the significance of this problem has not always been recognized by the public sector. The first sign that this issue had reached the level of national politics appeared in 1960 when John F. Kennedy, during his presidential campaign, issued a statement acknowledging that "traffic accidents constitute one of the greatest, perhaps the greatest, of the nation's public problems."[3] Since that time, attention has been directed toward raising public awareness about this sizable problem, while concurrent efforts have been made to identify fundamental elements that would render the nation's health care delivery system more responsive to the needs of those who have sustained traumatic injury. To date, only minimal effort has been focused on preventing injury. This is an area in need of further attention.

THE MILITARY EXPERIENCE

Many of the advances in the care of the critically injured before the 1960s were made by the military. The injuries sustained by military personnel and civilians during times of war were the primary focus of studies of traumatic injury and shock, which became the initial source of information regarding traumatic injuries.

The concepts guiding medical personnel in their attempts to care for the wounded during the Civil War (1861 to 1865) and the Spanish-American War (April 1898 to August 1898) were vague at best. Before World War I a variety of theories regarding traumatic injury and its treatment had been advanced, but there was a tremendous need to generate hard data to describe what became known as the "shock state" following injury.

In 1916, during World War I, the United States National Research Council of the National Academy of Sciences formed a Committee on Physiology, whose Subcommittee on Traumatic Shock began to collect, review, and analyze objective data regarding the physiology of circulation and its relationship to the various models that had been defined for the study of shock.[4] This was the first coordinated prospective work project organized for the purpose of obtaining a better understanding of the body's responses to severe trauma. The information from these studies was discussed at formal meetings and conferences, which resulted in more widespread dissemination of knowledge about shock resulting from traumatic injury. Although by the mid-nineteenth century the term *shock* began to be applied to the clinical state of individuals who had sustained severe trauma, the nature of clinical shock remained a mystery.[4]

It has only been since World War II that the nature of shock has been better understood and that the treatment regimen has become more clearly defined. During World War II, the care of trauma patients improved significantly. This was due largely to the prompt application of information obtained by the Medical Board for the Study of the Treatment of the Severely Wounded. This 22-member board was appointed on September 3, 1943, by the Theater Commander, Lt. General Jacob B. Devers, and was made up of medical officers, nurses, technicians, and support personnel who worked as a research team.[4] This team responded to any medical request from the field and compiled casualty data during an 8-month period in Italy. The data from observations of 186 military casualties comprised the first volume of the historical series by the Medical Department of the United States Army. It was titled *Surgery in World War II: The Physiologic Effects of Wounds.*[5] The information obtained by the board was disseminated not only in the field hospitals that were treating and studying the wounded but also throughout the front-line and base hospitals. The study results were impressive and led to a change in policy regarding the treatment of wound shock. Resuscitation practices improved, as hemodynamic alterations became better understood and knowledge about posttraumatic renal failure, an often-fatal complication of severe shock, emerged.

A similar but more extensive program was established during the Korean War (1950 to 1953) and later during the Vietnam War (1957 to 1975). The research efforts put forth during World War II by the Medical Board for the Study of the Treatment of the Severely Wounded continued and were strengthened by a newly established Surgical Research Team. This was made possible in part by the support services that had been made available from stateside organizations and institutions in the form of high-tech equipment sent to the combat zone. The emergence of the research team represented a significant achievement of the military medical efforts during the twentieth century and contributed to the further refinement of the care delivered to trauma patients during the Korean War. Through these efforts, progress was made in the clarification of the hemodynamic disturbances that occur with different forms of traumatic injury, and much knowledge was gained about organ function and the metabolic disturbances in shock and acute circulatory failure.

The pressing demands of war surgery, coupled with the advances in medical care that occurred during the previous century, contributed in part to the high level of performance that was realized during the Vietnam War. Improvements in field resuscitation, increased efficiency of transportation, and aggressive treatment of war casualties proved to be major factors contributing to lifesaving endeavors. The death rates of war casualties reaching designated facilities decreased from 8% in World War I, to 4.5% in World War II, to 2.5% during the Korean War, to less than 2% in the Vietnam War.[6]

THE MILITARY INFLUENCE

Based on what had been learned by the military during war regarding the significant impact of time on saving lives, coupled with scientific knowledge regarding the human physiologic response to injury, it became apparent that changes within our health care delivery system were necessary.

Many have questioned with dismay why the information learned about the care of the injured during our nation's military experiences was so delayed in being applied to injuries occurring in civilian life. This is indeed baffling because changes in patient care delivery that occurred during the Civil War and that were refined and improved during each subsequent military conflict were known to be responsible for the favorable trends in injury survival. The need for an effective system to care for the severely injured was just as pressing in the civilian sector as in the military arena. Yet this civilian need was not generally recognized or, if recognized, not accepted. As had been demonstrated consistently during wartime, rapid evacuation of the seriously injured from the battlefield to advanced treatment stations (mobile army surgical hospital units), which were equipped with necessary supplies and staffed with highly skilled personnel, saved lives. Although long overdue, the principles on which this system was designed have since been found to be easily transferable to, and as effective in civilian life.

The modern era of a civilian systems approach, which focused on more efficient emergency health care for the injured, began in 1966 with the publication of a document by the National Academy of Sciences, National Research Council. This document, *Accidental Death and Disability—The Neglected Disease of Modern Society,* was a far-sighted approach to the development of an effective emergency medical services system throughout our nation. It was the product of a 3-year study conducted by a committee on trauma, shock, and anesthesia in conjunction with special task forces from the Division of Medical Sciences, the National Academy of Sciences, and the National Research Council. The results were compiled after representatives from health care organizations reviewed the status of initial emergency care provided to individuals following "accidental" injury. The study groups reviewed a broad spectrum of factors, including ambulance services, voice communication systems, hospital emergency departments, and intensive care units, while incorporating research results in shock, trauma, and resuscitation. Based on identified deficiencies, the general areas of consideration recommended by the committee and outlined in the published document[7] included the following:

- "Accident" prevention
- Emergency first aid and medical care
  - Ambulance services
  - Communications
  - Emergency departments
  - Interrelationships between the emergency department and the intensive care unit
- Development of trauma registries
- Hospital trauma committees
- Convalescence, disability, and rehabilitation
- Medicolegal problems
- Autopsy of the victim
- Care of casualties under conditions of natural disaster
- Research in trauma

The national effort for establishing an improved emergency health care system and much of the basic framework on which the nation's emergency medical services (EMS) system has subsequently been built were presented in this document. This classic white paper represented the first major governmental report acknowledging that significant numbers of people were killed or disabled as a result of unintentional injuries in the civilian population, which was costing the nation billions of dollars each year. Contributing significantly to the high mortality and morbidity rates were the inefficiencies in the nation's emergency health care delivery system. Unskilled health care personnel working with inadequate transportation and communication system policies and guidelines were taking the injured to facilities that were not sufficiently prepared to treat them. It became apparent that the problems of initial care and management of injured persons were similar in kind, although different in magnitude and scope, to those encountered by the military during war. The time was right for the application of new knowledge and skills in caring for the injured.

EARLY PIONEERING EFFORTS

During the late 1960s and early 1970s, the need for a systematic approach to the care of the seriously injured patient became apparent. The initial efforts to design and develop emergency medical clinical delivery systems were based on the care requirements of specific types of injury (e.g., trauma, burns, and spinal cord injuries).[8] The conceptual design of a systems approach required that effective medical and surgical treatment regimens be applied in situations other than the traditional in-hospital setting. This necessitated the reorganization of preexisting health care structures, the implementation of new technologies, and the development of educational programs so that clinical treatment modalities proven effective in the hospital environment could be applied and tested in the prehospital and interhospital phases. Physician-supervised educational programs and extrahospital emergency care programs began to emerge, with emergency medical technicians-ambulance (EMT-A) and advanced life support emergency medical technicians-paramedic (EMT-P) assuming key roles.[8]

In several parts of the country, hospitals were categorized regionally, and those with demonstrated expertise were designated as trauma, burn, or spinal cord injury centers. In Illinois, for example, the regionalization of emergency care for multiple and critical injuries was initiated and developed statewide in 1971. As the Illinois trauma program began to develop and mature, a program of patient transfer and burn center care also was initiated for the four burn units and major burn center (Cook County Hospital) in Chicago, which utilized a patient distribution program and central bed registry.[9]

In 1972, in collaboration with the Illinois trauma program, representatives from the Midwest Regional Spinal Cord Injury Care Systems at Northwestern Memorial Hospital and the Rehabilitation Institute of Chicago (McGaw Medical Center, Northwestern University) formulated a macroregional catchment program for acute spinal cord injuries.[10] In 1973 the shock-trauma program of the University of Maryland, supported by the Maryland state government, was expanded statewide and became the Maryland Institute for Emergency Medicine (MIEM).[11]

These pioneering efforts were significant because they represented working models for further regional trauma/EMS systems development. The apparent successes resulting from these system designs became the catalysts for a more intense national effort to plan and implement improved trauma/EMS systems. The overall age-adjusted death rate from injuries and adverse effects for Maryland has been declining steadily since the implementation and maturing of the statewide emergency medical system and trauma care system. The rate declined from 29.8 in 1988 to 21.6 in 1997.

In comparison, the national figures for the same years were 35 and 28.9, respectively.[12]

FEDERAL SUPPORT OF TRAUMA/EMS SYSTEMS

Federal support of emergency medical services started during the early 1970s, when congressional hearings were held to promote the development of a comprehensive EMS law. In 1973 the Emergency Medical Services Systems (EMSS) Act was passed, which contained guidelines and specific technical measures that would support a nationally coordinated and comprehensive system of emergency health care accessible to all citizens. The identification of fundamental elements of the EMS system deemed necessary for the comprehensive care of the critically ill and injured was accomplished with this mandate. Included in the EMSS Act were 15 requirements (listed below) that would assist EMS system project planners and health care professionals in establishing comprehensive, area-wide, and regional EMS programs:[13]

1. Provision of manpower
2. Training of personnel
3. Communications
4. Transportation
5. Facilities
6. Critical care units
7. Use of public safety agencies
8. Consumer participation
9. Accessibility to care
10. Transfer of patients
11. Standard medical record keeping
12. Consumer information and education
13. Independent review and evaluation
14. Disaster linkage
15. Mutual aid agreements

The 1973 EMSS Act, with its subsequent changes in 1976, is considered one of the most important factors influencing the development of EMS systems throughout this country. This act focused on improving the nation's emergency death and disability statistics by mandating that the emergency medical care programs that were federally funded by the Department of Health and Human Services (DHHS) must plan and implement a systems approach on a regional basis for emergency response and immediate care provisions. Although many emergency medical conditions had been identified, the seven critical target patient care areas for regional EMS systems planning were major trauma, burns, spinal cord injuries, poisonings, acute cardiac conditions, high-risk infants and mothers, and behavioral emergencies. In-depth knowledge of the incidence, epidemiology, and clinical aspects associated with these categories is considered essential for appreciating a systems approach to regional planning and delivery of care. Much of this information, specifically that related to multiple traumas, spinal cord injuries, and burns, is explored in greater detail in this book in the respective chapters.

The federal government withdrew from its lead role in

EMS development in 1981 with the passage of the Reconciliation Act, which integrated the EMS program into the Health Prevention Block Grants and gave responsibility back to the states for direction and development of EMS. The General Accounting Office (GAO) report of 1986[14] disclosed the effect of this transition of EMS system programs from federal to state leadership under the block grant program, concluding that a major sector of the United States (more than 50%) lacked the universal phone access number 911, advanced life support ambulance services were lacking or limited in rural areas, and many areas had not developed trauma care systems at all. Senators Alan Cranston and Edward M. Kennedy first introduced legislation to address the recommendations of the 1986 GAO report in the 100th Congress in January 1987.

This legislation was finally signed into law as Public Law 101-590 by President Bush on November 16, 1990. This legislation, titled the Trauma Care Systems Planning and Development Act of 1990, is significant because it provided federal assistance for the development of emergency/trauma care systems throughout the United States. This act amended the Public Health Services Act by adding a new title, Title XII. The act authorized DHHS, through the Health Resources and Services Administration (HRSA), to make grants to states for trauma systems planning and development. The major provisions of this act include the following:[15]

1. *A council on trauma care systems.* The purpose of the council is to report needs of the trauma care system and how states are responding to such needs. This council has 12 public members, including two nurse positions (one critical care position and one emergency medical training position).
2. *A clearinghouse on trauma care and EMS.* This is to be established by contract to serve as a collection, compilation, and dissemination point for information relating to all aspects of emergency medical services and trauma care.
3. *Programs for improving trauma care in rural areas.* Grants will be authorized for public and private nonprofit entities for research and demonstration projects that will improve the availability and quality of emergency medical/trauma care in rural areas.
4. *Formula grants with respect to modification of state plans.* Most of the appropriated funds (80%) will be allotted by formula for each state and territory. Beginning in the second fiscal year that states receive funds, they must make a matching nonfederal contribution (in cash or in kind) in specified ratios.
5. *State plans and modifications.* Each state must submit to the Secretary of Health and Human Services the trauma care component of the state's EMS plan. The funds allotted for each state may be used only to make such modifications to the state plan as are necessary to ensure access to the highest quality of trauma care.

6. *Trauma care standards and a model trauma care plan.* Each state must adopt standards for designating trauma centers and for triage, transfer, and transportation policies. In addition, the Secretary must develop in the first year of this act a model trauma care plan that may be adopted for guidance by the states.

7. *Data and reporting requirements.* Each state must report annually to the Secretary the number of severely injured patients; the cause of injury and contributing factors; the nature and severity of the injury; monitoring data sufficient to evaluate the diagnoses, treatment, and outcomes of such trauma patients in each trauma center; and expenditures.

8. *Technical assistance and supplies and services in lieu of grant funds.* The Secretary shall provide technical assistance with respect to planning, development, and operation of any program carried out with the allotted funds, at no charge to the state.

9. *Waiver.* Under certain limited conditions, the Secretary may allow a state to use a percentage of allotted funds to reimburse designated trauma centers for uncompensated care.

The Trauma Systems Planning and Development Act was first funded at $5 million in fiscal year 1992 and for the following 4 years; however, in 1995 the 104th Congress rescinded most of the funding and did not provide any funding for fiscal year 1996. Senate Bill 1745 was passed in 1998, reauthorizing a number of public health programs, including the Trauma Systems Planning and Development Act. This legislation authorizes the program through fiscal year 2002 and provides $6 million in funding for states to plan and develop organized systems of trauma care.

As mandated by the Trauma Systems Planning and Development Act, a model trauma care plan was developed and published by HRSA as a template that states could use to design a local trauma system. This plan contained mandatory components necessary to meet the needs of all injured patients who require the services of an acute care facility. The plan stressed two important concepts: (1) the need for a trauma care system to be integrated into the overall EMS system and (2) the incorporation of existing EMS resources.[16] The plan classifies the components as "administrative" and "operational and clinical." The administrative component includes leadership, system development, legislation, and finance. The operational and clinical component includes public information/education and prevention, human resources, prehospital care, EMS medical direction, triage, transport, definitive care facilities, interfacility transfer, medical rehabilitation, and evaluation.[16]

Trauma/EMS System Development

As EMS systems have developed, the design seems to represent a composite of individual and unique systems of care for the particular patient group (e.g., multiple trauma, spinal cord injury, burns). Although it is necessary for these

TABLE 1-1	Key Components of a Clinical Emergency Medical Services System

Trauma
Facilities categorization
Trauma center designation
Transfer agreements and triage protocols

Cardiac Emergency
Patient access (911)
Citizen cardiopulmonary resuscitation (CPR)
Advanced cardiac life support (ACLS) paramedic response

Poisonings
Information specialists
Toxicologic information and treatment protocols
Telephone-directed home care and physician consultation

From Boyd DR, Edlich RF, Micik S: *Systems approach to emergency medical care*, Norwalk, Conn, 1983, Appleton-Century-Crofts.

systems to utilize common EMS components, such as transportation, communications, and specially skilled prehospital health team members, the care, resources, and facilities must be specifically designed for each patient group. EMS system components must be adapted to address and accommodate specific clinical needs if accurate and effective planning is to occur. For example, unlike EMS systems planning for cardiac emergencies or poisonings, the key EMS components for the trauma patient population are facilities categorization and trauma center designation (Table 1-1). For trauma patients, the establishment of triage and transfer protocols is critical so that immediate interventions are consistent and decisions regarding transfer to a designated trauma facility for definitive care are facilitated. Thus it is of utmost importance that regional trauma/EMS systems plan and develop clinically sound trauma care programs on a geographic basis. Because of the complex requirements, the care of the trauma patient has provided an excellent model from which to design a basic health care delivery system. This has since been expanded to include other types of emergency medical conditions.[17]

The clinical significance of the systems approach in developing a regional trauma/EMS system was clearly identified by the Division of Emergency Medical Services of the Department of Health and Human Services and reflected in their program guidelines. In congressional testimony, representatives of this agency described the unique clinical requirements of the multiple trauma patient, the need for a regionalized system of care, and the key EMS system components crucial to a successful and efficient trauma care program (i.e., facilities, critical care units, and transfer of patients). Although it was felt that a trauma/EMS system must respond adequately to all declared emergency calls within its designated geographic region, which included nonemergency cases (80%), truly emergent cases (15%), and critical cases (5%),[18] emphasis was placed on the need to identify effectively the critical patient whose chance of survival desperately depended on a competent trauma care delivery system. It was toward increasing the chance of survival for these critical patients that conceptual system planning and initial program development were directed.

In 1987 the American College of Emergency Physicians' Trauma Committee published "Guidelines for Trauma Care Systems."[18] The ACEP guidelines state that "trauma care represents a continuum that is best provided by an integrated system extending from prevention through rehabilitation and requiring close cooperation among specialists in each phase of care."

FACILITIES CATEGORIZATION.   In the 1976 report "Optimal Hospital Resources for Care of the Seriously Injured,"[19] the Task Force of the Committee on Trauma of the American College of Surgeons called for hospitals to commit personnel and facility resources to caring for seriously injured patients. The original proposal, presented in the 1966 landmark document *Accidental Death and Disability: The Neglected Disease of Modern Society,* suggested that the categorization of facilities should be based on the individual institution's capacity to handle a broad spectrum of emergency conditions.[7] This plan—the implementation of a variety of categorization schemes—proved to be unsuccessful, and a more detailed set of guidelines was provided by the Task Force of the Committee on Trauma of the American College of Surgeons in 1979. This revised document, "Hospital Resources for Optimal Care of the Injured Patient," replaced the 1976 report.[20] Emphasis was placed on special problems of geography, population density, availability of community and regional resources and personnel, and the pervasive demands of cost effectiveness, with the most significant element being commitment, personal and institutional. Institutional commitment was defined as the immediate availability of capable personnel and accessibility to sophisticated equipment, laboratory and radiologic facilities, operating rooms, and intensive care units. The personal commitment of hospital trustees, administrators, physicians, nurses, and other health care professionals also was imperative, because the responsibility for providing optimal hospital resources for the care of the seriously injured patient rests with these individuals.

TRAUMA CENTER DESIGNATION.   In the 1979 report[20] optimal standards for categorization of trauma care facilities were expanded and refined. Three distinct levels of trauma care services were identified, with functional responsibilities, capabilities, and comparable nomenclature outlined for the three levels. These were intended to serve as a guide for assessing an institution's potential for trauma center designation.

In the 1999 edition of the American College of Surgeons' Committee on Trauma report, "Resources for the Optimal Care of the Injured Patient,"[21] the emphasis is on the trauma system rather than a single trauma center. For optimal trauma care, a community must develop an all-encompassing systems approach to provide the appropriate level of trauma care. This system of care involves a lead governing agency for development and oversight, a prehospital emergency care system, and a network of hospitals that provide a spectrum of care to all injured patients. The definitive care network of hospitals is identified by Levels I through IV, depending on the depth of resources.[21] A Level I trauma care facility is a tertiary teaching hospital that takes a lead role in education, research, and system planning in a regional trauma care system. Level I trauma centers are usually located in metropolitan areas. The volume performance expectation is highest for a Level I center. Level I trauma centers are expected to admit at least 1200 trauma patients annually, with 20% of these patients having an injury severity score (ISS) of 15 or greater or with each trauma surgeon treating 35 or more trauma patients with an ISS of 15 or greater.[21] A Level I institution must make a firm commitment to furnish the personnel, facilities, and equipment necessary to provide total care for every aspect of injury through the phases of care from prevention through rehabilitation.[21]

A Level II trauma care facility is most likely a tertiary institution that may or may not be an academic center. A Level II trauma center should provide initial definitive trauma care for all levels of injury severity; however, because of limited resources it may not be able to provide the same comprehensive care as a Level I trauma center.[21] The role of the Level II trauma center in a regional trauma system varies depending on its location and proximity to a Level I trauma center. If the Level II center is located in a population-dense area with a short ambulance transport time to the closest Level I trauma center, the Level II would supplement the clinical activity and expertise of the Level I center. It is expected that the Level I and Level II trauma centers would work together to optimize resources in the region to provide the appropriate level of care for all injured patients. When the Level II trauma center is located in a more rural setting or is the only tertiary hospital in a region, it serves as the lead trauma facility for that region.[21]

A Level III trauma center is most often a community hospital in an area that lacks Level I and Level II hospital facilities. It must make a strong commitment to the optimal care of the trauma patient. Clear and concise transfer protocols are essential. These centers must have the capability to resuscitate and manage the initial definitive care of most injured patients. However, timely transfer of injured patients to higher level trauma centers must be provided when a patient's needs exceed the resources of the Level III center.[21]

An additional Level IV standard has been added to the revised ACS "Resources for Optimal Care of the Injured Patient."[21] A Level IV hospital is generally a small hospital in a rural area. This center is part of a regional trauma care network and will have transfer agreements with Level I and II centers. The Level IV center provides timely resuscitation and transfer of most injured patients.

Many other hospitals, both large and small, that have emergency department capabilities but have made no official commitment to an organized approach to the care of the seriously injured patient are encouraged to upgrade their trauma care. This type of institution is an implied fourth level of trauma care and requires strict treatment protocols and transfer agreements with higher-level facilities.

The intent of the guidelines outlined in the "Resources" document is to encourage each hospital to constantly monitor its capabilities as a trauma care facility and continue to strive to upgrade its resources. Ideally, if the guidelines are actualized, the severity of injury should be matched equally with appropriate facility resources and personnel expertise. Health care professionals working within a hospital who have an interest in trauma care, are educated and skilled in managing the special problems of trauma patients, and assume a well-defined role on a trauma team organized especially to provide optimal care will produce more favorable patient outcomes than those who view trauma care as another general service.

Although there is a distinct difference between the categorization of hospital emergency and critical care capabilities and the more formal process of selecting and designating certain facilities for specialty clinical services, the categorization of all hospitals within a particular trauma/EMS region is beneficial in two respects. First, categorization allows assessment of the hospital's general emergency department capabilities to care for seriously injured patients and of its overall critical care capabilities for specific patient groups. This is considered an integral part of the planning activity helpful in documenting the existing resources and in identifying deficits that may ultimately lead to appropriate improvements in trauma/EMS systems. This information is considered when decisions are made concerning the official designation of specialty care centers. Second, once designated, these specialty referral centers are held accountable for maintaining their capabilities.

TRANSFER AGREEMENTS AND TRIAGE PROTOCOLS. The relationship of a regional trauma/EMS system to the overall EMS system is an important consideration when planning a comprehensive systems approach to trauma care. EMS and trauma/EMS systems involve a complex series of events that must be coordinated effectively to provide a consistent mechanism for efficient health care delivery. Clinical research has provided a deeper understanding of the natural course of traumatic disease and has demonstrated that time is of the essence in treating these diseases. A standard mortality curve clearly shows that if a medical emergency is measured against time, death will eventually result if effective emergency care is not initiated promptly. The time constraints that exist for the seriously injured patient have served as the impetus for creating more effective care systems in an attempt to reduce mortality and morbidity.

Experience has shown that the outcome of traumatic injury is more favorable if resuscitation and stabilization efforts are initiated early and sustained. Although the time of patient death varies depending on the magnitude and variety of the traumatic pathology, a prompt trauma/EMS

system response, the provision of initial basic field care, the use of a sophisticated communications system, and the rapid and safe transport of the patient will save valuable time, and eventual death may be prevented. Each phase of EMS activity has a critical effect on mortality. Every single act can save time. Rescue squads and first responders are prepared to perform basic life-support skills in the field. In many parts of the country, more sophisticated and advanced measures are being taken by EMT-paramedics in caring for critically injured patients both during extrication efforts and during transport within the EMS system.[22]

The EMS process begins when notification is received by EMS system operators that an injury incident has occurred; an ambulance team is dispatched to the scene. The patient's condition is assessed, and resuscitation and stabilization efforts are initiated in the field. Their level of educational preparation and certification dictates the interventions and skill levels of the ambulance team members and field personnel. A sophisticated communications system allows the field personnel to contact authorized personnel at an appropriate trauma center for instructions concerning triage and treatment and provides the receiving hospital with an estimated time of patient arrival. Measures are then taken to transfer the patient to the most appropriate facility. This decision must be guided not only by the patient's condition and injury type but also by the geographic dynamics of that area. Thus each regional trauma/EMS system must be organized in such a way as to accommodate the unique needs of the area. Because there are distinct differences between urban and rural areas, three sociogeographic regional trauma/EMS models have been proposed for incorporation into the planning of trauma/EMS systems throughout the country[8]: the urban-suburban model, the rural-metropolitan model, and the wilderness-metropolitan model. When developing these sociogeographic models, population density, trauma care resources, and geography were considered.[8] Although some absolute examples of these models exist within regional trauma/EMS systems, most systems have more than one type model, as seen in Maryland, Oregon, Pennsylvania, Virginia, and San Diego County, California. Generally, attempts are made to centralize designated trauma or specialty care facilities within regional trauma/EMS systems to facilitate timely and efficient primary triage or secondary transfer of patients, if necessary. Protocols for field identification, triage, resuscitation, and transportation to designated trauma centers have been adopted and have become operational in many communities. These protocols not only facilitate consistency within the trauma/EMS system but also ensure that injured patients are taken to hospitals capable of continuing and expanding life-support measures initiated in the field. A sophisticated systems approach to triage, communication, and transport is of little avail if clinical expertise of the highest quality does not await the injured patient's arrival.

The trauma facility notified of a pending admission has the responsibility of alerting the in-house trauma team, whose members will report to the designated resuscitation area to prepare for the patient's arrival. Staff specialists and expert clinicians, equipment, supplies, and ancillary support systems must be immediately available if the complex problems of the seriously injured patient are to be managed in a timely fashion. Effective resuscitation and stabilization efforts are based on the implementation of a predetermined series of activities performed simultaneously by appropriate trauma team members. Once the patient is stabilized, priorities are established for definitive care. Depending on the type, magnitude, and severity of the patient's injuries, subsequent treatment may include additional diagnostic studies, surgical intervention, intensive care management, medical/surgical unit, or long-term rehabilitation.

In summary, the trauma/EMS system by design must provide immediate and appropriate care at the scene of an incident, safe and efficient transportation to the trauma center, definitive diagnostic and surgical interventions, critical care management, acute care (medical/surgical unity), and rehabilitation services. This broad scope of capabilities may be available within the respective geographic region. If not, the trauma/EMS system must respond by transferring patients out of that region to a distant trauma care facility where their specific needs can be met. It has become apparent that all EMS systems throughout the country need a stratified, or graded, echelon system of trauma/EMS care so that flexibility within the emergency health care system is guaranteed. In order to support an effective trauma care system, integration of and cooperation among all hospitals treating injured persons in a region are crucial. An inclusive systems approach can minimize geographic and geopolitic constraints, allowing efficient and effective use of resources to provide optimal trauma care to all injured persons served by the region and reduce the overall cost of care.[22-24]

The challenge for future trauma system development and maturation will depend on society's commitment of resources and the ability of the health care system to justify these resources based on the cost and benefit. Outcomes of the trauma system's performance must have data-driven multidisciplinary evaluation that looks not only at mortality rates but also includes functional patient outcomes and the efficient use of resources to achieve the optimal outcome. A major effort to facilitate trauma systems outcome evaluation was initiated by Dr. Mullins and Dr. Mann, who organized and directed the Skamania Conference in July 1998.[25] They invited trauma care experts from all regions of the United States to attend this 2-day conference for the purposes of (1) reviewing currently available data that has been used to evaluate the effectiveness of trauma systems, (2) assessing the strengths and usefulness of prior trauma system effectiveness studies, (3) defining the characteristics of a valid assessment of trauma system effectiveness, and (4) identifying the direction, format, and goals for future research.[25] The Skamania Conference was supported by two federal agencies, the National Center for Injury Prevention and the National Highway Traffic Safety Administration. A supplement to the *Journal of Trauma: Injury Infection and Critical Care* published in September 1999 focused on the Skamania Conference and outcomes research for trauma systems.[25]

THE EVOLUTION OF TRAUMA NURSING

HISTORIC BACKGROUND

Nurses have long been challenged by the complexity of the health care needs of seriously injured patients and their families. Because wars have been responsible for producing traumatic injuries in epidemic proportions, nurses have gained experience in caring for the wounded. Although no clear records exist, perhaps the first organized nursing effort focusing on battlefield injuries was pioneered during the Crimean War (1854), when Florence Nightingale, Lady Superintendent-in-Chief of female nursing in the English General Military Hospitals, led a group of women in caring for war casualties.[26] For approximately 2 years, this group of nurses provided makeshift hospital facilities; bathed and dressed wounds; and painstakingly sought proper sanitation, hygiene, and control of infection. In October of 1861, Nightingale was asked by the United States secretary of war for advice on setting up military hospitals for the Union Army, and her suggestions were widely adopted throughout the course of the Civil War (1861-1865).[27] Clara Barton, the first woman clerk of the U.S. Patent Office, served as a nurse caring for wounded men on the battlefield after the outbreak of the Civil War in 1861 and later during the Franco-Prussian War (1869). In 1881, after her return to the United States, Barton organized the American Red Cross, a volunteer society that was modeled after the International Red Cross (established in 1863 by Jean Henri Dunant).[28]

In subsequent wars, nurses have cared for the wounded on and off the battlefield, seeking new ways to manage the devastating injuries resulting from the ever-increasing power of weaponry. Under the most adverse circumstances, combat nurses worked to help salvage mutilated extremities, tried to replace massive losses of blood, and attempted to administer appropriate medications, when available, to those with severe clinical complications. All actions were taken to prolong life; even if initial efforts proved to be successful, death as a result of infection following a complicated clinical course was always a possibility.[29]

Enormous problems existed for the nurses who cared for the wounded. They found that the scars of battle extended far beyond those from burns or bayonet or bullet wounds. The psychologic implications for nursing care were just as pervasive as the physical demands; the mind and spirit were scarred as well. While caring for the wounded, nurses came to understand that the long-term effects and difficulties their patients faced as a result of war were far greater than the bullets, bombs, or missiles.

Violetta Thurstan, an English military nurse who served in World War I, writes in her *Textbook of War Nursing:*

Since the war, times and seasons have lost their meaning. Sometimes half one's life seems to have been crushed into a space of a very few hours, sometimes each day is so drawn out that it is an eternity in itself. August 1914, seems a dim, far-away epoch and those who played their part in the early days are veterans now. In many ways nursing was more interesting in the early days of the war, when everything had to be improvised or adapted, than later on when the excitement and the first rush were over, organisation brought to an undreamt-of pitch of perfection, and all necessaries amply and even lavishly supplied....Who shall say how many lives and limbs were saved by the nurses' ready inventiveness and clever fingers?

There was of course another side to this, the tragedy which no one who worked at that period will ever be able to forget, of seeing precious lives ebbing away for the want of some necessary that might have saved them if only it had been there.[29]

The knowledge gained from the experiences of the front-line nurses has provided valuable information in helping to understand trauma in civilian life. Moving from the war zone to the home front awakens us to the realities of our modern lifestyle. Influenced by the evolution of wounding forces unique to different historic periods, the occurrence of death and disability in our nation is astounding, and the effects are far reaching.[29-32]

CHANGES WITHIN THE HOSPITAL SETTING

During the 1970s, because of improved access to emergency medical services, the expanded educational preparation of emergency medical technicians, the development of sophisticated communication systems (including telemetry), and the use of more efficient means of transportation (including air evacuation), more viable patients were being brought to hospital facilities. During this same 10- to 15-year period of improved prehospital care, however, commensurate changes were not necessarily being made in the hospital. Reports indicated that basic errors in assessment and treatment of seriously injured patients were occurring with alarming regularity.[32-35] These errors, coupled with inadequate preplanning on the part of the hospital and poor mobilization and organization of hospital resources, often resulted in unnecessary death. The task of overcoming these unfavorable statistics presented a tremendous challenge to nurses, physicians, other health care professionals, and hospital officials.

EVOLUTION OF THE TRAUMA RESUSCITATION TEAM

Categorization of hospital facilities had been one strategy demanded by the federal government in an attempt to ensure that patients were taken to institutions capable of caring for their injuries. Unfortunately, in most parts of the country this change was occurring very slowly, if at all. However, a few facilities throughout the country began to make tremendous advances in caring for seriously injured trauma patients. Because these institutions cared for a large number of injured patients, they developed a staff of physicians and nurses proficient in caring for complex injuries. Statistical trends began to indicate that mortality and morbidity were substantially lower in these designated hospitals, which had more

qualified and experienced personnel and more extensive facilities.[36] The success of the nurses and physicians was dependent on a number of factors, including the implementation of an interdisciplinary team approach to care, which facilitated the coordination of resuscitation efforts, evaluation, and definitive management plans. The success of the trauma team depended not only on the knowledge base and skill level of each physician and nurse but also on the consistency and repetition of their practices as a team. Proven in both military and civilian settings, a dedicated trauma team approach is the most effective and efficient means to care for the critically injured trauma patient. The predetermined delegation of specialized role responsibilities to each nurse and physician team member fosters the efficient organization of talents, which decreases the time between the patient's arrival and the onset of definitive care. Thus the hospital trauma team's efforts to save lives continues to support the life-sustaining activities initiated during the prehospital phase of care.

The development of rapid and more efficient transport systems was instrumental in reducing the precious time interval between the onset of injury and the patient's arrival at the hospital. This time factor underlies many of the principles on which the initial care of the trauma patient was based. A firmer understanding of the volume requirements for circulatory resuscitation on the part of nurse and physician team members also had a significant impact on the team's approach to care. Success during the resuscitation phase of care increased the number of patients who then needed to be monitored closely and managed in an environment that provided continuity of intense nursing supervision and care. The extent of the patient's injuries, compounded by the potential for postresuscitation complications (e.g., respiratory insufficiency, renal failure, sepsis, coagulopathy), represented a new phase that required critical care medical and nursing management.[37]

TRAUMA NURSING

The critical care phase of nursing has provided unique challenges for nurses as new concepts of physiology and biochemistry have been applied. Concurrently, new evaluation techniques and management therapies have been introduced, which contributed to the advances made in the care of the seriously injured trauma patient. With the advent of miraculous technologic advances affecting physiologic monitoring and improvements in diagnostic procedures and medical treatments, trauma nursing faced a new frontier. One of the natural outcomes of this rapidly expanding technology was the nurse's increasing responsibility for complex decisions.

The introduction of innovative diagnostic methods and tools contributed to greater efficiency in the clinical evaluation process. The strengths of peritoneal lavage as a diagnostic tool were recognized, sparing many trauma patients unnecessary operative procedures. The computed tomographic (CT) scanner allowed precise diagnosis of intracranial injuries and provided more exact diagnoses for vertebral, acetabular, mediastinal, and some abdominal injuries. Simultaneously, advances in angiography provided a mechanism for precise diagnosis of vessel injuries in the chest, pelvis, and extremities. Advances in technology continue to aid in more accurate, timely diagnosis of injuries. The use of ultrasound to detect abdominal injury, spiral CT, and magnetic resonance imaging (MRI) during the resuscitation phase are examples of recent diagnostic advances.

Because of the complex care required by the critically injured patient, many trauma specialty fields within medicine began to emerge. These specialty services included traumatology, neurosurgery, orthopedic surgery, thoracic surgery, plastic surgery, oral surgery, critical care, and infectious disease medicine. With this trend came the potential for these specialists to care for the patient by focusing on the area of their expertise in partial or complete isolation from the patient's other health care problems. The unfavorable consequences of this fragmented approach to care became obvious. Because they provided bedside care on a 24-hour basis, nurses were in a position to facilitate the coordination of multidisciplinary patient care activities. They appropriately began to take measures to incorporate a comprehensive approach to planning care for the critical trauma patient. The role of the trauma nurse expanded as problem-solving and decision-making responsibilities increased, leading to a new era in collegial relationships. Nurses who cared for trauma patients in the emergency department, operating room, postanesthesia care unit, intensive care unit, and medical-surgical unit needed to develop special knowledge and skills to provide optimal care for trauma patients. As the trauma nursing theory and specialty practice was being developed, advanced practice roles emerged for nurses. The trauma coordinator and trauma clinical specialist roles were created in the late 1970s along with the early hospital trauma program development. Because of financial pressures from hospital cost containment efforts in the 1980s, the role of the trauma nurse case manager was developed to manage the hospital stay and discharge of trauma patients. The goal of this role is to move the trauma patient through the hospital care phase as quickly as possible in order to avoid denied hospital days by the insurance companies and Medicare. In the 1990s, as financial pressures on hospitals continued, the nurse case manager role in some trauma centers evolved to the use of acute care trauma nurse practitioners as active care providers and case managers for trauma patients within the hospital and to provide ongoing follow-up care.

TRAUMA REHABILITATION NURSING

During previous decades, as advances in the care of the seriously injured patient were made and incorporated into the resuscitation and critical care cycles, more lives were saved, and another phase of trauma care was recognized. As trauma patients emerged from intensive care settings, it became apparent that their medical and nursing care needed to take a new focus. Intensive care stays have shortened for most patients in the past 10 years. For the trauma patient, this early move to the medical-surgical unit meant that the nurses on these units had to deal with the complex acute care needs of these patients, as well as their rehabilitation needs. The trauma patient's rehabilitation needs had to be identified early in the acute phase of care. Appropriate care that addressed these rehabilitation needs was initiated while the patient was in the intensive care unit and continued through the hospital stay, and a discharge plan for ongoing rehabilitation in an inpatient or outpatient rehabilitation program was created. Attention also needed to be placed on assisting patients as they prepared for reintegration into their homes, jobs, and social groups. The nursing care during this intermediate or rehabilitation phase required the acquisition of new knowledge and skills in areas such as patient-family teaching, cognitive retraining, occupational and physical therapy, and discharge planning.

The evolution of effective rehabilitation methods and procedures has improved the clinical care of trauma patients. Failure to incorporate such advances into the plan of care for trauma patients results in avoidable yet significant societal health care costs. The socioeconomic impact of this unfortunate trend is believed to be so great that, for every dollar spent on rehabilitation services, it is estimated that between $6 and $35 could be saved by state and federal agencies.[38,39] More widespread application of the knowledge and skills associated with advanced rehabilitation practices may result in substantial economic savings and a more productive and improved quality of life for the trauma patient population.

To minimize the trauma patient's social and economic disability, it is essential that the rehabilitation components of care begin immediately. Appropriate interventions in managing the critically injured patient from injury through return to home enhance clinical outcomes (reduced disability and mortality), promote personal autonomy, and because an independent noninstitutional lifestyle is fostered, may shorten inpatient stays. Rehabilitation within this framework represents a process whereby the patient and family collaborate with nurses, physicians, and other specialists to identify mutual goals and plans to assist the trauma patient in achieving an optimal level of recovery. By striving to overcome limitations in functional cognition, communication, self-care, mobility, hygiene, vocation, family role, and coping abilities, a multidisciplinary rehabilitation system can provide all trauma patients with the opportunity to achieve maximal physical, social, psychologic, and vocational recovery.

In an effort to provide empiric data for effective rehabilitation, several studies were conducted on patients with severe lower extremity fractures. These studies have shown that a patient's ability to return to maximal function is complex and involves factors other than the physical disability, such as the physical, social, and economic environments.[40-42]

TRAUMA NURSING—THE FOCUS OF CARE

In response to changes in incidence, magnitude, and severity of injuries, the complexity of the therapeutic needs of the trauma patient population, and thus the demands on the entire health care system, the specialty field of trauma nursing has carved its niche. Influenced by a rapidly expanding body of knowledge focusing on how the human system responds to traumatic injury and which factors may make a difference in improving care, trauma nursing has expanded beyond the traditional practice mode. The effects of stress and adaptability on the course of illness, factors traditionally recognized by nurses, have become more readily valued as critical variables in the trauma patient's recovery. This is supportive of the holistic approach to patient care—attention on the whole individual, which is easily contrasted with a fragmented approach that focuses on specific pieces of information without acknowledging that these pieces are woven in an intricate fashion into the human fabric. The emphasis of trauma nursing is addressing the needs of the injured patient, which can be encompassed in five spheres: (1) support of vital life functions, (2) support for physiologic adaptation, (3) promotion of safety and security, (4) support for psychologic and social adaptation, and (5) spirituality. Holistic care of the trauma patient requires continuity in the delivery of expert nursing care that addresses all five spheres of patients' care needs. Several significant factors must be considered if this continuity is to be accomplished.

THE HUMAN RESPONSE TO TRAUMATIC INJURY. The impact of trauma on the individual can be viewed from various angles, including physiologic, psychologic, spiritual, and socioeconomic perspectives. The biologic makeup provides the human species with miraculous capabilities for maintaining itself in a relative state of homeostasis. As insults such as infectious agents, foreign bodies, and/or traumatic injuries are imposed on the human system, various physiologic components are activated in an attempt to counteract the insult and its effects. The human system has the function of maintaining a sense of equilibrium or balance; this function or process is often referred to as the "natural healing power" of the human species. This healing energy exists within all of us in some form to varying degrees. The biologic response of the individual to insults such as traumatic injury is in part dependent on the human organism's natural ability to adjust or adapt physiologically. How and to what degree the individual is able to adapt can be determined by observing behavioral responses, as well as monitoring certain physiologic parameters. These findings can often be translated by nurses and used as measurable therapeutic tools to predict outcomes.

The human organism cannot, however, be viewed simply from a biologic perspective. To do so would defy the laws of nature. No organism can be understood completely by studying only one aspect of it without acknowledging the effects of others on the composition of the entire system. This is not to say that scientific studies cannot be organized so that separate bodies of knowledge are identified and developed according to established processes. However, the scientific exploration of one human parameter in isolation, without considering the effects on the total human configuration, results in fragmented, useless information.

In keeping with this theme, the individual human response to traumatic injury also must be examined from the psychologic, spiritual, and socioeconomic perspectives. In order to provide efficient and effective nursing care that encompasses all realms of human response, the trauma nurse must employ a systematic means of observing and assessing the patient to elicit care needs in all five spheres. Part of the challenge for trauma nurses is to identify negative adaptation responses, behaviors, and attitudes and to help the patient adapt more positively.

Trauma patients face other hazards in addition to the physiologic effects of injury. They also must face the effects of traumatic insult on their thought patterns and attitudes. These conditions also may be worsened by deprived sensory systems, a situation that frequently occurs in an intensive care setting or from a prolonged hospital stay. In making compensatory adjustments, the mind may create illusions, hallucinations, and visions. When the patient is unable to cope with or to adapt independently to increasing tension, the trauma nurse must apply energies to provide emotional, psychologic, and physical support until the patient regains enough energy to resume independent functioning. This requires that the nurse formulate a plan of action based on open communication, especially important in the emotional atmosphere of an acute care environment. Thus, at the first available opportunity, the nurse should encourage the trauma patient to communicate fears, frustrations, and anxieties about the traumatic incident, the injuries sustained, the medical and nursing management regimen, and the future course of events. The patient's spiritual needs are assessed by obtaining information about religious orientation, culture, beliefs, and values and the patient's sense of belonging or connectedness with family, friends, and community.

Following comprehensive assessment, the nurse must choose appropriate nursing actions to enhance the forces of adaptation by redirecting the dynamic processes in a positive direction. The nurse can assist the patient in developing a new future based on assessment of the past and appraisal of realistic goals or limitations in the present. Ideally the trauma nurse's support and understanding will help the patient to accept the limitations caused by the traumatic injury.

In developing a comprehensive plan of care, the trauma nurse also must be alert to socioeconomic dynamics. Trauma has an impact on the social groups of which the patient is a member. In addition to the family system, these groups include work and church groups, as well as clubs and other social affiliations, all of which have an effect on the individual trauma patient. In order to enable the trauma nurse to assist the injured patient effectively in adapting, the reactions and expectations of family members and friends must be considered. Generally, the way in which injury and disability are viewed depends on a variety of factors, including the type of injury, previous personal experience with illness or injury, norms and values of the individual and particular social groups, and the perceived expectations for social reintegration. Understanding the social dynamics unique to each patient's situation will assist the nurse in identifying appropriate resources within the hospital and community that will help in planning for the patient's discharge. Understanding social dynamics is critical to the nurse's management of the patient's care plan, facilitation of hospital discharge to rehabilitation services, and follow-up during the recovery phase of care.

The effect of an injured family member on the entire family structure must not be overlooked. Considered an important and essential component in the nursing care plan, the family must receive attention and support from the trauma nurse. It is important and essential that the trauma nurse establishes a firm base of knowledge and develops skill in interacting with the patient's family members. The nature and severity of the impact of trauma on the members of the family will vary as a function of (1) the type of traumatic injury, (2) the phase or point at which the family is observed, (3) the family structure, (4) the identity of the injured person (e.g., mother, daughter, grandfather), (5) the point at which the traumatic injury occurs during the course of the individual's life, and (6) the point at which it occurs in the life of the family. The family's response to a sudden and traumatic injury that represents a crisis event is dynamic and interactive. To understand the family system and its individual members, the nurse should assess the crisis response in all family members or other significant relationships.[43,44]

Family function may be affected in different ways by the sudden traumatic injury of a family member. As the impact of the traumatic injury on the patient is considered from the biologic, psychologic, spiritual, and socioeconomic perspectives, so may the impact on the family structure.

The biologic functions of a family unit include the nurturing and physical care of a family member: feeding, cleaning, and tending to the injury or illness. This may include identifying, preventing, and attempting to cure health threats and determining when advice or assistance from others outside the family unit is necessary. Trauma nurses should identify themselves as supportive resources to family members so that open lines of communication are established, thus fostering the sharing of valuable information between the patient's family and the trauma health care team.

The development and maintenance of the patient's self-image and self-esteem are among the psychologic functions of the family system. This is accomplished through emotional communication patterns, which involve the expression of fear, anger, anxiety, frustration, joy, excitement, and contentment. The conditions under which these emotional expressions are permitted, not permitted, or controlled also must be identified by the family within the context of the culture with which the family identifies.

Included among the family's social functions are the tasks of defining group membership and group boundaries and establishing norms for relationships within the group, as well as outside the group. The family is also considered within the context of the formal or informal societal structure and is viewed as a wage-earning, product-consuming, help-giving, tax-paying unit within our socioeconomic system.

Each of the functions described represents an important component for assessing how well the family unit is fulfilling biologic, psychologic, emotional, and social functions.[44] The trauma nurse must be alert to the patterns of family system functions and incorporate the unique characteristics of patient-family lifestyles into the comprehensive plan of care.

NURSES' ROLE IN PREVENTION

An examination of the impact that trauma has on the community raises issues that must be addressed. In most communities, unintentional injuries are taken for granted. Perhaps a major problem relates to the knowledge, or lack of it, that communities have about injury and the effects not only on the individual and family but also on the community as a whole. The cost of trauma to the community must be seen in health care costs, as well as in the monetary expenditure resulting from reduced worker hours. As responsible members of the health care community, nurses should take responsibility for disseminating information about the nation's trauma problem. Health care professionals and consumers need to be alert to the causes of unintentional injuries and how they can be prevented.

As with many health care problems today, the cause of injury cannot be reduced to a single factor but must be viewed within the context of a broad spectrum of related factors. The predominant factor is human error. In 1990, 78% of vehicular crashes resulting in fatal or nonfatal injuries were caused by improper driving practices. A much smaller percentage was caused by vehicle defects or poor road conditions. Exceeding the posted speed limit or driving at an unsafe speed was the most common error reported in injuries of all severities in rural areas and in fatal injuries in urban areas. Right-of-way violations predominated in the occurrence of urban motor vehicle injuries.[2] Alcohol is a factor in approximately 41% of fatal motor vehicle crashes,[2] and illegal drugs and many legally prescribed medications can slow reaction time, thus contributing to the occurrence of injury.

The home can be a dangerous place as well. In 1990 mishaps that occurred in and around the home resulted in 28,400 deaths and 6,800,000 disabling injuries. With an injury total of this magnitude, it is estimated that 1 in 39 U.S. citizens was disabled one or more days by injuries received in home mishaps. Falls, poisonings, fires, criminal violence (including child abuse, domestic violence, and injuries from bullets and bombs), and sporting injuries, although representing a smaller proportion of the total number of deaths or cases requiring hospitalization each year, should alert the public to the importance of prevention.

Many injuries are both predictable and preventable in the same way that many impairments are treatable and the resulting disabilities preventable. The development of effective trauma prevention programs can provide countless opportunities for addressing the trauma problem as it currently exists in our society. Likewise, the ample availability of rehabilitation programs can create a proliferation of opportunities for thousands of trauma patients. Yet despite these common truths, a passive societal posture seems to prevail. It has been described as a "pervasive fatalistic attitude that equates impairment with disability and concludes that accidents just happen and nothing can be done to prevent them."[45]

Consumer involvement is imperative in gaining legislative support for issues pertaining to health, safety, and the prevention of unintentional injury. Unfortunately, the beneficial economic impact of trauma prevention has not been adequately and effectively translated into compelling public policy. The following situation serves as a case in point. A general feeling of optimism prevailed after Tennessee enacted a child restraint law, making it the fiftieth state to do so. Optimism continued as a similar trend with regard to general safety belt use laws seemed to emerge. Yet safety belt laws were reversed for a period of time (and have since been reenacted) in Massachusetts and Nebraska, despite supportive evidence that shows the savings in health care costs afforded by routine safety belt use are substantial.[45]

Trauma nurses have spoken out and should continue to do so as they assume a leadership role in influencing issues of injury prevention and control, refusing to accept the grim statistics regarding trauma in our society. A considerable number of currently active prevention programs have been initiated and maintained by trauma nurses throughout the country—courageous testimony to the energy, interest, and accountability exemplified by nurses on behalf of the public. Although a complete list of such programs is not available and a program-specific description and an in-depth discussion are beyond the scope of this chapter, it is important to note that trauma nurse-activists are addressing issues regarding alcohol and drug abuse and their implications for every injury mechanism and etiology; highway safety issues, including safety belt use, child restraint, and helmet laws; and domestic violence issues, including child abuse, firearms, and environmental influences.[46,47] Most importantly, trauma nurses continue to voice the strong belief that, in matters pertaining to trauma care, those who have assumed an intricate role in meeting the complex needs of the trauma patient population should play a key role in shaping policy.

TRAUMA NURSING TODAY

When considering the evolution of the trauma nursing specialty, one must understand several significant developments and events of the past three decades. A review of

TABLE 1-2   Milestones Of Trauma Nursing

1961 First shock trauma nurses. Elizabeth Scanlan, RN, and Jane Tarrant, RN, pioneered the nurse's role in the first two-bed shock/trauma research center with R. Adams Cowley, MD, at University of Maryland Hospital, Baltimore, Maryland.

1963 National Research Center awarded a first-of-a-kind grant to the University of Maryland in Baltimore to establish a center for the study of trauma.

1966 Cook County Hospital in Chicago opened a trauma unit with Robert Freeark, MD, as medical director and Norma Shoemaker, RN, as nursing supervisor.

1966 *Accidental Death and Disability: The Neglected Disease of Modern Society* (white paper on trauma) published, citing needs of trauma population. This led to federal funding of trauma centers.

1971 First trauma nurse coordinators hired for Level I trauma centers in Illinois. David Boyd, MD, hired Theresa Romano, RN, to direct the education and training of nurses working in the designated trauma centers in Illinois.

1973 Federal contracts awarded to Texas Women's University, University of Cincinnati, and University of Washington to begin graduate nursing programs in burns. These programs were the model for the first graduate trauma nursing programs.

1975 Maryland state EMS system established trauma nurse coordinator position for training, designation, and evaluation.

1982 ATLS for nurses (pilot program) taught in conjunction with physician course. Nursing track was developed by MIEMSS Field Nursing, Baltimore.

1983 Trauma nurse network organized to provide communication link for trauma nurses.

1986 TNCC course, Emergency Nurses Association.

1987 First national census forum on Development of Trauma Nurse Coordinator Role, Washington, DC.

1989 Society of Trauma Nurses formed.

1993 The inaugural issue of the *Journal of Trauma Nursing* is published by the Society of Trauma Nurses.

2000 Society of Trauma Nurses collaborates with the American College of Surgeons COT and ATLS Committees to provide the Advanced Trauma Care for Nurses course.

Modified from Beachley M, Snow S, Trimble P: Developing trauma care systems: the trauma nurse coordinator, *JONA* 18(7,8):34-42, 1980.

pertinent factual information in congressional testimony, technical reports, and the literature has established a historical perspective of the development of trauma/emergency medical services systems* (Table 1-2). The proliferation of designated trauma care facilities and the increasing regularity of formal meetings and conferences joining major organizations and professionals together are measures of the progress in recognizing trauma patients as a unique population requiring specialty services. These

*References 3, 5, 7, 13, 16, 19, 20.

professional gatherings are indicative of the need for increased coordination, and clearly defined responsibilities are needed if each group—nurses, physicians, paramedics, and other allied health care professionals—is to deliver effective and efficient care.

In the past 30 years, achievements and advances in this direction have been monumental and drastically surpass all efforts made during the preceding century. The technologic advances, the unquestioned recognition of need, and the impetus from many concerned individuals and professional groups have made this possible. These factors have resulted in support from local, state, and national governments for regional planning and implementation of efficient trauma care services. It is essential that nurses become involved in this regional trauma EMS planning, implementation, and evaluation locally, nationally, and internationally.

Many of the goals of the white paper *Accidental Death and Disability—The Neglected Disease of Modern Society*[7] have been attained or at least movement toward them has begun. An increasing number of institutions specialize in the care of the severely injured patient. The development and designation of such institutions may be viewed as a natural evolution as a result of the dramatically increasing magnitude of the trauma problem and the demands of the trauma patient population on the entire health care system.

Likewise, the demanding clinical needs of the critically injured trauma patients, coupled with trauma nursing's crossing of established boundaries within the traditional nursing educational structure, have led to the natural evolution of trauma nursing as a specialty field within the larger emergency health care system. As with all systems that change over time, trauma nursing continues to develop toward a higher level of organization. As trauma patient care requirements have become more complex, nurses have emerged as coordinators capable of integrating the actions of other health care professionals. This process has allowed the integration of the total care regimen, including all trauma specialty fields, which potentiates the process of unified action. Several expanded roles have been established as a means of meeting the special care needs and complexities of the trauma patient population and their families, among them the trauma nurse coordinator, trauma nurse practitioner, and trauma case manager.[48-52] This book presents a working body of knowledge based on principles from traditional nursing models and from the theoretic frameworks of medicine, psychology, physical science, education, and behavioral and social sciences. Perhaps it is this broad spectrum of required knowledge that has attracted a pioneering breed of nurses to accept the challenge of contributing the integral components of a multidimensional and holistic focus in caring for the trauma patient. The nature of severe injuries resulting in multisystem disruptions requires the trauma nurse to comprehend extensive scientific data; to synthesize care in life-threatening emergencies; and to lead, assist, and support the patient and family on the long journey toward recovery. Daily, this group of caregivers is bombarded with uncharted pathophysiologic phenomena and unceasing psychologic and emotional crises. For the nurse to function efficiently in this situation, high levels of energy and stamina are required. To do this, each nurse must take responsibility for periodically examining his or her stress levels while constantly being alert to the stress levels of others. This fosters an atmosphere of caring, not only for the patients and families but also for one another.

THE TRAUMA CYCLE—CONCEPTUAL DEVELOPMENT

In closely examining the cycle of events that occur throughout the many phases of trauma care—from the time of injury; through the resuscitation, critical, intermediate (medical-surgical unit), and rehabilitation phases of care; to the return to home and community—a wealth of information can be derived and added to the existing body of knowledge and skills of trauma nursing. This process of continued growth and development will determine the future direction of trauma nursing practice.

Although a traumatic injury occurs within a very short time frame, it has long-term effects. Trauma can therefore be viewed as a disease process with far-reaching consequences. Many of the changes that occur during and after a traumatic incident are a direct result of the individual's ability to adapt to the injured state. For this reason, this book is organized with the subject content presented in the context of time and space. In other words, we believe that it is beneficial to look at the individual's traumatic incident and subsequent care as it occurs in a cyclic pattern. What happens to an individual when an injury occurs will be described in blocks of time, or phases within the trauma cycle. This method takes into account what circumstances existed before the injury, which may or may not have precipitated the incident; what occurs at the exact time of the incident, with consideration of the biomechanics of the injury and the circumstances that may have contributed to its nature and extent; and what changes occur after a traumatic injury. This exploration of events will begin with time representing the resuscitation phase and will continue through the operative, critical care, and intermediate and rehabilitation phases to the time at which the individual is integrated into the community. At any time during this cyclic pattern, valuable information can be learned that will assist the skilled nurse in assessing and planning, implementing, and evaluating a special plan of care for the trauma patient and his or her family.

Reflected throughout the book is the view that the care of the trauma patient is not performed on a linear continuum with a beginning and an end but instead throughout a cyclic process. The trauma cycle represents a series of changes that leads back to its starting point; the patient enters the emergency health care system from the community and at some point reenters the community. As the individual returns to the community, the cycle is completed, yet the potential always exists for the cycle to be repeated—there is no end point. Accordingly, prevention is a concept that must receive prime consideration when caring for patients throughout the process. Based on the strong belief that prevention is better than cure, much emphasis will be placed not only on the prevention of traumatic injury but also on the prevention of complications, disability, and maladaptive adjustments on the part of the patient and family once a traumatic injury has occurred. The trauma sequel represents a complete cycle of phenomena and operations—changes that lead toward the restoration of a state of well-being. Helping patient and family return to a healthy state is the goal of the trauma nurse—and the target of all interventions.

REFERENCES

1. Trinkaus E, Zimmerman MR: Trauma among the Shanidar Neanderthals, *Am J Phys Anthropol* 57:61-76, 1982.
2. National Safety Council: *Injury facts,* Chicago, 1999.
3. U.S. Department of Health, Education and Welfare: *Report of the Secretary's Advisory Committee on Traffic Safety,* Washington, DC, Feb 29, 1968, U.S. Government Printing Office.
4. Simeone FA: Studies of trauma and shock in man: William S. Stone's role in the military effort (1983 William S. Stone Lecture), *J Trauma* 24:181-187, 1984.
5. The Board for the Study of the Severely Wounded, Medical Department, United States Army: In Beecher HR, editor: *Surgery in World War II: the physiologic effects of wounds,* Washington, DC, 1952, U.S. Government Printing Office.
6. Heaton LD: Army medical service activities in Vietnam. *Milit Med* 131:646, 1966.
7. U.S. Department of Health, Education and Welfare: *Accidental death and disability: the neglected disease of modern society,* Rockville, Md, 1996, Division of Medical Sciences, National Academy of Sciences, National Research Council.
8. Boyd D, Edlich RF, Micik SH: *Systems approach to emergency medical care,* Norwalk, Conn, 1983, Appleton-Century-Crofts.
9. Ogilivie RB: *Special message on health care,* Springfield, Ill, April 1, 1971, State of Illinois Printing Office.
10. Meyer P, Rosen HB, Hall W: Fracture dislocations of the cervical spine: transportation assessment, and immediate management, *Am Acad Orthop Surg* 25:171-183, 1976.
11. Cowley RA: Trauma center—a new concept for the delivery of critical care, *J Med Soc NJ* 74:979-986, 1977.
12. Maryland Department of Health and Mental Hygiene: *Maryland vital statistics annual report,* Rockville, Md, 1997.
13. U.S. Congress: *Emergency medical services systems act,* Public Law 93-154, Pub No SB2 410, Washington, DC, Nov 16, 1973, U.S. Government Printing Office.
14. U.S. General Accounting Office: *States assume leadership role in providing emergency medical services,* Pub No GAO/HRD-86-132, Washington, DC, 1986, U.S. Government Printing Office.
15. U.S. Congress: *Trauma care systems planning and development act of 1990,* Public Law 101-590, 104 Stat 2915, Washington, DC, Nov 16, 1990, U.S. Government Printing Office.
16. U.S. Department of Health and Human Services, Health Resources and Services Administration: *Model trauma care system plan,* Rockville, Md, September 30, 1992, Bureau of Health Services Resources, Division of Trauma and Emergency Medical Services.
17. Division of Emergency Medical Services, Health Services Administration, Bureau of Medical Services Administration: *Emergency medical services systems program guidelines,* DHHS Pub No (HSA) 75-2013, Washington, DC, 1975.
18. American College of Emergency Physicians' Trauma Committee: Guidelines for trauma care systems, *Ann Emerg Med* 16(4):459-463, 1987.
19. Committee on Trauma of the American College of Surgeons: Optimal hospital resources for care of the severely injured, *Bull Am Coll Surg* 61:15-22, 1976.
20. Committee on Trauma of the American College of Surgeons: Hospital resources for optimal care of the injured patient, *Bull Am Coll Surg* 64:43-48, 1979.
21. American College of Surgeons' Committee on Trauma: *Resources for the optimal care of the injured patient,* Chicago, 1999, American College of Surgeons.
22. U.S. Department of Transportation and National Highway Traffic Safety Administration: *Emergency medical technician: basic national standard curriculum,* Washington, DC, 1994, U.S. Government Printing Office.
23. Miller T, Levy D: The effect of regional trauma care systems on costs, *Arch Surgery* 130:188-193, 1995.
24. U.S. Department of Health and Human Services, Public Health Services, Centers for Disease Control, Trauma Care Systems Panel: Injury control, Position paper in the Third National Injury Control Conference, Washington, DC, April 1992, pp 377-426.
25. Skamania Symposium: Trauma systems supplement, *J Trauma* 47:3, Sept 1999.
26. Nightingale F: *Notes on nursing: what it is and what it is not,* New York, 1969, Dover.
27. Huxley EJ: *Florence Nightingale,* New York, 1975, Putnam.
28. *History of American Red Cross nursing,* New York, 1922, Macmillan, ch 1 & 2.
29. Thurstan V: Active Science. In Thurstan V, editor: *A textbook of war nursing,* London, 1917, GP Putnam's Sons.
30. Mays ET: *Clinical evaluation of the critically ill,* Springfield, IL, 1975, Charles C Thomas.
31. Oakes AR: Trauma: twentieth-century epidemic, *Heart Lung* 8:918-922, 1979.
32. Von Wagoner FH: Died in hospital: a three year study of deaths following trauma, *J Trauma* 1:401-408, 1961.
33. Gertner HR, Baker SP, Rutherford RB, et al: Evaluation of the management of vehicular fatalities secondary to abdominal injury, *J Trauma* 12:425-431, 1972.
34. Foley FW, Harris LS, Pilcher DB: Abdominal injuries in automobile accidents: review of care of fatally injured patients, *J Trauma* 17:611-615, 1977.
35. Houtchens BA: Major trauma in the rural mountains west, *J Am Coll Emerg Phys* 6:343-350, 1977.
36. Frey CF, Huelke DF, Gikas PW: Resuscitation and survival in motor vehicle accidents, *J Trauma* 9:292-310, 1969.
37. Allgöwer M, Border JR: Advances in the care of the multiple trauma patient: introduction, *World J Surg* 7:1-3, 1983.
38. Committee on Trauma Research Commission on Life Sciences, National Research Council and the Institute of Medicine: *Injury in America: a continuing public health problem,* Washington, DC, 1985, National Academy Press.
39. Hammerman SR, Maikowski S: The economics of disability from an international perspective, *Annu Rev Rehabil* 3:178-202, 1983.
40. Mackenzie EJ, et al: Physical impairment and functional outcomes six months after severe lower extremity fractures, *J Trauma* 4:528-538, 1993.

41. Mackenzie EJ: Return to work following injury: the role of economic, social, and job-related factors, *Am J Public Health* 11:1630-1637, 1998.

42. McCarthy ML, et al: Correlation between the measures of impairment, according to the modified system of the American Medical Association, and function, *J Bone Joint Surg* 80-87:1034-1042, 1998.

43. Leske JS: Treatment for family members in crisis after critical injury, *AACN Clin Issues* 9(1):129-139, 1998.

44. Tuck D, Kerns R: *Health, illness and families: a life span prospective,* New York, 1985, Wiley.

45. Maull K: Dispelling fatalism in a cause-and-effect world (1989 EAST presidential address), *J Trauma* 29:752-756, 1989.

46. Ernal Ségal: Straight Talk on Prevention (STOP) Program, *Maryland EMS Newsletter* 17(10):1-2, 1991.

47. Dearing-Stuck B: Trauma prevention. In Cardona G, editor: *Trauma nursing,* Oradell, NJ, 1985, Medical Economics Press.

48. Beachley M, Snow S, Trimble P: Developing trauma care systems: the trauma nurse coordinator, *JONA* 18(7,8):34-42, 1988.

49. Spisso J, et al: Improved quality of care and reduction of house staff workload using trauma nurse practitioners, *J Trauma* 30(6):660-663, 1990.

50. Gantt D, Price J, Pollock D: The status of the trauma coordinator position: a national survey, *J Trauma* 40(5):816-819, 1966.

51. Keough V, et al: A collaborative program for advanced practice in trauma/critical care nursing, *Crit Care Nurse* 16(2):120-127, 1996.

52. Daleiden A: The CNS as trauma case manager: a new frontier, *Clin Nurse Specialist* 7(6):295-298, 1993.

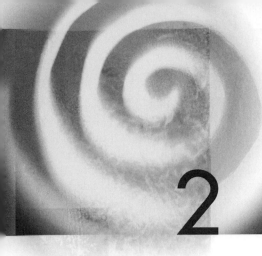

2

ECONOMIC ISSUES IN TRAUMA CARE

Connie A. Jastremski

Trauma exerts financial stresses on patients, hospitals, and society. It currently ranks second to cancer in costs of care but, as for any disease, medical care accounts for only a small portion of the total costs. Lost wages, property damage, and indirect costs are extremely high for traumatic incidents.[1] The total cost of fatal and nonfatal unintentional injuries in 1997—$478.3 billion—includes employee costs, vehicle damage cost, fire losses, wage and productivity losses, medical expenses, and administrative and employer costs (Table 2-1). These costs do not include the additional burden that intentionally inflicted injuries such as gunshot wounds, abuse, and other violent acts can impose.[2] The rise in urban violence has led to an increased prevalence of penetrating trauma, primarily from firearms. More than one million American civilians have been killed by firearms since 1993.[3] The use of firearms adds additional medical costs of $1.9 billion to $2.7 billion each year.[4] Approximately $10 billion is spent annually to cover physician and hospital costs alone, with the average trauma admission costing approximately $12,000.[5]

Much has been published regarding the efficacy of trauma care systems in reducing death and disability since publication of the 1966 white paper by the National Academy of Sciences, identifying trauma as the "neglected disease of modern society."[6] The financial burden placed on the trauma system and trauma centers continues to be a deterrent to expansion of comprehensive trauma systems. As of 1992, 92 trauma centers that had been accredited by their state or the American College of Surgeons (ACS) have closed.[7] It is estimated that only 25% of the United States population has access to organized trauma care.[8] An in-depth understanding of the economic issues that surround the provision of high-quality trauma care is essential to continuing development of trauma systems and to proactively implement changes that will increase the ability to provide the needed care.

As part of the health care system, trauma systems and trauma centers are facing the same turbulent economic times as the rest of the health care arena. Trauma care is both labor and resource intensive, and the financing of health care overall is shrinking. In addition, the care provided to many of the victims of trauma is uncompensated care, either self-pay or no funding. These economic forces, joined with the high cost of providing care to the injured, are conspiring to further compromise the delivery of high-quality trauma care in the United States.

This chapter focuses on the economic issues that surround trauma systems and trauma care delivery. The first part of the chapter discusses the financing of health care and the effect of recent economic changes on trauma care. The second section explores the cost of trauma care associated with special populations. The third part of the chapter describes strategies that have been attempted to confront the changing economic forces.

HEALTH CARE FINANCING

A historic review of the financing of health care is not only interesting but also contributes to our understanding of the dilemma that trauma care faces today. The system of financing health care parallels the system of the industrial revolution in this country. As production systems formed in the United States, the need for the management of health care became important. These changes were coupled with an economic explosion unmatched elsewhere in the world.

The sudden appearance of a great deal of surplus wealth at the turn of the twentieth century resulted in the development of "personal health" services structured for the individual buyer. The system that evolved was not based on equity and was not formulated to serve the masses. Private hospitals were built to serve the affluent and depended on religious and philanthropic contributions. Physician charges were based on the patient's ability to pay. The poor were the residuals of the system, and their care was generally provided in a charity hospital set up on a local or state level. These charity hospitals were built to buffer the voluntary, nonprofit hospitals that were growing in numbers.

Except for mental health, public safety, and the Veterans Administration, the federal government stayed clear of involvement in the evolution of the early health care system. The government purchased health care from the private sector. Thus before 1930 almost all health care services were purchased by individuals.[9]

TABLE 2-1	Costs of Unintentional Injuries, 1997	
Class of Injury	**Approximate Cost (Billions of Dollars)**	
Motor Vehicle	200.3	
Work	127.7	
Home	99.9	
Public	66.1	

Source: National Safety Council Data.

The period between 1930 and 1965 was marked by the development of third-party payment plans. The conception of prepaid health insurance was fueled by the Great Depression and the need for guaranteed payment of the rapidly rising costs of hospitalization. The rapid expansion of medical knowledge combined with increasing technology drove the costs of hospitalization to extreme heights at the time. Unpaid hospital bills threatened to impair the future growth of the health care industry. In response to the demands to pay a higher price for health care, hospitals developed what later evolved into the Blue Cross plans, and a group of entrepreneurs organized other private health insurance. Physicians who were worried about nonpayment of bills developed prepayment plans to ensure payment for their services. The passage of the Hill-Burton Act in 1946 fueled the growth and expansion of hospitals. This act provided support to the private, voluntary, not-for-profit hospitals that were losing their philanthropic financing. The development of large hospitals and increased technologies were encouraged by a retrospective payment structure defined by the third-party payers and supported by the federal government.

By the 1950s the general economy was growing steadily, but health services were propagating at an unimaginable rate. The provision of disease care progressively consumed a greater and greater portion of the gross domestic product (GDP). The common perception at that time was that there were too few hospitals and physicians. The cost of health care on a per capita basis began to rise exponentially around 1965. The health care industry was the second largest employer in the United States.[9] The third-party payers (not including the federal government) were covering 40% of the costs of hospital operations and 30% of the charges for physician services. The government was paid 50% of the hospital costs and 20% of the physician charges. It appeared that costs for health care were of no consequence.

In the mid 1960s the purchasers of health care began to express alarm at the pace at which the costs of health care were increasing. Employers (most of whom paid for their employees' health insurance) and the government were distressed by the dollars being spent. The federal government had become the single largest purchaser of health care. At the time, it was predicted that the percentage of the GDP related to health care would rise at a slope of 0.22% per year (as it had from 1960 to 1985) and reach a level of 14% by 2000. That percentage was attained in 1995 despite measures to contain health care costs.[10]

The most pervasive role of government in the payment of health care is as a third-party payer. This role is primarily the result of Titles 18 and 19 of the Social Security Act of 1965. These laws created Medicare and Medicaid, which commenced in 1966.[10] Under Title 18 the federal government administers an insurance program (Medicare) for the elderly and permanently disabled. It is divided into two separate elements, referred to as Part A and Part B. Part A is the program that provides payment for hospital care. It is financed by taxes on earnings and, the way the fund for Part A is designed, cannot be supplemented to any great extent. Part B, the medical care portion of the program, is optional and is financed by premiums from potential patients. The amount of payments to hospitals and physicians is determined at the federal level and has been dwindling over the past several years.

Title 19 created the federal government's program for the medically indigent, Medicaid. This program is a combined federal and state program, with increasing responsibilities being shifted to the state level. The percentage of federal contributions and the services provided under this plan vary from state to state.

With the extraordinary growth of the costs of health care, the government found itself in the alarming position of facing rapid extinction of the social security trust fund. It responded first by attempting to regulate the rate of growth through controls on expansion of services via elimination of "unnecessary" duplication of services. It attempted to accomplish this through the certificate of need (CON) mechanisms that put controls on these processes at the local level. However, these mechanisms failed to control the skyrocketing costs of health care.

Following an experiment to control health care costs in New Jersey, the federal government initiated the first prospective payment form of reimbursement. The plan was based on schedules on the average costs of care for 472 diagnosis-related groups (DRGs). This method of reimbursement to control hospital costs was directed originally at the elderly and the poor, whose care was being provided through Medicare and Medicaid. Other third-party payers quickly followed suit, and prospective payment plans became the way for health care reimbursement. With prospective payment, the health care organization had incentive to reduce costs of care and change the length of care delivered in order to make money. Anticipating the reimbursement allowed practitioners to determine how to manage patient care for less than the total to be paid. Any amount not used could be kept by the hospital. It was thought that this would be a "win-win" for the payers and the hospitals. The intended impact of the prospective payment system was to minimize the length of stay and thus decrease resource consumption.[11] The flaw in the plan was that the payment was based on "average" costs of care. If the patient had other illnesses (co-morbidities) or was just not "average," the hospital could lose a lot of money on a case-by-case basis. In

TABLE 2-2	**Effects of Managed Care on Health Care Insurance Plans**			
Parties	**Subscribers**	**Physicians**	**Hospitals**	**Employers**
HMOs	Restricted choices	Limited access	Limited access	Reduced cost
	Generous benefits	Discounted reimbursement or capitation	Discounted charges, per diems, case rates or capitation	
		Utilization Review (UR) requirements	UR	
PPOs	Choice from panel of providers	Access by contracting	Limited access	Reduced cost
	Co-pays	Discounted charges or fee schedule	Discounted charges or per diem	
	Out-of-network care with reduced benefits and higher cost	UR—mostly hospital based	UR	
	Broader benefits			
Indemnity	Free choice	All participate	All participate	Expensive but provides the most freedom for employees
	Deductible and 80/20 co-pays	Paid charges	Paid charges	
	Major medical benefits			
	Limited outpatient coverage			

addition, employers began demanding more reasonable rates for health care insurance for their employees. Almost three fourths of all health insurance is provided through employers, which explains their vested interest in the cost of health care.[10]

The push to find ways to control spending has given rise to a number of approaches. Most prominent among them is the concept of health maintenance organizations (HMOs), preferred provider organizations (PPOs), and managed care. *Managed care* refers to forms of insurance coverage in which enrollee utilization patterns and provider service patterns are monitored by the insurer or an intermediary with the aim of containing costs.[10] Managed care is most frequently associated with HMOs and PPOs because these types of organizations were the first to try to control the utilization of care. More recently, indemnity insurers have begun to introduce regulatory controls over providers, such as second-opinion requirements for surgery and length-of-stay reviews.[10] Paying on a per-case basis with a capitated rate allows the payers control over the practitioners by creating limits on reimbursement. Managed care is no longer a choice but a requisite for survival and a way to control costs. Table 2-2 summarizes the attributes of various types of insurance plans and the effects of managed care on their constituents.

THE FINANCING OF TRAUMA CARE

In 1966 the National Academy of Sciences and the National Research Council published a landmark report, *Accidental Death and Disability: The Neglected Disease of Modern Society.*[6] This report created the recognition that trauma is a disease and that improvements in care of the injured could make a difference in the survival rates of trauma victims. It also prompted the development of organized trauma systems.

The emerging trauma system concept involved the tenets of treating the patient within the "golden hour"[12] and getting the "right patient to the right place at the right time."[13] Federal funding for the development of trauma systems was made available by the Highway Safety Act of 1966 and the Emergency Medical Services Act of 1973. Supported by guidelines developed by the American College of Surgeons Committee on Trauma, the American College of Emergency Physicians, and the American Association for the Surgery of Trauma, trauma centers and systems began to develop.[14]

In 1979 West and associates produced the seminal study comparing preventable deaths in a trauma system with those in a geographic area without trauma centers.[15] The study was an additional catalyst for the development of trauma care systems.[14] Subsequently, multiple studies verified as much as a 50% reduction in preventable deaths (i.e., deaths that would not have occurred with prompt and appropriate care) after the initiation of regionalized trauma care, as well as a reduction in morbidity.[16-18] Despite the evidence that a systematic approach to care was best, the monies to support such systems were not forthcoming. A follow-up report by the National Academy of Sciences in 1985 concluded that insufficient progress had been made in injury control since the original study 20 years earlier.[19] The legislative response was the Trauma Care Systems Planning and Development Act of 1990, which awarded state grants for the implementation of statewide trauma systems.[14] This act prompted action to develop trauma systems, especially in areas that had none.

Trauma centers, the nuclei of the trauma systems, are under intense financial pressure. A consensus statement

TABLE 2-3	Financial Profiles of Trauma Centers: Profits and Losses Based on Reimbursement (1994)*		
	Urban	**Suburban**	**Rural**
Aggregate	−11.7%	−5.7%	+3.7%
Self-pay/other	−49%	−58%	−21%
Commercial (health, auto, workers' comp)	+23%	+25%	+26%
Managed care	−1%	+7%	+19%
Medicare	−17%	−22%	−18%
Medicaid	−40%	−39%	−24%
County	−39%	−48%	−49%

From Eastman AB, Bishop GS, Walsh JC, et al: The economic status of trauma centers on the eve of health care reform, *J Trauma* 36(6):835-844, 1994.

*Figures represent percent of profit or loss reported by type of hospital from payers for trauma care in 1993.

from the Third National Injury Control Conference of 1992, sponsored by the Centers for Disease Control, concluded that the financing of trauma centers was inadequate. It actually predicted the closure of trauma centers if changes were not made in the availability of financial support.[20] Trauma centers close for many reasons, but closures are generally perceived to result from inadequate reimbursement and high costs.[21] The Trauma Center Economic Study by Eastman et al, published in 1991, supported the assertion that uncompensated care is a major problem for trauma centers and indicated that inadequate reimbursement is a multifactorial problem.[8,22] These results were based on reports from 25 centers. In a second phase of the study, a comprehensive questionnaire was sent to 635 hospitals that were identified by the John C. Lincoln Hospital trauma center registry as likely serving as trauma centers. Responses were received from 313 hospitals in 48 states. The data, published in 1994,[8] assisted in further determining the causes of financial problems for trauma centers, as reported by the centers themselves.

One interesting finding of the cited study was that financial reimbursement problems were not limited to urban trauma centers. Among the centers serving suburban regions, 46% reported serious financial problems and 31% reported physician support problems, either of which can lead to trauma center closures. Fifty-seven percent of the rural centers also reported financial difficulties. In addition, 53% of the physicians in rural settings reported lack of enthusiasm about trauma care. These findings suggest that public policy designed to support organized trauma care needs to be applied broadly, rather than just targeted to urban areas. Table 2-3 shows a financial profile by reimbursement type, indicating percent gained or lost by urban, suburban, and rural trauma centers, as reported in 1994.[8]

Although rural trauma centers have been affected by the same issues as urban centers, their financial outcomes appear to be better. The net reimbursement for rural trauma is higher secondary to injury patterns, the lower severity of injury, and the favorable payer mix. Rogers et al[7] reported that more fee-for-service patients were admitted to their rural center in 1995. Patients' lower severity of injury demands less resource utilization. The authors stressed that specific policies and measures had been implemented to reduce the costs of caring for trauma patients. Examples of these changes in practices is discussed later in this chapter.

The problems of reimbursement have increased with prospective payment plans, lower payments from the government (Medicare and Medicaid), and increasing numbers of uninsured patients. This inadequate reimbursement threatens the organization of trauma care. Although Level I facilities have enjoyed a high level of physician support because of their teaching resources, financial pressures are particularly acute for teaching hospitals as managed care plans become dominate players in evolving patient referral patterns. It is anticipated that this pressure, coupled with a reduction in the number of residencies producing specialists, may create a very serious problem for organized trauma care in Level I centers.[8]

Physician reluctance to become involved in trauma care can contribute to the closure of a trauma center.[23] As physicians lose interest in providing trauma care, the quality of care diminishes. A component of this physician problem is the physician reimbursement system, the resource-based relative value scale (RBRVS) implemented by the Health Care Financing Administration in 1992. This system was developed in an attempt to reform Medicare's physician reimbursement policy. The payment system lumps together fees paid to physicians. Despite the active participation of surgeons on the RBRVS review boards, the scales still undervalue the efforts expended on critically injured patients.[24]

The general surgeon is the surgeon most often in house 24 hours a day, yet only 12% to 13% of blunt trauma patients have a general surgery operation. Evaluation/management reimbursement is inappropriately low for trauma resuscitation, and critical care reimbursement does not necessarily reflect the work involved.[24] This level of reimbursement for general surgeons, nationally considered the primary admitting physician, discourages their participation in trauma care. Another issue that discourages physician participation in trauma care is the fear of increased malpractice litigation. This concern has not proven to be valid.[14] As a matter of fact, it appears that the protocol-driven care utilized in most trauma centers is an effective way of preempting viable claims of negligence. This is especially true for perceived COBRA violations; organized trauma systems are effective in protecting the physician, hospital, and patients.

It is clear that trauma centers are in financial trouble for many reasons, the major ones being the cost of uncompensated care, the high operating cost of caring for the critically injured, and inadequate reimbursement from government medical assistance programs.[20] Without significant financial support from outside sources, it is clear that more trauma systems will disappear or consolidate their services and that more trauma centers will close.

Trauma Care Costs for Special Populations

Some trauma patient subpopulations use excess resources and thus place extreme financial burdens on the trauma center. A few of these populations are presented here as examples of additional considerations in the financing of trauma care.

Elderly Trauma

The population of the United States is aging. It is estimated that by the year 2040, more than 20% of the American population (68,000,000) will be older than 65 years of age. Trauma is the fifth most common cause of death in people older than 65 years, and many trauma centers are seeing an increase in the number of elderly trauma patients brought to them for treatment.[25] The costs of health care for the very old are proportionately higher than for the population as a whole.[26] The elderly are covered by the federal Medicare program, but as mentioned previously, Medicare reimbursement rates are often inadequate and are being cut every year. Medicare pays using the DRG prospective payment system. As the population ages, attention must be paid to the outcomes of these patients and the financial burden they may present. A study done at the University of Virginia examined the care of elderly trauma patients to determine if their outcomes were different from those for other trauma patients and the financial burden they represented. The data were obtained from patients admitted to the trauma service between July 1, 1994, and July 1, 1997. The two groups examined were divided by age: 18 to 64 years and 65 years and older. Despite higher injury severity and lower survival probability for the elderly, the length of hospital and intensive care unit days and the percentage of admissions to the intensive care unit (ICU) were similar. The per capita cost of hospital care was lower for the elderly than for the younger patients, which was a surprising finding. Also, the reimbursement was higher, primarily because 98% of the elderly patients were insured by Medicare, whereas many of the younger patients were uninsured or underinsured.[25] Although Medicare reimbursement may be low, it does pay some of the costs, whereas uncompensated care is a total loss.

Despite the findings of this study, there remains concern that as the elderly population grows the financial burden to the trauma center for their care when injured will increase. The education of the elderly regarding this pending health care crisis will be necessary to avert a disaster. Aggressive lobbying of Congress to modify Medicare DRG payment systems of trauma reimbursement by the well-organized and powerful elderly lobbies represents the best chance to correct this problem.[26]

Multiple Extremity Injuries

Patients with multiple extremity injuries are another special group within the trauma population. They consume a disproportionate share of health care resources during the initial phases of care and then face protracted periods of postinjury morbidity. One study[27] demonstrated that, despite nearly identical injury severity scores, the patients with multiple extremity injuries differed from the general trauma population in regard to several measures of resource utilization and outcome: length of stay, return to work, and subjective assessment of health-related quality of life. This study emphasizes the need for tools to better predict the needs of patients with multiple extremity injuries and to plan for them. It also emphasizes the need to use resource utilization data to determine the true costs of care and influence the reimbursement for these patients.

Minimally Injured Patients

Minimally injured patients are often overtriaged and overtreated, and this presents unique challenges in terms of reimbursement. As managed care organizations have encouraged decreased hospital length of stays and decreased utilization of resources, these minimally injured patients can be a component of the reduction of trauma care costs. One organization has developed a 24-hour observation critical path to guide the care of these patients.[5] The trauma team feels they have been successful in identifying the trauma victims suitable for observation using the 24-hour critical pathway. In addition, study of the common variances in the pathway may be used to further modify the anticipated outcomes for this group of patients without compromising care. Reducing resource utilization and length of stay are ways of improving efficiency in the trauma center while providing the appropriate level of care.

Severe Traumatic Brain Injury

Severe traumatic brain injury (TBI) is a major source of morbidity and mortality. In addition, patients with blunt TBI incur enormous hospital expenses as a result of frequent complications, including pneumonia and other infections, respiratory failure, and deep vein thrombosis.[28] Hospital and ICU lengths of stays tend to be longer in these patients, which automatically drives up the costs of care. The utilization of a clinical pathway focused on establishing an "optimal time table" for managing major patient care events to decrease the complications associated with TBI may be one strategy for controlling costs in these patients. At one center, the use of such a pathway resulted in significant reduction in ventilator days, ICU days, and hospital length of stay.[28] These reductions resulted in significant cost savings, which increased the financial viability of the trauma center.

Specific strategies for reducing cost and resource utilization for trauma patients do not increase reimbursement for trauma care, which is a major health care and public policy issue. It will take a great deal of consciousness raising and lobbying to increase politicians' attention to trauma care and to determine the future of trauma reimbursement provided by the federal government.

STRATEGIES FOR CONTROLLING COSTS IN TRAUMA

The managed care focus has forced hospitals to evaluate their delivery of care systems and processes surrounding the continuum of care. In performing this review, many organizations developed cost-effective methods for delivering trauma care. Rather than wait (and hope) for increased reimbursement, systems have attempted to change their performance through internal means. Many centers started by defining the costs associated with trauma care.[29] To understand these costs, three categories must be defined: fixed costs, variable costs, and marginal costs.

Fixed costs do not vary with input into the system. We often think of these costs as overhead (e.g., the costs to turn on the lights, for heating or air conditioning, to pay salaries, and to meet the mortgage).

Variable costs do vary with input. They include tests ordered, medication costs, length of stay, and treatments ordered. This is the component of cost over which we have the most control. Most studies done on cost reduction and increased efficiency focus on decreasing the variable costs.

The incremental marginal costs are associated with putting one more patient through the system. Marginal costs are usually negligible in health care unless caring for the patient creates an increase in fixed costs, such as requiring overtime.

In addition to understanding the costs associated with the delivery of care, it is important to identify the services that constitute the cost centers to determine the variable costs contributed by each center. These were identified by one trauma center as nursing, emergency department services, surgical services, laboratory, radiology, and pharmacy.[29] After the centers are identified, focused cost-reduction measures can be implemented. Cost containment is one approach to reducing cost while maintaining the quality of care.

One issue in determining the cost reduction/containment strategy that will be most effective revolves around the ability to identify true costs. Organizations are beginning to utilize cost accounting systems, but most still base decisions on charges rather than costs. This use of charges as a surrogate for costs can create difficulties when attempting to initiate cost reduction projects. The focus should be on reducing true costs and not the charges associated with the activities. A center can charge anything it wants for a particular activity, but with fixed reimbursement, the payers will pay only a fixed amount that hopefully will cover the true costs of the activity.

DECREASING DIAGNOSTIC TESTING

The wide spectrum of diagnostic modalities available to the traumatologist aids in the care of the injured victim. Early in the evolution of trauma care, it was assumed that more was

better, so all patients with blunt trauma underwent a standardized set of diagnostic tests. The "just-in-case" tests were ordered to prevent a missed diagnosis. Now it appears that ordering tests only when the patient presents symptoms is more appropriate. Many organizations are avoiding protocol-driven diagnostic workups and instead are tailoring the workups to the individual patient's clinical presentation and history. Not only are these tests cost effective, they also give the clinician the appropriate information to make subsequent clinical decisions.[20,30]

CONTROLLING SUPPLIES

A unit-specific evaluation of the use of supplies and the type of supplies can also be conducted to save costs.[8,20,30] Nurses can evaluate the products available at the bedside to determine what is necessary for the delivery of care. A concerted effort to limit stockpiling of resources at the bedside may decrease wastage of items when patients are discharged.[30] The cost effectiveness of reusable items and disposable items should be compared.

ATTENDING SURGEON COVERAGE

In Level I trauma centers the presence of an attending trauma surgeon at all trauma resuscitations is one way to decrease cost, improve efficiency, and improve quality of care. Educating physicians about the importance of cost reduction to the survival of the trauma center usually will increase their "buy-in." The in-house attending trauma surgeon can influence resource use by making appropriate patient-directed decisions based on physiologic presentation rather than anatomic or mechanism of injury guidelines.[5,31] A change in practice to require 24-hour in-house attending coverage reduced one institution's costs by improving patient movement through the resuscitation bay, avoiding unnecessary testing and unnecessary hospitalization.[31] It may also be possible to decrease the size of the trauma response team based on revised trauma activation criteria using a graded system.[8,20]

EXPANDING ROLES FOR NURSING

The role of the trauma nurse coordinator (TNC) continues to change to meet the needs of the trauma center. One center has added to the role of the TNC the duty of reviewing all discharge charts to ensure that the ICD 9 CM coding is accurate.[7,30] This activity, combined with the employment of a dedicated billing person for the trauma service, has enhanced the accuracy of billing and thus increased reimbursement. In addition, the TNC educates all new members of the trauma team about the importance of cost effectiveness as a criterion of care.

Many organizations have introduced the role of trauma case manager (CM)[6,7,26,27] to provide better continuity of care for trauma patients. The case manager reviews care on a daily basis to identify appropriateness of care and avoidance of unnecessary care. Case managers are also responsible for monitoring critical pathways for adherence or variances that can effect length of stay. Coordinating ancillary services for timely delivery of care and assisting the team in determining the timing of transfer are the biggest assets the CM can bring to cost-reduction issues.

The trauma nurse practitioner (TNP) is a new role in the acute care arena, serving as a midlevel practitioner who provides high-quality care within cost-containment constraints.[32] TNPs have a variety of responsibilities as a part of the trauma team. Their major role is direct patient care along with facilitating collaboration, coordination, and communication between the trauma surgeon and other subspecialty services. More specifically, the TNP's responsibilities include care of the trauma patient from the resuscitation bay to the ICU and to the floor through discharge and clinic follow-up.

As the number of residency programs in the specialties decreases, the TNP can fulfill some of the responsibilities formerly performed by less well-prepared residents. Level I trauma standards require a surgeon to be in house 24 hours a day, and at most institutions, a senior-level resident fulfills this requirement. If the number of residents is inadequate to provide such coverage, consideration can be given to the TNP supporting the surgeon's role in providing 24-hour trauma care.[32] The TNP can manage the stable in-house trauma patients, allowing the trauma surgeon time to rest or operate on new trauma patients. It affords the surgeon peace of mind knowing that the previously admitted, stabilized patients are being monitored appropriately. If multiple trauma patients arrive simultaneously, the TNP can assist with the resuscitation. The TNP can be a very valuable member of the trauma team and reduce the overall costs to the trauma center.

A study published in the *Journal of Trauma* in 1990 (early in the TNP movement) demonstrated the value of TNPs on the trauma team. Spisso et al[33] retrospectively examined the use of nurse practitioners in a tertiary care center. Outcomes were measured for 12 months before and after implementation of the TNP role. The findings demonstrated the value of the TNP, including decreased length of stay for the trauma patients, increased documentation of quality of care, decrease in patient complaints, and documented time savings for house staff.[33]

CONSOLIDATION OF TRAUMA SERVICES

Managed care has brought an era of mergers, acquisitions, and consolidations. Because of reduced reimbursement and increased competition for managed care contracts, organizations are more frequently considering a merger or consolidation of services. In some areas, consolidation is an outcome of competition in an area that has too many trauma centers.[34]

Mergers and acquisitions also create the venue for consolidation of services. When large hospitals combine to form a new entity or are bought by another entity, decisions to cut costs are high on the lists of the new owners. In many instances, competing trauma centers are now integrated[35] or one program has closed. In the integrated model, a unified trauma service can develop shared responsibility for trauma care. The sharing of personnel and other resources allows major cost savings to be realized. Further network savings can be achieved by eliminating or combining air medical support, educational programs such as advanced trauma life support courses, quality improvement efforts, and research under one system.[35] The largest savings comes from reducing duplication of services in two facilities.

NEGOTIATING MANAGED CARE CONTRACTS

As stated at the beginning of this section, it is important to know the costs of caring for trauma patients in order to be able to negotiate a contract with managed care organizations. For years hospitals did not provide cost data to the providers of care, mostly because they did not know the costs and used charges as the proxy to determine the dollars spent on delivery of care. Charges will no longer suffice as a good proxy for costs. Each organization needs to develop a good methodology for gathering actual cost-per-case data. In addition, accurate knowledge of cost data can help the trauma team determine where changes in practice are warranted to reduce unnecessary costs.[11]

Cost-accounting techniques must reflect information that will assist the hospital with contract negotiations in the managed care environment. It is possible to think of the trauma service as a profit center.[11] When the trauma service becomes a profit center there are incentives for both the hospital and the trauma physicians. For the hospital, trauma patient referrals and hospital networking to enhance capacity utilization is beneficial. Physical plant improvements and investing in emergency services can become priorities. Physician involvement in the operations of the hospital is of paramount importance for the success of the system. Physicians must have substantial and credible input on curbing the indirect costs associated with trauma care because these costs are responsible for half the cost associated with the care of trauma patients.[11] It is much easier to negotiate a contract with a managed care organization when the hospital has a track record of cost-effective care.

A center may want to examine insurance denial data and decreased level of reimbursement data to look for practitioner practices that are costly to the trauma service. The data can be collected for each provider on the trauma team by a trauma case manager or utilization review nurse. Each key physician activity can be examined to determine appropriateness of intervention. In addition, the documentation of key activities can be reviewed to see if the documentation is affecting the denial rates. This activity can lead to educational programs on maximizing clinical and financial outcomes through appropriate documentation and the adoption of best practices. There is a great deal of incentive for physicians to change behavior through this type of analysis of financial loss. For physicians, a service that generates a positive operating margin can justify new opportunities in funding for the service. Being identified as a profit center enhances the influence one has in the system as well.

SUMMARY

The financial aspects of trauma care are extremely complex. On the public policy side is the continued lack of recognition of the tremendous economic burden that injury, accidental or intentional, has on the public welfare of this country. On the hospital practitioner side is the tremendous financial burden of providing high quality care to these patients. Addressing these problems requires a multi-pronged approach.

More effort is needed toward prevention of injuries. Prevention is the single most important way to cut the cost of trauma care.[35] Increasing efforts aimed at primary prevention of intentional and unintentional injuries offers the best hope for the future.[20] Significant strides have been made in prevention techniques during the past two decades, but even more can be done. Lobbying for improved reimbursement from government programs that provide coverage for health care is of continued importance. As the population ages, more Medicare dollars will be spent on health care. Active lobbying of local and state legislatures is also necessary to ensure support of trauma systems. Letters and testimony can influence the process of legislating changes in reimbursement laws.

As practitioners of trauma care, we must assume our responsibility in controlling the costs of care. Examining the costs of providing trauma care is the first step in identifying changes that can be made. Improving the cost efficiency of diagnostic and therapeutic procedures, implementing a case management approach to care, working across the continuum of care, and changing the delivery of care can make a significant difference in the viability of the trauma service. Practitioners must learn more about health economics, a discipline concerned with determining the best way of using available health care resources to maximize the health of the community. Economic evaluations use analytic techniques to systematically consider all possible costs and consequences of potential clinical actions.[36] Although they do not form the sole basis for decision making, economic evaluations offer useful information at different levels of decision making.

REFERENCES

1. Cales RH, Heilig RW: *Trauma care systems: a guide to planning, implementation operation and evaluation,* Rockville, Md, 1986, Aspen Publishers.
2. *National Safety Council accident facts,* www.nsc.org/irs/statinfo/al4.htm, Sept 25, 1998.
3. Schwab CW, Frykberg ER, Bloom T, et al: Violence in America: public health crisis—the role of firearms, *J Trauma* 38(2): 163-168, 1995.
4. Miller T, Cohen M, Wiersema B: Medical care costs of injury and violence and the savings achievable through prevention. Presented to the Senate Finance Committee hearing on the Consequence of Social Behavior on Health Care, Washington, DC, Oct 19, 1993.
5. Cowell VL, Ciraulo D, Gabram S, et al: Trauma 24 hour observation clinical path, *J Trauma* 45(1):147-150, 1998.
6. U.S. Department of Health, Education and Welfare: *Accidental death and disability: the neglected disease of modern society,* Rockville, Md, 1966, Division of Medical Sciences, National Academy of Sciences, National Research Council.
7. Rogers FB, Osler TM, Shackford SR. Financial outcomes of treating trauma in a rural environment, *J Trauma* 43(1):65-73, 1997.
8. Eastman AB, Bishop GS, Walsh JC, et al: The economic status of trauma centers on the eve of health care reform, *J Trauma* 36(6):835-844, 1994.
9. Birnbaum M, Walleck CA: Rationing health care: impact on critical care. In Fein AI, editor: Critical care unit management, *Crit Care Clin* 9(3):585-602, 1993.
10. Jacobs P: *The economics of health and medical care,* ed 4, Gaithersburg, Md, 1997, Aspen Publications.
11. Taheri PA, Butz DA, Watts CM, et al: Trauma services: profit center? *J Am Coll Surg* 188(4):349-354, 1999.
12. Cowley RA: Trauma center: a new concept for the delivery of critical care, *J Med Soc NJ* 74(11):979-986, 1977.
13. Taylor B: Seen by the right people with the right patient in the right facility. Close encounters of the Cowley kind: an inclusive journal interview with R. Adams Cowley, MD, Director of the Maryland Institute for Emergency Medical Services, State of Maryland, *MD State Med J* 27(6):35-49, 1978.
14. Hammond JS, Breckenridge MB: Longitudinal analysis of the impact of a level I trauma designation at a University Hospital, *J Am Coll Surg* 188(3):217-224, 1999.
15. West JG, Trunkey DD, Lim RC: Systems of trauma care: a study of two counties, *Arch Surg* 114(3):455-460, 1979.
16. Eastman AB: Blood in our streets: status and evolution of trauma care systems, *Arch Surg* 127:677-681, 1992.
17. Eggold R: Trauma care regionalization: a necessity, *J Trauma* 23(3):260-262, 1983.
18. Clemmer TP, Orme JF, Thomas FO, et al: Outcome of critically injured patients treated at a level 1 trauma center versus full service community hospitals, *Crit Care Med* 13(5):861, 1983.
19. Committee on Trauma Research, Commission on Life Services, National Research Council, Institute of Medicine: *Injury in America: a continuing public health problem,* Washington, D.C., 1985, National Academy Press.
20. Elliott DC, Rodriguez A: Cost effectiveness in trauma care, *Surg Clin North Am* 76(1):47-62, 1996.
21. Champion HR, Mabee MS: *An American crisis in trauma care reimbursement: an issue analysis monograph,* Washington, D.C., 1990, The Washington Hospital Center.
22. Eastman AB, Rice CL, Bishop GS, et al: An analysis of the critical problems of trauma center reimbursement, *J Trauma* 31(7):920-925, 1991.
23. Richardson JD, Miller FB: Will future surgeons be interested in trauma care? Results of resident survey, *J Trauma* 32(3):229, 1992.
24. Trunkey DD: The positive features of trauma center designation, *J Am Coll Surg* 188(3):315-316, 1999.
25. Young JS, Cephas GA, Blow I: Outcome and cost of trauma among the elderly: a real life model of a single payer reimbursement system, *J Trauma* 45(4):800-804, 1998.
26. Sartorelli KH, Rogers FB, Osler TM, et al: Financial aspects of providing trauma care at the extremes of life, *J Trauma* 46(3):483-487, 1999.

27. Fern KJ, Smith JT, Zee B, et al: Trauma patients with multiple extremity injuries: resource utilization and long-term outcome in relation to injury severity scores, *J Trauma* 45(3):489-494, 1998.

28. Spain DA, McIlvoy LH, Fix SE, et al: Effect of a critical pathway for severe traumatic brain injury on resource utilization, *J Trauma* 45(1):101-104, 1998.

29. Taheri PA, Wahl WL, Butz DA: Trauma service cost: the real story, *Ann Surg* 227(5):720-724, 1998.

30. Flynn MB, Luchcinger J: Trauma care strategies for changing economic forces, *Crit Care Nurse* 17(6):81-89, 1997.

31. Imami ER, Clevenger FW, Lampard SD, et al: Throughput analysis of trauma resuscitations with financial impact, *J Trauma* 42(2):294-298, 1997.

32. Cupuro PA, Alperovich CG: Letters to the editor, *J Trauma* 43(6):988, 1997.

33. Spisso J, O'Callaghan C, McKennan M, et al: Improved quality of care and reduction in house staff workload using trauma nurse practitioners, *J Trauma* 30(4):660-665, 1990.

34. Haugh R: Consolidation: trauma trouble, *Hospitals and Health Networks* 73(1):20,22, 1999.

35. Trooskin SZ, Faucher MB, Santora TA, et al: Consolidation of trauma programs in the era of large health care delivery networks, *J Trauma* 46(3):488-493, 1999.

36. Heyland DK, Gafni A, Kernerman P, et al: How to use the results of an economic evaluation, *Crit Care Med* 27(6):1195-1202, 1999.

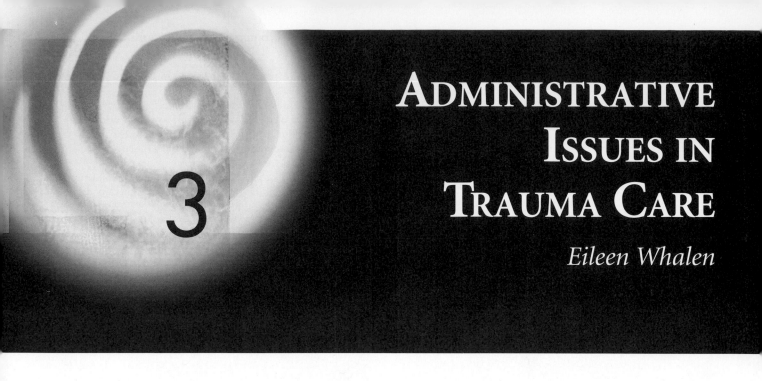

ADMINISTRATIVE ISSUES IN TRAUMA CARE

Eileen Whalen

The successful management of any area of health care requires skill, talent, and creative leadership. Knowledge of current health care issues, such as changes in reimbursement practices, legal and political implications of such changes, and personnel management, is essential in administration. A clear understanding of social and political motivating factors is critical to every health care administrator. Health care is a business, requiring managers to provide a businesslike approach in their decisions, keeping cost containment as a goal while still maintaining optimal provision of care. Almost every activity needs to be questioned in order to evaluate its outcome and justify its expense. Innovative approaches to management are greatly valued, and leaders in trauma care have been at the forefront of ensuring quality patient outcomes while responding thoughtfully to institutional and national fiscal concerns.

THE ROLE OF ADMINISTRATION IN A TRAUMA CARE DELIVERY SYSTEM

Health care is in transition, and trauma care is no exception. Historically the direction of trauma care has been toward the development of trauma centers, using a rational approach based on the concept of centralization, or tertiary care.[1] Since the inception of organized trauma care, care has been provided in regional systems driven by the most severely injured, major trauma patients, requiring treatment at a designated trauma center.[2] The paradigm has shifted to an inclusive model of trauma care. Emphasis has changed, recognizing that few individual facilities can provide all resources to all comers in all situations. Trauma systems should be designed to match each trauma care provider or facility's resources to the needs of the injured patient. The trauma center is an integral player in a trauma system that encompasses all phases of care from out of hospital through rehabilitation and reentry into society. Each medical facility should have a role in the regional system. Trauma systems

must be fully integrated into emergency medical services (EMS) systems and attempt to meet the needs of all injured patients regardless of the severity of injury.[3]

Given the inclusive model of trauma care systems, administrators of trauma centers can no longer focus on the trauma center only. Trauma center administrators must be involved in multiple components of the trauma system to ensure the efficacy of the system and thereby the success of their own center within the system. The administrative components of a trauma system consist of leadership, authority, planning and development, legislation, and finances.[2] As these components are essential for the success of a trauma system; they are fundamental to the success of a trauma center as well.

The Model Trauma Plan developed by the U.S. Department of Health and Human Services describes the leadership role in a trauma care system from multiple perspectives. On a statewide level, there needs to be a lead agency with the authority to provide overall system development. This typically falls to the state Department of Health, with some notable exceptions. In California, individual counties or groups of counties have developed trauma systems based on authority granted by state statue. In Pennsylvania, the state agency has delegated the authority for system development and management to the Pennsylvania Trauma Foundation. In Florida and Massachusetts, state and regionally based agencies share authority for the development and operation of trauma systems.[4,5]

Typically, the lead agency in any region is responsible for establishing standards for system performance. The lead agency serves as the arbitrator to ensure integration of the trauma system and the EMS system and ensures cooperation across state lines with no thought to geographic boundaries. The lead agency must have established authority based on enabling legislation and, ideally, legislation that provides funding for the system. Key provisions of enabling legislation include: plan development, integration of trauma and

EMS systems, adoption of standards for trauma care, organization of data collection systems, system evaluation, confidentiality protection for performance improvement activities, and authorization for funding.[1,2]

On a local level, many states (e.g., Montana, Oregon, and North Dakota) have developed a regional trauma committee structure typically led by a Level I or Level II trauma center. These committees are developed geographically based on referral patterns. They function to develop regional treatment and transfer guidelines, conduct performance improvement activities, share collective resources to develop public and professional education programs, and coordinate injury prevention activities. These committees are integrated with local EMS functions and serve as the conduit for communication among providers for local, state, and national changes. Many regional committees report to a state trauma advisory committee, the functions and membership of which are set by statue.

Because system development and ongoing changes occur at the regional or state committee level, it is imperative that senior administrators of the trauma center actively participate on these committees. Decisions regarding catchment areas, trauma center standards, funding of indigent care, and changes in legislation can dramatically affect the survival of an individual trauma center. Senior management must not delegate this role to the trauma nurse coordinator (TNC) or even the trauma medical director (TMD). Typically, subcommittees are developed to look at project-specific clinical issues, education, and performance improvement. The TNC or TMD best performs these types of subcommittee activities. The administrator's participation at local and state lead agency meetings is a major strength to a program and an obvious measurable indication of the institution's commitment to the trauma system.

State and local trauma care committees are frequently composed of members appointed by professional associations, such as the state hospital association or medical association. To this end, it is essential that senior administrators not delegate this responsibility if they are invited to represent their own peer group.

ORGANIZATIONAL CULTURE

Distinct cultures exist within organizational boundaries, which define the arenas in which individuals and groups function. These boundaries impose fiscal, behavioral, intellectual, and philosophical constraints while at the same time providing guidelines for success within the environment. An understanding of both the organizational culture and how to interact with it successfully is essential to all managers regardless of level or department.

The culture of an institution that provides care to trauma patients typically is very different from that of other health care organizations. There is often a greater tendency to manage with anticipation and preparation rather than with reactions after a problem or need is recognized. Strategic planning is essential for trauma services and for other major

health care programs. Forward thinking is apparent through the active sharing of information about anticipated changes and the provision of opportunities for involvement of personnel from all disciplines and levels in planning. Management is often aggressive, with attention given to streamlining services and making them readily available while limiting redundancy. Trauma patients require the services of almost every department within a hospital, which can create a natural common bond among these departments, as well as improve the working relationships among personnel.

The trauma service composition and function will depend largely on the culture of an organization, available resources, and the commitment of the organization to the highest quality of trauma care.

ADMINISTRATIVE COMPONENTS OF A TRAUMA PROGRAM

The success of any organization largely depends on the planning and vision of the leaders. Trauma programs must be planned strategically to ensure their initial success and maturation within the regional system and the institution. In the late 1970s and early 1980s and to some degree today, the administration of the trauma program within an institution was delegated largely to the TNC and the TMD. These two individuals ensured the quality of care, monitored adherence to regulatory standards, and facilitated public and professional education. Strategic planning for the program was never considered, and administrators were rarely involved with its maturation. The TNC was a middle-level manager responsible for a product line within the organization. The institution as a whole did not share in the planning, evaluation, or accountability of the program.

In today's health care environment, it is essential that the administration of any trauma center be integrally involved with the trauma center developmental plan. This plan should be determined by available resources, community needs, and socioeconomic factors and driven by consensus of the medical staff and administration, including nursing. The plan should be motivated by outcome goals common to the organization and fully integrated with areas of excellence already established within the institutional culture. The hospital board of trustees or directors must be fully committed to the trauma center developmental plan and provide necessary support. The planning process should be influenced by available data and should involve key clinical leaders and medical staff visionaries. The process should begin with an assessment of community needs, followed by an analysis of the appropriate trauma center standards to begin the determination of resources available within the organization. Hospitals must decide where their organization best fits within the regional trauma system and determine what level of service is appropriate for their organization. An assessment of current capabilities compared with the required standards will give the management team the opportunity to identify deficiencies and create opportunities for improvement. Once a decision is made as to what level of service will be provided, educational forums should be executed to convey accurate information to all key players. Financial barriers must be addressed. Medical staff commitment must be assessed. Strengths and weaknesses must be analyzed realistically, and threats to the organization must be addressed whether they are real or perceived. A work plan should be developed to address the deficiencies and a budget prepared to commit resources in a way that will guarantee the success of the trauma program. This level of planning and decision making requires administrative leadership and will not be successful if delegated to a well-meaning trauma nurse coordinator.

The trauma center developmental plan should be reassessed and refined at various stages during the life span of the trauma center. Certainly before and after an accreditation process an evaluation should occur, and it should be repeated subsequently in 3- to 5-year increments. As the program matures, the performance improvement process should guide the evolution of the plan.

The administrative structure of a trauma program defines institutional support and organizational commitment. The structure must include an accountable administrator, a medical director, and a trauma program manager (TPM). (In many organizations, the title of trauma nurse coordinator has been replaced to best reflect the responsibilities of the role.) The medical director and program manager must be given the power and authority to administer the trauma program. The program must be positioned strategically within the organizational structure so that it may interact with equal authority with other departments that provide patient care services.[3] There should be written resolutions by the administration/board and medical staff supporting the trauma program. Typically a management council or executive planning committee meets on a regular interval to manage the administrative policy, marketing, and overall health of the program. This committee determines the resources necessary to adhere to regulatory demands and to support the fiscal wellness of the program. The peer review committees of the trauma program deal with clinical performance improvement issues and should have direct reporting linkage to the hospital executive committee and or quality councils.

Without strong administrative leadership and vision, the planning and implementation of a trauma program within an organization and subsequently within a region will be jeopardized.

TRAUMA CENTER ACCREDITATION

The majority of health care institutions currently participate or have participated with the Joint Commission on Accreditation of Healthcare Organizations (JCAHO). Through a voluntary accreditation process, organizations can receive recognition for the standard of services they provide and receive guidance for evaluating and improving the quality of those services. JCAHO standards for accreditation are updated and published regularly and include guidelines for all essential departments within differing types of health care organizations. Accreditation occurs through a site-survey review process that compares existing services with JCAHO standards and rates them on the basis of scoring guidelines.

Trauma accreditation systems have been developed to meet the unique needs of trauma systems and trauma centers within the systems. Similar in some ways to the JCAHO process, the regulatory entity in a region or state will design a system to determine if trauma hospitals are meeting the criteria written in their trauma systems plan. Typically, states either adopt the current standards published by the Committee on Trauma of the American College of Surgeons or, through a committee process, write their own standards based on the College's criteria. These standards are customized to meet the unique needs of the individual state based on available resources. Only the regulatory entity has the legal authority to designate a trauma hospital. Enabling legislation discussed previously in this chapter is the basis of this authority.

In the past, trauma center accreditation was an option for hospitals wishing to demonstrate consistent compliance with recognized standards of trauma care. Today, some states and localities have established systems to reimburse physicians and hospitals for some portion of indigent trauma care. Regulatory agencies have required hospitals to achieve and maintain trauma center accreditation in order to access this funding.

Trauma center accreditation usually occurs in one of two ways. The first is through the verification and consultation program of the American College of Surgeons. The program may be conducted in a two-part process. Members of the Committee on Trauma conduct a consultation visit at the request of the hospital, community, or state authority. The purpose of the consultation is to assess current trauma care and to prepare the facility for a subsequent verification visit.[3] The consultation visit is typically conducted by a team of two general surgeons and results in a written list of recommendations for program improvement based on the latest version of the *Resources for Optimal Care of the Injured Patient.* Through trauma center verification the College verifies that a hospital is performing as a trauma center and meets established criteria.[3] The College's process of verification is one method utilized by states to ensure that trauma centers are meeting the standards specified in the state trauma plan.

The other method of verifying trauma centers' compliance to written standards is the use of independent reviewers hired by the regulatory agency to verify that the trauma care provided meets the standards as written. Typically this process utilizes a multidisciplinary team approach. The teams are comprised of an experienced trauma surgeon, a trauma nurse, a trauma center administrator, an EMS administrator, and possibly a neurosurgeon, orthopedic surgeon, or emergency medicine specialist, depending on the needs of the regulatory agency. The team is asked to substantiate for the regulatory agency that the hospital is in compliance with the approved trauma center standards for the region.

Regardless of the approach, there are cost implications, both direct and indirect, associated with the trauma center accreditation process that need to be considered in the trauma center budget. Because of the political and fiscal implications to the trauma center, administration must be intricately involved in the planning for the site review and must participate on the day of the verification visit. It is important that managers at all levels have an understanding of both the JCAHO standards and the trauma center standards so that the implications for their own departments are clear.

After successful completion of the accreditation process, most regulatory authorities will formally designate trauma hospitals for a period of time. Typically, if the hospital substantially meets the criteria, it is awarded a 3-year contract for service. This period varies depending on the maturity of the trauma system. Trauma center accreditation processes usually contain an appeal method to allow the hospital the right to resolve disagreements.

TRAUMA PROGRAM RESOURCE ALLOCATION

PERSONNEL RESOURCES

Budget planning includes several factors, most of which fall in the category of either personnel (concerned with individual workers) or nonlabor (related to supplies and capital equipment). When a new program is introduced into an organization, the unique demands of that program must be analyzed so the program can be resourced appropriately. A trauma program is complicated by the fact that the requirements for service must be available at all times, 24 hours a day, 7 days a week. A trauma program affects every department within the hospital in some way, from prehospital care to rehabilitation, including every support service. The most expensive allocation of any trauma program is the professional and ancillary personnel required to staff it. Staffing of the program depends on the level of service provided. In many Level I or II trauma centers, nursing and ancillary services are staffed 24 hours a day to meet the demands of existing programs such as emergency services, cardiac surgery, labor and delivery, and critical care. This may not be true of centers desiring to increase their level of service or of rural centers.

In anticipation of preparing a budget demonstrating personnel costs, several issues specifically related to trauma nursing must be considered. These include: (1) the forecasted workload, which is the number of patient days anticipated for the unit; (2) nursing's number of hours budgeted for trauma patient care on a daily basis; (3) planned productive and nonproductive time for individual workers; (4) the productivity goal for both the specific patient care area that is preparing the budget and the entire nursing department; and (5) the episodic nature of trauma. Summer, weekends, and nights are times of greatest resource consumption and are indicators to be addressed in budget planning.

The forecasted workload, or budgeted patient days, is most frequently determined by the hospital finance department through review of retrospective budget data, with addition of anticipated changes that may affect workload. Nurse managers of trauma units are influential in decisions about workload because they recognize changes that need to be considered when determining workload. Increases or reductions in medical services can directly affect patient days, as can the installation of a new process, such as a clinical or management information system. New services of any type, even those intended to streamline a function, will slow work to some degree and require time for the staff to learn the new system.

Each trauma program requires, at a minimum, a trauma program manager and a trauma medical director. The program manager at a Level I or II facility is typically a masters-prepared nurse working in a full-time capacity. In high-volume Level I and II centers, it is necessary to budget additional support to the TPM such as: case managers, additional trauma coordinators, nurse practitioners, injury prevention coordinators, clinical nurse specialists, and educators. It is important to understand the additional requirements of a Level I or II center as it relates to: performance improvement (PI), professional education, public education, injury prevention activities, and research. For PI activities at a busy level I or II center, depending on volume, one to three trauma registrars may be required to manage data reporting requirements. Many organizations use existing resources within their nursing or professional education departments to meet the educational demands of the trauma program. In some instances, these resources do not exist and must be added. However the functions are assigned, it must be realized that trauma center care has unique requirements for professional education, which must be considered during planning and budgeting. Trauma outreach and injury prevention has become an exciting new frontier for trauma professionals. Many Level I centers have taken a leadership role in the development of exciting programs fully integrated within existing community special interest groups and programs. Case management lends itself well to trauma programs because it greatly improves concurrent performance review and enhances cost containment with decreased length of stays while increasing patient satisfaction.[6]

Depending on trauma patient volume, the program manager in a Level III or IV center may perform other duties, such as working as the nurse manager of the emergency department or critical care area. Because the hospital's commitment to public education, professional education, outreach, research, and injury prevention are substantially less or nonexistent at this level, the staff requirement can be adjusted accordingly. Typically, a secretary or trauma registrar assists the program manager, or a part-time medical record technician is committed to the trauma registry.

The trauma medical director must be a general surgeon regardless of the level of service provided. His or her time commitment to the program varies according to the level of service, that is, Level I versus Level IV. The number and variety of compensation programs for surgeons and specialists are as varied as the number of trauma centers. Compensation for surgeons at Level I centers differs greatly from that at private facilities because the surgeons usually are salaried professionals. In the current environment, practically all trauma centers requiring unencumbered surgeons pay them in a private practice setting. The actual dollar amounts have been lowering in favor of other methods of improving the surgeon's and sometimes the subspecialist's compensation (e.g., billing services). Administrators should be cognizant of the fact that it is customary to pay an annual administrative fee to a medical director and compensate the surgeons providing unencumbered call. Contracts for service should comply with kickback statues or inurement issue standards required by state and federal law. Payment without clear expectations regarding scope of service and performance may be risky for the hospital and the physician.

In a busy Level I program, it is not unusual to find a director, five to seven full-time surgeons, and two or three surgical teams each with four to six residents. The requirements for surgical subspecialists such as orthopedics, neurosurgery, emergency medicine, and anesthesia must be considered. Level II and III facilities are typically covered with private-practice physicians rotating call. These scenarios vary, again depending on the culture of the organization and the resources at hand. Regardless of the level of service, each program will have secretarial demands that need to be addressed accordingly.

Because of the nature of the trauma business, ancillary staffing must be able to anticipate the 24-hour needs of the program and its projected volume. The clinical laboratory and radiology suite must be staffed accordingly. In addition, it is frequently necessary to develop callback systems for nursing, radiology, laboratory, and surgical personnel. Administrators should have a good understanding of the program demands related to personnel resources and should plan accordingly.

The budget for the trauma program should reflect the positions specifically designated for the program, such as TMD, TPM, all additional staff, and surgeons. Many hospitals charge on-call pay for nurses and technicians or additional education pay to the trauma program because the cost of these services would not be necessary if it were not for the trauma program.

SUPPLIES AND EQUIPMENT

Most trauma centers allocate costs for clinical supplies related to patient care through the department where the service is rendered. Budgeting supplies for an entire fiscal year requires an understanding of how to project trends in supply use, census, and inflation. Trauma patients use supplies at differing rates, depending on their reason for and length of hospitalization. Programs that are successful in managing unit costs for supplies allow two things to occur with ease: the stocking of adequate supplies on the unit and the activation of a patient charging system at the time the

supplies are used. Budgeting for supplies and equipment needs to consider these issues.

Trends in the annual use of supplies and in the charges for supplies can be calculated as follows: Determine either figure for each year during a 4- to 5-year period and the actual patient days for each year. Calculate the average of both. Divide the average number of supplies by the budgeted patient days for the new fiscal year. A specific rate of inflation can then be added, which typically is determined by the hospital's fiscal management group based on anticipated contractual increases. It is important to anticipate any changes (e.g., new technology) that may influence the need for supplies in the coming year. Newly implemented services and the opening or closing of other patient units may cause significant fluctuations in census or types of patients. In addition, unusual expenses that may occur on a one-time only basis during the year also need to be anticipated and added into budget projections. This method is far from exact, but it builds an annual projection through use of accurate historic information. The trauma program budget should also reflect specific supplies and equipment related to: computer hardware, software, office supplies, educational equipment, and programs.

CAPITAL EQUIPMENT

As in any hospital budget, capital equipment is defined by the dollar amount of the purchase. The threshold changes based on the institution. Budgeting for capital equipment expenditures typically requires significant justification because of the costs involved. Priorities in capital expenses are set on the basis of several factors. Equipment that will contribute to the revenue of the hospital will most likely receive high priority in the budget process. Ideally, the costs of the equipment and the anticipated annual operating costs will be either less than or, at a minimum, balanced against the revenue. Equipment necessary for patient safety and quality care is also given high priority in budgeting even though no revenue is anticipated directly from its use. Trauma program capital equipment is often allocated to the department where it will be housed or for which it will be charged, such as operating room, radiology, or critical care areas.

PERFORMANCE IMPROVEMENT

In any health care organization, three areas of major responsibility are essential to survival: (1) patient results or outcome, (2) organizational performance, and (3) profit potential.[7] Individual employee behavior (performance) can impact both patient outcome and patient satisfaction, but usually organizational systems have more direct influence, either in a positive or a negative manner. Both patient outcome and consumer satisfaction (including third-party payers) determine organizational profit and market share. Standards for all areas of hospital operation are used to provide guidelines for and define a desired level of performance and patient outcome. These standards form the basis of a total quality management program and emphasize continuous performance improvement.

The commitment to performance improvement is exceptional as it relates to modern trauma care. As previously addressed in this chapter and elsewhere in this text, one must anticipate the personnel needs of the performance improvement program and allocate resources appropriately.

PROFESSIONAL EDUCATION

Each trauma center is committed to some level of participation in professional education. The standards for professional education are rigorous, and meeting them can be costly. The standards span the continuum of: trauma care, encompassing prehospital providers, nurses, physicians, and ancillary personnel. Many hospitals provide: paid educational days, free continuing education opportunities within the organization, tuition reimbursement, and advanced training in specialty areas or certification within professional groups. Each trauma center must be cognizant of the educational requirements of the level of service they seek to provide and must develop a written plan as to how the requirements will be met. Inherent in the plan should be a commitment to funding commensurate with the level of care the hospital will provide.

Residency training programs enhance a trauma center and the trauma system as a whole. A surgical residency program should have a written curriculum and supervision within the trauma program. Trauma residents should be introduced to the service and have weekly educational conferences with the attending surgical staff.[3]

Trauma education is multidisciplinary in keeping with the fundamental idea of a team approach. The PI program should set priorities for ongoing continuing educational offerings. Funding of professional education within the trauma center is an objective measurement of institutional commitment to the trauma program and the system as a whole.

INJURY PREVENTION

Trauma centers play an important role in reducing the occurrence of injury by providing or participating in injury prevention activities. Data from the trauma registry can be used to identify the patterns, frequency, and risks of injury. In many states, regional trauma committees aggregate data to prioritize needs. The development and maintenance of injury prevention programs can be costly, so the ability to work collaboratively within a region, optimizing the integration of existing community coalitions, is critical for success.

Injury prevention activities do not happen just from the kindness of volunteers in the trauma center. Every trauma center, regardless of resources, has a commitment to injury prevention. Anticipating the cost of fulfilling this commitment is imperative when writing the injury prevention portion of the trauma center development plan. The plan must be evaluated periodically and changed as the type and frequency of traumatic events change in the community and during the maturation of the trauma program.

RESEARCH

Ideally, all trauma centers will participate in research activities as their resources and patient population allow. Traditionally, the requirement to conduct research to advance knowledge in trauma care and trauma systems has distinguished a Level I trauma center from other trauma centers. Research requires funding, and the administration of Level I centers should contribute to the effort with financial support of facilities and personnel. The level of funding dedicated to research activities is another objective measurement of institutional commitment to the trauma program.

SUMMARY

Because administration is an interpersonal process, it relies greatly on managers to influence, motivate, catalyze, and facilitate activities that lead to fulfillment of the organization's mission. The challenge of trauma care provides an unparalleled opportunity for innovative managers to effect system changes. Although the challenges presented to the administrator are constantly changing and evolving, the astute individual uses this opportunity to design innovative systems that support quality outcomes. In today's trauma milieu, it is imperative that administrators participate on regional trauma planning committees. The successful trauma program relies on aggressive administrative leadership and planning processes that are evaluated constantly and changed to respond to the needs of the community, institution, and the unique needs of the trauma program.

REFERENCES

1. Cales RH, Heilig RW: *Trauma care systems,* Rockville, Md, 1986, Aspen.
2. U.S. Department of Health and Human Services, Health Resources and Services Administration: *Model trauma care system plan,* Washington, DC, Sept 30, 1992, US Government Printing Office.
3. American College of Surgeons' Committee on Trauma: *Resources for the optimal care of the injured patient,* Chicago, 1999, American College of Surgeons.
4. Brazzolo G: *Inventory of trauma systems,* Chicago, 1993, Hospital Research and Educational Trust.
5. Bass RR, Gainer PS, Carlini AR: Update on trauma system development in the United States, *J Trauma* 47(3 Suppl): S15-S21, 1999.
6. Spisso J, O'Callaghan C, McKennan M, et al: Improved quality of care and reduction of housestaff workload using trauma nurse practitioners, *J Trauma* 30(6):660-663, 1990.
7. Hoesing H, Kirk R: Common sense quality management, *JONA* 20(10):10-15, 1990.

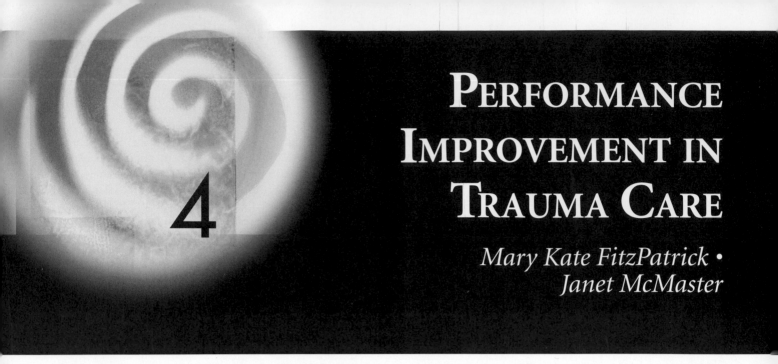

PERFORMANCE IMPROVEMENT IN TRAUMA CARE

4

Mary Kate FitzPatrick •
Janet McMaster

HISTORICAL PERSPECTIVE OF PERFORMANCE IMPROVEMENT IN TRAUMA CARE

A universal condition of trauma center accreditation is that specified injury data must be collected, analyzed, and maintained. In addition, the data must be monitored routinely by the trauma program in an effort to improve performance. The standards published by the American College of Surgeons' (ACS) Committee on Trauma in *Resources for Optimal Care of the Injured Patient* are the foundation for performance review in trauma centers.[1] These standards have gone through several revisions and continue to evolve.

The terms and principles related to quality have gone through many changes in recent times. "Quality assurance," "quality improvement," "continuous quality improvement," "total quality management," and "performance improvement" are all approaches to quality review that have been used in the past.[2] A major conceptual shift in these approaches has been the movement from a punitive quality assurance model to the more accepted system/process review. The health care industry continues to evolve its methodology for quality review, and the days of the "ABCs of morbidity and mortality" (accuse, blame, and criticize) are fading. This system/process performance improvement model is focused on outcomes, benchmarking, and performance of the system as a whole and moves away from emphasis on reviewing an individual's practice as a root cause.

Typically, hospital performance improvement and quality improvement have been service-line or unit specific. Depending on the institution, specific performance or quality committees would develop and implement projects, quite often following the Joint Commission on Accreditation of Healthcare Organizations' (JCAHO) accepted format, the performance improvement cycle (Figure 4-1). In the trauma care arena, there are standards that outline the basic type of performance review that trauma centers need to complete. Included in these standards are recommendations for performance indicators (including definitions) that should be monitored over time. Because of the strict standards set forth by trauma center accrediting agencies, often it is the trauma program that leads performance improvement efforts in hospitals.

Health care practitioners struggle to understand and operationalize the concepts of what we now call performance improvement. The popular literature on quality, which includes the works of pioneers like Juran and Deming, is focused on industrial settings. W.E. Deming, considered one of the leading figures in the movement to measure quality in industry, developed theories that are widely published. His work has been applied to multiple venues outside the traditional business world, including health care. *Out of the Crisis* (1986),[3] considered one of Deming's major works, provides anecdotes and examples of how to put his theories into practice.

A particular challenge to health care practitioners is determining how to apply techniques and principles designed for more "constant" industrial environments to the unpredictable and dynamic practice of medicine. The current environment in health care has presented additional challenges in the quest to operationalize performance improvement. Human and financial resources are lean and patient demographics are changing. To our advantage, however, are modern technologic advancements and the power of computerization in the maintenance and analysis of patient data.

TRAUMA PERFORMANCE IMPROVEMENT PLAN

Trauma programs should establish a written trauma performance improvement plan that addresses basic operational

IMPROVING ORGANIZATION PERFORMANCE FUNCTION

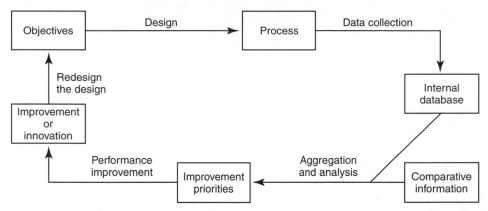

FIGURE 4-1 JCAHO **Performance Improvement cycle.** (From Joint Commission on Accreditation of Healthcare Organizations: *Joint Commission accreditation manual,* Oakbrook Terrace, Ill, 1998, The Commision.)

details and contains an overview of the process. This plan should be the result of a multidisciplinary effort and should be a dynamic document that is reevaluated periodically and updated to encompass key changes within the hospital trauma system and trauma care standards. Recommended distribution of the plan might include hospital quality improvement staff, nursing leadership, physician leadership from medical divisions involved in trauma care, and trauma program staff. This plan could be used as part of the orientation process for new hospital leadership who will be responsible for trauma patient care. The performance improvement plan should include the following:

- Overview of the process—issue identification.
- Personnel involved and their roles.
- Performance improvement forums/committees.
- Link to hospital/system performance improvement.
- Performance indicators (dynamic).
- Data maintenance methods.
- Guidelines for determining peer review judgment decisions (accountability).
- Performance improvement reports/provider profiles.
- Performance improvement loop closure (reevaluation).
- Provision for protection of confidentiality.

The performance improvement plan should consider state, regional, and national standards related to trauma care. The American College of Surgeons document titled *Trauma Performance Improvement, A How to Handbook* provides practitioners with an operational manual for establishing and maintaining a trauma performance improvement program.[4]

Integration of Trauma Performance Improvement With Institution and System Performance Improvement

Trauma programs lead the way in many institutions in terms of the depth, scope, and sophistication of performance improvement reviews. It is important that trauma programs be integrated into the overall hospital or system quality structure. Many health care organizations have adopted service-line teams to oversee performance improvement-related projects. Trauma crosses over and affects many service lines of the hospital structure, including nursing, emergency medicine, neurosurgery, anesthesia, orthopedics, rehabilitation services, radiology, laboratory services, perioperative care, critical care, nutrition, and blood bank. It is challenging to devise a single initiative that coordinates the activities of the multiple service lines through which care is provided to trauma patients. There must be some means of overseeing ongoing projects and determining areas of overlap, mutual benefit, and level of impact. For example, many hospitals collect intensive care unit (ICU) data; this data could be stratified to look at trends specifically within the trauma patient group. Conversely, data maintained by the trauma program may be stratified by phases of care and reported through the hospital performance improvement structure. Analysis of various levels of data from hospital departments can generate specific institutional projects. Projects that have the highest return on investment should be selected. Projects that target key areas or have strong potential to impact outcomes, patient satisfaction, or cost should be prioritized.

Many hospitals have adopted JCAHO guidelines to structure hospital performance improvement projects. The most recent format suggested by JCAHO is the performance improvement cycle. This process can be used to organize a project and is widely accepted (see Figure 4-1).[5] This format is applicable to trauma projects as well. Hospitals should have a written overall performance improvement plan, and this plan should be referenced in the trauma performance improvement plan.

Health care organizations are required by JCAHO to respond to sentinel events, defined as unexpected occurrences involving death or serious physical or psychologic injury, or any event that carries a significant chance of a serious adverse outcome. Appropriate responses include the following:

- Conducting a thorough and credible root cause analysis, focusing on systems and processes, not individual performance.
- Implementing improvements to reduce risk.
- Monitoring the effectiveness of those improvements.

The trauma performance improvement program must have a mechanism in place to report any identified sentinel events to the hospital department or committee responsible for JCAHO compliance.

PATIENT/ISSUE IDENTIFICATION

Identifying patients for trauma performance improvement review can be challenging. In hospitals without a designated trauma service, patients can be admitted to any one of a number of surgical or medical services. To help identify patients admitted with injury-related diagnoses, hospital information systems can produce reports with diagnoses, injury codes, and reasons for admission. The emergency department or admission log can be used to identify trauma patients.

Information for performance improvement review comes from many sources. Prehospital records, including fire, rescue, or ambulance run sheets and flight records from air ambulances, can provide information about the scene conditions, treatment rendered, and length of time at the scene. The patient's medical record is the main source for identifying performance improvement issues. The emergency department and trauma flow sheets should be designed to capture the timing and sequence of the resuscitation easily because this is key to evaluating care. Parts of the medical record that provide important performance improvement information may include the following:

- Physician documentation on progress notes or consultations.
- Operating room records, including anesthesia notes and postanesthesia care notes.
- Nurses' notes.
- Radiology and laboratory reports.
- Physical and occupational therapy notes.
- Social work or case management notes.
- Transfer records for patients transferred from another facility.

Because many hospitals are converting to electronic records, it will become essential for the person responsible for performance improvement to have access to the entire medical record, including electronically stored documents.

In addition to review of the medical record, it is helpful to have a mechanism for health care providers in all areas of the hospital, on all shifts, to contribute to the performance improvement process. They can report issues via a confidential, dedicated phone "hotline" or through issue identification forms, which can be submitted confidentially.

Significant issues that impact patient care should also be reported to risk management through appropriate institutional channels.

Videotapes of trauma resuscitations can identify opportunities for improvement that may not be evident through medical record review. Examples are provider noncompliance with standard body substance precautions or proper technique during procedures such as urinary catheter placement.

Other departments in the hospital may be a source of information regarding performance improvement issues. Infectious disease reports can identify patients with complications such as urinary tract infections or pneumonia, supporting or validating trauma performance improvement. Postdischarge records are a source of information regarding outcomes because they may identify missed injuries, delayed diagnoses, readmissions, or patient satisfaction issues. Postdischarge information can be obtained from outpatient records, feedback from rehabilitation facilities, follow-up from home care agencies, or autopsy reports. The medical examiner or coroner can often provide additional valuable data at mortality review forums.

TRAUMA PERFORMANCE IMPROVEMENT PROCESS: LEVELS OF REVIEW

There are many ways to structure a review of clinical care. Having both concurrent and retrospective features is ideal. Key steps should be established and should be modified based on the specific features of the trauma program (size, volume, resources, etc.). Key elements in the performance improvement process are diagrammed in Figure 4-2.

Data collection for performance improvement can occur concurrently with abstraction of data while care is being provided (primary review). The person in charge of concurrent review, usually a nurse (either the trauma coordinator, trauma performance improvement coordinator, or trauma case manager), uses various mechanisms to identify and follow up on issues as they occur. Patient care rounds, chart reviews, and direct staff and patient interaction are among the sources of data for concurrent review. The major advantages of concurrent review are that it allows (1) changes to occur in the patient's plan of care, which can influence outcome immediately, and (2) prompt feedback to providers regarding quality of care issues. One disadvantage is that it precludes an overview of the entirety of the case with all patient data from dictated radiology reports, discharge information, and postdischarge follow-up. Retrospective review occurs after the patient has been discharged, with data abstracted from medical records, registry reports, and so on (secondary review).

Retrospective review provides a comprehensive assessment of overall care and affords the opportunity to see trends in data and to compile statistics on groups of patients for analysis. The limitations of performing only retrospective reviews are (1) feedback to individual providers is delayed, (2) incidents must be reconstructed from memory, and (3) patient care cannot be affected in "real time." A

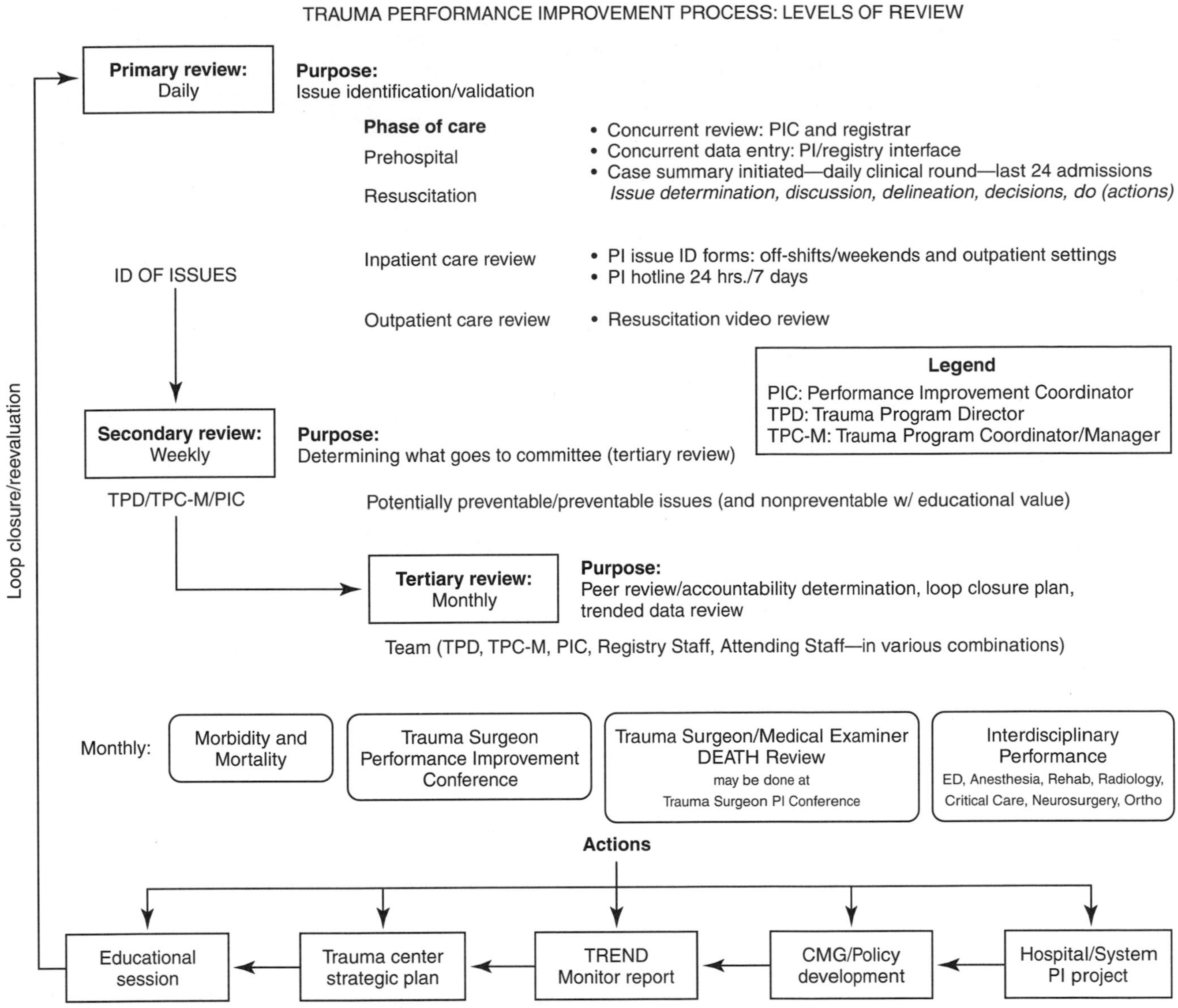

TRAUMA PERFORMANCE IMPROVEMENT PROCESS: LEVELS OF REVIEW

FIGURE 4-2 **Trauma Performance Improvement Process: Levels of Review.**

mature, comprehensive performance improvement program will have components of both concurrent and retrospective reviews.

PERFORMANCE IMPROVEMENT FORUMS

CASE SELECTION GUIDELINES FOR TERTIARY REVIEW

Criteria for determining which cases need to be discussed at a trauma performance improvement committee (tertiary review) must be established. This will vary based on volume and on local and state standards related to trauma performance improvement. Many institutions may review only cases that meet criteria for submission to the state and regional trauma registry (e.g., ICD-CM 800-995.9: deaths, ICU admissions, hospital length of stay [LOS] more than 48-72 hours, pediatrics). Depending on resources available, an institution may opt to review only clinical sentinel events,

cases with unexpected outcomes and those that involve preventable or potentially preventable occurrences. Other issues can be reviewed as aggregate data, and focused audits should be performed when data trends reflect significant fluctuations. Review of systems issues should be included in performance improvement committees. Appropriate hospital or system staff should be included in the forums when system issues will be discussed.

Ensuring attendance at performance improvement forums can be difficult. To facilitate attendance, a set calendar of meetings should be established on a routine day and time that are convenient for team members considering their clinical responsibilities. It may be helpful to incorporate trauma performance improvement committees into existing hospital and departmental forums like departmental morbidity and mortality conferences. There should be records of attendance (an ACS standard for participation in multidisciplinary peer review forums), and confidential files should be kept on the topics, patients, and participants at performance improvement forums. Preparation prior to meetings should include compiling a roster of cases to be presented, obtaining the medical records (when possible), and gathering the performance improvement case files. The guidelines for reaching peer review decisions and summary trauma registry data on individual cases should be available at performance improvement committee meetings. Using technology to enhance interactivity can be beneficial. Projecting patient case summaries during performance improvement meetings is one method that has been used to improve team participation in performance improvement discussions.

A key component of the performance improvement process is the provision of a peer review forum to discuss individual cases, trends in data, and comparative data related to system performance. Peer review forums should involve key trauma program/hospital staff (Table 4-1). Performance improvement committees can be structured in a variety of ways depending on the resources available, the volume of cases, and the local, state, and regional rules related to performance improvement reviews.

There are many options for designing the forum(s) in which trauma performance improvement issues will be reviewed. Surgeons taking trauma call could meet at a designated forum along with the trauma coordinator, trauma director, and registry staff, for example. In addition, there should be (based on the 1999 ACS standards) an interdisciplinary forum to review cases in which multiple services were involved or cases in which a single subspecialty was involved (e.g., neurosurgery, orthopedics, emergency medicine) but trauma surgeons or general surgeons taking

TABLE 4-1	**Performance Improvement Roles of Trauma Program Staff in a Level I Trauma Program**
Personnel	**Role in Performance Improvement**
Trauma Performance Improvement Coordinator RN	• Identifies issues concurrently. • Creates case file. • Selects cases for performance improvement committees. • Validates registry data. • Reports on clinical management guideline compliance. • Monitors trends in performance improvement reports/provider profile development. • Tracks loop closure/resolution. • Maintains performance improvement data.
Trauma Performance Improvement Medical Director	• Selects cases for performance improvement committees. • Moderates performance improvement committee meetings. • Performs chart review. • Analyzes performance improvement trended data/provider profiles. • Coordinates generation of correspondence for performance improvement follow-up. • Leads peer review judgment discussions with trauma director.
Trauma Program Manager/ Coordinator	• Analyzes trended performance improvement reports. • Participates in peer review judgement discussions. • Manages follow-up on performance improvement system issues. • Oversees development & implementation of performance improvement/registry plans. • Provides back-up coverage for performance improvement coordinator. • Validates trauma registry data. • Facilitates interdisciplinary performance improvement team. • Oversees clinical management guideline process: development implementation & surveillance. • Directs loop closure—practice/policy changes/educational changes. • Links to hospital/system performance improvement structures.
Trauma Program Director	• Facilitates the performance improvement committee discussions. • Moderates peer review decision/judgment determinations. • Directs development of performance improvement plan with trauma program manager. • Performs chart reviews. • Facilitates interdisciplinary performance improvement team. • Directs evidence-based clinical management guideline development. • Directs "loop closure"—practice/policy/educational changes. • Links to hospital performance improvement system.
Trauma Registry Staff	• Performs concurrent data abstraction & maintenance of trauma registry database. • Prepares performance improvement summaries from the trauma registry to facilitate data validation. • Participates in performance improvement committee meetings. • Oversees EMS documentation and autopsy report retrieval. • Prepares monthly standing registry reports.
Trauma Surgeons/Fellows & Interdisciplinary Liaisons	• Participates in performance improvement committee meetings. • Participates in peer review decisions/judgments. • Performs chart reviews.

trauma call were not involved. Finally, decisions must be made regarding how death cases should be reviewed and whether additional personnel such as the coroner or medical examiner should be included.[6]

Trauma performance improvement discussions can occur in forums with an emphasis on education. Multidisciplinary trauma conferences (morbidity and mortality conferences, video review conference, and journal clubs) may have elements of performance improvement review. The performance improvement aspects should be captured and filed appropriately.

PERFORMANCE INDICATORS: AUDIT FILTERS, OCCURRENCES, AND COMPLICATIONS

Performance improvement indicators are screens or triggers that are designed to activate review of potential risk-associated clinical or sytem occurrences. The ACS published trauma audit filters that became the national standard for trauma programs. The utility of current audit filters has not been determined definitively. Research has been done on whether the audit filters have consistent links to improved outcome.[7] Literature suggests that although some have found existing audit filters to be useful, others have found them labor intensive and costly.[8] Trauma programs should focus their resources and time on institution-specific filters that provide the most meaningful measures of patient outcome. This is an area that clearly requires continual review and analysis.

There are national recommendations regarding the types of clinical complications (now commonly referred to as "occurrences") that a trauma performance improvement system should monitor. The ACS provides a list of occurrences and definitions for performance improvement tracking. Many states and regions have developed their own list of occurrences based on the ACS standards. Universal definitions are paramount. In order to assess or compare trauma clinical care at a state or national level, there must be conformity in the definitions of occurrences tracked. This conformity ensures that incidence rates of a given occurrence are truly comparable (e.g., what one institution calls pneumonia is the same as what another institution classifies as pneumonia).

The comprehensiveness of the performance improvement program will depend on many factors: center maturation, volume, resources, and local and state requirements. The utility of reviewing certain trauma performance indicators for trauma has been studied.[9,10] Trauma programs should strive to routinely review the occurrences and filters used to monitor quality outcomes. One approach to analysis of performance indicators is a rate-based methodology (frequency of occurrence/denominator of total cases). The stage of the trauma program in its evolution and development will affect an institution's ability to review rate-based indicators. Performance indicators that prove to be ineffective measures of outcome (through rate-based measurements or other types of trending) should not be prioritized. One way to approach performance indicator review is to group indicators into categories such as "discretionary" and "nondiscretionary." Nondiscretionary indicators are mandated through local and state trauma rules. It often is these nondiscretionary audit filters that programs prioritize. Discretionary indicators may be the institution-specific audit filters and occurrences. There are opportunities in terms of continued research studies for reviewing the use of audit filters and determining a definitive link between certain trauma performance indicators and desired patient outcomes.

A key component of reviewing performance indicators is a systematic approach to determining peer review judgments. In reaching peer review judgments related to occurrences (complications), the following questions can facilitate consensus:

- Were accepted protocols and policies followed?
- Were clinical management guidelines adhered to?
- Was the case managed in accordance with Advanced Trauma Life Support (ATLS) guidelines?
- If occurrence involves a resident or student, was there evidence of adequate supervision?
- Was the system response optimal? Examples of system shortfalls include prolonged prehospital time, communications problems, failure of the paging system, delays in internal response, blood bank delays, and equipment malfunctions.
- Did the patient have preexisting medical conditions that contributed to the occurrence (e.g., diabetes, cardiac condition, or age extreme)?
- Was the occurrence evident before hospitalization (e.g., hypothermia, arrhythmia, or urinary tract infection)?

Example: A 35-year-old man was involved in a front-end motor vehicle crash. His medical history was unremarkable. He was the unrestrained driver of a compact car; the airbag deployed on impact. Pneumothorax and evidence of blood in the abdomen were detected by use of sonography. The patient was taken to the operating room for exploratory laparotomy. A review of the resuscitation videotape clearly shows a break in sterile technique during the insertion of the indwelling urinary catheter by the trauma resident. On hospital day three, the patient's temperature is elevated, and it is determined that he has a urinary tract infection (Table 4-2).

OUTCOMES

Evaluation of outcomes is an essential component of performance improvement in a trauma center. Outcomes can include quality of life indicators, measured by patient satisfaction surveys, and functional outcomes, measured by functional independence measure (FIM) or by collecting information regarding a patient's ability to return to work. Hospitals and insurance providers are interested in financial outcomes, measured by costs, readmissions, denied days, LOS, and ICU LOS. Other outcome measures include deaths, complications, delayed diagnoses, and missed injuries.

TABLE 4-2 **Performance Improvement Analysis of an Early Urinary Tract Infection**			
Determinants of Preventability	Responses	Discussion	Determination
Were accepted policies/procedures followed?	No	Proper technique for insertion of indwelling urinary catheter was not followed	
Were clinical management guidelines adhered to?	N/A		
Was management done as per ATLS guidelines?	Yes	Indwelling urinary catheter required for this patient	
If complication involves a resident or student, was there evidence of adequate supervision?	No		
Was the system response optimal?	Yes		
Did the patient have preexisting medical conditions that contributed to the occurrence?	No		
Was the occurrence/complication evident prior to hospitalization?	No		
DETERMINATION			• **Error in technique** • **Supervision deficiency**

One starting point for evaluating care is the use of the Trauma and Injury Severity Score tool (TRISS) to review cases ending in the death of the patient. In short, TRISS methodology is based on the following:

- Physiologic parameters, including respiratory rate (RR), Glasgow Coma Scale (GCS) score, and systolic blood pressure (SBP).
- Age (<15, 15-55, >55).
- Mechanism of injury (blunt or penetrating).
- Anatomic scoring of injuries by Injury Severity Score (ISS).

Based on these parameters, the probability of a patient's survival is calculated, and the outcome is expressed as expected death, unexpected death, or unexpected survivor. TRISS is useful in identifying unexpected outcomes, and it offers a standardized way to compare outcomes with those in other trauma centers, other states, and other populations. However, it has some limitations that reduce its usefulness in performance improvement review. Because TRISS depends on physiologic parameters on admission, patients who arrive intubated, without a recorded respiratory rate, are excluded from analysis. Similarly, intubated patients lack the verbal component of the GCS, which excludes them from analysis.[11] Additionally, patients who arrive dead may have no injuries recorded; therefore, no ISS can be calculated. These patients are excluded from TRISS analysis until final anatomic diagnoses are determined from autopsy results. Another weakness of TRISS analysis is that it is based on the ISS. The ISS was initially developed as a way to standardize severity of injuries for patients who were involved in motor vehicle crashes and had injuries to multiple body areas. The ISS is less accurate at classifying patients with multiple injuries to one body region, a disadvantage when calculating scores for patients with penetrating injuries.

Over the years, investigators have evaluated TRISS, and tried to improve the method of evaluating trauma care objectively.[12-16] Some of the more recent innovations based on ICD-9-CM coding have the advantages of being more cost efficient to calculate because they are based on injuries identified by medical record coders rather than specialized trauma registrars. In addition, they can be used to predict outcomes such as morbidity and length of stay, not just mortality. Another proposed method, the New Injury Severity Score (NISS), enhances ISS by including all the most serious injuries, not just the most serious in one body area.[17] These new methods need to be tested and validated on a large scale before they become widely accepted. No one method can replace a critical evaluation of patient care in a multidisciplinary forum using a framework for reaching peer review judgments. In this setting, the reviewers make determinations of whether the deaths are nonpreventable, preventable, or potentially preventable. Questions that need to be asked to determine preventability include the following:

- Was the death an expected outcome based on TRISS? (Despite its limitations, TRISS is widely used to predict outcomes and provides a starting point for review.)
- Are the patient's injuries considered nonsurvivable (i.e., ISS = 75)?[18] Examples:

  Head: Crush injury of skull or brain or massive destruction or penetration of brainstem.
  Thorax: Major laceration, perforation, or puncture of ventricle.
  Spine: Complete spinal cord injury with quadriplegia at C3 or higher.
  Abdomen and pelvis: Hepatic avulsion, Grade VI.

- Were standard procedures and protocols followed? Did patient care follow guidelines, such as in ATLS or

TABLE 4-3 **Performance Improvement Analysis of a Nonpreventable Death**				
Determinants of Preventability	**Responses**	**Discussion**		**Determination**
Was the death an expected outcome based on TRISS?	Yes	Expected death		
Are the patient's injuries considered nonsurvivable?	Yes	Probability of survival 0.004		
Were standard procedures and protocols followed?	Yes			
Was the care provided appropriate?	Yes			
Was the system response optimal?	Yes			
Was the outcome affected by the patient's preexisting conditions?	Unknown			
DETERMINATION				**Nonpreventable**

hospital-specific protocols? Keep in mind that guidelines do not replace clinical judgment, and there are situations when deviation from the guidelines is appropriate. If this is the case, the reason must be clearly documented.

- Was the care appropriate? Provider errors that could contribute to a patient's death include missed injuries, delayed diagnosis of injuries, technical errors, errors in judgment, and errors in management.
- Was system response optimal? Examples of system issues include prehospital transport time, communications problems, failure of the paging system, internal response issues, blood bank delays, equipment malfunctions, delays in final reading of radiographs, or nonavailability of operating room staff.
- Did the patient have preexisting medical conditions that contributed to the outcome? Preexisting conditions that contribute to a higher mortality rate include cirrhosis, coagulopathy, cardiac disease, renal disease, and malignancy.[19,20]

NONPREVENTABLE DEATHS

If the response to all these questions is yes, the death can be considered nonpreventable. However, even though the patient's injuries are considered nonsurvivable and the death nonpreventable, the remainder of the care should still be evaluated to identify areas for improvement.

Example: A 24-year-old male arrived at the trauma center within 10 minutes after being stabbed in the chest. The trauma team had prenotification of his arrival and was in the trauma bay. The patient's initial SBP was 60 and his GCS score was 8. He was intubated and resuscitated with intravenous (IV) fluids and packed red blood cells, which were readily available. A chest tube drained an initial 1000 ml of bright red blood, which was autotransfused. His subsequent SBP was 90, and he was taken to the operating room within 18 minutes after arrival. Thoracotomy revealed that he had exsanguinated from a laceration of the right ventricle and could not be resuscitated (Table 4-3).

PREVENTABLE DEATHS

If the response to the previous questions is no, the death is considered preventable. This indicates that the patient's injuries were considered relatively minor and survivable, but there were errors in judgment or management or technical errors that directly caused the patient's death.

Example: A 28-year-old male was transported to the emergency department by rescue services after falling from a curb. He was reportedly unconscious at the scene but was awake and responsive on arrival, with stable vital signs and a minor head laceration. Because he was apparently intoxicated and agitated, he was medicated with a sedative to calm him and placed in a room to "sleep it off." After a few hours, he was found to be unresponsive. A computed tomography (CT) scan was requested, but there was a delay in obtaining the scan because of a change of shift and personnel. Finally the CT scan showed a large epidural hematoma, and the neurosurgeons, who had left for the day, had to be called back to perform an emergency craniotomy. Despite their efforts, the patient did not recover, and he continued to be unresponsive until his death a few weeks later (Table 4-4).

POTENTIALLY PREVENTABLE DEATHS

The categorization of potentially preventable death requires an unbiased, critical review by the team. Determining that a death was potentially preventable indicates that the injuries and preexisting conditions were serious but the patient had the potential to survive if all other conditions were optimal. Errors in technique, errors in management, delays in care, or deviations from standard of care may have contributed to the patient's death.

Example: After a fall from a height, an elderly woman was admitted with a combination of injuries, including pelvic fractures, evidence of a closed head injury and intraabdominal injuries, and lower extremity fractures. Her initial vital signs were stable, but she quickly became hemodynamically unstable, requiring massive resuscitation with crystalloids and blood for hemorrhagic shock. During the resuscitation, she developed cardiac arrhythmia and ventricular fibrillation and could not be resuscitated. Review of her trauma flow sheet revealed that her admission temperature was 34° C (93.2° F), yet fluids and blood products were administered without the use of warming devices (Table 4-5).

MISSED INJURIES

Missed injuries and delayed diagnoses can be a significant cause of morbidity or mortality. Diagnoses not made during the initial assessment or during the tertiary survey can be labeled "delayed." Injuries not diagnosed until after the

TABLE 4-4   Performance Improvement Analysis of a Preventable Death

Determinants of Preventability	Responses	Discussion	Determination
Was the death an expected outcome based on TRISS?	No	Unexpected death by TRISS	
Are the patient's injuries considered nonsurvivable?	No	Probability of survival 0.924	
Were standard procedures and protocols followed?	No	Incomplete evaluation of potential head-injured patient with impaired neurologic evaluation	
Was the care provided appropriate?	No	Inadequate monitoring of potentially head-injured patient Administration of sedatives Delay in diagnosis	
Was the system response optimal?	No	Delay in CT scan, delay in neurosurgery response	
Was the outcome affected by the patient's preexisting conditions?	No	Intoxication affected his evaluation but should not have affected his outcome	
DETERMINATION			**Preventable**

TABLE 4-5   Performance Improvement Analysis of a Potentially Preventable Death

Determinants of Preventability	Responses	Discussion	Determination
Was the death an expected outcome based on TRISS?	N/A	Unable to calculate TRISS, intubated prior to arrival	
Are the patient's injuries considered nonsurvivable?	No	Injuries potentially survivable	
Were standard procedures and protocols followed?	No	Institutional guidelines to prevent hypothermia were not followed	
Was the care provided appropriate?	No		
Was the system response optimal?	Yes		
Was the outcome affected by the patient's preexisting conditions?	No		
DETERMINATION			**Potentially preventable**

patient's discharge can be categorized as "missed." Approximately 10% to 15% of all patients with multiple injuries will have a delayed or missed diagnosis.[21,22] Some missed injuries are unavoidable. Circumstances that contribute to missed or delayed diagnosis of injuries include the inability to assess patients thoroughly for pain because of hemodynamic instability or shock, decreased level of consciousness caused by head injury or alcohol intoxication, intubation, and the use of chemical paralytics. It may not be possible to examine patients with closed head injuries for pain, and extremity injuries may show up much later during rehabilitation. Nurses can play a role in revealing injuries by reporting swelling, bruising, or signs of discomfort when moving patients.

Some missed injuries may be prevented if the health care providers maintain a high level of suspicion. For example, patterns related to mechanism of injury should be appreciated. A person who has fallen from a height, landed on a hard surface, and sustained bilateral calcaneal fractures could also have fractures of the knees, hip, or thoracic spine, caused by the force transmitted up the skeletal system. Additionally, at the end of a fall, the victim usually has outstretched hands, causing bilateral Colles' fractures of the wrists ("Don Juan" syndrome). Unrestrained drivers or front-seat passengers involved in motor

vehicle crashes who have sustained a posterior dislocation of the hip should also be evaluated for knee injury, caused when the knee hits the dashboard. Lower right-sided rib fractures can be associated with liver lacerations. Lower left-sided rib fractures can be associated with splenic lacerations. Fractures of the neck of the fibula can cause a stretch injury of the peroneal nerve.

Provider-related issues that may contribute to missed or delayed diagnosis of injuries include failure to appreciate signs of injury, failure to complete a thorough physical examination, or failure to read x-ray films correctly. It is beneficial to have a system in which "rereads" by a radiologist are communicated to the trauma team directly so that a delay in diagnosis does not lead to further delay in care. Data regarding missed injuries or delayed diagnosis of injuries can be gathered from the patient's medical records, radiology reports, readmission data, outpatient records, and follow-up from rehabilitation hospitals. Autopsy reports may identify injuries that remained undiagnosed during the patient's hospitalization.

ACCOUNTABILITY

Most performance improvement issues are related to inadequacies in the system. Most complications are related to

TABLE 4-6 Monthly Provider Summary

Provider #	1	2	3	4	5	6	7	Trauma Team	Totals
Total Admissions	15	10	9	8	13	20	18		93
Deaths	1			1	3	2			7
Preventable									0
Potentially preventable					1				1
Nonpreventable	1			1	2	2			6
Complications									
Wound infection	1				1				2
Urinary tract infection							2		2
Pneumonia								2	2
Deep vein thrombosis								1	1
Pulmonary embolism								1	1
Enterocutaneous fistula				1					1
Technical Issues									
Pneumothorax s/p central line	1						1		2
Iatrogenic bowel injury			1		1				2
Retained foreign body					1				1
Missed diagnosis						1			1
Delayed diagnosis									0
Total Complications, Issues	2	0	1	1	3	1	3	4	

patient disease and are thought to be unavoidable. It is occasionally necessary to assign to a specific provider the responsibility for an error in management or technique, a missed or delayed diagnosis of an injury, failure to follow standard protocols or guidelines, or a complication. If the patient was being managed by a group of physicians rather than a specific provider, the responsibility should be assigned to the "team." If a patient has an unrecognized esophageal intubation, then the provider who was in charge of intubating and confirming airway placement is responsible, and the error in technique is assigned to the specific provider. If a patient develops an upper gastrointestinal bleed after a long ICU stay and if on review it is determined that the patient had never received appropriate prophylaxis, who was responsible is not as clear cut. The team of physicians responsible for that patient's care, whether it is the critical care service or the trauma service, is responsible, and the failure to follow guidelines is assigned to the appropriate team.

The issue of supervision should also be addressed in academic centers that provide learning experiences for students, residents, and fellows. Ultimate responsibility for the care of patients must be linked to a supervising attending physician and means of monitoring this role in the performance improvement process should be considered.

Resources for Optimal Care of the Injured Patient mandates an evaluation of provider-specific mortality rates, complication rates, compliance with continuing education, resource utilization, and participation in guidelines and protocols. The performance improvement program will be required to demonstrate that there is a systematic mechanism in place to collect objective data regarding performance and to provide feedback to individual providers.

Sample reports are provided in Tables 4-6 and 4-7 and Figure 4-3.

CORRECTIVE ACTION PLAN

Once system- or provider-related issues are identified, corrective actions should be taken, with the goal of improving patient care, not merely to be punitive. Possible actions include the following:

- Collection of data for a period of time to determine if the variation represents a trend or an isolated occurrence.
- Change in or better enforcement of policy or procedure.
- Development of clinical management guidelines.
- Presentation of the issue as a topic in an educational setting.
- Physician/provider counseling.
- Mandatory continuing education.
- Probation or suspension of staff members who have varied from accepted standards of care.
- Notification of risk management.

REEVALUATION (LOOP CLOSURE)

As mentioned previously, the performance improvement process can be viewed as a cycle, as per JCAHO's guidelines. One very important activity in closing a performance improvement case is to ensure that the recommended actions are implemented and that the actions have the desired effect of improving patient care, or "closing the loop." Strategies to ensure resolution include a paper "tickler" file, or a field in a database to indicate unresolved issues. This continuous reevaluation of the outcome guaran-

TABLE 4-7 Trauma Service Provider Summary

Provider	All Patients	Deaths	Percent Deaths	Unexpected Deaths	Preventable	Potentially Preventable	Nonpreventable	Unexpected Survivors	Blunt	Penetrating	Mean ISS	ISS >16
1	6	0	0.00	0	0	0	0	0	3	3	12	2
2	298	19	6.38%	0	0	2	14	0	208	90	9.08	46
3	94	5	5.32%	2	0	0	5	0	19	75	16.192	10
4	187	9	4.81%	1	0	0	6	0	125	62	10.395	39
5	206	21	10.19%	3	0	1	17	2	140	66	11.143	46
6	91	5	5.49%	0	0	0	5	0	64	27	12.06	23
7	136	7	5.15%	0	0	1	6	2	103	33	9.847	33
8	198	20	10.10%	0	0	0	18	1	141	57	12.271	48
9	33	1	3.03%	0	0	0	1	0	25	8	12.375	8
10	241	20	8.30%	5	1	2	16	0	153	88	11.257	49
11	176	11	6.25%	2	0	0	9	2	120	56	10.583	31
12	84	4	4.76%	1	0	0	4	0	17	67	14.81	6
13	109	9	8.26%	2	0	2	5	0	71	38	9.202	18
14	43	2	4.65%	0	1	0	1	0	36	7	9.805	7
15	147	11	7.48%	2	0	0	11	1	96	51	10.874	31
16	100	4	4.00%	1	0	0	4	1	67	33	9.375	19
Totals	2149	148	6.89%	19	2	8	122	9	1388	761	11.33	416

PEER REVIEW JUDGEMENTS: TRAUMA DEATHS

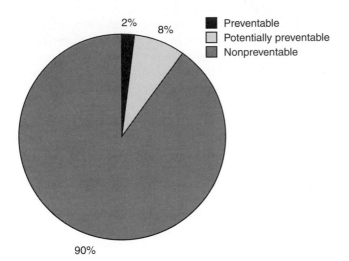

FIGURE 4-3 **Peer Review Judgments: Trauma Deaths.** Data con fabulated to provide example for reader.

tees that the performance improvement process remains dynamic and responsive to the changing environment in medicine.

RECORDKEEPING

Each state has regulations regarding the confidentiality of performance improvement or peer-review documents, but some guidelines regarding recordkeeping are universal. Patient identification should be limited to numbers or initials. Full names should be avoided if possible. Providers should be identified by a number rather than by name, and the list matching providers to numbers should remain confidential. Reports that are distributed at performance improvement meetings should be clearly marked "confidential" or "for peer review only." Any handouts for review at performance improvement meetings should be counted and then accounted for at the close of the meeting. Extras should be destroyed. Issues discussed at performance improvement forums must not be made public, and documents must not be published and distributed to others. Documentation must be limited to objective statement of the facts. As long as the information is not made public or distributed to others, it is usually protected from legal discovery. Attendants at performance improvement forums must have a professional or legitimate reason to be present.

It is important that performance improvement documents remain separate from medical records and not referenced in the patient chart because medical records can be requested in a subpoena. Performance improvement documents kept on file must be maintained in a secure manner, for example, in locked cabinets. If data are stored in a computer, the files must be password protected with access limited to those with a legitimate reason to view the documents. It is tempting to use the convenience and speed of e-mail or fax to communicate performance improvement

TABLE 4-8	**Steps in the Development of Clinical Management Guidelines**

- Monitor current performance.
- Collect input from multiple disciplines.
- Review published literature on the topic.
- Educate staff members affected by the guideline about the upcoming change.
- Implement the new guideline.
- Maintain surveillance and routine reporting of compliance.

information, but this practice should be discouraged unless strict guidelines regarding confidentiality are maintained.

There must be institution-specific, written guidelines regarding the handling of videotapes of trauma resuscitations. Tapes should be stored behind locked doors with limited access. They should be viewed only by those who have a professional reason to view a trauma resuscitation. There must be a specific time frame in which the tapes must be erased and reused or destroyed. Having the hospital legal department review the procedures of the performance improvement program to ensure compliance with approved state regulations regarding confidentiality of peer review documents is ideal.

A typical performance improvement file will include the following:

- Case summary.
- Registry data, including TRISS data.
- Issue identification forms.
- All correspondence sent and received.
- Supporting documents related to follow-up and closure.
- Autopsy reports, if applicable.

CLINICAL MANAGEMENT GUIDELINES

Standardizing (where appropriate) the approach to the care of injured patients has become an important goal of trauma programs. One strategy employed to standardize aspects of trauma care is the use of clinical management guidelines. The Eastern Association for the Surgery of Trauma has published templates of clinical management guidelines for injured patients, which have been modified and adopted by trauma programs across the country.[23]

There are key steps that are recommended in developing clinical management guidelines successfully (Table 4-8). One important step is to link them to the trauma performance improvement program. Clinical management guidelines should be evidence based (e.g., review of literature on clinical outcomes related to specific approaches). The trauma performance improvement program should guide development of clinical guidelines through analysis of trends in practice patterns and patient outcomes. When developing guidelines that affect several disciplines, input should be collected from the staff members who will be affected by the change. For example, a change in the procedure for clearing a trauma patient's cervical spine should be reviewed by representatives of radiology, neurosurgery, trauma, nursing, physical medicine, and rehabilitation services. A key element of a successful clinical management guideline program is education of all involved in implementing the guideline. Operational issues that could arise as a result of a new guideline should be determined during the planning stage, not after implementation.

Surveillance is probably the most critical element of a successful clinical management guideline program. There must be some identified mechanism to track and report compliance with guidelines. Measures to enhance compliance should be investigated, for example, inserting computerized prompts into physician order entry systems or providing pocket guides that remind providers of guidelines. Several surveillance models can be employed, using the trauma coordinator, registry staff who are performing concurrent abstraction, advanced practice nurses or trauma nurse clinicians, or if one is in place, a trauma performance improvement coordinator.[24]

REGISTRY: PERFORMANCE IMPROVEMENT INTEGRATION

A requirement of *Resources for Optimal Care of the Injured Patient* is that data be maintained on injured patients who are evaluated and managed at the trauma center. Based on local protocols and state statutes, data requirements may differ slightly. The trauma registry is a fundamental component of the center or trauma system. Only through the collection and analysis of data can the center and system develop and improve.

Many commercial trauma registry software packages are available. The type of registry package selected should be based on the desired features sought. Some key elements to consider when choosing a trauma registry package include database networking possibilities, report writing capabilities, compatibility/interface capability with other standard hospital information systems (e.g., radiology, laboratory, hospital registration systems), and compatibility with popular commercial personal computer platforms such as Microsoft Windows.

There should be a close interface between the trauma registry and the trauma performance improvement programs. Depending on the program's size, resources, and organizational structure, there may be overlapping roles and responsibilities for a single team member related to the registry and performance improvement functions.[25] In this era of lean program resources, reducing duplicate abstraction and streamlining information flow should be the goal. Hospitals should investigate the possibility of interfacing existing hospital data sources to minimize duplicate data entry and better use personnel.

Key systems for the trauma program to access would include the hospital admission database, the radiology system, laboratory system, operating room scheduling and tracking system, and computerized portions of the medical record. It is also suggested that, when feasible, trauma registry staff be integrated into the overall trauma administrative team. This is difficult when the trauma registry is physically housed in medical records or another location physically separate from the trauma program office and staff. Measures to incorporate the registry staff and to validate the accuracy of abstraction need to be determined. The registrar role in the trauma performance improvement program will enhance the overall process. Having the registrar(s) participate in performance improvement forums serves several purposes: It strengthens the issue identification process, allows validation of the information entered into the registry, and enhances registrar job satisfaction and sense of contribution. Registrars strengthen performance improvement discussions by providing insight into the coding of injuries, a unique understanding of the scoring methodologies commonly used in trauma care, and explanation of the criteria for audit filter and occurrence (complications) capture. The registry staff can be instrumental in the generation of reports that are essential to the performance improvement process. In addition, the registry staff can provide guidance on customization of the registry database for tracking performance-improvement-related data. In terms of day-to-day operations, the movement toward concurrent data collection presents new opportunities to strengthen the integration of registry and performance improvement programs.

In the future, the development and maintenance of a national trauma data bank should be the goal. There are many operational issues that have been encountered with current efforts to make this a national reality. Technologic advancements and the new and rapidly expanding field of health information management can make this goal obtainable.

TECHNOLOGY

Computerization can enhance the performance improvement process. Records can be stored in a database program and evaluated in a spreadsheet. Most spreadsheet programs display the data in graphs or charts for presentation, demonstrating trends over time or comparing performance by provider. Merging the information in the performance improvement database with templates in a word processing program produces letters that give feedback to referring physicians, request medical records from transferring institutions, request follow-up information from rehabilitation facilities, or refer patient cases to other physicians for review. Using an LCD projector to display data or case summaries on a screen during performance improvement meetings enables the presenter to make additions, corrections, or deletions; encourages participation; and makes the meetings interesting and interactive.

LOOKING TO THE FUTURE

Technology advancements will lead to challenges in the future. Traditionally, *CPR* has stood for cardiopulmonary resuscitation. This acronym now takes on an additional meaning in the age of information technology advances: computer-based patient record. The advent of full or partial electronic medical records will minimize issues of storage and retrieval of paper records, eliminate legibility issues, and perhaps decrease duplicative efforts within hospital systems. In addition, technology advancements will allow for easy communication of data between departments and interfaces between existing hospital systems. The potential exists for laboratory, radiology, and patient registration information to be electronically downloaded into the trauma registry database. Other technology improvements to look for in the future (perhaps in use in some places now) include the following:

- Voice recognition charting documentation.
- Web links for interhospital data transfer.
- Palm technology for prehospital and hospital data collection.
- Clinical decision support systems.

The elements of and format for trauma performance improvement reviews continue to evolve. As technology continues to develop, efforts need to be directed at the creation of a national trauma data bank that will help guide policy practice patterns for injury care. This will require a standard data collection format and the involvement of other data sources (e.g., law enforcement, coroners) in addition to the trauma centers. Much emphasis has been given to development of benchmarking trauma clinical outcomes. The University Health Consortium (UHC) has begun to study a subset of the nation's trauma centers for comparing clinical outcomes. This process is still in development and only compares the outcomes from university-based trauma centers. UHC is an alliance of the clinical enterprises of academic health centers. Although focusing on the clinical mission, UHC supports research and education missions. As an idea-generating and information-disseminating enterprise, UHC assists members to pool resources, create economies of scale, improve clinical and operating efficiencies, and influence the direction and delivery of health care.

The issue of limited health care dollars is another factor that must be considered as trauma performance improvement continues its evolution. Using data to streamline and improve care effectiveness while maintaining positive outcomes will be a priority for trauma care clinicians in the new millennium.

Transition to a national trauma data bank, a goal of the American College of Surgeons' Committee on Trauma for years, will greatly enhance the ability to perform meaningful trauma benchmarking. Including data from hospitals with 24-hour emergency departments (non-trauma centers that treat injured patients) would provide a very powerful source of injury information, which could then guide public health and safety initiatives to prevent injury, the ultimate in loop closure.

REFERENCES

1. American College of Surgeons, Committee on Trauma: *Resources for optimal care of the injured patient,* Chicago, 1999, American College of Surgeons.
2. Wright JE: The history of the surgical audit, *J Qual Clin Pract* 15:81-88, 1995.
3. Deming WE: *Out of the crisis,* Cambridge, Mass, 1986, MIT-CAES.
4. American College of Surgeons, Committee on Trauma: *Trauma performance improvement, a how to handbook,* Chicago, 1999, American College of Surgeons.
5. Joint Commission on Accreditation of Healthcare Organizations: *Joint Commission accreditation manual,* Oakbrook Terrace, Ill, 1998.
6. Nayduch D, FitzPatrick MK: The application of forensic findings to the trauma quality management process, *J Trauma Nurs* 6(4):98-102, 1999.
7. Cryer HG, Hiatt JR, Fleming AW et al: Continuous use of standard process audit filters has limited value in an established trauma system, *J Trauma* 41(3):389-395, 1996.
8. Rhodes M, Sacco W, Smith S: Cost effectiveness of trauma quality assurance audit filters, *J Trauma* 30:724-727, 1990.
9. Nayduch D, Moylan J, Snyder BL et al: American College of Surgeons audit filters: an analysis of outcome in a statewide trauma system, *J Trauma* 37:565-575, 1994.
10. Hoyt DB, Hollingsworth-Fridlund P, Fortlage D et al: An evaluation of provider-related and disease-related morbidity in a level I university trauma service: directions for quality improvement, *J Trauma* 33:586-601, 1992.
11. Offner P, Jurkovich G, Gurney J et al: Revision of TRISS for intubated patients, *J Trauma* 32:32-35, 1992.
12. Baker SP, O'Neill B, Haddon W et al: The Injury Severity Score: a method for describing patients with multiple injuries and evaluating emergency care, *J Trauma* 14:187-196, 1974.
13. Champion HR, Sacco WJ, Cornazzo AK et al: A revision of the trauma score, *J Trauma* 29:623-676, 1989.
14. Sacco WJ, Copes W, Staz C et al: Status of trauma patient management as measured by survival/death outcomes: looking toward the 21st century, *J Trauma* 36:297-298, 1994.
15. Rutledge R, Osler T, Emery S et al: The end of the Injury Severity Score (ISS) and the trauma and injury severity score tool (TRISS): ICISS, an international classification of diseases, the ninth revision-based prediction tool, out performs both ISS and TRISS as predictors of trauma patient survival, hospital charges, and length of stay, *J Trauma* 44:41-49, 1998.
16. Al West T, Rivara F, Cummings P et al: Harborview assessment for risk of mortality: an improved measure of injury severity on the basis of ICD-9-CM, *J Trauma* 49(3):530-541, 2000.
17. Hoyt DB: Is it time for a new injury score (commentary)? *Lancet* 44:580-582, 1998.
18. Boyd CR, Tolson MA, Copes W: Evaluating trauma care: the TRISS method, *J Trauma* 27:370-378, 1987.
19. Morris JA, Mackenzie EJ, Edelstein SL: The effect of preexisting conditions on mortality in trauma patients, *JAMA* 14: 1942-1946, 1990.
20. Milzman D, Boulanger B, Rodriguez A et al: Pre-existing disease in trauma patients: a predictor of fate independent of age and injury severity score, *J Trauma* 32:236-244, 1992.
21. Sommers M: Missed injuries: a case of trauma hide and seek, *AACN Clin Issues* 6:187-195, 1995.
22. Enderson BL, Reath DB, Meadors J et al: The tertiary trauma

survey: a prospective study of missed injuries, *J Trauma* 30:666-669, 1990.

23. Pasquale M, Fabian TC: Practice management guidelines for trauma from the Eastern Association for the Surgery of Trauma, *J Trauma* 44(6):945-946, 1998.

24. Frankel HL, FitzPatrick MK, Gaskell S et al: Strategies to improve compliance with evidence-based clinical management guidelines, *J Am Coll Surg* 189(6):533-538, 1999.

25. FitzPatrick MK, Heliger L, McMaster J et al: Integration of concurrent trauma registry and performance improvement programs, *J Trauma Nurs* 7(4):92-97, 2000.

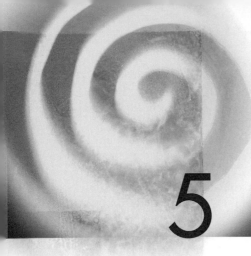

LEGAL CONCERNS IN TRAUMA NURSING

5

Robert W. Heilig

Trauma nursing has undergone a rapid evolution, as is evident by the nursing, medical, and scientific content of this book. Before the 1950s any nursing book that dealt with the law could do so in the context of ethical or administrative considerations only. Up to that time, the law for nurses was subordinate to the law for physicians, as was the nurse's role in patient care.

The legal notion of independent judgment by nurses was established during the late 1950s and early 1960s.[1,2] Today the nurse in a trauma setting performs highly skilled functions in the care of patients, including the coordination and delivery of services, the monitoring of complex physiologic data, the diagnosis of psychologic and physical states, and the operation of sophisticated life-saving equipment. The performance of such functions mandates the regular exercise of independent judgment without the supervision of a physician.[3]

This increased sophistication and the added authority bring additional responsibility. This in turn requires that the nurse have greater knowledge of medical, scientific, and especially legal issues. Trauma nursing takes place against the backdrop of a legal system growing increasingly complex and vigilant of professionals.

The purpose of this chapter is to provide trauma nurses with a survey of the primary legal issues that affect their professional lives. Its main themes are the patient's right to control over his or her body and life and the nurse's obligation to act reasonably and prudently according to current standards of nursing care. This chapter does not substitute for the advice of an attorney. It will provide nurses with a working knowledge of those subject areas in which they or their patients have specific rights and responsibilities.

SOURCES OF LAW

United States law is divisible into four main areas: common law, statutory law, administrative law, and constitutional law. These divisions correspond to the three branches of government at the federal and state level: judicial, legislative, and executive. Constitutional law deals with those rights and protections granted by our Constitution.

Common law results from decisions of the courts. The judiciary is given the responsibility to seek the facts in particular cases and controversies and to apply the law to reach a decision. *Statutory law* derives from acts passed by legislatures. The legislatures (Congress at the federal level and legislative bodies at the state level) are empowered to pass laws dealing with subjects for whom the respective constitutions have granted them authority. *Administrative law* stems from the rule-making process and results in regulations promulgated by the executive branch. The President of the United States and the governors of individual states preside over the operation of executive or regulatory agencies that have been given specific authority to make rules by acts of the legislatures. All three branches of federal and state government are restricted by the "higher" law of the Constitution of the United States. Constitutional law, in particular the first 10 amendments (the Bill of Rights), set forth many of the rights of patients and nurses (as employees). Actions that are contrary to its provisions cannot be incorporated into common, statutory, or administrative law. State governments are also restricted by any additional provisions contained in the constitutions of the individual states.

Each of these sources of law influences the legal issues discussed in this chapter. These issues are undergoing change as the law evolves. The methods by which the law is created and the manner in which it changes will be discussed in the following section.

COMMON LAW

Common law is the term used to describe the body of principles that arise from court decisions. More generally, it is known as *case law* and consists of the accumulation of judicial opinions prepared by judges at the trial and appellate levels from lawsuits initiated by parties (litigants) to a controversy. Common law traces its roots back to eleventh-century England. The underlying principle of the common law is *stare decisis,* which means the law will provide continuity by deciding cases consistent with the precedents set by earlier cases. This means only that controversies between two litigants that are the same factually and that raise the same legal issues will be decided the same way. This continuity is dependent on there being no changes in statutory law and no changes in public policy. Because both evolve as society changes, common law also evolves. The reliance on precedent in judicial decrees generally guarantees controlled change in the common law on which the public can rely.

Over the years judges have recognized the existence of a number of rights that are necessary for the orderly operation of society. Many of these have been embodied in the law of torts. For nursing, the area of common law that is most relevant is *tort law,* which is more commonly known as malpractice, assault and battery (unauthorized and unprivileged contact between two people), and the judicially recognized right to privacy.

Torts are civil (as opposed to criminal) "wrongs" committed by one person against another. Typically these wrongs can be "righted" through an action brought before a judge and jury. For example, hundreds of years ago courts established the individual's right to be free of the negligent acts of another that cause harm, and it established the right to the remedy to this harm (i.e., monetary compensation to the injured party). Whereas civil law speaks to the relations between people, criminal law speaks to actions prohibited by society as a whole. Legal actions under civil law are between private parties; actions under criminal law are brought by the government (society) against individuals (or corporations).

STATUTORY LAW

Statutes are the acts of Congress and state legislatures that regulate the lives of the people. Unlike common law, statutory law does not change through time and evolution but rather by the deliberate acts of the legislatures to create, amend, or repeal statutes. Statutory law deals with such diverse topics as taxation, interstate commerce, and regulation of professions, which is pertinent to nursing.

Trauma nursing, like all nursing, is affected by state laws that define the minimum standards required of a licensed nurse. These laws, generally called *Nurse Practice Acts,* exist to protect citizens from untrained or incompetent persons who offer to practice nursing.[4,5] They regulate nursing by defining the types of acts that licensed practical nurses (LPNs) and registered nurses (RNs) can perform and by providing a mechanism to exclude from the profession those who are incompetent.

Trauma nursing is also affected by statutes dealing with brain death and by laws requiring that nurses report incidents of child or spousal abuse, abuse of the elderly, and certain criminal acts. Other legislative acts prescribe the manner in which criminal evidence must be handled in order for it to be admissible in a criminal action. These statutes have been the subjects of many judicial proceedings over the past 40 years, so the law relative to the handling of criminal evidence is grounded in common law and statutory law.

ADMINISTRATIVE LAW

Administrative law is created when a regulatory agency is empowered by the legislature through a statute to make rules to control the actions of a class of individuals. These rules and regulations are the clarification of statutes passed by the legislature or Congress and must be consistent with the intent of the legislature.

Administrative law is a relatively modern and uniquely a U.S. form of law. Rules and regulations can be and are changed by the executive agencies that administer them as the circumstances underlying them change. The administrative procedure statutes of the state and federal governments control the process for developing and changing regulations. This means that regulatory agencies are empowered to make rules and to change them only after the class of individuals affected has had the opportunity to comment on the changes. The purpose of these requirements is to ensure that regulations reflect the reality of, for example, nursing practice and that they not be unreasonable. Furthermore, the rules cannot be made in an arbitrary or capricious manner. Regulations change not exclusively as a result of societal evolution and not exclusively by the act of a legislative body. Rather they are the result of statutory changes and changes in the work of the people regulated.

Trauma nursing is affected by administrative law through the state boards of nursing. They exist as a result of the legislature empowering the boards to regulate nursing through Nurse Practice Acts.[4] These boards establish and enforce the rules that define requirements for licensure, but they also are empowered to further define allowable nursing acts and the education requirements for nurses. State boards of nursing decide cases involving violations of the professional standards of care embodied in these regulations or set forth in the enabling legislation. The board of nursing can discipline nurses if they violate the standards established for practice. These standards do vary slightly from state to state, and the reader is encouraged to investigate the particulars of the state in which he or she is licensed. Some of the bases for disciplinary action common to all states include fraud in obtaining or in using a nursing license; conviction of a felony or other crime involving moral turpitude (acts involving abusive behavior, dishonesty, or immodesty); knowingly failing to file a required record or report; knowingly filing a false record or report; and drug or alcohol addiction or other physical or mental condition rendering the individual nurse incapable of acting as a nurse. The grounds for disciplinary action also may include refusing to provide, withholding of, denial of, or discrimination in providing nursing services to patients who have tested positive for the human immunodeficiency virus (HIV).[4] One's license is likely to be suspended or revoked for a serious violation of the standards of practice or for repeated violations.

Another area of law that may significantly affect trauma nurses is local ordinances. In many regions the trauma system is controlled locally. That is, a county may be empowered to designate and adopt rules regulating trauma centers. These local rules (ordinances) frequently contain reporting and educational requirements for nurses.

Law affects the lives of all professionals. The types of laws and the manner in which they come into being have been explained. What remains is to relate these concepts to the specific aspects of trauma nursing practice.

LEGAL ISSUES OF TRAUMA NURSING

The issues of law that affect trauma nursing derive from the three sources of law and the actions of the corresponding branches of government. The general legal concepts discussed in the following sections contain both the pertinent elements of the law and their relevance to nursing actions. Many of these concepts are interwoven with ethical considerations discussed in Chapter 6.

CONSENT TO TREATMENT

The nature of trauma practice requires that nurses touch patients and administer therapeutic care. The law, on the other hand, has as a basic principle the right of the individual to determine who shall touch him or her and in what manner and that the competent individual can refuse to be treated. Violation of this right of the individual is a violation of common law.[6]

Every human being of adult years and sound mind has a right to determine what shall be done with his or her own body. A professional who provides treatment without the patient's consent commits an assault for which he or she is liable in damages.[7] About this right the law is quite rigid, and failure to obtain consent for a treatment may subject the professional to a lawsuit.

Three elements must be present if consent is to be valid: (1) capacity, (2) information, and (3) voluntariness. *Capacity* refers to the right of the patient to give consent. Minors and incompetent adults lack the capacity to give consent. *Information* refers to the sufficiency of the patient's understanding of what is being consented to. If the descriptions of treatments given on consent forms or made verbally fail to state clearly what is to be done in a way the patient can understand, then consent is not valid. *Voluntariness* refers to lack of coercion. Consent obtained by trick or by threat is not valid.

The requirement to obtain consent applies to all treatments done to a patient. Specific consent for invasive procedures must be obtained by the person performing the procedure, generally the physician. Nurses frequently are involved in obtaining consent for such procedures on behalf of the physician. Although the nurse is not directly responsible for the performance of these procedures and the particulars of such consent are not required of nurses, it is prudent to be aware of them. For nursing practice separate from physician practice, the reasonable act for the nurse is to inform the patient of any touching to be performed and the reason for the touching and to obtain the patient's consent.

Violations of common law for obtaining valid consent require that the patient shows that the treatment caused some harm and that the treatment would not have been permitted if the possibility of this harm were known. This is true even if there is no lack of care in administering the treatment. It is therefore *critical* to obtain consent to stay within the law. Note that harm does not necessarily equate to injury, and nonconsensual contact, even if beneficial to the health of the patient, is not permitted under the law.

INFORMED CONSENT

Over the years, the concept of consent has been refined so that it is now referred to generally as *informed consent*. The adjective *informed* is not superfluous in this concept. It exists because the courts mandate that consent can be given only if the patient is knowledgeable about the effects of the treatment and has made an affirmative decision to receive the treatment.

Hospitals and trauma centers all require patients to sign a consent to treatment form upon admission. Nurses should look on this form as constituting consent by the patient to be taken care of in the facility and not as consent to all procedures, treatments, and therapies. Each time the patient is to be touched, the action involved should be explained, and either verbal or written agreement or some action demonstrating willingness to participate in the treatment should be received from the patient. Consent forms that specifically list the procedures to be performed and the risks or consequences are gaining increasing favor under the law. Note, however, that a signed consent form obtained from a patient who does not understand its contents is not valid consent.

The general rule of consent is that the patient should be told everything that is to be done each time something is to be done to or for the patient and that the patient should agree to the treatment or procedure. The patient should be informed of the nature of the treatment, its benefits and risks, and any reasonable alternatives. Furthermore, the explanation should be couched in terms *understandable* to patients, because courts tend to favor what the "reasonable patient would expect to know to make an informed decision regarding consent for treatment" as opposed to the prior practice of relying on what a "reasonable practitioner" would tell the patient.

Of course, not all patients are capable of giving consent. The law has permitted exceptions to the requirement of informed consent.

EMERGENCY DOCTRINE

The first such exception is one that has great application in trauma care. When a patient is unconscious or otherwise incapable of giving consent, treatment may proceed under the *emergency doctrine*, which implies consent. This implication frees the nurse from liability for violation of common law. *Implied consent* means that the patient would have consented to the treatment required to maintain health had that patient been able because the alternative would have been death or serious disability. The law assumes that the patient would act reasonably, and the maintenance of bodily integrity is a reasonable act. Note, however, that the emergency doctrine's implication of consent terminates as soon as the patient's disabling condition (e.g., unconsciousness) abates.

COMPETENCY TO GIVE CONSENT

A second exception to the informed consent rule relates to competency. Consent is legally valid only if it is given by someone who is recognized as being of "adult years and sound mind."[7] This means that someone not of legal age or who is judged to be in some way incompetent cannot give the consent that would constitute a valid defense to a lawsuit for battery. A parent or legal guardian must give consent for the treatment of a minor. Even in an emergency, an attempt to contact a parent or guardian must be made and some notation that the parent or guardian was unavailable should be made in the chart. A listing of the steps taken to find the parent will be critical in the event a lawsuit is filed.

There are further considerations to this exception to the informed consent rule. A minor is generally considered to be anyone under the age of 18. In some states an individual under the age of 18 who is married, has a child, or is otherwise emancipated from the parents is considered an adult for purposes of giving consent to medical treatment.[8] Additionally, some states permit a minor to consent to emergency medical treatment without a parent's consent.[8] Most hospitals have written policies and procedures that specifically deal with many of these circumstances. A second consideration, and one that bears some watching, is consent by the state as legal guardian. The majority of the states protect parents from criminal liability for denying life-saving medical care to their children on religious grounds. Although uncommon, the state may consent to the treatment of a minor after the parents have refused consent. The reason is that some states, in order to protect the child's rights, will consent to the life-saving treatment when the parents will not. This will most likely occur when the parents' religious beliefs preclude the use of blood transfusions or other medical techniques. This type of consent is not common and is given only under extreme circumstances because the states are typically loathe to interfere in the parent-child relationship. The consent, when given by the state, is effective in the same way as described previously.

Some patients, although not minors, may not be competent to give consent. The concept of being of sound mind is the second half of the competency equation. Any person who is not competent because of some mental disability (e.g., lack of mental capacity or senility), chronic alcoholism, drug addiction, or physical disability or disease that renders the individual incapable of making reasoned judgments should be under the control of a guardian.[8] Another common cause of incompetency is the injury that caused the patient to be brought to the hospital. Examples are shock, severe pain, severe emotional distress, head injuries, and the presence of mind-altering drugs (legal and illegal). In cases where there is no guardian, one may have to be appointed by the court. Consent for this type of patient is obtained in the same manner as for minors, with the guardian substituting for the parent. Consent is implied by law for such patients when emergency medical treatment is required.[8] Where there is no guardian and no durable power of attorney relative to medical care (a document by which a person grants a designated other person the authority to make health care decisions in the event of the person's incapacity to make decisions), state law may provide that the consent of a spouse, adult child, adult sibling, adult grandchild, or a grandparent be substituted.[8,9]

Issues of consent must be considered before each treatment or procedure is commenced, whether in the resuscitation, operative, critical care, or intermediate and rehabilitative phase. It is important that the nurse be knowledgeable about consents obtained by or for physicians because the primary nurse is the consistent coordinator of patient care.

REFUSAL OF TREATMENT

One of the reasons that consent should be obtained separately for each treatment or procedure is that the patient has the right to control all touching of the body not only through consent but also through refusal of treatment. The nurse needs to be aware of the consent obtained by the physician so that a patient's subsequent refusal of treatment can be identified. The withdrawal of consent or any other refusal of treatment must be documented properly in the chart and, because it is often against medical advice, should be witnessed by several people. Again, hospital policy should dictate how this must be documented and by whom. Readers are encouraged to investigate and become familiar with the policies regarding these issues at their institutions. Any treatment or procedure done after a patient refuses treatment is a violation of that patient's legal rights and may become the subject of a successful lawsuit, even if the treatment has beneficial results.

ASSAULT AND BATTERY: FAILED CONSENT

Assault and *battery* are common-law torts that protect the individual from the threat of contact and from unpermitted contact, respectively. They are intentional torts, distinguished from negligent torts. The legal elements of battery are that the person committing the action intends to cause a harmful or offensive contact and that the act is unpermitted and unprivileged. Assault is similar except actual contact is not required; only the immediate apprehension of a harmful or offensive contact is needed. The good intentions of the nurse do not justify action constituting assault or battery.[10] The nurse may have the patient's best interests in mind, but if the contact is not consensual, a lawsuit may follow.

In a nursing context, failure to obtain informed consent followed by the performance of a procedure is battery. Continued treatment after the patient's refusal of treatment is also battery. Although this may seem bizarre in the face of successful treatment or the saving of the patient's life, a patient's deeply held belief may make the contact sufficiently offensive to take the matter to court.

PATIENT CONFIDENTIALITY AND THE RIGHT TO PRIVACY

Nurses, by ethical code and through the policies of hospitals, are required to keep the identity and condition of their patients confidential. In law this concept of confidentiality is expressed as the common-law right to privacy. It has been called the "right to be let alone" and was introduced in U.S.

law in 1890.[11] There is no clearly recognized right to privacy under the federal constitution, but many states have explicitly enacted a privacy clause in their constitutions or by statute.

An action for invasion of privacy can be brought for monetary damages. Such action is divided into four major themes: (1) appropriation of the individual's name or picture without consent, (2) intrusion into the person's seclusion (as in a hospital bed), (3) public disclosure of private facts, and (4) placing the individual in a false light in the public eye.[12] The first three are particularly relevant to the trauma nurse.

Hospital policies generally require that consent be obtained from a patient before photographing injuries for use in a professional journal. Appropriation of the patient's picture or name is outside the law. The second theme, intrusion into the patient's seclusion, involves the unauthorized entry of a person such as a member of the press into an area where the patient has an expectation of privacy. This doctrine forms the legal basis for visiting policies. The third forms the legal basis for hospital policies that restrict employees from discussing patients with the press or public.[13] The confidentiality of diagnoses, treatments, test results, and procedures takes on added significance for patients with AIDS because it is almost certain that they will require hospitalization at some time during the course of their illness.[14]

The right to privacy applies to the whole continuum of trauma care. During resuscitation or critical care, information about the patient may be increasingly sought by distant relatives, friends, and business associates. Nurses must be particularly careful to avoid divulging information from a patient's medical record or committing unwarranted intrusions into the patient's personal affairs. Pressure from the press and public may be most intense at the beginning of an incident involving a prominent person; however, the right to privacy remains throughout the patient's stay. Although it is a regular practice of researchers to use a series of photographs of the progress of a patient's treatment in scholarly works, consent must first be obtained.

Trauma nurses are frequently involved with patient chart reviews. Not all these reviews take place within the confines of the hospital or among the medical staff. Typically, medical staff review of patient charts (care) is structured so that the confidentiality of the patient is maintained. Where this becomes a problem for some trauma nurses and centers is the system review of trauma patient care. It is not unusual for a regional trauma committee to have a multidisciplinary trauma outcomes committee. Trauma centers are required to bring patient charts to the committee and discuss the care provided.

Two significant legal concerns arise out of this process. First is the requirement for the members of the committee to maintain patient confidentiality. It is not uncommon for members of these committees to be emergency medical services (EMS) personnel who may not be familiar with patient confidentiality issues nor have any obligation to maintain confidentiality. An agreement to maintain confi-

dentiality should be drawn up by an attorney familiar with such documents and signed by all committee members on a regular basis.

The second, even larger concern relates to the discoverability of the patient's chart and any discussions of patient care during a committee meeting. Most states have laws that protect the information discussed in similar meetings that take place in hospitals by their medical staffs. However, the vast majority of these protections do not extend to discussions outside the hospital and its staff.

Several states have revised their laws in order to encourage regional performance improvement committees by extending the protection from discovery to these committees and their members. Participants in these types of committees are encouraged to determine what, if any, protections are in place to protect committee discussions from discovery.

As with most of the legal rights and responsibilities detailed so far, there are exceptions to the stringency of the privacy right. Society has determined that the individual's right to privacy is secondary to the prevention and prosecution of spousal, child, and elderly abuse. Nurses therefore are empowered by statute to report incidents of abuse without fear of liability in a civil action for invasion of privacy. Mandatory reporting requirements relative to abuse and other prohibited acts are described next.

MANDATORY REPORTING

Mandatory reporting requirements exist in the law to identify actions that society abhors. The general rule stated earlier is that the facts of a patient's injuries and treatments are confidential and protected by the right to privacy. That right is superseded by mandatory reporting requirements because public policy dictates that these reportable actions are illegal.

Reporting laws require that hospitals, doctors, and nurses notify the appropriate state agency when certain incidents occur. They also protect the individual reporting the incident from liability for an inaccurate report unless a false report was made with knowledge of its falsity. There is a flip side to this protection from liability: If a nurse or doctor fails to report an incident and a further injury occurs from the same proscribed action, that individual may be held liable for the failure to report it.[15]

The trauma or emergency nurse must see if the trauma was the result of an act proscribed by law. Examples include child and spousal abuse. Many states have reporting requirements when such abuse is identified. When injuries resulting from abuse are discovered, the nurse must take two actions: (1) notify the physician in charge of the patient's case and any other person identified by hospital policy and (2) make sure a report is filed with the appropriate agency. Failure to follow these two steps in the reporting of an abuse may subject the nurse to liability even though all internal policies have been followed.

Additional examples of incidents with mandatory reporting requirements are abuse in nursing facilities; attempted suicide; and injuries resulting from violence, illegal abortions, animal bites, and motor vehicle crashes. As noted earlier, most hospitals have extensive policies and procedures in place regarding these issues.

NEGLIGENCE/MALPRACTICE

The main theme of the common law that pervades the legal issues discussed thus far is that of reasonableness. Patients expect that their injuries and conditions will be explained to them in a manner that they can reasonably be expected to understand. A patient incapable of giving consent because of injuries will consent to the course of life-saving treatment because it is reasonable to do so, or so the law presumes. The patient has the right to have reasonable expectations of privacy protected by the nurse.

The issue of law discussed in this section also focuses principally on this notion of reasonableness. Suits for malpractice, or professional negligence, are actions brought by patients against nurses because the nurse is seen by the patient as not having exercised reasonable care in the treatment of the patient's injuries.

The law of negligence, simply stated, is the breach of a duty owed by the nurse to the patient that results in injury to the patient. Four elements are identified in the law: (1) a duty of care, (2) breach of this duty, (3) a causal connection between the flawed conduct (act or failure to act) and injury, and (4) the injury or damage suffered by the patient.[16] The crux of the action for negligence is that the nurse did not use reasonable care, and an injury resulted.

When applied to professionals, *negligence* is referred to as *malpractice.* The law measures the professional's duty of care differently than the duty of care owed by nonprofessionals. This one distinction separates ordinary negligence from malpractice. It is mentioned here because, although it is generally accepted that nurses exercise independent professional judgment and should be treated as professionals, not all states allow nurses to be sued for malpractice. Such states hold nurses to the standard of negligence only.[17]

In daily life, individuals must act with reasonable caution so as not to cause harm to others. Drivers are expected to exercise reasonable care. Failure to do so (such as when a car runs a red light, strikes a pedestrian, and breaks his leg) is a failure to use reasonable care. It is negligence because (1) the driver had a duty to drive carefully, (2) the driver breached that duty by running the red light, (3) the pedestrian was struck by the car, and (4) the pedestrian suffered a broken leg.

ESTABLISHING THE NURSE'S LIABILITY.   The nurse has the duty to provide competent care to patients. If that care is provided in a less than competent manner and the patient is injured as a result, malpractice occurs. The critical definition is of the duty of care and its measurement by the law. The causal connection between the nurse's conduct and the injury must then be established and damages assessed.

Duty of care in negligence is defined as what the reasonably prudent person would do in the same or similar circumstances. This is a fiction recognized by the law

because there is no person or group of people identifiable as the "reasonably prudent person." It is not what the average person does, but what the law thinks the average person should have done. Due care requires that people not engage in conduct that involves unreasonable danger to others. Critical to the understanding of this duty is that it is conduct being evaluated, not state of mind.[16]

In states that do not have malpractice standards for nurses, the duty of nursing care is based on what the reasonably prudent person (not nurse) would do.[17] The specialized training and knowledge of the nurse are not considered when the standard of care is measured in negligence suits in these states.

Malpractice differs from negligence for precisely this reason. The knowledge and training of the nursing profession define the standard for malpractice. This means that nursing as a profession establishes certain minimum qualifications of education through, for example, the licensure requirements of the boards of nursing. All nurses must meet such professional standards to be considered "reasonably prudent nurses." An action that falls below these minimum qualifications and causes injury is malpractice. In addition, specially qualified nurses (e.g., CCRNs) must maintain educational and practice requirements set down by the boards and, in addition, may be held to a standard for all such specialty qualified nurses on a national basis.[18] These requirements form the basis for the duty of care required of such a certified nurse over and above the qualifications of all nurses.

A description of emergency nursing, which shares many common traits with trauma nursing, helps to illustrate these qualifications. Emergency nursing practice is the nursing care of individuals of all ages with perceived physical or emotional alterations that are undiagnosed and may require prompt intervention. Emergency nursing care is unscheduled and most commonly occurs in a specific care setting, such as an emergency department, a mobile unit, or a suicide prevention center. Thus the nursing care is episodic, primary, and acute in nature.

The scope of emergency nursing practice encompasses nursing activities directed toward health problems of various levels of complexity. A rapidly changing physiologic or psychologic status, which may be life-threatening, requires assessment of the severity of the health problem, definitive intervention, ongoing reassessment, and supportive care to significant others. The level of physiologic or psychologic complexity may require life-support measures, appropriate health education, and referral. The scope of emergency nursing practice encompasses not only nursing activities directed toward health problems presented by the individuals but also knowledge of and the observance of legal aspects, such as reporting an incident to governmental agencies (e.g., police or public health departments) when a situation calls for such action. Emergency nursing practice is affected by the brevity of patient interaction with the nurse, the stressful climate created by lack of control over the number of individuals seeking emergency care, and the limited time frame in which to evaluate the effectiveness of intervention.

In emergency settings, nurses have assumed an increasingly independent, professional role. With this change comes the added burden of legal responsibility for their actions. One particular legal problem that may confront the nurse in the field occurs when an injured victim is treated on the scene with physician support provided only through radio communication. If the doctor orders treatment that will be harmful to the patient, the nurse can be held responsible (and the trauma center vicariously) if the orders are followed and the nurse knew or should have known that the harm would occur.[19] This is a dilemma for the nurse at the scene. If the prescribed treatment fails, the doctor will be subject to a malpractice action. However, the increased knowledge and ability of nurses exposes them to liability if their compliance with the doctor's orders result in an injury.

Particularly important is the responsibility of the trauma nurse to document operative events accurately and thoroughly. The rush to prepare the patient for surgery often requires deviations from standard protocols. Compromises in required nursing routines expose the professionals to liability if uncorrected later in the patient's course of recovery.

Many trauma operations last 12 hours or more, resulting in nursing shift changes and rotation of other staff. Ideally, all sponges, needles, and instruments are accounted for after an operation. In lengthy surgeries with multiple concurrent procedures, the tracking of these accoutrements of surgery may be faulty. Where there is a discrepancy, it should be documented in the nurse's notes. A radiograph should be ordered at a later time to determine if the discrepancy is a counting error or the missing sponge or instrument is still in the patient's body. Recovery of such an intruder in the patient will mitigate, if not eliminate, the liability of the hospital and of the surgical team.

Another area of exposure to liability for the nurse involves cautery burns from inadequately grounding the patient. Even in the face of an emergent surgical procedure, the law may not be understanding of injuries caused by improper procedure. The best course of action for the operative nurse remains to ensure that the ground is in place to lessen exposure to malpractice liability.

Particularly critical in the immediate aftermath of an operation is the responsibility to record and document procedures and their future implications to the course of care of the patient. Exposure to infection, for example, is important to the later phases of care, and failure to record these exposures may adversely affect the patient's recovery. These complications expose the operative nurse to liability for malpractice if not properly documented. The length and complexity of trauma surgery compounded by difficulty in achieving proper patient positioning can result in the development of peripheral nerve damage and ischemic tissue injury related to pressure. Proper care mandates that the patient's body is padded at weight-bearing points; however, skin breakdown may still occur later. The nurse's

responsibility in this event is to document complications so those nurses in the postoperative care phase can initiate treatment.

Standards of reasonable nursing care are required of nurses at all stages of the patient's treatment. This is particularly true in managing the discharge process. A patient being prepared for discharge must be thoroughly educated in, for example, wound care and the use of pharmaceuticals. Reasonable care mandates that the patient be given oral and written instructions explaining how to perform the daily tasks that will promote recovery. Where appropriate, the patient must have demonstrated the ability to perform these tasks. In all cases the patient's understanding of the instructions must be demonstrated clearly to the nurse. The patient's support system, whether it is family, home health care providers, or a rehabilitation facility, must be prepared to care for the patient.

ELEMENTS OF A MALPRACTICE SUIT. In a patient's suit for malpractice, what constitutes due care is established through the testimony of expert witnesses. An expert is qualified in court through educational credentials and experience and is then permitted to state an opinion about what is or is not proper care. No one other than a duly qualified expert is permitted to give opinions about what is the duty of care in a court of law. This expert will, in all likelihood, be a nurse who will give testimony about what constitutes proper care for nursing. Physician experts also may be called to differentiate between the duties of physicians and nurses' practice, especially where a nurse is claimed to have exceeded the limits of nursing practice.

As with duty of care, the proximate cause of the injury is established in court by the expert witness. The patient's experts can be expected to state that the injury was a result of the nurse's failure to follow proper practice protocols. The nurse's experts will, of course, state that the injury occurred in a different way. Although this creates a "battle of the experts," this process has been deemed necessary by the judiciary because the knowledge of professional practice is not within the common knowledge of laypersons serving as jurors.

Expert witnesses are needed in proving the nexus, or connection, between the care and the injury because the patient as plaintiff has the burden of proof to show that malpractice occurred. There is an exception to the rule that only experts can prove the causal nexus between action and injury; it is rarely applied but bears noting. Some injuries are considered to be of a type that most likely does not happen in the absence of malpractice. This narrow class of injuries shifts the burden of proof to the defendant without the need for expert testimony for the patient. The legal concept is *res ipsa loquitur,* which translated literally is "it speaks for itself." The nurse as defendant in these cases must prove that the injury did not occur from the treatment.

Once the first three elements of malpractice are established, damages must be proved in order for the nurse to be liable to the patient. Damages are characterized as either compensatory or punitive. *Compensatory* damages are the monies necessary to make the patient "whole." They include the medical expenses associated with the injury, past and future; lost earnings and earning potential; pain and suffering; and loss of consortium (inability to function as a spouse). The injury is viewed as a continuum beginning at the time of injury and extending until cured. If the elapsed time between these points is short, damages are assessed for only that brief time. If, however, the resulting injury is permanent, damages are estimated for the patient's estimated life span. Damages awarded to pay for pain and suffering are usually the largest part of the award, although some state legislatures have acted to place a cap on the amount of this type of award. Damages awarded are to pay for what the patient must endure as a result of the nurse's breach of the professional duty of care.

Punitive damages are monies awarded in excess of compensatory damages to punish the nurse for his or her conduct. Because there is this element of punishment, punitive damages are rarely awarded and then only in cases involving "gross negligence," where the nurse acted maliciously or in reckless disregard of the patient's life. Many states either limit or prohibit punitive damages in medical negligence cases.

RESPONDEAT SUPERIOR AND VICARIOUS LIABILITY. The law of malpractice does not view the nurse's actions in isolation. A trauma nurse is generally an employee of a hospital (trauma center). The employer-employee relationship is established when the employer has the ability to control and direct the performance and duties of the employee. The nurse's actions, by this definition, are considered to be those of an employee if they are within the scope of employment.

If all the conditions of an employer-employee relationship are satisfied, the negligence of the nurse will be imputed to the hospital as well. This is the doctrine of *respondeat superior*. Respondeat superior applies only to employees, not independent contractors. Courts recognize that a hospital employs nurses to work for it rather than merely providing a place where nurses can act of their own volition. This means that the trauma center is liable for the negligence of its nurses who are operating within the scope of their employment.

The only complication in the application of respondeat superior occurs when, for example, the nurse is assisting a surgeon who is not a "house officer" (employee of the hospital). A surgeon employed and paid by the trauma center is an employee of that center in the same way the nurse is. Respondeat superior applies equally to both because they share the same "master," the trauma center. The difficulty arises when the surgeon is not an employee of the hospital but is reimbursed by fees charged directly to the patient. In states that apply this distinction to a lawsuit, the doctrine of the "borrowed servant" applies. This rule states that the negligence of the nurse is imputed to the surgeon even though the surgeon does not employ the nurse. Furthermore, the liability of the surgeon for the nurse's negligence accrues only if the negligence occurred when the surgeon exercised control over the nurse's actions. The accepted rule in states that apply the borrowed servant doctrine is to hold the hospital liable for the nurse's negligence and to hold the surgeon jointly liable. Vicarious liability does not extend to the nurse supervisor for the malpractice of subordinates because a true employer-employee relationship does not exist. The supervisor is an employee of the trauma center, as is the staff nurse. Nurse supervisors can be held liable, however, if acts of commission or omission in supervising (negligent supervision) cause a patient's injury.

Although the discussion of vicarious liability and respondeat superior has centered on the nurse's malpractice, these concepts apply equally to the other torts previously discussed. Like malpractice, they occur during the course of the nurse's duties and are therefore imputed to the employer.

GOOD SAMARITAN RULE. As with many of the legal issues discussed in this chapter, there is an exception to the law of malpractice where a negligent nurse may not be held liable. The trauma nurse who becomes involved in the care of the victim of a car crash or of a violent crime during off-duty hours is not liable for negligent acts. When an off-duty nurse happens to be at an incident scene, there is an ethical and moral, if not legal, duty to stop and render assistance. To encourage professionals to help injured victims, the legislatures of all states have passed statutes that grant nurses (and generally all medical professionals) immunity from liability for negligent acts. These statutes, named after the biblical Good Samaritan, state that health care professionals who stop and aid injured victims without compensation for that help will not be liable for their acts, even if negligent.[5,20]

There is also, however, an exception to the Good Samaritan rule. The law will not exempt the nurse from acts that constitute gross negligence, acts that manifest a reckless disregard for the life of the patient.[21] The rule is that if the care was rendered in good faith and an emergency existed, the nurse will be free from liability. The nurse who is a member of an emergency team sent to the scene of an incident is not covered by the Good Samaritan rule. The professional duty of care is required of this type of nurse.

LAW OF DEATH AND THE DYING PATIENT

BRAIN DEATH. *Brain death*, simply stated, is the irreversible cessation of brain activity, as determined in accordance with reasonable medical standards. The essence of brain death statutes is that the traditional definition of death—cessation of respiration and heart action—still holds true but that death may occur even if the body is kept alive by mechanical means in the absence of brain activity.

Trauma nurses need to understand brain death for two reasons. First, the families of patients who have suffered extensive head injuries must be counseled about the death of their loved ones. Second, trauma patients are often organ donors because they are frequently young and were healthy before being injured. Many organs remain viable for transplantation.

There is no single law in the United States that defines when death occurs, yet a number of states and the District of Columbia have adopted the Uniform Determination of Death Act. This statute states that an individual is dead when, based on accepted standards of medical practice, either irreversible cessation of circulatory and respiratory function or irreversible cessation of all function of the entire brain, including the brainstem, occurs.

Clinical criteria for establishing brain death have been developed. The reasonable and prudent approach incorporates clinical tests that ensure all brain function, including brainstem function is irreversibly absent. Clinical findings that indicate absence of brain function include:

1. No response to stimuli, including noxious stimuli
2. No pupillary response to light
3. No eye movement in response to head turning (oculocephalic or Doll's eyes reflex) or irrigation of the ear with ice water (oculovestibular or caloric reflex)
4. No corneal reflexes
5. No gag or cough reflex
6. No spontaneous respirations even with the paCO$_2$ in excess of 60 mmHg[22]

Potentially reversible disorders that may obscure the neurologic examination (e.g. hypothermia, metabolic imbalance, presence of neurodepressant drugs or neuromuscular blocking agents, shock) must be ruled out. An isoelectric (flat) electroencephalogram tracing or cerebral blood flow study indicating no brain perfusion are examples of test results that may be used to confirm brain death.[22] Special considerations must be observed when declaring brain death in children.

The brain death statutes are all couched in terms of the cessation of brain activity as determined by reasonable medical standards. The language of the laws permits changes in the determination of death as medical techniques improve. Trauma nurses need to stay informed of these changes, so they can fulfill their role in family support as well as remain alert to appropriate opportunities for organ procurement. A discussion of the law can do no more than state that medical techniques underlie the standards for the determination of death. Independently, nurses must keep abreast of changes in the state where they practice. Again many hospitals have written policies detailing how these procedures should be carried out and who is responsible for carrying them out.

ANATOMICAL GIFT ACT. A corollary to the brain death statutes is the organ donation laws now in existence in many states. These laws include the Uniform Anatomical Gift Act, which specifies how an organ donation, an anatomic gift,

can be made by a patient. The law includes a requirement of written authorization from the patient. Notice that whether a patient is an organ donor may be included on a driver's license so long as an affirmative statement of intent to donate was obtained when the license was issued. Usually, the act also states that the physician or surgeon who pronounces death is prohibited from removing or transplanting the donated organs.[23]

LIVING WILLS. Legal issues in caring for a dying patient center on two key concepts: living wills and withdrawing or withholding treatment, including cardiopulmonary resuscitation. The issues raised here recently gained added importance to trauma nurses through the federal Patient Self-Determination Act. Under this law, health care providers now are required to provide information to patients about living wills and other similar proxy documents.

Increasingly, states are accepting directives made by patients long before they were ill or injured. These laws specifically state that the decision to withhold or withdraw treatment for a terminally ill patient resides with that patient. These wills outline patients' wishes in the event that they become comatose or otherwise mentally incapacitated and dependent on extraordinary means of life support. These directives are called *living wills* (Figure 5-1). Their purpose is to state the patient's desire that extraordinary care be withheld or discontinued in the event that it would be fruitless and to relieve the emotional burden on the families of these patients.[8,23]

DECLARATION

On this (date) day of (month, year), I (person's name), being of sound mind, willfully and voluntarily direct that my dying shall not be artificially prolonged under the circumstances set forth in this declaration:

If at any time I should have an incurable injury, disease, or illness certified to be a terminal condition by two (2) physicians who have personally examined me, one (1) of whom shall be my attending physician, and the physicians have determined that my death is imminent and will occur whether or not life-sustaining procedures are utilized and where the application of such procedures would serve only to artificially prolong the dying process, I direct that such procedures be withheld or withdrawn, and that I be permitted to die naturally with only the administration of medication, the administration of food and water, and the performance of any medical procedure that is necessary to provide comfort care or alleviate pain. In the absence of my ability to give directions regarding the use of such life-sustaining procedures, it is my intention that this declaration shall be honored by my family and physician(s) as the final expression of my right to control my medical care and treatment.

I am legally competent to make this declaration, and I understand its full import.

(Signature)

(Witnesses' signatures)

FIGURE 5-1 **Sample Living Will.** (Modified from Annotated code of Maryland, sec 5-602c.)

The underlying concept for these wills is that adults of sound mind (see earlier discussion under Consent) have the right to determine which treatments they will consent to and which they will refuse. The wishes of the patient are of paramount importance. It is no surprise, then, that a method of prospectively stating the individual's will about use of life support has been created.

The use of living wills has not reached all the states.[22] However, they are sufficiently pervasive that trauma nurses should be familiar enough with them to be able to identify a living will if one is presented to them.

WITHHOLDING OR WITHDRAWING TREATMENT. Many courts have grappled with the problem of withholding or withdrawing treatment from a dying patient. There is, at present, no set of legal doctrines that apply to all clinical situations or to all states. The basis of common-law decisions permitting the patient to die is the same as for giving informed consent. The patient may consent to have treatment withheld or withdrawn.[24]

In the 1990 *Cruzan* case, the Supreme Court of the United States held that a state's policy favoring continuation of life support supersedes the opinions of a patient's close family members when there is no clear and convincing evidence of the patient's wishes to withhold or withdraw treatment. The court held that the states may indicate the kind of evidence required to establish a patient's wishes.

In this case the family of Nancy Cruzan stated that they believed she would not want treatments to continue after they had become futile. The state of Missouri refused to recognize these opinions as Nancy Cruzan's wishes and instead required that life support be continued. Missouri's public policy is to continue life support unless a written directive from the patient states otherwise.

Cruzan does not say that all states must follow Missouri's policy of continuing life support, only that the states *may* do so. It also does not state that written directives are required to discontinue life support for a patient, but it does state that individual states such as Missouri may so require, whereas others may apply different evidentiary standards.

Cruzan may cause the unfortunate consequence of "jurisdiction shopping." Because the Court recognized that individual states may act as the final arbiter in maintaining or withdrawing treatment, there will be large differences in these policies. As a result, family members seeking to have treatment withdrawn from a patient may attempt to move the patient from a state that requires maintaining treatment to one that leaves the decision to the family. Isolated cases of family members seeking to move patients to states with more liberal rules for withholding or withdrawing treatment have occurred since the *Cruzan* decision.

Although the right of the individual to terminate extraordinary (or life-sustaining) care is well established, what constitutes such care is less clear. In the case of Karen Ann Quinlan, the court distinguished between what constituted ordinary and extraordinary care. A respirator, in this case, represented extraordinary care for a comatose patient in a persistent vegetative state with no hope of recovery. The guardians were permitted to have the respirator withdrawn.[25]

The distinction between ordinary and extraordinary care depends on the individual situation and the judgment of those involved. Gerald Kelly, a Roman Catholic ethicist, however, formulated a widely quoted definition. It states:

Ordinary means all medicines, treatments and operations which offer a reasonable hope of benefit and which can be obtained and used without excessive cost or other inconvenience. Extraordinary means are all machines, treatments and operations which cannot be obtained or used without excessive expense, pain or other inconvenience, or if used would not offer a reasonable hope of benefit.[26]

A *life-sustaining procedure* has been defined as any "medical procedure, treatment, or intervention which uses mechanical or other artificial means to sustain, restore, or supplant a spontaneous vital function or is otherwise of such a nature as to afford a patient no reasonable expectation of recovery from a terminal condition and which, when applied to a patient in a terminal condition, would serve to secure only a precarious and burdensome prolongation of life."[8]

Withholding or withdrawal of extraordinary treatment does not eliminate all duties owed the patient. Ordinary supportive care must be continued. There are still differences of opinion regarding supportive care, especially special mechanisms for feeding, although many living wills specifically state that nutrition is to be discontinued.

DO NOT RESUSCITATE ORDERS. Living wills express the individual's wish that extraordinary means not be used to prolong the life of the body when such action will be fruitless. This wish is a form of a do not resuscitate (DNR) order from the patient. Although living wills are not used universally, a DNR order usually originates from the attending physician in consultation with the patient or family members. Ensuring that the order is based on a correct legal foundation is imperative so that there are no adverse ramifications.

DNR orders must be written on an order sheet, and an accompanying note should appear in the progress notes with the rationale for the order. A written order documents the fact that a decision has been made and by whom. It ensures that the decision is clearly communicated to all nurses so that cardiopulmonary resuscitation (CPR) is not initiated inappropriately. It also acts to assure nurses that they can withhold CPR without fear that they have neglected the patient.

DNR orders take on different character depending on the physician who enters the order. The order may simply state that CPR not be initiated should the patient suffer cardiac arrest. This is recognition that death is imminent and that CPR will not save the life, only temporarily prolong it. An alternative order is one that continues life support, such as feeding and ventilatory support, but that orders no additional initiation of therapeutic treatments. The distinction between an order that terminates existing treatments and one that does not initiate new therapies often is based on the practitioner's ethical framework and has no legal significance. The legal importance centers on the existence of a DNR order rather than the order's clinical characteristics.[22] All hospitals must have policies for dealing with DNR orders, and such policies are the best source of information for the trauma nurse.

The principal issue in the use of DNR orders is what would be the wishes of the patient. Living wills eliminate this concern because the patient has clearly stated what should be done. In all other cases consent must be obtained from someone who is substituting judgment for that patient. The next of kin (spouse or children, for example) and the patient's legal guardian (parents or court-appointed guardian) are prime examples. Hospital policies as a reflection of state law also may permit the physician in charge of the patient's case, an administrator, or the hospital attorney to act as this substitute.[22] The nurse who receives a DNR order from a physician must be conversant with the current law in the state in which she or he practices.

PHYSICAL EVIDENCE AND CHAIN OF CUSTODY

Chain of custody of physical evidence is particularly applicable in cases in which the injury resulted from a violent crime such as a shooting or rape although it also has application in civil matters. Chain of custody consists of two parts: a documentation component and a handling component. The first mandates meticulous recording of all evidence discovered (or samples taken), where it came from, when, and to whom it was given. Receipts should be maintained as each piece of physical evidence or sample is given by the nurse to, for example, a laboratory technician. These receipts should list what was given, who gave it, to whom it was given, and the date and time of the transfer of possession.

The handling component speaks to the need for purity in a sample and the need to keep physical evidence in its original condition. Potential contaminants should be kept away from tissue samples. A gun should not be handled unless it is absolutely necessary so that fingerprints are retained.

PROTECTION OF PATIENTS' PROPERTY

When a patient is brought into a trauma center, the trauma nurse is engaged in many activities that may involve resuscitation and preparation for surgery. The protection of a patient's property can be forgotten easily. Although this may seem a relatively mundane concern in comparison with resuscitation, surgery, or critical care, property loss and damage frequently result in monetary claims against the hospital. The law underlying the responsibility to protect the patient's personal possessions is a bailment.

The patient entrusts the trauma center through the trauma nurse to hold property and clothing until it is reclaimed at a later time. Property should be marked and stored so that it can be returned to the patient upon request or discharge or, upon death, to the family. The patient is the only person authorized to determine its disposition. Proper documentation is therefore necessary.

ANTIDUMPING ISSUES

Perhaps the most complicated, if not convoluted, area of law facing nurses in trauma care is the Emergency Treatment and Labor Act (EMTALA). This law, passed in 1986, was originally known as the Consolidated Omnibus Budget Reconciliation Act (COBRA). Today these Acts are known more commonly as the antidumping laws.

Under EMTALA, Medicare-participating hospitals (most hospitals receive some federal monies) are required to provide a "medical screening exam" and, if necessary, stabilizing treatment to all individuals who "come to the hospital" and request evaluation or treatment for a medical condition. The definitions of "medical screening exam" and "come to the hospital" have been the subject of numerous hearings.[27]

On November 10, 1999, the Health Care Financing Administration (HCFA) and the Office of the Inspector General (OIG) of the Department of Health and Human Services issued a final special advisory bulletin on the antidumping statute.[28] After reviewing numerous comments, HCFA/OIG issued an advisory bulletin stating that their purpose was "to provide clear and meaningful advice with regard to the application of the antidumping law."[28] The advisory bulletin, in and of itself, does not have the force of law, but HCFA surveyors, OIG attorneys, and others involved in the enforcement of the law rely heavily on the document's recommendations.

A major purpose of the advisory bulletin was to address issues created by managed care. The managed care phenomenon was still in its formative stages when the law was passed in 1986. Issues related to managed care specifically addressed by the HCFA/OIG document includes delay in treatment while obtaining authorization and dual staffing arrangements.

Many states have enacted statutes similar to EMTALA, some of which carry criminal sanctions. In at least one case a New York nurse was held to have individually violated the state antidumping statute, which constituted a criminal offense.

Furthermore, there are specific guidelines regarding the reporting of known or suspected violations of the law. A nurse could be found to have violated the act if she or he knew a patient's transfer was a clear violation of the act and did not report the violation.

The Balanced Budget Act of 1997 (BBA) contains numerous provisions specifically related to managed care. More specifically, the BBA defines "emergency services" and what a managed care organization (MCO) must pay for if the MCO contracts with a state to provide care for Medicaid patients.[29]

From the trauma center perspective, this provides some reimbursement for the care mandated under EMTALA. The BBA is being implemented through a series of letters (22 as of April 2000) from HCFA to its regional administrators.

DISCUSSION

Given the obligation of advising nurses with a single phrase, an attorney would most likely say, "Act reasonably." Although this phrase is fundamentally true, it provides the nurse with only a general framework for guarding patient's rights and for protection from professional liability. Handling the day-to-day legal dilemmas inherent in the practice of trauma nursing requires both this framework of reasonableness and specific knowledge of common points of law as applied to the patient-oriented situation in question.

Acting reasonably means that patients should be consulted at all possible times, so they are aware of the nature and rationale of nursing interventions. This will promote the patient's cooperation in recovery, which is critical to the nurse's protection against subsequent legal actions.

Acting reasonably means knowing and following standing orders and protocols for the assessment and care of the patient at the time of arrival in the emergency department. These protocols ensure that medically appropriate assessment and triage are performed even in the absence of a physician. Clearly, standing orders do not take the place of nursing judgment and are not to be followed blindly when additional injury to the patient may result. Objective self-assessment is also inherent in reasonable practice. Tasks and procedures for which the nurse is inadequately trained should not be done without seeking help from a senior nursing colleague, supervisor, or physician.

There is no complete protection from malpractice litigation, and recent trends suggest that nurses suffer expanded susceptibility to lawsuits. However, liability can be limited through a number of actions. Because nurses are often in a position in which they possess exclusive patient information, the importance of proper documentation and communication of this information takes on great significance. It must be stressed that the entire medical record plays a crucial role as evidence in determining the standard of care provided by the nurse. It also can be used by the nurse during a lawsuit to help recall the details of actions taken in the patient's care long ago. Documentation must be accurate and complete, describing the patient's changing condition, nursing diagnoses, plans and actions, and reports to physicians and other professionals. Effective verbal and written communication provides continuity among nurses and between nurse and physician.

Incident reporting is a specific type of documentation that is reasonable in the eyes of the law. A well-written incident report states facts rather than conclusions without supporting observations. Hospital policies detail the steps to follow in reporting an incident such as a patient fall or the injection of the wrong drug or an incorrect dosage. The policies should include how an incident report is prepared and who is responsible for its disposition. Incident reports are important to the hospital as indicators of areas of potential liability. As employees, nurses are required to report incidents promptly and thoroughly. The reports can mitigate the nurse's liability to the patient. They also can limit the nurse's potential liability to the hospital if the nurse is sued by the hospital to recover judgments against it based on the nurse's negligent actions.

Maintaining current and adequate levels of malpractice insurance is another prudent and protective action. Hospitals may provide malpractice insurance for their nurses. Nurses should be aware of the extent of this coverage, as well as any exclusionary clauses present in the insurance agreements that leave them open to personal liability for adverse judgments. Nurses must be aware of the relevant periods covered by the policies. There are two types of malpractice insurance. The first covers claims made during the period of coverage. The second covers claims resulting from occurrences during the period of coverage, even if the claim is made after the policy's expiration date.

Being aware of new medical and scientific issues through continuing education is also important. Nursing supervisors and administrators must be responsive to the need of nurses to remain current on hospital policies and changes in state laws that affect their practice.

These reasonable acts, coupled with adherence to the standards of quality nursing care, will generally keep trauma nurses free from legal liability for their actions. Although such acts may not always keep the nurse out of court, they will significantly reduce the chance of an adverse judgment in a lawsuit.

CONCLUSION

The legal issues of this chapter identify areas of exposure of the trauma nurse to liability. They also speak of responsibilities that nurses have to society, to the hospital where they are employed, and to themselves. In the future, trauma nurses' actions will be subject to increasing scrutiny. There may be changes so that emergency and critical care nurses are granted a different license endorsement to practice based on higher educational and experience requirements. Higher standards of professional conduct will, in turn, be expected. Trauma nurses as expert witnesses will become more commonplace as their professionalism is more widely recognized by the law. By offering the court the benefit of years of special training, skill, and education, trauma nurses may perform a valuable service in advocating for the nursing specialty and bringing about changes in the law that reflect the realities and expertise of trauma nursing practice.

As has been noted throughout this chapter, there are or should be many hospital policies and procedures relating the subjects discussed herein. Without a doubt there is significant protection available to nurses if they follow hospital protocols. Failure to be aware of or follow existing policy may place the nurse out on a legal limb by himself or herself. It is incumbent on nurses to make themselves aware of hospital policies and procedures that relate to their areas of work.

Central to United States jurisprudence and the legal issues presented in this chapter is the right to control one's own life and to expect others to act in a reasonable fashion. Trauma patients, despite their incapacitation, are accorded these rights by the laws of the United States and of the individual states. Trauma nurses must operate within this framework to be legally effective.

The law need not be viewed as the nurse's adversary. A rapport can be established easily in which nurses maintain respect for the rights of patients while exercising their judgment about types of treatment and quality of care. Knowledge of the law and legal responsibilities can enhance the nurse's relationship with patients.

REFERENCES

1. *Goff v. Doctors General Hospital,* 333 P2d 29 (Cal App 1958).
2. *Darling v. Charleston Community Hospital,* 33 Ill 2d 326, 211 NE 2d 253 (1965), *cert denied,* 383 U.S. 946 (1966).
3. Louisell DH, Williams H: *Medical malpractice,* New York, 1985, Matthew Bender, p 16A-2.
4. Health Occupations Article, *Annotated Code of Maryland,* sec 8.
5. West's Annotated California Code Business and Professions, sec 2725, 2727.5.
6. *Nancy Beth Cruzan v. Missouri,* 497 U.S. 261, 269 (1990).
7. *Schloendorf v. Society of New York Hospital,* 211 NY 125, 105 NE 92 (1914).
8. Health–General Article, *Annotated Code of Maryland,* sec 5, 20-102, 107
9. *Anonymous v. State,* 17 App Div 2d 495, 236 NYS 2d 88 (1963).
10. Prosser WL: *Handbook of the law of torts,* ed 5, St. Paul, Minn, 1984, West-Wadsworth Publishing, pp 28-34.
11. Warren S, Brandeis L: The right to privacy, *Harvard Law Rev* 4:193, 1890.
12. Prosser WL: *Handbook of the law of torts,* ed 5, St. Paul, Minn, West-Wadsworth Publishing, 1984, pp 790-800.
13. American Hospital Association: *A patient's bill of rights (Management and Advisory Series),* Chicago, 1992.
14. Wold JL: AIDS testing: an ethical question, *J Neurosci Nurs* 22:258, 1990.
15. *Landeros v. Flood,* 551 P2d 389, Cal Sup Ct (1976).
16. Prosser WL: *Handbook of the law of torts,* ed 5, St. Paul, Minn, West-Wadsworth Publishing, 1984, pp 101-135.
17. Morris WO: The negligent nurse: the physician and the hospital, *Baylor Law Rev* 33:109, 1981.
18. Rocereto LR, Maleski CM: *The legal dimensions of nursing practice,* New York, 1982, Springer, p 99.
19. Connors JP: Nursing errors. In Mackauf SH: *Hospital liability,* New York, 1985, Law Journal Seminars Press, pp 33-66.
20. Courts and Judicial Proceedings Article, *Annotated Code of Maryland,* sec 5-309.
21. *Black's law dictionary,* ed 7 (rev), St. Paul, Minn, 1999, West-Wadsworth Publishing, p 1103.
22. Kaufman HH: Brain death following head injury. In Narayan RK, Wilberger JE, Povlishock JT, editors: *Neurotrauma,* New York, 1996, McGraw-Hill, pp 819-833.
23. West's Annotated California Health and Safety Code, sec 7182, 7188.
24. *Nancy Beth Cruzan v. Missouri,* 497 U.S. 261, 277, 1990.
25. *In re Quinlan,* 70 NJ 10, 355 A 2d 647, *cert denied sub nom. Garger v. New Jersey,* 429 U.S. 922 (1976).
26. Rhodes AM, Miller RD: *Nursing and the Law,* ed 4, Rockville, Md, 1984, Aspen Systems.
27. First Supreme Court decision on patient dumping, *Law Watch* 99:9, March 2, 1999.
28. HCFA/OIG issue final special advisory bulletin on patient dumping, *Law Watch* 99:54, Nov 23, 1999.
29. *Social Security Act,* sec 1932(b)(2).

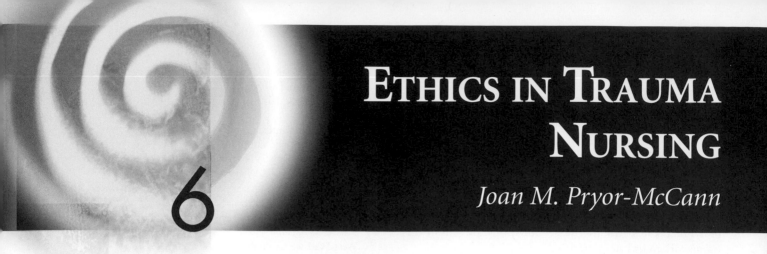

ETHICS IN TRAUMA NURSING

6

Joan M. Pryor-McCann

Many ethical questions confront nurses in their every-day practice. Trauma nurses, however, face a unique set of problems that make the resolution of ethical issues more difficult than in other nursing settings. For example, patients admitted to trauma units often have not chosen to be admitted there. Usually these persons have experienced a medical emergency requiring immediate health care intervention and admission. A trauma-induced hospital visit differs markedly from an elective surgery hospital admission or even an admission in which the patient walks into the emergency unit under his or her own power. If a voluntarily admitted patient has a cardiac arrest, the nurse can reasonably infer that the patient sought and wanted care, but in the event of a cardiac arrest in a nonvoluntarily admitted trauma patient, this inference cannot be made.

Not only is it unknown whether the trauma patient wants care, but often the trauma nurse cannot ascertain what the patient's wishes are regarding particular treatment options. For example, the trauma patient's decision-making ability is commonly incapacitated by an altered level of consciousness or is impaired by severe pain, anxiety, anger, or drugs. Sometimes such alterations are amenable to reversal with short-term treatment, and direction for care can then be obtained from the patient. More often than not, however, crucial life-or-death decisions must be made immediately, before these conditions can be reversed, in which case temporary alterations in decision-making ability are as problematic as any long-term ones. Community health nurses or hospital floor nurses are generally familiar with their patients' wishes and those of their families, but the trauma nurse is often not, and gaining speedy access to such information can be difficult or impossible.

At the same time, experienced trauma nurses are all too familiar with the practical implications of their ethical decisions. For example, they are keenly aware that if they place a 75-year-old patient with chronic obstructive pulmonary disease (COPD) on a ventilator, that person may never be able to be weaned from the machine. They also know that many people survive initial trauma but are unable to obtain or afford quality rehabilitative care.

The trauma setting is fast-paced compared with other health care settings. Trauma settings require quick decision making and allow very little time for information gathering, deliberation, or weighing alternatives. This, of course, is part of the reason emergency care guidelines for particular health care interventions are necessary in such settings. Yet whereas trauma nurses usually have clearly delineated procedures to follow during the resuscitation phase, there are no similar guidelines to assist them in making crucial ethical decisions. Frequently treatment decisions involve both issues. The decision whether or not to code a patient, for example, is an ethical and a health care decision.

This chapter attempts to provide the trauma nurse with some guidance for making ethical decisions. Knowledge of nursing's code of ethics, as well as knowledge of moral principles and theories, will help trauma nurses resolve troublesome ethical issues that arise in this setting. It is vitally important that the trauma nurse become familiar with these aspects of ethics so they can make sound ethical decisions in their practice.

THE DIFFERENCE BETWEEN ETHICS AND LAW

Some nurses believe that when their legal obligation is clear, their ethical obligation is also clear. Some nurses claim even more—that is, that their legal obligation always coincides with or determines their ethical obligation. In other words, these nurses hold that when a nurse knows that a doctor's orders call for a code to be initiated, this fact alone ends any deliberation about whether or not it is ethical to code the patient in question. Although this may sometimes be true, it is certainly not always true. Several crucial distinctions must be made between ethical and legal decisions.

First of all, ethics and law are not the same thing. The former deals with moral behavior and the latter with legal behavior. Admittedly, ethical choices are often reduced by pressures of the moment to worries about legal risk, but compliance with the law does not guarantee ethical behavior, nor is it an excuse for ignoring the ethical aspects of a decision.[1] For example, slavery was once legal in parts of the United States, but even at that time many persons questioned its morality, and most of us would agree today that slavery is ethically unacceptable. Similarly, abortion is now a legal alternative for pregnant women, but many persons question the morality of abortion. Laws themselves are not necessarily ethically sound. In fact, laws themselves are properly the subjects of ethical appraisal and evaluation. Therefore the assumption that if nurses do their legal duty and follow doctors' orders they will also be performing their ethical duty is not necessarily correct.

Another difference between law and ethics is evident in the fact that existing laws do not always give direction for particular ethical problems. The law often lags behind current ethical questions. For example, it took years for legislatures to enact statutes accepting brain death criteria as part of the legal definition of biologic death, yet nurses were faced with ethical decisions about the care of such patients long before these laws were enacted. The status of living wills is another legal issue that remains unresolved in some states, but ethical questions about the care of people who express their wishes in living wills must be addressed now. Ethics, then, is broader and more inclusive than law, and the nurse is not always able to gain direction for current ethical difficulties by consulting the law.

On the other hand, law is not irrelevant to ethics. Difficult ethical decisions can often be clarified by referring to the reasoning employed by courts and legal scholars on the issue in question or related issues. This is true because legal reasoning reflects our society's perceptions on a subject and because the law has its roots in public acceptance and its adherence to fair and reasonable procedures for decisions on issues. Some ethicists also claim that knowledge of one's legal obligations, although not decisive for answering ethical questions, is necessary for discerning one's ethical obligation.[2] Such obligations are often taken to be limited by the risks of legal liability or financial loss that an agent might incur secondary to a particular choice. For example, should nurses consider the legal risks they would be taking if they do not act consistently with their legal obligation to follow a doctor's orders to code a patient? This is certainly not the only information they should consider, but it is information that is clearly relevant to whether or not they should code their patients.

Curiously, nurses often consider physicians who make treatment decisions based on considerations of legal risk as morally pernicious. Interestingly, nurses usually do not apply the same negative assessment standard to themselves. What if a nurse conducts a code on his patient merely because the doctor ordered it, in spite of his own ethical concerns about such an intervention? Is he also without principles or perhaps immoral? One could argue that the nurse and the doctor are in somewhat different positions, and, of course, to some extent this is true. For example, the doctors write the orders, and the nurses are legally bound to follow them. However, in assessing a nurse's or a doctor's moral culpability for ordering or initiating a code out of sole regard for their own legal risks, it is apparent that the two seem to be on equal footing. If the assessment of the physician is valid, then, logically speaking, a similar assess-

ment of the nurse is required. The truth of the matter is that it is unclear whether any doctor or nurse acts immorally merely because he or she is concerned with legal risks. Legal risks are relevant data to consider when making moral decisions, and more analysis of a case is needed before moral culpability can be judged. The process of analyzing ethical decisions is discussed later in this chapter, but there is an important lesson to be gained from the point made here. Nurses must be more careful and more consistent in their assessments of the ethical implications of both their own actions and those of other health care workers.

In order to approach such assessments properly, nurses need more knowledge. Clearly compliance with the law is not enough to guarantee morally correct decisions, so many nurses look for guidance to the ethical code proposed by their professional association. The next section will discuss this document.

THE CODE FOR NURSES

In 1950 the American Nurses' Association adopted a code of ethics to guide professional nursing practice.[3] This document codifies nursing's traditional involvement with the obligations that health care workers owe to those under their care.[4] After several revisions, the code is now known as the *Code for Nurses with Interpretive Statements.*[5] (Hereafter it is referred to as the *Code for Nurses,* or simply the *Code.*) The *Code* serves as a public declaration of the standards and values by which all professional nurses are expected to practice. The *Code* has "performative force" because of its influence on nursing licensure, institutional accreditation, and curricula, as well as its use in court cases as the document representing accepted professional values and standards.[6]

Professional codes of ethics are always mixtures of creed and commandments (beliefs and rules). The belief aspects of the *Code for Nurses* can be found in the preamble, and the rule aspects are delineated in the 11 statements and their interpretations that follow. Although the ethical codes of some health professions have been criticized as paternalistic and limited, the nursing code has garnered much praise for its comprehensiveness and the emphasis it places on the autonomy of the patient.[7] In addition, the *Code* provides protection for clients by explicitly prohibiting behaviors that Jameton and others have called "the dark side of nursing," such as the labeling, stereotyping, or stigmatizing of patients by word or deed.[8] Every professional nurse should familiarize herself with the *Code for Nurses* because its ideals are those deemed by the profession as essential for ethical nursing practice.

The *Code for Nurses* also serves to inform the public that nurses acknowledge their unique position of care and assures the public of the standards and values by which all nurses are expected to function.[6] Duties such as veracity (truth telling) and advocacy are mentioned explicitly in the code. The preamble speaks to nurses' regard for the moral principles of beneficence (doing good), autonomy (patient self-determination), and justice (fairness).[9]

However, as impressive and important as the *Code* is, it cannot provide a specific answer to all the ethical questions that arise in nursing practice. Like other professional codes, the *Code for Nurses* provides general guidelines that must be applied in specific situations. Making this shift from the general to the specific is especially difficult in trauma settings, where treatment decisions often have to be made quite rapidly, where patients may be either upset or unresponsive, and where adequate information about the patient and the patient's life situation is lacking.

For example, Section 1.1 of the *Code for Nurses* states, "Clients have the moral right to determine what will be done with their own person, to accept, refuse or terminate treatment." How should a trauma nurse respond to a very anxious and despondent battered woman who insists, "Don't you dare treat me. I just want to die"? Does this patient's statement constitute a refusal of treatment? Should the trauma nurse abide by this woman's expressed wishes? Can a trauma nurse always get permission to render necessary life-saving treatment? If the patient ends up in the trauma unit after a suicide attempt, does the suicide victim have the right to refuse emergency life-saving treatment? Clearly the *Code for Nurses* does not address these complex questions in which the nurse's obligations and duties conflict and a resolution is not immediately apparent.

The same section of the *Code* states, "Truth telling and the process of reaching informed choice underlies the exercise of self-determination, which is basic to respect for persons." Should a trauma nurse tell a mother that her baby has just died if the nurse knows that the mother has stated that she will stop any life-saving treatment for herself if her baby dies? This is a classic case of a conflict of duty. The nurse has both the duty of veracity (to tell the truth) and the duty of beneficence (to do good for her patient). The *Code for Nurses* expects nurses to maximize these duties, but in the preceding case it seems that both cannot be maximized. The interpretive statements do say that the nurse should always tell the truth to the patient unless telling the truth will do more harm than good. The difficulty for the nurse in the preceding case is determining whether this particular situation qualifies as one of the latter exceptions. One can see that the *Code for Nurses* does not completely answer this difficult yet crucial question.

Trauma nurses also must make decisions about triaging patients and distributing scarce resources. The *Code for Nurses* simply does not provide much direction for these essential activities. In fact, Section 1 of the *Code* directs nurses to "provide services . . . unrestricted by considerations of social or economic status, personal attributes, or the nature of the health problems." Taken at face value, this requirement seems to undermine the very practice of nursing itself. Currently it is unquestionably understood that prognosis and illness are valid considerations for triage decisions, but obviously little guidance is provided by the *Code for Nurses* about how this process should be carried out.

Admittedly, no professional ethical code could capture all the myriad of ethical questions that arise within the scope of that profession's practice. The limits of the *Code for Nurses* illustrate that strict adherence to it is not enough to guarantee ethical behavior on the part of professional nurses. More important, however, is the fact that practicing nurses need to evaluate the *Code for Nurses*. Just as laws should be evaluated in light of ethical principles, so too should practicing nurses ethically critique the *Code for Nurses*. Is the current accepted *Code for Nurses* the very best code of ethics for a nurse to practice by? Can nurses always act ethically if they adhere to the beliefs and rules included in the *Code*? What general standards or principles can be used to evaluate the *Code for Nurses*? In order to gain expertise to answer these questions, one needs to explore both moral principles and ethical theories.

ETHICS

Ethics can be defined as the philosophic study of moral conduct, whereas morals or morality is understood philosophically as dealing with what is right and what is wrong in a practical sense.[10] In this chapter, as in common usage, the terms *ethics* and *morals* are used interchangeably. Likewise theories about ethics are sometimes referred to as moral theories or as ethical theories. In addition, the morality of an action is explored by looking at the ethical or moral justifications for the action. Ethics, then, involves a systematic appraisal of moral situations using moral principles and ethical theories to justify resolution of the question What, all things considered, ought to be done in this situation?[11]

Ethics is a human enterprise that requires one to look at one's own obligations and provide justification for one's own actions. Nursing ethics requires nurses to look at their professional obligations and explore how these obligations coincide with or are justified by general ethical principles and theories.

Trauma nurses need to deal with myriad ethical issues in their everyday practice. Some of these issues are clear and easily answered by referring to the *Code for Nurses;* however, many issues are ambiguous and difficult to answer. An ethical dilemma occurs either when there is no obvious answer to the issue at hand or the available alternative actions are each somewhat morally justifiable or are all morally undesirable. Olesinski and Stannard conclude that the overall nature of the ethical dilemmas confronted by critical care and emergency department nurses lies in the disparity between actual and ideal nursing practice.[12] Gaul[13] clarified the nature of such ethical dilemmas by analyzing responses of 270 nurses from 39 different states. She identified what she called the "four major causes of ethical suffering" in these nurses. These include situations in which (1) the patient's interests conflict with the treatment plan, (2) the nurse's responsibility to the family conflicts with those owed to the patient, (3) the nurse has opposing moral responsibilities, or (4) the nurse experiences a sense of powerlessness and lack of control over the elements of the ethical dilemma. The *Code for Nurses* cannot and should not be expected to resolve all these kinds of cases. Each one has numerous facets and considerations to take into account. Despite the complexity and uniqueness of each individual case, however, there are some commonalties on which the nurse can and should base her ethical decisions. These are the general moral principles that provide the foundation for ethical nursing practice.

MORAL PRINCIPLES

Ethicists discuss four basic moral principles that affect nursing practice. The first is the principle of *beneficence*, which requires that the nurse "ought to do good for and prevent or avoid doing harm to" her patient.[14] This latter obligation, that of avoiding harm, is called *nonmaleficence*, and in general ethics it is usually considered more binding than the duty to do good.[14] However, given the nurse's specialized education and training, coupled with the reasonable expectation by the public that nurses can resolve or ameliorate many health care problems, professional nurses do have responsibilities of beneficence and nonmaleficence to their patients. Sometimes a nurse cannot avoid causing some harm to a patient while properly performing her professional responsibilities. For example, nurses give injections or deliver other types of painful treatments such as debriding burn wounds or changing nasogastric tubes. These treatments are considered ethically acceptable only if the harm is minimized as much as possible and the benefit to be gained is worth the pain. One great difficulty with the principle of beneficence involves determining just what constitutes good or worthwhile gain for a particular patient. For example, is it beneficent to withhold food and water from a patient who has no likely chance of recovering from a terrible head injury and remains comatose? Withholding food clearly does constitute some harm, but does the good of allowing nature to take its course and letting the patient die outweigh the harm of not feeding him or her? Some nurses and ethicists reason that it does, whereas others claim that it does not. How should this issue be resolved? Perhaps investigating other moral principles will provide some guidance.

Autonomy is another moral principle that has gained prominence in health care settings as patients' rights and informed consent issues have arisen.[15] It has a long history in general ethics, most notably in Immanuel Kant's writings. *Autonomy* refers to the freedom to rule oneself. It includes the right of informed consent, the right to accept or refuse treatment, and the right to confidentiality. The principle of beneficence often conflicts with the moral principle of autonomy. For example, when a patient chooses not to have a recommended treatment needed to save his life, the nurse must decide whether to override the patient's decision in order to do the beneficent thing and administer the treatment or abide by the patient's refusal. Which principle should have the most weight for the trauma nurse in such a situation, the principle of autonomy or the principle of beneficence? Most ethicists today agree that autonomy has more weight in moral decision making than beneficence, but

despite this, nurses often take a paternalistic stance vis-à-vis their patients.

Benjamin and Curtis[16] point out how difficult it is to justify any paternalistic actions with adults. They list three criteria that must be met in order to decide ethically to carry out any paternalistic action:

1. *The autonomy condition:* when the patient is, under the circumstances, irretrievably ignorant of relevant information or the patient's capacity for rational reflection is significantly impaired.
2. *The harm condition:* when the patient is likely to be significantly harmed unless interfered with.
3. *The ratification condition:* when it is reasonable to assume that if the patient regained greater knowledge or recovery of his or her capacity for rational reflection at a later time, the patient would ratify the decision to interfere by consenting to it.

These are strong criteria, and they require much justification to warrant any overriding of a patient's autonomy. Often trauma nurses restrain patients against their wishes for safety reasons or out of legal or medical concerns. In cases in which patients are awake and alert enough to make decisions and refuse to be restrained, if the nurse continues with the restraining, he or she clearly is choosing to override the patient's own autonomous wishes. The more difficult case is one in which the patient is refusing, but the nurse has reason to think that his or her capacity to decide is impaired. The criteria listed above require more than this to justify overriding the patient's wishes such as knowing that the harm is significant and that there is reason to assume that the patient would authorize the restraining if he or she could reason better. If these conditions are met, the restraining is justified. Use of placebos also can be contrary to a patient's autonomy rights, and yet some health care workers continue to try to justify the use of placebos solely on the basis of beneficence.

Most ethicists agree that the autonomy rights of a patient override the professional's beneficence obligations in usual cases.[17-20] For example, the moral and constitutional legitimacy for withholding or withdrawing life-sustaining treatment at the request of the patient appears well settled in the United States.[21] Even when a patient is in a coma and the question is whether or not to continue nutrients and water, many think the issue is resolved if a living will made by the patient requests such withdrawal. This is because most regard living wills as akin to the patient exercising his or her autonomy, and they agree that such autonomy should be respected. Unfortunately, many people do not have a living will, or the document itself may be unclear on this issue. In such cases the nurse is in a difficult position in trying to determine what action beneficence requires, since the patient's autonomous wishes are unclear. In such cases decisions regarding whether to withdraw certain forms of treatment often fall to the family.

Ozuna[22] encourages nurses to be knowledgeable about aspects of the patient that the family may be most interested in such as whether the patient can experience pain or suffering or whether the patient is capable of responding meaningfully to stimuli. Sharing such information with families repeatedly and with compassion helps them to accept the realities of the patient's current status. Unfortunately, sometimes this precise information cannot be determined by current technology, in which case the nurse is unable to meet the family needs and is left with ambiguity about how to maximize the beneficent interests of the client.

The third ethical principle is *justice,* which requires that nurses treat all their patients fairly. This does not necessarily mean that each and every patient is treated exactly alike, but rather that equals are treated equally and that those who are unequal should be treated differently according to their differences.[23,24] This means that patients with similar health care problems deserve the same care, and those who have different needs should be attended to according to those needs. It also means that the nurse should take into consideration a patient's cultural and religious preferences. However, when one looks at the way the general principle of justice functions in mainstream ethics, a possible problem does arise for the nurse.

General ethics requires everyone to be fair to everyone. When justice is limited in scope to a particular nurse's patients, duty to those patients may conflict with general ethical duty to everyone at large. This issue rears its head vociferously when scarcity of resources comes into play. Consider a case in which a trauma nurse is to receive a large number of patients from a disaster site. Does the nurse owe a duty to the patients he or she already has, to the ones he or she might get, or to both?[25] What if the duties seem to conflict? This difficult issue will occur more and more as health care resources become increasingly scarce. Can the trauma nurse justify using current resources on patients who have a lower chance of recovery rather than saving those resources for potential patients who will have a better chance to recover? What if the latter patients never arrive? The answers to these questions remain unclear, especially when one acknowledges the special obligation nurses have to patients already in their care.[26] Furthermore, if the public decides that nurses have obligations of justice to persons not included in the nurses' current patient load, this decision would have profound implications for the principle of fairness in future health care decisions. It is unclear whether the nurse could ethically function under such a requirement because of the traditional nursing commitment of special duties owed to current patients. These issues are only part of the conundrum of gray areas currently under consideration in the arena of public and professional ethics.

The last moral principle, *fidelity,* may shed some light on the appropriate actions of a nurse in promise-making situations. Fidelity involves being faithful to one's promises. What are the promises nurses implicitly make to patients in their care? Minimally, nurses promise that they will do no harm to that person, and it is hoped that they will do as much good for their patients as they can. Note that this promise is made implicitly to patients already under the nurses' care. However, this principle does not provide very clear directions for what obligations (if any) the nurse owes to any potential or future patients. What is clear is that if a nurse makes an individual promise to a patient, then he or she has an obligation to follow through on it. The proper content of any promise a nurse should make to a patient, however, is still a gray area. Should a nurse remain faithful to a promise not to code a patient even if a physician has ordered such a procedure? What if this nurse needs her job to feed her five children and has reason to believe that if she resists the order she could be fired? Considerations about the nurse's own risks in making certain choices seem relevant to the moral weight of her promise, but to what extent should they prevail? Should the trauma nurse withhold pain medication from a patient because of persistent low blood pressure readings, despite the nurse's explicit promise to try to relieve the patient's pain? These complex questions are not entirely resolvable using only moral principles as guidelines. Perhaps a review of ethical theories will help to clarify the nurse's obligations in these complex cases.

MORAL THEORIES

Moral or ethical theories are more general than rules and principles and provide the most basic foundation for ethical decision making, especially when rules or principles conflict. Theories set priorities on which rules or principles override others in specific instances.[27] There are two major types of moral theories: teleologic and deontologic. The term *teleology* is derived from the Greek word *telos,* meaning "goal" or "end." Teleologic moral theories are consequentialist theories because they hold that the rightness or wrongness of an act is determined solely by the consequences the act produces or is foreseen to produce. All consequentialist theories are alike in that they require that a moral agent's actions maximize the good; however, they differ in what they consider the good to be. Such theories view no particular act as morally wrong in and of itself; only the consequences determine the morality of any action. Thus a particular act can be right in one situation and wrong in another situation as long as the consequences of the act differ in terms of the amount of good they produce.[11]

The term *deontology* is rooted in the Greek word *deon,* meaning "duty." Deontologic theories deny what consequentialist theories affirm. Deontologic theories claim that the morality of an act is determined by more than the consequences of that action. The moral status of an act is a result of other relevant factors such as the nature of the act itself. Using this type of theory to evaluate the morality of actions involves looking at established rules and principles that govern human conduct such as the Ten Commandments, the *Code for Nurses,* or other procedures for determining formal duties.[10]

Although there are many different kinds of consequentialist or deontologic theories, the most familiar ones are utilitarian consequentialism and Kantian deontology. These two kinds of theories illustrate the reasoning often offered in discussions of ethical questions facing trauma nurses.

UTILITARIANISM

Classic utilitarianism has its roots in the early nineteenth century works of Jeremy Bentham and John Stuart Mill. Despite the variations in their particular theories, both held that actions are to be judged by the amount of happiness or unhappiness that results from the action and that no one person's happiness or unhappiness counts any more than another's. Each person's welfare is equally weighted in the utilitarian calculus.

The power of utilitarianism lies in two important points. First, promoting the "most good overall" has strong intuitive appeal. It certainly seems like a laudable thing to do and may be the very best that one can hope to accomplish in the complex cases that face trauma nurses. Second, utilitarianism offers an objective way (in theory) to determine the answer to any and every ethical dilemma. One merely assesses the consequences of the various alternatives and chooses the one that leads to the greatest happiness. In effect, utilitarianism does away with every ethical dilemma, and all cases have a decisive, determinative best way to proceed.

Despite the obvious advantages of utilitarianism, there remain some grave difficulties for nurses who accept this as their sole theory of morality. Beneficence, autonomy, justice, and fidelity are accepted principles that apply to nursing practice. These principles cannot be accommodated in their appropriate weight for proper ethical decision making of nurses in a utilitarian framework. This is because utilitarianism gives no moral status to any principle beyond that it accords to the principle of utility, that is, maximizing overall good.[9]

Here is an example showing the type of difficulty that a nurse might face by accepting utilitarianism as the appropriate ethical theory to guide his or her actions. Suppose a wealthy, famous patient was admitted to the trauma unit from the scene of a car crash, and imagine that all the currently available nursing resources were lavished on this patient, while other needy patients went unattended. Such an action would clearly seem to be unethical and violate the basic principle of fairness. However, if this patient subsequently gave a huge donation to the trauma center, which resulted in equipment being available for a greater number of patients than those left unserved originally, the actions of the nursing staff would be judged as right using utilitarian standards. This is because a greater good resulted from the lavishing of resources on this one patient than would have occurred if the nurses had not done that. Surely this is an unacceptable outcome of moral decision making. Nurses do believe that unfair treatment of patients is morally wrong, just as the *Code for Nurses* claims. Thus utilitarianism falls short of capturing some of the basic moral principles that nurses incorporate into their professional practice in this case. It does not have the theoretic flexibility to allow for the special duties that nurses believe they owe to their patients.

However, utilitarianism does have some insights to offer nurses when considering ethical questions. It does seem that consequences should have some bearing on ethical decisions. Although it is apparent that nurses cannot consider consequences as the only relevant moral factor, it remains to be determined just how much weight should be given to consequences by the nurse. An exploration of deontology will shed some light on this difficult question.

DEONTOLOGY

Immanuel Kant,[28] an eighteenth-century philosopher, believed that morality consisted of following absolute rules no matter what the consequences. His primary test of whether a rule should be followed was to apply the categorical imperative of universality to the considered action. Whether or not the action was moral did not depend on the desire of the agent or the consequences of the action, but rather on whether one's duty was to perform the action as determined by his moral test, better known as the *categorical imperative.* Kant explored several applications of his categorical imperative in assessing the morality of lying, stealing, and suicide. These have been studied intensely and nearly uniformly rejected by later ethicists. For example, Kant concluded that stealing and suicide are always wrong and one must always tell the truth in all circumstances. However, the appeal of Kantian ethics remains for persons who believe that acting on principle rather than because of good results is an important ethical insight. Kant places a high value on autonomy and respect and can accommodate the special duties that nurses are thought to owe their patients. Most contemporary deontologists think Kant went too far in concluding that morality requires absolute rules that do not take into account any consequences of actions. His theory is also limited in that it cannot adjudicate cases in which more than one duty applies but no alternative action can maximize both. Conflicts-of-duty situations are common in nursing practice, but Kant's ethics offers no way to resolve them. Several ethicists have tried to remain faithful to the spirit of Kantian ethics while trying to accommodate these commonsensical, well-established aspects of morality.

W.D. Ross[10] proposes a theory that provides some guidance in this regard. He claims that duties originate from the social relationships one finds oneself in and that eventually these duties are coalesced by humans into general duties. Ross claims that general duties have *prima facie* status and are overridable only in very particular circumstances. Furthermore, any overriding of a *prima facie* principle requires its own justification. He lists fidelity, reparation, gratitude, justice, beneficence, and nonmaleficence as *prima facie* duties owed to others. Ross does not prioritize these duties but says that some apply more stringently than others and all can be overridden at times. Presumably, circumstances and possible consequences play a role in defining the proper kind of justification for overriding a general principle. Thus Ross's theory manages to support some of the special duties of a nurse while allowing for mitigating circumstances such as the consequences of the act to be considered. Unfortunately, however, Ross's theory gives little direction about the way that justification is to proceed. He offers no rules or procedures to use in weighing the stringency of application of a particular principle in a specific moral situation nor any ways to justify one principle being applicable over another. So although Ross allows for more flexibility regarding rules and consequences than Kant, his theory is incomplete in that it provides little guidance for deciding difficult cases.

W.K. Frankena,[29] another modern deontologist, posits a theory in which the principles of beneficence and justice are considered to be the most basic of all moral principles. Thus, for Frankena, in cases in which there is a conflict between one of these primary principles and autonomy or fidelity, the right moral action will be the one that maximizes the basic principle. In a nursing situation in which justice and autonomy conflict, justice prevails, or if beneficence and fidelity conflict, beneficence triumphs. However, a major problem persists, for how is a case of conflict between beneficence and justice to be decided? Some of the cases discussed previously involving scarcity of resources and duties owed to very ill patients with questionable prognoses have this exact issue at their heart. If two patients have equal need to go to the intensive care unit (ICU) but there is only one ICU bed available, how does one decide which patient to send? Frankena's theory does not provide specific guidance for these difficult yet pressing cases.

As can be seen, both the utilitarian and deontologic theories have their own unique contributions to moral reasoning and their own sets of difficulties. In fact, no moral theory is without some problems. All moral theories fall short of some commonsensical and well-accepted portion of ethical judgment. This does not necessarily mean that any one of the moral theories is itself in error, because it could also be the case that more than one moral theory is needed to deal with new and complex issues in health care settings. It should also be noted that each theory provides the nurse with some very important ethical insights and therefore can offer guidance for the nurse when dealing with difficult ethical problems.

THE ETHICS OF CARING

Some nursing ethicists and theorists, such as Gadow,[30] Benner,[31] Bishop,[32] Watson,[33] and others,[6] have described the ethic of nursing as the "ethic of caring." Gaul, Olesinski, and others opt for Gilligan's term, calling the ethical theory of nursing practice the "ethic of care."[13,34] Although definitions vary, *care* and *caring* are associated most often with the principle of beneficence. Some say care and caring are the same thing as beneficence. Others believe that the nurse's obligation to care for patients (to be caring) is merely supported by the principle of beneficence. As discussed previously, this emphasis on beneficence has its problems. Paternalism has often clouded the moral ideal of "doing good," and the ethic of care or caring is vulnerable to this difficulty. Perhaps this is why advocacy is so often linked by nursing scholars to the ethic of care or caring. But Winslow[35] and Trandel-Korenchuk[36] point out several complex difficulties inherent in the concept of advocacy. Much of the difficulty lies in the need to clarify exactly what advocacy requires. For example, is advocacy *doing* for a patient, *assisting* a patient, *defending* a patient, or some combination of these actions?

Other problems involve clarifying *what* is to be advocated; that is, should the nurse advocate the patient's actual wishes or rather what is in the best interest of the patient? Furthermore, who is to define what constitutes the "best interest" of the patient? Should it be the patient, his or her family, the most expert health care professional, or someone else? How do the rules change with patients of different ages, competencies, or levels of consciousness?

Gadow[30] describes a model of "existential advocacy" that she claims avoids paternalism while maintaining the nurse as an involved, caring participant in the patient's decision-making process, but aspects of her model remain controversial.[35] For example, Gadow states that, as advocates, nurses should answer patients directly if asked their opinion about treatment options. Yet many question whether nurses can ever recommend a course of action for patients without interfering with the patients' autonomy by inadvertently manipulating or coercing them. Others question Gadow's claim that nurses gain ethical knowledge about where the boundary between benefit and harm lies for patients based on the nurse's special role as the touching, ministering caregiver.[30]

Bandman and Bandman[6] point out that the caring ethic has its roots in both the history of philosophy and the contemporary work of Carol Gilligan,[37] and Gaul notes that current literature in philosophy, feminist studies, and nursing have devoted much attention to the ethic of care.[13] However, Bishop and Scudder[32] claim that nursing's caring ethic belongs primarily to nursing's own history and practice.[22] Whatever the basis of the caring ethic, it offers important insights for nurses who seek to practice ethically. For example, the caring ethic describes the orientation nurses should have toward their patients; it demands empathy and compassion. It provides a basis for explaining the special duties that nurses owe their patients, such as beneficence and advocacy. Many authors regard the ethic of caring as a virtue theory of ethics because it deals primarily with the required moral excellence of nurses' character, demanding that nurses be caring toward their patients.[13,34] However, difficulties arise when one attempts (as Gadow[30] and Gilligan[37] do) to use the ethic of caring as a theory of moral obligation, that is, a theory that determines what actions are morally permissible, impermissible, or required. One difficulty is that the ethic of caring seems to be based on feelings, values, and intuition in such a way that the charge of pernicious relativism and subjectivism is hard to defend.

Recently, Gastmans and colleagues attempted to give a fuller account of the morality of nursing practice.[34] They claim that moral nursing practice requires three components: a caring relationship between nurse and client, an episode of caring behavior toward the client that integrates the virtue of care with expert activity, and the goal of "good care" as the aim for the nursing activity. The "virtue of care" requires the acceptance of a "caring attitude" by the nurse and the performance of caring behaviors inspired by this attitude. This affective involvement of the nurse in the well-being of the patient is distinguished from other kinds of feelings such as those that may occur when attracted to certain personal features of a person. The former kind of affectation is required for moral nursing practice whereas the latter is not. It is not clear whether this amended version of the ethic of caring avoids the problems of relativism and subjectivism mentioned earlier. But even if it does, Gastmans and colleagues point out another limitation of their theory and one that would seem to plague any other ethic of caring theory. It involves the scope of the theory. Ethic of care theories require a relationship between the nurse and the patient, so they can only be used to justify the ethical nature of direct patient contact types of nursing practice. Gastmans and colleagues agree that other kinds of nursing practice that do not involve a relationship between patient and nurse may have moral significance, but they admit that their ethic of caring cannot provide any support, explanation, or guidance for such areas of practice.[34] This limitation might not be a problem for a caring ethical theory if no other sorts of nursing had moral significance, but that seems not to be the case.

McDaniel, for example, claims that the work of nurse managers has a moral component. She holds that nurse managers are required ethically to create work environments that provide opportunities for nurses to engage in discussions about ethical concerns, that support nurses in their quest to provide ethical nursing care, and that develop policies and procedures that sustain nurses' ethical care with clients.[38] Likewise, Aroskar and Corley[39,40] claim that nurse managers have a moral responsibility to support collegial and collaborative relationships within nursing and between nursing and medicine because research has shown that positive patient outcomes and compassionate nursing care are dependent on such relationships. The ethic of care cannot provide any direct support for these claims, yet most nurses agree that nurse managers have moral obligations of this sort.

As has been seen, although the ethical theories and principles discussed thus far offer some direction regarding the moral dimensions of nursing practice, none is without significant limitations. Whereas ethical decision making requires a process that considers all the relevant moral factors, it is not endless, nor is it arbitrary. How should a nurse decide important ethical questions? How should a nurse adjudicate between the ethical insights offered by the various moral theories and principles in order to act responsibly? The next section provides some direction in this regard.

ETHICAL DECISION-MAKING APPROACHES

DeGrazia,[41] Baker,[42] and others[13] have pointed out various problems with using a foundationalist approach to ethical decision making. In this approach, a specific ethical theory or principle is used as the first premise in a deductive logical argument, and the pertinent facts about the ethical case are used as the second one. The ethically correct action is then deduced from these two premises. This method of ethical decision making has been criticized as not being sensitive enough to the complexity of the facts involved in ethical

cases and for assuming a specific cultural value perspective. In addition, this approach is not very comprehensive. It gives little direction for new or unusual cases, yet these are just the sorts of cases that trauma nurses deal with all the time.

Callahan,[43] Curtin,[44] Degrazia,[41] and others support a more "coherentist" approach to ethical justification. A Harvard philosopher named John Rawls[45] has proposed such an approach in his theory of justice. He calls it "wide reflective equilibrium." Degrazia tests what he calls "specified principles" using the process of wide reflective equilibrium; and Gaul, following Arras,[13,45] also suggests using wide reflective equilibrium to decide ethical questions, but in combination with a case-based method called *casuistry.* The wide reflective equilibrium process can help nurses clarify their own moral framework by comparing and contrasting three important ethical databases—their own beliefs, values, and considered moral judgments—to moral principles and ethical theories. It is the preferred decision-making process for nurses to use when making ethically supportable choices in health care settings. The usefulness of this process is well illustrated by Benjamin and Curtis[16] in their book on nursing ethics when they discuss the justification process that leads to the acceptance of using brain death criteria as a definitive way of establishing a person's death.

When beginning the reflective equilibrium process, the nurse should clarify the pertinent facts of the case at hand, the ethical question it presents, and the possible alternative actions that are available. Minimally the facts include the patient's medical status, prognosis, stated wishes (if any), and current mental status. There may be more than one ethical issue involved in the case, but often there is only one clear dilemma—for example, whether or not to code a patient. Finally, the nurse should list the alternative actions available, such as calling a code; not calling a code; beginning some but not all code actions; or discussing the patient's code status with the patient, family, or doctor. Then, while considering each alternative in turn, the nurse should clarify his or her own moral judgments about the alternative by exploring background beliefs and considered moral reasoning and then cross-referencing these with known and accepted moral principles and theories. Such deliberation might proceed something like this:

Considering the first alternative (i.e., calling a code), the nurse should initially identify his or her values and beliefs about the morality of calling a code on the patient in question. If the nurse has concerns about calling a code on this patient, it is likely that he or she has some moral compunction against taking this action. However, this alone is not enough to assure that the nurse's moral judgment in this case is ethically sound. The nurse must then examine that judgment for validity by comparing it with accepted moral beliefs, principles, and theories. The nurse might find that some people question the rightness of coding the kind of patient in question, whereas others do not. The nurse should then further consider the action of calling a code.

In reflecting on the principle of beneficence, the nurse should consider his or her obligation not to harm the patient and his or her responsibility to do good. The nurse therefore needs to clarify whether or not calling a code is good in this situation and whether the harm that might be incurred by conducting a code is ethically warranted. If the nurse thinks that death is a more desirable end in this case than coding the patient, he or she needs to test the initial judgment by looking for further verification from the moral theories of utilitarianism and deontology.

Utilitarianism might confirm the nurse's tentative conclusion that coding the patient is wrong if the good of not coding outweighs the bad of coding. Things to consider are the consequences for the patient; the outcomes for society in terms of resource use and other payoffs; and the possible legal, financial, and other results that such a decision may cause for the nurse, doctor, family, and hospital. In utilitarianism the possible legal difficulties for the health care team count in this assessment just as much as the actual outcome for the patient. Depending on the good or bad consequences that might occur for the nurse, patient, and others, utilitarianism might lead to the conclusion that the coding of the patient in question is the right moral action or the wrong moral action.

Given the status of the principle of beneficence in their systems, the deontologic theories of Frankena and Ross would support the coding of a patient if it was in the patient's best interests to survive. However, these theories could also support the decision to not code the patient if it was in the patient's best interest to end the patient's suffering and this was only possible by dying. Thus the difficulty here lies in determining what is in the patient's best interest, and this is often very difficult to do. If the patient's autonomous wishes about coding are known, given the status of autonomy in deontologic frameworks it is likely that those wishes would prevail. When a patient's wishes are not known, there is still some disagreement about who should decide whether or not a code should be called in any particular case. Clearly the expertise of the physician is relevant to such a decision, but in most cases the decision cannot be made definitively on a purely medical basis. At this point in the analysis, the coding of the patient would be considered an ethically supportable action if the patient desired it or if the patient's best interests demanded it. On the other hand, it would not be morally supportable to call the code if the patient did not want such action or if the patient's best interests boded against such action. After conducting this inquiry concerning the first of the possible alternative actions, the nurse should go on to do a similar analysis of all the other possible actions available to resolve the ethical issue in question.

Obviously this type of analysis is very thorough and as such gives much credence to the decisions made. It is the preferable approach when the nurse has the time for prolonged deliberation. However, this process is time consuming, and it is not feasible in situations that require quick decision making.

Kenneth Iserson[46] has suggested another approach to ethical decisions when a rapid appraisal is needed, such as in many emergency and trauma situations. He claims that one should begin by asking if the ethical problem at hand is similar in type to any other ethical problem for which one has already worked out a rule about how to proceed. If so, he suggests that the individual follow that rule, not because it is necessarily correct, but rather because it is more likely than not to be an ethically acceptable action, given that the individual has used it before and discussed it with others. In addition to Iserson's guidelines, the rule should be an ethically comfortable stance for the nurse, and the nurse should already have clarified the facts, the moral question, and the alternative actions available in the situation. If the rule is ethically unacceptable for the nurse, or if the nurse has no rule for this type of situation, then any option that would buy time for further deliberation without excessive risk to the patient must be considered. If there is such an option, the nurse should take it. If there is no available option, then the nurse should perform three quick moral assessment tests on the alternative action under consideration:

1. *Impartiality test:* The nurse asks if he or she would be willing to have this action performed if the nurse were in the patient's place.
2. *Universalizability test:* The nurse asks if he or she would be willing to have this action performed in all relevantly similar circumstances.
3. *Interpersonal justifiability test:* The nurse asks if he or she is able to provide good reasons to justify his or her actions to others.[46]

The first test is not infallible, but it is a good way to correct one obvious source of moral error, that of partiality or self-interested bias. The second test is also designed to eliminate a moral decision difficulty, shortsightedness. It enables the nurse to evaluate the action by considering whether it should be followed as a general practice in all similar circumstances. This is important because, although one may approve of the action in the particular situation, it may not be an acceptable practice to follow in similar circumstances. Moral rules are supposed to apply generally, and it is this that the nurse is assessing with this test. The final test requires that the nurse has reasons for proceeding in the way decided on and, further, that others would approve of the reasons for this action. This ensures that the nurse has considered the decision thoughtfully and that his or her reasons are sound and nonidiosyncratic.

All ethical stands should be reviewed periodically for relevance and credence. Sometimes this process results in rule adjustments, whereas at other times it merely confirms the nurse's preexisting stance. Whatever way it goes, the review process will help to clarify and reinforce sound ethical decision making on the part of the nurse. Schroeter and Taylor[26] identify several strategies that nurses in critical care environments can use to address the ethical issues that they confront in practice. Becoming familiar with typical issues that arise is an important first step. Nurses should discuss such issues with resource persons such as ethicists, ethics committee members, administrators, and peers. Nurses also need to keep abreast of the literature on familiar and new ethical issues and seek out the opinions of other health care professionals, especially physicians, on these issues. Nurses should form groups to support each other in ethically ambiguous situations and to help brainstorm about the means to deal with such issues. Trauma nurses should know and understand the policies of their institutions regarding such things as brain death criteria, non-heart-beating organ donation, and the status of living wills and durable power of health care attorney documents. If nurses have questions about these policies, it is their duty to seek clarification and to bring problems to the appropriate person. In addition, departmental processes should be put into place to address common ethical problems and to acknowledge the suffering that nurses experience in such situations.[26] Although there is no way to eliminate or totally resolve all ethical questions in practice, having a structure in place to assist the staff nurses in dealing with ethical dilemmas will go a long way toward resolving the ethical difficulties that nurses face.

In addition, trauma nurses themselves can be prepared to deal with ethical problems if they are knowledgeable about nursing's code of ethics; general moral principles; ethical theories, including the ethic of caring; and ethical decision-making processes. Armed with these guideposts, they have at their fingertips the tools they need to make sound ethical decisions in nursing practice.

REFERENCES

1. Capron AM: Legal setting of emergency medicine. In Iserson KV, Arthur B, Sanders MD, editors: *Ethics in emergency medicine,* ed 2, Tucson, 1995, Galen Press.
2. Buchanan AE: What is ethics? In Iserson KV, Arthur B, Sanders MD, editors: *Ethics in emergency medicine,* ed 2, Tucson, 1995, Galen Press.
3. Veins DC: A history of nursing's code of ethics, *Nurs Outlook* 37(1):45-49, 1989.
4. Yeaworth RC: The ANA code: a comparative perspective, *J Nurs Scholarship* 17(3):94-98, 1985.
5. American Nurses Association: *Code for nurses with interpretive statements,* Kansas City, Mo, 1976, 1985.
6. Bandman E, Bandman B: *Nursing ethics through the life span,* ed 3, Norwalk, Conn, 1995, Appleton & Lange.
7. Reich WT, editor: *Encyclopedia of bioethics,* rev ed, Tappan, NJ, 1995, Macmillan.
8. Corley MC, Goren S: The dark side of nursing: impact of stigmatizing responses on patients, *Sch Inq Nurs Pract* 12(2):99-122, 1998.
9. Pryor-McCann J: Ethical issues in critical care nursing, *Crit Care Nurs Clin North Am* 2(1):1-13, 1990.
10. Feldman F: *Introductory ethics,* Englewood Cliffs, NJ, 1978, Prentice-Hall.
11. Rachels J: *The elements of moral philosophy,* ed 3, Burr Ridge, Ill, 1998, McGraw-Hill.
12. Olesinski N, Stannard D: Commentary on casuistry, care, compassion and ethics, *AACN Nurs Scopes Crit Care* July-Sept 1996.
13. Gaul AL: Casuistry, care, compassion, and ethics data analysis, *Adv Nurs Sci* 17(3):47-57, 1995.
14. Mitchell C, Achtenberg B: *Study guide for code gray film,* Boston, 1984, Fanlight Productions.
15. Fry ST: Ethical principles in nursing education and practice: a missing link in the unification issue, *Nurs Health Care* 3(9):363-368, 1982.
16. Benjamin M, Curtis J: *Ethics in nursing,* ed 3, New York, 1991, Oxford University Press.
17. Davis AJ, Aroskar MA, Liaschenko J: *Ethical dilemmas and nursing practice,* ed 4, Englewood Cliffs, NJ, 1997, Prentice Hall.
18. Jameton A: *Nursing practice: the ethical issues,* Englewood Cliffs, NJ, 1984, Prentice Hall.
19. Thompson JE, Thompson HO: *Bioethical decision-making of nurses,* New York, 1995, Appleton-Century-Crofts.
20. Veatch RM: *Medical ethics,* ed 2, Boston, 1996, Jones & Bartlett.
21. Gostin LO: Deciding life and death in the courtroom, *JAMA* 278(18):1523-1528, 1997.
22. Ozuna J: Persistent vegetative state: important considerations for the neuroscience nurse, *J Neurosci Nurs* 28(3):199-203, 1998.
23. Beauchamp TL, Walters L, editors: *Contemporary issues in bioethics,* ed 5, Belmont, Calif, 1999, Wadsworth.
24. Beauchamp T, Childress JF: *Principles of biomedical ethics,* ed 4, New York, 1994, Oxford University Press.
25. Reverly S: An historical perspective. In Mitchell C, Achtenberg B: *Study guide for code gray film,* Boston, 1984, Fanlight Productions, pp 20-21.
26. Schroeter K, Taylor GJ: Ethical considerations in organ donation for critical care nurses, *Crit Care Nurse* 19(2):60-69, 1999.
27. Bandman EL, Bandman B: Ethical aspects of nursing. In Flynn JB, Heffron PB, editors: *Nursing from concept to practice,* ed 2, Norwalk, Conn, 1988, Appleton & Lange.
28. Kant I: *Fundamental principles of the metaphysics of morals,* New York, 1949, Liberal Arts.
29. Frankena WK: *Ethics,* ed 2, Englewood Cliffs, NJ, 1973, Prentice Hall.
30. Gadow S: Ethical dimensions. In Beare PG, Myers JL, editors: *Principles and practice of adult health nursing,* St. Louis, 1990, Mosby.
31. Benner P, Tanner CA, Chesla CA: *Expertise in nursing practice: caring clinical judgement and ethics,* New York, 1996, Springer.
32. Bishop AH, Scudder JR: *The practical, moral, and personal sense of nursing,* Albany, 1990, State University of New York Press.
33. Watson J, Ray MA, editors: *The ethics of care and the ethics of cure: synthesis in chronicity,* New York, 1988, National League for Nursing Publication no. 15-2237.
34. Gastmans C, Dierckx de Casterle B, Schotsmans P et al: Nursing considered as moral practice: a philosophical ethical interpretation of nursing. *Kennedy Inst Ethics J* 8(1):43-69, 1998.
35. Winslow GR: From loyalty to advocacy: a new metaphor for nursing, *Hastings Cent Rep,* June 1984.
36. Trandel-Korenchuk D, Trandel-Korenchuk K: Nursing advocacy of patients' rights: myth or reality? *NLN Publ* (20-2294):111-120, June 1990.
37. Gilligan C: *In a different voice,* Cambridge, Mass, 1982, Harvard University Press.
38. McDaniel C: Ethical environments: reports of practicing nurses, *Nurs Clin North Am* 33(2):363-371, 1998.
39. Aroskar MA: Ethical working relationships in patient care: challenges and possibilities, *Nurs Clin North Am* 33(2):313-324, 1998.

40. Corley MC: Ethical dimensions of nurse-physician relations in critical care, *Nurs Clin North Am* 33(2):325-337, 1998.
41. DeGrazia D: Moving forward in bioethical theory: theories, cases and specified principalism, *J Med Philos* 17(8):511-539, 1992.
42. Baker R: A theory of international bioethics: multiculturalism, post-modernism, and the bankruptcy of fundamentalism, *Kennedy Inst Ethics J* 8(3):201-231, 1998.
43. Callahan JC, editor: *Ethical issues in professional life,* New York, 1988, Oxford University Press.
44. Curtin LL: Nursing ethics: theories and pragmatics, *Nurs Forum* 17:4-11, 1978.
45. Rawls J: *A theory of justice,* rev ed, Cambridge, Mass, 1999, Belknap Press.
46. Iserson KV: An approach to ethical problems in emergency medicine. In Iserson KV, Arthur B, Sanders MD, editors: *Ethics in emergency medicine,* ed 2, Tucson, 1995, Galen Press.

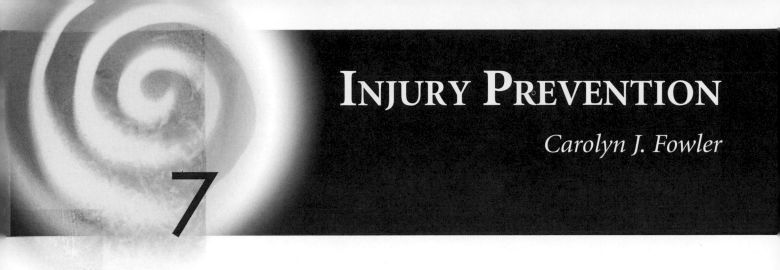

INJURY PREVENTION

Carolyn J. Fowler

7

Injury is the most underrecognized public health problem facing the nation today. Overall, unintentional injuries, homicides, and suicides together constitute the fourth leading cause of death in the United States, accounting for 146,941 deaths in 1998 (6% of the total).[1] Unintentional injury alone is the fifth leading cause of death across all ages in the United States.[1] In younger members of the population, those between the ages of 1 and 44 years, injury is the leading cause of death.[2] Before the age of 35, injury accounts for more deaths than all other causes combined (Table 7-1).[2,3] Unintentional injury alone (without the contribution of homicide and suicide) is the leading cause of death in people 1 to 34 years of age.[4] Among adolescents and young adults, 8 of every 10 deaths are injury related. Injury causes the premature death of many young people and thus is the leading cause of years of potential life lost (YPPL) before the age of 75.[2] Indeed, injury is responsible for more years of potential life lost than cancer, heart disease, or acquired immunodeficiency syndrome (AIDS). In the United States motor vehicle crashes alone have claimed more lives than all of this nation's wars.[5]

The societal cost of injury is enormous. Health care charges for the treatment of injury represent only a portion of the total financial burden. Other costs include those associated with loss of income, productivity, and property. Social costs are harder to measure but include pain, suffering, reduced quality of life, lost human potential, and disrupted families. In 1995 the estimated total lifetime cost resulting from injury in the United States in that year was estimated at $260 billion (in 1995 dollars).[6,7]

Injury is perceived to be a condition that affects young people disproportionately, yet trauma continues to be a major health problem throughout life. Despite the obvious importance of injury as a cause of premature death, the highest injury-related death rates are experienced by the elderly (65 years and older), a sector of the population that is expected to increase from 13% to 22% by the year 2030.[8] Similarly, our oldest citizens (those over 75 years of age) experience death rates nearly three times those of the general population; this group is expected to rise from 5% to 9% of the population in the next three decades.[8] Nonfatal injuries in the elderly are also a major concern. For many older adults, a hip fracture may begin a downward spiral of immobility-related morbidity, an end to independent living in the community, and shortened life span. Indeed, half of all elders who are hospitalized for a hip fracture are unable to return home or live independently after the injury.[9] Unless we are able to reduce death and injury rates among people over the age of 65, it is estimated that by the year 2030 this group will sustain more than one third of all injury-related deaths and hospitalizations. The social impact of this cannot be overstated.

Injury can be prevented or controlled at three levels. Primary prevention involves preventing the event, such as the car crash, that causes the injury. Secondary prevention involves preventing an injury or minimizing its severity during that crash. Tertiary prevention is optimization of outcome through medical treatment and rehabilitation. Trauma nurses will be most familiar with tertiary prevention and to a lesser extent with secondary prevention. Development of emergency medical services and systems and expert trauma management has improved, and will continue to improve, the outcomes for injured patients. However, these advances will never be enough to reduce the toll of injury-related death significantly. Why? The majority of deaths from traumatic injury occur early. It is estimated that, because of the severity of the injuries, half of all trauma deaths cannot be prevented with even the best medical management.[10] For those who survive their injuries, the sequelae may be profound and, in some cases, increase that individual's chance of re-injury.[10] Achieving a significant reduction in trauma-related mortality and morbidity therefore must include attention to primary prevention. Indeed, during Trauma Awareness Month and at other community events, the American Trauma Society promotes the concept that the best trauma management is prevention.[11]

At some time, all trauma nurses will ask, "Could this have been prevented?" Why then has injury prevention received so little attention in trauma training programs and trauma services? Trauma, it seems, is so endemic in our society that we fail to realize the enormity of its financial and social costs or our potential as a society to reduce its toll. In 1988 Dr. William Foege, former director of the Centers for Disease Control and Prevention, called injury "the principal public

TABLE 7-1	Ten Leading Causes of Death by Age Group in the United States, 1998				
					Age Groups
Rank	<1	1-4	5-9	10-14	15-24
1	Congenital Anomalies 6,212	**Unintentional Injuries 1,935**	**Unintentional Injuries 1,544**	**Unintentional Injuries 1,710**	**Unintentional Injuries 13,349**
2	Short Gestation 4,101	Congenital Anomalies 564	Malignant Neoplasms 487	Malignant Neoplasms 526	*Homicide 5,506*
3	SIDS 2,822	*Homicide 399*	Congenital Anomalies 198	*Suicide 317*	*Suicide 4,135*
4	Maternal Complications 1,343	Malignant Neoplasms 365	*Homicide 170*	*Homicide 290*	Malignant Neoplasms 1,699
5	Respiratory Distress Synd. 1,295	Heart Disease 214	Heart Disease 156	Congenital Anomalies 173	Heart Disease 1,057
6	Placenta Cord Membranes 961	Pneumonia & Influenza 146	Pneumonia & Influenza 70	Heart Disease 170	Congenital Anomalies 450
7	Perinatal Infections 815	Septicemia 89	Bronchitis, Emphysema, Asthma 54	Bronchitis, Emphysema, Asthma 98	Bronchitis, Emphysema, Asthma 239
8	**Unintentional Injuries 754**	Perinatal Period 75	Benign Neoplasms 52	Pneumonia & Influenza 51	Pneumonia & Influenza 215
9	Intrauterine Hypoxia 461	Cerebrovascular 57	Cerebrovascular 35	Cerebrovascular 47	HIV 194
10	Pneumonia & Influenza 441	Benign Neoplasms 53	HIV 29	Benign Neoplasms 32	Cerebrovascular 178

From National Center for Injury Prevention and Control: Ten leading causes of death, 1998, Atlanta, 2000, Centers for Disease Control and Prevention, www.cdc.gov/ncipc/osp/data.htm.

health problem in the United States today."[12] One year later Surgeon General C. Everett Koop testified that "if some infectious disease came along that affected children [in the proportion that injuries do], there would be a huge public outcry and we would be told to spare no expense to find a cure and to be quick about it."[13] Much progress has been achieved in the ensuing years, but the commitment of the public, and of the health care profession, to injury prevention is still woefully inadequate—a symptom of society's "general tendency to underinvest in programs designed to prevent social problems."[14] Why? Three answers come to mind: (1) injury is underrecognized and, as such, grossly underfunded and studied relative to other health problems of similar magnitude; (2) injury prevention is relatively young as a field of scientific inquiry and professional practice; and (3) training in injury prevention methods is lacking.

Trauma nurses know all too well how a few seconds can alter the course of a healthy young person's life forever. They have witnessed the effects of alcohol and other substance abuse and access to lethal weapons as risk factors for injury;

they recognize predictable trauma case histories; they know that certain days, times, and weather conditions are associated with increased caseload. Fortunately, many have also witnessed the protective effects of interventions such as seat belts, helmets, and improved vehicle design. Clearly, trauma nurses possess the awareness and many of the attributes needed by injury preventionists and can make valuable contributions to injury prevention. The goal of this chapter, therefore, is to enable the trauma nurse to think about injury in a critical and systematic way. Traumatic injury is approached as a health problem to be solved. A public health problem-solving paradigm[15] and two related conceptual frameworks for problem diagnosis and decision making are introduced.

AN OVERVIEW OF INJURY PREVENTION

Although traumatic injury has been a problem throughout the ages, injury prevention is a relatively new field of scientific inquiry. Historically, injuries (often called *accidents*) have been viewed as the result of human error, fate, or

25-34	35-44	45-54	55-64	65+	Total
Unintentional Injuries 12,045	Malignant Neoplasms 17,022	Malignant Neoplasms 45,747	Malignant Neoplasms 87,024	Heart Disease 605,673	Heart Disease 724,859
Suicide 5,365	**Unintentional Injuries 15,127**	Heart Disease 35,056	Heart Disease 65,068	Malignant Neoplasms 384,186	Malignant Neoplasms 541,532
Homicide 4,565	Heart Disease 13,593	**Unintentional Injuries 10,946**	Bronchitis, Emphysema, Asthma 10,162	Cerebrovascular 139,144	Cerebrovascular 158,448
Malignant Neoplasms 4,385	*Suicide 6,837*	Liver Disease 5,744	Cerebrovascular 9,653	Bronchitis, Emphysema, Asthma 97,896	Bronchitis, Emphysema, Asthma 112,584
Heart Disease 3,207	HIV 5,746	Cerebrovascular 5,709	Diabetes 8,705	Pneumonia & Influenza 82,989	**Unintentional Injuries 97,835**
HIV 2,912	***Homicide 3,567***	*Suicide 5,131*	**Unintentional Injuries 7,340**	Diabetes 48,974	Pneumonia & Influenza 91,871
Cerebrovascular 670	Liver Disease 3,370	Diabetes 4,386	Liver Disease 5,279	**Unintentional Injuries 32,975**	Diabetes 64,751
Diabetes 636	Cerebrovascular 2,650	HIV 3,120	Pneumonia & Influenza 3,856	Nephritis 22,640	*Suicide 30,575*
Pneumonia & Influenza 531	Diabetes 1,885	Bronchitis, Emphysema, Asthma 2,828	*Suicide 2,963*	Alzheimer's Disease 22,416	Nephritis 26,182
Liver Disease 506	Pneumonia & Influenza 1,400	Pneumonia & Influenza 2,167	Septicemia 2,093	Septicemia 19,012	Liver Disease 25,192

bad luck. Injury prevention efforts reflected and inadvertently supported this belief by encouraging people to adopt safe and responsible behaviors or by blaming the victims for the events that led to their injuries or deaths. Most attempts at injury prevention focused on training individuals to be more careful, a preoccupation with what Leon Robertson called "[a] basic cultural theme . . . that sufficient education will resolve almost any problem."[16] The concept that injury, like disease, is the product of the interaction of a human host and an agent within the environment and can therefore be examined using epidemiologic methods first appeared in the public health literature in 1949.[17] More than a century after epidemiologists knew that explaining the development of epidemics as the consequence of individual behaviors was inaccurate and ineffective for the development of preventive strategies. This and later developments in injury control are discussed in a comprehensive article by Julian Waller.[18] Dr. Waller, a pioneer of the injury field, is one of many who advocated for the removal of the term *accident* from discussions of injury.[19] This was promoted to draw attention to the fact that injuries do not exhibit the randomness conveyed by the term *accident* and that injuries can be explained using scientific methods common to public health.[20]

The late Dr. William Haddon, considered by many to be the father of injury epidemiology, refined the understanding of the role of energy as the agent of injury. Injury, as now defined within the injury community, is "any unintentional damage to the body resulting from acute exposure to thermal, mechanical, electrical, or chemical energy or from the absence of such essentials as heat or oxygen."[21] For an energy transfer (or energy deprivation) to occur, a human host and the agent of injury must interact within an environment. Interaction of host, agent, and environmental factors produces both the injury and the eventual outcome from that injury. This pivotal work of identifying the agent of injury and the vehicle (or carrier of the energy) and refining the relationships of host, agent, and environment in producing injury and its outcomes resulted in the development of the Haddon Phase-Factor Matrix.[22] This tool is still an important and frequently used conceptual framework in injury epidemiology and is explained in detail later. Despite these contributions, and later efforts to reject "accident proneness" as an explanation for childhood injuries,[23] the tendency to look at human behavior as the root of the injury problem and to focus prevention efforts on changing those behaviors is still pervasive. Individual knowledge, attitudes, beliefs, and behaviors are very important factors in injury prevention, as is the role of education and health behavior change; but to develop effective, sustainable injury prevention strategies, we must expand our field of vision beyond the individual. In short, we must subject injury problems to thorough scrutiny before we act.

IDENTIFYING AND DEFINING THE INJURY PROBLEM

The focus of trauma management is on the individual and his or her unique combination of injuries. The focus of injury prevention is much broader. Injury is a health problem of populations and, as such, must be identified on more than a case-by-case basis. Thereafter, it may be grouped and defined in several ways. Knowing how a problem was identified and how it has been defined is critical at all levels of injury prevention. For example, a trauma nurse interested in an area of tertiary prevention, such as optimizing functional outcome following severe head injury, may decide to review articles about management protocols and patient outcomes. The patients in Study I may seem to do much better than those in Study II. The nurse may decide to further investigate or even consider implementing the management protocols used by Study I. However, to implement these protocols would be unwise; essential preliminary information has been ignored. We cannot begin to compare differences in outcome unless we understand the differences in input. How are the hospitals and the patient populations in Studies I and II similar and different? What were the criteria used to determine the severity of injury in the study? Were penetrating head injuries included or excluded? Were all deaths reported, or only those that occurred after admission and within a defined time frame after injury? What was the average time to admission? If Study I included many cases that were transfers from other centers, early deaths in the transfer population are essentially excluded, thus reducing the total case fatality rate. What was the average age of the patients? What were the causes of the head injuries in the two studies? Were the patients comparable in terms of total injury severity? These considerations apply throughout all levels of prevention. For example, studying the protective effect of bicycle helmets or child passenger restraints in populations receiving trauma care fails to reveal those persons who are protected so effectively that they do not require any medical management. The issue of assessing exposure remains a great challenge to the injury prevention community. It is therefore important not only to gather information about the injury problem, but also to be familiar with the source of that information and how the injury population of interest was defined.

Even more important to trauma professionals is the awareness that the quality of the trauma team's documentation influences the quality and value of sources of injury data. Hospital records and death certificates are important sources of data. Health professionals must realize that the information they document in the trauma facility will find its way into aggregate data sets that are used for research and policy development. For example, our national injury fatality data are based on vital statistics data. These, of course, are derived from information reported on death certificates. Other important research data sets such as the Fatal Analysis Reporting System (FARS) of the National Highway Traffic Safety Administration also use vital statistics data. Data errors or omissions originating in the hospital can therefore affect the ultimate quality of our national data. Even more important is the fact that injury coding and classification systems use data contained in patients' records. Illegible, ambiguous, inaccurate, contradictory, or missing information compromises our ability to develop and maintain accurate data systems. An elderly patient who succumbs to pneumonia after sustaining a hip fracture will appear as a "natural death" in vital statistics data if the initiating event, the fall, is not clearly documented in medical records and on the death certificate. Information from emergency medical providers, such as the circumstances of a car crash or the use of restraints, will be lost if not documented. Careful and thorough reporting of information available on the etiology, clinical course, and outcome of the injury is in itself a contribution to injury prevention.

Definition of the injury problem of interest is a critical—and often ignored—step that must precede attempts to survey, measure, investigate, or prevent injuries. An injury problem can be defined in many different ways, and it is important that all stakeholders involved in the prevention initiative understand and agree on the working definition before action is taken. Although an injury problem definition may include clinical variables such as severity, it may be a purely social or political definition such as "injuries occurring in the uninsured." The following section presents examples of variables used in defining injury problems.

Most commonly, injuries are reported by severity: fatal, severe, moderate, minor. Surrogates for actual injury severity (e.g., hospital admissions, emergency department visits, ambulatory care visits, length of stay) are also common in the injury literature. Trauma nurses are familiar with identifying injuries by body region (head injury, spinal cord injury, maxillofacial injury, lower extremity injury) or by the nature of injury (burns, penetrating injuries, blunt force injury). Injury can also be defined using statements of the population at risk: the pediatric population, the elderly, adolescents, pregnant women, construction workers, urban populations, rural populations, minority groups, and gender groups. The setting or circumstances in which injury occurs may also be used to define the injuries of interest. Sport and recreational injuries, injuries in school or day care, occupational injuries, injuries occurring in nursing homes, injuries occurring between intimate partners, and injuries in the home are examples of such definitions.

An important way of classifying injury is by intent: unintentional or intentional. Unintentional injury, sometimes referred to in lay terms as "accidental" injury, includes: motor vehicle and other transportation injury, drowning, fire and burn injury, falls, sport and recreational injury, and other injuries, such as needle stick injuries, that occur unintentionally. Intentional injuries are the result of intended actions. This does not necessarily mean that the final result was intended. For example, one person may strike another intentionally without intending to kill that person. Of course, there are many intentional injuries for which both the final outcome and the action were intended. Intentional injuries may be self-inflicted (completed suicide, attempted suicide, and other self-destructive behaviors such as self-mutilation) or inflicted on another. This latter category, assaults and homicides, receives much public attention. Although this is entirely appropriate and necessary because firearm injuries have become the leading cause of death in some groups and areas of the nation, many health care providers may be surprised to realize that firearm suicides outnumber firearm homicides or that, overall, intentional injuries are far less common than unintentional injuries.[2,4,24]

For some types of injuries, intent is hard to determine. Examples are carbon monoxide poisoning, drowning, and drug intoxication. When confronted with a person who has died as a result of a drug overdose, there is a possibility that this is an unintended overdose. It could also be a suicide or even a homicide if the supplier contaminated the supplied substance intentionally. Many factors are considered when determining the manner of death ("accidental," suicide, homicide, or undetermined). For almost all injury deaths, whether early or late, determining manner of death is the responsibility of the medical examiner or coroner. The criteria used to do this vary slightly by jurisdiction and must therefore be understood by those wishing to identify categories of deaths, especially if deaths in several jurisdictions are to be compared.

One of the problems with identifying and defining deaths by intent is that it may break out, and therefore diminish, the apparent magnitude of deaths from the same mechanism. Reporting injuries and deaths using a matrix approach that places primary emphasis on the cause (or mechanism) of injury and only secondary emphasis on intent is a recent development in the injury field, one with great value for injury prevention policy development.[2] For example, in 1998 firearms accounted for 68% of homicides and 58% of suicides but only 1% of unintentional injury deaths.[24] The social burden of firearms is most apparent when one focuses primarily on the proportion of all injury deaths that are the result of firearm injury. In 1995 firearms accounted for 24% of all injury deaths, second only to motor vehicles at 29%.[2]

The role of alcohol is an example of a problem that is magnified as one looks beyond individual mechanisms of injury. Approximately 40% of an annual 100,000 alcohol abuse-related deaths result from trauma.[25] The relationship between alcohol consumption and motor vehicle crashes is well described in the scientific literature and kept in the public eye by the tireless efforts of the country's most successful grassroots advocacy organization, Mothers Against Drunk Driving (MADD).[26] Less well known by the public is the association between alcohol consumption and numerous other types of injury such as boating; and drowning deaths, violence, domestic violence, and recreational injury.[27,28] Trauma has been called a "symptom of alcoholism," an opinion supported by numerous investigators.[27,29-31] Alcohol intoxication on initial admis-

sion is also associated with a 2.5-fold increase in the likelihood that the patient will be readmitted for trauma in the future.[30] Although alcohol involvement in trauma has decreased by approximately 25% in the past decade, conservative estimates still implicate alcohol and illicit drugs in 19% of the estimated 2.2 million trauma patients hospitalized each year.[28] A recent study of seriously injured trauma center patients found that a high percentage of patients were at risk for a current psychoactive substance use disorder and that this group's prevalence of current alcohol dependence was nearly three times higher than estimates for US residents 15 to 54 years of age.[31] Detecting and managing alcohol-related problems in trauma patients poses an enormous challenge to the trauma care system.

Defining the injury problem is a difficult step in program development, but injury prevention programs developed without adequate definition will flounder. If we pursue a medical analogy, problem definition is the beginning of the diagnostic process. A 70-year-old woman has presented to your emergency department with a hip fracture after a fall. Fall-related hip fractures in elderly women are a common and well-identified injury problem. But fall-related hip fractures occur in very different circumstances. A broad definition of the problem may be useful when measuring the total burden of fall-related hip fractures in elderly women, but it is inadequate as the basis for an intervention. We wish to prevent falls in the elderly in relation to the following:

- Group (age range, gender, community-dwelling, patients with existing disabilities such as visual impairment, frequent fallers)
- Region (the country, the state, a community, a residential facility)
- Environments (individual homes, nursing homes, recreational facilities, the street, the work place, unfamiliar environments)
- Circumstances (ice, rain, on stairs, when getting up at night, in the shower, when taking certain medications, during dementia transitions)
- Severity (any fall, any injury, any fracture, hip fracture, traumatic brain injury)
- Consequences (injury requiring hospitalization, disabling injury, injury requiring that the person be placed in an elder-care facility, falls that cause elders to restrict their activities from fear of subsequent falls)
- Other social considerations (falls in the uninsured, falls in patients of a certain health maintenance organization [HMO], falls in persons with a history of falls, falls that result in litigation)

Careful definition of the problem is the foundation for all future analyses. It may help to ask yourself this question: "What is the specific problem I need to solve, and why?" If the answer is not clear, an intervention cannot be focused adequately. Definitions of injury problems may also evolve over time as our knowledge, awareness, and social practices change. The area of child passenger safety is one such example. At one time the problem definition for deaths and injuries to child motor vehicle occupants might have been that child passengers were unrestrained in cars. An early study by another pioneer of the injury prevention field, Professor Susan Baker, defined a specific problem: disproportionately high injury and death rates in infant passengers. Her work laid the foundation for the development of rear-facing infant seats.[32] Next came the realization that children needed special restraints, but the public's awareness of this fact was low. Attention was given, appropriately, to building public awareness, passing child restraint laws, and making child safety seats available. As safety seat usage rates increased, so did awareness of a new problem: restraint misuse. It was not enough that people knew they should restrain their child in a safety seat, that they purchased a seat, or that they used it all the time. New problems were defined: car seat-vehicle incompatibility, high levels of incorrect use, and the problem of rear-facing infant seats placed in front of an air bag. Most recently, there is growing realization that our almost exclusive attention to the youngest children (up to 4 years of age) and our nonspecific "Buckle Up" message for older children has left the 4- to 8-year-olds inadequately protected in vehicles.[33] National attention is now focused on increasing booster seat use in children in the 40- to 80-pound weight range (4- to 8-year-olds), who cannot be restrained adequately by adult seat belts.[34]

Evolving problem definitions require similar evolvement of injury prevention initiatives. For example, 24 years after the first statewide child passenger safety law was passed in Tennessee, Washington State's Anton Skeen Law (HB 2675) will take effect on July 1, 2002.[35] This bill, signed into law during the 2000 legislative session, is the first state law in the United States to require booster seat use. Members of the trauma and emergency medical communities played active advocacy roles to help ensure passage of the law. Other child passenger safety laws and prevention initiatives of yesterday will have to be revised to keep pace with the changing understanding of what is required to protect this age group in motor vehicles. The critical lesson here is that problem definitions are not universally relevant. Time invested in this problem definition stage of the problem-solving process will reduce subsequent frustration and enhance the potential for success.

MEASURING THE INJURY PROBLEM

Once identified and defined, the injury problem should be measured. Measurement is important for several reasons, including resource procurement and allocation, intervention planning and delivery, and evaluation. The choice of measurement criteria is influenced by data availability, time, and needs. When presented with an injury problem, begin with some triage questions:
What is the magnitude of this injury?

- Incidence (the number of new cases of an injury that occur during a specified period of time in a population at risk for that injury)[36]

- Prevalence (the number of affected persons with a particular injury present in the population at a specified time divided by the number of persons in the population at that time)[36]

What is the severity of the injury?

- High case fatality (such as firearm injuries or suicide attempts)
- Low case fatality (such as playground injuries) in high numbers
- High morbidity (such as traumatic brain injury, spinal cord injury, severe lower extremity injury, hip fracture in the elderly, and burns)

How preventable is the injury?

- Do we have proven interventions that can be used to prevent this injury (e.g., bicycle helmets, seat belts, product modification)?
- Are there distinct clusters of injuries (clustering of injuries suggests that specific environmental risk factors are present)?

What are the costs of this injury?

- Are there direct costs such as financial costs of medical care (both acute and long term) and other nonmedical goods and services related to the injury (e.g., "costs for home modifications, vocational rehabilitation, administrative costs for health and indemnity insurance")?[37]
- Are there indirect morbidity costs (i.e., "the value of foregone productivity due to injury-related illness and disability") and mortality costs (i.e., "the value of foregone productivity due to death at an early age")?[37]
- Do additional costs include those associated with property damage, police and fire services, and legal fees related to compensation; and social costs such as pain, suffering, quality of life, lost human potential, and disrupted families? [37]
- Is some group disproportionately affected (e.g., young, urban African-American men; elderly women; children in custody; health care workers)?
- What is the public's interest in this injury problem (e.g., will the public support stronger child passenger safety laws; are they aware that firearms are used more frequently in suicides than in homicides; do they care whether a child's playground is safe and well maintained)?
- What are the consequences of not acting to prevent this problem (e.g., with a rapidly aging population, can we afford to ignore the problem of injuries in the elderly)?

Answering these questions adequately often involves significant training and effort. A complete discussion of measurement methods is beyond the scope of this chapter. Nevertheless, much time, money, effort, and expertise is devoted to measuring the burden of injury, and there are many valuable data resources available to those interested in determining the magnitude of an injury problem. A list of such resources is included later in this chapter.

Even without extensive resources, it is possible to work through the checklist (previously listed), as one might work through a triage situation, to guide decision making about optimal use of resources. When, for example, a high-profile injury death triggers public interest and demands that action be taken, should we respond with a prevention initiative? Is this one of many similar deaths and injuries? If so, we may use the heightened awareness to generate support for prevention initiatives. If this turns out to be a relatively rare but emerging injury problem, we would be wise to invest our resources in learning more about the injury through data collection and surveillance before we intervene. If, however, this is a truly rare event, can we justify allocating any resources to this problem at the expense of other more significant problems?

Measurement is important to determine the extent of the injury problem, but it is also critical to our ability to evaluate the effectiveness of interventions or any shifts in injury patterns that may be occurring as a result of interventions. Careful measurement of the injury problem is a wise investment.

IDENTIFYING KEY DETERMINANTS

Having identified, defined, and measured the injury problem, one must begin the diagnostic process required to determine the causal factors associated with the problem. Injuries do not occur in a vacuum. In order to prevent injuries, or reduce their severity, one must understand the circumstances in which they happen. As with infectious and chronic diseases, the six basic questions of epidemiology apply: *what* is happening to *whom; when, where, why,* and *how*? These supposedly simple questions are problematic because what we see when we examine a situation is a function of where and how we look. If, for example, we are convinced that teenage drivers are fundamentally unsafe, we may assume on hearing of a single-vehicle crash in which a teenage boy died that the crash was the result of human error—another tragic example of teenage risk-taking. But what if we were to visit the crash site and find that the road was narrow, winding, and lined with trees? What if we were to look at police crash records or newspaper reports and find that several other single-vehicle crashes involving drivers of different ages had occurred in this location? What if several other similar crashes had occurred but drivers of small-sized vehicles were the only ones to die? Most injuries occur within environments that human beings have made; understanding the contribution of environmental factors is therefore essential.

Typically, numerous factors interact to produce an injury and its outcome. In focusing prevention efforts on the most obvious factor—usually human behavior—we ignore other critical factors that may in fact be more modifiable than human behavior. The history of efforts to prevent child

pedestrian injury is one such example. The road environment is complex; navigating it safely requires significant cognitive ability not present in children before the age of 9 years.[38,39] Despite this understanding, when a 5-year-old child is killed or injured as a pedestrian, it is not uncommon to read the phrase "pedestrian error" on the police report. Even when an unsupervised child runs into a road at 10 pm, the incident is frequently called "accidental." Over the years the majority of pedestrian safety programs have focused on persuading and training children to be safer pedestrians and have shown little success. But why should an exclusively child-focused approach work? If we pause to look beyond the victim, we will see numerous other factors that contribute to these injuries: design of the road, traffic speed, traffic density, signage, visibility, size and design of the vehicle, driver training, driver awareness and behavior (including substance use), supervision of children, presence of distractions (e.g., dogs, balls, other children), child's level of exposure to the traffic environment, level of traffic enforcement, and legal and social consequences of hitting a child pedestrian. Individually each of these factors may influence the child's risk of injury. Together their interaction produces a set of circumstances that either supports or discourages the likelihood of pedestrian injury. Examining the presence and interactions of these factors in a systematic way is an important problem-solving step.

Factors that are important precursors of a public health problem, and therefore possible targets for prevention initiatives, may be referred to as *key determinants*.[15] Key determinants may be numerous. It is important therefore that one employ an organizational framework to examine these multiple factors and their interactions in a logical manner. Usually organization of key determinants begins by grouping factors. The organizational framework used most commonly in injury problem solving is the Haddon Phase-Factor Matrix. As shown in Table 7-2, the Haddon Matrix is a 3 × 4 table. The four factors of the matrix are human (individual) factors, agent (and carrier) factors, physical environmental factors, and social environmental factors.[40] Identifying these factors and assessing their relative importance is crucial to the development of effective prevention strategies. A second important concept is that, although the energy transfer occurs quickly, it is only one part of a dynamic process. Haddon described three phases representing stages in a time continuum that begins before the injury occurs and ends with the outcome. These phases are known as the *pre-event*, the *event*, and the *post-event* phases.[40] The interaction of factors in the *pre-event phase* determines whether an event (such as a car crash) that has the potential to cause injury will occur. Factors interacting in the *event phase* influence whether or not an injury will result from this event and what the type and severity of that injury will be. Finally, the interactions in the *post-event phase* determine the consequences (short- and long-term outcomes) of the injury.

The Haddon Matrix can be used in several ways. Most commonly it is used to think about the factors involved in an injury problem. Becoming familiar with the literature on the

TABLE 7-2	The Haddon Phase-Factor Matrix: Factors Associated with Motor Vehicle Crashes			
FACTORS→ ↓PHASES	Human (Individual Factors)	Agent and Vehicle	Environment: Physical	Environment: Social
Pre-event	Age, gender, visual acuity, alcohol or other substance use, fatigue, distraction, cell phone use, risk-taking behavior, driving skill and experience, reaction time, exposure (frequency of travel)	Vehicle design (road-holding ability, rollover risk, braking capacity) and maintenance, condition of tires, visibility (e.g., daytime running lights)	Design and maintenance of roadway, traffic density and flow, condition of road surface (wet, icy, oil slick, etc.), weather, visibility, traffic control (signals, lights, signage), animals and other obstacles in roadway	Speed limits, licensing laws and restrictions, impaired driving laws, motor vehicle occupant restraint laws (for all ages), regulations limiting driving hours for truck drivers, regulations limiting cell phone use, vehicle maintenance regulations, road rage
Event	Restraint use, age-related health status, preexisting conditions such as osteoporosis, position in vehicle	Speed, size, and crash-tolerance of vehicle; type of restraint systems (seat belts, air bags, child safety seats); interior surface hazards (e.g., protruding handles)	Roadway design: median dividers, guardrails, breakaway poles, roadside hazards (e.g., trees, parked vehicles)	Enforcement of speed limits and restraint laws
Post-event	Age and preexisting co-morbidities that may influence clinical course	Integrity of fuel system, vehicle design-related barriers to extrication	Urban/rural location, distance from emergency medical services, barriers to extrication and emergency management	Good Samaritan laws, bystander assistance, planning, and delivery of emergency medical services, quality of trauma care and re-habilitation, insurance and compensation practices, psychosocial support structure, job retraining

injury problem of interest before filling out the matrix will help identify possible risk factors that may otherwise be ignored. Not only does the Haddon Matrix help us to think outside the box (the *blame the victim* box), but it also helps us identify what we need to find out about the problem. For example, do we have reliable data on restraint use? Do we know how many of the children who do not wear bicycle helmets already own a helmet? The value of the Haddon Matrix is that it illustrates the multifactorial etiology of injury. A potential problem it creates, however, is that one may feel lost in a maze of causal factors. Faced with so much information, some preventionists complain that it is difficult to know what to target. To overcome this problem, it is necessary to take another step. Look at all the factors listed in the matrix and ask, Which of these factors is (are) controllable? For example, we cannot change an elderly woman's age, but we may be able to enhance her general health status, her muscle tone, or her balance. Next look at the list of modifiable factors and consider which of these changes is

the most likely to be accomplished. For example, which of the following is most likely to be accomplished: teaching 16-year-old drivers to drive safely or limiting their crash exposure through graduated licensing programs? Look at this final list to determine whether altering the variable would change the outcome significantly. For example, emergency medical services (EMS) response time is modifiable, but some injury mechanisms, such as firearm injury and drowning, result in such severe injuries that enhanced EMS alone does not have the potential to reduce the death toll significantly. This process forms the basis of causal thinking, which is critical to intervention and evaluation planning and is discussed in the next section.

IDENTIFYING POTENTIAL INTERVENTION STRATEGIES

Once the problem is diagnosed and the factor(s) to be targeted with intervention(s) identified (the change targets), the mechanism that will be used to achieve the desired

TABLE 7-3   **The Haddon Strategies Applied**
1. **Prevent creation of the hazard.**
Do not manufacture three-wheeled all-terrain vehicles (ATVs), certain types of ammunition and certain poisons; ban human pyramids
2. **Reduce amount of the hazard.**
Limit pills per container, decrease water temperature in homes, limit contact drills in football
3. **Prevent release of the hazard.**
Provide handrails for the elderly, improve braking capability of vehicles, reduce alcohol use by drivers
4. **Alter release of the hazard.**
Blister packaging of pills, child safety seats and seat belts to control deceleration forces, release bindings on skis
5. **Separate person and hazard in time and space.**
Bike and pedestrian paths, remove trees near roadways, evacuate hurricane paths
6. **Place barrier between the person and the hazard.**
Bike helmets, childproof closures, four-sided pool fencing, protective goggles, insulation of electric cords
7. **Modify basic qualities of the hazard.**
Breakaway poles near roadways, energy-absorbing surfacing, shatterproof glass in windshields
8. **Strengthen resistance to the hazard.**
Prevent osteoporosis, promote muscle conditioning in athletes, apply earthquake and hurricane building codes
9. **Begin to counter damage done.**
Early detection: smoke detectors, road-side phones, early warning systems, emergency response systems
10. **Stabilize, repair damage, and rehabilitate.**
Treatment, rehabilitation, vocational and self-care retraining, modification of environment for disabled

Modified from Baker SP, O'Neill B, and Ginsburg MJ et al: *The injury fact book,* ed 2, New York, 1992, Oxford University Press; and Haddon W Jr: The basic strategies for preventing damage from hazards of all kinds, *Hazard Prevent* 16:8-12, 1980.

change must be identified. The danger at this point is a "knee-jerk" response when selecting an intervention. The easiest, most obvious, most affordable, or most acceptable strategy is seldom the most effective. As is the case when selecting treatment modalities for injured patients, one's knowledge of the range of potential injury prevention strategies is critical when choosing prevention options. Another legacy of Dr. William Haddon is his list of 10 injury control strategies that can be applied to all types of injury.[40-42] These strategies address the control of hazards with the potential to cause injury, but each targets a different point along a continuum between creation of the hazard and the final outcome. These strategies, with examples of their application, are presented in Table 7-3.

The Haddon strategies describe the countermeasures that must be put in place to prevent the occurrence of injury, reduce its severity, or achieve the best possible outcome from the injury. In essence, they describe an *end* we wish to achieve. The *means* we take to achieve that end may vary. For example, when faced with the problem of young children being poisoned when they ingest multivitamins containing

iron, we may decide to implement Haddon strategy two: *reduce the amount of the hazard.* We eliminate strategy one, *prevent creation of the hazard,* as an option because iron-containing vitamins exist for valid health reasons, and we cannot justify not producing them. Because a major group of users of these products, pregnant and lactating women, are also likely to have children of ages at high risk for ingestion, we must accept that exposure to the hazard (iron-containing vitamins) is probable. The strongest possible (most upstream) intervention is therefore necessary. Strategy two is much more upstream than the now widely used strategy six: *placing a barrier between the child and the hazard* with childproof closures or use of safe storage such as locked cabinets. It also addresses the dose-response nature of iron-ingestion poisoning. Having selected *reducing the amount of the hazard* as our strategy, we must identify means to that end. An educational approach might be to educate mothers (and grandparents) of young children to buy small containers of the medication. A technologic solution might be to manufacture vitamins with lower unit doses so that a child would have to ingest greater quantities of the pills before reaching a toxic dose. A regulatory approach might be to mandate warning labels on containers or limited dose dispensing of the vitamins or to restrict their over-the-counter distribution. Often we combine approaches for maximum effect. For example, we may limit over-the-counter availability of the vitamins, require that they be dispensed in a child-resistant container, and provide educational materials about the risk of iron-containing vitamins to those who purchase them.

In general we aim to intervene as early in the causal chain as possible. An analogy used in the injury prevention community is finding multiple people drowning in a river. Do we focus our efforts downstream on pulling them out of the water one by one and attempting resuscitation, or do we walk upstream to find out why they are all falling (or being pushed) into the river? In the acute care setting, the trauma nurse is the rescuer downstream. Nurses who embrace (directly or indirectly) a primary prevention role move upstream to deal with the factors that led to the trauma epidemic. Fortunately for injury prevention, some trauma professionals have found it possible to do both. Indeed, for accreditation purposes, some trauma services are required to demonstrate involvement in prevention.[43] Comprehensive prevention requires work at all levels of the continuum. Investing all our efforts and resources downstream will never be enough to control the injury epidemic. Furthermore, if we fail to monitor activities and trends *upstream,* we cannot equip ourselves to deal with future consequences *downstream.*

Perhaps the greatest challenge to identifying effective primary prevention strategies is preoccupation with the individual: the *blame the victim, train the victim* paradigm. It has been said that "no mass disorder afflicting mankind was ever brought under control or eliminated by attempts at treating the individual."[44] Injury is, indeed, a mass disorder requiring urgent preventive action. To control this problem we must move beyond talking to individuals about safety and embrace the wide range of intervention options available to us.

Intervention strategies fall into four main categories, sometimes called the Four Es:

1. Education (and behavior change)
2. Engineering (and technology)
3. Enforcement (and legislation)
4. Economic approaches (incentives and disincentives)

Each of these approaches is described in the following sections.

Education encompasses a wide range of strategies that range from one-on-one education to initiatives that educate society and eventually influence social norms. Health education and health promotion, although criticized by some in the past as ineffective, have much to offer the field if used strategically. We must, however, move beyond a preoccupation with reaching individuals with brochures, fliers, posters, and overcrowded informational displays. Effective prevention frequently requires modification of the nature of the hazard or of the physical or social environment, which is usually the purview of *engineering* or *enforcement*. This has led to suggestions that we should focus on engineering solutions rather than educational approaches. In reality there is no place for either/or; we need both.[45] Little is accomplished in our society without the commitment and involvement of groups of people. Mobilization of this valuable resource—be it parents, health care providers, legislators, law enforcement agencies, the media, product manufacturers, or funding agencies—requires the ability to influence knowledge, attitudes, beliefs, and behaviors. The behavioral sciences can also help us identify barriers to change and those factors that predispose, enable, or reinforce change, whether at the individual or national level. Trauma nurses who wish to present educational programs are encouraged to identify, and consider as a resource, professional health educators and behavioral scientists in their organizations and communities.

Engineering involves *engineering out the hazard* (such as designing safer products and safer roadways) or using engineering and technology to protect the person in an energy-transfer situation (helmets, restraint systems, crumple zones in cars, automatic sprinkler systems). After injury has occurred, engineering approaches include the development of technology to enhance early warning and emergency response and, of course, the technology associated with management, rehabilitation, and reintegration of the injured person into society. Many of the injury hazards in today's world are the result of products or environments that we have created with technology. It is not surprising, therefore, that technology is an important part of the solution. Engineering interventions to prevent injury are so pervasive in our society, however, that we may not notice them, take them for granted, and forget how relatively recent these achievements are. The fact that safety sells, so evident in current motor vehicle advertising campaigns, is a very recent development in our society and the result of years of injury prevention and consumer advocacy. Indeed, each step forward in road design, product modification, product labeling, policy and legislation, and changed social norms about injury has been hard won.

Enforcement is an oversimplified term for a wide-ranging area that involves the development and enforcement of law, regulation, and policy. Federal, state, and local laws and regulations have been used to advance injury prevention in numerous and varied ways.[5] For example, laws and regulations have been used to establish and fund federal safety programs; create a mandate for emergency medical services systems development; mandate E-coding in 23 states; require the use of seat belts, car seats, bicycle helmets, and other safety equipment; establish speed limits and traffic control regulations; regulate the manufacture and distribution of consumer products; set safety standards for schools, school buses, child care facilities, health care settings, and the workplace; control high-risk behaviors such as drunk driving; establish building codes; set standards for vehicle design and performance; and create trauma registries and other data systems. Tort law or private litigation has been used successfully to protect the public from unsafe products.[5] This has been achieved in several ways, including seeking compensation for victims of negligence and deterring, through liability, negligent practices by companies.[46,47]

Despite numerous successes, gaps in some existing laws compromise both coverage and effectiveness.[5] Additionally, the effect of any law, regulation, or policy is closely linked to its enforcement. Challenges to enforcement are not limited to inadequate law-enforcement resources. Those responsible for enforcing a law or policy must believe in the law, their ability to enforce it, and the utility of that enforcement. Building support for enforcement may be as important as creating public support for the law if it is to be implemented. Many injury prevention laws encounter powerful opponents and are challenged or overturned. Achieving passage of and defending injury prevention legislation usually requires extensive and prolonged advocacy efforts and compelling data. In 1981 Lawrence Berger suggested six conditions to be met when contemplating the implementation of injury legislation. These are that one

---

be thoroughly convinced that the bill addresses a strikingly important issue. One should have evidence that the bill's action can be effective; support from judges and police officers that the law can be enforced expeditiously; economic estimates that excessive costs will not be involved; legal counsel confirming the constitutionality and compatibility of the proposed law with existing legislation and ordinances; and broad-based support from constituents.[48]

Clearly, writing, passing, and implementing injury prevention laws is not the sole responsibility of lawyers, legislators, and the law-enforcement community.[49] Elizabeth McLoughlin, a tireless injury prevention activist, has documented many of the lessons learned in California's prolonged efforts to achieve legislation requiring the use of helmets by motorcyclists.[50] One valuable advocacy lesson, which she continues to develop and apply in other areas of injury prevention, is the power of using "the authentic voice of survivors and family members who have been affected" in support of legislation.[50,51] Because of their expertise and personal experience of caring for trauma victims, trauma nurses can make valuable contributions when they join efforts to develop and advocate the passage and implementation of injury prevention laws.

Economic incentives—or in many cases disincentives—are employed to persuade people or organizations to adopt safe practices or behaviors. Examples include fines for traffic offenses, increased insurance premiums, withholding of federal funds, and financial penalties imposed by courts on the manufacturers of unsafe products. Positive incentives include lowered insurance premiums for safe drivers or those buying safer vehicles and incentives to corporations that provide safe working environments.

To be effective, interventions must target the risk factors. The relationship between the chosen intervention and the risk factor we hope to change must be stated explicitly. For example, if an identified risk factor for adolescent bicycle-crash-related head injury in your community is that teens do not own helmets, helmet distribution would be a logical intervention choice. Helmet distribution would not be a logical choice if the identified risk factor is teenagers' refusal to wear helmets even if they have them.

The Haddon Matrix can be used in a second way to assist in the identification of possible interventions. This is accomplished by thinking about what interventions might be used to address risk factors present in different cells of the matrix. Pre-event phase interventions attempt to reduce the number of events with the potential to cause injury: prevent car and bike crashes, falls, house fires, ingestion of poisons, assaults, and so on. Examples of such interventions would

be graduated licensing programs for teenage drivers, limiting the number of hours driven without rest by truck drivers, enforcing speed limits, passing legislation that penalizes people caught driving while intoxicated, putting traffic-calming measures in place in areas with many pedestrians, mandating use of safety harnesses for construction workers, enforcing building standards in nursing homes, and closing beaches when there are strong currents.

Event phase interventions attempt to reduce the number and severity of injuries that occur in these events. Examples include seatbelts and air bags, enhanced vehicle crashworthiness, bicycle helmets and handlebar design, bulletproof vests for police officers, smoke detectors and automatic sprinkler systems, controlling access to lethal weapons, prevention of osteoporosis, and physical conditioning of athletes.

Post-event phase interventions attempt to prevent complications and optimize outcome. Those most familiar to the trauma nurse include emergency medical management, medical care, and rehabilitation. Others include improving the integrity of vehicle gas tanks to reduce the chances of post-crash fires, early detection and notification of injury, preventing entrapment, improving health insurance status and social support structures (to optimize rehabilitation), and job retraining.

Injury prevention also employs active and passive strategies. An *active* strategy is one that requires a person to act each time he or she, or the person he or she hopes to protect, is to be protected. A *passive* strategy will afford protection without action on the part of the person to be protected. All intervention strategies lie on a continuum from entirely active to entirely passive. Seat belts, for example, are not entirely active. They require that a person fasten the seat belt each time he or she gets into the vehicle, but, once fastened, the belt will protect the person for the duration of the trip. Figure 7-1[52] illustrates the relationship

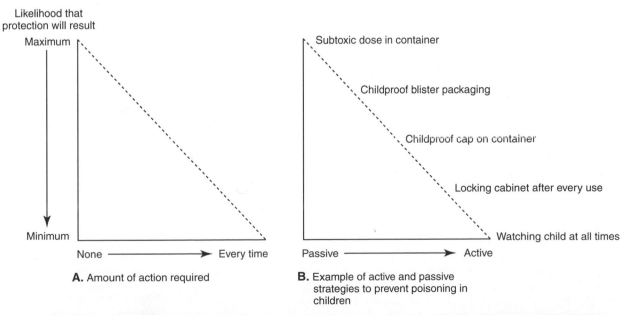

FIGURE 7-1 The Relationship Between the Amount of Action Required and the Likelihood That Protection Will Result. (Modified from Baker SP: Childhood injuries: the community approach to prevention, *J Public Health Policy* 2(3):235-246, 1981.)

between the type of strategy and the likelihood of prevention effectiveness.

An inverse relationship is observed: Prevention effectiveness increases as the need for action decreases. For this reason, whenever possible, injury prevention specialists will try to implement an intervention that is passive. In most cases, achieving passive strategies—such as modification of an unsafe product or environment—requires that some infrastructure be established. This infrastructure might be public support for a law or policy, designated funds for road improvement, legal and/or financial penalties for the manufacture of products that lead to injury, or an energetic advocacy effort.

Trauma nurses who feel uncomfortable with the idea of engineering or law and policy approaches may find it helpful to realize that they can contribute to these efforts in other ways. Increasingly, injury prevention efforts include comprehensive or multicomponent approaches and interdisciplinary collaborations. The *spectrum of prevention* (Table 7-4)[53,54] is a tool that has been used to encourage comprehensive programs that move beyond a purely educational approach. The six levels of the spectrum represent areas in which prevention initiatives can be implemented. The critical concept, however, is that the levels are synergistic; prevention effectiveness may be enhanced by creating strong linkages between the components. Level 3, *educating providers,* is of particular relevance to trauma nurses. Cohen and Swift emphasize that "providers have influence within their fields of expertise and opportunities to transmit information, skills and motivation to clients, and colleagues. It is essential, therefore, that they receive education to improve their own understanding of prevention." They go on to comment that certain professionals (such as trauma nurses) "can be highly effective advocates for policy changes related to their job experience."[53] When used with the Haddon Matrix, the spectrum can suggest systematic approaches to an injury problem.

Possible intervention strategies can be identified in many ways. The injury prevention literature is a rich source of information. Several injury prevention texts[5,9,21,41,55] devote chapters to different types of approaches. The excellent Web site of the Injury Control Resource Information Network (ICRIN) at the University of Pittsburgh (www.injurycontrol.com/icrin) can be searched by topic area and provides extensive links to other sites. Through it the trauma nurse can access the Center for Injury Prevention and Control of the Centers for Disease Control and Prevention (CDC), CDC-funded injury control research centers, federal agencies, and a wealth of injury prevention resources. Another valuable source of information on the effectiveness of injury prevention interventions—systematic reviews of childhood injury prevention interventions—can be found at the Web site of the Harborview Injury Prevention and Research Center in Seattle (depts.washington.edu/hiprc/childinjury). Trauma nurses are encouraged to browse the Web sites listed in Table 7-5 for further information about injury and injury prevention.

The range of possible interventions and access to information about them expand constantly. The main challenge to identifying intervention options is not a lack of information; it is failure to consider this information-gathering step an important part of the problem-solving process.

TABLE 7-4   The Spectrum of Prevention

Influencing Policy and Legislation
Developing strategies to change laws and policies
Changing organizational practices
Adopting regulations and shaping norms
Fostering coalitions and networks
Convening groups and individuals for greater impact
Educating providers
Informing providers who influence others
Promoting community education
Reaching groups with information and resources
Strengthening individual knowledge and skills
Enhancing individual capacity

Modified from Cohen L and Swift S: The spectrum of prevention: developing a comprehensive approach to injury prevention, *Inj Prev* 5(3): 203-207, 1999; and The Prevention Institute: [Prevention] tools and frameworks, www.preventioninstitute.org/tools.html.

TABLE 7-5   Selected Web Sites Containing Injury Prevention-Related Information.

Organization	Web Address
Injury Control Resource Information Network	www.injurycontrol.com/icrin
National Center for Injury Prevention and Control (CDC)	www.cdc.gov/ncipc
WISQARS (Scientific data and injury statistics from the National Center for Injury Prevention and Control)	www.cdc.gov/ncipc/osp/data.htm
American Trauma Society	www.amtrauma.org
Children's Safety Network	www.edc.org/hhd/csn
Consumer Product Safety Commission	www.cpsc.gov
Insurance Institute for Highway Safety	www.highwaysafety.org
National Highway Traffic Safety Administration	www.nhtsa.dot.gov
National Safe Kids Campaign	www.safekids.org
The Prevention Institute	www.preventioninstitute.org
The Trauma Foundation	www.tf.org

The sites listed here contain numerous links to other sites. Many have sophisticated search capability.

SELECTING A STRATEGY TO IMPLEMENT

At first the range of potential strategies may be intimidating. Recognizing the importance of technologic or regulatory strategies may cause a nurse comfortable with one-on-one patient encounters to feel inadequate. Even injury prevention specialists feel at times that the obstacles to achieving such interventions are insurmountable, causing some to retreat to easier, more familiar, or more immediate interventions. The Intervention Decision Matrix[56] is a simple tool designed to identify intervention options and choose between them (Table 7-6). It can also identify long-term goals and intervention options that support each other.

Seven elements of the Intervention Decision Matrix are used as decision criteria when selecting an intervention:

Effectiveness
Feasibility
Cost feasibility
Sustainability
Political acceptability
Social will
Possible unintended consequences

Effectiveness refers to the likelihood that the intervention will do what it is intended to do. Specifically, will the intervention reduce the number and/or severity of injuries? As discussed previously, a passive injury prevention strategy is more likely to be effective than an active strategy.

Feasibility refers to the likelihood that an intervention will happen. Is it technically possible, practical, achievable, and viable? Are safer products and technical solutions possible and available? Do they work? This is not a recommendation to choose low-risk and easily achieved interventions, for these are seldom effective. Rather, it cautions the enthusiastic preventionist to avoid trying to change the essentially unchangeable, such as the road-crossing abilities of 4-year-old pedestrians. Some of our most effective interventions have taken numerous years to achieve. Through the efforts of others, what was not feasible 10 years ago is feasible today.

Cost feasibility refers to the affordability of an intervention. At a time of limited resources, cost considerations are an important factor in intervention selection. The danger is that cost becomes the only consideration, to the detriment of effectiveness. Selecting an intervention with low effectiveness because it is the least expensive alternative squanders all resources. No matter how "affordable" an intervention appears to be, if it yields very low injury prevention returns, the cost per protected person will be enormous.

Sustainability refers to the potential for continued effect. It can be thought of in two ways:

1. Will the effect persist after the intervention is completed? For example, will driving in excess of the speed limit return to preenforcement levels when the police leave the site?
2. Will the intervention become institutionalized? For example, will it become the social norm that people wear seat belts? Will a community assume responsibility for the maintenance of a newly renovated playground?

Political acceptability can also be viewed in two ways:

1. Is the intervention ethical? Is it equitable? Is it constitutional? Does it violate human rights? Is it unreasonably intrusive? These, of course, are critical issues that must be weighed carefully when considering any intervention.
2. What is the prevailing political mood about this intervention? For example, it is often easier to pass legislation that requires protection of children than that protecting adults. Many areas of injury control are impeded by the fact that the political process creates barriers to interventions that compelling

TABLE 7-6 The Intervention Decision Matrix: Comparison of Interventions for Bicycle-Related Head Injury

INTERVENTIONS→ ↓DECISION CRITERIA	Bicycle Helmet Laws for Cyclists of All Ages	Bicycle Helmet Laws for Children	Education Campaign to Promote Bicycle Helmet Use	Road Design (Bike Paths, etc.)
Effectiveness	Moderate	Moderate	Low	Moderate
Feasibility	High	High	High	High
Cost feasibility	High	High	High	Low
Sustainability	Moderate	Moderate	Low	High
Political acceptability	Low	Moderate	High	Moderate
Social will	Low	Moderate	Moderate	Moderate
Potential for unintended consequences	Moderate	Low	Low	Moderate
INTERVENTION PRIORITY	**LOW**	**MODERATE**	**LOW**	**MODERATE**

Source: Fowler CJ and Dannenberg AL: *The intervention decision matrix*, rev ed, Baltimore, 1999, The Johns Hopkins Center for Injury Research and Policy.

scientific evidence and, in many cases, public opinion support. An intervention that has low political acceptability faces a major obstacle and alerts us to the need for awareness building. But, and this is important to remember, political obstacles of this type are not insurmountable.

Social will is the key to building constituent support and challenging political barriers. Low social will indicates the need to generate support for the initiative. This may be achieved in various ways but requires that the factors contributing to the low social will be assessed. People may be unaware of the problem, unconcerned about it, resistant to change, afraid of the cost or inconvenience of interventions, or too busy to care. Each reason requires a different remedial approach. The key issue is that, with time, social will and ultimately political barriers may be changed. If however low social will is a barrier to prevention, understanding and addressing the causes of this should be a priority. Attempting to implement interventions in settings where social will is low is like swimming against the current. Coalitions and informal networks that bring together diverse sectors of the community may help build social support for prevention initiatives.[53] As often-quoted social anthropologist Dr. Margaret Mead once said, "Never doubt that a small group of thoughtful, committed citizens can change the world. Indeed, it is the only thing that ever has."

Possible unintended consequences may be positive or negative and may result from any intervention. An important principle in injury control is, as in medicine, "First, do no harm." Some interventions with the potential to protect may also have the potential to cause harm. A recent example is the airbag-related deaths of approximately 70 children.[57] High school driver education courses that increased the driving exposure of 16-year-olds led to increases in motor vehicle crash involvement and death rates in this group. When courses were discontinued[58,59] or driving curfews imposed,[59,60] crashes were reduced substantially. In April 2000 the American Academy of Pediatrics issued a policy statement (RE 9940) discouraging swimming programs for children under the age of 4 years.[61] Many potentially harmful unintended consequences of early training were noted in the discussion, such as the fact that early lessons did not translate into higher levels of swimming proficiency; removal of a child's fear of water may inadvertently encourage an unsupervised child to enter the water; parents of trained children may develop a false sense of confidence in their child's ability; the lack of an established relationship between safety training and observed safety skills; and the potentially tragic consequences of even a brief lapse in supervision.[61]

PLANNING THE IMPLEMENTATION

A familiar saying, "Those who fail to plan, plan to fail," is wise counsel to anyone implementing injury prevention programs. Time invested in implementation planning will save time, resources, and frustration. Ideally, implementation and evaluation (discussed below) should be planned together. A prudent first step is to review factors that are key to successful implementation of education, engineering, and enforcement strategies. These factors, summarized in Table 7-7, are compiled from a comprehensive discussion of injury prevention by Sleet and Gielen.[62]

Next it is time to plan the implementation. Before taking any intervention actions, one should consider and document the following:

1. The project goal
2. Project objectives
3. Action steps (sometimes called process objectives)
4. The intended audience for each step
5. The methods/strategies to be used for each step
6. The indicators of success for each step
7. Evaluation methods for each step (discussed below)
8. A project timeline
9. A person (or group) responsible for each action step

The *project goal* is a statement of your project's destination. Ideally it should be specific and measurable within a reasonable time frame. It is not always practical to define outcomes as reductions in deaths and injuries. Although reducing the burden of injury is our ultimate goal, it may be

---

TABLE 7-7   Key Factors for Successful Implementation of Injury Prevention Strategies

For successful implementation of education and behavior strategies, the target group must:

Be exposed to the appropriate information

Understand and believe the information

Have the resources and skills to make the proposed change(s)

Derive benefit (or perceive a benefit) from the change

Be reinforced to maintain the change over time

For successful implementation of engineering and technology solutions, the technology must:

Be effective and reliable

Be acceptable to the public and compatible with the environment

Result in products that dominate in the marketplace

Be easily understood and properly used by the public

For successful implementation of legislation and law enforcement strategies:

The legislation must be widely known and understood

The public must accept the legislation and its enforcement provisions

The probability, or perceived probability, of being caught if one breaks the law must be high

The punishment must be perceived to be swift and severe

Modified from Sleet D and Gielen A: Injury prevention. In Gorin SS and Arnold J, editors: *Health promotion handbook*, St. Louis, 1998, Mosby.

wiser to define a more attainable goal such as "to reduce the number of vehicles that run red lights in Hazard City by 25% within the next 12 months."

Project objectives are the map to your destination. They provide a set of outcomes that will need to be reached if the project goal is to be achieved. Remember the word *DOTS* as you write objectives. Objectives should be **D**iscreet, **O**utcome focused, **T**ime framed, and **S**pecific. Each criterion is described below:

- *Discreet* means that each desired outcome should have its own objective. Writing "Increase overtime funding and levels of enforcement at high risk intersections" combines two objectives. This is a problem because the two desired outcomes pose different intervention challenges.
- *Outcome focused* implies that something will change and that the change will be measurable. For example, "Funds will be obtained to cover the cost of 100 hours of overtime enforcement activity."
- *Time framed* means that the stated objective should include a date by which the outcome will be achieved. "By October 1, 2002, funds will be obtained to cover the cost of 100 hours of overtime enforcement activity." Typically, program objectives are short-term objectives.
- *Specific* refers to how, and to what extent, the outcome will be achieved. "By October 1, 2002, X dollars will be obtained through a grant from the Magnanimous Foundation to cover the cost of 100 hours of overtime enforcement activity."

Action steps (sometimes called process objectives) are the actions one takes to achieve the program objectives. These may include securing letters of support for a grant application, ordering incentive items, convening an advisory group that includes members of partner agencies, developing educational materials, organizing media events, gathering data to identify hazardous intersections, and conducting training of field workers.

The *intended audience for individual action steps* is not necessarily the same as that stated in the program goals and objectives. Organizing a media event will involve one group of people, planning enforcement schedules another, targeting repeat offenders yet another. Being specific about the group involved in each step conserves resources and helps identify the partners you will need to involve in program implementation.

The *methods/strategies to be used for each step* represent the bottom line: How will this happen? Writing down each step may seem unnecessary but it protects from errors of omission. Additionally, it provides the basis for a realistic estimate of time and resources needed to complete the project.

The *indicators of success for each step* determine how you will know the process objective (action step) has been achieved. This is what you hope to find when you evaluate this part of the process. For example, what will indicate to you that the activity has increased law enforcement's willingness to do enforcement?

Evaluation methods identified for each step are the key to good program management and evaluation throughout the life of the program. Many methods are quick and affordable. The benefits of evaluation are discussed below.

A *project timeline* is most useful if it is written down using real dates instead of week markers such as weeks 12-16. This alerts project staff to potential conflicts, such as meetings scheduled for public holidays, a training session planned for the week of Thanksgiving, and so on.

A *lead person (or group) should be designated as responsible for each step*. This enhances resource management, project monitoring, and staff accountability. In summary, implementation planning will help:

- Eliminate planning gaps
- Keep you focused and on track
- Manage resources wisely
- Make objectives attainable

PROGRAM EVALUATION

Evaluation is a valuable part of any injury prevention program. Contrary to popular opinion, evaluation is not a personal judgment of the program staff, nor is it used to trick unsuspecting programs into revealing their flaws; it is not something to be undertaken only if funding absolutely depends on it. Evaluation is a tool that, if used well, can build better programs. Evaluations may be simple or complex depending on one's needs, resources, training, and professional perspective. Real-world program evaluations need not be exhaustive or complex to provide valuable information about the program and should be considered prevention partners rather than adversaries. There are only four categories of information that evaluation can reveal about the program: good things that you have already identified, good things that you have not identified (a bonus), bad things that you have identified, and bad things that you have not yet identified. Fear of discovery in this latter category deters many from doing evaluations, yet most of us would like to know as early as possible if we had a malignant tumor. In the same way that early detection and management of a malignancy may enhance the chances for a good outcome, early detection and management of program problems enhances the chance of a good outcome. Evaluation is therefore an excellent management tool if integrated into the program from the very beginning.

There are many practical reasons to perform evaluations and to continue performing them throughout the life of the program[63,64]:

1. **Determine whether the planned program objectives are adequately defined and measurable.**
   When planning an evaluation, it is essential to clearly define the program goals and objectives to be measured. Early evaluation planning will iden-

tify overly broad or vague intervention objectives that put programs at risk of failure.

2. **Identify the program preferences of your target group and program partners.**

    Once the desired intervention has been identified (e.g., building community support to modify an unsafe playground near the hospital), evaluation can help you determine which approaches are most likely to be acceptable and productive.

3. **Ensure that program materials and program messengers are suitable for and acceptable to the recipients.**

    This is one of the most important reasons to evaluate programs. So many programs produce materials that are entirely unsuitable for the people who will receive them. Common problems include: a reading level that is too high; too much information; vague information (e.g., all children should buckle up); culturally inappropriate language, pictures, or messages; cluttered or overcrowded materials; and incorrect idiom for the age group. This extends beyond written materials. For example, program presenters must have credibility with the target audience, and a program venue in a community where few people own cars must be easily accessible via public transportation during the hours the program will be offered.

4. **Determine whether what you plan to do is feasible.**

    Many programs flounder because they are too ambitious. Others fail because planning occurred in a vacuum. Many factors can affect your ability to deliver the program. Potential barriers to implementation should be assessed carefully and the program plans modified accordingly. Successful programs tend to be focused and well defined. Start with small, achievable programs and build your experience, credibility, and support base.

5. **Monitor whether program activities are happening as planned.**

    No matter how well conceived a program is, it cannot be effective if it does not happen. For example, are the activities happening, are people attending events, are coalition members delivering the information necessary for drafting the proposed legislation? These important questions must be answered: Is it happening? If not, why? How can it be improved? Did that work?

6. **Have an early warning system for unintended consequences of your intervention.**

    As discussed previously, interventions to prevent injuries may have side effects. These unintended consequences may be positive or negative. It is important to identify both. Negative consequences are critical, because they may increase risk of injury to certain members of the population or create a new risk entirely. Positive effects may help support

the current intervention or similar initiatives in the future.

7. **Determine whether program objectives are being met and you are progressing toward the stated goal.**

    If, for example, your program objective is to achieve passage of legislation, there are several interim objectives that will need to be accomplished during the process. Each should be considered an outcome to be measured. In your journey toward legislation, these outcomes are the mileposts that will let you know whether you are moving in the right direction and whether you are covering enough miles each day to get to your destination on time. For example, did the bill get to the house committee on time? Missed preliminary deadlines may mean a year's delay, lost social support momentum, or an end to funding.

8. **Provide baseline data for future projects.**

    Injury prevention gains are often achieved incrementally; seat belt or bicycle helmet use rates that were considered successes 5 years ago are only starting points for new initiatives. Information we gather about our target community for a current project may help identify future priorities or approaches. If planned and conducted carefully, evaluation and needs assessment form part of the same information cycle, thus conserving valuable resources.

9. **Determine whether the intervention is effective.**

    This is the most well-known reason to perform an evaluation and one frequently tied to program funding. Did the program work? Did it make a difference? Can we demonstrate an association between our program and the observed changes?

10. **Identify factors that may limit the effectiveness of such interventions.**

    Many factors may limit the effectiveness of apparently successful interventions. Failure to sustain the intervention effect is an important factor. Programs that demonstrate short-term successes, such as increased bicycle-helmet use or the presence of a working smoke detector, may find that over time these gains are lost. Educational and enforcement campaigns that are intensive but of short duration should, if at all possible, include a long-term evaluation component. Other factors that may limit effectiveness include decreased funding for over-time needed to enforce a law, the emergence of cheaper and unsafe alternatives to safe products, or challenges to policy and law.

11. **Justify resource allocation and qualify for funding in the future.**

    Increasingly, prevention programs are required to demonstrate the benefits that result from investment of resources. Assessments of the cost-effectiveness and cost-benefit of programs may be used to determine whether a program is fiscally responsible and whether it should be funded or continued.[65] It can also be used to determine, in times of multiple priorities and resource limitation, where and how prevention dollars should be invested. Cost-effectiveness analysis examines the relationship between program costs and program outcomes when those outcomes (e.g., lives saved) are not measured in dollars.[66] Cost-benefit analysis expresses the relationship between program costs and program benefits in dollars (e.g., X dollars invested in prevention results in Y dollars saved).[66] Although the nurse may never be asked to conduct such an analysis, one practical step toward such an evaluation should always be taken: the monitoring and documentation of resources obtained and expended during the program. Monitoring the budget is only part of this task. Resources invested may be more than money: volunteer time, in-kind services, discounted prices on safety equipment, use of personal vehicles, and so on.[5] All should be considered when calculating program cost.

12. **Develop your own experience and self-efficacy in conducting evaluations.**

    When asked why they do evaluations, many people answer, "because we must to get funded." This illustrates the lack of confidence people have in their ability to conduct evaluations and, more importantly, their failure to realize what evaluation can do for them. Even a simple evaluation can provide valuable information about the program. The hardest evaluation is the first.

13. **Promote the viability and commitment of your program team.**

    At some time, every trauma nurse will experience the frustration that results when, having invested considerable time and energy in an activity, she or he receives no feedback about the outcome. Unlike the immediate reward that may be apparent when a trauma nurse helps save a life in the clinical setting, it has been said that the rewards for prevention are more "ethereal."[67] Stephen Teret, a prominent injury preventionist, notes that "if the preventionist is highly successful, the individual who was spared injury . . . may never even know that he or she was at risk."[67] Given the absence of immediate feedback, evaluation can help prevent burnout by demonstrating to those involved in the project the early, tangible outcomes that result from their actions. In its role as a management tool, evaluation also enhances the likelihood that a program will be focused, well organized, and implemented. This in itself promotes the viability of the team.

14. **Prevent, through dissemination of negative findings, replication of ineffective programs.**

    The worst program outcome is not a program that fails but a program that fails in silence. News of successful interventions are published and reported in many ways; it is not so with the negative findings. If an intervention fails, the program team should have access to enough information from the evaluation to determine, at least in part, why. This information can help the team—and others considering implementation of similar programs—to overcome these problems in the future.

15. **Contribute to the body of knowledge about the effectiveness of interventions to prevent injury.**

    Trauma nurses will be familiar with the term *evidence-based medicine*.[68] Although growing, the body of knowledge about the effectiveness of interventions to prevent injury is limited. Evaluations of intervention effectiveness therefore enhance our ability to practice evidence-based prevention.

16. **Increase community support.[53,69]**

    This may seem to be a peripheral reason to evaluate, but it has several program benefits. Evidence of early program successes may decrease resistance to the initiative; releasing information to stakeholders may increase their awareness of, support of, and trust in the project; and coalitions that are kept involved and informed are more likely to function effectively. A well-integrated program evaluation can enhance the overall health of the program.

Evaluation can be divided into four distinct stages:

1. Formative
2. Process
3. Impact (short-term outcomes)
4. Outcome (longer-term outcomes)

Formative evaluation is pilot testing (of intervention components) or troubleshooting (when something changes or goes wrong). It is done for quality assurance and to ensure that program materials are suitable for the target audience. Examples of formative evaluation questions might include the following:

- When is the best time to offer training sessions?
- Do teenage mothers understand the educational materials that are available for new mothers?
- How is our community different from community X?
- Do kids prefer yellow or green helmets?
- Is this instructor suitable for this audience?
- How difficult is it to install a rear-facing infant seat correctly?

Formative evaluation is very affordable and should be done during program planning and when any situation (e.g., the trainer) changes.

Process evaluation is used to determine whether the intervention activities are happening as planned. Ideally, it should be done throughout the life of the program. Examples of process evaluation questions include the following:

- How many people attended the health fair?
- What percentage of coalition members attend all meetings?
- How many bicycle helmets were distributed?
- Have we identified a sponsor for the proposed legislation?

Process evaluation is an early warning system for things that may go wrong. Use the information to enhance the implementation.

Impact (or short-term outcomes) evaluation measures the short-term impact the program has on the participants. It is determining whether the intervention had any effect on the audience. Where possible, it should be done after each encounter with the target group. Examples of short-term outcomes evaluation questions are listed below:

- How many people left the car seat check with correctly installed seats for each child?
- After the presentation, did parents' awareness of their child's need to ride in a booster seat increase?
- Did the audience's knowledge of risk factors for falls increase?
- Did vehicle speed decrease during the enforcement period?

Outcome evaluation or longer-term outcomes evaluation assesses whether the program made a measurable difference: Did it work? Examples of outcome evaluation questions include those listed below:

- To what extent have injuries to 4- to 8-year-old motor vehicle occupants decreased?
- By what percentage have bicycle helmet use rates increased?
- Have resources for youth programs increased as a result of this advocacy effort?
- Have we reduced the number of crashes associated with running red lights?

Repeat evaluations may be necessary to demonstrate that the intervention effect is real, sustained, and generalizable. Unfortunately, because of the cost involved, few interventions are evaluated this rigorously.

The choice of evaluation design will influence the strength of the conclusions and the value of information available to the program team and others. Poor quality data, the wrong data, or the wrong conclusions will undermine your evaluation. Pick the strongest design you can afford and, when in doubt, discuss your plans with an expert. Ideally the program should be evaluated by an outside investigator, but few projects have funds available to hire an evaluation consultant for more than a few hours. The following suggestions are offered to make evaluation more affordable:

- If you are able to contract an evaluation expert, do so

during the design phase of the intervention. No matter how skilled a statistician the evaluator is, she or he will be unable to produce good answers from bad data.
- Try to establish relationships with local universities, colleges, or research organizations. These may provide lower-cost or in-kind technical assistance.
- Decide what your evaluation objectives are. What do you need to know and why? The evaluation should meet the needs of your project.
- Establish a database for formative and process evaluation data at the beginning of the project. In this way resources are conserved as program management and evaluation activities merge.
- Never underestimate the power of information. Look at the data regularly. They are collected to inform and improve program implementation. Discuss any concerns with someone you trust who is experienced in your area.
- Recognize that assessment and evaluation form part of the same cycle. Time invested in careful planning of data collection will conserve valuable resources now and in the future.

It is beyond the scope of this chapter to describe evaluation methods in more detail. Readers are encouraged to read the referenced resources for additional information. Evaluation is much more than an inconvenient requirement imposed by funding agencies. It is a critical component of successful injury prevention programs and a valuable prevention partner.

CHALLENGES TO IMPLEMENTATION

As many injury researchers search for new and innovative solutions to complex injury problems, we should not forget that for some problems we have effective solutions. Bicycle helmets work,[70] occupant restraints work,[71,72] regulating hot water heater temperature works,[73] modification of household and infant products works, child-resistant packaging works,[74] graduated licensing works,[75] and many other interventions and approaches work. Why then are there so many injuries from causes for which we have solutions? The answer is warehousing—not delivering the interventions to the population at risk. In some cases we plan to deliver the intervention (the product leaves the warehouse), but it is not delivered intact and in time.

Implementation of effective injury prevention strategies may be our greatest challenge. No matter how well conceived and planned a program is, it will not be effective if it does not happen, if it is implemented inadequately, or if the intervention time frame is too short. Prevention program planners with limited resources are advised to look at the literature (and Web sites listed in Table 7-5) and select proven interventions whose implementation is well documented. So many resources are wasted as the same mistakes are made again and again. When considering an intervention, the nurse who reads or hears about a similar program should not hesitate to contact the people running the program. A phone call or e-mail correspondence can yield valuable, practical information not readily available elsewhere.

Fractionation of effort is a major impediment to program implementation. Essentially it is as though we were to hire a team of people to build a house, each with responsibility for a different piece of the project but without any team planning or communication before, during, or after the project. If in fact this house were ever built, it is likely that it would be flawed, over-budget, and behind schedule. It is not uncommon to find several groups or organizations within a community working on aspects of the same injury problem in isolation from each other. Institutional and organizational mandates, real or imagined traditional roles, and interagency politics may reinforce this fractionation. To optimize resource utilization and the chances for success, fractionation of effort must be challenged. Coalitions and collaborative initiatives are energizing prevention efforts in many areas of injury control. If well managed, coalitions can increase the visibility of the issue, funding opportunities, and the skill base of the participants. Readers interested in coalitions are encouraged to visit the Web site of the Prevention Institute, www.preventioninstitute.org, for more information on coalition building for injury control.

It is important that the trauma nurse be aware of several modifiable barriers to implementation of effective programs. These include the following:

1. Inadequate or absent evaluation
2. Overly broad problem definition
3. Incomplete problem diagnosis
4. Unrealistic goals
5. Poorly defined program objectives
6. Working in a vacuum
7. Turf wars
8. Planning and implementation gaps
9. Cruise control and tunnel vision
10. Burnout

Reference has been made to each of these previously. Of all 10 problem areas, the first one, *inadequate or absent evaluation,* is the most important. To understand why, the trauma nurse is encouraged to reread problems 2 through 10 and ask if evaluation throughout the life of the program could have prevented, or reduced the severity of, this problem. The answer for all nine is yes. Investing limited resources, energy, and expectations in poorly designed and implemented programs will lead to failure, frustration, and burnout. Even well-planned prevention efforts may take years to bear fruit, and they face numerous challenges along the way. Persistence and patience, combined with a continued sense of urgency, are notable attributes of successful preventionists. Get to know your opponents and your supporters. Start small and build your prevention skills. Nothing breeds success like success.

Battling obstacles to effective prevention programs may be demoralizing at times, but it is not nearly as demoralizing as watching again and again as young lives are lost to injuries that could have been prevented. Adopting a problem-solving approach to injury control does not guarantee program success, but it will assist readers to think about injury problems—and the trauma nurse's role in injury prevention—critically, systematically, and creatively.

REFERENCES

1. Centers for Disease Control and Prevention: Deaths/mortality, 1998, www.cdc.gov/nchs/fastats/deaths.htm, 2000.
2. Fingerhut LA, Warner M: *Injury chartbook. Health, United States, 1996-1997,* Hyattsville, Md, 1997, National Center for Health Statistics.
3. Centers for Disease Control and Prevention, National Center for Injury Prevention and Control: Scientific data, surveillance & injury statistics, www.cdc.gov/ncipc/osp/data.htm, 2000.
4. Centers for Disease Control and Prevention, National Center for Injury Prevention and Control: Ten leading causes of death, United States 1997, all races, both sexes, www.cdc.gov/ncipc/osp/states/10lc97.htm, 1998.
5. Christoffel T, Gallagher SS: *Injury prevention and public health: practical knowledge, skills, and strategies,* Gaithersburg, Md, 1999, Aspen Publishers.
6. Rice DP, MacKenzie EJ, Jones AS et al: *Cost of injury in the United States,* San Francisco, 1989, Institute for Health and Aging, University of California, and the Injury Prevention Center, Johns Hopkins University.
7. Miller TR, Pindus NM, Douglass JB et al: *Databook on nonfatal injury: incidence, costs and consequences,* Washington, DC, 1995, The Urban Institute Press.
8. www.census.gov/population/projections/nation/nas/npos1530.txt, April 5, 2000.
9. National Center for Injury Prevention and Control: *Working to prevent and control injury in the United States: fact book for the year 2000,* Atlanta, 2000, Centers for Disease Control and Prevention.
10. Mackenzie EJ, Fowler CJ: Epidemiology. In Mattox KL, Feliciano DV, Moore EE, editors: *Trauma,* ed 4, New York, 2000, McGraw-Hill.
11. American Trauma Society: Trauma Awareness Month bookmark, www.amtrauma.org/programs/mrc/bookmark.cfm.
12. Institute of Medicine: *The future of public health,* Washington, DC, 1988, National Academy Press, 23.
13. Koop CE: *Surgeon General's statement before the Subcommittee on Children, Family, Drugs, and Alcoholism,* Washington, DC, February 9, 1989, U.S. Senate.
14. Institute of Medicine: *Reducing the burden of injury: advancing prevention and treatment,* Washington, DC, 1999, National Academy Press, ix.
15. Guyer B: A problem solving paradigm for public health. In Armenian H, Shapiro S, editors: *Epidemiology and health services research,* New York, 1997, Oxford University Press.
16. Robertson LS: *Injuries: causes, control strategies, and public policy,* Lexington, Mass, 1983, Lexington Books.
17. Gordon JE: The epidemiology of accidents, *Am J Public Health* 39:504-515, 1949.
18. Waller JA: Reflections on a half century of injury control, *Am J Public Health* 84(4):664-670, 1994.

19. Waller JA, Klein D: Society, energy, and injury—inevitable triad. In National Institute of Child Health and Human Development: *Research directions towards the reduction of injury in the young and old,* DHEW Publication no. (NIH) 73-124, Bethesda, Md, 1973, The Institute.

20. Grossman DC: The history of injury control and the epidemiology of child and adolescent injuries, *Future Child* 10(1): 23-52, 2000.

21. The National Committee for Injury Prevention Control: *Injury prevention: meeting the challenge,* New York, 1989, Oxford University Press, 4.

22. Haddon W Jr: The changing approach to the epidemiology, prevention, and amelioration of trauma: the transition to approaches etiologically rather than descriptively based, *Am J Public Health* 58:1431, 1968.

23. Langley J: The "accident-prone" child—the perpetration of a myth, *Aust Ped J* 18:243-246, 1982.

24. Hoyert DL, Kochanek KD, Murphy SL: Deaths: final data for 1997, *Natl Vital Stat Rep* 47(19), 1999.

25. Stinson FS, De Bakey SF: Alcohol-related mortality in the United States, 1979-1988. *Br J Addiction* 87:777-783, 1992.

26. Hamilton WJ: Mothers against drunk driving—MADD in the USA, *Inj Prev* 6:90-91, 2000.

27. Smith GS, Branas CC, Miller TR: Fatal nontraffic injuries involving alcohol: a metaanalysis, *Ann Emerg Med* 33(6): 659-668, 1999.

28. Li G: Epidemiology of substance abuse among trauma patients, *Trauma Q* 14(4):353-364, 2000.

29. Clark DE, McCarthy E, Robinson E: Trauma as a symptom of alcoholism, *Ann Emerg Med* 14(3):274, 1985.

30. Rivara FP, Koepsell TD, Jurkovich GJ et al: The effects of alcohol abuse on readmission for trauma, *JAMA* 270(16): 1962-1964, 1993.

31. Soderstrom CA, Smith GS, Dischinger PC, et al: Psychoactive substance use disorders among seriously injured trauma center patients, *JAMA* 274:1043-1048, 1997.

32. Baker SP: Motor vehicle occupant deaths in young children, *Pediatrics* 64:860-861, 1979.

33. Winston FK, Durbin DD: Buckle up! is not enough: enhancing protection of the restrained child, *JAMA* 281(22):2070-2072, 1999.

34. Boost America: Raising kids with safety in mind, www.boost-america.org, October 21, 2000.

35. Office of the Governor of Washington State: Locke signs bill to strengthen seat belt law for safety, access.wa.gov:80/news/article.asp?name=n0003195.htm, March 28, 2000.

36. Gordis L: *Epidemiology,* Philadelphia, 1996, W.B. Saunders.

37. Institute of Medicine: *Reducing the burden of injury: advancing prevention and treatment,* Washington, DC, 1999, National Academy Press, 55.

38. Sandels S: Young children in traffic, *Br J Educ Psychol* 40:111-115, 1970.

39. Vinje MP: Children as pedestrians: abilities and limitations, *Accid Anal Prev* 13(3):225-240, 1981.

40. Haddon W Jr: Advances in the epidemiology of injuries as a basis for public policy, *Public Health Rep* 95:411-421, 1980.

41. Baker SP, O'Neill B, Ginsburg MJ et al: *The injury fact book,* ed 2, New York, 1992, Oxford University Press.

42. Haddon W Jr: The basic strategies for preventing damage from hazards of all kinds, *Hazard Prevent* 16:8-12, 1980.

43. Committee on Trauma, American College of Surgeons: *Resources for optimal care of the injured patient:* 1999, Chicago, 1998, American College of Surgeons.

44. Albee GW: Psychopathology, prevention and the just society, *J Prim Prevent* 4:5-40, 1983.

45. Shield J: Have we become so accustomed to being passive that we've forgotten how to be active? *Inj Prev* 3(4):243-244, 1997.

46. Teret SP: Injury control and product liability, *J Public Health Policy* 2(1):49-57, 1981.

47. Teret SP: Litigating for the public's health, *Am J Public Health* 76:1027-1029, 1986.

48. Berger LR: Childhood injuries: recognition and prevention, *Curr Probl Pediatr* 12(1):24, 1981.

49. Christoffel T: The misuse of law as a barrier to injury prevention, *J Public Health Policy* 10(4):444, 1989.

50. McLoughlin E: The almost successful California experience: what we and others can learn from it. In Bergman AB: *Political approaches to injury control at the state level,* Seattle, 1992, University of Washington Press, 57-67.

51. The Trauma Foundation: Channeling grief into policy change: survivor advocacy for injury prevention, *San Francisco General Hospital Injury Prevention Network Newsletter* 13, 2000.

52. Baker SP: Childhood injuries: the community approach to prevention, *J Public Health Policy* 2(3):235-246, 1981.

53. Cohen L, Swift S: The spectrum of prevention: developing a comprehensive approach to injury prevention, *Inj Prev* 5(3): 203-207, 1999.

54. The Prevention Institute: [Prevention] tools and frameworks, www.preventioninstitute.org/tools.html.

55. Committee on Injury and Poison Prevention: *Injury prevention and control for children and youth,* ed 3, Elk Grove Village, Ill, 1997, American Academy of Pediatrics.

56. Fowler CJ, Dannenberg AL: *The intervention decision matrix,* Baltimore, 1999, The Johns Hopkins Center for Injury Research and Policy.

57. Centers for Disease Control and Prevention: Notice to readers: warning on interaction between air bags and rear-facing child restraints, *MMWR* 42:280-282, 1993.

58. Robertson LS, Zador PL: Driver education and fatal crash involvement of teenaged drivers, *Am J Public Health* 68(10): 959-965, 1978.

59. Robertson LS: Crash involvement of teenaged drivers when driver education is eliminated from high school, *Am J Public Health* 70(6):599-603, 1980.

60. Preusser DF, Williams AF, Zador PL et al: The effect of curfew laws on motor vehicle crashes, *Law and Policy* 6:115-128, 1984.

61. American Academy of Pediatrics Committee on Sports Medicine and Fitness and Committee on Injury and Poison Prevention: Swimming programs for infants and toddlers, *Pediatrics* 105(4):868-870, 2000.

62. Sleet DA, Gielen AC: Injury prevention. In Gorin SS, Arnold J, editors: *Health promotion handbook,* St. Louis, 1998, Mosby.

63. Dannenberg AL, Fowler CJ: Evaluation of interventions to prevent injuries: an overview, *Inj Prev* 4:141-147, 1998.

64. Thompson NJ, McClintock HO: *Demonstrating your program's worth: a primer on evaluation for programs to prevent unintentional injury,* rev ed, Atlanta, 2000, National Center for Injury Prevention and Control.

65. Miller TR, Levy DT: Cost outcome analysis in injury prevention and control: a primer on methods, *Inj Prev* 3:288-293, 1997.

66. Patton MQ: *Utilization focused evaluation,* ed 3, Thousand Oaks, Calif, 1997, Sage Publications.

67. Teret SP: Postponing appointments: in praise of preventionists, *Johns Hopkins Public Health* (Spring):5, 1999.

68. Gray JAM: *Evidence-based health care. How to make health policy and management decisions,* London, 1997, Churchill Livingstone.

69. Capwell EM, Butterfoss F, Francisco VT: Why evaluate? *Health Prom Pract* 1(1):15-20, 2000.

70. Rivara FP, Thompson DC, Thompson RS et al: The Seattle children's bicycle helmet campaign: changes in helmet use and head injury admissions, *Pediatrics* 93(4):567-569, 1994.

71. Evans L: The effectiveness of safety belts in preventing fatalities, *Accid Anal Prev* 18:229-241, 1986.

72. National Highway Transportation and Safety Administration: The effect of a standard seat belt use law, www.nhtsa.dot.gov/people/injury/airbags/seatbelt/effect.htm, May 27, 2000.

73. Erdmann TC, Feldman KW, Rivara FP et al: Tap water burn prevention: the effect of legislation, *Pediatrics* 88:572-577, 1991.

74. Walton WW: An evaluation of the poison prevention packaging act, *Pediatrics* 69:363-370, 1982.

75. Foss RD, Evenson KR: Effectiveness of graduated driver licensing in reducing motor vehicle crashes, *Am J Prev Med* 16(1 Suppl):47-56, 1999.

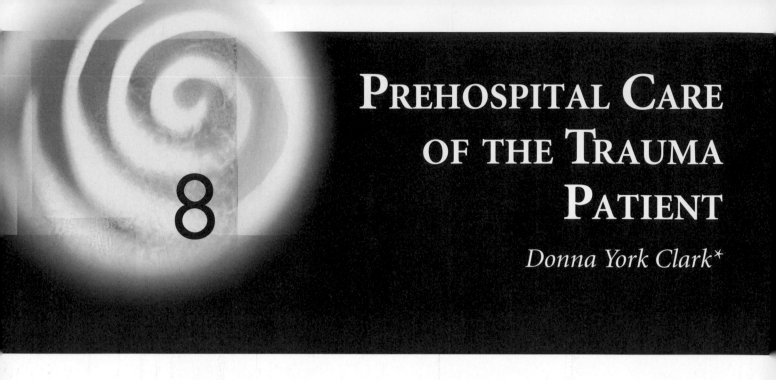

8

PREHOSPITAL CARE OF THE TRAUMA PATIENT

Donna York Clark*

Traditionally the role of nursing in the care of the trauma patient has been confined to the hospital. Other than in military nursing or public health, nursing's role in the prehospital environment has been limited. In the early 1970s civilian nurses began working outside the hospital in air medical helicopters. With the increase in advanced care delivery, tertiary care centers, critical care ground transport, and air medical services, the role of nursing outside the hospital is rapidly expanding. This chapter focuses on the importance of the integration of nursing into the emergency medical services (EMS) system and the changes necessary to care for patients in the field.

THE PREHOSPITAL CARE TEAM

Trauma directly affects approximately 60 million people per year in the United States, and 150,000 of those injured die.[1] The significance of this problem has led to the development of specialized systems to respond to the injured, with the goal of decreasing mortality and morbidity. Teamwork is an essential determinant in the outcome of trauma care, for there are few individual successes and even fewer individual failures.[2] Each member of the team is dependent on the others, and successful outcome is based on teamwork.

Effective teamwork among health care providers must begin in the prehospital setting in order for the patient who has sustained injury to achieve optimal outcomes. "Prehospital" describes the phase when health care providers attend to the needs of the patients outside the hospital. Others may use the phrase "out of hospital" to describe the same subject.

Traumatic injury can generate chaos. This chaos may envelop all participants at the scene of the incident, including those injured, family members, bystanders, and the prehospital and public safety personnel who respond. Routine activity comes to a standstill. There is a need to bring order to the situation. In many locations, dialing 911 is the point of access to order.

The three-digit number 911 was set aside by Congress in the late 1960s to provide a simple method for accessing assistance from public safety personnel. Currently 911 systems exist in approximately two thirds of the United States. Calls to 911 are received by emergency dispatchers, who are trained in emergency medical dispatch or priority medical dispatch.[3]

These dispatchers are a critical component of the prehospital care team. A 911 communications center receives requests for help, determines the type of resources to dispatch, and documents all activity related to a particular incident.

Determining the most desirable use of prehospital resources—police, fire, paramedic unit, air medical helicopter—is a complex process. Each prehospital system has protocols fine-tuned to the availability of resources for the area in order to guide the dispatcher's decision-making process. The dispatcher will solicit key initial information such as the type of incident, the number of individuals involved, and the location of the incident.[4] This information will direct the dispatcher to activate the appropriate team members to facilitate the delivery of care and restore order to potentially life-changing situations. The dispatcher will also give prearrival instructions to the caller. The types of available prehospital care resources vary slightly from region to region. This chapter discusses, in general, the basic scope of practice for each (Table 8-1).[5]

INCIDENT COMMAND SYSTEM

In the early 1970s the incident command system (ICS) was adopted by fire and police services in the United States.[6] The purpose of the ICS was to formalize job descriptions and

*The author would like to extend an incredible thank you to Nanette Trias, Administrative Assistant, Stanford Hospital and Clinics, for her assistance in the preparation of this chapter.

TABLE 8-1 Team Members and Training

Team Member	Training and Primary Role in Trauma Scene Response
Firefighter	Trained in fire science, fire suppression, extrication, BLS, and emergency first aid; certified, nonlicensed
Emergency medical technician (EMT)	Basic level of emergency responder trained to complete basic assessments, initiate oxygen therapy, and provide advanced first aid; certified, nonlicensed
Emergency medical technician-paramedic (EMT-P)	Advanced-level emergency responder trained to complete advanced assessments, initiate IV therapy, and institute airway management, including endotracheal intubation and drug administration; practices as a physician extender; all practice directed by standing orders and protocols or via on-line physician order; certified, licensed in some states
Mobile intensive care nurse (MICN)	Specially trained RN who provides on-line consultation to prehospital personnel; participates in destination choices; licensed provider
Flight nurse	Specially trained RN with broad experience in emergency and critical care nursing; routinely an expanded practice role; practice involves use of a helicopter or fixed-wing aircraft; advanced assessments and interventions including but not limited to endotracheal intubation, rapid sequence induction intubation, central line placement, chest tube placement, and pharmacologic intervention; practice directed by physician medical director and authorized program-based protocols; licensed provider
Flight paramedic	Specially trained paramedic with broad experience in prehospital care and transport; most flight nurses and flight paramedics receive the same flight-specific training; many perform similar skills, including advanced assessments and intervention such as endotracheal intubation, rapid sequence induction intubation, central line placement, chest tube placement; practice directed by physician medical director and authorized program-based protocols; in some areas practice may be limited by state-defined paramedic scope of practice; licensed in some states, certified in others
Flight physician	Physician serving as an air medical team member; 4% of flight programs in the U.S. routinely use a physician as part of their crew; level of experience varies from intern to well-seasoned, board-certified physician specialist; licensed provider[5]
Medical director	Multifaceted role, varies system to system; provides medical direction in policy and procedure formation as well as on-line advice to responding teams; most agencies involved in prehospital response have assigned physicians for this role; ensures quality care delivery

ensure effective, clear, concise communications in chaotic situations such as the response to a building fire or a roadside crash. The intention was to create a mechanism that brings order to chaos.

The ICS is a field management tool that is flexible enough to be exercised in a variety of incidents. The ICS is organized around five major activities: command, operations, planning/intelligence, logistics, and finance/administration. This system requires the designation of an incident commander (IC) who is responsible for all functions required at the response. The IC may choose to delegate authority to others during the incident; however, this does not relieve the IC from overall responsibility. ICS incorporates the principle of unified command, which allows all agencies that have jurisdictional or functional responsibility (e.g., state-based highway patrol and a local fire agency responding to a multiple vehicle crash on a state road) to jointly develop a common set of incident objectives and strategies. Unified command ensures that no single agency loses authority or accountability[7] (Table 8-2).

ICS is more than organization; it is a common language used in emergency response systems. For some incidents, only a small number of the ICS elements may be necessary. If the incident enlarges, the ICS system has the capability to incorporate many more individuals to meet the needs of the incident. The objective is to have clear goals and job descriptions for all involved—a universal response to aid those who are injured.

COMMUNICATIONS

Communication is the cornerstone to an effectively run response and is essential for a successful EMS system.[8] Effective communications systems are all encompassing; they include: the public, EMS units, fire, police, air operations, and medical direction. The tools used for effective communication include: mobile data terminals (MDT), two-way radios, cellular/digital/satellite phones, and pagers.

Radios are a mainstay of EMS communications. In this era of high technology, every agency and municipality involved in EMS response has internal and external radio communication capabilities. Like telephone numbers, radio frequencies are dedicated to certain agencies by the Federal Communication Commission and, unlike traditional phone lines, can be designated for specific activities. For example, a certain frequency may be designated as a tactical frequency, and all responders from agencies participating in an extrication will be directed to that frequency, but medical operations may use another frequency. Radio channels are divided into bands and frequencies. Table 8-3 outlines the available radio frequencies and the pros and cons associated with their use.

It is essential that people who are active in an EMS system

TABLE 8-2	Incident Command System: Function Overview
Functions	**Responsibilities**
Command	Coordinates all activity; a command is present for all incidents
Operations	Directs activity (resources, machinery, personnel) required to meet incident goals
Planning/Intelligence	Collects, evaluates, and displays incident information; maintains status of resources; prepares incident action plan and incident-related information
Logistics	Provides adequate services and support to meet needs of incident resources
Finance/Administration	Tracks incident-related costs, including personnel and equipment

Modified from State of California, Office of Emergency Services: *Standardized emergency management system field course module 2—principles and features of ICS,* Sacramento,1995, OES.

have a clear understanding of the communications equipment available to them and the ability to troubleshoot technical and tactical challenges. Communication is the key element to the success of the EMS team and a critical tool in the safety of the operations. It also can be the weak link that precipitates failure.

THE TRAUMA SCENE

The goal of prehospital response is to deliver high-quality care to the patient and maintain the safety of the responders. The cycle begins with the specific incident. For example, when a pedestrian is struck by a motor vehicle, many people react: the people directly involved, the passersby, those who stop to help, and the public servants whose services are requested. The situation can be described in many ways and "calm" is never part of the description.

ACTIVATION OF THE EMS RESPONSE

The EMS response is usually initiated by a civilian who calls 911. The caller describes the incident to the EMS dispatcher. From the description of the incident, the dispatcher gleans many important facts: the number of victims, the exact location of the incident, the general age of the victim(s), and an estimation of the kinetic energy involved, which is

TABLE 8-3	Radio Channel Frequencies and Bands	
Frequencies	**Pros**	**Cons**
Very high frequency (VHF)—low band	Long range Effective in wide areas Possible to transmit and receive on the same frequency	Often disrupted Difficult to use in metro areas Commonly monitored by civilians
VHF—high band	Less easily disrupted Possible to transmit and receive on same frequency Useable in metro areas Covers large area Cost effective	Difficult to transmit within structures Commonly monitored by civilians
Ultra high frequency (UHF)	Least susceptible to interference Possible to transmit and receive simultaneously Possible to add repeaters or relays to extend service area	Cost increases because of repeaters and equipment required Commonly monitored by civilians
800-megahertz band	Suited for metro use Possibility of sharing frequencies among agencies Can be integrated with computerized dispatch systems Less commonly monitored by civilians	Shorter range of service Unable to transmit telemetry Cost may increase because of equipment required
Cellular/digital/satellite phones	Costs are decreasing User friendly Allows one-on-one communication Option in some radio dead zones Relatively private	Unable to monitor multiple agency transmission Cannot be used for air-to-ground communications Cell sites may be overwhelmed in a disaster
Mobile data terminals (MDT)	Allows readable, secure text information Recallable	Costly Mandates close proximity to unit
Pagers	Cost effective User friendly	One-way or two-way transmission of information

derived from the estimated speed of the vehicle. With this information the prehospital care providers arrive at the scene with expectations regarding the types of injuries they may encounter.

The prehospital/EMS provider's response is activated by the dispatch service. Most EMS systems require providers to adhere to time limits, such as response times and time at the scene, to ensure appropriate rapid response to victims. Acceptable response times in urban and suburban settings range from 4 to 8 minutes (measured from the time dispatch takes the call until the arrival of the first responder), whereas response times in rural areas may be much longer. As a result of varying geography, population, roadways, and resources, acceptable response times will vary from area to area.

SAFETY AT THE SCENE

Regardless of the level of responder, the first arriving individual assesses the scene for safety. A primary goal during all EMS response is to do no further harm to victims and to maintain the safety and well-being of all responders involved. Safety requires constant attention. Safe practices are one of the most critical components of an emergency response system's success, because unsafe practices breed further injuries.

It is critical to eliminate the potential for additional injuries. The scene must be evaluated for fire sources, potential for explosion, continuing gunfire, "hot" electrical wires, unruly crowds, and other hazards. First responders alter traffic patterns to limit risk of further incident and call for additional resources as indicated. If the incident involves a vehicle, it must be determined if the vehicle is secure. Is the vehicle at risk of rolling down an embankment? If the vehicle struck a tree, is that tree strong enough to serve as a brace? If the vehicle is not secure, it must be secured with cribbing (wood blocks or air bags) to ensure stability.

Hazardous materials (substances capable of posing unreasonable risk to health, safety or property) present a significant threat to prehospital operations. Their involvement can elevate an incident that affects one individual to a catastrophic event affecting an entire metropolitan area. It is the responsibility of the emergency response team to suspect hazardous materials when responding to incidents involving trucks, railcars, industrial buildings, or unmarked containers and to take appropriate precautions.

The approach to a hazardous materials scene is one of caution and investigation. Fire and other public safety personnel should enter the scene in a coordinated fashion. Responding teams should ascertain the name and chemical number of the material if possible. This information may be collected from the truck's "bill of lading" and material safety data sheet (MSDS) or other written material accompanying the driver. If this information is available, the prehospital care provider may obtain more information about the material from the United States Department of Transportation or the Chemical Transportation Emergency Center (CHEMTREC).[9] CHEMTREC, a public service of the Chemical Manufacturers Association, supports a 24-hour telephone number (800-262-8200) allowing access to databases that assist in identifying hot zones and decontamination priorities. Another source of advice related to hazardous materials is the regional poison control center for the local area.

"Hazardous material" is not a misnomer. Such a substance can add more hazard and risk to the rescue, extrication, and transport of an injured individual. If the victim has had contact with a hazardous substance, a specific course of action is advocated (Table 8-4) to minimize the physiologic effects and to protect medical personnel in the prehospital and in-hospital phases of care. The objectives of scene safety are to keep the patient and crew safe and to complete the job at hand. Once the scene has been secured, patient care may begin.

INITIAL CARE OF THE TRAUMA VICTIM

First responders are often police officers or fire/rescue personnel (EMTs) trained in basic life support; in most cases responders trained in advanced life support (ALS) (e.g., paramedics) are not part of the first responder team.[10] Therefore, first responder care typically involves basic life-saving techniques. Initially, the victim's airway must be assessed and opened with chin lift or jaw thrust. In trauma cases the jaw thrust is the maneuver of choice. The goal is to ensure airway patency while maintaining cervical spine integrity. Simultaneously, pressure is applied to areas of gross bleeding.

Paramedics are trained in more extensive patient evaluation techniques and are capable of performing advanced patient care procedures. Recent trends in paramedic education stress the importance of rapid assessment and the performance of only those interventions required to maintain survival en route to a trauma center. The "load and go" mantra of the 1960s has been revised to allow airway control, proper immobilization, and then rapid transport. Additional procedures such as placement of intravenous lines and splinting are done en route.

TABLE 8-4 **Interaction With Hazardous Materials**
Set up safety zones for hazardous material response as outlined in the ICS guidelines.
Protect rescuers by applying nonporous personal protective clothing and goggles.
Move the victim to safe area upwind with fresh air.
Support ventilatory efforts, apply oxygen if indicated.
Initiate CPR if indicated; follow triage guidelines.
If toxic material contacts skin or eye, vigorously flush areas with water (contain runoff if possible).
Remove contaminated clothing and footwear.
Isolate contaminated items.

MODE OF TRANSPORT

When determining the appropriate mode of patient transport, paramedics should consider the following:

- The acuity level of the patient
- Time of day and traffic patterns
- Trauma plan of the municipality and location of the closest appropriate trauma center
- Potential difficulties (e.g., airway management in a combative child)
- Other available resources

The widespread availability of air transport with highly trained medical team members gives many EMS responders an important tool in the care of the trauma patient. Like any intervention, air transport should be used appropriately, because it has inherent risks and benefits. In many areas of the country, a medical helicopter is activated by paramedics or first responders based on preestablished launch criteria; therefore, the vehicle and advanced medical team members are available soon after the arrival of paramedics and secondary responders. If it is determined that the helicopter and its team are not needed at the scene, the request can be canceled.

As stated earlier, protocols vary from region to region. It is essential that all prehospital providers have a clear understanding of available resources and local protocols.

Air medical transport should be considered for critically injured patients in situations that require prolonged extrication, extended ground transport to the appropriate trauma center, or protracted manual transport out of a remote area.[11] The National Association of Emergency Medical Services Physicians developed guidelines to promote effective and consistent use of air medical services (Table 8-5).

When using air medical resources, one of the most significant considerations is the ability to land the aircraft near enough to the patient to allow rapid and uncomplicated access but distant enough to prevent the patient and caregivers from being affected by the noise and rotor-wash of the helicopter. When landing an air medical helicopter at an injury scene, there are many things to consider in preparing the landing zone (LZ). General guidelines for selecting a LZ are described below; however, it is important to confirm these with local operators before initiating practices. Select a landing site that is at least twice the overall length and width of the aircraft, with a firm level surface, usually 75 feet by 75 feet. The slope of the ground should be less than 10 to 15 degrees to prohibit anyone from walking uphill into a spinning blade and to avert rotor blades from dipping and making contact with the ground. A landing zone must also have approach and departure paths that are clear of obstructions (wires, trees, towers, etc.) and that allow flight into the wind. Finally, the LZ must have a coordinator, someone with a radio to immediately communicate to the pilot trauma crew regarding pertinent issues.

TABLE 8-5	Clinical Indicators and Operational Situations in Which Air Medical Transport Should Be Considered

I. Specific Clinical Indicators
   a. Spinal cord or spinal column injury or any injury producing lateralizing signs
   b. Partial or total amputation of an extremity (excluding digits)
   c. Two or more long-bone fractures or a major pelvic fracture
   d. Crushing injuries to the trunk or head
   e. Major burns
   f. Patients less than 12 or more than 55 years of age
   g. Patients with near-drowning injuries, with or without existing hypothermia
   h. Adult patients with any of the following vital sign abnormalities:
      1. systolic blood pressure <90 mm Hg
      2. respiratory rate <10 or >35 per min
      3. heart rate <60 or >120 bpm
   i. Patient unresponsive to verbal stimuli
II. Operational Situations
   a. Mechanism of injury
      1. Vehicle rollover with unbelted passengers
      2. Vehicle striking pedestrian at >10 mph
      3. Falls from >15 ft
      4. Motorcycle victim ejected at >20 mph
      5. Multiple victims
   b. Difficult access situations
      1. Wilderness rescue
      2. Ambulance access or exit impeded at the scene by road conditions, weather, or traffic
   c. Time and distance factors
      1. Transportation time to the trauma center >15 min by ground ambulance
      2. Transport time to local hospital by ground longer than transport time to trauma center by helicopter
      3. Patient extrication time greater than 20 min
      4. Use of local ground ambulance leaves local community without ground ambulance coverage

Modified from National Association of Emergency Medical Services Physicians: Air medical dispatch: guidelines for scene response, *Prehosp Disaster Med* 7(1):75-78, 1992.

EXTRICATION

Extrication is the removal of a trapped victim. A person may be pinned by an automobile, a motorcycle, or roadside obstructions—the possibilities are infinite. A basic principle of extrication is that a few designated prehospital care providers should remove the entrapped victim rather than having all providers enter the area of entrapment.[12] Although all activities are time critical, the safety of responders and the injured is paramount.

Once the area in which the victims are trapped is determined safe to approach, the locations of the injured are determined. If any are in imminent danger, they are removed in the safest, most efficacious manner. The goal is

TABLE 8-6 Extrication Tools

Tool Type	Function
Hand tool	Any common hand tool such as a hammer or screwdriver
Portapower	Hand-driven hydraulic cylinder/hand-powered spreader and cutter
Sawzall	Hand saw that cuts through metal and glass
Torch	Cuts through rebar or other metal debris; mostly seen in building collapse situations
Saw	Cuts through sheet metal, wood, or other material
Spreader/Cutter	Pries open vehicle doors and hinges Cuts sheet metal and pillars
Ram	Pries open doors and peels back roofs

to cause no further harm. All efforts are made to protect the victim's airway and spine during this process.

The entrapment/extrication issue becomes complicated when the patient cannot be removed by routine maneuvers. An example is an unrestrained driver involved in a head-on collision at freeway speeds whose lower extremities are entangled in the pedals and flooring of the car. Removal of this traumatically injured person requires more than lifting: It requires tools and expertise in extrication.

The experts in extrication in most United States municipalities are fire departments. Although equipment may vary, fire department personnel have expertise and training in extrication. As noted in earlier discussion, fire services should be a resource in all EMS plans. These services are often mobilized by the 911 dispatcher seconds after the call is received.

Fire department personnel size up the scene for safety and establishment of requirements to accomplish removing the victim. Then the extrication process begins. The rescuers can access the victim through the vehicle's doors (if they are operable), by breaking glass and entering through window openings, or by using tools to cut or pry the vehicle apart.

The extrication team will use the tools that most effectively and efficiently accomplish the job. The choice depends on the mechanism of injury, vehicle, and location. Different situations require different tools. Sometimes the goal will be to pry a door open, whereas other times the goal may be to remove the roof of a car. Tools used in extrication are listed in Table 8-6.[13]

TREATMENT

Once access to the victims has been gained, the rescuers will rapidly triage them. As outlined in *Flight Nursing: Principles and Practices*, the care delivered should include the following[12]:

1. Establish an airway with cervical spine precautions.
2. Provide artificial ventilation without oxygenation. Oxy-

gen use *may* be deferred if nearby petroleum-based products present the possibility of ignition or fire.
3. Control external hemorrhage.
4. Initiate cardiopulmonary resuscitation (CPR) as indicated. (CPR may be ineffective, depending on patient position and location.)

PREHOSPITAL TRAUMA CARE: HOW MUCH AND WHEN?

The priorities of assessment and treatment are based on the ABCs—airway, breathing, and circulation.

AIRWAY

Evaluation of the airway begins with an assessment for patency. The question to be answered in this assessment is whether the patient can move air through the passageway. If the answer is yes, the provider moves on to the next phase of evaluation. If the answer is no, further evaluation and intervention are warranted.

When patency is in question, airway adjuncts such as nasopharyngeal tubes or endotracheal tubes may be used to support airway integrity (Table 8-7). Intervention will be dictated by the ability to maintain the airway and to meet the body's physiologic needs.[14] In some cases the prehospital care provider's decision to intervene or not will be determined by the potential for complication, not the presentation alone. Two examples of when a decision to intubate will require careful consideration are the patient with thermal injury and the individual with a cervical spine injury.

Burned patients have great potential for development of complete airway obstruction.[15] This obstruction is caused by inflammation of burned airway tissue from exposure to steam heat, inhaled gas, or fire. As resuscitation fluids are administered, the risk for airway obstruction increases. The prehospital care provider must assess the burned patient's airway carefully. This evaluation should include but not be limited to assessing for the presence of carbonaceous sputum; the presence of a reddened or enlarged tongue; hoarseness of voice; difficulty swallowing; and tightening throat as described by the patient. All these symptoms are indications of airway swelling and, if they are not managed early, could result in complete airway obstruction. Early endotracheal intubation is recommended for the severely burned and for patients with burns involving their airway and/or circumferential neck or chest.

The Head and Spinal Cord Injury System Data Bank reports that spinal cord injury is sustained by approximately 30 to 40 per million people each year.[12] Most trauma patients are suspect for spinal injury and should be treated accordingly. This treatment includes maintaining in-line stabilization of the cervical spine and placing the victim on a long backboard with a stiff cervical collar and adequate strapping.[1] Airway integrity should be assessed, and the initial intervention for maintenance should be the jaw thrust maneuver. If further airway intervention is required, consistent alignment of the cervical spine must be maintained. Recommended airway interventions may include nasotra-

TABLE 8-7 Airway Adjuncts		
Adjunct	**Uses**	**Contraindications/Risks**
Suctioning	Removes debris or blood	
Nasopharyngeal airway	Maintains open airway in stuporous or comatose patient	Head/facial trauma
Oropharyngeal airway	Prevents tongue from obstructing airway; used only in unconscious patients	Conscious patients; may induce vomiting
Laryngeal mask airway	Provides unsecured airway; easy to position for placement; limited use in EMS at present; used only with unconscious patients	Aspiration
Intubation	Provides secure airway, avenue for artificial ventilation	Esophageal intubation; high degree of skill required
Rapid sequence intubation	Delivery of sedative and paralytic to facilitate orotracheal intubation	Failure of intubation; removal of patient's ventilatory drive
Needle cricothyroidotomy	Short-term, rapid airway security	Penetration of the airway; high training competency requirements; difficult to find landmarks in bloody or edematous patient
Surgical cricothyroidotomy		High training requirements

cheal intubation in the absence of maxillofacial trauma because of the reduced neck movement with this procedure. In many areas of the country, rapid sequence intubation (RSI) is the airway intervention of choice for cervical spine-injured patients.[16] Spinal cord injury and its potential direct many of the airway choices of the prehospital provider.

In most incident responses ALS providers are secondary responders and will receive the patient from firefighters, EMTs, or other BLS providers. The paramedics begin their care by confirming the primary survey. The objective of the primary survey is to identify any life-threatening issues and address them immediately.[1]

The initial focus of care is airway management. Insertion of an oral airway may be attempted, but success will be limited if the patient has a clenched jaw. Endotracheal intubation may or may not be an option at this time. The presence of trismus precludes direct laryngoscopy. In most states the paramedic scope of practice does not include the use of sedatives or neuromuscular blocking agents to facilitate intubation. If intubation is impossible or unsuccessful, bag-valve-mask ventilation is the only option available. In states where paramedic care does include paralytic administration or where air medical services (including nurse or physician team members) are used, RSI may be used to augment the accomplishment of definitive airway control. RSI has become the standard of care in air medical prehospital practice to secure airway control for severely injured patients.[17,18] RSI is the consecutive administration of a sedative and a neuromuscular blocking agent to induce paralysis and unconsciousness for the purpose of fostering laryngoscopy followed by endotracheal intubation.[19] A sample air medical provider's RSI protocol is presented in Table 8-8. The flight crew, working in concert with the other prehospital providers, ensures that an intravenous line is established to allow drug administration so that the RSI process can begin. In most scenarios a cardiac monitor with pulse oximetry is applied. Within minutes the RSI agents are administered and the airway secured.

At times intubation is not possible. This may be due to patient condition, position, or anatomy. However, the critical need for airway stabilization remains. Advanced providers in some EMS systems and most air medical crews would proceed to more advanced interventions. These advanced airway adjuncts include insertion of a needle cricothyroidotomy or a surgical cricothyroidotomy.

BREATHING

Evaluation of the patient's breathing includes: assessment of his or her level of consciousness, respiratory rate, chest excursion, chest symmetry, skin color, and oxygen saturation levels. Not all prehospital care providers have access to pulse oximeters as an assessment tool.

Once an initial assessment has been completed, oxygen is administered. As outlined earlier, the environment must be evaluated and all risks associated with oxygen administration must be ruled out before its application. In most trauma cases high-flow oxygen delivered by a nonrebreather mask is administered. Further oxygenation support may be required and may include the use of bag-valve-mask ventilation or intubation to allow mechanical ventilation.

Alteration in breathing and effective oxygen delivery may be caused by a loss of chest wall integrity or the loss of pleural space integrity as a result of thoracic injury. Chest wall or pleural space injuries may require some prehospital intervention, such as needle thoracostomy or chest tube placement. Tension pneumothorax may be caused by blunt or penetrating mechanisms of injury. Signs and symptoms

Stanford Hospital and Clinics Life Flight
Rapid Sequence Induction Intubation

I. Purpose
Rapid sequence induction (RSI) is a specific method of inducing general anesthesia and endotracheal intubation, which combines sedation to induce unconsciousness (induction) with muscular paralysis. This method minimizes the risk of aspiration in nonfasting patients with complex airway emergencies.

II. Equipment
Refer to Oral Endotracheal Intubation Procedure
Medications required for RSI are the following, given intravenously:
Lidocaine
Atropine
Midazolam
Etomidate
Succinylcholine
Vecuronium
Morphine sulfate

III. Procedure

Interventions	Key Points
1. Follow Routine Medical Care Protocol.	RSI technique is particularly useful for a patient who has a full stomach or increased intracranial pressure (ICP).
2. Evaluate need for RSI.	
3. Assess upper airway anatomy for likelihood of unsuccessful intubation.	
4. Assess for patient movement before administering paralytic agents.	
5. Apply cricoid pressure throughout procedure to occlude esophagus until placement is ensured.	Avoids gastric insufflation.
6. Preoxygenate with high-flow oxygen per bag-valve-mask.	
7A. *For head injured/increased ICP with systolic blood pressure (SBP) >90:*	
a. Administer lidocaine 1.5 mg/kg.	Lidocaine may blunt the increased ICP associated with laryngoscopy. If possible, allow 90 seconds before proceeding with succinylcholine.
b. Give etomidate 0.2-0.3 mg/kg.	Give etomidate over at least 20 seconds to decrease risk of myoclonus.
c. If a child <5 years old, premedicate with atropine 0.02 mg/kg (0.1 mg minimum) unless significantly tachycardic.	Pretreatment with atropine will antagonize vagal responses in children. Observe for arrhythmias.
d. Give succinylcholine 1.0-1.5 mg/kg.	Succinylcholine induces a transient potassium efflux and should not be administered if serum potassium is >5.5 mEq/L.
e. If succinylcholine is contraindicated, attempt intubation without paralytics.	Contraindications to succinylcholine: • burns older than 8 hours • massive crush injuries • organophosphate poisoning
7B. *For head injured/increased ICP with SBP <90:*	
a. Administer lidocaine 1.5 mg/kg.	
b. If a child <5 years old, premedicate with atropine 0.02 mg/kg (0.1 mg minimum).	
c. Give succinylcholine 1.0-1.5 mg/kg.	
d. If succinylcholine is contraindicated, attempt intubation without paralytics.	
7C. Actual or potential respiratory failure, airway protection:	
a. Liberally spray lidocaine or Cetacaine spray for topical anesthesia of tongue and oropharynx if available.	
b. Sedate with etomidate 0.05-0.10 mg/kg.	
c. Attempt to intubate without paralytics.	
d. If patient response precludes intubation (i.e., trismus, gag reflex or combative), consider paralytics listed below.	

Continued

TABLE 8-8	**Sample Policy and Procedure for Rapid Sequence Induction Intubation—cont'd**

Interventions	Key Points
e. If a child <5 years old, premedicate with atropine 0.02 mg/kg (0.1 mg minimum). f. Give succinylcholine 1.0-1.5 mg/kg. g. Intubate patient per Intubation Protocol after the onset of adequate relaxation.	If intubation attempt is unsuccessful and O_2 saturation is decreasing, ventilate with bag-valve-mask with continuous cricoid pressure and attempt intubation again.
8. If a second dose of succinylcholine is required because of lack of adequate relaxation, pretreat with atropine 0.02 mg/kg (0.1 mg minimum) if <16 years old and administer second dose of succinylcholine.	If unable to intubate after repeated attempts, then assist ventilations with bag-valve-mask and continue cricoid pressure until patient resumes spontaneous respirations. If unable to intubate and unable to adequately support ventilations with bag-valve-mask (i.e., decreased SaO_2 or heart rate), then surgical airway is necessary.

9. Reassess movement of extremities before administration of long-acting paralytics.
10. Obtain chest radiograph on interfacility patients after intubation.
11. For sedation and paralysis of intubated patients:
   a. Give midazolam 0.05-0.1 mg/kg and/or morphine sulfate 0.1 mg/kg (or other medication as directed) if SBP >90. Titrate to effect.
   b. Give vecuronium 0.1 mg/kg.
Repeat as needed for continued sedation and paralysis as indicated by movement, tachycardia, or elevated blood pressure.
12. Each time patient is moved, reassess position of endotracheal tube (ETT).
	By documenting "ETT placement $\sqrt{} \times 4$" the endotracheal tube placement has been verified with positive $ETCO_2$ color change, symmetrical chest movement, mist in tube, and easy compliance of chest wall.

13. Auscultate breath sounds on arrival at receiving hospital.
14. If any doubt as to ETT position, direct laryngoscopy is indicated.
15. Document:
   a. Indications for intubation
   b. Size of ETT
   c. Position of ETT at lip in cm
   d. Description of breath sounds after intubation and on arrival at receiving facility
   e. Absence of epigastric air movement
   f. Vital signs pre- and post-ETT placement
   g. $ETCO_2$ detector and SaO_2 monitor readings
   h. "ETT placement $\sqrt{} \times 4$" after each time the patient is moved
   i. Presence of blood, vomitus, or foreign body in airway
   j. Appropriate grade of laryngoscopic view
   k. Extremity movement before initial short- and long-term paralytic administration and after intubation
   l. Medications, doses, routes, and patient response
	Use the Cormack and Lehane grading system.

of a tension pneumothorax include respiratory distress, tracheal deviation away from the affected side, neck vein distention (if patient is euvolemic), no breath sounds or decreased breath sounds on the affected side, hyperresonance to percussion, and shock.

A diagnostic and interventional maneuver for tension pneumothorax is needle decompression (needle thoracostomy).[1,20] A 14- or 16-gauge angiocatheter (2½ inches or greater) or a long spinal needle is placed at the second or third intercostal space at the mid-clavicular line on the af-

fected side. When a tension pneumothorax is present, as the needle enters the pleural space a rush of air, ease in ventilatory pressure, and/or a rise in blood pressure may be noted. Each of these occurrences indicates a release of pressure from the pleural space and allows more effective gas exchange.

Chest tube insertion in the field has been a topic of discussion for many years. Many EMS administrators and trauma care specialists believe that it is a critical prehospital skill. Other experts feel that it is an intervention that should only be performed in the hospital.[21,22] In many areas of the country, prehospital chest tube insertion is performed by specially trained transport teams, which in most cases include nurses or physicians.

Another significant thoracic injury that requires prehospital intervention is the open pneumothorax or sucking chest wound. An open pneumothorax allows communication of outside atmospheric pressure with pleural space pressure. Signs and symptoms of an open pneumothorax include respiratory distress, subcutaneous air on the affected side, decreased or absent breath sounds on the affected side, tracheal deviation, and hemodynamic decompensation.[23] Prehospital interventions for a patient with an open pneumothorax include airway management, oxygen administration, application of a three-sided dressing, and possibly insertion of a chest tube. All these interventions must be performed rapidly and can be accomplished during transport to the receiving center.[1]

CIRCULATION

Prehospital evaluation of circulation is accomplished by the following: assessment of the patient's level of consciousness, the presence or absence of gross bleeding, skin color, capillary refill, pulse (rate and quality), blood pressure, and cardiac monitor tracing. All ALS providers have access to cardiac monitoring devices.

Initial intervention includes application of pressure to areas of gross bleeding. Once bleeding is slowed, initiation of volume replacement is a priority. Intravenous access with multiple large-bore catheters should be accomplished as long as obtaining access does not slow transport. The American College of Surgeons Committee on Trauma's *ATLS Instructors Manual* states that all adult patients should rapidly receive 2 L of crystalloid solution. This should be restricted only if the patient shows signs or symptoms of heart failure. In the pediatric population ATLS guidelines direct prehospital administration of 20 ml/kg as a fluid bolus.[1,24] These guidelines are well practiced; however, they are still controversial.

Research has challenged the practice of early rapid administration of crystalloids by demonstrating worse outcomes in victims of penetrating trauma who received early prehospital fluid resuscitation compared with similar patients who did not receive aggressive fluid resuscitation in the prehospital phase.[25,26] It is essential to analyze this information carefully before prehospital practice is changed. It is critical to note that this research was performed in an urban setting with short transport times. It may be appropriate to consider altering fluid resuscitation in patients with penetrating trauma, but the need to adjust fluid delivery to others has not yet been validated. It is essential for prehospital care providers to discuss this with their on-line medical advisor if questions arise.

After airway, breathing, and circulation have been established, the prehospital care provider evaluates the patient for other injuries that may compromise life or limb. The team begins the secondary survey, which is a head-to-toe assessment of the patient. The objective of the secondary survey is to identify all potentially life-threatening or complicating factors. The secondary survey is often done while in transport to the receiving hospital. At times this survey may not be completed before arrival and should not delay transport.

TRAUMATIC BRAIN INJURY

Annually approximately 1.6 million people experience traumatic brain injury (TBI). The impact of these injuries is significant to both the individual and society. It is critical to initiate appropriate care for the TBI patient as soon after the injury as possible. The Brain Trauma Foundation describes prehospital care as "the first critical link in providing appropriate care for individuals with severe brain injury."[27]

It has been established that episodes of hypoxemia and hypotension in the prehospital setting are commonly associated with poor outcomes from TBI. Focusing on adequate oxygenation and hemodynamic stability in the field is critical for these patients. In its recent publication, *Guidelines for Prehospital Management of Traumatic Brain Injury*, the Brain Trauma Foundation recommends the following[27]:

- All patients should be reassessed every 5 minutes because of the rapid changes possible in TBI patients.
- All verbally unresponsive patients who demonstrate extensor posturing or flaccidity in response to noxious stimuli should have an airway secured if possible and be hyperventilated (20 bpm/adult, 30 bpm/child, and 35 bpm/infant).
- All verbally unresponsive patients who demonstrate abnormal flexion in response to noxious stimuli but have asymmetric pupils should have an airway secured if possible and be hyperventilated as described previously.
- All TBI patients should have their oxygen saturations maintained at greater than 90%.
- Systolic blood pressure (BP) should be monitored and maintained at greater than 90 mm Hg for adults and those 12 to 16 years of age; greater than 80 mm Hg for those 5 to 12 years of age; greater than 75 mm Hg for those 1 to 5 years of age; and greater than 65 mm Hg for infants less than 1 year.
- Patients should be transported to a trauma center if their Glasgow Coma Scale (GCS) score is 13 or less.

Rapid recognition and correction of airway, breathing, or circulation compromise and transport to a definitive care facility are essential for the brain-injured patient to have the greatest chance for optimal recovery.

ORTHOPEDIC INJURIES

Orthopedic injuries are not the primary focus of the prehospital caregiver. Once the primary assessment and interventions are completed, the focus is on moving the patient to the most appropriate trauma receiving center.

Extremities may be evaluated while en route to the trauma center. If extremities have obvious fractures, pulses are evaluated serially. If pulses are present, extremities are

TABLE 8-9	Orthopedic Adjuncts	
Device	Indication	Comments
Splint	Maintain placement Decrease pain	Wide variety available (e.g., cardboard, metal, and plastic)
Pneumatic trousers	Pelvic fracture Provide tamponade effect	Rapid removal in hospital may result in severe drop in blood pressure
Traction	Splints apply traction to reinstate positioning for adequate blood flow	Include Hare traction and Sager splints

splinted as they are seen. If no pulses are present, the extremity is positioned physiologically and the pulses reassessed. The presence or absence of the pulse will dictate further intervention. The goal of all prehospital care related to orthopedic injuries is to preserve what remains and do no further harm. Adjuncts available to aid the prehospital provider in caring for orthopedic injuries are found in Table 8-9.

TRANSPORT OF THE TRAUMA PATIENT

HOW TO TRANSPORT

Once safe access to the injured patient has been accomplished, the focus of the team is on delivery of the injured to the appropriate receiving center. How is the patient to be transported? The options are by ground, by air, or by water. Factors to consider include: the number of patients, the location of the patient(s), the location of the receiving center(s), the care required of the patients en route, and the scope of care of the transporting prehospital care providers.

The ground options include transport by a BLS ambulance and crew or transport by an ALS ambulance and crew. In most areas of the country, the BLS crew's scope of practice allows delivery of first aid and administration of oxygen and CPR during transport. BLS providers can deliver oxygen, place nasal and oropharyngeal airways, and apply and maintain splints. If the patient requires any advanced intervention, including intubation or intravenous fluid administration, an ALS scope of practice is required and the patient should be transported by an ALS ambulance and crew.

If the incident has required activation of an air ambulance, whether because of the number of patients, the location of the patient, or the acuity of care required, it is important to note the reason. Helicopters and crews have diverse capabilities and skills depending on classification and training.

Each area of the United States has a different method of determining how air providers are classified and how scope of practice is defined. For example, in California air medical providers are defined under Title 22 of the state Code of Regulation.[28] In this document a rescue helicopter is defined as "an aircraft whose usual function is not prehospital emergency patient transport but may be utilized, in compliance with local EMS policy, for prehospital emergency patient transport." An air ambulance is described as "any aircraft specially constructed, modified or equipped and used for the primary purpose of responding to emergency calls and transporting critically ill or injured patients whose medical flight crew has at a minimum two attendants certified or licensed in advanced life support." The state of California has additional classifications: ALS rescue aircraft, BLS aircraft, and auxiliary rescue aircraft. These types of aircraft carry different crews who meet specific requirements and have specific medical care capabilities.

In this chapter air medical transport is discussed using the Commission of Accreditation of Medical Transport Systems (CAMTS)[29] requirements that define the scope of care and type of caregiver.

In situations where air medical transport is used, the entire team participates in preparing the patient for transport. Injured patients are transported on a long backboard with a cervical collar in place. The patient is secured with safety belts to prohibit movement and maintain stability in flight or during ground transport. In all transport situations everyone involved has a specific responsibility, which keeps things running smoothly and precludes oversight of critical activities. In most air medical crew role delineations, one individual is responsible for the essential role of patient airway management. The same crew member is responsible for maintaining the airway and directing movement to be sure that any artificial airway (e.g., endotracheal tube) is not dislodged. In helicopter operations, one crew member is specifically responsible for directing others' activity around the aircraft to ensure safety and to limit confusion during loading or off-loading.

Safety in operation is a vital focus in all air medical activities. The most critical phases of flight are takeoff and landing. During these times the entire crew focuses their attention outside the aircraft, looking for wires, flying debris, or anything else that would interfere with a safe, unobstructed flight path. In most air medical operations, takeoffs and landings are considered "sterile cockpit" times. This means that only mission safety-specific discussions are held by the crew via the intercabin communication system or radio. During this time air medical crews will not routinely give information over the radio or respond to calls. This "sterile cockpit" heightens awareness and directs attention.

During this entire time the patient's heart rate, blood pressure, oxygen saturation, and (in many cases) end tidal CO_2 levels are monitored. Other interventions are performed as directed by the patient condition and clinical protocol. In some areas of the United States, blood is transfused in the prehospital setting. The crew focuses on the patient and safety simultaneously.

A critical component of the transport phase is making hospital contact. The goal is to give the receiving hospital as much information as possible to allow adequate preparation for the delivery of the critically injured person. Time is of the essence, and the succinct delivery of information may be the difference between life and death.

WHERE TO DELIVER THE PATIENT

In most areas of the United States, critically injured patients are delivered to dedicated trauma centers. The objective of a trauma system is to have necessary resources immediately available to meet the needs of the injured patient.

In *Resources for Optimal Care of the Injured Patient: 1999*,[30] the American College of Surgeons states that the care of the trauma patient requires an organized, systematic approach with preset plans and protocols that ensure rapid access to care by dedicated and expert personnel at specialized facilities. Trauma care requires a significant commitment of personnel and resources. The goal is to be ready for any type of patient presentation at any time. Trauma centers are designated by the American College of Surgeons as Level I, II, III, or IV. Level I and II trauma centers are required to have 24-hour availability of general and neurologic surgery, emergency medicine services, and in-house anesthesiology. Further differentiation of these centers is beyond the scope of this chapter. For further information, contact the American College of Surgeons.

In systems where the receiving hospital is not a trauma center, it is necessary for the accepting hospital to have policies and practices in place to foster the rapid transfer and transport of an injured patient whose needs outweigh the capabilities of that hospital to a trauma care facility.

In situations where an air ambulance is used, determination of a safe landing zone must be considered. Most trauma centers have helipads designated to receive these patients. Each state has different regulations regarding landing of emergency medical helicopters; it is critical to evaluate these rules and procedures before the event.

At the discretion of the air medical program, the aircraft may be unloaded "hot" (with engines/rotor blades turning) or "cold" (after the blades have stopped turning and engines are shut down). Regional differences and program philosophies influence this choice. Some believe hot off-loading saves critical minutes; others counter that cold off-loading is safer because it limits movement of staff and equipment under moving rotor blades.[31,32]

DELIVERY OF THE PATIENT

TRANSFER OF CARE

In all situations the transporting crew transfers the care of the injured individual soon after arrival at the receiving hospital. The members of this crew deliver information and the patient. It is the responsibility of the crew delivering the patient to verify before leaving the facility that the accepting team has a clear understanding of the patient's recent event, vital signs, and all other assessment and intervention data. The exact time of transfer has been the subject of debate.

A guiding principle is a team focus on delivering the best care to the patient, which is facilitated by communication and interaction.

TRANSPORT DOCUMENTATION

All events, assessments, and interventions must be documented accurately and descriptively. The patient care record must be clear, objective, and succinct, containing an accurate accounting of the care provided and the circumstances of the transport. In general, documentation must be legible and free of unrecognized abbreviations. It is recommended that documentation be completed as soon as possible after the conclusion of patient care. Most EMS and air medical systems have documentation forms in a checklist format to ensure that all significant areas are addressed. It is critical to fill in all areas of the documentation form; no blank areas should remain.[33] If there are nonapplicable areas, the caregiver draws lines through them to prevent late additions by others. Documentation marks the close of the prehospital phase of patient care. It is critical that it is a true reflection of events.

SUMMARY

Effective delivery of care in the prehospital environment is essential to enhance the outcomes of the 60 million people injured each year. As is discussed in this chapter, success is affected by the cohesiveness of the multidisciplinary prehospital team, communication flow, and appropriate care delivery.

The prehospital environment is different from other health care settings. In no other practice area is safety of the provider such an essential component in minute-by-minute decision making. At times it is without lights, electricity, or other adjuncts and support systems of which in-hospital providers are easily assured. Nurses have a strong role in this arena as caregivers and team members. It is appropriate that nurses participate in a system that ensures the injured patient receives the best possible care in the field.

The definition of appropriate prehospital care must be critically evaluated. There are many practice approaches that lack a strong research base, which has led to regional practice variations. Included in these differences are scope of practice requirements, airway management techniques, and fluid resuscitation, to name just a few. Additional research and continued refinement of prehospital care is necessary to improve the ultimate outcome of those injured.

REFERENCES

1. American College of Surgeons' Committee on Trauma: *Advanced trauma life support manual*, Chicago, 1997.
2. Patruras JL: The EMS call. In Pons P and Cason D, editors: *Paramedic field care: a complaint-based approach*, St. Louis, 1997, Mosby, 27-34.
3. Dernocouer K: Safety and the field/dispatch connection, *Emerg Med Serv* 27(8):23-24, 1998.

4. Clawson J: *Emergency medical dispatch priority card system,* Salt Lake City, 1979, Salt Lake City Fire Department.

5. Rau W, Lathrop G: 1998 Medical crew survey, *Air Med* (4)5:22-27, 1998.

6. Johnson JC: Multiple casualty incidents and disasters. In Pons P and Cason D, editors: *Paramedic field care: a complaint-based approach,* St. Louis, 1997, Mosby, 629-642.

7. State of California, Office of Emergency Services: *Standardized emergency management system field course module 2—principles and features of ICS,* Sacramento, 1995, OES.

8. Finerty TR: Emergency medical services systems. In Krupa D, editor: *Flight nursing core curriculum,* Park Ridge, Ill, 1997, National Flight Nurses Association, 737-750.

9. Public Service of the Chemical Manufacturers Association, CHEMTREC, (800) 262-8200, Arlington, Va, 2000.

10. National Association of Emergency Medical Technicians: *Pre-hospital trauma life support: basic and advanced,* ed 3, St Louis, 1994, Mosby.

11. National Association of Emergency Medical Services Physicians: Air medical dispatch: guidelines for scene response, *Prehosp Disaster Med* 7(1):75-76, 1992.

12. Holleran RS: Extrication and scene management. In National Flight Nursing Association: *Flight nursing: principles and practice,* ed 2, St. Louis, 1996, Mosby, 37-48.

13. Stewart C, Conover K, Terry M: General principles of rescue. In Pons P and Cason D, editors: *Paramedic field care: a complaint-based approach,* St. Louis, 1997, Mosby, 616-627.

14. Walls RM, editor: *Advanced emergency airway management,* Dallas, 1997, American College of Emergency Physicians.

15. American Burn Association: *Advanced burn life support provider's manual,* Lincoln, Neb, 1996, The Association.

16. Simon B: Pharmacologic aids in airway management. In Dailey RH, editor: *The airway: emergency management,* St. Louis, 1992, Mosby, 145-170.

17. Mageau AP: Airway management/oxygen therapy. In Krupa D, editor: *Flight nursing core curriculum,* Park Ridge, Ill, 1997, National Flight Nurses Association, 69-95.

18. Sing RF, Rotundo MF, Zonies DH et al: Rapid sequence induction for intubation by an aeromedical transport team, *Am J Emerg Med* 16(6):598-602, 1998.

19. York D: Rapid sequence induction for intubation. In Proehl J, editor: *Emergency nursing procedures,* ed 2, Philadelphia, 1999, WB Saunders, 26-30.

20. Patrick VC: Emergency needle thoracentesis. In Proehl J, editor: *Emergency nursing procedures,* ed 2, Philadelphia, 1999, WB Saunders, 130-132.

21. Barton ED, Epperson M, Hoyt D et al: Prehospital needle aspiration and tube thoracostomy in trauma victims: a six year experience with aeromedical crews, *J Emerg Med* 13(2):155-63, 1995.

22. York D, Dudek L, Larson R et al: A comparison study of chest tube thoracostomy: air medical crew and in-hospital trauma services, *Air Med J* 12(7):227-229, 1993.

23. Bravo AM: Trauma and burns. In The Johns Hopkins Hospital Department of Pediatrics, Barone M, editor: *The Harriet Lane handbook,* ed 15, St. Louis, 2000, Mosby, 73-75.

24. Trunkey D: Prehospital fluid resuscitation. In Trunkey D and Lewis F, editors: *Current therapy of trauma,* ed 4, St. Louis, 1999, Mosby, 129-130.

25. Bickell WH, Wall MJ, Pete PE: Immediate versus delayed fluid resuscitation for hypotensive patients with penetrating torso injuries, *N Engl J Med* 331(17):1105-1109, 1994.

26. Demetriades D, Chan L, Cornwall E et al: Paramedic vs. private transportation of trauma patients: effect on outcome, *Arch Surg* 131(2):133-138, 1996.

27. Brain Trauma Foundation: *Guidelines for prehospital management of traumatic brain injury,* New York, 2000, National Highway Transportation Safety Administration.

28. State of California: California code of regulation, Title 22, Div 9, 2000.

29. Commission on Accreditation of Medical Transport Systems: *Accreditation standards of CAMTS,* ed 3, Anderson, SC, 1997, CAMTS.

30. American College of Surgeons' Committee on Trauma: *Resources for optimal care of the injured patient: 1999,* Chicago, 1998.

31. Deimling D, deJarnett R, Rouse M et al: Helicopter loading time study: hot versus cold, *Air Med J* 18(4):145-148, 1999.

32. Criddle LM: The hot loaded patient: review and analysis of 1 year experience, *Air Med J* 18(4):140-144, 1999.

33. Krupa D: Legal. In Krupa D, editor: *Flight nursing core curriculum,* Park Ridge, Ill, 1997, National Flight Nurses Association, 819-826.

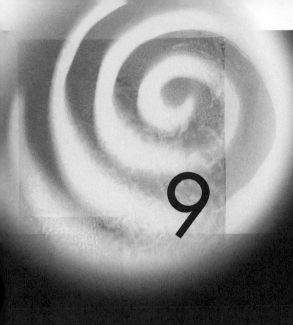

9 NURSING PRACTICE THROUGH THE CYCLE OF TRAUMA

Kathryn Truter VonRueden •
Robbi Lynn Hartsock

Traumatology is now fully recognized as a specialized branch of general surgery. Concurrently, because of the uniqueness and complexity of patients with multiple injuries, trauma nursing also has evolved as a specialized field.

One of the most challenging aspects of caring for trauma patients is the development of a plan of care that addresses each component of the patient's needs in a logical, organized fashion to ensure continuity and coordination of all care disciplines. Formulation of such a plan requires incorporation of the five components of the nursing process: assessment, diagnosis, planning, implementation, and evaluation. In addition, the nursing plan of care is inextricably intertwined with and reflective of the plans of other trauma team members as the overall plan of care is developed and implemented throughout the cycle of trauma care.

This coordination of patient care requires individuals with a wide range and breadth of knowledge and skills. Trauma nurses must have an understanding of the significance of the impact of the traumatic injury on the patient, the patient's family, and society. They must be adept at sophisticated monitoring and at caring for the intense physiologic needs, and they must be able to respond to the psychologic and social demands of the patient. They also must be able to assist the family in coping with the stress and emotional devastation that accompany a sudden traumatic event. Patient and family recovery is heavily dependent on the skills of the nurses as caregivers, communicators, collaborators, and coordinators throughout the cycle of trauma.

TRAUMA NURSING PRACTICE

In 1961 Dorothy Johnson defined nursing practice in terms of three major components: nursing care, delegated medical care, and health care.[1] The nursing process is incorporated into each of these components and provides a framework for bringing the three components together. In describing the overall purpose of *nursing care,* she stated, "The achievement and maintenance of a stable state is nursing's distinctive contribution to patient welfare and the specific purpose of nursing care. The change of any magnitude toward recovery from illness or toward more desirable health practice depends on the periodic achievement and maintenance, perhaps only for a short time, of this stable state."[1]

Delegated medical care refers to the care given by the nurse, which contributes to the development and implementation of medical care plans. *Health care* refers to the service that has the promotion and maintenance of desirable health practices as its purpose.

When developing a plan of care for the multiply injured patient, all three of these components are relevant. During the initial phase of care immediately after injury and during the stabilization phase, it is vital that the focus include both nursing care and delegated medical care components. As patients enter the rehabilitative phase, the health care component takes on more significance because they learn ways to live with residual impairments from their injuries and they become reintegrated into society.

Health care also implies the education of the public in the area of injury prevention. Trauma nurses have an essential role in the educational process by providing information to people of all ages.

Throughout the cycle of trauma care, specialized expertise is required to provide quality care and to achieve optimal outcomes for this complex patient population. Credentialing of trauma nurses is a way to ensure accountability in practice and competence in performance. Competency-based orientation and periodically required cognitive and psychomotor certifications are a means to this end. In addition, annual competency verification updates staff on new or revised procedures and complex or high-risk procedures, and it provides trauma center designation-required educational content.

PROFILE OF THE TRAUMA PATIENT

Several characteristics of the multiply injured contribute to the complexity of this unique patient population:

- Traumatic injuries are sudden. Unlike the patient who is hospitalized for elective surgery, the trauma patient and family have no warning. The injury is an unexpected, severe interruption of normal life. There is no time to plan or prepare; one must simply cope with the injury once it occurs.
- Drug and alcohol abuse commonly plays a causative role in injury. The multiply injured patient whose history includes substance abuse is typically more difficult to initially assess and later to manage effectively. Often family members' feelings of guilt because the inability to convince the patient to seek help for a drug or alcohol problem may affect their ability to cope effectively with the family member's injury.
- Because of the severity and complexity of injury, most trauma patients require long-term rehabilitative care. Systemic sequelae and physical handicaps also may result. Learning to cope adequately, both physically and psychologically, is a process that must begin early after hospitalization.
- Psychologic sequelae are extremely common in multiply injured patients. Many experience posttraumatic stress syndrome and grieving after the injury. Depending on the individual's existing support systems and coping mechanisms, adaptation to severe injuries may be difficult.
- Trauma is a disease of the young. The average age of the multiply injured patient is between 15 and 34 years.[2] Their inexperience with life crises, developmental stage, and level of maturity create special needs that must be considered when planning effective interventions.
- The number of elderly trauma patients is increasing and will continue to do so with the "graying of America." In 1995 unintentional injury was the third leading cause of death in patients 45 to 65 and the seventh leading cause of death in patients 65 and older.[3] This population has unique needs that necessitate alterations in the typical approaches to resuscitation, critical care, and rehabilitative practices.
- Many critically injured patients who do not survive are potential subjects of a medical examiner's investigation. This is due to the fact that their injuries are a result of violence or unintentional injury. Therefore legal implications must be considered before a plan of care can be developed. Once the plan of care is developed, it may be subjected to greater scrutiny by staff, hospital administrators, criminal investigators, attorneys, and patients' families than the plan for a patient admitted for elective surgery.
- Serious injuries are often subtle. Many injuries are obvious, and they often mask others that may be even more life threatening. Nursing assessment is of greater significance when the occurrence of subtle injuries is considered because the diagnosis may be delayed.
- The multiply injured patient has tremendous potential for developing complications during the hospitalization phase. In collaboration with the trauma surgeon, the nurse is largely responsible for preventing, detecting early, and minimizing the consequences of such complications.
- Initial injuries or their required treatments create additional problems that greatly influence care planning for multiply injured patients. Many are immobilized because of hemodynamic instability, severe respiratory dysfunction, or orthopedic or neurologic injury. Communication is often difficult if an endotracheal tube or a tracheostomy tube is necessary for ventilatory support. Infection is prevalent in many of these patients because of the nature of their injuries, multiple invasive procedures, and exposure to the numerous trauma team members who provide care for them.
- Because multiple injuries affect several body systems, implementation of standard and accepted methods of treatment for each injury is often difficult or contraindicated. For example, the existence of a severe brain injury may prohibit routine repositioning and chest physiotherapy treatments ordinarily required by a patient with thoracic injuries. Alternative methods of treatment that do not compromise the patient's existing injuries must be explored.
- The treatment of critically injured patients often imposes serious economic burdens on their families. The cost of critical care and rehabilitative care can be staggering.

These characteristics and the necessarily complex treatment modes make planning care for the multiply injured patient a difficult and challenging task.

Implementation of a philosophy of care that focuses on a well-communicated and organized approach to the delivery of trauma care and medical expertise is essential. The Committee on Trauma of the American College of Surgeons suggests the following requirements for that approach[4]:

1. Rapid identification of the injury followed by easy access to the emergency medical system (EMS)
2. A central emergency dispatching system such as 911
3. Appropriately trained and appropriate level of EMS provider available to respond to the scene, that is, basic versus advanced life support
4. Prehospital triage protocols that authorize the EMS providers to make triage decisions *before* the patient is taken to a hospital
5. A communication system that allows direct conversation between the prehospital providers, trauma center personnel, and the physicians who provide medical direction

6. A designated trauma center with immediate availability of specialized surgeons, anesthesia providers, nurses, and emergency resuscitative equipment and radiologic capabilities

7. A trauma system that coordinates care among all levels of trauma centers and an interfacility transfer process that allows for prompt transfer of the patient to a higher level of care

8. Access to rehabilitative services in both the acute and long-term phases of recovery

CRUCIAL CONSIDERATIONS WHEN PLANNING CARE

COLLABORATIVE PRACTICE

When initiating the plan of care for the multiply injured patient, collaborative practice is crucial. This concept is a common theme in current medical and nursing literature. It describes the ideal working relationship between the physician, nurse, and personnel from other disciplines, resulting in higher-quality care. The purpose of collaborative practice is to integrate care regimens into a comprehensive approach to patient needs. It is a relationship in which professionals define specific roles and jointly determine a relationship that is most beneficial to the patient.

Collaborative practice may significantly affect morbidity and mortality of the critically ill.[5] Critical care units in large educational institutions do not always have the lowest mortality rates or the most effective care. Highly coordinated systems for patient management that result in quality patient care are often lacking. Excluding other variables, investigators have concluded that the *process* of care is essential to reduce morbidity and mortality. Inherent in the process is the positive interaction and collaboration of physicians and nurses in achieving optimal results and the adherence to established protocols and procedures to guide their care. Collaborative practice, when used in treating the multiply injured patient, includes all members of the trauma team, from prehospital to rehabilitative care, working together toward a common goal—providing the best possible trauma care. Without collaborative practice, this common goal and optimal patient outcomes cannot be realized.

Hope for the survival of the multiple trauma patient rests with the collaborative efforts of the trauma nurses, physicians, technicians, and therapists who constitute the trauma team. Paramedics, nurses, and physicians labor together to resuscitate, stabilize, diagnose, and treat the severely injured patient.

Optimal care of trauma patients, which implies minimal errors and complications and maximal efficiency and continuity, is provided by a team that accurately and consistently communicates, beginning with the field providers and subsequently with the nurses and physicians who follow the patient from admission throughout the resuscitative and operative phases. In a collaborative environment, care becomes directed and focused. Communication and collaboration must continue throughout the cycle of trauma care.

PATIENT ADVOCACY

The role of the trauma nurse as a patient advocate is critical in many situations during the cycle of trauma care. The patient may be comatose, paralyzed, sedated, or in pain. These conditions alter the ability to participate actively in decision making. Such conditions also may contribute to a communication deficit, increasing the potential for care to become disjointed among the many involved services and personnel. Through the advocacy role the trauma nurse participates with the patient, family, and colleagues to develop processes of care that restore optimal function of the patient.

DEVELOPING AN INTEGRATED PLAN OF CARE

A specialized plan of care is clearly a necessity for the multitrauma patient. Regardless of the facility (a designated trauma center versus a community or large university hospital), mechanisms to address the trauma patient's needs must exist.

MECHANISMS TO ASSIST IN PLANNING QUALITY CARE

Highly specialized trauma care requires several mechanisms for guidance and direction. Policies and protocols specifically addressing the care of trauma patients must be developed and based on current modes of therapy. They must be followed and consistently updated as new therapies, equipment, and research dictate. It is imperative that the established protocols, policies, standards, and procedures be reviewed on a consistent basis and changed to reflect and incorporate new modes of therapy and current research findings. They should be consistent with the guidelines set forth by organizations such as the American College of Surgeons' Committee on Trauma, the Eastern Association for the Surgery of Trauma, the Society of Trauma Nurses, the American Association of Critical Care Nurses, and the Society of Critical Care Medicine.

From these guidelines trauma nursing standards are developed to facilitate the implementation of these policies and protocols. These standards should reflect an aim for the highest levels of care, yet they must be realistic and based on the resources available to implement them. These standards also form the basis for nursing care evaluation. In addition, nursing procedures must be written to implement the policies, protocols, and standards. It is important to note that if the standardized guidelines and procedures promulgated by the preceding organizations are used, they must be tailored to meet the needs of the individual patient. For example, a procedure outlining the proper use of the hypothermia blanket (a standard procedure in most critical care units) must include special precautions in relation to aspects of the trauma patient's care, such as its use in spinal cord-injured patients whose thermoregulation mechanisms may be significantly impaired. In addition, a procedure manual, preferably on-line, should be readily available as a resource in the patient care area.

SYSTEM OF CARE DELIVERY

A system of nursing care delivery capable of providing highly specialized care must be established. One system that best facilitates the coordination of specialized care is that of primary nursing, where the nurse in each phase serves as the patient's care coordinator. Primary nursing facilitates goal-directed coordination of the many teams of trauma care providers that are necessary to provide the highest quality of care. Other systems of care delivery may be equally effective as long as they ensure nursing accountability for goal-directed care and for communication and coordination of the trauma team.

One member of the trauma team should be in charge of coordinating this care, and the primary nurse who cares for the patient on a consistent basis is ideal for orchestrating this process. Ensuring that treatment plans and interventions from the various disciplines are congruent with the overall plan of care is the primary function of this role. The trauma nurse's level of assessment skills, accountability, and educational preparation combine to make the primary nurse's role an excellent one to assume this level of complicated care coordination.

To further ensure collaboration and continuity of trauma patient care, a case-management system is implemented in most trauma centers and is generally a requirement for trauma center verification or designation. Typically the trauma case manager is a master's-prepared clinical nurse specialist or trauma nurse coordinator. The case manager is responsible for the daily review and coordination of multidisciplinary services, efficient use of resources, patient disposition through the system, and arrangement of follow-up care. The trauma case manager role is absolutely essential in trauma centers where a strong primary nursing system is not in place.

A philosophy of trauma nursing must exist that encompasses beliefs about the trauma patient's care from prevention through reintegration into the community. All nurses caring for these patients must adopt this philosophy as care is planned and delivered.

In addition to a philosophy of trauma nursing, nurses caring for these patients must also possess a strong pathophysiologic knowledge base. This is needed to assess the patient and to plan and direct care throughout the phases. Particularly for the resuscitation and critical care phases, it is advantageous for the trauma nurse to have significant experience in emergency and critical care nursing before caring for patients whose injuries may involve many body systems and whose psychologic responses are often complex.

THE PLAN OF CARE

The written plan of care is a vital component of the trauma patient's care. The Joint Commission on Accreditation of Healthcare Organizations (JCAHO) requires a documented plan of care that addresses physiologic, psychologic, and environmental factors.[6] The care plan for the trauma patient must not be written only with the idea of satisfying this requirement but rather must be looked on as the link between injury and readaptation—the base from which all care is delivered. This plan should be developed by, familiar to, and used by *all* members of the trauma team. It must be succinct and reflect changes in care as they become necessary. The plan also should be evaluated and revised at regular intervals, dictated by patient acuity and specific goals or outcomes.

PROBLEMS IN ACTUALIZING PLANS OF CARE

The complex nature of the multitrauma patient necessitates an involved plan of care. For many reasons, it is often difficult to develop a written plan. Time is a limitation; however, it is important not to lose sight of the value of the written plan even when time constraints are inevitable.

Educating the nursing staff on how to develop and write an effective plan of care is essential. Workshops given at specified periods each year are one possible avenue, but staffing constraints may prevent their feasibility. Alternative means of education (e.g., learning modules and videotapes) must be explored.

It is also necessary to ensure that the plan of care is followed, evaluated, and revised when the primary nurse is not available. Ideally a consistent "relief nurse" should assume this responsibility in the absence of the primary nurse. However, widespread use of temporary nurses (i.e., float pool or contract nurses) makes this difficult, if not impossible, to accomplish.

CRITICAL PATHWAYS

In the past decade, critical pathways and practice guidelines have been developed to save time and ensure quality care for trauma patients. Critical pathways prescribe day-to-day multidisciplinary activities such as interventions, consultations, diagnostic testing, and patient and family education for trauma patients with common physiologic alterations or those with similar injuries. Developed and agreed on by a multidisciplinary group, critical pathways concretely direct the efforts of all services. These are extremely beneficial when planning care for the trauma patient and may be used throughout the phases. Many trauma patients exhibit the same responses in relation to specific injuries; therefore, standardized pathways and guidelines addressing these responses have several advantages. They conserve valuable time and promote continuity and consistency of care.

The reluctance of some physicians and nurses to use these standardized plans usually stems from the concern that patient individuality will be lost. However, there is no substitute for sound clinical judgment, which prevails over a "cookbook" approach.

Regardless of the type of plan of care chosen by an institution, it must have the following characteristics:

- Be based on physiologic priorities
- Provide an organized, logical approach to trauma patient care
- Identify specific goals or outcomes and interventions

- Be developed and used by the multidisciplinary trauma team
- Have utility throughout the cycle of trauma care

PHASE I: FIELD STABILIZATION AND RESUSCITATION

The ultimate goal in the prehospital phase is to stabilize and transport the multiply injured patient to the appropriate level trauma center via the safest and most rapid transport mode. Accomplishing this requires collaboration that begins at the scene where the patient is injured. An effective EMS system provides a means for specially trained paramedics to communicate with trauma physicians at the receiving hospital and a centralized communications center to assist in planning the appropriate mode of transport for that patient. Conditions at the scene also may require calls for additional personnel to help with extrication or additional law enforcement officers to assist with crowd control or to direct traffic to prevent further injuries. In addition to the indispensable role of the paramedic, the role of the nurse and physician in the field can be of great value, as the concept of "go teams" (physicians and nurses who go from the hospital to the scene) has illustrated. In addition, flight nurses (and physicians in some programs) who staff hospital-based helicopter programs are in widespread use across the country. See Chapter 8 for a complete discussion of the prehospital phase of trauma care.

ASSESSMENT AND DIAGNOSIS

The advanced trauma life support (ATLS) guidelines for initial assessment provide a standardized approach.[7] When communicating assessment findings to the receiving hospital, it is imperative that a common language and approach be used, such as a specific trauma injury scoring system or the Glasgow Coma Scale.

In the field or at the scene of any injury, the priorities are always the ABCs: airway, breathing, and circulation. Establishing an airway at the scene is often difficult. The injured individual may be trapped inside a vehicle with a steering wheel crushed against the chest or may have been ejected from the vehicle, resulting in serious head and facial injuries with severe bleeding causing airway obstruction. EMS personnel should suspect the trauma patient of having a cervical spine injury until proved otherwise, and an airway should be established with this possibility in mind.

Immediately following attention to the ABCs, the neurologic status should be assessed. The baseline neurologic status (level of consciousness and pupillary size and reaction) of the trauma patient is of such a critical nature that it must be included as part of the primary assessment.[8] Once the primary survey has been completed, a secondary survey is performed to establish the presence of further injuries.

External evidence of trauma should alert the caregiver to the possibility of internal injury. These signs may be easily overlooked in the presence of obvious hemorrhage or other significant wounds. Abrasions, contusions, and pain on movement can be observed at the scene and may lead to early recognition of occult injuries. Back and neck pain may suggest spinal injury. Abrasions and contusions of the chest and abdomen may herald occult internal injuries and concomitant head injury. Deformity and pain suggest extremity injury. All patients should be managed as though they have sustained serious injuries until a thorough examination can be made at an appropriate trauma center. If the patient is unresponsive, it should be assumed that spinal, thoracic, and abdominal injuries are present until proven otherwise. In this phase the mechanism of injury is always considered when assessing for signs of obvious or occult injury. It is essential that EMS personnel provide as much information as possible about how the injury occurred and relate specific assessment findings to the receiving facility.

DEVELOPING AND IMPLEMENTING THE PLAN

Assessment, diagnosis, and initiation of planned interventions are simultaneous activities. As quickly as alterations in the ABCs are identified, treatment is instituted. Several basic principles are followed at the scene of an injury:

1. Ensure that the scene is secure (i.e., EMS personnel should not enter a scene that poses obvious risk to their own safety).
2. Remove the patient from a hazard only when the risk (e.g., fire) outweighs the danger.
3. Establish an airway, maintaining cervical spine neutrality.
4. Initiate cardiopulmonary resuscitation (CPR) as indicated.
5. Control obvious hemorrhage with direct pressure.
6. Establish intravenous access.
7. Immobilize the neck (with a cervical collar) and spine (with a long backboard) if the mechanism of injury dictates.
8. Splint extremity injuries.
9. Transport to the closest, *most appropriate* facility as soon as possible.

A primary objective of care in the field is to prevent further injury. Care in extricating and transporting patients to avoid further damage in spinal cord injuries cannot be overemphasized. Attention to limb position and to the handling and splinting of fractures may decrease the possibility of neurovascular damage and/or fat emboli. Further contamination of open wounds must be avoided to decrease the incidence of overwhelming infection at a later stage.

In the prehospital phase, effective triage is vital to ensuring that the patient is sent to the most appropriate facility based on the injuries present. Specific guidelines for making these decisions must be in place and rigorously followed. Triage protocols are defined within each jurisdiction or state EMS system.

Once the appropriate level of trauma center is identified, decisions about which mode of transport will be used are the next priority. Transporting the patient from the scene to the hospital requires selection of the method best suited to avoid or reduce complications.

The communication system used during the prehospital phase must be clear, accurate, rapid, and cost effective. Depending on the EMS system, biomedical telemetry systems, radio transmitters, standard or cellular telephones, or telemedicine may be used. Once the patient arrives at the hospital, a more detailed account of the mechanism of injury, assessment findings, and treatment administered at the scene is given to the hospital's trauma team.

Documentation from the field is crucial to the plan of care. EMS records should include information on: patient status, vital signs, mechanism of injury, therapy received, and present medical history (if relevant). Any relevant social history (e.g., involvement of other family members) is also documented. Injury data should include time of injury, geographic location, and any other pertinent data. These prehospital written records should be placed with the patient's medical record and kept because the data from them are essential in completing data requirements for trauma registries and databases. In addition, most trauma center verification or designation standards also require that the prehospital sheets be present in the medical record.

EVALUATION

During the prehospital phase, ongoing evaluation of the treatment and transport plans is imperative. Continuous assessment of the patient's condition is vital to detect any signs of deterioration that may necessitate a change in plans. If the patient's condition worsens, transport to the *closest* hospital for stabilization with subsequent transfer to an appropriate level trauma center may be required. If delays in the planned transport mode occur, alternate transport might be necessary to save time and the patient's life. Changes in the patient's condition also must be relayed to the receiving facility to allow alternate orders for treatment to be issued. In situations in which EMS personnel require assistance in treatment or triage decisions, the existence of some means for consultation with a trauma physician is essential. This dedicated radio or telephone allows field personnel to communicate directly with a trauma physician as vital decisions are made.

After the patient has reached the trauma facility, it is important that the trauma team reviews the prehospital care. Any identified concerns from the prehospital phase of care (e.g., esophageal intubation, inappropriate triage or treatment decisions) should be communicated back to the prehospital jurisdictional leadership or appropriate persons. This is essential in improving quality in the trauma system as a whole.

In summary, an effective plan of care for the injured victim begins at the scene of the injury. Assessment, treatment, and communication during this phase will impact all subsequent stages of the patient's care. Dr. R Adams Cowley, father of the "golden hour" concept, found that multiple trauma patients who received definitive care within 60 minutes of their injuries had the best chance for recovery. The overall mortality rate of 15% to 20% doubled for every hour lost in receiving that care.[9]

PHASE II: IN-HOSPITAL RESUSCITATION AND OPERATIVE PHASE

Because the patient often arrives at the receiving facility from the scene with little of the golden hour remaining, immediate life-saving measures are required. A coordinated, collaborative, unified approach is the cornerstone of trauma patient care in the resuscitation unit. Philosophically, all trauma patients are in critical condition until proven otherwise. Advanced preparation to allow immediate access to equipment, supplies, and personnel is essential. This is made possible by notification of the patient's pending arrival at the trauma center.

PREPARATION AND INITIAL CONTACT

The resuscitation nurse plays a vital role even before the patient arrives. Requisite equipment for treating all injury priorities is established by the American College of Surgeons' Committee on Trauma in the ATLS manual.[7] This equipment should be located in the area where the trauma patient arrives and should be readily accessible. In some institutions proximity of the patients in the resuscitation area to the operating room is prohibitive; therefore, the trauma resuscitation area must be able to support major surgical procedures. The design of some small resuscitation areas and emergency departments makes this a challenge, but it must be recognized that every second lost as a result of disorganization decreases the patient's chance of survival. Having received prior notice of a patient's arrival allows preparation of routine equipment and supplies and acquisition of any unusual equipment required for specific injuries. Preassembled sterile instrument trays should be readily available to save valuable time.

Members of the trauma team are notified and must be present when the patient arrives. In major trauma centers this team usually consists of an attending (trauma surgeon or emergency medicine physician), a trauma fellow, one or two emergency medicine or surgery residents, one or two nurses, and a variety of other personnel. Response times and presence of these individuals is dictated and monitored by the trauma center verification or designation process. Preparation also includes donning of appropriate protective attire (goggles/face shield, mask, gloves, and impermeable cover gown) before the patient's arrival.[10] Each member of the team is assigned a specific role during the resuscitation, which is determined before the patient arrives.

ASSESSMENT

The resuscitation nurse plays a vital role in the quick assessment and stabilization of patients on admission. After the notification of a pending admission, trays should be opened, suction apparatus and overhead lights turned on, and intravenous (IV) lines primed with the appropriate fluids. Additional equipment is prepared based on specific information obtained from the field personnel. Trauma patients who arrive at the trauma facility by helicopter should be met by some members of the trauma team, ideally the resuscitation nurse and a person trained in emergency airway techniques. The comprehensive plan of care for the hospital phase is initiated on the helipad by performing a rapid primary survey to ensure that the ABCs are intact. If the patient is conscious, the nurse may also obtain a brief initial history at this time.

While assessing the patient, therapeutic communication is a priority. The nurse meeting the patient at the helipad, at the ambulance entrance, or in the emergency department establishes verbal communication and continues the exchange throughout this phase of care. "While steps to protect the patient's life obviously take highest priority, the nurse needs to begin to address the patient's emotional and mental state as well. By orienting [the patient] to reality and providing support, you can do much to relieve . . . anxiety and assist [the patient] toward resolution of [the] crisis."[11] The trauma patient is frightened and confused and may be experiencing pain or hypoxia. Although the emphasis during this phase is on assessment and stabilization of the patient's physical condition, full recovery demands that the patient's emotional state also be considered. Psychologic support to calm the patient, prepare him or her for what is ahead, and establish trust is important during this stage.

On arrival in the resuscitation area from the helipad or ambulance entrance, the nurse provides the trauma team with a succinct report of the assessment and clinical findings. The initial assessment and resuscitation activities are protocol driven and should be "indelibly ingrained" in the minds of all team members.[8] Throughout the resuscitation and stabilization phase, the physician team leader and admitting nurse coordinate procedures not only to carry out the established protocols for treatment but also to individualize care when appropriate. Specialists are consulted when appropriate, sedation is given so that a thorough medical examination may be obtained, and priorities of treatment are established.

Documentation is critical during this phase of care. Records used must contain vital information that is crucial to the plan of care. Vital signs and hemodynamic stability must be monitored continuously to detect subtle changes in the patient's condition. Particular attention must be paid to intake and output. Overloading the patient initially may appear inconsequential at this stage of care; however, it may predispose the patient to severe pulmonary dysfunction within a few hours. The nurse must be certain that accurate intake and output records are kept so that problems such as volume overload are either avoided or acknowledged, in which case appropriate treatment may be initiated to avoid complications. Continuous monitoring following the collection of baseline data is done to detect changes in the patient's condition as early as possible. Recording vital signs and electrocardiographic changes as often as every 5 minutes may be necessary.

The team approach is the most important factor during both the assessment and treatment of the patient. Following established protocols, the trauma nurse and physician approach the assessment of the patient in a systematic, organized fashion.

The assessment must be done quickly and efficiently. Priority-based trauma protocols provide the framework for detecting and treating life-threatening injuries. The first priorities focus on the traditional ABCs of airway, breathing, and circulation and are expanded to include D for neurologic disability, and E for exposing all injuries and for environmental control (thermoregulation).[8] Secondary priorities identify less evident but still life-threatening respiratory or cardiovascular dysfunctions. Third priorities are to detect and evaluate more subtle injuries that may contribute to morbidity and mortality but that are not necessarily life threatening.

DEVELOPING AND IMPLEMENTING THE PLAN

Appropriate patient management consists of the rapid assessment and treatment of life-threatening pathology. Logical sequential treatment priorities are established on the basis of overall patient assessment in any emergency involving a critical injury to the patient. Patient management consists of a rapid initial evaluation, resuscitation of vital functions, more detailed secondary and tertiary assessments, and, finally, the initiation of definitive care. Prevention of irreversible tissue hypoxia is the essence of trauma resuscitation. Treatment of life-threatening respiratory and cardiovascular instability, brain injury, and spinal cord injury *before* definitive diagnosis is often essential in the management of the multiply injured patient. The time taken to establish a firm diagnosis before life-saving measures are instituted may mean the difference between life and death.

HISTORY.   The resuscitation nurse obtains as accurate a database as possible if the patient is alert. In addition to physical symptoms, initial information includes: allergies, significant medical history, current medications, age, religion, and weight. A brief history can be accomplished rapidly by an "AMPLE" history: A, allergies; M, medications currently being taken; P, past illnesses; L, last meal; E, events preceding the injury.[7]

Information regarding these aspects of the patient's medical background is vital for the trauma team and must be known before initiating treatment. It is often impossible to obtain such a history when families are not available and the patient is comatose. The belongings of the patient are examined for medic-alert cards delineating allergies or medical problems, or prescription medications that might give a clue to underlying medical conditions. The Patient Self-Determination Act (1990) requires that the hospital also seek information regarding any advanced directives that the patient may have made. This information may be useful to the trauma team in making ethical decisions regarding treatment.[12]

DIAGNOSIS.   The resuscitation nurse must be aware of the actual or suspected medical diagnoses to begin the plan and the care. One of the first steps is to establish a trauma database that will help to guide patient care. The aim of the database is to organize facts concerning the causes and the nature of injury and the degree of trauma sustained. The data collected provide a basis for both medical and nursing care.

Evaluation of prehospital status and care is essential to the database. This provides an understanding of the mechanisms of injury, the initial physical findings, and other clues important to the management of the patient. Evaluation of a critical patient's status and the ultimate medical and nursing management are dependent on analysis of vital signs, fluid resuscitation, and other critical data entered in the trauma database. Establishing and maintaining an accurate database are key responsibilities of the resuscitation nurse. Accuracy of diagnosis, therapeutic medical and nursing plans of care, and patient outcomes depend on this function.

DIAGNOSTIC STUDIES.   The multiply injured patient may require several diagnostic studies before accurate medical diagnoses can be made. The nurse plays a vital role in preparing the patient and in coordinating these studies. Portable radiography equipment should be available in the trauma resuscitation area, but often additional studies must be done in a main radiology department. Transporting the patient in a safe and timely manner is the responsibility of the trauma resuscitation nurse. During transport, patient care should be maintained at the same level as that provided in the resuscitation unit. This is a team effort that often requires a trauma physician, nurse, and respiratory therapist to participate in the transport. A multipurpose cart equipped with the materials required for resuscitating and maintaining patients during transport can be developed for this purpose. Portable monitoring equipment (electrocardiograph [ECG] and pressure monitors) should be available and used during transport when appropriate. Blood products may also be transported safely with the use of an insulated container.

Appropriate laboratory tests are drawn (with typing and crossmatching or screening for blood receiving first priority). After these initial measures and a secondary survey, treatment of less serious injuries and more thorough radiographic studies are initiated.

After the initial stabilization procedures and the secondary assessment, nursing interventions are continued based on priorities of care. Continuous monitoring is carried out, psychologic support is continued, and appropriate treatments are administered.

STABILIZATION OF LIFE-THREATENING CONDITIONS.   The immediate objective in this phase of care is the stabilization of life-threatening conditions. The concept of "treatment prior to diagnosis" is crucial during this phase and based on establishment of an airway, adequate ventilation, and perfusion. Control of hemorrhage and initiation of fluid resuscitation must be accomplished rapidly.

A chest tube may need to be inserted rapidly to relieve a tension pneumothorax or hemothorax. The amount of chest drainage must be monitored closely to assist in determining blood replacement needs and the need for surgical intervention. Type-specific blood may be given until crossmatching has been completed. In a life-threatening emergency, uncrossmatched O-negative blood may be administered until laboratory results are complete.

Trauma resuscitation nurses use the principles and techniques of ATLS.[7] Although in most trauma centers nurses do not intubate or insert central venous lines, they prepare equipment for and assist with these procedures in addition to understanding their priority in resuscitative care. Trauma nurses must be familiar with and adept at setting up and performing an autotransfusion. After the patient is stabilized and emergency procedures are completed, a more thorough secondary survey can be done. Focused assessment sonography for trauma (FAST) or peritoneal lavage may be performed to determine the need for exploratory abdominal surgery. Additional radiologic studies may be obtained. Obvious or suspected fractures are immobilized with the use of splints or backboards if these are not already in place. Relief of pain becomes a consideration, but management must be considered judiciously before the administration of any medication. Medication can make accurate neurologic assessment difficult and may cause hypotension in an underresuscitated patient. On the other hand, if a patient arrives in a combative or severely restless state that hinders airway control and thorough examination, anesthetic or paralyzing agents may need to be used. Nursing management during this phase is first directed by established protocols and then by priorities of care. The overall assessment of the patient by the physician and nurse will guide the plan of care as it evolves. Throughout this phase the nurse must continuously anticipate and assess changes in the patient's condition, prepare equipment, and assist the trauma team with procedures aimed at stabilization.

CARDIAC ARREST

Most patients who arrest during the resuscitation phase following traumatic injury do so secondary to profound intravascular volume depletion.[8] Thus closed chest massage in many cases is not sufficient to maintain an effective stroke volume. An arrest caused by hypovolemia requires massive volume infusion with red blood cells and manual compression of the ventricles via open thoracotomy.

The nurse on the trauma team must ensure the accessibility of the necessary equipment for open or closed CPR and assist the trauma surgeon accordingly. Successful resuscitation requires a well-organized, collaborative effort on the part of the trauma team.

The potential for sudden cardiac arrest remains a priority into the critical care phase and, although less likely to occur there, into the intermediate and rehabilitation phases. In the critical care phase, cardiac arrest may result from: overwhelming sepsis, arrhythmias secondary to myocardial damage, multiple organ failure, respiratory failure, tension pneumothorax, or pulmonary embolization. In the intermediate and rehabilitative phases, a pulmonary embolus or complications from long-term care may precipitate an arrest.

Because cardiac arrest is often a sudden event that can occur in any phase of care, standardized protocols that address resuscitation are imperative. Although arrest protocols will vary with each institution, they should address the following components:

1. Physician coverage and the process for notification of the physician
2. Identification of team members
3. Specific role responsibilities for each team member (e.g., who is in charge, who is responsible for ventilating the patient)
4. Coverage of the remaining patients in the area
5. Control of traffic in the area
6. Restocking of emergency drugs and supplies

COMMUNICATION WITH THE FAMILY DURING THE RESUSCITATION PHASE

The initial communication with the patient's family occurs during the resuscitation phase of care. Family members are generally in a state of crisis, having had no time to prepare for the suddenness of an injury to their loved one. The trauma nurse and physician together provide information concerning the patient's injuries and condition. The initial patient and family histories are obtained. The nurse thereafter serves as a liaison to the patient's family, keeping them updated on their family member's condition as often as time will allow. The initial approach with the family often sets the tone for the entire hospital stay of the patient.

Joy[13] suggests the following guidelines for communicating with the family in crisis:

1. Recognize that the traumatic event affects everyone associated with the injured person, including the family, neighbors, friends, co-workers, and community associates.
2. Acknowledge that family members in crisis may each express their reactions in unique ways. These include: crying, fighting among themselves, being disruptive, showing anger or guilt, or being silent.
3. Overcome language barriers by obtaining appropriate interpreters to allow the family to be fully informed and fully heard.
4. Avoid using medical jargon when speaking to family members unless they are health care providers who have a full understanding of the terminology. Technical words provide little information to the family and serve more to confuse and frighten them.
5. Acknowledge the family's concerns related to the financial impact and potential legal ramifications related to the traumatic event. Offer them the appropriate resources to answer their questions.

6. Be an attentive listener. Attempt to secure a quiet place to talk with the family so that other things happening in the clinical setting do not distract from the discussion.

PSYCHOLOGIC SUPPORT

Psychologic support for the patient is also a priority throughout this phase of care. Patients are in as much a state of crisis as their family members. Even though the total systems approach to trauma is used to guide treatment, it is essential to recognize that the total system being dealt with is a human being. The patient has had no time to anticipate the injury. Attempts to cope with this fact are often worsened by pain or hypoxia. The rapid sequence of unfamiliar activities, beginning with rescue, impairs the patient's ability to perceive events realistically.

For full recovery, the patient's emotional state must be addressed from the beginning. The nurse should introduce himself or herself and provide the patient with a brief description of the surroundings and an explanation of procedures as they are performed. These explanations should be short and concise and may need to be repeated. Patients in the resuscitation phase feel powerless. They have little control and a significant amount of fear of the unknown. Keeping them informed aids in reducing these feelings.

SPIRITUAL CONSIDERATIONS

The spiritual component is also vital to the multiply injured patient's plan of care. The nurse must consider the patient's spiritual practices as soon as that information is available because these practices may have a significant impact on the plan of care. For example, if the patient is critically injured and death is imminent, the need for a priest to administer the sacrament of the sick to a Catholic patient must be addressed. Often it is the nurse who calls a priest, especially if the family has not yet arrived in the emergency area. If the patient is identified as a Jehovah's Witness, the treatment plan typically requires some modification, particularly during the resuscitation and critical care phases. Each trauma facility should have a clear policy covering the withholding or administration of blood for these patients.

EVALUATION AND TRANSITION

During this phase of care, continuous assessment is required to reevaluate the appropriateness and effectiveness of medical and nursing interventions. As the patient's condition stabilizes or changes, the plan of care is reevaluated and altered to accommodate the changing profile. Determination of the patient's readiness to move into another phase is a collaborative decision. Clear communication is essential. Provision of pertinent information regarding injuries, treatments, psychosocial issues, and the plan of care is necessary to facilitate patient transition to the next phase.

OPERATIVE PHASE

Many traumatic injuries require surgical intervention. Once the patient has been resuscitated and it is determined that operative procedures are warranted, the work of the nurse in the trauma operating room begins. Many aspects of this role include the traditional responsibilities of any operating room (OR) nurse. In addition to these, however, the operative needs of the multiply injured patient make the nurse's role more complex and demanding.

Operating rooms in major trauma centers require fully staffed teams around the clock and the ready availability of at least one suite for direct admissions into the OR. In other facilities the operating room team must be prepared to react promptly when the trauma patient arrives. Trauma patients may require repeated surgical procedures to treat their injuries successfully. Rooms must be available for these elective procedures without sacrificing ready availability of rooms for emergent cases.

ASSESSMENT. The role of the perioperative nurse, which traditionally includes a preoperative assessment and interview of the patient, may be drastically altered during the resuscitation phase for any of the following reasons:

1. The patient may be comatose or unable to communicate effectively if an endotracheal tube or a tracheostomy is in place.
2. The emergency care necessitated by the instability of the patient may render him or her inaccessible to the operative nurse until arrival in the operating room.
3. The patient may have required induction of anesthesia immediately on arrival in the resuscitation area to allow implementation of resuscitative and diagnostic measures.
4. If the patient is awake, the physiologic and psychologic impact of injury may be so overwhelming as to preclude any assimilation of information given.

In these situations the priorities for the trauma nurse in the perioperative phase include the following: ascertaining the urgency of the need for surgical intervention, arranging for the availability of a room, preparing the necessary equipment for the procedures to be performed, and coordinating the participation of the various specialty surgical teams who will be operating on the patient. Any data collection needed is obtained from the resuscitation trauma nurse or physician. The OR nurse must obtain a detailed summary of what occurred during resuscitation. As the patient progresses past the critical care phase, elective surgical procedures may be necessary to restore maximal function. In these cases the OR nurse plays a vital role in establishing trust and in providing the appropriate patient education.

DIAGNOSIS. From a medical standpoint the trauma patient who arrives in the operating room is far different from the patient undergoing elective surgery. The latter has been diagnosed preoperatively, and surgical intervention has been prescribed to correct the disorder. The multiply injured trauma patient, on the other hand, often arrives in the operating room without a specific diagnosis. FAST may have identified the presence of a hemoperitoneum, but the specific organs injured will not be known until an exploratory laparotomy is performed.

DEVELOPING AND IMPLEMENTING A PLAN. As the multiply injured patient is transported into the operating room, the specialized plan of care continues. The nurse's role during the actual operative phase remains crucial. In collaboration with the surgical teams and anesthesiologist, continuous assessment of the patient's hemodynamic stability is a priority. Meticulous documentation continues. The circulating trauma nurse plays a major role as coordinator. Multiply injured patients often require procedures performed by several different specialty teams either simultaneously or sequentially. Equipment for all these procedures must be readily available and properly placed for easy access. Coordination between the teams is essential. The nurse must be able to set up equipment that might be needed to repair injuries that were totally unsuspected until surgical exploration identified them. The OR nurse and the surgical services that will be performing the procedures generally determine the order of surgical procedures based on time and priority of surgical intervention. If conflict arises, the attending trauma surgeon makes the decision about which procedure has priority. A patient who has a hemoperitoneum, an open ankle fracture, a deep chin laceration, loose teeth, and multiple facial fractures might be treated in the following manner: One team of surgeons will perform the exploratory laparotomy, while the oral surgeon extracts teeth and applies arch bars. On completion of these procedures, the orthopedic surgeon may set the ankle, while the plastic surgeon closes the laceration of the chin.

Because of the necessity for multiple surgical procedures, the patient may be on the OR table for many hours. The effects of prolonged positioning on the table and administration of anesthesia must be addressed. Pressure sores can occur even before the patient arrives in the critical care unit if vulnerable areas have not been protected. Decreased circulation from blood loss, hypothermia, and prolonged administration of anesthesia all contribute to this problem.

It may be difficult to maintain accurate sponge counts because emergent situations may not allow time for a preoperative count. Radiographic confirmation is often the only choice to ensure that a sponge has not been left inadvertently in the patient.

Blood and blood products must be readily available to the trauma operating rooms. Many trauma centers have established separate refrigerators in the OR area for the storage of blood and blood products. To prevent severe hypothermia, all blood and intravenous fluids should be warmed by whatever equipment the individual facility has chosen for that purpose.

The anesthesia providers have additional responsibilities when the trauma patient undergoes anesthesia for emergency surgery versus those when elective surgery is performed. These patients must be monitored accurately, often for prolonged periods. Constant vigilance is an absolute requirement. Assessment of hemodynamic and pulmonary status, maintenance of multiple intravenous lines, administration of appropriate medications and fluids, and preparation for sudden, unexpected deterioration of the patient are responsibilities that make the trauma anesthesia provider unique.

EVALUATION AND TRANSITION.   After surgery the patient must be scrutinized and prepared for transport to the postanesthesia care or critical care unit. An accurate report to the receiving unit is required before transport to allow the nurses in the next phase to prepare for the admission. The initial communication with the receiving unit should, however, occur soon after the patient's arrival in the OR. Periodic updates related to the patient's condition or disposition status assist other units to prepare for the patient's arrival. Often critical care units need to alter current patient assignments and obtain specific supplies and equipment to accommodate the needs of a postoperative trauma patient.

The multiply injured patient is often admitted directly to the critical care unit postoperatively. On arrival in the unit, a survey of vascular access sites, fluids and medications being infused, and drainage tubes by both the OR nurse or anesthesia provider and the receiving trauma nurse in the critical care unit is good practice. An accurate report of the resuscitation efforts, surgical procedures performed, vital sign trends, fluid balance, estimated blood loss, and medications and anesthesia administered ensures continuity in the plan of care.

Severely injured patients often require additional surgeries to treat injuries or complications that may have developed after primary surgery. Many of these occur while the patient still requires critical care and maximal technologic support. The OR nurse has the responsibility, in conjunction with the critical care nurse and respiratory therapist, to transport the patient safely.

COMMUNICATION WITH THE FAMILY.   Another primary responsibility of the OR trauma nurse is family intervention. Every attempt should be made to keep the family informed both before and during the surgical procedures. Before surgery the information conveyed to them should include: suspected injuries, planned surgical procedures, estimated time the patient will be in surgery, and potential for death. When operative procedures are prolonged, consistent communication with family members is imperative. Information given intraoperatively should include the following: an update on the current status of the patient, what the family can expect postoperatively, the surgeon's name, necessary phone numbers to obtain information postoperatively, and the reiteration of the time estimate for completion of surgical procedures. After the procedure the trauma surgeon should explain which operative procedures were performed, the stability and prognosis of the patient, and the unit to which the patient will be admitted.

Comfortable waiting areas for families should be available as close to the OR floor as possible. Beverages, a telephone, and pillows make their wait less unpleasant. Often during this phase the family members are at a loss to know what they can do to help. Sometimes the suggestion that they or their friends can donate blood to help replace that given to their loved one provides them a purpose during this time of waiting and uncertainty.

PHASE III: CRITICAL CARE

The critical care phase for the patient with multiple system injuries requires the skills and collaboration of a variety of health care professionals. Because of the wide spectrum of physiologic, psychologic, and sociologic derangements encountered after severe traumatic injury, coordination of the health care team is integral to management of trauma patients in the critical care phase. The efforts of the health care team must be synchronized to provide optimal care, to minimize the physiologic and psychologic stress of the injuries, and to provide cost-effective care with appropriate resource use. It is essential that one physician and nurse be designated to coordinate the many disciplines involved in the critical care phase. Depending on the trauma care management model embraced by the institution, the physician coordinator may be the admitting trauma surgeon or a critical care intensivist. When multiple services are involved, coordination by a critical care intensivist has been shown to provide more efficient, cost-effective care delivery with improved patient outcomes.[14] Similarly, the nurse coordinator may be an advanced practice nurse such as the trauma coordinator, trauma case manager, clinical nurse specialist, or acute care nurse practitioner; in other models the coordinating nurse may be a staff-level primary nurse. Regardless of the title, the nurse designated to coordinate the patient's care has the responsibility to remain abreast of the status and progress of the patient, activities and plan of care of the multidisciplinary team, flow of information between team members, and interactions with the family members.

ASSESSMENT

Just as the resuscitation area nurse prepares for the emergency admission of a multitrauma patient, the critical care nurse must identify and anticipate the many needs of the patient and prepare for arrival in the critical care unit (CCU). The resuscitation nurse, the anesthesia provider, or the postanesthesia care unit nurse gives the CCU nurse a thorough report, including the physical aspects of the patient's injuries, interventions, current status, family information, and any special equipment that will be needed. For example, monitoring, ventilatory, warming, and emergency equipment should be available and checked for proper functioning before the patient's arrival. Anticipation of physiologic derangements is necessary to prepare for the admission of a potentially unstable hypotensive, bleeding, hypothermic patient.[15,16] The scope and fundamental principles of critical care assessment of trauma patients are similar to those for other critically ill populations.

GENERAL CONSIDERATIONS.   Admission of the severely injured patient to the critical care unit directly from the operating room is usually preferable because it enhances the continuity of care and avoids an additional transport that might put the critically ill patient at risk. In addition, a CCU typically has more readily available support services and resources than a postanesthesia care unit (PACU).[17] If a PACU is used, continuity in the plan of care and family contact is essential. On admission to the critical care area, the patient is immediately connected to monitoring equipment and placed on a ventilator. Infusions of IV fluids or blood products are noted, and the site for each is identified immediately. The position and patency of drains; the condition of wound dressings; and the location, type, and status of skeletal traction are established.

After establishing that vital physiologic functions are intact, the CCU nurse continues receiving a detailed report from the previous care providers (Table 9-1) and conducts a thorough assessment. This information is documented to provide a baseline for assessing changes in patient status and family interactions and for initiating interventions during the critical care phase.

PHYSICAL.   A total systems assessment is conducted and documented completely, system by system, in the nursing record at least once every 24 hours. Use of a standardized assessment form or computer documentation system decreases time needed for recording. Frequent reassessment and documentation of changes are ongoing responsibilities.

TABLE 9-1   Information Required from Anesthesia, Operating Room, or Resuscitation Area Personnel after Patient Transfer to Critical Care Unit

Admitting trauma surgeon
Mechanism of injury
List of injuries
Diagnostic tests completed and results
Resuscitation area interventions
Hypotensive episodes before or during admission
Surgical procedures, findings, and complications
Type of anesthesia and medications administered
Current infusions
Type and volume of blood products received
Estimated blood loss
Fluid balance
Drains, intravenous catheters
Most recent vital signs and trends
Family information
    Notification
    Name of spokesperson
    What they have been told about the patient's injuries
    If they have seen the patient
    How they can be reached

Most often the nurse at the bedside identifies changes in the patient's condition that warrant notification of the medical team for corresponding changes in treatment.

Near constant evaluation of the multiply injured patient is vital during this phase for many reasons. The body responds to the stress of trauma with many physiologic and emotional changes. The trauma patient may deteriorate and fail to achieve physiologic stability as a result of systemic inflammatory response syndrome (SIRS) from the initial injuries, as a sequelae of massive fluid resuscitation, or from injuries that may have been missed on admission. Possible life-threatening complications that often occur in this phase demand early detection for prevention or treatment to increase chances of survival. Ongoing assessment data act as validating criteria for accurate diagnoses and interventions. The patient's tolerance of and response to prescribed medical and nursing therapies must be monitored.

Throughout the phase of critical care, one of the major values of ongoing assessment is the early detection of actual or pending complications. For example, the patient with a severe pulmonary contusion may go on to develop adult respiratory distress syndrome (ARDS); early recognition of this condition allows early therapeutic intervention. A primary objective in the early detection of complications following traumatic injury is anticipation by the nurse of potential complications that are associated with specific injuries, surgical procedures, and volume resuscitation. During assessment the nurse must keep in mind the injuries that the patient has sustained and the complications commonly associated with them.

DIAGNOSTIC STUDIES.   Critically ill trauma patients typically require multiple and frequent diagnostic studies. Although most often appropriate, periodic evaluation of practice protocols is important to ensure cost-effective care and resource use. Opportunities to reduce the number of diagnostic procedures a patient is subjected to without impacting the quality of care delivered should be explored.[18] Examples include careful scrutinization of the need for complete blood laboratory panels versus individual tests, routine chest radiographs after over-the-wire central venous catheter change, or follow-up computed tomography (CT) scans.

During the critical care phase, serial laboratory studies have a role in the evaluation of the patient's status and are used with other data to alter the treatment plan. Protocols for obtaining these tests ensure that appropriate monitoring takes place.[19] Protocols include the types of tests to be drawn and their frequency, the type of container to be used for each test, and where they are to be sent for analysis or if they should be done using bedside technology.

Blood samples for serial hematocrit, hemoglobin, coagulation profile, serum lactate level, electrolytes, and arterial and venous blood gases should be drawn based on clinical pathways reflecting the patient's condition. Routine complete panels are often not necessary, and laboratory diagnostic studies that do not trigger an intervention should be avoided.[20] Although laboratory studies provide necessary data for assessment, the volume of blood drawn must be minimized. Unnecessary blood sampling affects the patient and the resource consumption and costs.

Multiple trauma patients who are hemodynamically compromised and require a high level of ventilatory support may be too unstable to risk an unnecessary transport for diagnostic studies in areas outside the critical care unit. Interruption of traction devices also may be detrimental to a patient. In these cases, bedside studies may be necessary. These studies (e.g., evoked potentials, ECG) are often time consuming and involve large pieces of equipment. The nurse caring for the patient should coordinate proper timing of the tests so they do not interfere with other needed treatments or the patient's rest or sleep schedule. While a test is being done, monitoring of the patient must not be interrupted. Care should be scheduled so that necessary treatments may be completed just before or immediately after a test.

PSYCHOSOCIAL.   The ongoing evaluation of a trauma patient's psychologic adjustment to injury is as important as ongoing physical assessment. It is a vital component of holistic care. The psychologic response to trauma may fluctuate dramatically as adjustment to the injuries occurs. One moment the patient may demonstrate signs of adjustment to the injury; the next moment the patient may succumb to depression or anger and lash out or not cooperate with treatment.

Trauma patients' psychologic responses are often totally unpredictable. A 40-year-old patient with paraplegia secondary to a thoracic spine injury may adjust better than a 16-year-old boy whose severely fractured femur will keep him from fulfilling his life's dream of playing professional football. A continuous psychologic assessment will enable the primary nurse to plan interventions that will help a trauma patient deal with the injuries more effectively. Knowledge of the patient's existent, or nonexistent, support systems, how the patient usually reacts to stressful situations, and the patient's previous coping mechanisms will enable the nurse to develop a more individualized plan of care.

FAMILY.   Beginning on the first day of a patient's admission, the critical care unit primary bedside nurse and, if appropriate, the advanced practice nurse must assess the family members for their knowledge of the patient's injuries and for their ability to interpret and accept what has been communicated to them.[13] Coping mechanisms and support systems that they use to deal with crisis should also be identified and documented. All such family information and the planned interventions and strategies to assist them are documented for all caregivers to refer to in the patient record.

Families in crisis often latch on to a single piece of information, and unless it is clear to all those caring for the patient what the family has been told, family members may receive mixed messages. On initial contact with the family members, a spokesperson is identified so that all communication relating to the patient's condition can be relayed to that one person to avoid the possibility of varied interpretations by several different family members. To prevent inaccurate or inconsistent information from being delivered to the family, regular communication by the primary or coordinating nurse or physician with the spokesperson is important. Early assessment and appropriate interventions such as providing information, active listening, facilitating flexibility in visiting, and family caregiver conferences are key to effective management of families of trauma victims.

DEVELOPING AND IMPLEMENTING THE PLAN

During the critical care phase the concept of collaborative practice, begun in the resuscitation phase, becomes even more important. Many different medical services may be involved in the care of the multiply injured (e.g., orthopedics, neurosurgery, plastic surgery, infectious disease, and critical care). Respiratory therapists, physical therapists, nutritionists, and others who have daily contact with the patient assume integral roles in the care plan. The primary nurse or case manager is the individual with a global view of all the services involved; therefore the nurse's role as coordinator is of great significance. The trauma patient is dependent on the nurse at this stage of care. The patient looks to the nurse as the coordinator, decision maker, and advocate. It is beyond the scope of this chapter to address all nursing care concerns during the critical care phase. In caring for trauma patients, however, there are particular aspects of critical care nursing practice that have special relevance to this phase of care.

MULTIDISCIPLINARY APPROACH

All aspects of the plan of care for the critically ill trauma patient involve multiple disciplines. Coordination of these disciplines to ensure common patients goals is uniquely the responsibility of the primary care nurse. Daily multidisciplinary rounds facilitate sharing of information and objectives, reviewing variances on clinical pathways, and developing short- and long-term plans; the primary nurse, or designee must be part of these interactions and decisions. Integration of the clinical pathways, management guidelines, and protocols facilitates the coordination of disciplines and promotes achievement of positive patient outcomes.[18,21-23]

In very complex cases, holding multidisciplinary conferences every 2 to 3 weeks allows all disciplines to discuss their perspectives and agree on priorities and specific long-term goals. This plan should be documented for reference by all the disciplines. Subsequent conferences focus on evaluation of progress and revising the plan. Participants in caregiver conferences include representatives from all the specialty areas and services involved in the patient's care.

EMERGENCY PROCEDURES

The multitrauma patient has the potential for developing sudden life-threatening complications. Critical care trauma nurses require the cognitive and psychomotor capabilities to deal with emergent situations. The need for emergency equipment is unpredictable; thus accessibility is essential. The availability of up-to-date emergency equipment in good working condition is required at all times. Seconds count: Patients' lives may depend on the anticipation of critical events and the readiness of emergency equipment. Nursing orientation programs and skills updates need to include competency-based education and training on emergency equipment and supplies such as internal and external temporary pacemakers, surgical trays for opening a patient's chest or abdomen, and intracranial pressure monitors.

Bedside operative procedures are not unusual, and the critical care nurse should be prepared to facilitate these. The nurse coordinates the efforts, obtains necessary equipment, ensures the presence of appropriate personnel (e.g., an anesthesia provider and OR nurses), maintains continued high-level care and monitoring, serves as the patient's advocate, and maintains communication with the family.

DOCUMENTATION

The physiologic monitoring that occurs in the critical care unit generates a large amount of data that, together with the clinical picture of the patient, provides the basis on which to prescribe treatment. Identifying trends from these data is crucial to detecting subtle changes in patients' conditions and to altering therapy accordingly. To identify these trends in a timely and objective manner, documentation must be thorough and must allow for visual examination of various categories of data in relation to other sets of data. For example, whether a computer or a flow sheet is used, it is important to be able to look at all parameters, interventions, and the patient's response to interventions (e.g., vital signs, oxygen delivery and uptake, intake and output, medications, and neurologic status) simultaneously over a given time in the patient's course of treatment.

Electronic records are very useful for documenting physiologic data. Automatic physiologic monitoring capabilities, IV drug calculation programs, and recording of laboratory data are helpful adjuncts to the development of specialized and individualized plans of care. The computer allows data gathered by various disciplines involved in trauma patient care to be accessed and used by care providers at any given time and from various locations.

TRANSPORTING CRITICAL CARE PATIENTS

Effective diagnostic procedures and therapies for the multitrauma patient often depend on information obtained through special tests such as CT or nuclear medicine studies. An already compromised, critically injured patient may have to undergo the additional stress of transport to other areas of the hospital. When the patient is multiply injured or unstable, the potential problems and the nurse's responsibilities increase in direct proportion to the number and severity of life-threatening injuries already present. To ensure patient safety before, during, and after the transfer, the trauma nurse must use advance planning to coordinate care requirements, personnel, backup equipment, and sup-

plies. The level of patient monitoring and care should not change during transport.[24]

Once the risks have been weighed against the necessity of the test, the nurse assumes responsibility for the coordination of the transport. Patient needs during transport are many and include: respiratory support, medications (routine and emergency medications and premedications for diagnostic tests) that must be given while out of the unit, IV fluids, and adequate monitoring.

During any transport the nurse has the responsibility to protect and preserve all IV and monitoring catheters, cables, and drains. Unintentional dislodgment of these may pose significant risks to the patient and in some cases may be life threatening.

The number and type of personnel accompanying the patient must also be decided. A transport policy should provide guidelines for these decisions. If it is necessary to transport blood with an unstable trauma patient, an insulated container with a temperature indicator to monitor the temperature range of the blood should be used. Any equipment specific to the individual patient must also be taken. The nurse must be aware of the nearest emergency equipment cart en route and at the destination.

After all plans have been made, a final checklist ensures that all aspects have been covered and often alerts the nurse to facts that may affect the procedure for which the patient is being transported. For example, a patient with a Hoffman device in place may need that device adjusted before transport to enable the patient to fit into the CT scanner, and some very large patients may not fit into the CT scanner. If such factors are overlooked, they may cause cancellation of the test at the last minute after the patient has already undergone the risk of transportation.

SPECIAL CONSIDERATIONS

EVIDENCE-BASED INTERVENTIONS.   Patient care that is driven by research-based protocols and guidelines enhances patient outcomes, allows measurement of outcomes by reducing practitioner preferences, and increases cost effectiveness of care and resource use.[22,23] For example, protocols for suctioning, tracheal lavage, tracheostomy care, tracheostomy changes, and chest physiotherapy should be integrated into the pulmonary care regimen for all patients. Prone positioning, institution of kinetic therapy, and early mobilization are evidence-based interventions that reduce the risk of nosocomial pneumonia and improve oxygenation and ventilation.[25-27]

The use of specialty beds and mattress overlays has become common practice in the care of the multiply injured patient. When prescribed appropriately, they can enhance the patient's recovery process. The placement of a patient on one of these beds should be a collaborative nursing and medical decision based on specific criteria. Guidelines for placing patients on these beds prevent unnecessary or inappropriate use and expenditures. For instance, kinetic therapy beds have proven to be efficacious in reducing the incidence of nosocomial pneumonia and other immobility-related complications when instituted within 72 hours of admission and rotated for 15 hours per day.[26] Air-fluidized beds relieve interface pressure and enhance healing of large wounds. Low-air-loss beds decrease interface pressure and reduce the risk of pressure sore development.[28] These are appropriate for patients who are at high risk for skin breakdown as determined by a risk assessment such as the Braden scale.[29,30]

The belief that rehabilitation begins on admission has long been accepted, but it is particularly relevant when planning care for the trauma patient. At the time the patient enters the critical care phase, rehabilitation needs are addressed according to protocol to minimize the impact of immobility on all systems and lessen the possibility of delayed recovery. Attempts to reduce musculoskeletal alterations begin in the critical care phase. Early splinting of extremities when appropriate, active and passive range of motion exercises, and frequent repositioning aid in prevention of serious contractures and other musculoskeletal problems arising from immobilization.[31] Literature also supports the application of pneumatic leg compression devices early after hospital admission to deter the development of deep vein thrombosis related to extremity injury and immobility.[25,32]

VISITING CONSIDERATIONS

Family visits are a vital part of the overall plan of care and can influence patient outcome. Visiting by family members and others should be encouraged during the critical care phase. Patient and family needs are important considerations in the nurse's individualization of visiting practices. Flexible visiting policies that include the family, friends, children, and even pets have been implemented successfully in a number of institutions.[33-35] Visits provide the nurse with an opportunity to assess the family's understanding and perception of their loved one's injuries and to provide information. Families who are restricted from visiting a critically ill member often suffer fear, anxiety, hopelessness, and helplessness. These may be displayed as hostility and anger toward the staff in an attempt to appear in control of the situation.

IMPACT OF PHARMACEUTIC AND TECHNOLOGIC ADVANCES

Nursing care during the critical care phase has become increasingly specialized and complex. Pharmacologic and technologic advances continue to improve the care of critically ill trauma patients. As new drugs and devices become available and are incorporated into patient care, nurses are challenged to maintain a high level of expertise and keep abreast of the indications for use, desired physiologic effects, side effects or complications, and other related implications. For example, administration of agents such as perfluorocarbon, nitric oxide, inflammatory mediator receptor antagonists, and monoclonal antibodies is increasingly common. The clinical pharmacist, as a trauma team member, is a valuable resource to the nurses and physicians,

not only as new pharmacologic agents are introduced but also in the routine management of the patient receiving multiple medications.

The use of sophisticated technology in trauma care requires a high level of expertise and competence. Nurses and other staff members must be properly educated and credentialed before assuming the responsibilities of caring for patients supported by sophisticated life-support devices. Extracorporeal lung assistance and renal replacement therapy are examples of therapies in which the nurse must monitor the device's function and the patient's response and manipulate multiple variables (e.g., gas flow rates, blood flow rates, and fluid and electrolyte replacement) accordingly.

A system of equipment evaluation and control is important. For example, it is advantageous to have all units use the same monitoring system or emergency equipment so that the entire staff can become familiar with and secure in its use. Evaluation, acquisition, and integration of new technology are important aspects of trauma/critical care nursing. Participation in the technology assessment process, developing specific criteria for use and establishing outcome measures, and planning the integration and education processes are important aspects of the critical care nurse's role (Table 9-2).[36,37]

When using highly technical equipment, computer systems, and other devices, the critical care nurse should know

---

TABLE 9-2 Template for Technology Assessment[36]

What is the basic science underlying the technology?
What are the indications for its use claimed by the manufacturers?
What are the common secondary indications claimed by frequent users?
Does the technology provide the basic function claimed by the manufacturer? by the frequent user?
What are the efficacy data available to support its use?
Are there any appropriate data available?
Data to consider:
  Survival
  Morbidity
  Length of stay
  Benefits
  Complications
What are the costs of using the technology?
  Initial capital outlay
  Ongoing operating costs
  Labor impact
  Resource requirements
  Indirect costs (e.g., special hospital space or program displacement)
  How is the total cost of patient care affected?
Should there be any special user requirements (e.g., knowledge base or experience) for safe and effective use of the technology?

that an important role is humane caring. Naisbitt's theory[38] of "high tech, high touch" is relevant to the trauma patient's care and should be incorporated in the plan of care. This formula describes the way we have responded to technology. Whenever new technology is introduced into society, there must be a counterbalancing human response—that is, high touch—or the technology is rejected. High technology is inherent and ever-expanding in the trauma/critical care field.

Naisbitt acknowledges that there is no way to keep humans from devising new tools, but we must also take care not to use these tools as the sole solution. "When we fall into a deep trap of believing or hoping that technology will solve all of our problems, we are actually abdicating the high touch of personal responsibility. The more high technology around us, the more the need for human touch."[38] As the need for more high-touch care increases, ensuring consistent patient care is essential to provide holistic care and optimize patient outcomes. In addition, consideration of the critical care environment is important to minimize the untoward effects of a high-tech critical care unit. Strategies to promote physical and psychologic healing for the patient and family include: reducing extraneous noises, using dim and indirect lighting, using soft colors, hanging pictures and photographs, and playing music of the patient's choice.[39]

CLINICAL RESEARCH

Because of the complexity of traumatic injury, the multidisciplinary approach to trauma care is a rapidly evolving field, and efforts are continuously made to encourage trauma practitioners to conduct research to increase the scientific basis of nursing and medical care. Studies of the characteristics of the trauma population and multiple therapeutic interventions should continue to refine the process and improve outcomes of trauma care.

The multitrauma patient may suddenly become the vehicle for a number of simultaneous medical and nursing research endeavors that can improve care and clinical operations. A trauma center must have an established multidisciplinary committee for reviewing all proposed research studies and existing protocols to protect the patient (and family) yet facilitate both nursing and medical research projects. Exploring the trauma patient's responses to injury and the effectiveness of specific treatments is vital to developing evidence-based patient management; therefore, conducting and implementing research are essential components of high-quality patient care as long as established protocols for scientific investigations are followed.

THE DYING PATIENT

Caring for a dying patient is not an uncommon situation in the field of trauma nursing. The definition of nursing expressed by the International Council of Nurses[40] addresses the nurse's role in the care of the dying: "The unique function of the nurse is to assist the individual, sick or well, in the performance of those activities contributing to his health his recovery, or the peaceful death that he would perform unaided if he had the necessary strength, will or knowledge."

Occasionally, conflicting opinions among the medical staff, nurse, and family regarding the continuation of aggressive treatment arise. In these situations the nurse must assume the role of coordinator and patient advocate. The nurse's roles include: working with all team members; involving appropriate resources such as the chaplain or ethics committee to assist in decision making and emotional support of the family and the health care team; participating in development of a final plan of care that is implemented consistently; and documenting the decisions in the patient's medical record.

Traumatic injury, especially severe head injury, often creates the potential for organ donation. Trauma patients are frequently young, with many healthy organs suitable for donation. The potential organ donor patient requires a specialized plan that involves physiologic management, and the family requires intense emotional support. Critical care nurses are in a position to aid family decision making regarding requests for organ donation. Specific education addressing not only the care of patients who are potential organ donors but also supporting a family decision to consent is an especially important aspect of the orientation of critical care trauma nurses.[41]

Once the patient has been identified as a potential donor, the local organ/tissue procurement organization is contacted. These groups often assume responsibility for many aspects of care of the family and patient. The staff are highly trained experts, skilled and sensitive in requesting the gift of organ donations from grieving families and in providing specific guidelines for patient management in preparation for organ donation.[42]

The dying patient, whether eligible as an organ donor or not, has the right to an individualized plan of care that integrates "caring" as the most vital component. The transition from life to death is a voyage that requires the company and quiet reassurance of another. The potential exists, in these moments, for the exchange of many human gifts and values that otherwise go unnoticed.

EVALUATION AND TRANSITION

The evaluation component of the nursing process is ongoing during the critical care phase. During the initial postoperative period, emphasis is on physiologic stabilization as the body attempts to regain homeostasis following the stressor of traumatic injury. Just as assessment is continuous and appropriate interventions are based on the assessment, the evaluation of the patient's response is also a continuous process to allow timely alterations in interventions. During this phase, adjustments in the plan of care are based on the patient's response to therapy, development of complications, or emergence of SIRS. The coordinating nurse and physician have the responsibility to monitor and reevaluate the patient's status.

As the patient stabilizes, assessment again becomes a critical factor to prepare the patient for transfer to a less critical care environment. Planning for discharge begins early in the critical care phase. Often the need for a rehabilitation facility or long-term ventilator unit is evident early in this phase. Collaborative discussions and plans with the family, discharge planner, case manager, and other health care providers should take place to identify the suitable and desired facility and expedite transfer when the patient is healed sufficiently.

The transition from critical care to a less intensive care unit may be difficult for the patient and family, who have for days or months depended on the critical care primary nurses and formed strong relationships and trust. Early planning for transfer will assist the patient and family to make the transition. Discussions related to patient readiness and characteristics of the new unit or rehabilitation facility help the patient and family to prepare. Ideally this takes place as far in advance as possible and may serve as a motivator for the patient. Notifying and communicating with the receiving unit nurses in advance, identifying the next primary care nurse, reviewing the plan of care and personal details with her, and introducing the patient to the nurse facilitates the transition and maintains continuity of care. Particularly in cases of long-term stays on the critical care unit, the preassigning of a primary nurse is useful to ease the transition. The nurse on the intermediate care unit can begin to establish a trusting relationship by visiting the patient and family before transfer from the critical care unit. These pretransfer visits also serve as early assessment opportunities and may elucidate special needs of the patient or family. The patient and family also need to be prepared for the necessity of a move to another unit related to other patient acuity changes or the need for the critical care unit to emergently accept new admissions.

PHASE IV: INTERMEDIATE CARE

Many trauma patients do not require critical care and are admitted directly to the immediate care unit from the resuscitation unit, emergency department, or postanesthesia care unit. These patients and their families have unique physical and psychologic needs that should not be minimized because the patient is not injured severely enough to require critical care.

An integrated approach to care continues to be a vital concept as the patient progresses to an intermediate care level. Many health team members continue to be involved in assessing the patient's progress and in planning and implementing different aspects of care. The roles of the coordinating nurse and physician are significant in this phase to maintain continuity of patient care. Many of the concepts previously presented in the critical care phase continue to

apply to nursing care of trauma patients in the intermediate phase.

ASSESSMENT

PHYSICAL. Patients admitted to the intermediate care unit from the resuscitation or postanesthesia care unit may not be considered "critically ill"; however, they still require very close observation, especially during the first 72 hours. Initially, undiagnosed injuries may become evident and require rapid interventions on the part of the nurse and physician team. In addition, intermediate care units are admitting more acutely ill patients from the critical care area as a result of improved resource use and the need for critical care beds.[43,44] Complications, commonly related to immobility, infection, and sepsis, may develop within this time. Astute assessment of vital signs, sensorium, physical signs and symptoms, laboratory values, and ECG changes allows early identification of problems and interventions, which may substantially reduce patient morbidity.

The immediate phase of care still requires a high level of vigilance because physiologic and psychologic complications may occur. Ongoing assessment is vital. The nurse performs and documents a complete systems assessment once every shift. Any unexpected physiologic changes must be reported promptly to the appropriate individual, be it the physician, nurse practitioner, or physician assistant. During this phase the trauma patient often appears to be doing well. Seemingly insignificant changes noted during the assessment have the potential of being overlooked or viewed as unimportant when, in fact, they may be signaling the onset of complications. A high index of suspicion alerts the nurse to subtle changes in physiologic status and more intensive investigation of the cause of the change. Complications after traumatic injury may occur unexpectedly and on a delayed basis in the postcritical phase. Dislodgment of a deep vein thrombus with embolization to the pulmonary vasculature is a far too common example.

PSYCHOLOGIC. Trauma patients may exhibit significant psychologic changes from their baseline personality. The changes may be related to the psychologic effect of the injuries or to latent effects of mild brain injury. Distinguishing between these is essential to implement appropriate strategies to aid the rehabilitation process. During the critical phase, a predominant concern is whether the patient will live or die. Once the patient recognizes that the immediate crisis is over and he or she is going to live, the emotional trauma manifested by psychosocial problems may begin to surface. For example, the patient may exhibit disproportionate sick-role behavior or have difficulty in expressing grief. Anger, blaming, and withdrawal are also signs of altered or ineffective coping. This reaction frequently occurs when the patient realizes that the incurred injuries require a long period of rehabilitation for complete recovery.

These are just a few examples of psychological problems that may surface during this phase. Continuous assessment for symptoms that signal the actual or potential presence of altered coping mechanisms facilitates institution of preventive measures and interventions. The families of these trauma patients experience similar shock and disbelief. The nurse must assess the family's ability to cope with the crisis of sudden injury.

REHABILITATIVE. During the intermediate care phase a more vigorous assessment of rehabilitation takes place. Anticipating and assessing for potential complications that may prolong rehabilitation is essential. The patient whose tibial fracture heals well with external fixation but who develops footdrop as a result of inconsistent splinting, range-of-motion therapy, and exercise is at risk for prolonged hospitalization, additional rehabilitation, and possibly additional surgery to correct the problem. Early in this phase of trauma care, the coordinating nurse, case manager, discharge planner, or trauma coordinator evaluates the patient for the need for extensive rehabilitation at a specialty center. Assessment of patient and family requirements for a rehabilitation facility and assessment of available rehabilitation centers is important to determine which facility is most appropriate to meet the needs of the patient and family. Early identification of rehabilitation needs is essential to facilitate referral and timely placement in a rehabilitation facility.

DEVELOPING AND IMPLEMENTING A PLAN

One of the most effective means of planning care in the intermediate phase is the patient-centered multidisciplinary conference. Conferences include all the disciplines involved with the trauma patient's recovery. In addition to medicine and nursing, representatives from speech, occupational, and physical therapy should be involved. Needs assessments are presented, outcomes are established, and a specific plan is determined. As a plan is established, the patient is included in mutual goal setting. A flexible plan allows the patient to take an active part in identifying long- and short-term goals and in outlining how these goals will be reached. Monitoring patient progress toward achievement of desired goals and outcomes is the responsibility of the coordinating nurse. Subsequent conferences should focus on evaluation of progress and identification of additional strategies to expedite the patient's recovery and discharge.

ACTIVE PATIENT INVOLVEMENT. As the patient recovers from his or her physical injuries, the plan of care focuses on maintaining physiologic stability, preventing complications, and facilitating emotional recovery. Interventions become more consistent but continue to be outcome driven. Outcomes are often more predictable during this phase and should be documented on a timeline. The patient must be included and given responsibility for a more active role in planning and participating in care. A primary objective in the intermediate phase is to move the trauma patient from a dependent role to a more independent one, striving toward regaining optimal function. Interventions that aid the patient and family in adapting to the residual effects of the injuries and functioning independently are a priority.

Even an immobilized patient needs to be involved in making choices about his or her care. Initially, patient involvement may be limited to the opportunity to make simple choices, such as deciding when to bathe. Or, for example, if there are three activities of daily living that must be relearned, which one is personally important to the patient to learn first? Allowing the patient some choices in care and collaboratively developing schedules provide the patient with some control and encourage the patient to assume a more active role and strive toward independence.

REHABILITATION NEEDS

The familiar statement "rehabilitation begins on admission" takes on greater relevancy when formulating the plan of care for the trauma patient, especially the multisystem injured patient. During the resuscitation, operative, and critical care phases, rehabilitation needs are addressed; however, the emphasis of patient care is clearly on achieving physiologic stability. In the phase of intermediate care, the rehabilitative focus assumes greater significance. The patient learns to take increasing responsibility for his or her care and activities of daily living. Often specific plans are required for the patient to relearn activities of daily living. This is especially true of patients with neurologic dysfunction related to injuries or the long-term effects of paralytic agents used in the critical care phase. The overall long-term plan for rehabilitation needs is developed during this phase of care.

Preparation for transfer to a rehabilitation facility requires collaborative planning and communication with the multidisciplinary team, the patient, the family, and the receiving center. All must be involved in the decision-making process and informed of the time line and potential date of transfer to facilitate patient preparation and a timely, smooth transition.

FAMILY INVOLVEMENT

During this phase, family members begin to be less concerned about the physiologic problems of the patient and start to focus more on what needs to be accomplished before discharge can occur. They begin to want to be involved with the patient's care. They no longer ask, "Will the patient live?" but now ask, "How long will it be before the patient can go home?"

In this stage family involvement in patient teaching is important. Many patients continue to require dressing changes, pin care, or tracheostomy and airway care after their discharge. After teaching family members a procedure, part of the learning process includes return demonstrations and reinforcing the teaching by having the families administer care during their visits. This not only allows the nurse to evaluate how well the family member performs the care but also gives the family member confidence in the new skills and a sense of self-satisfaction from actually assisting in the patient's care. This also may increase the patient's feelings of acceptance by family members, especially if disfiguring injuries are present.

The family-centered conference is an integral component of this phase. The family should be made aware of the goals that have been formulated and the plan of care that has been developed to meet these goals. The need for family members' involvement in the development and implementation of the plan is emphasized, and appropriate resources should be mobilized to assist them in this role. The family may be faced with helping to find and/or choose an appropriate rehabilitative facility for the patient. The coordinating nurse, or an advanced nurse practitioner with the assistance of the family service or social service counselors, can assist the family by providing them with information to make this decision. The specific type of rehabilitation needed by the patient may require placement in a facility far from home. This can be a difficult decision for the family if they are not helped to understand the importance of a proper rehabilitation center placement. Financial counselors, visiting nurse associations, and self-help groups are resources commonly needed by the family and patient to aid the transition from acute care to a rehabilitation center or home.

Unique Considerations During the Intermediate Care Phase

Adjustment to Injury. Patients experience interrelated physical, cognitive, and personal responses to their traumatic injuries. The nurse needs to appreciate the full extent of the cognitive and personal aspects of the patient's physical recovery. Understanding the wide range of responses to trauma allows the nurse to "harness the patient's natural healing ability and promote optimal recovery."[45]

When these responses are identified as maladaptive, a specific, consistent care plan that mobilizes all resources must be developed. As the patient physically feels better, attempts to manipulate health care personnel may be made, often resulting in a delayed progression toward discharge, especially if leaving the security of the hospital environment is frightening. Depression may occur as the sequelae of the injuries are recognized by the patient. This can lead to resistance or noncompliance with the therapeutic regimen or delayed progression through the grief process.

Difficulties coping with alterations in body image often surface during this stage. It is important to recognize behavior patterns that may signal that the patient is having problems preserving or adjusting to his or her body image after traumatic injury. If it is identified early, therapy to assist the patient in dealing with changes in body image can be planned and implemented. Family service counselors or a psychiatric liaison nurse are valuable participants of the health care team when patients begin to elicit maladaptive responses to their injuries. A visit by a former trauma patient or an amputee (if the patient has lost a limb) may prove beneficial.

Immobilization. Even though many multitrauma patients are immobilized intentionally by orthopedic devices, pharmacologic agents, or personal protective devices, the side effects of immobilization linger and assume greater significance during the intermediate phase of care. By the time the patient reaches this stage of care, he or she may already have been immobilized for a significant time, and complications of immobility may be apparent. Some of these include: muscular and cardiac deconditioning; ventilation and perfusion abnormalities; orthostatic abnormalities; alterations in ingestion, digestion, and elimination; and development of deep vein thrombus with embolization.[31] The prevention and treatment of complications from immobility are priorities in the plan of care.

Early and aggressive mobilization is beneficial and necessary to prevent sequelae from immobility. Some techniques of fracture management, such as the use of intermedullary rods, plates, screws, or external fixator devices, allow earlier mobilization of patients with multiple fractures. However, even patients in traction may be mobilized if creative methods for maintaining the traction are used. For example, hanging the traction rope and weights over a straight-backed chair may maintain sufficient tibial traction so that the patient may sit up in a chair several times a day. The patient with turning restrictions who needs chest physiotherapy to prevent or treat atelectasis can still be treated if the nurse works with the physician to select the safest way to position the patient. Prophylaxis against deep vein thrombus is imperative, even when mobilizing patients, using external pneumatic compression devices, plantar plexus pulsation devices, or low-dose or low-molecular-weight heparin.[32]

Evaluation

As in previous phases, nursing and medical interventions need to be evaluated continuously for effectiveness. Overall evaluation is directed at the patient's progression toward discharge to home or a rehabilitation center. The discharge from acute care that occurs at the end of this phase should not be sudden. Goals that were set by the health care team must be met, and documentation of such should be present. Discharge needs to be a predicted and planned event, so when it does occur, the patient and family members look forward to it and feel comfortable rather than frightened or insecure.

Phase V: Rehabilitation

It is difficult to address rehabilitation as a phase separate from the others because, as previously discussed, it begins on admission and continues throughout the patient's acute care hospitalization. Once physiologic stability is achieved, emphasis of care progresses to recovery and adaptation. The primary nursing objectives in the rehabilitation phase are to assist the patient in overcoming disabilities or adapting to his or her environment within the confines of permanent disabilities resulting from trauma. This involves dealing with the total psychosocial and physical needs regardless of whether the disabilities are temporary or permanent. The family is an integral part of the care in reorientation, teaching, and discharge planning and in helping to reintegrate the patient into the family system and the community. Nursing must be accountable for recruiting and mobilizing patient and family resources.

ASSESSMENT

As previously discussed, rehabilitation begins on admission. Even during resuscitation and operative phases of care, assessment for and prevention of potential problems that prolong the period of rehabilitation must occur. For example, improper positioning on the operating room table for extensive and multiple surgical procedures may cause skin breakdown even before the patient reaches the critical care area or intermediate care unit. During the critical care phase, assessment is crucial to recognizing conditions that may ultimately lead to prolonged rehabilitation. For example, a patient receiving pharmacologic paralysis to facilitate mechanical ventilation may need bilateral foot splints to prevent footdrop, a preventable complication that can prolong and complicate rehabilitative efforts.

Assessment continues to be a mainstay of nursing care in the rehabilitation phase. Assessment in this phase includes determining the patient's psychologic response to injury, evaluating the patient's potential level of function, ascertaining the availability of support mechanisms to assist the patient in injury adjustment and eventual reintegration into society, and coordinating the various community resources and health disciplines that facilitate a smooth rehabilitative process.

The patient's and family's economic situations must be assessed early during acute care so that, by the time the patient is ready for rehabilitation treatment, a plan can be developed that places the lowest economic burden on those involved. Insurance coverage and the patient's and family's economic resources are vital considerations when determining which rehabilitation center will be best for the patient. The center not only must meet the patient's physical needs but also be economically feasible.

DEVELOPING AND IMPLEMENTING A PLAN

If rehabilitative needs have been assessed as the patient moved through the initial and intermediate phases of care, a well-developed plan should be in place (with the ultimate goal of returning the patient to an optimal level of functioning) by the time the patient moves into the rehabilitative phase. During this phase a goal is for the patient to regain control—to become the decision maker with the support of the health care team. The care plan in this phase would allow for resumption of normal cycles of activity, rest, and increased interaction with family and friends. Mutual goal setting, providing an atmosphere so that the patient can work toward community reentry, and ensuring that he or she remains medically stable are essential components of the plan. Each patient uniquely adapts to traumatic injury; thus planning care requires creativity and persistence.

The patient must be and perceive himself or herself as an integral part of the rehabilitation process. The plan should address physical, psychologic, and teaching needs of both patient and family. Family members may need assistance from social service counselors if they begin to feel they will be unable to cope with an injured family member's care or disability once they return home. During the rehabilitation phase, encouraging family members to participate as much as possible in the plan of care is important and will assist them to effectively deal with the reality of residual disabilities.

A consistent, planned approach is the essential component of the care plan during this phase. All members of the health team must be working toward the same defined goals on an outcome-oriented time line and each should be aware of other members' roles as they strive to achieve these goals. The roles of physical therapists, speech therapists, and occupational therapists are vital to the care plan and must be included in its development and evaluation. Thorough discharge planning is crucial.

During the rehabilitation phase the patient may exhibit a cycle of progression/regression. The patient may be fully cooperative and demonstrate consistent progress 1 day or for a period of several weeks, only suddenly to become uncooperative, depressed, and unwilling to comply with the care plan he or she helped develop. These periods of setback are not uncommon because the patient struggles to adapt to the injury and the lifestyle changes it has imposed.

EVALUATION

Consistent weekly evaluation of the plan of care or rehabilitation critical pathway is vital during this phase. Assessment of patient response to interventions that address physical and psychologic needs may indicate a need to alter those interventions to meet the set goals effectively. The nurse's role as coordinator of the health care team takes on even more importance during the rehabilitation phase because more team members and outside resources become involved actively in the care plan.

The rehabilitation phase continues when the patient is discharged to home or to a rehabilitation center. The process is not complete until the patient is reintegrated successfully into the community. Reintegration is actually the final phase, and all resources that are available to assist the patient toward the goal should be used. Rehabilitation is an integral part of trauma nursing care and significantly affects the patient's potential for maximal recovery.

POSTDISCHARGE PHASE

Assessment of the trauma patient does not end at hospital discharge; rehabilitation also includes caring for the patient's physical and psychologic status after leaving the hospital. This process must take into account the patient's family as well. Trauma patients, especially those requiring extended care, often develop significant support systems and "significant other" relationships while hospitalized. If these relationships are interrupted suddenly, patients often face additional readjustment problems in their homes. As demonstrated by war victims whose injuries have resulted in body image changes (such as amputation), trauma patients often display a facade of total acceptance of their injury while hospitalized, but after discharge they experience severe depression or loss of motivation when they reenter society. As long as their environment includes patients with similar injuries, they often do well psychologically. When they return home, however, they begin to feel "different" from the healthy, so-called normal people who surround them.

Postdischarge patient assessment can occur by several means: return clinic visits, home visits from a visiting nurse association or public health home referral, or home visits from trauma nurses who cared for the patient (if the facility provides for this). Assessment factors critical to the evaluation of the patient, such as coping mechanisms, response to family and friends, and general mood and effect, should be identified in a nursing discharge summary or a visiting nurse referral form.

PHASE VI: PREVENTION

The trauma nurse has an essential role in all levels of injury prevention—primary, secondary, and tertiary. In addition, designing and implementing effective public education programs is a required standard in most trauma center verification or designation processes.

Programs that are data-driven from the hospital-based or statewide trauma registry ensure that the message delivered to the community focuses on the most common mechanisms of injury for that population and age group. For example, in an urban community where pedestrian injuries as the results of running red lights are a major cause of injury, safety campaigns focused on farm injuries will have no impact. Similarly, red light running awareness programs in a rural community with no traffic lights are equally as ineffective.

There are numerous national, state, and local organizations whose primary mission is injury prevention and public education. These include: the American Trauma Society, SAFE KIDS, the National Highway Traffic Safety Administration (NHTSA), Emergency Medical Services for Children (EMSC), and the Centers for Disease Control and Prevention's Injury Control Division. These organizations are only a few of the many that work collaboratively to educate the lay public on the causes of injury and methods to prevent it. Underlying all injury prevention efforts is the belief that trauma is no accident; therefore the use of the word *accident* is discouraged because it implies random and unpreventable injury.

A thorough discussion of the principles of injury prevention is beyond the scope of this chapter; refer to Chapter 7 for that content in its entirety.

SUMMARY

The trauma patient is unique because of the nature of injuries, the suddenness of the traumatic event, and the multiplicity of health care professionals required to organize and implement an effective plan of care from the scene of injury through reintegration into the community. The hope for survival and the physical and emotional recovery of the trauma patient depends on the collaborative efforts of the trauma nurses, physicians, therapists, and others who constitute the trauma team.

Three essential components are necessary to ensure high quality care and the best possible outcomes for multiply injured patients: collaborative practice; use of evidence-based protocols, procedures, and plans of care; and the often indefinable art of nursing and medicine.

Coordination of care by a primary nurse, nurse practitioner, trauma coordinator, or other advanced practice nurse is an effective model for delivering efficient and high-quality care to the trauma patient through collaborative practice. "Best practice, best care" for the multiply injured, to maximize resources, minimize and reduce complications, and optimize continuity and outcomes, is provided by a physician-nurse team that follows the patient from admission and resuscitation through hospital discharge and then periodically follows the patient and family in the rehabilitation and postdischarge phases. The multidisciplinary approach to trauma care ensures the ready availability of needed experts. Inherent in this approach is the significant involvement of numerous services and individuals. The strength of the multidisciplinary approach is the expertise that each group brings to the care of the patient. Essential are a coordinating physician and a coordinating nurse as key links to continuity and early collaborative care planning.

Florence Nightingale described the role of the nurse as having "charge of somebody's health," based on the knowledge of "how to put the body in such a state to be free of disease or recover from disease."[46] The nurse who coordinates the plan of care for the multiply injured patient exemplifies this historical definition.

Finally, in addition to the science of providing quality trauma care, the art of trauma care is an essential component through all the phases. For it is this art, the undefined humanistic element, the finely developed "sixth sense" of experienced trauma nurses and physicians, that often determines whether a multiply injured patient lives or dies. The multiply injured patient is truly complex and challenging. Through collaborative teamwork, quality care can be planned and delivered from resuscitation to reintegration into society.

REFERENCES

1. Johnson DE: The significance of nursing care, *Am J Nursing* 61:63-66, 1991.
2. Jacobs BB, Jacobs LM: Epidemiology of trauma. In Feliciano DV, Moore EE, Mattox KL, editors: *Trauma,* ed 3, Stamford, Conn, 1996, Appleton and Lange, 15-30.
3. Davis JW, Kaups KL: Base deficit in the elderly: a marker of severe injury and death, *J Trauma* 45:873-877, 1998.

4. American College of Surgeons' Committee on Trauma: *Resources for optimal care of the injured patient: 1999,* Chicago, 1999, The College.
5. Baggs JG, Ryan SA, Phelps CE et al: The association between interdisciplinary collaboration and patient outcomes in a medical intensive care unit, *Heart Lung* 21(1):18-24, 1992.
6. Joint Commission on Accreditation of Healthcare Organizations: *Comprehensive accreditation manual for hospitals,* Oakbrook Terrace, Ill, 1999, The Commission.
7. American College of Surgeons' Committee on Trauma: *Advanced trauma life support,* ed 6, Chicago, 1997, The College.
8. Dunham CM, Cowley RA: *Shock trauma critical care manual,* Gaithersburg, Md, 1991, Aspen Publications.
9. Cowley RA: Trauma center: a new concept for the delivery of critical care, *J Med Soc N J* 74(11):979-986, 1977.
10. Occupational Safety and Health Administration, U.S. Department of Labor: Intro to 29 CFR 1910.1030, occupational exposure to bloodborne pathogens, Washington, D.C., March 5, 1992, Government Printing Office.
11. Groves M: Initial communication with trauma patients. In Cardona V, editor: *Trauma nursing,* Montvale, NJ, 1985, Medical Economics, 15-18.
12. US Congress: Patient self-determination act, Washington, DC, 1990, Government Printing Office.
13. Sister Agnes Mary Joy: Psychosocial complications. In Mattox KL, editor: *Complications of trauma,* New York, 1994, Churchill Livingstone, 313-328.
14. Hanson C, Deutschman C, Anderson H et al: Effects of an organized critical care service on outcomes and resource utilization: a cohort study, *Crit Care Med* 27:270-274, 1999.
15. Mikhail J: The trauma triad of death: hypothermia, acidosis, and coagulopathy, *AACN Clin Issues* 10:85-94, 1999.
16. Von Rueden K, Dunham C: Sequelae of massive fluid resuscitation in trauma patients, *Crit Care Nurs Clin North Am* 6:463-472, 1994.
17. American College of Critical Care Medicine: Critical care services and personnel: recommendations based on a system of categorization into two levels of care, *Crit Care Med* 27:422-426, 1999.
18. Flynn MB, Luchsinger J: Trauma care strategies for changing economic forces, *Crit Care Nurse* 17(6):81-89, 1997.
19. Pilon C, Leathley M, Landon R et al: Practice guideline for arterial blood gas measurement in the intensive care unit decreases numbers and increases appropriateness of tests, *Crit Care Med* 25:1308-1313, 1997.
20. Namias N, McKenney G, Martin L: Utility of admission chemistry and coagulation profiles in trauma patients: a reappraisal of traditional practice, *J Trauma* 41:21-22, 1996.
21. Clemmer T, Spuhler VJ: Developing and gaining acceptance for patient care protocols, *New Horiz* 6(1):12-19, 1998.
22. Rhodes M: Practice management guidelines for trauma care: presidential address, 7th Scientific Assembly of Eastern Association for the Surgery of Trauma, *J Trauma* 37:635-644, 1994.
23. Fuss MA, Pasquale M: Clinical management protocols: the bedside answer to clinical practice guidelines, *J Trauma Nurs* 5:4-10, 1998.
24. Transfer Guidelines Task Force: Guidelines for the transfer of critically ill patients, *Am J Crit Care* 2:189-195, 1993.
25. Von Rueden K, Harris J: Pulmonary dysfunction related to immobility in the trauma patient, *AACN Clin Issues* 6:212-228, 1995.
26. Choi S, Nelson L: Kinetic therapy in critically ill patients: combined results based on a meta-analysis, *J Crit Care* 7:57-62, 1992.
27. Chatte G, Sab J-M, Dubois J-M et al: Prone position in mechanically ventilated patients with severe, acute respiratory failure, *Am J Respir Crit Care Med* 155:473-478, 1997.
28. Inman K, Sibbald W, Rutledge F et al: Clinical utility and cost-effectiveness of an air suspension bed on the prevention of pressure ulcers, *JAMA* 269:1139-1143, 1998.
29. Bergstrom N, Braden B, Laguzza A et al: The Braden scale for predicting pressure sore risk, *Nurs Res* 38:205-210, 1987.
30. Panel for the Prediction and Prevention of Pressure Ulcers in Adults: Pressure ulcers in adults: prediction and prevention, Clinical practice guideline #3, AHCPR publication no. 92-0047, Rockville, Md, May 1992, Agency for Health Care Policy and Research, Public Health Service, US Department of Health and Human Services.
31. Szaflarski N: Immobility phenomena in critically ill adults. In Clochesy JM, Breu C, Cardin S et al, editors: *Critical care nursing,* Philadelphia, 1996, WB Saunders, 1313-1334.
32. Clagett G: Prevention of postoperative venous thromboembolism: an update, *Am J Surg* 168:515-522, 1995.
33. Simon S, Phillips K, Badalamenti S et al: Current practices regarding visitation policies in critical care units, *Am J Crit Care* 6:210-217, 1997.
34. Pierce B: Children visiting in the adult ICU: a facilitated approach, *Crit Care Nurse* 18:85-90, 1998.
35. Proulx D: Animal-assisted therapy, *Crit Care Nurse* 18:80-84, 1998.
36. Technology Assessment Task Force of the Society of Critical Care Medicine: A model for technology assessment applied to pulse oximetry, *Crit Care Med* 21:615-624, 1993.
37. Ahrens T: Impact of technology on costs and patient outcome, *Crit Care Nurs Clin N Am* 10:117-125, 1998.
38. Naisbitt J: *Megatrends: ten new directions transforming our lives,* New York, 1982, Warner Books, 39-53.
39. Jastremski C, Harvey M: Making changes to improve the ICU experience for patients and their families, *New Horiz* 6:99-109, 1998.
40. Potter P, Perry A: *Fundamentals of nursing,* St. Louis, 1985, Mosby.
41. Evanisko M, Beasley C, Crigham L et al: Readiness of critical care physicians and nurses to handle requests for organ donation, *Am J Crit Care* 7:4-12, 1998.
42. Stark J, Coolican M, guest editors: Dying, death, donation and bereavement care, *Crit Care Nurs Clin N Am* 6:545-632, 1994.
43. American College of Critical Care Medicine of the Society of Critical Care Medicine: Guidelines on the admission and discharge for adult intermediate care units, *Crit Care Med* 26:607-610, 1998.
44. Zimmerman J, Wagner D, Knaus W et al: The use of risk predictions to identify candidates for intermediate care units—implications for intensive care utilization and cost, *Chest* 108:490-499, 1995.
45. Fontaine DK: Physical, personal, and cognitive responses to trauma, *Crit Care Nurs Clin North Am* 1:11-22, 1989.
46. Nightingale F: *Notes on nursing: what it is and what it is not,* New York, 1860, Harrison and Sons.

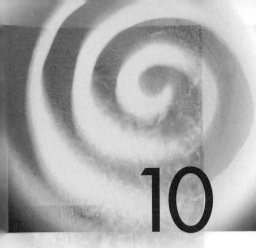

TRAUMA REHABILITATION

Karen Klender Heist

The evolution of the specialty of trauma during the past 30 years has been accompanied by great strides in medical technology. Emergency services have become highly sophisticated, creating the ability to save the lives of even the most severely injured people. The introduction of rapid transport from the scene of injury, often involving air evacuation, along with our increasingly mobile and active society have resulted in a new population of injured people who probably would have died several decades ago.

Highly effective emergency and critical care services have created a demand for services that restore quality of life to people who have survived severe injury. The result is the specialty practice of trauma rehabilitation. Although the ramifications of disability after injury are well understood, the long-term needs of the injured have not been fully met. Needs continue to be identified and services designed to complete the cycle of trauma care.

Trauma rehabilitation begins the instant that health care services are provided to a trauma patient. At first the focus is on preventing further injuries by thorough assessment and stabilization. As the patient stabilizes, the focus changes to restoring and maximizing function. Rehabilitation attempts to meet the patient's physical, intellectual, and psychosocial needs at each point throughout the trauma cycle.

An understanding of the philosophy of rehabilitation is essential for all nurses engaged in the trauma cycle of care, from those in the emergency departments and critical care units to those in rehabilitation hospitals or transition teams and in-home care agencies. Nurses must think as rehabilitation professionals throughout the trauma cycle in order to support the patient and family system toward optimal return to function.

DEFINITION OF REHABILITATION

Rehabilitation is a dynamic team process that maximizes an impaired individual's function by minimizing deficits to achieve the highest quality of life possible.[1] It further involves prevention of secondary injury and compensation and adaptation to disability, leading to reintegration into community life.

Among the many factors that affect patient outcome, the one most influential is the patient's motivation. It is the role of the rehabilitation professional to support trauma patients until they assume full responsibility for themselves.[2,3] For example, depression following a spinal cord or brain injury may prevent the patient from setting his or her own recovery goals.

HISTORY OF TRAUMA REHABILITATION

The focus of rehabilitation following trauma has changed through its development. In its early stages, rehabilitation was referred to as "physical medicine," primarily referring to restoration of motor skills and adaptation by compensation following physical disability.[4] Today an emphasis on motor recovery continues within rehabilitation. Most early benefits in rehabilitation were seen in patients with acute diseases, such as polio, and in veterans, many of whom sustained disabling spinal cord injuries or lower extremity amputations. Other forms of rehabilitation—such as for psychiatric problems; substance abuse; traumatic brain injury; stroke; and behavioral, learning disability, and developmental disorders—received far less attention and treatment. Therefore most of the early rehabilitation programs were oriented to the treatment of the physically disabled.

Vocational rehabilitation emerged as a need following the success of individual adaptation to a physical disability. Vocational rehabilitation programs initially involved evaluation of the patient's physical capacity followed by vocational testing, training, and placement. Subsequently, emphasis was placed on neuropsychologic assessment to identify cognitive factors related to work performance. The complex interrelationship among physical, cognitive, and psychosocial rehabilitation remains underappreciated by professionals, patients, families, society, legislators, and third-party payers.

During the 1980s greater attention was given to the development of rehabilitation programs for people recovering from severe brain injury. More than any other disabled population, brain-injured survivors require treatment from professionals in all disciplines working with them on cognitive, physical, and psychosocial issues. For example, it is difficult for a physical therapist to treat a gait disorder and ignore impaired attention and memory. It is impossible for a speech pathologist to help a person overcome a severe dysarthria while ignoring motor control problems that prohibit the person's use of an augmentative communication system. The brain-injury rehabilitation model has expanded rehabilitation from its limited focus on physical and vocational disability to include cognitive, behavioral, and psychosocial disability.

The knowledge gained and techniques learned from the treatment of psychiatric disorders, including substance abuse, have also been integrated into trauma rehabilitation. Substance abuse is becoming more common as a coexisting factor among the injured, requiring addiction treatment to be more available in the rehabilitation process. Many patients with brain and spinal cord injury have preexisting learning disabilities that need to be considered during their recovery. Improvements in rehabilitation programming better meet the needs of all trauma patients. There is heightened sensitivity among health care professionals to identify all the rehabilitation needs of the trauma patient.

There has been a proliferation of rehabilitation services and settings in response to the demand for rehabilitation, yet access to services remains inconsistent, particularly in the community reintegration phase. Appropriate services are not conveniently available to all trauma patients because of poor understanding of what specialized services are required, decreased appreciation for recovery potential, and lack of funding. Infrequently, disabled patients must go out of state for rehabilitation programs. This does not support continuity from the trauma center to a rehabilitative environment. It is important that the full continuum of services be available within the patient's community if possible.

The Balanced Budget Act of 1997 reduced reimbursement, particularly Medicare reimbursement, for rehabilitation services.[5] The first phase reduced rehabilitation provided in skilled nursing facilities and through home care agencies; reimbursement to acute rehabilitation hospitals follows in subsequent years.[6,7] A dramatic impact has already been experienced by health care providers.[8,9] In response, numerous rehabilitation providers have eliminated staff, sold their practices, or closed in recent months. Without funding to support rehabilitation services, the availability of care will decline significantly. The government's goal is to eliminate overuse and abuse of services. Whether or not this change is cost effective remains to be seen. It will be a primary topic for study in the next few years.

TRAUMA POPULATIONS THAT REQUIRE REHABILITATION

Most trauma patients require some rehabilitation services. Services may be as basic as patient and family education done by the emergency department staff on identification of postconcussive symptoms and the availability of follow-up services for a patient with a mild brain injury. Provision of this rehabilitative teaching can avoid unnecessary patient suffering. More severely injured persons require specialized rehabilitation services based on their diagnosis. Patterns of services have been established for many disabilities. The most common specialized rehabilitation programs in trauma are for spinal cord injury, brain injury, orthopedic and soft-tissue injury, and multiple trauma. Pediatric and adult rehabilitation are distinct subspecialties. Each group benefits from different rehabilitation program components, including unique facilities, equipment, mix of professionals, and approaches to treatment. The Commission on Accreditation of Rehabilitation Facilities provides standards for comprehensive inpatient rehabilitation, spinal cord injury, brain injury, postacute rehabilitation, comprehensive outpatient rehabilitation, pain rehabilitation, and various other specialized rehabilitation programs. These standards are considered an expected level of practice by today's rehabilitation providers.[10]

Programs for people with spinal cord injuries focus on life-changing physical disability. Emphasis is placed on relearning physical activities and using compensatory methods and adaptive devices. A large portion of the program involves patient teaching. It requires a motivated patient with enough self-direction to become independent and avoid complications. Psychosocial support is a major component. To be rehabilitated successfully, the patient must learn to adapt to the disability physically and psychologically.[2,11] Advances in computer technology, electrical muscle stimulation, and research in nerve cell growth are shaping the future of spinal cord injury rehabilitation. (See Chapter 22 for additional information.)

The head-injured population requires a different focus. Their rehabilitation program depends on the degree of deficit resulting from the injury.[12] Patients in coma require multisensory stimulation and prevention of physical complications caused by immobility. Confused patients or those displaying inappropriate behavior need specific behavioral modification and therapeutic behavioral approaches, sometimes including secured settings. All team members address improvement in cognitive function and social awareness. The physical effects of brain injury are as varied as the cognitive deficits. (See Chapter 19 for information specific to the brain-injured patient.)

The patient education component of brain injury rehabilitation is also unique. Because of the patient's cognitive and behavioral deficits, most of the teaching about the injury, its effects, and management of problems is provided to the patient's family and support systems. As the patient recovers enough insight to learn and use the information, more teaching is provided. This is also true in the provision of psychosocial support. Rehabilitation research relates ongoing support to improved long-term outcome.[13] Societal acceptance and community reintegration are key areas of brain injury rehabilitation programming for the future.

Patients with orthopedic or soft-tissue injuries and those with multiple system trauma need a rehabilitation program with both medical and surgical emphases. Complex injuries may require an extended time for recovery because of multiple surgeries. Attention is given to prevention of infection and other complications during tissue healing. Amputees may require the use of prosthetic or adaptive devices. Psychosocial support addresses changes in body image, loss of independence and control, and lower self-esteem. Health education commonly emphasizes the patient's physical needs and should expand to address psychosocial issues.

COMPONENTS OF REHABILITATION

Although certain trauma populations require a specialized rehabilitation program for the best outcome, several components are common to all programs regardless of the setting. Two key elements are the team approach to maximizing the patient's potential and the development of an individualized rehabilitation plan.

REHABILITATION TEAM

Not unlike other specialties in health care, trauma rehabilitation requires a team approach. The concept of a team as a group of specialists working toward a common goal is simplistic, yet it is implemented quite literally in the rehabilitation setting. Also inherent in team philosophy is congruency in goals, consistency in approach, and communication among all team members.[14] Most teams treat a specific group of patients exclusively. They usually meet weekly to discuss the patients' progress and set new, achievable weekly goals.

Early rehabilitation teams were called multidisciplinary, with each specialty having separate goals and approaches. This method offered the benefit of input from many specialties to the patient's plan of care, but each discipline had individual goals. Fragmentation of care became a major problem.

The use of an interdisciplinary team avoids fragmentation. Each member of the team focuses on a particular area of expertise and blends with the expertise of other team members. In an interdisciplinary approach, patient goals are developed by the team rather than by each discipline. An example of this is the cooperative effort of behavior modification strategies for a brain-injured patient's agitation. Consistent approaches to patient behavior may include reduction of external stimuli, avoiding patient fatigue, and providing treatment in a quiet area.

A growing approach in team dynamics, the transdisciplinary team,[15] is similar to the interdisciplinary team in the method in which mutual goals are formed. Team members bring their special expertise to the group. The distinguishing characteristic in this model is that each member is responsible for sharing observations about all aspects of the patient's rehabilitation, particularly when the team meets to review progress. An observer of the team would find it more difficult to determine each member's primary discipline based on his or her verbal input during a team conference.

Disciplines may approach therapeutic treatments collectively rather than individually. Physical and occupational therapists may have joint therapy sessions with the patient to establish the most appropriate custom wheelchair for proper positioning. A speech pathologist, occupational therapist, and rehabilitation nurse may schedule a mealtime session with the dysphagic patient to assess and establish team approaches to feeding.

Each team specialist has the responsibility to address the overall functional goals for the patient. It takes mature professionals to let go of the traditional territory associated with each discipline, allowing team members to make observations across disciplines while understanding the perspectives of fellow team members.

COMPOSITION OF THE TEAM. The team is composed of those who have input to the rehabilitation plan, including family members. The team can number from just a few to a large group of specialists. Team membership is determined by two factors: the diagnosis and the phase of the trauma cycle (Table 10-1). Rehabilitation for specific injuries requires a typical complement of appropriate specialists who are able to meet the comprehensive needs of the patient. In some cases the mix of team members reflects more physical rehabilitation emphasis in the early phases (e.g., a comatose patient on a ventilator). Often the cognitive and psychosocial components of rehabilitation are implemented further along in the cycle. By the time the patient is in the reintegration phase, the physical impairments may have been largely resolved, leaving the team focused primarily on psychosocial adaptation after injury.

All members of the team are equally essential to the patient's success. Some disciplines, such as nursing and social services, remain involved with the patient throughout the continuum of care, but the focus of their involvement may change. Other primary team members are involved for limited periods, working with the patient through the intermediate and rehabilitation phases. For example, physical, occupational, speech, and respiratory therapies are intensively active during the periods of acute or rehabilitation hospitalization.

The most important member of the rehabilitation team is the patient. It is the responsibility of the professionals on the team to help the patient understand his or her active role in rehabilitation. In many outpatient rehabilitative settings, patients are referred to as "clients," reflecting the cooperative investment between the injured person and the rehabilitation professionals. As the patient moves through the cycle, he or she sheds the patient role and returns to a status of self-responsibility.[16]

To ensure that the most appropriate and individualized team is organized, a team leader assumes a holistic view of the patient's rehabilitative process and expected outcome. The team leader defines a realistic expected outcome for each patient. In addition, the team leader, either directly or indirectly, determines which specialists will be needed on the team.

TABLE 10-1	Changes in Team Membership and Focus Throughout the Trauma Cycle			
	Critical Care Phase	**Intermediate Phase**	**Rehabilitation Phase**	**Reintegration Phase**
Rehabilitation Focus	Life saving is priority; focus on prevention of further injury or debilitation	Prevention of complications from injury and immobility	Restoration of function and compensation for disability	Adaptation to abilities and disabilities in community/home life
Team Member and Role				
Patient, family, significant others	• Passive and dependent role (may be in crisis), provide database for patient	• Support physical healing • Learn about injury, potential problems, and process of rehabilitation • Psychosocial support system • Active input to plan of care	• Determine goals with team • Process of learning skills, practicing and testing new situations • Make realistic plans for future	• Self-determining • Utilize team as resource consultants • Establish lifelong plan
Physician(s)	• Emergency stabilization and treatment	• Promote physical healing • May involve many specialists • Initiate physiatry consult	• Physiatrist primarily, with medical consultants	• Follow up as indicated; lifelong physical adaptation
Nurse	• Stabilization • Physical treatment • Support in crisis	• Promote healing • Holistic assessment of recovery process • Patient and family teaching	• Integrate therapy gains into 24-hour daily routine • Patient and family teaching	• Screening • Assessment for areas of difficulty in adaptation
Social worker	• Crisis intervention • Collect psychosocial database	• Psychosocial support, grieving • Financial process • Referral planning	• Planning for reintegration process • Resources for family and patient	• Support and referral during adaptation • Peer support groups
Physical therapist		• Initial assessment of rehabilitation potential • Prevent immobility problems	• Active restoration • Compensation • Adaptation	• Consultant role or single service provider
Occupational therapist		• Initial assessment of rehabilitation potential • Prevent immobility problems • Begin self-care	• Active restoration • Compensation • Adaptation	• Consultant role or single service provider
Cognitive, speech, and audiology specialists		• Initial assessment of rehabilitation potential • Alternative communication, swallowing, cognitive remediation	• Active restoration • Compensation • Adaptation	• Consultant role or single service provider
Vocational counselor		• Consultant • Early assessment	• Assessment • Retraining • Job placement	• Consultant
Therapeutic recreation		• Consultant	• Integration of new skills into a quality leisure lifestyle	• Consultant
Possible consultants	• Variety of medical specialists • Clergy • Respiratory therapy	• Respiratory therapy • Psychologist-neuropsychologist • Financial planner • Medical specialists • Nursing specialists • Dietitian	• Same as for intermediate phase plus: • Prosthetics • Orthotics • Biomedical engineering	• Potentially any health care provider • Based on long-term patient and family need
Payer	• Informed of initial injury • Authorization for services	• Insurance specialist may plan for transfer to acute and other rehabilitation programs • Authorization for services	• Find most cost-effective rehabilitation gains • Authorization for services	• Lifelong plan for finances • Responsibility shifted to patient

TEAM LEADERSHIP.   Another aspect of the team is its form of leadership. Various models of leadership—the physician-led team, the multidisciplinary team, the rehabilitation coordinator role, and the case manager role—are discussed in this section.

Early team models were based on physician leadership. The physician ordered rehabilitation therapies and progress reports from the therapists to establish patient goals. The advantage of this model was consistency of goals for all members. But by limiting the input and influence of a variety of disciplines, this structure yields goals based only on the physician's perspective. In the early years of trauma rehabilitation, most rehabilitation goals were mobility and self-care achievements, often neglecting cognitive, linguistic, and psychosocial needs. This scope of rehabilitation reflected the priorities the physician chose for the patient's outcome. Many of the physicians attending to trauma patients had limited knowledge of and experience in the specialty of rehabilitation. Currently, in most rehabilitation settings, the physicians who lead the teams have broader experience in rehabilitation, and often they are highly specialized in the rehabilitative needs of their patients.

As specialization developed among rehabilitation professionals, the therapy disciplines gradually assumed a stronger role. Members of each discipline reported their own observations and treatment plans to the physician and the other team members. Goals were formulated by each discipline. This provided greater input from team members, but the problem of fragmentation became apparent. At times the goals of the disciplines were divergent.

Rehabilitation Coordinator.   Clinical managers of rehabilitation programs throughout the country established the role of rehabilitation coordinator to blend the fragmented, multidisciplinary efforts of the team. Today this model is in place in many rehabilitation settings. Team meetings are led by either the physician or the rehabilitation coordinator, and the goals of all team members are blended into interdisciplinary goals for the patient. A comprehensive rehabilitation plan is established that addresses physical, cognitive, and psychosocial issues; defined rehabilitation potential; and a safe discharge plan. Members of the team are accountable to the rehabilitation coordinator in their work of meeting the clinical needs of the patient but are not directly supervised by the rehabilitation coordinator. The rehabilitation coordinator often uses informal influence over the other members of the team while ensuring a quality, individualized rehabilitation program for the patient.

Case Manager.   The role of case manager was introduced when managed care sought to save costs by streamlining care. Managed care initiated the use of external case managers—that is, clinicians, who do not provide direct care but who review and manage catastrophic cases with high costs to insurance companies and are employed or contracted by the insurer.[17] Many of these cases involve traumatic injuries. Facility-based case management has become the standard of practice for many rehabilitation programs.

Most case managers are registered nurses with rehabilitation or critical care experience. Case managers oversee the clinical progress and treatment of patients who have experienced catastrophic events and are undergoing rehabilitation. They coordinate a rehabilitation plan that is clinically advantageous to the patient but also extends the patient's health care funding to the best use of coverage and clinical benefit as projected over the long-term course of recovery.[18] Some case managers, often those employed by third-party payers, follow the care during the patient's lifetime, spanning multiple clinical settings.[19] Case managers working for medical care providers do not follow the patient on a long-term basis; however, they do consider the future impact of health care decisions.

The case manager's role is to coordinate the most appropriate rehabilitation strategies based on the assessment of the patient and the experience of the clinical team. The case manager works with the physician to implement a cost-effective rehabilitation plan for the patient. For example, if a therapist requests a custom wheelchair for the patient, the physician evaluates the clinical benefit and the case manager evaluates the cost-benefit ratio. This might include a projection of wheelchair cost against the length of time the chair would be appropriate for the patient. For a patient who is making successive physical gains, an adaptable chair might be the wiser choice. On the other hand, a patient who is functionally stable might maximize the use of a custom chair designed for his or her current status. An analysis of purchase versus rental may also enter into the decision. By selectively using funds, the patient actually receives more effective rehabilitation because it is given at the most appropriate time for maximal gain. In this way the patient's funds are extended over time as opposed to an intensive short-term program that exhausts funds and leaves the patient with no long-term benefits. This model of cost management is more common with worker compensation funds or litigation settlements. Most managed care or insurance policies contain costs by medical review and authorization for specific diagnostic evaluations, procedures, or treatment approaches.

Case managers who work for the payer may require that all durable medical equipment, tests, and treatments be preauthorized by the insurer to ensure payment. Often the treatment is authorized for a specified time, usually a specific number of days, and reauthorization is required based on the patient's clinical improvement and potential for further progress. A provider-based case manager frequently is the contact with the patient's insurer for all authorizations and clinical updates.

The case manager role is similar to the rehabilitation coordinator role, with the focus on effecting quality of care through the design and management of the patient's therapeutic plan. A facility-based case management workload is typically as high as 24 patients, depending on the severity and complexity of the cases. A large rehabilitation program may have several case managers, each responsible for leading team conferences. Case management changes the physician's role on the team. In a truly collaborative approach, the physician, providing specialized medical input, becomes a partner with the clinical team in developing a rehabilitation plan.

Both the case manager and the rehabilitation coordinator roles have been excellent career opportunities for rehabilitation nurses. These roles demand a rehabilitation professional that can step beyond his or her clinical discipline and function with a holistic clinical and financial perspective as the patient's advocate. The nursing profession lends itself to a role of this nature; however, case managers and coordinators practice with a variety of professional backgrounds. In settings without case management, staff nurses may identify this as a new opportunity, resulting in improved patient care, cost savings, and an elevated level of function for the nurse. An additional benefit to nurses with case management experience is the opportunity for employment with third-party insurers and managed care organizations.

The patient gradually becomes more involved in decision making as he or she becomes more physically, cognitively, and psychosocially independent, regardless of team leadership styles. Patient decision making is as important a goal as functional independence in a quality rehabilitation process.

REHABILITATION PLAN

REHABILITATION POTENTIAL. Thorough assessment and evaluation of the patient's rehabilitation potential are the first steps following trauma. Although it is difficult to predict a final outcome after trauma, there are parameters that help to determine the amount and rate of a patient's potential progress. These factors represent the patient's strengths and weaknesses in the areas of physical, cognitive, and psychosocial functioning.[2,20] Other factors that influence rehabilitation potential are the patient's age, length of time since injury, premorbid health, support systems, secondary complications, and availability of resources.

Physical Factors. For some disabilities there are well-established outcomes. These outcomes may change as technology develops to compensate for impairment. Thirty years ago a C6 quadriplegic patient would not have been able to feed himself or herself. Today this is possible. Perhaps in the future there will be fewer physical limits because medical technology will be able to replace, rebuild, or stimulate the growth of a new spinal cord. It is important that rehabilitation professionals maintain their awareness of current research so that their patients can benefit when new products becomes available.

Concurrent diagnoses also influence rehabilitation outcome. Many trauma patients have multiple injuries, preexisting conditions, or complications of trauma that significantly impact their potential to recover.

As the population ages, the incidence of trauma in the elderly is rising. Individuals are physically active well into their 80s and beyond and thus are subject to the risks of an active adult lifestyle. The effects of normal aging and a higher likelihood of concurrent medical conditions, such as diabetes, complicate healing and may seriously reduce rehabilitation potential.[21]

Cognitive and Psychosocial Factors. If physical impairment were the only factor determining rehabilitation potential, two patients with similar injuries would have comparable outcomes. Cognitive and psychosocial factors influence rehabilitation outcome as well. Cognitive factors include the patient's ability to learn new things, solve problems, and make appropriate judgments and decisions; educational level; readiness to learn; prior experiences; and many other complex factors.[22] Psychosocial factors, including income, family support, lifestyle, mood, relationships, personality, and coping ability, all affect the patient's potential. A highly motivated patient with sufficient financial resources and a supportive family living nearby is not the common scenario after trauma. Many trauma patients have a history of substance abuse, unemployment, poor education, and unhealthy lifestyle.[23]

Evaluating Rehabilitation Potential. Each professional working with a trauma patient needs to evaluate the patient's rehabilitation potential. The clinician first defines the rehabilitation outcome that would be typical for the patient's injury. Then the outcome is further analyzed by assigning a probability factor or percentage of predicted success to the estimated outcome. A patient who has had a traumatic below-the-knee amputation may have excellent potential to return to work and be independent in the actives of daily living using a prosthesis. However, when the evaluator considers that the patient is 53 years old, is developmentally disabled, lives alone, and has sustained multiple infections and stump revisions during the acute phase, the potential for independent living and return to work becomes significantly lower. Recognizing these probability factors provides rehabilitation professionals with a clearer picture that the patient either will need significantly greater resources or may not be able to reach the standard desirable outcome.

Rehabilitation potential should not be a question of yes or no or good or poor. Not all evaluators apply percentages of success to the case. The important point is that the rehabilitation assessment summarizes the strengths that will support rehabilitative efforts and considers strategies to work with or around the negative aspects to prevent a failure. Nearly every patient has some potential for improvement, but the potential must be weighed against what is both cost effective and a reasonable expectation for patient success.

Successful rehabilitation was traditionally defined as a return to work and home life. This outcome was expected to occur despite the time constraints of the relatively few rehabilitation program options—acute physical rehabilitation along with vocational counseling and training. Perspectives regarding successful rehabilitation have expanded. A desirable outcome is one that achieves improvement in the patient's quality of life within appropriate cost parameters. Time frames for a successful program are subject to a combination of patient need and funding limitations. From a quality of care perspective, an individual's expected outcome and rate of recovery dictate the type of rehabilitation program that is best for the patient. Because health care costs increase and treatment options multiply, cost-benefit analysis is a critical element in the formulation of rehabilitation program recommendations following the evaluation of potential. The ability of the rehabilitation industry to measure its success and failure with clinical and functional outcomes will greatly influence future decisions.

Realistic goals are set for the patient, and an estimated time for achievement is established. If these goals are individualized and sensitive to the patient's strengths and weaknesses, any patient should have good rehabilitation potential for his or her unique goals.

GOAL DEVELOPMENT. The development of long-term and short-term patient goals is a collaborative process. The goals are adjusted based on the patient's progress and should reflect the uniqueness of the patient. Long-term goals reflect a phase of the patient's recovery after hospitalization. Short-term goals are the achievable steps toward the overall long-term goal. Goals should be functional, such as dressing or transferring, and directed toward overcoming the impairment, such as strengthening elbow flexors. Goals can be developed for family education, such as education on range-of-motion techniques, for a patient who is in a persistent vegetative state after a severe brain injury. Increased range of motion alone is not a functional goal. However, the resulting improved positioning when seated in a chair benefits the patient's quality of life and prevents complications by increasing stimulation, improving hygiene, reducing spasticity, and preventing decubiti and contractures. To establish a functional goal, the team considers the most realistic and appropriate outcomes for an individual patient. Ambulating for 20 feet is a measurable goal. The ability to get to and from the bathroom focuses on function and is measurable. All goals should be measurable and reproducible. The appropriateness of specific goals should be meaningful to the patient's functional independence.

For successful rehabilitation, mutuality of goals between the patient and the rehabilitation specialists is essential.[16] Mutuality is a concept defined as a unified acceptance and agreement by both parties of what will be achieved. It should be based on the patient's value system, not that of the professional. Often a trauma patient begins treatment with a fairly passive position in the plan of care. The patient usually agrees to follow the regimen or to allow treatments to be conducted without much thought or question. As the crisis period subsides, the patient becomes more interested and actively involved in decision making.

The assumption that a compliant patient is an ideal patient is misleading. Even the term *compliance* suggests that the decision and plan are created and enforced by outside sources. It is the patient, not the staff, who has the ultimate responsibility for outcome. The patient should be included as an equal partner in the decision-making process. Values play a major role in the functional goals set by both the staff and the patient. A conflict in values should be recognized openly, and mutual goals should be sought. Education in values clarification is helpful to staff members working in rehabilitation to prepare for resolution of these conflicts.

IMPLEMENTATION OF THE PLAN. Individualized strategies are developed for the achievement of functional goals.[10] Any strategy to be used should be understood by all team members to avoid incongruent techniques that could erode functional gains. Strategies used to achieve restoration of function are different from those used to compensate for disability.

Therapy implementation has traditionally been provided through one-on-one sessions. In recent years therapists have used other approaches, including group treatment and co-treatment by professionals from two disciplines working with one patient. This frequently occurs in the rehabilitation or reintegration phases of the cycle.

In the first option, functional goal groups are created, such as social skills, mobility, and self-care skills. Patients with common goals are gathered together to follow a specific program to achieve that goal with the benefit of group dynamics and peer feedback. The use of group technique improves application of rehabilitation strategies in the real world. Society revolves around interactions with others in one-on-one, small group, and large group situations. To approximate society, various interactive strategies are used. This prepares the injured patient to function in society, builds coping skills, and allows the patient to test his or her adaptation to injury in a supportive group setting. It is appropriate for the rehabilitation nurse to participate in this therapy and, in some situations, direct it.

Co-treatment sessions allow several specialists to work with one patient at the same time. An example might be a daily mealtime session with the occupational therapist, speech pathologist, and nurse to improve a dysphagic patient's ability to feed himself or herself. The team members become more integrated because they focus on functional, rather than discipline-specific, goals. The interactive nature of co-treatment enhances the evaluation and treatment process, resulting in an outcome that is more effective than can be gained through individual sessions with each of the component disciplines. Therapy disciplines that experience a consistent need to work together should consider joint evaluation sessions in anticipation of these needs.

Reimbursement practices continue to affect clinical practice in rehabilitation. Many funding sources, both government and private, require authorization for special treatment sessions or impose specific guidelines for their use. Co-treatment may be viewed as too costly, and the payer may reimburse for only one of the disciplines providing treatment. Because of the need for cost containment, less co-treatment is done in today's rehabilitation programs, often with the focus on evaluation. The use of group treatment has increased in recent years and has proven to be cost effective. Payers may have specific guidelines for the staff-to-patient ratio for authorized group therapy treatment. Payment for any rehabilitation treatment option is best supported and measured by outcome data systems.

REHABILITATION OUTCOME

One of the most important components of rehabilitation is the accurate, comprehensive measurement of patient outcome.[20,24] Literally hundreds of outcome scales exist. Most rehabilitation programs collect outcome data relevant to their own program. It is difficult to compare programmatic outcomes because the evaluation tools collect data by different methods and at varying times. Specific measurement systems have improved for comparison of outcomes in similar settings, but they remain lacking in sensitivity for comparison outcomes across various rehabilitation settings, including: acute rehabilitation, subacute care, home care, and outpatient programs.

What constitutes a quality outcome? Functional gains that are not retained over time initially may give the appearance of an inflated outcome. An example of good outcome measurement includes measures of function done at the time of admission to and discharge from a rehabilitation program, followed by measures at 6 months and 1 year after discharge. Postdischarge interval measurements are used to document functions that have been sustained. Exorbitant expenditures to achieve a slightly higher outcome may not be the wisest use of the patient's financial resources. Clinical and functional outcome measures related to rehabilitation costs are most influential to support funding for rehabilitation.

Third-party payers continue to drive the rehabilitation system toward more cost-effective alternatives. Through their ORYX initiative, the Joint Commission on Accreditation of Healthcare Organizations (JCAHO) now requires facilities to select and implement specific outcome measurement systems as part of their accreditation process.[25] Many of these measurement systems are used nationwide, usually by purchase or subscription.

One of the most widely used outcome data systems associated with trauma rehabilitation is the Uniform Data System for Medical Rehabilitation (UDSMR).[26] This and other standard functional measures can be applied easily at varying intervals before and after discharge. Guidelines and training for professionals using the assessments are available. These instruments also have the capacity to measure sustained outcome over time.

In July 2000 the Health Care Financing Administration (HCFA) began requiring a clinically-based measurement tool, the Minimum Data Set for Post Acute Care (MDS-PAC), to be used for reimbursement in acute rehabilitation hospitals.[27] The Balanced Budget Act of 1997 requires similar data systems for skilled nursing facilities and home care organizations. It appears that HCFA is adopting data systems not only for reimbursement purposes but also for demonstration of the clinical condition of the patient. Alternatively, a combination of measures may be used in HCFA's database.[28] Potentially these measures could be used to compare clinical populations across various rehabilitation settings. The resulting cost-benefit data would dramatically improve utilization and reimbursement for rehabilitation in the future.

The simplicity of such measures provides a basis for comparison of programs in terms of quality, cost effectiveness, time efficiency, and development of lasting outcomes. Measures such as these help to guide use of rehabilitation services by monitoring the best match between patient needs and the most appropriate rehabilitation setting at each point along the cycle.

AVAILABILITY OF REHABILITATION FOR THE TRAUMA PATIENT

Available rehabilitation options have become widely divergent. Traditional medical inpatient rehabilitation is now just one of many types of programs. Because the complex needs of trauma patients have been recognized, a full range of rehabilitation programs and services have been developed. One of the confusing aspects of understanding what types of rehabilitation options exist is defining the difference between rehabilitation programs and rehabilitation services. It is also necessary to recognize when each option is most appropriate to the patient's rehabilitation goals.

PROGRAMS AND SERVICES

A rehabilitation service is a single component in a rehabilitation program. An example is physical therapy services on an outpatient basis for a posttraumatic amputee needing prosthetic gait training. In this example the patient may not require other therapy or rehabilitative services, so the single service of physical therapy meets the patient's needs. Counseling or occupational therapy also would be available within the program.

In comparison, a rehabilitation program is much more than the cumulative effect of multiple rehabilitation services. It is the coordination and synergy of multiple disciplines. A program can exist in an inpatient, outpatient, or residential (home care) setting if the services are coordinated and if the approach is a team effort.

A successful rehabilitation program allows for cooperation and communication by the entire team assigned to the patient. An inpatient setting that provides nursing and medical care of the patient and offers physical, occupational, and other therapies does not automatically become a rehabilitation program. When multiple disciplines integrate their efforts toward mutual functional goals and carryover occurs from therapy to nursing care, the essence of a true rehabilitation program is being offered to the patient.

Discharge planning for the trauma patient involves understanding whether he or she requires a single service or a comprehensive program. Fragmentation of care is one of the primary risks for failure of rehabilitative efforts. The match of patients' needs and goals to appropriate programs or services maximizes outcomes. When evaluating rehabilitation programs, it is important to determine whether there is adequate coordination of services to provide integration rather than fragmentation of goals.

Severely injured patients in the late rehabilitative phase and reintegration phase of the trauma cycle could appropriately have their follow-up needs met by a single rehabilitation service. This depends on the complexity of injury, psychosocial supports, and intellectual ability of the patient and family to carry out the plan. Discharge planners should take into consideration that a highly motivated patient or family support system can provide a great deal of care coordination for home-based rehabilitation services. Each case must be evaluated on individual need.

CENTERS OF EXCELLENCE

Certain rehabilitation programs have elevated themselves to distinction through continual research in the specialty of rehabilitation and application of that research to practice. Often these facilities are known for a subspecialty in rehabilitation, such as spinal cord injury, brain injury, or burn rehabilitation. Some of them are known regionally, whereas others have a national reputation. Patients with extremely complex or unique injuries may require a facility of this level of expertise. Referral is determined by agreement among the referring medical acute care treatment team, a payer representative (often a case manager), the family, and the patient. Use of these facilities by patients from outside the local region or state has decreased because the specialty of rehabilitation has grown and managed care has put tighter controls on health care spending.

INFLUENCE OF MANAGED CARE

The availability of resources continues to be influenced by managed care. Managed care is defined as group of "systems that integrate financing and the delivery of appropriate health care services through: selected health care providers furnishing services to members, explicit standards for provider selection, quality assurance and utilization review programs, and financial incentives for members to use selected providers."[29] A payer selects preferred rehabilitation providers to deliver services for the patient population at different points in the cycle. These preferred provider arrangements sometimes limit alternatives for the patient. However, the coordination of services by managed care often is greatly improved. Case management, discussed earlier in the chapter, can be a component of a managed care system. Acute care trauma nurses may find themselves providing referral documentation to utilization review nurses, case managers, and other payer representatives to plan transfer to a rehabilitation facility.

CURRENT AND FUTURE REHABILITATION ALTERNATIVES

The future of rehabilitation delivery promises a full spectrum of programs and services ranging from acute inpatient rehabilitation to outpatient and residential settings. With an increased availability of cost-effective alternatives and continued pressure to cut health care costs for rehabilitation, the number of patients served by acute inpatient programs is expect to decrease significantly in the next decade.

Programs are carried out in three general locations: inpatient, outpatient, and home. Traditional rehabilitation has been provided predominantly through the inpatient setting, but outpatient and home-based rehabilitation alternatives are capable of providing the essential components of team approach and rehabilitation planning and achieving positive outcomes.

The following sections describe program options that may be provided to the trauma population. It is not an all-inclusive list; rather, it is an attempt to demonstrate the variety of programming available throughout the country. Not all these options are cost-effectively accessible to all patients, particularly in rural areas.

INPATIENT REHABILITATION

Comprehensive acute inpatient rehabilitation may be found as a dedicated unit within hospitals, freestanding hospitals, and skilled nursing facilities. The criteria of the Commission on Accreditation of Rehabilitation Facilities (CARF) for comprehensive inpatient rehabilitation[10] (often referred to as "acute rehabilitation") require that the patient must demonstrate functional gains at least every 2 weeks and that each patient must participate in therapy for a minimum of 3 hours per day. This is an extremely active program. Typically patients are in various individual and group therapies for the bulk of the day, with rehabilitation carryover by the nursing staff and specific therapeutic evening programs.

Patients who are ready to begin the transition to home and community may use a therapeutic leave of absence (TLOA). Each TLOA has specific individual goals. Included in the process are patient and family education and post-TLOA evaluation to determine the outcome.

Subacute rehabilitation, an alternative to "acute rehabilitation," has experienced a boom in the 1990s. This alternative setting meets the needs of patients who are not able to tolerate the daily intensity of an acute inpatient rehabilitation program and those who are making slower progress but still require the coordinated services of an interdisciplinary team. Subacute rehabilitation units may also be provided in a variety of bed licensing arrangements, including acute hospitals, long-term or chronic hospitals, and skilled nursing facilities.[30] In addition, many long-term care facilities provide therapy services to patients needing rehabilitation.[31] One of the critical factors that differentiates subacute rehabilitation in a skilled nursing facility from long-term care is that the subacute patient requires an active rehabilitation program by a coordinated team, rather than a residential placement utilizing rehabilitation services that are focused on maintaining the patient's current quality of life.

The similarities between acute and subacute inpatient rehabilitation cause a great deal of confusion. This is largely related to the fact that these programs may be operated under the same type of bed license with provision of the same list of services. The key difference is the intensity of the program and the expected rate of patient recovery. JCAHO has established standards for subacute rehabilitation to assist in clear understanding and evaluation of such programs.[32]

Transitional living programs focus specifically on community reintegration. The patient lives in a structured home environment, usually with 4 to 10 other patients. Social and behavioral adaptation skills are an important focus, in addition to the adjustment to physical disabilities in a home and community setting. The home environment is typically paired with a modified work or school setting in either the same or a nearby location. Transitional living provides inpatient rehabilitation for a specific length of time to achieve identified goals.[33] It is not a long-term residential placement, as the name indicates.

Structured living, on the other hand, is an extended placement that provides life skills and rehabilitation support services. It may also be called a group home or nonmedical residential rehabilitation.

OUTPATIENT REHABILITATION

Outpatient medical rehabilitation programs are among the most innovative rehabilitation alternatives. An outpatient medical rehabilitation program provides a wide range of therapeutic services and approaches by a coordinated team in both individual and group sessions. The patients require minimal medical and nursing care and are functionally independent enough to live at home and commute to their rehabilitation program. Depending on the intensity of need, patients are seen on a daily or intermittent basis. CARF has established a separate set of accreditation criteria to ensure consistency of outpatient medical rehabilitation programs.[34]

The number of "work-hardening" programs has grown in the past few years. Work hardening commonly is associated with an outpatient medical rehabilitation program and provides physical and cognitive strengthening of the patient's functional abilities. The program simulates components of the patient's actual or potential work functions, gradually increasing the complexity and repetition of tasks until patients are prepared to return to a work setting.

Patients in day treatment programs demonstrate significantly higher functional independence than those in inpatient rehabilitation settings. The focus of the day treatment program is geared to a specialized aspect of reintegration, such as social behavior, cognitive rehabilitation, and prevocational training. Day hospitals provide nursing, medical, and therapy services to a patient during daytime hours to improve the level of patient function or, in a day-care model, to relieve the family from 24-hour care.

Vocational programs may provide highly specialized services, including in-depth patient evaluation, work assessment, trial work settings, work hardening, supervised and assisted work settings, and training for new employment skills. A sheltered workshop is a supervised and structured work setting used as either a short-term rehabilitation approach or a job placement, depending on the rehabilitation potential of the patient.

HOME-BASED REHABILITATION

Home-based rehabilitation programs are possible if there is full coordination of the therapeutic services involved; however, they are usually not the most cost-effective option. The patient lives and participates in the program at home. The patient does not have to be independent and can require up to 24-hour-a-day nursing care. Home-based programs are an especially therapeutic approach if the family feels strongly about the patient being at home and if inpatient and outpatient programs are not readily available. It is also a good alternative if the patient's nursing care needs preclude the patient from benefiting from a more aggressive inpatient rehabilitation setting or if a transportation problem interferes with outpatient rehabilitation.

A high level of family input and involvement are characteristic of home-based programs. However, these programs may lack adequate social and behavioral rehabilitation because of isolation from the patient's peer group. A combination of home-based and outpatient programs is an effective option, especially when an inpatient program would be inappropriate. Home-based rehabilitation often is not a cost-effective option and is not used as frequently as other alternatives. Often the payer may require that the patient be homebound and unable to participate in rehabilitation through any other alternative. Some families opt to pay privately for services at home.

With such a variety of rehabilitation settings, careful consideration is necessary to match the patient's needs to services and programs. Rehabilitation providers must clearly distinguish between the types of programs offered so that the most appropriate setting can be identified.

What factors really determine placement? In theory the patient's needs are matched to program goals. In reality the factors of local program availability and funding play major roles in decision making. Within the limitations of funding, discharge decisions are driven primarily by the patient's medical stability, types and intensity of services needed, functional ability, and social and psychologic considerations.

FOCUS OF REHABILITATION THROUGHOUT THE CYCLE

Rehabilitation is the motivation that moves the patient through the entire cycle, although it often is referred to as a specific period within the cycle. Maximized patient function is the common goal of all health care providers.[1,14]

As the patient proceeds through the cycle, the focus of rehabilitation shifts. After the initial crisis of injury, the patient is medically stabilized. At this early stage the severely injured patient depends on family and professionals to anticipate complications and plan for future progress. Later the patient takes on a much more active role in the rehabilitation team, eventually determining all individual goals.

No clear distinction or key event marks the patient's departure from one phase and entry into the next. Depending on the complexity of the injury, complications, and the psychosocial system into which the patient tries to reintegrate, movement through the cycle may be at varying paces and intensities. Patients may need to return to earlier phases in the cycle during the course of recovery. Most rehabilitation protocols are diagnosis specific.

CRITICAL CARE PHASE

Beginning at the injury scene through resuscitation and immediate stabilization, the rehabilitation goal during the critical care phase is to prevent further injury and secondary complications. Delay in treatment, unidentified injuries, and unintended injury caused by emergency procedures can impose additional impairment, resulting in a lengthened and complicated recovery. Decreased functional recovery may be a consequence of preventable complications during the critical phase.

Life-threatening injury is the greatest concern in an emergency setting; however, the long-term effects of non-life-threatening injury may be the most disabling to the patient. For example, in a patient with multisystem injuries, such as multiple fractures, a pneumothorax, and abdominal bleeding, a brachial plexopathy may be undiagnosed. When the other injuries are resolved, loss of motor function and chronic pain from the brachial plexopathy may persist and interfere with the patient's productive return to work and home life. A trauma patient with a cervical spinal cord injury has a 10% to 15% risk of having an associated undiagnosed mild brain injury. The residual cognitive impairment, including poor attention and memory, and the behavioral effects, such as altered judgment and apathy, could greatly interfere with the learning process required in spinal cord injury rehabilitation. The patient could be misdiagnosed as noncompliant or depressed when he or she actually is in need of specific head injury rehabilitative techniques.

The severity of injury must be considered in context. A minor injury may have severe consequences. This is not to say that stabilizing the most life-threatening injury is not the priority. Rather, it implies that the emergency practitioner needs to be aware of all the patient's injuries, the potential concurrent injuries associated with the patient's condition, and the possible lifelong consequences of all injuries. This awareness by emergency professionals can foster prevention of further injury and appropriate follow-up of all injuries.

Another rehabilitation goal during in the critical care phase is to establish a baseline assessment of the patient's adjustment to the injury. Coping is an individualized process that depends on the perspective of the patient and family. People respond to injury in terms of the perceived loss or potential loss of function. A construction worker may be more devastated by the loss of a limb than a computer data processor because a source of income is threatened. A teenage girl may be more concerned about a facial laceration than internal injuries. Generalizations cannot be made, but a perceptive emergency practitioner can anticipate these priorities. Those who have initial contact with the family or with the patient, if appropriate, should note the initial reaction to suspected diagnosis. Documentation of such responses provides valuable insights into patient and family values and the impact each injury potentially has on the patient. Early assessment of social history provides another indicator of the type of psychosocial and rehabilitative support the patient has and will need in the future. Even at this early critical phase, this information can become the basis for an individualized rehabilitation plan.

INTERMEDIATE PHASE

The intermediate phase of rehabilitation includes the period of medical stabilization, which may occur in critical care, intensive care, progressive care, and other medical-surgical care units. During this period the focus is on acute treatment of injuries, including: surgery, multiple procedures, medications, and other complex care. Even though most emphasis is placed on medically treating the patient, the necessary rehabilitation focus for this phase is the prevention of complications. The critical care nurse should blend technical treatment expertise with application of such rehabilitation fundamentals as positioning for proper body alignment, providing psychosocial support and patient education, and minimizing the complications of immobility.[35,36]

Prevention of physical complications can avert interruption or delay of progress toward functional recovery, and it also can prevent additional cost for care of the patient.[37] Although it is only one of many complications, decreased mobility is common in severely traumatized patients. All body systems are at risk for complications from immobility (Table 10-2).[38-40] Specific nursing measures for minimizing the immobility include positioning to prevent pressure sores and contractures and ensuring proper nutrition for healing and prevention of skin breakdown.

Regardless of how complex the trauma, the nurse initiates mobilization techniques and compensatory strategies to prevent complications. The trauma nurse benefits from a thorough understanding of normal body mobilization and physiology of body systems. Many prevention techniques are based on approximating normal body function. For example, many new surgical treatments for serious fractures promote early weight bearing and ambulation. The trend is to eliminate the need for unnecessary immobilization and to promote a normalization of activity even through the intermediate phase of trauma.

In addition to physical complications, immobility has a number of psychosocial effects. Sensory deprivation, loss of control, and changes in body image and self-esteem are all related problems of the immobilized patient. An acute reaction could alter the patient's ability to adapt and to recover from the injury.

Support from the trauma nurse as a caregiver prevents or reduces psychologic overreactions of the patient. The nurse can use empathy and receptive listening to allow the patient to ventilate stress. Supporting communication and visitation by family and significant others helps to prevent social isolation. Encouragement of independence in daily activities, care-related decision making, and making choices

TABLE 10-2	Physical Complications Related to Immobility Commonly Seen in Trauma Patients		
Body System	**Complications**	**Pathophysiology**	**Prevention**
Neurologic	Potentially affects all body systems	Caused by decreased level of consciousness; injury to cortex, motor, or sensory systems	• Neurologic assessment • Specific focus on the effects seen in other body systems • Understand neurologic basis of complication
Respiratory	Fatigue, decreased productivity; infection, pneumonia, respiratory acidosis	Decreased respiratory movement, unable to mobilize secretions, alterations in blood gases	• Assessment of respiratory status and changes in level of consciousness • Mobilization of secretions by turning, coughing, and deep breathing; postural drainage, percussion, vibration, early ambulation, humidification
Cardiovascular	Orthostatic hypotension, fatigue, increased cardiac workload, thrombosis, embolus	Increased heart rate, cardiac output, stroke volume in supine position; loss of supporting muscle tone resulting in venous stasis; orthostatic neurovascular receptors cannot adjust to position changes; hypercoagulability and external pressure to vessels	• Cardiovascular assessment • Encourage mobilization, exercise, range of motion, positioning • Antiembolic stockings • Provide adequate hydration • Avoid Valsalva maneuver
Gastrointestinal	Anorexia, fatigue, malnutrition, constipation, impaction, bowel obstruction, diarrhea, dehydration	Negative nitrogen balance and protein deficiency; stress; decreased appetite creates bowel intolerance; muscle weakness; diminished ability to apply abdominal pressure needed for evacuation; psychologic factors and position for defecation may increase difficulty	• Assessment of GI functioning, including baseline history of nutrition, exercise, and bowel habits • Coordinate bowel plan with nutrition specialist • Adequate hydration • Positioning and privacy • Gastrocolic reflex timing factors, use of digital stimulation • Stool softeners, and suppositories for stimulation • Adjust tube feedings to avoid constipation or diarrhea • Small, frequent feedings to increase tolerance and decrease anorexia • Encourage intake of protein, fluids, bulk foods
Urinary	Urinary reflux, incontinence, urinary stasis, renal calculi, urinary tract infection	Loss of effect of gravity, urinary stasis in renal pelvis; increased calculi formation from urine sediment in renal pelvis; diminished coordination of sphincters and muscles in supine position; bladder distention, overflow incontinence	• Assess urinary tract function • Promote movement and exercise • Maintain fluid intake • Decrease calcium intake • Monitor distention and voiding patterns • Prevent incontinence • Use upright or sitting position for voiding if possible • Intermittent catheters preferred to indwelling
Musculoskeletal	Muscle atrophy, contractures	Muscles shorten and atrophy; loss of ROM as supporting ligaments, tendons, and capsule lose mobility; ROM becomes permanent; spasticity of antagonistic muscle with weakness of opposing muscle creates contracture	• Ongoing assessment • Passive, active, and active-assisted ROM exercises • Appropriate positioning and body alignment in both bed and chair

Continued

TABLE 10-2   Physical Complications Related to Immobility Commonly Seen in Trauma Patients—cont'd

Body System	Complications	Pathophysiology	Prevention
Musculoskeletal—cont'd	Osteoporosis, stress fractures, heterotrophic ossification	Normal bone-building activities are dependent on weight bearing and movement; increased destruction of bone, release of calcium; bone becomes porous and fragile; abnormal calcification over large joints may also occur	• Calcium supplement to diet is not recommended • Promote weight bearing
Integumentary	Skin breakdown; stage I to IV skin ulcers; secondary infection of skin ulcers, sepsis	Prolonged pressure to skin diminishes capillary blood supply and stops flow of nutrients to cells; necrosis of cells results in skin breakdown, allowing infection to enter body	• Assessment of skin integrity, nutritional status, and risk factors for breakdown • Reposition; shift pressure and patient weight frequently; "every 2 hours" rule may not be adequate • Check for changes in blanching, sustained redness • Keep off all red areas • Massage at-risk areas to promote circulation • Teach patient to inspect own skin and shift weight • Increase protein in diet • Take immediate, consistent action on any areas of breakdown

whenever possible promotes improved feelings of self-determination, self-esteem, and self-worth, which increase the patient's motivation to progress toward recovery. The trauma nurse should apply principles of adaptive and maladaptive coping and the process of grieving loss into the assessment of the patient's psychosocial status.[41] This same supportive role is required from the nurse by the patient's family.[42]

Patient and family education begins in the intermediate phase. The nurse, a readily accessible member of the trauma team, may be overwhelmed with questions from the patient and family. An understanding of their readiness to learn helps the nurse recognize the purpose behind these questions. In the early phases of trauma care, many families and patients are not ready to learn fully about the injuries and the consequences. They are more specifically searching for comfort and support. This is evidenced in the case of a family that asserts several weeks later that "no one ever told me this" in regard to information that was shared weeks earlier in response to questions. When the families and patients are under stress, they are not able to use their maximal learning potential.

Readiness for learning includes the right environment and motivation for learning and the ability to retain the presented material. When a family asks a question to find support and comfort, the technical answer often is lost, whereas the feeling of comfort is retained. With this in mind, the trauma nurse prepares to teach, repeat, and review

important information to validate that learning has taken place. The trauma nurse can be a key resource to the patient and family to prepare them for the cycle of care ahead and the prospective outcomes associated with the patient's type of injury.[36]

Rehabilitation specialists are introduced to the patient's treatment team early in the intermediate phase.[43] The decision of which rehabilitation specialties should be active on the care team depends on the diagnosis and effects of injury. During the intermediate phase, the trauma nurse coordinates closely with the clinical specialties working with an individual patient and makes appropriate recommendations to the physician for rehabilitation referrals.

Physical, occupational, and respiratory therapists are among the first rehabilitation specialists to evaluate and treat the patient. Largely focused on physical aspects of disability, they may begin treatment as early as in the critical care unit. Until the patient is medically stable enough to be seen in the therapy department or treatment area, they provide bedside interventions.

Physical therapists encourage mobility and prevent contracture of the patient through range-of-motion exercises, positioning techniques, and active exercise programs. Results of musculoskeletal evaluation suggest specific needs for movement and positioning in daily care. Physical therapists may also begin early transfer to a chair and weight-bearing activity.

Respiratory therapists or, in some instances, physical

therapists work on mobilization of respiratory secretions by percussion, vibration, and postural drainage. Physiologic monitoring of respiratory status through blood gas analysis, pulse oximetry monitoring, and pulmonary function testing provides measures of treatment benefit and need for further treatment.

Assessment of the performance of activities of daily living by the occupational therapist can begin while the patient is still bedridden. In addition to establishing functional goals, it promotes improved self-esteem and a sense of control within the patient. For those who are severely neurologically impaired, the occupational therapist may focus on maintaining upper-extremity position and mobility, which will allow functional use of limbs or muscle groups. Splinting of the extremities may be used for therapeutic positioning. The occupational therapist may also suggest specific adaptive equipment and techniques to be implemented by the nursing staff.

A speech pathologist is an appropriate early rehabilitation referral for trauma patients with brain injury, high cervical spinal cord injury, and facial injury. Any patient with an artificial airway, such as a tracheal or endotracheal tube, may also benefit from a speech or communication specialist. A speech pathologist can offer various techniques to promote stimulation from coma, cognitive rehabilitation, communication through alternative methods and devices, and improvement of perceptual deficits.

Dysphagia is a specific area of disability that may need to be evaluated and treated in the intermediate phase because the patient becomes ready for oral intake. The speech pathologist may use video fluoroscopy to assess the exact nature of a swallowing problem. Treatment of swallowing disorders often includes consultation by a speech pathologist, an occupational therapist, a rehabilitation nurse, and a respiratory therapist.

An early referral to a physiatrist, a physician specialized in rehabilitation medicine, expedites the implementation of rehabilitation care during the intermediate phase. In some settings a rehabilitation clinical nurse specialist or nurse practitioner can begin to plan and implement the rehabilitation process. Early assessment by rehabilitation specialists permits a projection of rehabilitation potential and an active plan for maximal recovery.

Rehabilitation may be a new concept for the patient and family. They may not realize that acute medical stabilization is just the beginning of recovery. Preparation for transfer to a rehabilitation program includes education about potential patient functional goals, identification and selection of appropriate programs, and support during the upheaval of the transfer process.

Transfer from the atmosphere of the intensive care unit, where the patient is given total care, to a rehabilitation unit that fosters independence can be a shock to the patient and family. There comes a point in the patient's acute hospital stay when the emphasis of care should begin to change, and the patient should be encouraged to be independent. Implementing strategies to promote independence as early as possible better prepares the patient for the process of rehabilitation.

REHABILITATION PHASE

A great deal of rehabilitation effort and expertise is necessary during the rehabilitation phase, especially for severely injured patients. However, this phase is only one facet of the continuing rehabilitation that occurs throughout the trauma cycle. If rehabilitation were ignored in the other phases, functional outcomes would be severely decreased.

Most rehabilitation occurs in an inpatient setting, such as a rehabilitation unit of an acute care hospital or a freestanding rehabilitation facility. Depending on the type and severity of the disability, the frequency and type of medical monitoring, family support systems, and patient motivation, an outpatient or home-based rehabilitation program could be appropriate if a comprehensive team approach is provided.

Key themes throughout the rehabilitation phase are restoration, compensation, and adaptation. The rehabilitation team evaluates each individual case for (1) the ability to recover normal function, (2) appropriate areas to replace normal function with other strategies (compensation), and (3) areas in which the patient must change his or her lifestyle, roles, and expectations to adapt to disability. This evaluation results in a rehabilitation plan, with setting of both long-term and short-term goals. Depending on the patient's progress, these goals may need periodic adjustment.

Active rehabilitation includes learning new skills, practicing them, and testing skills in the environment. This is why the rehabilitative process takes weeks to months to complete. Some patients may be in and out of rehabilitation programs for years, learning and further improving skills with each admission. Few people have the capacity for learning all that is necessary to adapt to injury at one time. Many goals spill over into the reintegration phase. Progress with each short-term goal may vary.

As medical stability and functional independence increase, the patient asserts his or her rights for self-determination. This issue is extremely frustrating at times to the trauma team, whose values may conflict with those of the patient they have worked so hard to help.

For example, a patient who had sustained a C4-5 injury with resulting quadriplegia was transferred to a rehabilitation hospital from an acute care setting. The acute care staff had made every effort to maintain function of all body systems. Specifically, the patient's upper extremity range of motion was outstanding. About 8 weeks after transfer the rehabilitation hospital provided the acute trauma nurses with a progress report on the patient. He was taking notably more control of his life and responsibility for his own actions. But the presence of upper-extremity contractures was a shock to the acute care staff. At first the acute care staff blamed the rehabilitation staff for neglect. Later they began to understand that this severely injured young man chose to maintain only enough range of motion to scratch his nose for comfort. He did not share the rehabilitation team's goal of self-feeding. His goal was control of his comfort and reserving his energy for activities other than self-feeding.[44]

The patient's values guide the course of rehabilitation. The challenge is understanding when a traumatized patient is ready to be released from the sick role and considered competent and sufficiently informed to make self-determining judgments. The trauma rehabilitation nurse strives to provide as many options as possible for maximized function, but the injured person makes the ultimate decision.

REINTEGRATION PHASE

Community reintegration strategies usually begin during the rehabilitation phase. One strategy is the use of a therapeutic leave of absence from an inpatient setting, which allows the patient and family to test the adapted function in the real world. This strategy is also used in modified reintegration settings that blend home care and outpatient programs. Of all areas in trauma rehabilitation, the reintegration process is the most limited in alternatives because of limited reimbursement avenues.

Reintegration is the process of applying therapeutic adaptation and compensation to the patient's premorbid lifestyle. A difficult question facing rehabilitation specialists is, When does rehabilitation end and lifelong health management begin? Trauma patients stay in the health care system for extended periods. Functional gains are achieved even years after injury. Rehabilitation programs strive for maximized patient potential. Who determines when a patient has reached his or her potential?

One of the most difficult barriers in rehabilitation is that the services provided are limited by what services are funded. Many patients are kept in the rehabilitation system for extended periods. This has both a positive and a negative effect. Positively, some continue to achieve goals at a slower pace, therefore reaching a higher outcome. Others remain in the rehabilitation system for a lifetime without making appreciable gains. Not enough lifelong care options exist because most health care insurance does not cover lifelong care. The patient often remains in the rehabilitation system unnecessarily or receives no services because there are no alternative settings or funding. If the patient receives ongoing care in a setting that lacks appropriate resources, much of the costly and difficult rehabilitation outcome may never be achieved.

In order for the trauma cycle to have a truly positive outcome, society needs to put the following pieces into place: (1) awareness and acceptance of the rehabilitated trauma patient in society, (2) provision of a complex variety of services that meet the specific reintegration needs of the trauma patient, and (3) financial support for the most appropriate alternatives at each phase of rehabilitation. It is only with these supported systems that each person who experiences injury can realize quality of life.

ISSUES IN TRAUMA REHABILITATION

FUNDING FOR REHABILITATION

The most challenging issue after trauma is the lack of funding for patients needing rehabilitation programs and services. The prospect of paying out of pocket for rehabilitation is extremely lofty for the average person. Because of inadequate private funding and limited federal and state reimbursement systems, many trauma patients never receive the rehabilitation that is appropriate for their disability. This is particularly true of rehabilitation during the reintegration phase of the cycle. Emergency and life-saving services are provided to many people who are not able to return to a fully functional role in society.

Private insurance sometimes provides benefits for rehabilitation but predominantly for physical therapy only. Rehabilitation services in an acute care hospital or rehabilitation hospital may be funded, but not such services provided in the home, as long-term rehabilitation, or in transitional living environments. The available coverage often does not provide for what could be the most appropriate and cost-effective program for the patient. Often the insurance benefits are exhausted and the patient and family are bankrupted early in the rehabilitative care of a catastrophic injury. The burden of ongoing care often falls back on state medical assistance programs, which have also seen steady cost-cutting measures in recent years.

Experts in the field of rehabilitation continue to provide data to third-party payers to increase funds available for care of the injured. Insurers are using the expertise of rehabilitation nurses as case managers to enhance the cost-effectiveness and appropriateness of rehabilitation admissions. An administrative waiver, in which a third-party payer agrees to a cost-effective plan of care not specifically covered by the patient's policy, is an alternative that can sometimes be negotiated on a case-by-case basis. Health care consumers continue to pressure the managed care industry for expanded benefits.

Until recently, federal and state funds for rehabilitation have been provided as reimbursement to providers based on a formula that projected the costs of care. This methodology left little financial incentive for facilities to care for the catastrophically injured. As a result, many rehabilitation programs have limited their admission of government-funded patients. This issue is particularly true of government funding for the nontraditional rehabilitation alternatives and for programs that support the patient's late-stage rehabilitation and reintegration. It is a vicious cycle that forces the increased use of less appropriate and costlier rehabilitation options, especially in the later stages of the cycle.

With the implementation of the Balanced Budget Act of 1997, HCFA replaced cost-based reimbursement with a prospective payment system (PPS) for rehabilitation hospitals, skilled nursing facilities, and community-based settings.[5] PPS manages cost by using a national standard for payment for similar services, adjusted by clinical need and geographic costs. Based on rate implementation to date, overall the reimbursement is lower than received in the cost-based system. Phase-in of PPS rates began for skilled nursing facilities in July 1998. At the time of this writing, rehabilitation hospitals are scheduled to begin prospective payment on October 1, 2000.

Over the past decade, some alternative rates for catastrophically injured people have been negotiated with some federal and state funding sources, based on cost-benefit analysis and projected overall savings in the cost of care. This practice is likely to decrease with the implementation of the PPS.

Managed care administration of medical assistance funds has occurred for various populations in most states. Implementation of state-funded managed care related to rehabilitation and long-term care remains in its infancy. It is unclear at this time how state funding for rehabilitation and catastrophic care will be funded under a managed care design.

Every avenue of rehabilitation funding is under pressure to reduce costs. Over the next 5 to 10 years we are likely to see the environment for rehabilitation greatly affected by managed care. The resulting reimbursement systems will determine which service alternatives will survive. In addition, we are likely to see significant reduction in the amount of rehabilitation services delivered per case. However, expectation for successful outcomes will remain high. There will be a great deal of pressure on the field of rehabilitation to reinvent itself to some degree if it is to remain financially viable.

ACCEPTANCE OF THE TRAUMA-DISABLED PERSON IN SOCIETY

Public awareness of trauma and its long-term consequences is slow to change, considering it is the leading cause of death and disability for young adults.[45] Long-term disability in such a young population leads to an ever-increasing percentage of people whose lives have been altered by trauma. The media have helped to enlighten society about physical disability. Disabled parking, curb ramps, and other accessibility-related standards, such as those defined in the Americans with Disabilities Act of 1990, are accepted and expected in daily life.[46] Adaptations in the workplace are becoming more visible. Disabled persons are depicted as role models in sports, business, and other areas of success. Society's acceptance of the physically disabled person is becoming a reality.

Unfortunately, not much progress has been made regarding awareness of the cognitive and psychosocial ramifications of injury. Cognitive and behavioral disabilities caused by head injury and injury-related psychologic trauma are poorly understood by the public. People who do not comprehend the nature of the problem and the needs of the cognitively and behaviorally disabled become anxious and reject them. There is an attempt to label people with behavior problems as mentally retarded, crazy, or rude. Mental illness has a long history of poor acceptance in society. As the mentally disabled population grows, more people will have contact with these individuals in work, home, and community settings. Efforts at public education and sensitization enhance the true reintegration of intellectually and behaviorally disabled people. This process is necessary for trauma-disabled people to return to a contributing role in society. However, it is unrealistic to think that all catastrophically injured people will return to the community, whether because of limited function or societal resistance.

TRAUMA PREVENTION

Issues related to rehabilitation would not exist if the initial trauma were prevented. Both media exposure and legislation by advocacy groups, such as Mothers Against Drunk Driving (MADD), have created nationwide support for the prevention of trauma.[47] The greatest focus has been placed on prevention of traffic accidents and drug- and alcohol-related trauma. Recent changes in child car seat safety, seat belt, and air bag legislation reflect a growing consciousness of prevention.[48] The debate over drug, alcohol, and handgun laws represents attempts to prevent traumatic injuries.

Trauma prevention is an educational process. As with any preventable problem, it is not that society does not want to prevent the trauma, but rather that it increasingly recognizes situations with a potential for injury. As awareness of trauma increases, so will legitimate public support for those actions that can prevent the injuries from occurring.

It is the responsibility of all health care professionals to support education through individual, family, and community teaching; media exposure; community interest groups; churches; schools; and other settings in the community. The public also expects health care professionals to act as role models of healthier and safer living.

Total prevention of traumatic injury is a worthy challenge to professionals and our society. It is a reasonable goal for society to work toward reduced incidence and severity of injury and disability in the immediate future.

SUMMARY

ROLE OF THE TRAUMA REHABILITATION NURSE

Rehabilitation of the trauma patient presents many exciting and expanding opportunities for nurses. New roles for rehabilitation experts benefit from nursing's holistic approach to the physical, cognitive, and psychosocial components of rehabilitation programming. Rehabilitation liaison and discharge planning roles in trauma centers effectively link the intermediate and rehabilitation phases of care.[1] Clinical nurse specialists and nurse practitioners support early initiation of rehabilitation techniques by awareness of the benefits of rehabilitation. In the rehabilitation and reintegration phases, nurses also contribute through their roles as rehabilitation coordinators and case managers.[18,49,50]

In addition to clinical practice, many nurses have blended rehabilitation specialization with administration, public relations, business, and research to provide a wealth of expertise and skill to health-related companies and insurers. Nurses are also effective in program development, management, marketing, and consulting roles.

Regardless of the trauma rehabilitation nurse's specific function, it is essential that all members of the profession involve themselves in the issues that rehabilitation will face in the future. Active participation in professional and disability-related organizations such as the Association of Rehabilitation Nurses, the American Congress of Rehabilitation Medicine, the American Association of Spinal Cord Injury Nurses, the Case Management Society of America, the National Association of Rehabilitation Professionals in the Private Sector, the American Spinal Cord Injury Association, and the Brain Injury Association and their local networks offers an opportunity for nurses to work creatively and constructively toward improved legislation and guidelines for practice, community awareness, and community support for the disabled population. Involvement in rehabilitation issues may occur on an individual basis or through activities by the employing facility or organization. Nurses in clinical practice with direct interaction with patients and families have the vital role of educating those most directly affected about rehabilitation issues. Through this comprehensive effort, issues can be resolved.

A wealth of personal and professional growth is available to nurses in trauma rehabilitation. The specialty continues to work through its new stages of development and welcomes creative ideas and expertise. For the person who longs to create an advanced practice role in nursing, trauma rehabilitation may offer this opportunity.

FUTURE RESEARCH

A great deal of research still needs to be conducted on the phases of rehabilitation after traumatic injury. Trauma rehabilitation has borrowed therapeutic approaches from many other specialties, including stroke and neurologic disease rehabilitation, psychiatry, normal and abnormal child development studies, and mental retardation. The areas in which clinical research can be conducted over the next decade are unlimited. The National Institute on Disability and Rehabilitation Research (NIDRR) funds research for eight key areas of impact.[51] These research areas include: emphasis on health and function of the disabled, application of technology, community reintegration and employment, and public education. Advocates for the injured are lobbying for a significant increase in federal funds for clinical research.

The cost-effectiveness of rehabilitation poses both ethical and pragmatic concerns. As of 1996 the estimated annual total cost to the nation for unintentional injuries alone was more than $444 billion.[52] Analysis by the House Subcommittee on Small Business, including private rehabilitation facilities, cited lifetime care costs for a severely brain-injured person to be more than $4 million.[53] Does society have the funds to rehabilitate everyone? The cost could be reduced by careful scrutiny of rehabilitation services provided on a case-by-case basis, or the funds might be made available only to those injured people who meet specified criteria and have the greatest potential outcome. How would society decide who has the greatest potential outcome?[54]

It is the responsibility of every rehabilitation practitioner and facility to closely examine and study the cost-effectiveness and benefits of treatments and practices. Many health care professionals assume that more care is better care. Future research could be directed toward identifying minimal standards that still result in high-quality outcomes. Over the next 5 years, federally mandated clinical outcome tools will provide a base of information across rehabilitation settings, perhaps initiating research and practice guidelines for the best alternatives in rehabilitation. Other studies may consider how often a specific treatment is needed. For example, what level of staff member is most cost effective for each aspect of clinical care? By creating practice based on innovation and recent clinical research, professionals in the specialty may be able to contain the skyrocketing costs of rehabilitation.[55]

Because outcome measurement for trauma rehabilitation is still developing, adequate data are not yet available to evaluate the long-term and lifelong needs of the traumatized population. Studies of the effects of aging and lifestyle on people who have experienced a catastrophic illness will also help the rehabilitation profession provide appropriate education, adaptation, and follow-up for lifelong support.

Clinical research toward heightened potential for recovery is a most exciting prospect.[48,52] Physiologic studies of central nervous system tissue support the theory that nerve cells are able to regenerate. Electrical stimulation of muscle groups supports the use of previously ineffective limbs. The potential for improved recovery is positive. To this end, the field of trauma rehabilitation and its patient population benefit from the research, education, expert clinical practice, and leadership of professional rehabilitation nurses.

REFERENCES

1. Association of Rehabilitation Nurses: *Role of the rehabilitation nurse in the trauma care system,* Glenview, Ill, 1991, The Association.
2. Brillhart B, Johnson K: Motivation and the coping process of adults with disabilities: a qualitative study, *Rehabil Nurs* 22:249-252, 255-256, 1997.
3. Krause JS: Prediction of long-term survival of persons with SCI: an 11 year prospective study. In Eisenberg MG, Glueckauf RL, editors: *Empirical approaches to psychosocial aspects of disability,* New York, 1991, Springer.
4. Stryker R: *Rehabilitation aspects of acute and chronic nursing care,* ed 2, Philadelphia, 1972, WB Saunders, 5-11.
5. Majority Staffs, House and Senate Committees on the Budget, U.S. Congress: *The Balanced Budget Act of 1997,* HR 2015, Washington, D.C., July 29, 1997, U.S. Government Printing Office.
6. Duchene PA: The Balanced Budget Act of 1997: Implications for rehabilitation nurses in skilled nursing facilities, *Rehabil Nurs* 23:210-211, 1998.

7. Hartmann J: The Balanced Budget Act of 1997: How the prospective payment system affects providers of rehabilitation services, *Rehabil Nurs* 23:263-264, 1998.

8. Lellis M: Industry study proves RUGs-III does not account for needs of subacute patients, *National Report on Subacute Care* 7:14, 5-9, July 14, 1999.

9. American Hospital Association: *The Balanced Budget Act and hospitals: the dollar and cents of Medicaid payment cuts,* www.aha.org/bba/LewinTOC.html, accessed May 10, 1999.

10. Commission on Accreditation of Rehabilitation Facilities: *Standards manuals and interpretive guidelines for medical rehabilitation,* Tucson, 1999, The Commission.

11. Krueger DW: Psychological rehabilitation of physical trauma and disability. In Krueger D, editor: *Rehabilitation psychology,* Rockville, Md, 1984, Aspen, 6-8.

12. Cobble N, Bontke C, Brandstater M et al: Rehabilitation of brain disorders: intervention strategies, *Arch Phys Med Rehabil* 4 (Suppl):324-331, 1991.

13. White MJ, Holloway M: Patient concerns after discharge from rehabilitation, *Rehabil Nurs* 6:316-318, 1990.

14. Dean-Baar S, editor: The purpose and function of the rehabilitation team. In Mumma CM, editor: *Rehabilitation nursing: concepts in practice, a core curriculum,* ed 2, Evanston, Ill, 1987, Rehabilitation Nursing Foundation, 345-372.

15. Lyth JR: Models of the team approach. In Fletcher GF, Banja JD, Jann BB et al, editors: *Rehabilitation medicine: contemporary clinical perspectives,* Philadelphia, 1992, Lea & Febiger, 225-242.

16. Byrne ML, Thompson LF: *Key concepts for the study and practice of nursing,* ed 2, St. Louis, 1978, Mosby, 103-126.

17. Wiener SM: Rehabilitation nursing in the private sector, *Rehabil Nurs* 8:31-32, 1983.

18. Heffner R: *The rehabilitation nurse's survival guide: a complete clinical quick reference guide,* El Paso, Tex, 1995, Skidmore-Roth.

19. Jaffe K: Facility-based case managers: the evolution continues, *Case Manager* 2(2):39-42, April 1991.

20. Rondinelli RD, Murphy JR, Wilson DH et al: Predictors of functional outcome and resource utilization in inpatient rehabilitation, *Arch Phys Med Rehabil* 72(7):447-453, 1991.

21. Dries DJ, Gamelli RL: Issues in geriatric trauma. In Dries DJ, Gamelli RL, editors: *Trauma 2000: strategies of the new millennium,* Austin, Tex, 1992, RG Landers.

22. Lambert J: Meeting the emotional needs of a patient, *Rehabil Nurs* 24(4):141-142, 1999.

23. McKinley WO, Kolakowsky SA, Kreutzer JS: Substance abuse, violence and outcome after traumatic spinal cord injury, *Am J Phys Med Rehabil* 78(4):306-312, 1999.

24. Faraci P, Leiter P, Weeks DK: Trends in lengths of stay, charges, and functional outcomes: implications for the rehabilitation industry, *J Rehabil Admin* 20(2):1996.

25. The Joint Commission on Accreditation of Healthcare Organizations: *ORYX,* www.jcaho.org/perfmeas_frm.html, accessed Aug 31, 1999.

26. Uniform Data System for Medical Rehabilitation (UDSMR): www.udsmr.org/, accessed Aug 31, 1999.

27. Health Care Financing Administration: *Minimum data set for post acute care (MDS-PAC),* www.hcfa.gov/medicare/hsqb/mds20/pacde.htm, accessed Aug 31, 1999.

28. Young M: An interview with Carl Granger MD, *Rehab Continuum Report,* July 13, 1999.

29. Masso AR: *Trends in managed care,* Medical Case Management Conference III, Individual Case Management Association, Dallas, Tex, July 18, 1991.

30. Friswell RJ, Radice J, Katz A: Rehabilitation: facilities target service to a changing market, *Provider* 16(11):8-13, 15, November 1990.

31. Murray PK, Singer ME, Fortinsky R et al: Rapid growth of rehabilitation services in traditional community-based nursing homes, *Arch Phys Med Rehabil* 80(4):372-378, 1999.

32. Joint Commission on Accreditation of Healthcare Organizations: *Standards for long-term care, subacute care programs, and dementia special care units,* Chicago, 1998, The Commission.

33. Jones M, Evans RW: Rating outcomes in post-acute rehabilitation of acquired brain injury, *Case Manager* 2(1):44-47, January 1991.

34. Commission on Accreditation of Rehabilitation Facilities: *Standards manuals and interpretive guidelines for outpatient medical rehabilitation programs,* Tucson, 1999, The Commission.

35. Sherburne E: A rehabilitation protocol for the neuroscience intensive care unit, *J Neurosci Nurs* 18(3):140-145, 1986.

36. Deering-Stuck B, Brunner Summey L: Rehabilitation of trauma patients. In Cardona VD: *Trauma nursing,* Oradell, NJ, 1985, Medical Economics Books, 221-231.

37. Deutsch PM, Sawyer HW, editors: *A guide to rehabilitation,* New York, 1986, Matthew Bender, Chapters 7 and 13.

38. Benda S, editor: Nursing diagnosis. In Mumma CM, editor: *Rehabilitation nursing: concepts in practice, a core curriculum,* ed 2, Evanston, Ill, 1987, Rehabilitation Nursing Foundation, 149-344.

39. Moore KA, Vassar TM: Mobility and rest in adults: new perspectives on old problems. In Funk SG, Tornquist EM, Champagne MT et al, editors: *Key aspects of recovery: improving nutrition, rest and mobility,* New York, 1990, Springer, 291-296.

40. Vallbona C: Bodily responses to immobilization. In Kotte EJ, Stillwell GK, Lehman JF, editors: *Krusen's handbook of physical medicine and rehabilitation,* Philadelphia, 1982, WB Saunders, 963-976.

41. Campion L: The nurse's role in the management of emotional problems. In Krueger D, editor: *Rehabilitation psychology,* Rockville, Md, 1984, Aspen, 213-220.

42. Care and support of the family. In Blumenfield M, Schoeps MM: *Psychological care of the burn and trauma patient,* Baltimore, 1993, Williams & Wilkins.

43. Boughton A, Ciesla N: Physical therapy management of the head injured patient in the intensive care unit, *Top Acute Care Trauma Rehabil* 1:1-18, 1986.

44. Ridley B: Tom's story: a quadriplegic who refused rehabilitation, *Rehabil Nurs* 14(5):250-253, 1989.

45. Peters KD, Kochanek KD, Murphy SL: Deaths and death rates for the 10 leading causes of death in specified age groups, by race and sex: U.S., 1996, *Natl Vital Stat Rep* 47:9, 1998.

46. Public Law 101-336, 101st Cong, July 26, 1990, *The Americans with Disabilities Act of 1990.*

47. Mothers Against Drunk Driving (MADD): www.madd.org, accessed Aug 31, 1999.

48. Perrin J, Wilkins J: Traumatic brain injury. Physiatric pearls, *Phys Med Rehabil Clin N Am* 7:527-538, 1996.

49. American Nurses Association and the Association of Rehabilitation Nurses: *Rehabilitation nursing: scope of practice, process and outcome for selected diagnoses,* Kansas City, Mo, 1986, ANA.

50. Association of Rehabilitation Nursing: *Role description of case managers,* Glenview, Ill, 1990, The Association.

51. The National Institute on Disability and Rehabilitation Research (NIDRR): www.ncddr.org/urlist.html, accessed August 31, 1999.

52. Eachempati SR, Reed RL II, St. Louis JE et al: "The Demographics of Trauma in 1995" revisited: an assessment of the accuracy and utility of trauma predictions, *J Trauma* 45(2): 208-213, 1998.

53. Office of United States Congressional Representative Ron Wyden (D-OR): Memo of 2/1/92 to House Subcommittee on Small Business on "silent epidemic"—Brain injury rehabilitation costs, *Long-Term Care Manag* :1, February 27, 1992.

54. Wennberg JE: Outcomes research, cost containment and the fear of health care rationing, *N Engl J Med* 323(17):1202-1204, 1990.

55. Dittmar SS: Future directions in rehabilitation nursing. In Hoeman SP: *Rehabilitation nursing: process and application,* St. Louis, 1989, Mosby.

PART II

CLINICAL MANAGEMENT CONCEPTS

MECHANISM OF INJURY

11

John A. Weigelt • Jorie D. Klein

In *Webster's Third New International Dictionary*, *trauma* is defined as "an injury or wound to a living body caused by the application of external violence." Injury is a public health problem of vast proportions. It is the leading cause of death for persons below the age of 44 years and the fourth leading cause for all ages. For ages 1 to 34, motor vehicle crashes (MVCs) are the most common cause of death. Injuries sustained in motor vehicle crashes, work and occupational injuries, injuries at home, and non-motor vehicle public injuries accounted for 92,200 deaths in 1995, which is a rate of 35.4 deaths per 100,000 population.[1] Traumatic injuries lead to 3.6 million hospital admissions each year, with an average of 7 days per hospital stay.[2] More than 4 million potential years of productive life are lost annually as a result of trauma, exceeding the loss resulting from heart disease, cancer, and stroke combined. The annual cost to our nation from injuries is staggering. MVCs are responsible for 50% of the costs related to the treatment of and recovery from traumatic injuries.

Injury results from acute exposure to different types of energy such as kinetic (as conveyed by crashes, falls, and bullets), chemical, thermal, electrical, or ionizing radiation. Injury also results from a lack of essential agents such as oxygen (e.g., drowning) and heat (e.g., frostbite).[3] The injury occurs because of the body's inability to tolerate exposure to the excessive acute energy. Wounds vary depending on the injuring agent. For example, damage from a gunshot blast is dependent on the missile's mass and velocity; degree of burn varies with temperature and duration of contact; injuries from deceleration depend on the victim's body mass, rate of deceleration, and area over which the energy is dissipated. Effects of an injury are also dependent on personal and environmental factors such as age, sex, nutrition, underlying disease processes, and geographic region (rural versus urban). These factors help define populations at risk for various types and severities of injuries.

RISK FACTORS

Risks of injury from different causes vary by age, sex, race, income, and environment, including factors such as alcohol abuse, geographic region, and temporal varia-tion. Identification of characteristics of different populations and subgroups at risk for injury allows prevention measures to be focused on high-risk groups. One way of subdividing injury groups is according to intentional and unintentional events. For example, ingestion of a toxic substance can be intentional, as in a suicide attempt, or unintentional, as in an inadvertent ingestion. The mechanism of injury is the same, but the events leading to the injury differ.

AGE

Death rates from injuries are highest in patients 75 years of age or older.[4] A contributing factor to this high death rate in the elderly may be secondary to associated medical conditions. The in-hospital fatality rate for this group is 15% to 30% compared with 4% to 8% in younger patients.[5] The number of elderly patients admitted for treatment of injury continues to increase. In 1993 and 1994 patients older than 75 years of age accounted for 412 trauma admissions per 10,000 population.[4,6] In 1996, 13.4% of patients admitted for injury were older than the age of 75 years.[6]

The highest injury rate occurs in persons between the ages of 15 and 24 years[7] because of their participation in high-risk activities. Poor judgment with the use of alcohol and drugs also contributes to the high injury rate. The lowest injury rate is for children ages 5 to 14.[7] The highest homicide rate occurs among people between 20 and 29 years of age. Suicide rates for both sexes show little variation with age. The incidence of domestic violence is highest among women between the ages of 16 and 24 years.[8]

SEX

Injury rates are highest for 15- to 24-year-old males.[9] The mortality risk for males is 4.6 times that for females,[4] possibly because of male involvement in hazardous activities. The unintentional injury death rate for males peaks between the ages of 20 and 24 years and again in the elderly years; suicide has similar peaks. The rate of homicide peaks between 25 and 30 years of age. In females the death rate peaks at 15 to 19 years for unintentional injury and at 20 to 24 years for homicide. Women in their late 40s have the highest suicide rate. Nonfatal injury rates for men and women do not differ significantly, suggesting that injuries to males are more severe than those to females.

Domestic violence is more often directed against females than males. In 1996, 75% of the approximately 1800 homicides perpetrated by an intimate partner involved a female victim. An intimate partner is responsible for 28.5% of homicides in females 18 to 24 years of age compared with only 2.5% of male victims.[8]

RACE AND INCOME

Injury death rates vary according to race and socioeconomic level. In a depressed economy the suicide and homicide rates increase and the number of MVCs decrease. Native Americans (Indians, Eskimos, and Aleuts) have the highest death rate from unintentional injury regardless of income. African Americans have the highest homicide rate. Caucasians and Native Americans have the highest suicide rate. Asian Americans (Chinese, Japanese, Koreans, Hawaiians, Filipinos, Guamanians) have the lowest death rates from unintentional injuries, homicide, and suicide. The unintentional injury rate is higher in low-income areas (71 per 100,000 population) than in the wealthiest areas (34 per 100,000 population). An inverse relationship exists between income levels and death rates for African Americans and Caucasians; that is, the higher the income, the lower the death rate.[4] This relationship is maintained for domestic violence.[10] For Asian Americans there is essentially no difference in death rates among all income groups.

ALCOHOL

Alcohol not only contributes to injury-producing events such as MVCs but also can increase the severity of injury, such as by preventing escape from a burning house.[9] Alcohol is a major factor in motor vehicle, home, industrial, and recreational injuries and in crime, suicide, and family abuse.[11] Automobile crash fatalities are alcohol-related 63% of the time in persons between the ages of 21 and 34 years.[12] Reyna and associates[11] showed that for 16- to 30-year-olds, alcohol-related emergency department trauma visits were twice as common as for patients older than 30 years. The incidence of alcoholism in the general population is believed to be approximately 5% to 10%.[11] Recent evidence suggests that alcohol interventions in a trauma center may reduce the risk of injury recurrence.[13]

GEOGRAPHY

Geographic comparison of injury rates demonstrates the diversity in our population and exposure to hazards. This is reflected in the high unintentional injury rate in rural areas and high intentional injury rate in urban areas.[14] Rural unintentional injuries are commonly caused by MVCs, lightning strikes, and exposure to chemicals. Urban unintentional injuries are most commonly poisonings. Homicide is highest in cities; suicides are highest in cities with populations of 250,000 to 1 million. Clearly the physical environment has an important influence on injury rate.

Terrorism is a new threat in the United States, and geography is a factor in the terrorists' choice of attack.

Urban environments are often targeted because they offer the possibility for the greatest number of casualties or greatest political effect.[15]

TEMPORAL VARIATION

Deaths from injury occur most frequently on weekends, with a Saturday peak. Suicide rates show less variation: Monday is the peak time, with the fewest occurring Friday through Sunday. Unintentional injuries are temporally related to times of high recreational activity. Injuries associated with swimming and motorcycle use are most common in warm weather months, whereas injuries associated with skiing and snowmobile use are seen during cold weather months.

EFFECTS OF INJURY ON SOCIETY

A health problem can be examined by its cost to society, but this cost does not encompass the grief, pain, and social disruption experienced by an individual and family. Death before 70 years of age is premature.[4] By considering the years of life lost prematurely because of health problems, it can be calculated that 4 million years of life are lost prematurely as a result of injury each year. Even when intentional injuries (homicide, suicide) are excluded, 3 million years of life are lost, which is greater than the loss from any other single disease.

Indicators used to compare the impact of health problems are cost to society, physician contacts, and hospital admissions. Injuries remain one of the most expensive health problems; their total cost to society is not known. The total cost estimate for injury in 1996 was $260 billion.[4] The total cost just for motorcycle crash injuries in California in 1991 was $98 million.[16] These injuries were associated with a lost productivity of $603 million. Another analysis in 1995 placed the total cost of motor vehicle crashes and unintentional injury at $441 billion.[1] In 1994 lifetime medical costs as a result of gunshot wounds were estimated to be $2.3 billion.[17] Three fourths of these costs were attributed to gunshot wounds associated with assaults. A disabling injury to a younger individual has great indirect costs because the disabled youth will require more medical care over a prolonged period based on life expectancy. This cost is borne by society, often with no financial input to society from the disabled individual.

Injury ranks first as the reason for physician visits and contacts for treatment. In 1995 there were 2.5 million hospital discharges related to injury and 37 million emergency department visits. Heart disease was second and respiratory disease third.[9] More than 25% of all emergency department or hospital clinic visits are for treatment of injuries.[1] Injuries account for approximately 3.6 million hospital admissions yearly, which is 1 of every 10 short-term admissions. The number of admissions for injury among all age groups is higher than for all other diseases except circulatory and digestive disorders. The elderly have the highest hospitalization rate for injury; a major cause is hip fracture. Other injuries accounting for a high number of hospitalizations include head trauma in 15- to 24-year-olds and back and neck sprains in the 35- to 44-year-old group.

Initial Assessment and History

In the initial evaluation of the trauma patient, a careful history of the events leading to the injury must be obtained. The practitioner must attend to urgent therapeutic needs along with the usual diagnostic evaluation.[18] Obtaining an accurate history—especially asking about the mechanism of injury—can reduce morbidity and mortality.

Answers to questions about the circumstances of the impact are helpful when assessing potential injuries sustained in a motor vehicle-related crash (such as automobile, motorcycle, and pedestrian injuries). At the site of the incident, prehospital care personnel should quickly survey the scene, noting the appearance of the vehicle(s) involved and the damage sustained to the passenger compartment.[19] It is important to know the speed of the vehicle, the point of impact, and the type of impact (single-vehicle, high-speed, front-end, rear-end, or T-bone intersection collision). The evaluating team should determine whether the patient was the driver or the passenger, whether safety devices (safety belt, child safety seat, and airbag) were used, and where the victim was found at the scene. Death of an occupant in the vehicle should alert the team to potential energy forces within the collision. Patients from a vehicle in which an occupant has died and patients who are ejected from a vehicle have a higher morbidity and mortality and warrant a thorough evaluation for injury.

Frontal-impact collisions that cause the vehicle to have a bent steering wheel or column, knee imprints in the dashboard, or a broken windshield are associated with head injuries, hemopneumothoraces, injuries to the spleen or liver, and dislocation of the patella.[19] Femur fractures with or without posterior fracture-dislocation of the ipsilateral hip must be considered. Deceleration injuries such as aortic rupture must be ruled out.

Side-impact collisions produce contralateral neck sprains, cervical fractures, head injuries, lacerations to the soft tissues, lateral rib fractures or flail chest, abdominal injuries, and pelvic and acetabular fractures.

Rear-impact collisions result in hyperextension neck injuries, and there may be rebound frontal-impact injuries. Ejection from the vehicle produces a multitude of injuries, such as penetrating impalement wounds, head injuries, cervical fractures, and road burns. The risk of injury is increased by 300% when the occupant is ejected.

Motorcycle crashes produce single or multiple impacts. The evaluating team must determine the type of collision (direct impact with stable object or impact with another vehicle), rate of speed, where the victim was found in relation to the cycle, and if protective devices were worn (helmet, gloves, and boots). Head injuries, long-bone fractures, pelvic fractures, and soft tissue injuries are common.

Pedestrians hit by vehicles may have many injuries. The prehospital team should identify (or estimate) how fast the vehicle was traveling, the type of vehicle, the point of impact, and whether the victim was thrown or dragged. Waddell's triad occurs when a pedestrian is struck by a car.[20] When the victim is a child, injuries are caused by three events: (1) the bumper and hood impact the femur and/or chest, (2) the victim is thrown upon impact, and (3) the contralateral skull is injured by the force of impact. One of the resulting injuries is often missed in the initial evaluation. Adult pedestrians receive a lateral impact from contact with the bumper and hood, injuring the lower and upper leg, because adults try to protect themselves by turning sideways (Figure 11-1). Fractures to this area are recognized, but ligamental damage in the other knee is often overlooked.

Penetrating trauma refers to any injury produced when a foreign object passes through the tissue. Energy is dissipated through the tissue, producing the injury. Injuries from penetrating trauma are more predictable than those caused by blunt trauma. It is important to identify the type of weapon (caliber of gun, length of knife blade), stance of the assailant, distance from the assailant to victim, and potential number of wounds.

It is not always possible and sometimes is impractical to obtain a detailed history, but information can be obtained from family members, paramedics, firefighters, police officers, onlookers, or eyewitnesses. Priority is obviously given to managing life-threatening injuries such as those that cause inadequate ventilation, hypoxia, or bleeding. After the patient is resuscitated and stabilized, the trauma practitioner should begin a detailed review of the patient's history, physical findings, and laboratory results to direct further investigations.

A quick, thorough physical examination must be performed during or immediately after resuscitation. It is important to systematically examine the undressed patient to avoid overlooking injuries. Injuries are easier to detect in patients with penetrating trauma than in those with blunt injury, because surface injury may or may not be present with blunt injury. Failure to diagnose the patient's injuries correctly is associated with a high mortality rate.[21] An index of suspicion for associated injuries based on the mechanism of injury must be maintained.

Some body areas do not lend themselves easily to physical examination, such as the cranium, vertebral column, and bony thorax.[22] Injury may exist without classic signs, but the mechanism of injury may raise suspicion enough to warrant further diagnostic examinations. Examples include computed tomography (CT) for diagnosis of brain

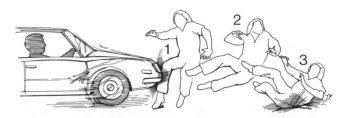

FIGURE 11-1 Waddell's triad in adult pedestrians. Impact (1) with the bumper or hood and lateral rotation (2) produces injury to the upper and/or lower leg (3).

injury, CT or angiography for blunt chest injury and possible aortic injury, and plain radiography for spinal column evaluation. All tests must be performed without placing the patient at risk of further injury. The patient is reexamined continually to identify changing physical findings.

Complete assessment of the trauma patient is aided by knowing the cause of injury. MVCs are the most common cause of injury, followed by falls.[21] Other causes of injury are pedestrian collision, drowning, fire, burn, explosion, poisoning, firearm, assault, aspiration, machinery, and sports activity. In some cases the cause can be related to patterns of injury, which indicate expected types of injury. For example, injury patterns include sports injuries after sudden deceleration (diving, falling), excessive forces (twisting, hyperextension, hyperflexion), or changes in momentum (boxing).[21] Because of repeated blows to the head in boxing, cumulative brain damage may occur, with resultant neurologic damage depending on the affected area. Spinal cord injuries can occur while participating in gymnastics or playing football. Head injuries can occur while playing football or while horseback riding. Skiing can produce fractures, and knee injuries are common with skiing and football. This information plus the events preceding the incident can provide clues to the practitioner regarding the patient's response, expected severity of injury, and possible occult or missed injuries. Common areas where injuries are missed include the extremities (hand and foot), upper extremities (forearm and upper arm), and skin (scalp lacerations).

MECHANISM OF INJURY

The mechanics of injury are related to the type of injuring force and subsequent tissue response. A thorough understanding of these two facets of injury helps in determining the extent and nature of damage. Injury occurs when the force deforms tissues beyond their failure limits. This can result in anatomic and physiologic damage. Anatomic damage, such as skeletal fractures, will usually heal, and function will return. Physiologic damage, such as central nervous system injury, may be permanent despite the healing process. The mechanism of injury can help explain the type of injury, predict eventual outcome, and identify common injury combinations. Knowledge of this information improves trauma patient management.

BIOMECHANICS

The principles of mechanics are used to investigate the mechanisms of physical and physiologic responses to force. The injuring force can be penetrating or nonpenetrating. The resultant injury depends on the energy delivered and area of contact. Penetrating injury usually involves a concentration of injury to a small body area; nonpenetrating injury distributes energy over larger areas. Injury can occur by slow deformation of tissue, such as in a wringer injury[23]; however, the predominant feature is usually speed and violence, such as the impact of the head against a windshield or a bullet's penetration into an extremity.

The field of biomechanics involves a variety of disciplines, including engineering, physiology, medicine, biology, and anatomy. Knowledge of injury mechanisms allows the appropriate biomechanical measurements to be made to characterize injuries. Many approaches are used in this field of inquiry, and research is best conducted with representatives of as many of the disciplines as possible. Detailed reviews from various aspects of basic biomechanical research are available but are beyond the scope of this chapter.

INJURY CONCEPTS

Among the factors that influence injury are velocity of collision, object shape, and tissue rigidity. Body tissue has inertial resistance as well as tensile, elastic, and compressive strength. *Tensile strength* equals the amount of tension a tissue can withstand and its ability to resist stretching forces. *Elasticity* is the ability of a tissue to resume its original shape and size after being stretched. *Compressive strength* refers to the tissue's ability to resist squeezing forces or inward pressure. Whenever the force exceeds maximum tissue strength, a fracture or tear occurs.[24]

Force is a physical factor that changes the motion of a body either at rest or already in motion. It is calculated by the following equation[25]:

$$\text{Force} = \text{mass} \times \text{acceleration}$$

The more slowly the force is applied, the more slowly energy is released, with less subsequent tissue deformation. If the same force is dissipated over a large surface area, the tissue disruption is further reduced. The forces most often applied are acceleration, deceleration, shearing, and compression. *Acceleration* is a change in the rate of velocity or speed of a moving body. As velocity increases, so does tissue damage. *Deceleration* is a decrease in the velocity of a moving object. *Shearing forces* occur across a plane, with structures slipping relative to each other. *Compressive resistance* is the ability of an object or structure to resist squeezing forces or inward pressure.[25]

Viscoelastic properties of tissue help absorb energy and protect vital organs from the effects of impact. If the energy transmitted to the tissue remains below the limit of injury, the energy will be absorbed without causing injury.[26] This phenomenon is used to protect against injury by using energy-absorbing structures and padding. These protective objects do not prevent deformation of tissues but can extend the duration and reduce the force of impact below the limit of injury.

When the tissues are deformed beyond the recoverable limit, injury occurs. Tissue or structure deformation can be measured according to changes in shape, commonly defined as a change in length divided by the initial length.[26] Another term for this change is *strain*. Two major types of strain are tensile and shear. A third type is compressive, which is less common and is responsible for crushing injuries. Tensile and shear strain applied to an artery is illustrated in Figure 11-2. Stretching of the artery along its longitudinal axis increases its length and tissue strain. If the strain or increase in length is too great, the tissue will break. An "all or none"

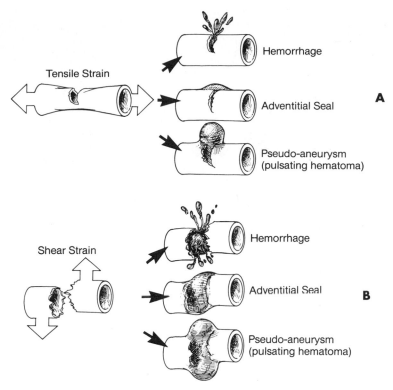

FIGURE 11-2 A, As the artery is stretched along its longitudinal axis, its length and amount of tissue strain increase. An increase in length that exceeds tensile strength causes the artery to break. The injury can result in a complete tear or can produce lower degrees of damage if the strain is less. **B,** Shear strain occurs when the force is applied 90 degrees to the longitudinal axis. Varying degrees of injury can occur with different levels of force. (Modified from Committee on Trauma Research, National Research Council and the Institute of Medicine: *Injury in America,* Washington, DC, 1985, National Academy Press, 52.)

phenomenon is not present, so the artery may completely or partially break. A similar result can be produced by a force applied at 90 degrees to the long axis of the artery. This shear strain occurs when the movement of tissue in opposite directions exceeds recoverable limits. Other examples of tensile strain injuries are femur and rib fractures. Shear strain injuries include hepatic vein laceration from differential movements of hepatic lobes and brain injury from movement of the brain within the skull. Compressive or deformation strain is a factor in contusion injury. This type of injury often leaves the surface of the tissue undamaged (Figure 11-3).

Another factor in strain injury is the loading or strain rate.[26] Tissue response depends on both strain and rate of strain application. Bony injuries can be used to demonstrate this principle. Compact bone will fail at lower strain values if the strain applied is at a rapid rate.[27] The same strain applied more slowly will not cause tissue failure. In general, the viscous tolerance of a tissue is proportional to the product of loading rate and amount of compression.[26] A tissue's tolerance to compression decreases as the rate of loading increases.

Our overall knowledge regarding injury mechanisms for specific organ systems continues to improve. The Crash Injury Research and Engineering Network (CIREN) has been instrumental in enhancing our knowledge regarding injuries in motor vehicle crashes. The mission of this program is to improve the prevention, treatment, and

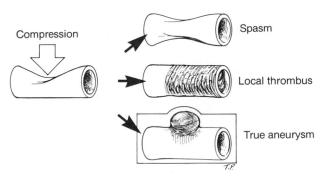

FIGURE 11-3 A crushing force can be applied over an artery, causing damage to the arterial wall. Little or no damage occurs to the overlying skin. The compression produces stretching and shear forces in the arterial wall, which cause injuries similar to those produced by a pure tensile or shear force. (Modified from Committee on Trauma Research, National Research Council and the Institute of Medicine: *Injury in America,* Washington, DC, 1985, National Academy Press, 53.)

rehabilitation of MVC injuries, thereby reducing deaths, disabilities, and human and economic costs. CIREN is sponsored by the National Highway Traffic Safety Administration and uses a multidisciplinary approach to investigate crashes. Information from this program demonstrates that proper seat belt restraint reduces head injury from frontal crashes but not lateral crashes.[28] Also, belts do not prevent abdominal injuries in lateral crashes, and contact intrusion injuries commonly cause brain, liver, and lung injuries.

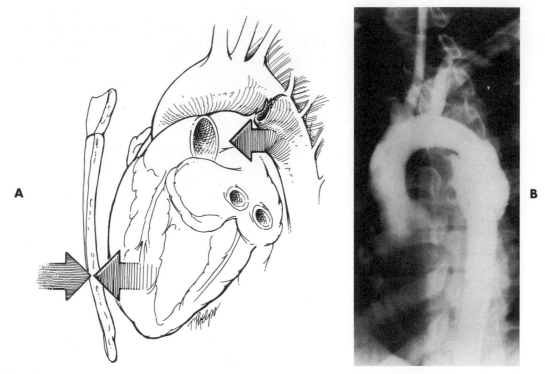

FIGURE 11-4 A, As the chest wall decelerates, the heart and aorta are still in motion. The aorta continues to move anteriorly after the chest wall has stopped, causing shear forces to be focused on the aorta at its point of attachment to the posterior chest wall. If the forces exceed tissue strength, an aortic laceration occurs. **B,** The aortogram reveals an aortic injury after a deceleration injury, with the dye column interrupted just beyond the aortic isthmus. Proper management dictates surgical repair as soon as possible.

Impact biomechanics is an important aspect of injury mechanisms, especially for motor vehicle crashes. Impact biomechanics has four principle areas of study: (1) understanding the mechanism of injury; (2) establishing levels of human tolerance to impact; (3) soliciting the mechanical response to injury; and (4) designing more humanlike test dummies and other surrogates.[29] The following discussion covers blunt forces, thermal injury, and penetrating trauma and various organ responses to these forces.

BLUNT INJURY

Blunt trauma is caused by a combination of forces: deceleration, acceleration, shearing, crushing, and compression. Multiple injuries are common. Blunt trauma is often more life-threatening than penetrating trauma because the extent of injuries is less obvious and their diagnosis is difficult.

Laboratory, radiographic, and invasive studies along with physical examination aid in the diagnostic process. Knowledge of tissue properties can help decide what diagnostic studies are needed. Explosion injuries can occur in air-filled organs such as the bowel and lung. The forces are transmitted in all directions; if pressure is not released, tissues will break or burst. Solid organs that have sustained crush injuries may display little external evidence of injury. Blunt abdominal trauma is responsible for only 1% of all trauma admissions but is associated with a 20% to 30% mortality rate. Much of this mortality rate is attributed to associated head and chest injuries.

Common causes of blunt-force injury include MVCs, falls, aggravated assaults, and contact sports. The automobile is responsible for at least 50% of these nonpenetrating injuries.[30] Direct impact causes the greatest injury and occurs when there is direct contact between the body surface and the injuring agent.[21] Indirect forces are transmitted internally, with dissipation of energy to the internal structure. The extent of injury from indirect forces depends on the transference of energy from an object to the body. Injury occurs as a result of energy released and the tendency for tissue to be displaced on impact.

Acceleration-deceleration forces are a common cause of blunt injury. An example is injury to the thoracic aorta. Rapid deceleration in MVCs can cause major vessels to undergo stretching and bowing. Shearing is produced when stretching forces exceed the elasticity of vessels. Shearing damage is seen in the vessel walls, causing them to tear, dissect, rupture, or form an aneurysm.[26] This shearing damage occurs in the vessels as they decelerate at a rate different from that in the areas they perfuse. The aorta is fixed tightest to the chest wall at the isthmus just below the origin of the subclavian artery. Movement of the aorta above and below this fixation point produces a shearing force, causing injury, which has a mortality of 80% (Figure 11-4). The lowest rate of aortic injury in MVCs is associated with use of three-point restraint belts and an air bag.[31]

HEAD INJURIES

Head injury is a major health problem in the United States, with a rate of occurrence ranging from 200 to 610 per 100,000 population.[32] Death is a common outcome; survivors often face debilitating sequelae. These results are especially sobering considering that the highest rate of injuries is in the 15- to 19-year-old age group. The three most common mechanisms of injury are motor vehicle crashes (114 per 100,000), falls (41 per 100,000), and aggravated assaults (23 per 100,000). The fatality rate is 5.2% for MVCs, 6.2% for falls, and 6.3% for assaults.

Head injury is produced by the initial impact, but the momentum imparted to the head and brain dictates the eventual type and degree of injury.[33] This concept is detailed for a number of injury types in Table 11-1.

When a head is struck and its velocity is changed from rest to 1.7 m/sec (38 mph), a positive pressure (approximately 1 atm) develops on the percussed side at the brain-skull interface.[34] Simultaneously a negative atmospheric pressure develops at the opposite pole. This vacuum produces transient cavitation, which is a factor in contrecoup injuries (injury to the brain directly opposite the site of the impact). The other factor in contrecoup injuries is produced by the brain sliding within the cranial vault. The inside of the skull is not a smooth surface, and the brain substance is torn and damaged by rigid protuberances as it slides over them.

Acute subdural hematoma (ASDH) is the most significant cause of death associated with head injury because of its high incidence (30%), high mortality (60%), and high severity of injury (Glasgow Coma Scale score of 3, 4, 5).[35] Three mechanisms of injury have been identified: (1) direct laceration of cortical arteries and veins with penetrating injury, (2) large contusions with extensive "pulping" of brain tissue, and (3) the most common type, tearing of veins that bridge the subdural space as they travel from brain to dura. This last mechanism is more likely to occur after a fall or an assault (72%) than after a motor vehicle crash (24%).[35] In contrast, diffuse brain injury has been found in 89% of victims of MVCs and in only 10% of victims of falls and assaults.[35]

Injury biomechanics can be used to explain this difference. The parasagittal bridging veins have strong viscoelastic behavior, which makes their response to force dependent on the rate at which the vessel is strained. The ultimate strain to failure decreases with increasing strain rate. When acceleration or deceleration occurs rapidly, the veins will fail. A person falling 25 feet and striking his or her head on concrete with a stopping distance of 0.1 cm has a deceleration force of 200 g with a duration of 3.5 msec. The equivalent deceleration would happen in a vehicle crashing into a rigid barrier at 40 mph. The dashboard deforms 10 cm and the duration is 35 msec. The longer deceleration time decreases the chance of ASDH but increases the chance of diffuse brain injury.[35]

Occipital skull fractures from backward falls have a high mortality.[36] This is related to direct injury to vital posterior fossa structures and to contrecoup injury in the frontotemporal area. A third of 134 patients in one report suffered contrecoup injuries.[36] This high incidence of severe contrecoup injuries is related to the forces applied, the momentum generated, and the bony irregularities in the anterior skull.

SPINAL CORD INJURIES

The muscular and articular supports of the spinal cord are insufficient to tolerate violent forces. Areas where injury is most often seen are the junctional regions between the cervical, thoracic, lumbar, and sacral spines. Mechanisms of injury involved with spinal cord damage include axial loading, flexion, extension, rotation, lateral bending, and distraction (Figure 11-5).[37]

Axial loading injury occurs when the force is applied upward or downward to the spinal column with no posterior or lateral bending of the spine.[37] A burst fracture of the vertebral body or disk extrusion results. This type of injury is common in MVCs when a person's head is thrown upward and strikes the roof of the car.

In a flexion injury the force causes extreme movement of the spine beyond the normal range. The head is bent forward on the cervical spine. Flexion with rotation produces a more severe injury. A vertebral body is thrown forward, and the cord is compressed. The wedging force placed on an adjacent vertebra crushes it and drives fragments of bone into the spinal canal. Flexion injury can occur with only a small amount of force. Posterior longitudinal or articular ligaments are torn, displacing the fracture forward into the lower vertebra (Figure 11-6).

In hyperextension injuries the cervical spinal cord is extended as the head is bent back sharply (see Figure 11-6). A downward force causes compression of the vertebral bodies. Fracture of the pedicles or lamina can be seen, depending on the direction and intensity of the force.[37] Posterior dislocation of the upper vertebrae on the lower occurs, further complicating the injury. Acceleration forces can cause hyperextension of the neck, producing what is commonly known as "whiplash injury."[24] These injuries can squeeze the spinal cord, supplying the main stress in the center of the cord, resulting in the syndrome of acute central cervical cord injury. In this syndrome there is greater motor impairment of the upper limbs compared with the lower because the nerve fibers supplying the lower limbs are more peripherally situated and suffer less damage. Distraction injury to the cervical spine, a separation of the spinal column with cord transection, is seen with hangings.[38]

Forces applied sufficiently to the anterior skull or face can displace the upper vertebrae backward, and the vertebral body above the distraction may separate.[24] This leaves the disc intact but strips the posterior longitudinal ligament from the vertebral body below. Spinal cord contusion against the lamina of the vertebra below can be seen.

FRACTURES

The biomechanics of fractures is an area in which knowledge is currently available.[27] Some basic definitions used to

TABLE 11-1   Head Injury: Relationship of Injuring Agent, Forces Applied, Pathophysiology, and Clinical Results

Type	Impact Velocity	Force* Momentum	Velocity Imparted† (Change)	Shear Strain‡	Damage To:					Clinical Effects
					Scalp	Bone	Vessels	Brain	Stem	
Stab	Low	Low	Small	Linear +	++	+	+	Local, mild	0	Specific, mild
Gunshot§	High	Low	Small	Linear +	++	++	Deep +++	Specific, variable	0	Specific, variable
Crush	Very low	Very low	None	Linear +	+++	++++	+	Diffuse, mild	0	General, mild
Blow, mild	Low	Low	Small	Linear + Rotary +	+	+	+	Local, mild	+	General, moderate
Blow, severe	Moderate	High	Large	Linear ++ Rotary +++	++	+++	++	Contrecoup	+++	General, moderate to severe
Fall, mild	Low	High	Large	Linear ++ Rotary +++	+	+	++	Contrecoup	++	General, moderate to severe
Fall, severe	Low	Very high	Very large	Linear +++ Rotary ++++	+++	+++	Surface +++	Diffuse, severe	++++	General, severe

Adapted from Walker AE, Ray CD, Laws ER et al: Injuries of the head and spinal cord. In Zuidema GD, Rutherford RB, Ballinger WF, editors: *The management of trauma*, Philadelphia, 1979, WB Saunders, 181-253.
*Forces are either acceleration (as with an object striking the head) or deceleration (as with a head in motion striking an object).
†Velocity change is relative to velocity before impact.
‡Shear strain forces are for the brain relative to the skull.
§For gunshot wounds, the variability of injury is related to the kinetic energy of the missile.

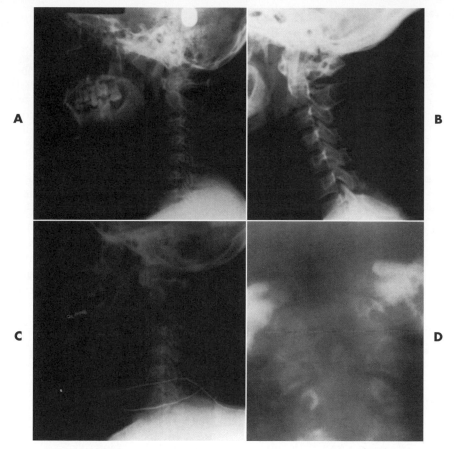

FIGURE 11-5 Flexion, extension, distraction, and axial loading injuries. **A,** Flexion injury with wedge compression of C5 with posterior retropulsion. **B,** Extension injury with teardrop extension avulsion of anteroinferior aspect of C2. **C,** Distraction injury with C2 disarticulated from C3 and a bilateral pedicular fracture of C2 with abnormal widening of spinous processes C1 and C2 (hangman's fracture). **D,** Tomogram showing a Jefferson fracture caused by axial loading. There is lateral displacement of the lateral masses of C1 in relation to C2, which is more marked on the right side.

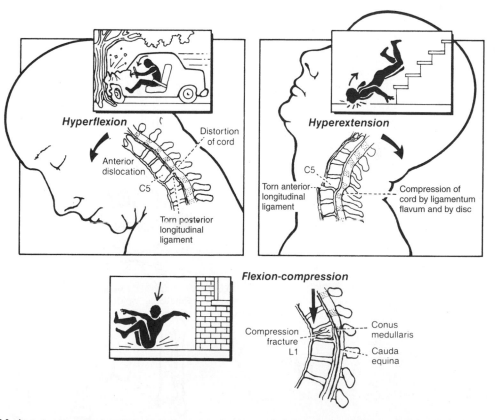

FIGURE 11-6 Mechanisms of injury for spinal column injuries. (From Black P: Common mechanisms of closed spinal injury. In Zuidema GD, Rutherford RB, Ballinger WF, editors: *Management of trauma,* Philadelphia, 1985, WB Saunders, 228.)

describe fracture biomechanics are helpful in understanding possible injuries. Force and strain have already been discussed and defined. Stress is defined as the internal resistance to deformation or the internal force generated from the application of a load[26]:

$$Stress = load/area \ on \ which \ the \ load \ acts$$

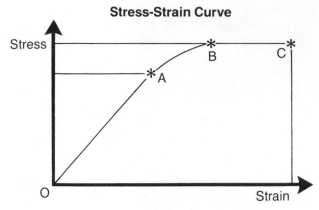

Stress-Strain Curve

FIGURE 11-7 Stress-strain curve. Strain increases proportionately with stress to point A. From point A to point B, the strain is greater than the stress. Point A is called the *yield point,* or *limit of proportionality,* and point B represents the *ultimate tensile strength.* Point C is the *break point,* or *breaking strain,* of the material. At C the material remains permanently deformed and does not recover its original shape.

Stress cannot be measured directly. It is measured in force per unit area and expressed as pounds per square inch (psi) or kilograms per square centimeter (kg/cm²). Other terms for force include *pound force, kilogram force,* and *dynes.*

Both extrinsic and intrinsic factors are important determinants of whether a bone will fracture when stress is applied. Extrinsic factors include magnitude, duration, direction, and rate of force application. Intrinsic factors are properties of bone that determine its susceptibility to fracture. These include energy-absorbing capacity, modulus of elasticity (Young's modulus), fatigue, strength, and density.[39] Energy-absorbing capacity is related to the strain characteristics of the bone. The energy absorbed to produce femoral neck failure is 60 kg/cm². Stress-strain curves (Figure 11-7), or Young's modulus, measure elasticity. Fatigue failure occurs when a material is subjected to repeated stresses that are below its breaking point but the cumulative stress results in failure. Bone strength is directly related to its density. As bone density is reduced by osteoporosis, the stress required to fracture the bone decreases.

Fractures can be classified by their mechanism of injury (Figure 11-8). Fractures caused by direct trauma are tapping, crush, low-velocity penetrating, and high-velocity penetrating.[26] Tapping injuries occur from kicks to the shin or blows with nightsticks to bony areas. Little energy is

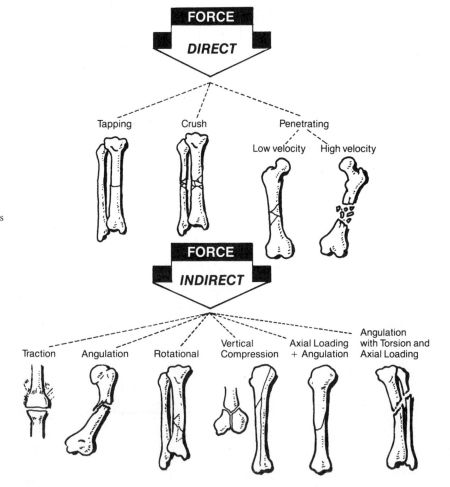

FIGURE 11-8 Types of fractures produced by various direct and indirect mechanisms of injury. (From Harkness JW: Principles of fractures and dislocations. In Rockwood CA, Green DP, editors: *Fractures,* Philadelphia, 1975, JB Lippincott, 4.)

absorbed by soft tissue. Crush and high-velocity injuries produce multiple comminuted areas as well as soft-tissue damage. Indirect trauma also can produce fractures.[26] Traction injuries usually involve tendons pulling pieces of bone away at their attachments, such as external rotation injuries of the ankle. Angulation fractures are explained by tension and compression stress (Figure 11-9). As a lever is angulated, the convex surface is under tension stress and the concave surface is under compression stress. The convex surface fails first, giving rise to a transverse fracture. Rotational fractures are rare because it is difficult to apply a true rotation force to a bone.[26] Compression fractures do occur and are explained by vector analysis. If a homogeneous cylinder is loaded axially until it fails, the fracture will

appear at an angle of almost 45 degrees (Figure 11-10). Because bones are not homogeneous, most axial loading produces T- or Y-shaped fractures at the lower end of the bone. Combinations of forces usually produce oblique or curved fracture lines.

Fractures in the thoracolumbar spine can present interesting clinical findings. Wedge or compression fractures are the most common fractures in this area of the spine. They result from acute flexion forces.[40] The injury can occur after a fall with feet landing first. An associated injury is an os calcis fracture. Burst fractures are produced when forces are applied perpendicularly to the spinal column. Spinous process fractures occur from direct force to the flexed spine or a violent muscle pull.

Pelvic fractures can be simple to manage or may produce life-threatening hemorrhage. Injury to the lower genitourinary tract should always be a concern with any pelvic fracture. Open pelvic fractures have a mortality rate four times that of closed fractures.[41] Traction fractures of the ischial tuberosity and anterior iliac spine represent stable simple pelvic injuries.[42] A shear fracture of the ilium is found in the motorcycle rider who is thrown forward and catches the iliac crest on the handlebars. Straddle fractures result from direct trauma to the perineum. Urethral injury should be sought in these patients, especially males. Patients with blood at the penile meatus, perineal or scrotal hematoma, or a nonpalpable prostate gland by rectal examination should not have a Foley catheter placed until a urethral injury is excluded by urethrogram. Malgaigne fractures are those with fracture lines through the sacroiliac joint and pubic rami on the same side (Figure 11-11). This allows the two sides of the pelvis to float free; the resultant vascular disruption can produce massive bleeding.

Acetabular fractures happen when the hip is flexed and

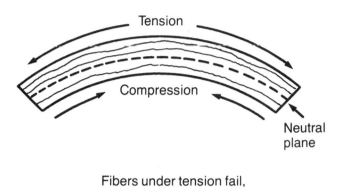

Tension

Compression

Neutral plane

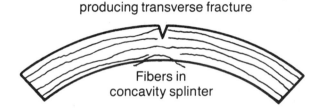

Fibers under tension fail, producing transverse fracture

Fibers in concavity splinter

FIGURE 11-9 Forces sustained to produce an angulation fracture. (From Rockwood CA, Green DP, editors: *Fractures in adults*, Philadelphia, 1984, JB Lippincott, 13.)

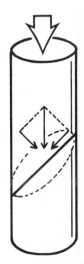

FIGURE 11-10 Vertical forces applied to a homogeneous cylinder will cause the structure to fail at an angle of 45 degrees to the long axis of the cylinder. The forces can be resolved into two forces, with the maximum shear force at 45 degrees to the long axis.

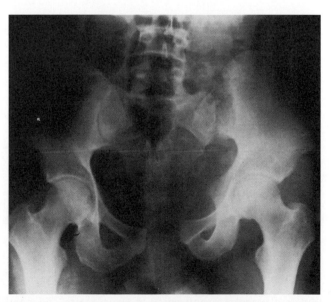

FIGURE 11-11 Radiograph of a Malgaigne pelvic fracture. Fracture line is through the sacroiliac joint and ipsilateral pubis, allowing the two sides of the pelvis to separate.

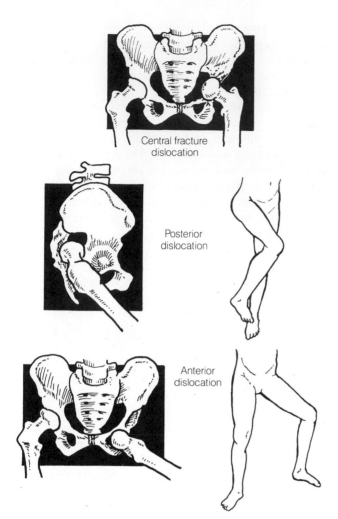

Central fracture
dislocation

Posterior
dislocation

Anterior
dislocation

FIGURE 11-12 Three types of hip dislocation. (From Hughes JL: Initial management of fractures and joint injuries. In Zuidema GD, Ballinger RB, Rutherford RB, editors: *Management of trauma*, Philadelphia, 1985, WB Saunders, 621.)

abducted during an MVC. The knee hits the dashboard during the forward body acceleration, and the femur is driven through the acetabulum.[43] If the thigh is crossed at impact, a posterior dislocation of the hip is produced.[44] The presence of these injuries should suggest the need for evaluation of the ipsilateral knee. An anterior dislocation of the hip is found when a posterior force is applied to an abducted, externally rotated thigh. Leg deformity in posterior and anterior hip dislocation is diagnostic (Figure 11-12).

One of the most common and potentially most serious upper extremity fractures is a supracondylar humeral fracture in children.[45] The anterior capsule and collateral ligaments are stronger than bone in children. Thus as the elbow is locked in extension, the forces applied cause the weakest area, the supracondylar bone, to fracture. Even if the fracture is not displaced, the potential for swelling around the elbow is great and can produce arterial obstruction and vascular insufficiency of the forearm and hand. Volkmann's ischemic contracture can occur if the blood supply is occluded.

ABDOMINAL INJURIES

The automobile is responsible for at least 50% of intra-abdominal injuries. The liver, spleen, and kidney are the most common organs injured after blunt trauma. The National Crash Severity Study found that with an Abbreviated Injury Score (AIS) of at least 3 and lateral impact, the organs most likely to be injured were kidneys (43%), spleen (33%), and liver (24%).[46] Animal experiments demonstrate that the risk of abdominal injury is a function of the impact velocity multiplied by the forced abdominal compression.[46,47] The mechanisms of blunt visceral injury include crushing, shearing, and bursting forces.[26] In low-velocity, high-compression injuries the mechanism is most likely due to organ motion and shearing forces. In high-velocity, low-compression mechanisms the likely cause is bursting.

A crushing injury is represented by a midbody laceration of the pancreas. This can occur when the force is applied anterior to posterior, causing the pancreas to be crushed against the vertebral body. A shearing injury can result from acceleration-deceleration forces acting on the hepatic small bowel mesentery or renal vessels. In both cases the momentum of the organ mass applies the force to the organ's vascular pedicle, causing injury. The apparent weight of the liver (actual weight, 1.8 kg) during a 36 km/hr impact would be 18 kg; a 72 km/hr impact, 72 kg; and a 108 km/hr impact, 162 kg.[48] It is easy to understand how vessels attaching this organ to its blood supply could be stretched and torn. Impact velocities for hepatic injuries have been studied. Significant hepatic contusion occurs at velocities above 12 m/sec. At 20 m/sec deep lacerations and transections are produced. A bursting injury can occur if the intestines are compressed in a closed loop formation, resulting in failure of the wall strength.

CAUSATIVE AGENTS IN BLUNT TRAUMA

MOTOR VEHICLE CRASHES. Automobile crashes cause approximately 50,000 deaths annually.[1] Seventy-eight percent involve automobiles, trucks, or motorcycles; 18% involve pedestrians; 2% involve bicyclists; and 2% involve collisions with trains.[49] Some factors affecting the risk of occupant injury or death are amount of highway travel, road characteristics, speed, vehicle size, and restraint use.[14] Road characteristics, speed, vehicle size, and restraint use can also affect the mechanism of injury.

Highway design can change the injury pattern. Crashes are reduced by separating opposing streams of traffic, eliminating intersections, removing obstacles from roadsides, using breakaway barriers, and surfacing roads with materials that decrease skidding. Successful examples of these changes include a death rate on interstate highways in 1979 of 1.6 per hundred million vehicle miles (mvm), whereas on rural, two-way roads it was 4.8 per hundred mvm.[26] Fatal collisions occur when roadside objects are struck within 40 feet of the road, emphasizing that road design should include a wide shoulder space free of obstacles.[14,26]

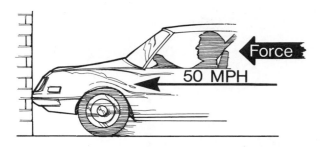

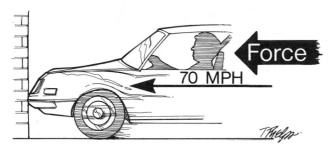

FIGURE 11-13 Force is increased approximately twofold when impact occurs at 70 mph in comparison with 50 mph.

Speed is also an important determinant of the likelihood and severity of injury. The energy dissipated increases with the square of the change in velocity. Thus the forces on a properly restrained occupant in a forward crash at 70 mph might be roughly twice the forces at 50 mph (Figure 11-13). It has been estimated that the 55 mph national speed limit saved 5000 lives annually.[14]

Vehicle size and design also change injury patterns. Small cars are involved in more crashes per mile and are associated with more deaths and injuries per crash than larger cars. The simple approach of making cars larger is not viable, because approximately 40% of occupant deaths occur in single-vehicle crashes. Changing vehicle design, especially interior design, can improve the safety of the occupants. Incorporating design changes that are used in automobile racing also would increase the likelihood of escaping a vehicular crash without injury.[50]

Before a collision the occupant is moving at the same speed as the vehicle. During the collision the vehicle and occupant decelerate to a speed of zero, but not necessarily at the same rate. The deceleration forces are transmitted to the body according to the following relationship[46]:

$$\text{Gravity} = \text{mph}^2/30 \times \text{stopping distance (ft)}$$

Three collisions actually happen. The first is the car into another object. The second collision is the occupant's body with the interior of the car. A third collision may occur when internal tissues impact against rigid body surface structures. An example is the fracture of ribs by the steering wheel from the second collision and lung perforation by the ribs from the third collision (Figure 11-14).

Unrestrained occupants are injured by contact with the steering wheel, instrument panel, or other car interior structures or by ejection. The most significant cause of death is ejection from the vehicle, which is fatal in 27% of cases.[50]

Other causes of mortality are impact with front or rear doors (18%), the steering assembly (16%), and the instrument panel (13%).[46]

Restraint systems allow occupants to decelerate with their vehicles rather than more abruptly when thrown against unyielding structures inside or outside the vehicles.[28,50,51] Injuries are reduced by preventing ejection of the occupant during crashes, prolonging deceleration time, and reducing severity of impact by the occupant against the car interior.[52,53] The interior design of the vehicle can make a difference in injury mechanisms. A stiff armrest is more damaging than a soft armrest for lateral impacts. Stiff armrests produce an injury with an AIS of 4 compared with an AIS of 2 when a soft armrest is in place.[54]

Properly worn restraints decrease the number of fatalities and severity of injury. Major head injuries fell from 43% to 34% in car passengers when laws were enacted requiring seat belt use.[14] A study by Volvo of Sweden showed no deaths under 60 mph when a harness-type restraint was worn.[55] Lap belts decrease the likelihood of ejection but not of impact with the vehicle interior. A three-point shoulder lap belt is the most effective restraint.[51] The harness belt reduces the impact of the second collision and thus reduces head and facial injuries, intraabdominal solid viscus injuries, and long-bone fractures.[53] One study found that the use of seat belts would have prevented 40% of deaths and lap belt/shoulder harnesses would have prevented another 13%.[53] However, crash victims who were restrained had an increase in the incidence of abdominal hollow viscus injury.[56] This could be a result of a sudden increase in intraluminal pressure or shearing of relatively fixed ligaments and mesenteric attachments by the deceleration forces against the restraining device. These are the same forces that may cause an intraabdominal aortic injury.[57] Patients with Chance fractures (vertebral body fracture extending through the pedicles of the spinous process, usually in the lumbar region) are commonly rear-seat passengers who are using only a lap belt. This type of restraint use is also found among patients who suffer a hollow viscus injury.[58]

The increase in seat belt laws may produce new injuries related to their misuse. Seat belts can be misplaced intentionally or unintentionally. Examples of intentional misuse include placing small children in a harness designed for an adult. Defining injuries specific to malpositioning of seat belts is difficult. Neck, chest, and abdominal injuries have been reported in association with improper use of seat belts.[59-61] Use of seat belts by pregnant women is always a concern. Proper application of a seat belt is associated with a decrease in maternal and fetal injury.[62,63]

Collapsible steering columns and high-impact-resistant windshields help decrease injury from the second collision. The latest attempt to prevent these second collisions in MVCs is installation of inflatable air bags that are activated on impact. This is a passive restraint mechanism.[64,65] It is clear that the addition of the air bag will reduce injuries. Heart injuries are very rare, and their occurrence in frontal

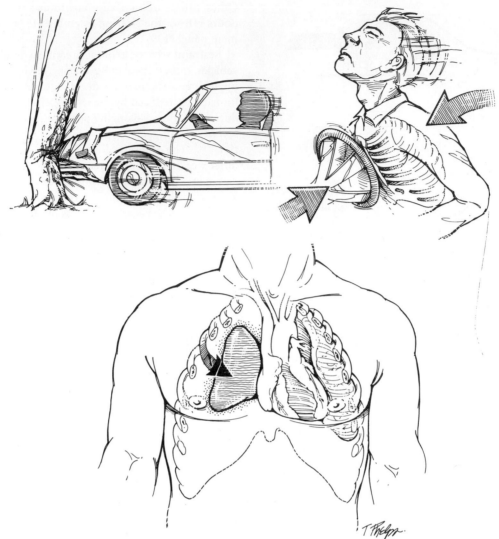

FIGURE 11-14 The three collisions of a head-on motor vehicle crash: The car hits an object, and the occupant's body impacts on some surface within the motor vehicle. The result is collision between internal tissues and the rigid body surface structures.

motor vehicle crashes is correlated with the type of restraints in use. A three-point restraint system has a heart injury rate of 0.15% compared with a rate of 0.03% for three-point restraints and an air bag.[66] As with any restraint device, airbags can also cause injury when improperly used. These injuries range from the mild to lethal.[67-69] Most injuries are minor (abrasions and fractures of extremities). In fatal injuries, car occupants have been in unusual positions or improperly restrained when the air bag is activated.

Other motorized vehicles can present different mechanisms of injury. One type of transportation that is of concern is the all-terrain vehicle, which is essentially a motorcycle.[70,71] Four-wheel all-terrain vehicles (ATVs) are now common, although three-wheel types are still seen. The three-wheel vehicle is a problem because there is a perception of safety from the wide tripod base. Injuries with either type of ATV are produced by two mechanisms: The rider strikes an unseen wire or branch or the rider flips the

motorcycle while turning or avoiding an obstacle. It is not uncommon for the vehicle to strike the rider after it flips. Few regulations concerning these vehicles are in force, although strong warnings from the manufacturers have been issued in response to consumer action.

Snowmobile injuries have increased over the years.[72,73] Most of these injuries appear related to human factors. These include inexperience, use of alcohol, excessive speed, driver recklessness, and poor adherence to manufacturer recommendations. Ejection from these vehicles with injuries to the head and extremities are common.

Personal watercraft injuries have increased fourfold since 1990.[74,75] Human error is again a common theme. Proper supervision and training is recommended as well as the use of personal flotation devices when using watercraft.

Another sports activity that is associated with increased injuries is inline skating. Fractures of the upper extremities from falls on to outstretched arms are common.[76] These and other common injuries can be prevented with use of simple safety equipment, including wrist guards, elbow pads, and helmets.[77]

FALLS: VERTICAL DECELERATION INJURIES.   Falls are the second leading cause of death as a result of trauma in the United States.[7] In falls the relationship between physical forces of deceleration and biomechanical factors of the organism determines the type and severity of injury. Energy of a body in motion is expressed by kinetic energy *(KE)*, which is a function of the body mass *(m)* and its velocity *(v)* expressed as $KE = mv2$. Mass, acceleration, and deceleration of the body in addition to the duration and area of application of the force are important when determining extent of injury sustained as the result of a fall.[25,78] Although the distance of a fall is often used to identify patients likely to have sustained major injury, it correlates poorly with injury severity.[79] Other factors can be related to the energy sustained in a fall.

Duration of force application relates to whether the force is applied slowly or rapidly. The following formula describes the kinematics of vertical deceleration:

$$W = KE \times k/TA$$

Wounding *(W)* is directly related to the kinetic energy of the body modified inversely by the time of deceleration *(T)* and area through which the energy is dissipated *(A)*.[25] The *k* is a constant for a tissue type or an organism. The velocity at impact for a fall of 1 second over a distance of 16 feet is 32.2 ft/sec, or 21.9 mph. If duration is increased to 6 seconds and distance to 580 feet, the velocity at impact is 193.2 ft/sec, or 131.7 mph. The velocity at impact can be used as a measure of the kinetic energy of the body, which is related to the severity of tissue injury.

Tissue elasticity and viscosity must be considered as biomechanical factors of vertical deceleration. Elasticity is the tissue's ability to resist stretching and resume its previous shape. If the tissue remains distorted, it is said to be *plastic.* Viscosity is the tissue's resistance to change in shape when there are changes in motion. The body's ability to withstand deceleration forces is a combination of these two tissue properties.[25]

Tissue disruption at impact is caused by the motion of the tissues. The body's ability to withstand this force increases if there is uniform motion of all tissues. Increasing stopping distance or time of deceleration and enlarging the area of energy dissipation can minimize the injury. These concepts are emphasized in a report of a woman who fell 50 feet and landed at a speed of 37 mph on her back and side, depressing the earth 4 inches. She had no loss of consciousness or signs of injury.[80] The magnitude of injury increases as tissue cohesion is overcome. Forces transmitted at impact include compression, stretching, and shearing, which can occur singly or in combination.[25]

Skeletal injuries, especially of the lower extremities, are common with vertical deceleration. Wedge or compression fractures of vertebral bodies with fracture-dislocation of the

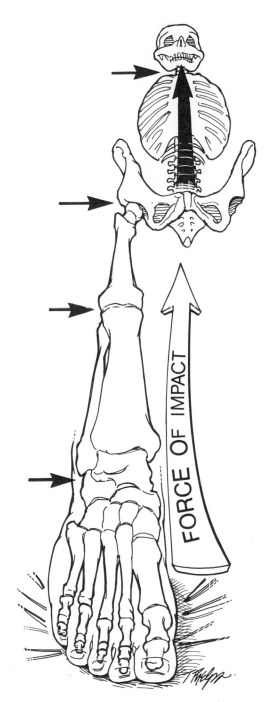

FIGURE 11-15 Forces resulting from a fall are transmitted up to the spine through the long leg bones and pelvis.

spine are caused by both flexion-compression and rotational injury forces. Torsion injury is also common and results from the force being transmitted to the feet and up the legs to the pelvis and supporting structures of bone, muscle, and cartilage (Figure 11-15).[78]

PENETRATING TRAUMA

Penetrating trauma refers to injury produced by foreign objects penetrating the tissue. The severity of injury is related to the structures damaged. The most commonly

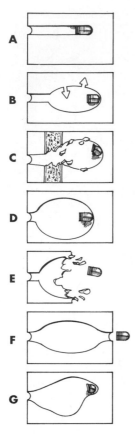

FIGURE 11-16 Patterns of injury in animal tissue secondary to variations in the ballistics of the missile and tissue characteristics. **A,** Low velocity, no cavitation, entrance and exit small. **B,** Higher velocity, formation of cavity, arrows show direction and magnitude of acceleration of tissue. **C,** Velocity as in **B,** but deformation of bullet and creation of secondary missiles after penetrating bone. **D,** Very high velocity, large cavity, and small entrance. Exit may be small. **E,** Very high velocity, thin target, large and ragged exit. **F,** Velocity, caliber, and thickness of tissue such that cavitation occurs deep inside and entrance and exit are small. **G,** Asymmetric cavitation as bullet begins to deform and tumble. (Modified from Swan KG, Swan RC, editors: *Gunshot wounds: pathophysiology and management,* Littleton, Mass, 1980, PSG Publishing, 9.)

involved organs are intestines, liver, vascular structures, and spleen.[81] The mechanism of injury with penetrating trauma is the energy created and dissipated by the object into the surrounding areas.[82] Evaluation of injury is often difficult and dependent on the type and characteristics of the injuring agent, energy dissipation, tissue characteristics, and distance from weapon to target (Figure 11-16).

The extent of injury is proportional to the amount of kinetic energy *(KE)* that is lost by the missile[83]:

$$KE = mass \times (V1^2 - V2^2)/2$$

*V*1 is impact velocity, and *V*2 is exit or remaining velocity. It should be noted that doubling the mass only doubles the energy, whereas doubling the velocity quadruples the energy. Rotational energy is also a factor, because most missiles are shot from barrels that are rifled, causing the bullet to spin. Total kinetic energy can be estimated by adding velocity and rotational energy. Velocity at impact depends on three factors: muzzle velocity, distance of weapon from target, and influence of air friction on the missile (Figure 11-16).

Low-velocity weapons at a range less than 50 yards and high-velocity weapons at less than 100 yards have impact velocities that equal muzzle velocities. To penetrate skin a missile must have an impact velocity of 150 ft/sec; a velocity of 195 ft/sec is required to break bone. Increase in mass can affect total energy (magnum shells will usually increase energy by 20% to 60%).[83]

The amount of kinetic energy lost by the missile is directly related to the tissue damage. The energy lost by the missile is transferred to the tissue. Factors that increase the amount of kinetic energy transferred effectively increase tissue destruction. As the missile penetrates, a tract is created that temporarily displaces tissue forward and laterally. This tissue acceleration creates a temporary cavity as tissues are stretched and compressed, a process called *cavitation.* Cavitation is directly proportional to the amount of kinetic energy transmitted to the tissue.[83] It commonly occurs with missiles traveling 1000 ft/sec or greater. The size of this cavity may be many times the diameter of the bullet. This phenomenon produces damage to structures outside the direct missile path and is commonly referred to as *blast effect.* The effect that cavitation has on wounding potential was illustrated by a wounding study that attempted to control the size of the temporary cavity.[84] The average tissue destruction was reduced by one third if the cavity size was limited by an external envelope.

The velocity of a missile determines the extent of cavitation and tissue deformation. Low-velocity missiles localize injury to a small radius from the center of the tract and have little disruptive effect. A low-velocity missile travels less than 1000 ft/sec, or 305 m/sec.[85] Low-velocity bullets cause little cavitation and blast effect. They essentially only push the tissue aside.

High-velocity missile injuries are more serious because of the amount of energy lost and cavitation produced. High-velocity missiles travel at more than 3000 ft/sec, or 914 m/sec.[85] Damage from high-velocity missiles is dependent on three factors: density and compressibility of tissue injured, missile velocity, and the primary missile's fragmentation.

High-velocity bullets compress and accelerate tissue away from the bullet, causing a cavity around the bullet and its entire tract. The cavity enlarges as the bullet transfers its kinetic energy to the tissue. A negative pressure is created behind the missile, contaminating the wound with foreign material. The diameter of the cavity might be 30 to 40 times the diameter of the bullet. This area is often devitalized and requires debridement. The cavity collapses and tissue recoils until all energy is dissipated. Tissue cohesiveness and elasticity resist expansion of the cavity. More cohesive and elastic tissues experience less damage. Dense tissue absorbs more kinetic energy, causing greater damage. This retarding factor can be related to tissue specific gravity. The higher the specific gravity, the more energy imparted and the greater the damage[83] (Table 11-2).

In injuries from high-velocity missiles, the exit wound through narrow structures or tissue such as an extremity will be larger than the entrance wound because all energy is not

TABLE 11-2 **Specific Gravity of Tissues**	
Tissue	**Specific Gravity**
Rib	1.11
Skin	1.09
Muscle	1.04-1.02
Liver	1.02-1.01
Fat	0.8
Lung	0.5-0.4

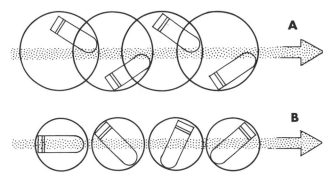

FIGURE 11-17 Effect of yaw on wounding potential. **A,** *Yawing* is the deviation of a bullet in its longitudinal axis from the straight line of flight. **B,** *Tumbling* is the action of forward rotation around the center of mass. (Modified from Swan KG, Swan RC, editors: *Gunshot wounds: pathophysiology and management,* Littleton, Mass, 1980, PSG Publishing, 11.)

dissipated at the exit point. Cavitation, along with yawing and tumbling, is still occurring. Through dense broad tissue the exit wound is small because energy is dissipated and cavitation is complete.[86] If bullet fragmentation occurs, there may be no exit wound. The need for debridement can be extensive with high-velocity missile damage. Amputation and mortality rates are high.[85,86] High-velocity missile injuries to the head are destructive because the cranial vault is fixed and not able to yield to the expanding temporary cavity created by the missile.

After velocity, tissue yaw is the second most important factor in tissue destruction (Figure 11-17). As a bullet's velocity increases, it becomes unstable in flight and may yaw or tumble.[86] *Yawing* is the deviation or deflection of the nose of the bullet from a straight path. The bullet strikes the body at an angle. With greater angles of yaw, the bullet is slowed and more kinetic energy is lost to the tissue. *Tumbling* is the action of forward rotation around the center of mass, a somersault action of the missile that can create massive injury.[83,85,86] Yawing and tumbling increase the area of the missile as it hits the target. Impact increases these motions, which increases the amount of energy released by the bullet, producing more damage.

Various types of bullets are made to alter (in most cases, increase) the amount of energy transmitted. A bullet that passes through tissue without deforming transfers little energy and causes less damage than the bullet that slows down or stops in the tissue. One way to increase the energy transferred is to allow the missile to alter shape on impact. Bullets with hollow points mushroom on impact and yield great amounts of kinetic energy. Soft-nosed and flat-nosed bullets have similar effects.[83,85]

Muzzle blast is another mechanism of injury for penetrating trauma. *Muzzle blast* refers to the cloud of hot gas and burning powder at the muzzle immediately after firing.[83] This is a factor when the gun is in contact with the skin or at close range (within 3 feet). The gas and powder enter the cavity and cause internal explosion by creating a burn. Cavitation is caused by combustion of powder and the forceful expansion of gases. This is common with a shotgun wound but is not seen with handguns because the amount of gas released is less and the wound is too small for it to enter. As the gas is trapped between skin and bone, a stellate tear results from the ballooning of skin out from the bone.[86] This injury does not occur if subcutaneous tissue is present, because of tissue cohesiveness and elasticity.

SHOTGUN INJURIES

Shotguns are short-range, low-velocity weapons that use multiple lead pellets encased in a larger shell for ammunition. Each pellet is considered a missile; there can be 9 to 200 small pellets, depending on the size of pellet and gauge of the gun.[87] A brief description of the mechanism of shotgun injuries, including the weapon, ammunition, and ballistics, is important in understanding the clinical findings in patients sustaining wounds from these weapons.[88]

Gauge designates the bore of the gun. Common gauges include 10, 12, 16, 20, 28, and .410.

The shotgun shell is made up of the primer, powder, wad, and shot, in that order. Shotgun powder is fast burning and creates a low chamber pressure. Common shot sizes range from size 2 through 9 and have a respective pellet diameter of 0.15 to 0.08 in. Ninety no. 2 shot pellets equal 585 no. 9 shot pellets in weight. Larger shot sizes include buckshot and BBs. Buckshot sizes are designated as 4, 3, 2, 1, 0, and 00. Each 00 buckshot is 0.328 inches in diameter. There are also single projectiles, called "slugs" or "pumpkin balls." The plastic or paper wad separates the pellets from the gunpowder. This wad of unsterile material increases the potential of infection in a shotgun wound.[87,88] The wad is expelled with the pellets but loses momentum and drops about 6 feet from the barrel. The pellets leave the barrel close together and separate as they move away from the barrel.

Wounding capacity is the function of mass and projectile velocity. Considering only ballistics, the shotgun is inferior to a single-projectile, high-velocity rifle such as the M-16. The average muzzle velocity of a shotgun is between 1100 and 1350 ft/sec. Rifle slugs have a muzzle velocity approaching 1850 ft/sec. The M-16, with a bullet weighing 55 grams, has a muzzle velocity of 3200 ft/sec. The kinetic energy of the M-16 at the muzzle is 1248 foot-pounds (ft-lb). A no. 6 shotgun pellet, 0.11 inches in diameter, has striking forces of 7.21 ft-lb per pellet at the muzzle and 3.88 ft-lb per pellet at 20 yards. A 12-gauge shotgun with 225 to 428 pellets in the load theoretically has 1694 ft-lb at the muzzle. Therefore, at point-blank or very close range a shotgun injury has the potential for creating extensive tissue damage, similar to a high-velocity missile injury.

The shot pattern is of clinical importance. The major factor affecting the nature of the shotgun wound is the range from the target at which the gun is discharged. Most significant wounds occur in a range up to 15 yards. At less than 6 feet a tight, dense pattern is produced with extensive damage from the muzzle blast and mass of pellets. At 3 to 6 feet the single entrance wound is 1.5 to 2 inches in diameter with scalloping at the edges.[88] There is extensive contamination from shotgun wadding, clothing, skin, hair, burning, and powder entering the wound. At greater distances a pellet does less damage because of the loss of velocity and energy.

If a 12-gauge shotgun loaded with no. 6 shot (275 pellets) were fired accurately at a distance of 40 yards into a 6-foot, 160-pound person, approximately 200 of the pellets would strike within a 30-inch diameter. This would be between the midthigh and the shoulders, across the trunk, and extending approximately 9 inches on either side. If the shot were absolutely evenly distributed, there would be approximately 2 inches between each pellet. At a range of 10 yards, this wound would be only 7 inches in diameter. These pattern changes are used by Sherman and Parrish to classify shotgun wounds.[89] Type 1 is a penetrating wound at a range of more than 7 yards. Type 2 is a perforating wound at a range of 3 to 7 yards. Type 3 is a massive point-blank wound inflicted at a range of less than 3 yards.

LOW-VELOCITY PENETRATING WOUNDS

Other types of penetrating wounds, such as stab wounds and impalements, are low-velocity wounds. These wounds are usually obvious, yet the patient must be undressed and inspected for entrance and exit wounds. If the offending agent remains in place, its trajectory can be traced and underlying trauma predicted. If removed, the gender of the assailant can be helpful in estimating the trajectory: Males tend to stab with an upward thrust and females with a downward thrust.[21] This assessment should not be considered absolute, because intentional injuries often follow no pattern.

Stab wounds are low velocity and therefore low energy; the injuries produced depend on the location of penetration. Little damage occurs to tissue except in the locale of the injury. It must be remembered that multiple body cavities can be penetrated by a single wound. In particular, the thoracic and abdominal cavities can be injured by a wound whose entrance is located over one or the other cavity. Lower chest wounds, from the nipples to the costochondral margin, are frequently found to injure abdominal contents because the diaphragmatic excursion extends superiorly up to the nipple line or fifth intercostal space during exhalation (Figure 11-18).

Impalement injuries usually result from a forceful collision between the object and patient during MVCs or falls or from falling objects. The spectacular nature of these injuries should not preclude proper management. The impaled object should be left in place until definite surgical therapy is

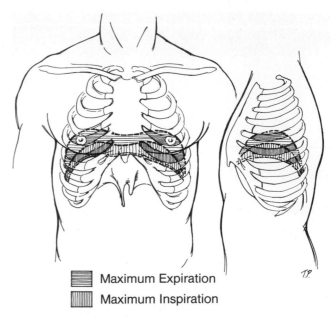

▤	Maximum Expiration
▥	Maximum Inspiration

FIGURE 11-18 Diaphragmatic excursion during inspiration and expiration and its possible effect on penetrating injuries to the lower chest and upper abdomen.

available.[90-92] This recommendation dates back to 1862 in a treatise about arrow wounds and the ability of the arrow to tamponade vascular injuries.[88] Removal of these foreign bodies can remove the vascular control, causing exsanguinating hemorrhage. Another concern with these injuries is bacterial and foreign-body contamination. Care should be taken to remove all foreign material from these wounds; occasionally, extensive wound debridement is required.

SMOKE INHALATION AND PULMONARY BURNS

Inhalation injuries occur when the respiratory tract is exposed to the products of combustion. The type and severity of injury are determined by the type of gases inhaled, their concentration, and the duration of exposure. Thermal injury to the respiratory tree is uncommon because the heat-exchanging efficiency of the respiratory tract is so high that even superheated air is cooled before it gets below the larynx.[93] Steam inhalation can produce thermal injury of the lower respiratory tract because steam has 4000 times the heat capacity of air. The presence of these injuries should be suspected if certain circumstances are present: (1) fire in a closed space, (2) unconsciousness or inebriation associated with smoke exposure, (3) fires involving plastics, (4) presence of carbonaceous sputum, and (5) steam explosions.[93]

The most immediate concern in a patient exposed to a fire is carbon monoxide (CO) intoxication. This is the most frequent immediate cause of death. Carbon monoxide has an affinity for hemoglobin 210 times that of oxygen.[94] The signs and symptoms of CO intoxication are related to blood carboxyhemoglobin (COHb) concentration (Table 11-3).

Inhalation of toxic constituents of smoke may damage alveolar epithelium and capillary endothelium. This results in increased permeability of the alveolar-capillary

TABLE 11-3	Signs and Symptoms Caused by Various Concentrations of Carboxyhemoglobin
Blood Saturation (% COHb)	**Signs and Symptoms**
0.3-10	None
10-20	Tightness across forehead; headache
20-30	Throbbing headache; abnormal fine manual dexterity
30-50	Severe headache; syncope; nausea and vomiting
60-70	Coma; convulsions; death

TABLE 11-4	Common Toxic Products of Combustion
Substance	**Toxic Products of Combustion**
Polyvinyl chloride	Hydrogen chloride, phosgene, chloride
Wood, cotton, paper	Acrolein, acetaldehyde, acetic acid, formaldehyde, formic acid
Petroleum products	Acrolein, acetic acid, formic acid
Nitrocellulose	Oxides of nitrogen, acetic acid, formic acid
Polyurethane	Isocyanate, hydrogen cyanide
Polyfluorocarbons (Teflon)	Octafluoroisobutylene
Melamine resins	Ammonia, hydrogen cyanide

membrane, which can produce noncardiac pulmonary edema and hypoxemia.[95] These toxic products also reduce bacterial clearance and mucociliary transport. Combustion of many common construction materials produces a large number of toxic byproducts capable of this type of injury (Table 11-4).[94]

Motor vehicles provide some unique mechanisms of injury for burns. Carburetor priming resulted in 4% of admissions to one burn center.[96] The burns most frequently involved are the head, neck, and upper extremities. Gasoline is often used to prime an engine that has run out of gas. This practice is unnecessary and dangerous because it can produce an explosion and fire, which may happen when the gasoline comes in contact with hot metal, an electrical spark, or retrograde ignition from too much gasoline in the intake manifold. Burns sustained during an MVC are a second mechanism type and occur in two patterns: (1) The person is trapped in a burning vehicle, receiving facial and upper extremity burns with associated inhalation injury; or (2) the person is thrown from the vehicle and sustains less severe burns and no inhalation injury. Motorcycle crash victims are common in this second group. Associated injuries, including fractures, are common but do not correlate with mortality.

The injury most commonly associated with mortality is inhalation injury (36%).[97]

EXPLOSIVE BLASTS

Explosive blasts are a result of detonated explosives being converted to large volumes of gases.[98] The pressure created ruptures the casing, and resultant fragments become high-velocity projectiles. The blast shock wave created by the remaining energy has three components: positive phase, negative phase, and mass movement of air. The blast shock wave's velocity is as high as 3000 m/sec (10,000 ft/sec), which decreases to the speed of sound within a variable distance.[98] This is dependent on the composition and amount of explosive used. The positive-pressure phase is the maximum pressure reached by the blast wave and is greatest next to the immediate explosion. Pressure falls as the wave moves away from the explosion source. The negative-pressure phase follows immediately and lasts 10 times as long.[98] An equal volume of air is displaced along with the expanding gas and travels behind the blast wave. The mass movement of air can actually cause disruption of tissue, traumatic amputation, and evisceration.[98]

Blast injuries in water are more severe than in air because the blast wave travels farther and more rapidly in water as a result of its greater density. Explosions in closed areas are more damaging than those in open spaces because of the toxic gases and smoke that are inhaled. Posttraumatic pulmonary insufficiency results and is reflected in blood gases with low Pao_2 and increased $Paco_2$.

Damage occurs most often at tissue-air interfaces. Damage in the lung is in the alveolar wall, with resultant hemorrhage and edema. The abdominal organs will show damage to the visceral wall, and the trauma may cause perforation.[98] These types of injuries are rare if the explosion occurs in the open and the victim is not close to the detonation point. In a study by Guy and colleagues, animals exposed to a thoracic blast of 100 psi demonstrated transient apnea, bradycardia, and hypotension.[99] The same blast applied to the abdomen produced no acute changes in cardiopulmonary parameters. The ear is the most sensitive organ to explosions; eardrums will rupture at about 7 psi.[98] Burns also can be seen if a fireball effect is present. Penetrating injuries can occur if projectiles are released.

TERRORISM

Recent events suggest that terrorism is a medical issue. Conventional weapons, such as bombs, could be used and would produce mechanisms consistent with blast injury, burns, smoke inhalation, and blunt and penetrating injuries. The threat of nuclear, biologic, and chemical (NBC) weapons cannot be ignored.[100] NBC agents are instruments of mass destruction and they represent new challenges to our medical system. These challenges come in many forms. Identification of the agents is the first step, followed by understanding their mechanisms of injury and then devel-

TABLE 11-5	**Differences in Chemical and Biologic Agents That Could be Used for Terrorism**	
	Chemical	Biologic
Onset	Rapid, minutes to hours	Delayed, days to weeks
Patient Location	Downwind from release point	Widely spread through geographic region
First Responder	Paramedics, police, firefighters	ED nurses and physicians, ID physicians
Decontamination	Critical	Not necessary
Treatment	Chemical antidotes	Vaccines, antibiotics
Patient Isolation	None after decontamination	Absolute with communicable diseases

ED, Emergency Department; *ID*, Infectious Disease
Modified from Henderson DA: The looming threat of bioterrorism, *Science* 283:1279-1282, Feb 26, 1999.

oping systems to deal with their results. In some cases our medical capabilities will be limited to control attempts because no treatment is known (e.g., Ebola virus). In others, early recognition and administration of treatments can be life saving (e.g., Sarin gas). Responses to chemical and biologic agents are different (Table 11-5).

Biologic weapons are especially frightening. They appear easy to obtain, easy to apply, and difficult to detect early enough to intervene successfully if at all.[15,101]

INJURY SCORING

An objective system for measuring severity of injury is helpful in triaging patients, allocating and evaluating medical resources, assessing quality of medical care, conducting institutional auditing, and preparing comparative studies of morbidity and mortality.[102] A number of severity indices are available; however, each has its problems and limitations.[103-105]

A commonly used system is the Injury Severity Score (ISS), which was developed by Baker and associates.[106] This system uses the AIS and is best applied to patients with blunt injuries. The AIS was first published in 1971 as a single comprehensive scale for injuries related to MVCs. The most recent edition is the AIS-90.[107] The system divides the body into seven regions and uses a severity code for each injury. One is a minor injury and six is a fatal injury. Mortality increases with the AIS grade of most severe injury; this increase is not linear but quadratic. AIS scores from the second and third most severely injured body regions also tend to indicate an increased risk of death and maintain the quadratic relationship. To calculate the ISS, the AIS scores from the three most severely injured body regions are used to define a number score that relates to severity of injury. Because the association of the AIS score to mortality is quadratic, the ISS is defined as the sum of the squares of the highest AIS grade in each of the three most severely injured areas. A problem with the ISS is that it is a retrospective tool. This score can only be calculated once all injuries are known.

The need for a prospective physiologic scoring mechanism produced the Trauma Score (TS).[103] The components of the Revised Trauma Score (RTS) are listed in Table 11-6. The Glasgow Coma Scale score is combined with simple physiologic measurements to derive a RTS between 1 and 12. Lower scores are associated with higher mortality. This severity index has considerable statistical support and can be combined with the ISS to yield the expected chance of patient survival (Figure 11-19). The resulting Trauma and Injury Severity Score (TRISS) method is based on regression equations, which consider patient age, severity of anatomic injury (ISS), and physiologic status of the patient (TS). These comparisons are useful in identifying individual patients with statistically unexpected outcomes, whether good or bad. Survivors above the 50% mortality line would be an unexpected favorable outcome, whereas deaths below the line would be an unfavorable outcome. TRISS also can be used to compare populations of trauma patients while controlling for severity mix.[106] Weaknesses of TRISS continue to be an underestimation of the outcome of patients with multiple injuries in one anatomic area.[108]

This problem is answered with a number of systems, including New Injury Severity Score (NISS), A Severity Characterization of Trauma (ASCOT), and ICD-9-Based Illness Severity Score (ICISS).[106,109] ASCOT was developed to improve on TRISS.[109] ASCOT works for penetrating and blunt mechanisms, as well as with different age groups. Most recently, ICISS emerged as another prediction tool.

The ICISS was developed to predict survival, length of stay, and hospital charges.[110] It has subsequently been compared with TRISS and found to be superior in predictive power.[111-113] However, despite calls for replacement of TRISS by ICISS, TRISS is still commonly used.[114] Although all these developments are proceeding, the value of administrative databases to predict outcome has now been questioned.[115]

Another development is a move to functional outcome measurements.[116-118] The Short Form 36 (SF36) and quality-of-life scales are commonly used.[116,119] These measures are especially important in assessing outcome from orthopedic injury.[120-122]

SUMMARY

With injury as our fourth leading cause of death and one of the United States' most expensive health problems, a thorough understanding of the circumstances that result in injury is necessary for all health care personnel. Mechanism of injury helps to identify the type, extent, and pattern of injury and even relates to potential complications and outcome. Mechanism of injury affords the practitioner an opportunity to suspect certain injuries in addition to the obvious ones, thereby improving delivery of patient care.

TABLE 11-6   Revised Trauma Score

Assessment	Method	Coding
1. Respiratory rate	Count respiratory rate in 15 seconds and multiply by 4	10 - 29 = 4 >29 = 3 6 - 9 = 2 1 - 5 = 1 0 = 0
2. Systolic blood pressure	Measure systolic cuff pressure in either arm by auscultation or palpation	>89 = 4 76 - 89 = 3 50 - 75 = 2 1 - 49 = 1 0 = 0

3. Glasgow Coma Scale score

Eye Opening	Best Verbal Response	Best Motor Response
Spontaneous = 4	Oriented = 5	Obeys command = 6
To voice = 3	Confused = 4	Localizes pain = 5
To pain = 2	Inappropriate words = 3	Withdraws to pain = 4
None = 1	Incomprehensible sounds = 2	Flexion to pain = 3
	None = 1	Extension to pain = 2
		None = 1

Convert Glasgow Coma Scale score as follows:
13 - 15 = 4
9 - 12 = 3
6 - 8 = 2
4 - 5 = 1
<4 = 0

To obtain the trauma score, add the final scores for respiratory rate, systolic blood pressure, and converted Glasgow Coma Scale score together.

Summary of Survival Probability in a Trauma Center

Trauma Score	12	11	10	9	8	7	6	5	4	3	2	1	0
Survival	.995	.969	.879	.766	.667	.636	.630	.455	.333	.333	.286	.259	.037

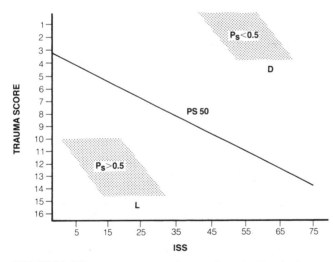

FIGURE 11-19 Trauma score plotted against the Injury Severity Score. The probability of survival above the PS 50 isobar is less than 50%, and the probability of survival below the isobar is greater than 50%.

Prevention of injury is also aided by knowing the mechanism of injury. Active involvement of the trauma practitioner in organizations and programs aimed at injury prevention should be sought so their firsthand knowledge can be used to educate the public in injury prevention. This knowledge must be used if successful programs are to be developed that will prevent injury and improve on the currently dismal statistics of injury in the United States.

REFERENCES

1. National Safety Council: *Accident facts, 1995,* Chicago, 1995, National Safety Council.
2. Haupt BJ, Graves E: *Detailed diagnostic procedures for patients discharged from short-stay hospitals: United States, 1979,* DHHS Pub No (PHS) 82-1274-1, Washington, DC, 1982, U.S. Department of Health and Human Services.
3. The National Committee for Injury Prevention and Control: *Injury prevention: meeting the challenge the national committee for injury prevention and control,* New York, 1989, Oxford University Press.
4. Bonnie RJ, Fulco CE, Liverman CT, editors: *Reducing the burden of injury,* Washington, DC, 1999, National Academy Press, 41-59.
5. Schwab CW, Kauder DR: Trauma in the geriatric patient, *Arch Surg* 127(6):701-706, 1992.
6. Eachempati SR, Reed RL, St. Louis JE et al: The demographics of trauma in 1995 revisited: an assessment of the accuracy and utility of trauma predictions, *J Trauma* 45(2):208-214, 1998.
7. Foege WH, Baker SP, Davis JH et al: Epidemiology of injuries: the need for more adequate data. In Grossblatt N, editor: *Injury in America,* Washington, DC, 1985, National Academy Press, 25-36.

8. Sisley A, Jacobs LM, Poole G et al: Violence in America: a public health crisis—domestic violence, *J Trauma* 46(6): 1105-1113, 1999.

9. Baker JP, O'Neill B, Karpf RS: *The injury fact book,* Lexington, Mass, 1992, Heath.

10. Centerwall BS: Socioeconomic status and domestic violence, *JAMA* 273(22):1755-1758, 1995.

11. Reyna TM, Maj NC, Hollis HW et al: Alcohol-related trauma, *Ann Surg* 201(2):194-197, 1985.

12. Centers for Disease Control and Prevention: Quarterly table reporting alcohol involvement in fatal motor vehicle crashes, *MMWR* 40(11):187-188, 1991.

13. Gentilello LM, Rivara FP, Donovan DM et al: Alcohol interventions in a trauma center as a means of reducing the risk of injury recurrence, *Ann Surg* 230(4):473-483, 1999.

14. Baker SP, Dietz PE: The epidemiology and prevention of injuries. In Zuidema DG, Rutherford RB, Ballinger WF, editors: *The management of trauma,* Philadelphia, 1979, WB Saunders, 794-821.

15. Slater MS, Trunkey DD: Terrorism in America, an evolving threat, *Arch Surg* 132(10):1059-1066, 1997.

16. Max W, Stark B, Root S: Putting a lid on injury costs: the economic impact of the California Motorcycle Helmet Law, *J Trauma* 45(3):550-556, 1998.

17. Cook PJ, Lawrence BA, Ludwig J et al: The medical costs of gunshot injuries in the United States, *JAMA* 282(5):447-454, 1999.

18. Lopez-Viego MA: *The Parkland trauma handbook,* St. Louis, 1994, Mosby.

19. Weigelt JA, Klein JD: Mechanism of injury. In Mancini B, Klein JD, editors: *Decision making in trauma management,* Philadelphia, 1991, BC Decker, 1-4.

20. Feliciano DV: Patterns of injury. In Feliciano DV, Moore, EE, Mattox KL, editors: *Trauma,* ed 3, Stamford, Conn, 1996, Appleton & Lange, 85-103.

21. Krantz, BE: Initial assessment. In Feliciano DV, Moore, EE, Mattox KL, editors: *Trauma,* ed 3, Stamford, Conn, 1996, Appleton & Lange, 99, 123-139.

22. American College of Surgeons' Committee on Trauma: Biomechanics of injury. In: *Advanced trauma life support course manual,* Chicago, 1997.

23. Golden T, Fisher JC, Edgerton MT: "Wringer arm" reevaluated: a survey of current surgical management of upper extremity compression injuries, *Ann Surg* 177(3):362-369, 1973.

24. Hyde AS: *Crash injuries, how and why they happen: a primer,* Key Biscayne, Fla, 1992, HAI, 45-62.

25. Maull KI, Whitley RE, Cardea JA: Vertical deceleration injuries, *Surg Gynecol Obstet* 153(2):233-236, 1981.

26. Foege WH, Baker SP, Davis JH et al: Injury biomechanics research and the prevention of impact injury. In Grossblatt N, editor: *Injury in America,* Washington, DC, 1985, National Academy Press, 48-64.

27. Rockwood CA, Green DP, editors: Fractures. In: *Rockwood and Green's fractures in adults,* Philadelphia, 1996, JB Lippincott.

28. Siegel JH, Mason-Gonzalez S, Dischinger P et al: Safety belt restraints and compartment intrusions in frontal and lateral motor vehicle crashes: mechanisms of injuries, complications and acute care costs, *J Trauma* 5(34):736-759, 1993.

29. King AI, Yang KH: Research in biomechanics of occupant protection, *J Trauma* 38(4):570-576, 1995.

30. Jacobs BB, Jacobs LM: Epidemiology. In Feliciano DV, Moore EE, Mattox KL, editors: *Trauma,* ed 3, Stamford, Conn, 1996, Appleton & Lange, 15-30.

31. Brasel KJ, Quickel RR, Yoganandan N et al: Seat belts are more effective than air bags in reducing thoracic aortic injury in frontal motor vehicle crashes (Abstract), Big Sky, Mont, 2000, Western Trauma Association.

32. Ommaya AK, Dannenberg AL, Salazar AM et al: Causation, incidence, and costs of traumatic brain injury in the U.S. military medical system, *J Trauma* 40(2):211-217, 1996.

33. Gikas PW: Mechanism of injury in automobile crashes, *Clin Neurosurg* 19:175-190, 1972.

34. Trunkey DD: Force in blunt trauma. In Trunkey DD, Lewis FR, editors: *Current therapy of trauma,* ed 2, Burlington, Ontario, 1986, BC Decker, 102-104.

35. Gennarelli TA, Thibault LE: Biomechanics of acute subdural hematoma, *J Trauma* 22(8):680-686, 1982.

36. Young HA, Schmidek HH: Complications accompanying occipital skull fractures, *J Trauma* 22(11):914-920, 1982.

37. Viano DC: Causes and control of spinal cord injury in automotive crashes, *World J Surg* 16(3):410-419, 1992.

38. Bucholz RW: Unstable hangman's fractures, *Clin Orthop* 154:119-124, Jan-Feb 1981.

39. Harkess JW: Principles of fractures and dislocations. In Rockwood CA, Green DP, editors: *Fractures,* Philadelphia, 1975, JB Lippincott, 1-90.

40. Przybylski GJ, Marion DW: Injury to the vertebrae and spinal cord. In Feliciano DV, Moore EE, Mattox KL, editors: *Trauma,* ed 3, Stamford, Conn, 1996, Appleton & Lange, 307-327.

41. Richardson JD, Harty J, Amin M et al: Open pelvic fractures, *J Trauma* 22(7):533-538, 1982.

42. Dalal SA, Burgess AR, Siegel JH et al: Pelvic fracture in multiple trauma: classification by mechanism is key to pattern of organ injury, resuscitative requirements, and outcome, *J Trauma* 29(7):981-1000, 1989.

43. Dakin GJ, Eberhardt AW, Alonso JE et al: Acetabular fracture patterns: associations with motor vehicle crash information, *J Trauma* 47(6):1063-1071, 1999.

44. Reigistad A: Traumatic dislocation of the hip, *J Trauma* 20(7):603-606, 1980.

45. Rockwood CA, Green DP, editors: *Fractures in children,* Philadelphia, 1996, JB Lippincott.

46. Rouhana SW, Lau IV, Ridella SA: Influence of velocity and forced compression on the severity of abdominal injury in blunt, nonpenetrating lateral impact, *J Trauma* 25(6): 490-500, 1985.

47. Miller MA: The biomechanics of lower abdominal steering-wheel loading, *J Trauma* 31(9):1301-1309, 1991.

48. Lau VK, Viano DC: Influence of impact velocity on the severity of nonpenetrating hepatic injury, *J Trauma* 21(2): 115-123, 1981.

49. Dolan WD, Gifford RW, Smith RJ et al: Automobile-related injuries, *JAMA* 249(23):3216-3221, 1983.

50. O'Day J, Scott R: Safety belt use: ejection and entrapment, *Health Educ Q* 11(2):141-146, 1984.

51. Newman RJ: A prospective evaluation of the protective effect of car seatbelts, *J Trauma* 26(6):561-564, 1986.

52. Bucklew PA, Osler TM, Eidson JJ et al: Falls and ejections from pickup trucks, *J Trauma* 32(4):468-472, 1992.

53. Wild BR, Kenwright J, Rastogi S: Effects of seat belts on injuries to front and rear seat passengers, *Br Med J* 290(6482): 1621-1623, 1985.

54. Viano DC, Andrzejak DV: Biomechanics of abdominal injuries by armrest loading, *J Trauma* 34(1):105-115, 1993.

55. Denis R, Allard M, Atlas H et al: Changing trends with abdominal injury in seatbelt wearers, *J Trauma* 23(11): 1007-1008, 1983.

56. Wisner DH: Injury to the stomach and small bowel. In Feliciano DV, Moore, EE, Mattox KL, editors: *Trauma,* ed 3, Stamford, Conn, 1996, Appleton & Lange, 551-571.

57. Dajee H, Richardson IW, Iype MO: Seat belt aorta: acute dissection and thrombosis of the abdominal aorta, *Surgery* 85(3):263-267, 1979.

58. Anderson PA, Rivara FP, Maier RV et al: The epidemiology of seatbelt-associated injuries, *J Trauma* 31(1):60-67, 1991.

59. Contosavios DL, Laposata EA: Sagittal liver transection: an injury from improperly worn shoulder harness seatbelts: a report of two cases, *J Trauma* 33(4):637-640, 1992.

60. Huelke DF, Mackay CM, Morris A: Vertebral column injuries and lap-shoulder belts, *J Trauma* 38(4):547-556, 1995.

61. McCarthy MC, Lemmon GW: Traumatic lumbar hernia: a seat belt injury, *J Trauma* 40(1):121-122, 1996.

62. Wolf ME, Alexander BH, Rivara FP et al: A retrospective cohort study of seatbelt use and pregnancy outcome after a motor vehicle crash, *J Trauma* 34(1):116-119, 1993.

63. Tyroch AH, Kaups KL, Rohan J et al: Pregnant women and car restraints: beliefs and practices, *J Trauma* 46(2):241-245, 1999.

64. Haddon W, Baker SP: Injury control. In Clark D, MacMahon B, editors: *Preventive medicine and public health,* Boston, 1981, Little, Brown, 109-140.

65. Insurance Institute for Highway Safety: *Background manual on the passive restraint issue,* Washington, DC, 1977.

66. Augenstein JS, Perdeck E, Williamson J et al: *Heart injuries among restrained occupants in frontal crashes,* 1996, SAE970392.

67. Maxeiner H, Hahn M: Airbag-induced lethal cervical trauma, *J Trauma* 47(6):1148-1151, 1997.

68. Duma SM, Kress TA, Porta DJ et al: Airbag-induced eye injuries: a report of 25 cases, *J Trauma* 41(1):114-119, 1996.

69. Perdikis G, Schmitt T, Chait D et al: Blunt laryngeal fracture: another airbag injury, *J Trauma* 48(3):544-546, 2000.

70. Golladay ES, Slezak JW, Mollitt DL et al: The three wheeler: a menace to the preadolescent child, *J Trauma* 25(3):232-233, 1985.

71. Krane BD, Ricci MA, Sweeney WB et al: All-terrain vehicle injuries, *Am Surg* 54(8):471-474, 1998.

72. Hamdy CR, Dhir A, Cameron B et al: Snowmobile injuries in northern Newfoundland and Labrador: an 18-year review, *J Trauma* 28(8):1232-1237, 1998.

73. James EC, Lenz JO, Swenson WM et al: Snowmobile trauma: an eleven-year experience, *Am Surg* 57(6):349-353, 1991.

74. Shatz, DV, Kirton OC, McKenney MG et al: Personal watercraft crash injuries: an emerging problem, *J Trauma* 44(1):198-201, 1998.

75. Branche CM, Conn JM, Annest JL: Personal watercraft-related injuries a growing public health concern, *JAMA* 278(8):663-665, 1997.

76. Calle SC, Eaton RG: Wheels-in-line roller skating injuries, *J Trauma* 35(6):946-951, 1993.

77. Schieber RA, Branche-Dorsey CM, Ryan GW et al: Risk factors for injuries from in-line skating and the effectiveness of safety gear, *N Engl J Med* 335(22):1630-1635, 1996.

78. Lukas GM, Hutton JE, Lim RC, et al: Injuries sustained from high velocity impact with water: an experience from the Golden Gate bridge, *J Trauma* 21:612-618, 1981.

79. Goodacre S, Than M, Goyder EC et al: Can the distance fallen predict serious injury after a fall from height? *J Trauma* 46(6):1055-1058, 1999.

80. DeHaven H: Mechanical analysis of survival in falls from heights of fifty to one hundred and fifty feet, *War Med* 2:586, 1942.

81. Fabian TC: Abdominal trauma, including indications for celiotomy. In Feliciano DV, Moore, EE, Mattox KL, editors: *Trauma,* ed 3, Stamford, Conn, 1996, Appleton & Lange, 441-459.

82. Graeber GM, Belville WD, Sepulveda RA: A safe model for creating blunt and penetrating ballistic injury, *J Trauma* 21:473-476, 1981.

83. Ordog GJ, Wasserberger J, Balasubramanium S: Wound ballistics: theory and practice, *Ann Emerg Med* 13:1113-1122, 1984.

84. Janzon B, Seeman T: Muscle devitalization in high-energy missile wounds, and its dependence on energy transfer, *J Trauma* 25:138-144, 1985.

85. Swan KG, Swan RC: *Gunshot wounds—pathophysiology and management,* Littleton, Mass, 1980, PSG Publishing.

86. Fackler ML: Wound ballistics. In Trunkey DD, Lewis FR, editors: *Current therapy of trauma,* ed 2, Burlington, Ontario, 1986, BC Decker, 94-101.

87. Deitch EA, Grimes WR: Experience with 112 shotgun wounds of the extremities, *J Trauma* 24(7):600-603, 1984.

88. Flint LM, Cryer HM, Howard DA et al: Approaches to the management of shotgun injuries, *J Trauma* 24(5):415-419, 1984.

89. Sherman R, Parrish A: Management of shotgun injuries: a review of 152 cases, *J Trauma* 3:76-86, 1963.

90. Bowsher WG, Smith WP: Severe facial injury by impalement, *J Trauma* 24(11):999-1000, 1984.

91. Horowitz MD, Dove DB, Eismont M et al: Impalement injuries, *J Trauma* 25(9):914-916, 1985.

92. Ketterhagen JP, Wassermann DH: Impalement injuries: the preferred approach, *J Trauma* 23(3):258-259, 1983.

93. Crapo RO: Smoke-inhalation injuries, *JAMA* 246(15): 1694-1696, 1981.

94. Fein A, Leff A, Hopewell PC: Pathophysiology and management of the complications resulting from fire and the inhaled products of combustion: review of the literature, *Crit Care Med* 8(2):94-98, 1980.

95. Herndon DN, Traber DL, Niehaus GD et al: The pathophysiology of smoke inhalation injury in a sheep model, *J Trauma* 24(12):1044-1051, 1984.

96. Klabacha M, Nelson H, Parshley P et al: Carburetor priming: a cause of gasoline burn, *J Trauma* 25(11):1096-1098, 1985.

97. Purdue GF, Hunt JL, Layton TR et al: Burns in motor vehicle accidents, *J Trauma* 25(3):216-219, 1985.

98. Owen-Smith M: Bullet wounds: explosive blast injuries. In Hughes S, editor: *The basis and practice of traumatology,* Rockville, Md, 1983, Aspen Publishing, 80-91.

99. Guy RJ, Kirkman E, Watkins PE et al: Physiologic responses to primary blast, *J Trauma* 45(6):983-987, 1998.

100. Cole LA: The specter of biologic weapons, *Scientific American,* pp 1-14, Dec 1996.

101. Inglesby TV, Dennis DT, Henderson DA et al: Plague as a biological weapon: medical and public health management, *JAMA* 283(17):2281-2290, 2000.

102. Wisner DH: History and current status of trauma scoring systems, *Arch Surg* 127(1):111-117, January 1992.

103. Champion HR, Sacco WJ, Carnazzo AJ et al: Trauma score, *Crit Care Med* 9(9):672-676, 1981.

104. Committee on Medical Aspects of Automotive Safety: Rating the severity of tissue damage. I. The abbreviated scale, *JAMA* 215(2):277-280, 1971.

105. Ornato J, Mlinek EJ, Craren EJ et al: Ineffectiveness of the trauma score and the CRAMS scale for accurately triaging patients to trauma centers, *Ann Emerg Med* 14(11): 1061-1064, 1985.

106. Senkowski CK, McKenney MG: Trauma scoring systems: a review, *J Am Coll Surg* 189(5):491-503, 1999.

107. American Association for Automotive Medicine: *The abbreviated injury scale (AIS), 1985 revision,* Des Plaines, Ill, 1985.

108. Brenneman FD, Boulanger BR, McLellan BA: Measuring injury severity: time for a change? *J Trauma* 44(4):580-582, 1998.

109. Champion HR, Copes WS, Sacco WJ et al: Improved predictions from a severity characterization of trauma (ASCOT) over trauma and injury severity score (TRISS): results of an independent evaluation, *J Trauma* 40(1):42-49, 1996.

110. Osler T, Rutledge R, Dies J et al: ICISS: an international classification of disease-9 based injury severity score, *J Trauma* 41(3):380-386, 1996.

111. Rutledge R, Osler T: The ICD-9-based illness severity score: a new model that outperforms both DRG and APR-DRG as predictors of survival and resource utilization, *J Trauma* 45(4):791-799, 1998.

112. Rutledge R, Osler T, Kromhout-Schiro S: Illness severity adjustment for outcomes analysis: validation of the ICISS methodology in all 821,455 patients hospitalized in North Carolina in 1996, *Surgery* 124(2):187-196, 1998.

113. Hannan EL, Szpulski Farrell L, Bessey PQ et al: Predictors of mortality in adult patients with blunt injuries in New York state: a comparison of the trauma and injury severity score (TRISS) and the international classification of disease, ninth revision-based injury severity score (ICISS), *J Trauma* 47(1): 8-13, 1999.

114. Rutledge R, Osler T, Emery S et al: The end of the injury severity score (ISS) and the trauma injury severity score (TRISS): ICISS, an international classification of diseases, ninth revision-based prediction tool, outperforms both ISS and TRISS as predictors of trauma patient survival, hospital charges, and hospital length of stay, *J Trauma* 44(1):41-49, 1998.

115. Hunt JP, Baker CC, Fakhry SM et al: Accuracy of administrative data in trauma, *Surgery* 126(2):191-197, 1999.

116. Kaplan RM, Ganiats TG, Sieber WJ et al: The quality of well-being scale: critical similarities and differences with SF-36, *Int J Qual Health Care* 10(6):509-520, 1998.

117. Brenneman FD, Wright JG, Kennedy ED et al: Outcomes research in surgery, *World J Surg* 23(12):1220-1223, 1999.

118. Wright JG: Outcomes research: what to measure, *World J Surg* 23(12):1224-1226, 1999.

119. Michaels AJ, Michaels CE, Smith JS et al: Outcome from injury: general health, work status, and satisfaction 12 months after trauma, *J Trauma* 48(5):841-850, 2000.

120. MacKenzie EJ, Cushing BM, Jurkovich GJ et al: Physical impairment and functional outcomes six months after severe lower extremity fractures, *J Trauma* 34(4):528-539, 1993.

121. Butcher JL, MacKenzie EJ, Cushing B et al: Long-term outcomes after lower extremity trauma, *J Trauma* 41(1):4-9, 1996.

122. Michaels AJ, Michaels CE, Moon CH et al: Posttraumatic stress disorder after injury: impact on general health outcome and early risk assessment, *J Trauma* 47(3):460-467, 1999.

12

SHOCK AND MULTIPLE ORGAN DYSFUNCTION SYNDROME

Thomas Vary • Barbara McLean • Kathryn Truter VonRueden

Shock is the hemodynamic manifestation of cellular metabolic insufficiency, resulting from either inadequate cellular perfusion, a basic biochemical inability to properly utilize oxygen and other nutrients, or an inappropriate or amplified stimulation of cellular signaling cascades. A state of hyperinflammation, hypoperfusion, and hypermetabolism may influence the critically injured patient's initial presentation. The common denominator is a decreased utilization of oxygen by the tissues. Prolonged deficits in oxygen utilization lead to tissue injury and organ dysfunction syndrome, which may progress to multiple organ failure and, if left unchecked, death. The etiologies of shock can be placed into four broad categories: reduction in cardiac pump function, decreased vascular tone, diminished circulating volume, and alterations in cell signaling.

CATEGORIES OF SHOCK

REDUCTION IN CARDIAC PUMP FUNCTION

In shock states secondary to cardiac pump failure (cardiogenic shock), the underlying pathogenesis is related primarily to the failure of the left ventricle to adequately pump blood to the systemic circulation. Heart failure, acute myocardial infarction, end-stage valvular disease, severe pulmonary hypertension, or multiple organ dysfunction syndrome (MODS) may cause cardiac pump failure. As the cardiac index diminishes, tissue perfusion becomes compromised. The major compensatory mechanism is an increase in heart rate and vascular tone in order to maintain essential organ perfusion. Cardiogenic shock is a combination of failure to mobilize venous volume, a loss of myocardial contractility, and a compensatory vasoconstriction response, which promotes a systemic shunt mechanism. The combination of failures creates a venous volume overload state with relative arterial hypervolemia as blood flow is redirected to the central organs.

Clinical Presentation. Signs and symptoms of shock states related to cardiac pump failure include hypotension, increased systemic vascular response (SVR), tachycardia, decreased stroke volume index (SVI), decreased urine output (UO) and increased ventricular volumes measured by the central venous pressure (CVP), right atrial pressure (RAP), and pulmonary artery occlusion pressure (PAOP). Refer to Table 12-1 for formulas and normal values of hemodynamic parameters.

DECREASED VASCULAR TONE

Shock may also occur when vascular tone is lost, resulting in massive vasodilation. In neurogenic shock, depression of the central nervous system diminishes sympathetic outflow causing a loss of vasomotor control. The loss of a vasomotor response leads to the pooling of blood in both the arterial and venous circulatory systems. The inadequate venous return (preload) decreases myocardial end-diastolic fiber stretch, reduces the cardiac index, and ultimately impairs tissue perfusion. The alteration in arterial tone leads to hypoperfusion. Neurogenic shock may be induced by deep general or spinal anesthesia; brain injury, particularly in the basal regions near the vasomotor center; and high cervical spinal cord injury close to the sympathetic spinal ganglia outflow tracts (usually above T1). Furthermore, the pain associated with severe multiple trauma inhibits the vasomotor center in the brain, thereby dilating the systemic vasculature and hindering the already compromised venous return.

TABLE 12-1   Hemodynamic Parameters

Parameter	Formula	Normal Values
CO	Heart rate × stroke volume	4-8 L/min
CI	CO/Body surface area	2.5-4 L/min/m^2
SVI	CI/Heart rate	33-47 ml/beat/m^2
RAP	Direct measurement	0-8 mm Hg
PAOP	Direct measurement	8-12 mm Hg
RVEDVI	$\dfrac{\text{Stroke volume}}{\text{RV ejection fraction}}$	60-100 ml/m^2
SVRI	$\dfrac{(\text{MAP} - \text{RAP}) \times 80}{\text{CI}}$	1360-2200 dyne/sec/cm^{-5}/m^2
PVRI	$\dfrac{(\text{MPAP} - \text{PAOP}) \times 80}{\text{CI}}$	<425 dyne/sec/cm^{-5}/m^2
LVSWI	SVI (MAP - PAOP) × 0.0136	40-70 gm-m/m^2/beat
RVSWI	SVI (PAP - RAP) × 0.0136	5-10 gm-m/m^2/beat

CO, Cardiac output; *CI*, cardiac index; *SVI*, stroke volume index; *RAP*, right atrial pressure; *PAOP*, pulmonary artery occlusion pressure; *RVEDVI*, right ventricular end-diastolic volume index; *SVRI*, systemic vascular resistance index; *MAP*, mean arterial pressure; *PVRI*, pulmonary vascular resistance index; *MPAP*, mean pulmonary artery pressure; *LVSWI*, left ventricular stroke work index; *RVSWI*, right ventricular stroke work index.

Loss of local vascular tone is also the underlying pathophysiologic mechanism of anaphylactic shock. The body reacts to a foreign substance by activating the immune system against an antigen. The inflammatory response to the antigen-antibody reactions directly damages the endothelial lining of the blood vessels, increasing vascular permeability. The antigen-antibody reaction also induces the release of histamine or histamine-like substances, which possess vasodilator properties. Histamines increase vascular capacity through venodilation, reduce arterial pressure by dilating arterioles, and increase capillary permeability, promoting a rapid shift of fluids into the interstitial spaces. Both neurogenic and anaphylactic shock can be treated acutely by rapid restoration of a euvolemic state and administration of sympathomimetic drugs, promoting vasoconstriction and increasing venous return and contractility.

Clinical Presentation.   Signs of neurogenic shock include hypotension, decreased SVR, bradycardia, decreased SVI, decreased UO, and decreased ventricular volumes, measured as low CVP, RAP, and PAOP. Signs of anaphylactic shock include hypotension, decreased SVR, tachycardia, decreased SVI, decreased UO, and decreased ventricular volumes, measured as low CVP, RAP, and PAOP.

DIMINISHED CIRCULATING VOLUME

HYPOVOLEMIC SHOCK.   Hypovolemic shock is caused by a reduction in circulating volume. Depletion of the effective circulating blood volume subsequently decreases cardiac index and therefore oxygen delivery. Inadequate intravascular volume leading to a shock state occurs in a number of conditions. Severe burns create loss of fluids and electrolytes through denuded areas, resulting in enormous ongoing losses of plasma volume and concentrating the red blood cells, which increases the viscosity of the blood, further altering cellular perfusion. Intestinal obstruction, ischemic

bowel, and gut injuries may cause third-space sequestration of fluid in the peritoneal cavity, leading to a significant decrease in circulating volume and cardiac index. The increased peritoneal volume may also lead to increased abdominal pressures, further decreasing distal arterial perfusion and decreasing venous return. High serum glucose levels can act as an osmotic agent, pulling fluids and electrolytes into the vascular compartment and subsequently, through osmotic diuresis, losing both.

Nonhemorrhagic trauma may induce a shock state. Severe contusion or crushing damage to soft tissues often sequesters blood and plasma in the interstitial space of the injured tissues. The net effect is diminished blood volume. Hypotension and shock may follow the fall in cardiac index that accompanies the decrease in venous return. The hypotension may not become evident until the patient's position is changed for diagnostic procedures such as chest radiographs because of the mechanisms that normally compensate for moderate intravascular volume loss. In all forms of hypovolemia, circulating volume is reduced, venous return decreases, cardiac index falls, systemic shunt is introduced, and a shock state ensues.

Clinical Presentation.   Signs of hypovolemic shock include hypotension, increased SVR, tachycardia, decreased SVI, decreased UO, and decreased ventricular volumes, measured as low CVP, RAP, and PAOP.

HEMORRHAGIC HYPOVOLEMIA.   Hemorrhagic hypovolemic shock affects the host in two ways: through a loss of circulating volume and a decrease in oxygen-carrying capacity. In addition to the loss of circulating volume, the acute decrease in red blood cells reduces both oncotic pressure and oxygen-carrying capacity. The oxygen transport deficit superimposed on the circulatory volume loss presents the characteristic features of hemorrhagic hypovo-

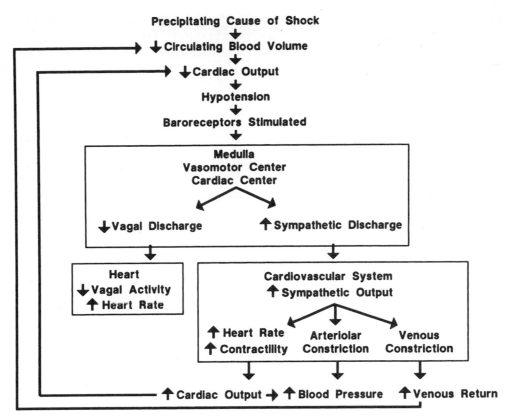

FIGURE 12-1 Compensatory mechanisms for the restoration of circulatory blood volume.

lemia: significant base deficit and lactic acidosis. The initial compensatory response is a profound tachycardia combined with a compensatory systemic shunt as long as central and local sympathetic tone are intact (Figure 12-1). The vasoconstrictor response may significantly and urgently place the nonessential organs (e.g., gut, kidney, skin) at risk.

Clinical Presentation.   Signs of hemorrhagic hypovolemic shock include hypotension; increased SVR; tachycardia; decreased SVI; decreased UO; decreased ventricular volumes, measured as low CVP, RAP, and PAOP; severe base deficit; and lactic acidosis.

COMMON SHOCK PATHWAYS

Regardless of the pathology, when tissue perfusion is inadequate to meet the tissue metabolic demands, a shock state can ensue. Hypoperfusion promotes a response heralded by a compensatory increase in circulating catecholamines, which augments oxygen delivery. The additional availability of oxygen supports an increase in cellular extraction of oxygen to meet higher metabolic requirements.[1-3] The response to increased circulating catecholamines causes an increase in venous return and thus preload, vasoconstriction of arterioles (increasing afterload), and increases in heart rate and myocardial contractility. Combined, these compensatory mechanisms also alter

the temporal myocardial balance of systole to diastole and increase myocardial oxygen demand and requirement for high-energy phosphate bonds.

The shock episode can be divided into three major phases: compensatory, progressive, and irreversible. In the compensatory phase, tissue perfusion is altered, but organ function is maintained via the compensatory mechanisms. An intact neuroendocrine compensatory response is essential to survival. Stress hormones are released, volume is preserved, and nonessential organs are bypassed. The increase in sympathetic discharge requires intact receptor sites, adequate neurotransmitters, functional thyroid hormones, and responsive fibers. As fibers respond, heart rate increases, arterioles and venules constrict at the nonessential tissue level, and perfusion pressure to essential organs is maintained. For a time the host is able to maintain function of essential organs. During the progressive phase, there is a decreased response to the compensatory mechanisms and arterial perfusion cannot be maintained. In the decompensated, irreversible stage, the patient becomes increasingly refractory to therapy.

The common underlying mechanisms of shock are oxygen deficiency, cellular hypoxia, ischemia, and anoxia. Oxygen deficit promotes a response heralded by increased circulating catecholamines, resulting in a compensatory increase in oxygen delivery (hallmarked by increasing heart rate and vasoconstriction of both arterial and venous beds) and an increased cellular extraction of oxygen.

If prolonged, the host may suffer an insurmountable oxygen debt.

As a result of injury, prolonged hypoxic and hypoperfused states, or overwhelming sepsis, complex inflammatory pathways are stimulated. These pathways, when overactivated or unregulated, may result in catastrophic consequences. Humoral and chemical mediators change the vascular structures and metabolic pathways to such a degree that the capillary blood flow and oxygen delivery mechanisms may be profoundly impaired, and a profound metabolic acidosis will ensue. Even if oxyhemoglobin is available in the arterial bed, metabolic dysfunction, altered capillary flow, and intracellular dysfunction may prevent the extraction of oxygen, leading to organ dysfunction and eventually organ failure.[4]

Early recognition of the cause of shock is essential in order to protect and preserve organ function. In traumatic, hemorrhagic hypovolemic shock, the major mechanisms of compensation present a predictable picture (hypotension, increased SVR, tachycardia, decreased SVI, decreased urine output, decreased ventricular end-diastolic volume [e.g., low CVP, RAP, and PAOP], severe base deficit, and lactic acidosis). Usually patients with this presentation can be resuscitated if shock is identified and controlled at initial presentation.

COMPENSATORY CHANGES TO HEMORRHAGE

Hemorrhage, regardless of its cause, results in a compensatory response designed to stabilize a life-threatening situation. Blood loss of less than 10% may occur without any significant effect on blood pressure or cardiac index. Blood loss greater than 10% initiates a powerful response designed to maintain perfusion of vital organs until the circulating volume and oxygen delivery are restored either by replacement of blood and fluid during resuscitation or through a redistribution of fluid volumes in the body. When more than 10% to 15% of the total blood volume is lost, cardiac index diminishes as a result of decreased venous return. Venous return is a major determinant of preload (stretch of ventricular fibers). A proportional relationship exists between preload (ventricular filling) and stroke volume. A reduction in preload progresses to diminished stroke volume. Failure to maintain cardiac index leads to decreased arterial pressure, which causes an increase in sympathetic discharge. The sympathetic stimulation increases the heart rate and promotes vasoconstriction, which may further limit ventricular filling and ejection. Hemorrhagic loss of more than 40% of the total blood volume precipitates a profound decrease in the cardiac index and renders the compensatory mechanisms ineffectual (Figure 12-1).

Clinical Presentation. Signs and symptoms of hemorrhage include hypotension to inaudible blood pressure, tachycardia to extreme tachycardia, and severe alteration in mental status, ranging from confused to comatose.

CIRCULATORY REFLEXES RELATED TO HEMORRHAGIC HYPOVOLEMIA

The circulatory reflexes triggered by all forms of shock, particularly acute hemorrhage, are designed to restore arterial pressure and blood flow to normal in order to prevent organ damage. An integrated response to blood losses greater than 10% of the total blood volume is initiated by the baroreceptors, which respond to the fall in blood pressure, and by the atrial type B receptors, which respond to a fall in blood volume. Hypotension stimulates the vasomotor center, increasing sympathetic outflow. The carotid artery chemoreceptors respond to decreases in the blood pH and a rise in Pco_2 and the metabolic acid H^+. Activation of the carotid body chemoreceptors stimulates the vasomotor center (Figure 12-2). The net effect of the baroreceptor response is an increased sympathetic discharge by the medullary vasomotor center, which is carried over the sympathetic efferent fibers to the heart, systemic arterioles, and adrenals. Increased sympathetic discharge has a positive inotropic effect on the myocardium that augments contractility. Improved myocardial performance results from the direct release of catecholamines at the cardiac sympathetic nerve endings in the proximity of myocardial β_1 receptors and by vasomotor center inhibition of vagal parasympathetic outflow. This change in the balance between the sympathetic and parasympathetic pathways increases atrial pacemaker activity and reduces atrioventricular conduction time, resulting in an increased heart rate. A heart rate greater than 120 beats/min may limit ventricular filling and decrease stroke volume.

Increased arteriolar constriction results in a systemic shunt, which redistributes blood flow away from nonessential organs with low oxygen requirements, such as skin and skeletal muscle. If the cause of the hypovolemia is not corrected, blood flow to the visceral organs will eventually be diminished. Despite a reduced blood volume, venous constriction in response to the sympathetic output tends to enhance venous return and prevent pooling of the blood in the venous circulation. Because the venous system has a capacitance of up to 60% of the circulating volume, venoconstriction can markedly increase venous return, ensuring adequate blood volume for maintenance of myocardial preload. Hemodynamic compensation by stimulation of the sympathetic nervous system is extremely efficient if the shock state is not allowed to continue for a long period and blood and fluid losses do not persist.

FLUID SHIFTS. To compensate for the reduced circulating blood volume, fluids shift from extravascular to intravascular spaces. The fluid shift occurs as a direct result of the decreased intracapillary hydrostatic pressure associated with the loss of blood volume. Normally the balance between hydrostatic pressure promoting filtration and the plasma oncotic pressure promoting reabsorption favors a small net loss of fluid into the interstitial space. In a shock state the reduction of blood pressure decreases the capillary hydro-

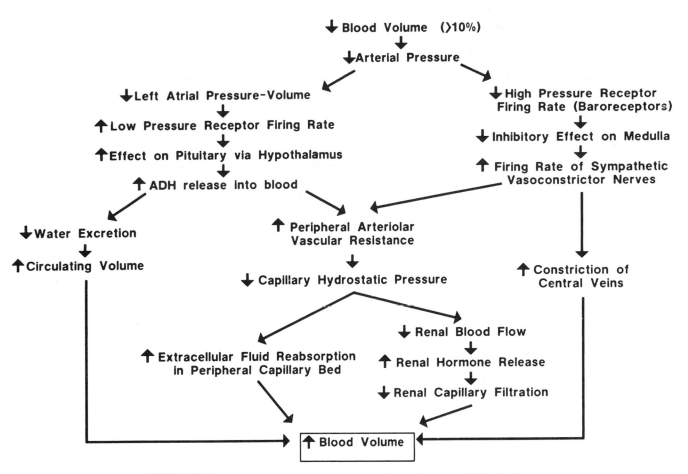

FIGURE 12-2 Compensatory mechanisms after loss of greater than 10% of blood volume.

static pressure, decreasing filtration. The net effect is an increased fluid volume in the capillaries. Decreased venous pressure and arteriolar vasoconstriction are separate factors contributing to the reduced capillary hydrostatic pressure and outward fluid movement into the vascular compartment.

In hemorrhagic shock the loss of red cells may cause a significant decrease in oncotic pressure. Coupled with an inflammatory process that alters vascular tone and endothelial permeability, there may be a significant loss of volume into the third space, further exacerbating arterial hypovolemia. If this "relative" hypovolemia is treated aggressively with volume resuscitation, the extravascular volumes may increase significantly.

Because the kidneys are considered nonessential, a reduction in renal blood flow is associated with hypovolemia. Decreased renal perfusion initiates efferent renal arteriolar vasoconstriction through the stimulation of the juxtaglomerular apparatus (a renal baroreceptor). Renin is subsequently released and is converted to angiotensin I and II by the endothelial cells of the lung and liver. Angiotensin II, a potent vasoconstrictor, raises arterial pressure and stimulates aldosterone secretion by the adrenal cortex. Aldosterone increases blood volume by increasing sodium and therefore water reabsorption in the renal tubules. The

responses to hypovolemia can occur within seconds, as occurs with increased sympathetic discharge, or can require days, as with kidney-mediated changes in water and salt excretion. All the compensatory mechanisms initially result in increased circulating blood volume in an attempt to increase stroke volume and oxygen delivery.

LIMITS OF COMPENSATION.   Blood loss can be so severe that the compensatory mechanisms cannot restore the system to normal (Figure 12-3). The most important factor in patient survival is arresting the hemorrhage. If the hemorrhage is not stopped or volume replacement is insufficient, myocardial performance deteriorates. When the arterial pressure falls low enough, coronary blood flow decreases below that required for adequate delivery of oxygen to the myocardium. The end result is deterioration of heart function. Myocardial ischemia secondary to inadequate coronary perfusion pressures reduces cardiac index, further lowering arterial pressure.

A positive-feedback cycle develops, and the initial hypovolemia leads to dire consequences. As cardiac index diminishes, cerebral perfusion is also reduced and the patient becomes increasingly obtunded. Eventually blood flow to the vasomotor center of the medulla is so depressed that the vasomotor center becomes progressively less active

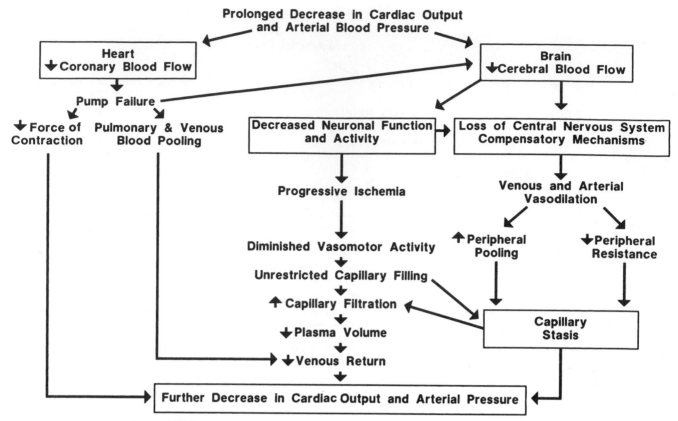

FIGURE 12-3 Negative effects of prolonged shock after loss of more than 10% of blood volume.

and finally fails. The systemic vasculature is no longer able to maintain its vascular tone; vasodilation and vascular collapse ensue. During this stage the vascular beds behave more as passive distensible tubes and no longer exhibit active adjustment to circulatory changes. Arterial vasodilation can lead to reduced blood flow to capillary beds in critical organs, whereas venous dilation causes blood to pool in the veins, decreasing venous return and further reducing cardiac index. Eventually this sluggish blood flow in the periphery leads to changes in the capillaries that increase permeability, and large volumes of fluid move out of the vascular spaces, further lowering blood volume. Unless this cycle and these conditions are reversed rapidly, survival of the patient is doubtful. Irreversible shock occurs when damage to the cells is sufficient to depress metabolic and structural functions. At this point, widespread cellular necrosis occurs in most tissues, leading to organ failure and death.

OXYGEN CONSUMPTION.   Normal cell function is dependent on the delivery of adequate oxygen and other substrates to ensure adequate adenosine triphosphate (ATP) production by the mitochondria. Delivery of oxygen (Dao_2) is dependent on the oxygen content in the arterial blood (Cao_2) and blood flow through the tissue beds (cardiac output [CO]). The hemoglobin content and oxygen saturation of hemoglobin in the arterial blood (Sao_2) and the

TABLE 12-2   Oxygen Delivery Parameters

Parameter	Formula	Normal Values
Cao_2	$(Hb \times 1.37 \times Sao_2) +$ $(0.003 \times Pao_2)$	20 ml O_2/dl
Cvo_2	$(Hb \times 1.37 \times Svo_2) +$ $(0.003 \times Pvo_2)$	15 ml O_2/dl
Dao_2I	$CI \times Cao_2 \times 10$	500-600 ml O_2/min/m^2
Dvo_2I	$CI \times Cvo_2 \times 10$	375-450 ml O_2/min/m^2

Cao_2, Arterial oxygen content; Hb, hemoglobin; Cvo_2, venous oxygen content; Dao_2I, arterial oxygen delivery index; Dvo_2I, venous oxygen delivery index; CI, cardiac index.

partial pressure of oxygen in arterial blood (Pao_2) determine Cao_2. Hemoglobin and Sao_2 are major determinants of Cao_2 because only a very small percentage of the total oxygen content of the blood is present in a dissolved state as measured by Pao_2. Table 12-2 summarizes the variables used for clinical evaluation of the adequacy of oxygen transport.

Oxygen consumption index (Vo_2I) is an indicator of tissue oxygen utilization. Vo_2I is affected by the adequacy of oxygen delivery and cellular ability to extract oxygen. In an afebrile, resting patient Vo_2I averages 140 ml O_2/min/m^2 (also calculated as 3.5 ml O_2/min/kg or 250 ml O_2/min).

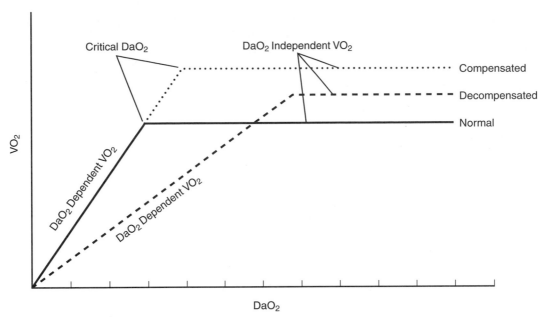

FIGURE 12-4 The relationship of oxygen delivery (Dao_2) and consumption (Vo_2), showing oxygen consumption as dependent on oxygen delivery and cellular extraction of oxygen up to a critical level where consumption becomes independent of oxygen delivery and is sustained by cellular oxygen uptake. Under normal oxygen demand conditions, increased Dao_2 is associated with a rise in Vo_2 *(solid line)*. In compensated SIRS/MODS, Dao_2 is increased to meet high oxygen demands and is also associated with a rise in Vo_2 *(dotted line)*. In decompensated SIRS/MODS, Vo_2 is insufficient to meet high oxygen demands because of altered cellular oxygen extraction, despite an increase in Dao_2 *(dashed line)*.

TABLE 12-3	**Oxygen Utilization Parameters**		
	Parameter	**Formula**	**Normal Values**
	Svo_2	Direct measurement	60%-80%
	Pvo_2	Direct measurement	35-45 mm Hg
	O_2 Extraction	Cao_2-Cvo_2	3-5 ml O_2/dl
	OER	Cao_2-Cvo_2/Cao_2	22%-30%
	Vo_2I	$(Cao_2$-$Cvo_2) \times CI \times 10$	120-170 ml/min/m^2
	pHa	Direct measurement	7.35-7.45
	BE/BD	Direct measurement	−2-+2
	Lactate	Direct measurement	0.5-2.2 mmol/l

OER, Oxygen extraction ratio; *Vo_2I*, oxygen consumption index; *pHa*, arterial pH; *BE/BD*, base excess/base deficit; for all other abbreviations see Tables 12-1 and 12-2.

The normal stress response to trauma, surgery, or well-controlled sepsis is associated with an increase in oxygen consumption of 15% to 35%.[5,6] In a critically ill, hyperdynamic patient, cellular failures of oxidative metabolism may occur even with increased perfusion and oxygen delivery (Figure 12-4). Table 12-3 summarizes the variables used for clinical evaluation of the adequacy of oxygen utilization.

In the absence of toxic metabolic failure, a mismatch between oxygen delivery and tissue demand is caused by reduced oxygen delivery in low perfusion syndromes.[7,8] Such a condition is caused by hypovolemic or cardiogenic shock, or underperfusion of localized tissue beds as a consequence of compensatory shunting of blood flow away from less essential organs and tissues. The loss of perfusion and systemic pressure causes a reduction in oxygen delivery and thus cellular Vo_2 (Figure 12-5).

Oxygen availability is the most important determinant of viable oxidative energy metabolism. Cellular oxygen consumption is influenced by the availability of oxygen delivered via the microcirculation and extraction of oxygen from the capillaries to meet cellular oxygen requirements. A reduction in oxygen delivery results in several characteristic changes. A decline in blood flow results in a greater extraction of arterial oxygen in an attempt to maintain oxygen consumption. Furthermore, a compensatory increase in sympathetic stimulation results in augmented stroke volume and/or heart rate as a mechanism to increase oxygen delivery. In hypovolemic and cardiogenic shock, an increase in proportional use of oxygen is noted. Inadequate oxygen delivery, cellular extraction, and consumption result in cellular conversion to anaerobic metabolism for energy substrate production that causes a concomitant increase in production and release of lactate. For example, after cardiac surgery, lactate concentrations rise when oxygen delivery falls below a critical value of 300 ml/min/m^2.[9] As patients progress into systemic inflammatory response syndrome (SIRS), proportional use of oxygen further decreases as cellular signaling produces metabolic failure when the cells lose their ability to extract oxygen.

CELL FUNCTION.   Maintenance of normal cellular structure and function depends on the cell's ability to synthesize large amounts of energy. The energy requirements of different cells and organs vary depending on their functions. Continuous demands for energy are dictated by cellular and subcellular membrane ion pumps necessary to maintain the internal cellular environment; by the rate of protein synthe-

sis, especially in cells with a high rate of protein turnover; and by mechanical work such as muscle contraction in cardiac and skeletal muscle (Figure 12-6). The energy reserves of the cell are limited, and the demand for energy is generally derived from the continual catabolism of various fuels, particularly glucose and fatty acids. The energy derived from metabolism of these fuels is stored in the form of ATP. ATP is synthesized by the phosphorylation of adenosine diphosphate (ADP) via three processes: oxidative phosphorylation using the mitochondrial electron-transport chain; substrate phosphorylation; and conversion of creatine phosphate to creatine, with the synthesis of ATP and ADP catalyzed by the enzyme creatine phosphokinase. Oxidative phosphorylation is by far the most important pathway for ATP synthesis, accounting for as much as 95% of the total ATP production over a wide range of ATP utilization rates in various organs.[4]

In well-oxygenated tissues the rates of oxidative phosphorylation and oxygen consumption are coupled tightly to the rate of ATP use. Mitochondrial ATP synthesis depends on a continuous supply of oxygen and substrates. Tissues cannot store oxygen; hence, effective perfusion is necessary to provide sufficient delivery of oxygen for maintenance of adequate ATP production. Thus any condition that compromises oxygen delivery to the tissues would tend to alter the mitochondrial capability to synthesize ATP via oxidative phosphorylation. The imbalance of oxygen and the ensuing anaerobic metabolic effect put the cell at risk for death.

SYSTEMIC INFLAMMATORY RESPONSE SYNDROME

PATHOPHYSIOLOGY

Systemic inflammatory response syndrome (SIRS) is both the creator and creation of shock states. SIRS is a sustained, intravascular inflammation resulting from an uncontrolled host response to multiple stimuli that continually evoke a

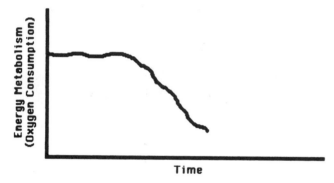

FIGURE 12-5 Oxygen consumption falls in hemorrhagic shock as the supply of oxygen to the body is reduced subsequent to the fall in circulating blood volume.

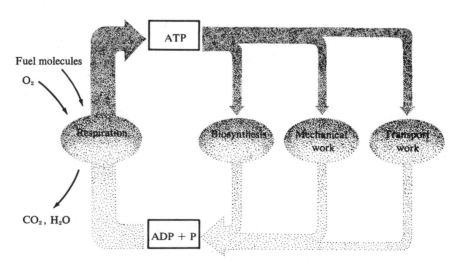

FIGURE 12-6 Relationship between energy production and energy use in maintenance of normal cell function. (From Lehninger AL: *Bio-energetics,* ed 2, Menlo Park, Calif, 1971, Benjamin, 13.)

series of cascades. These cascades create an imbalance of cellular oxygen supply and demand, which results in the hallmark oxygen extraction deficit. The presence of a bacterial invasion identifies a septic nidus and is termed septic shock, however; approximately 60% of patients will have clinical signs of sepsis without an apparent bacterial invader.[10,11]

The response to a noxious stimulus (e.g., trauma, pancreatitis, aspiration, or infection) evokes a cascade of mediator responses that in turn stimulate a secondary mediator response. Inflammatory mediators are designed to heal wounds and combat pathologic invaders through a controlled inflammatory response. However, a continuously stimulated response or a severe infection may result in a sustained inflammation (SIRS). Overwhelming SIRS occurs when the responders are continuously activated and upregulated.

Persistent inflammation is fueled by the disruption of, and further disrupts, aerobic cellular cycles, which oxidize metabolic fuels to produce ATP. As failure of these energy processes occurs, the cells become dysfunctional and can no longer maintain homeostasis. The cytokine cellular signal stimulates the immune-coagulation-inflammatory axis, which further perpetuates the hypermetabolic, hyperdynamic, and humoral response. More than 200 mediators are known. Changes in either cellular metabolism or vascular permeability can profoundly affect the delicate balance between oxygen delivery and extraction. The cells produce myriad of agents that alter vascular permeability and dynamics and cellular metabolism, promoting adhesion of molecules, catecholamines, chemotaxis, coagulation cascade, oxyradicals, and proteases.[12] The decrease in vascular resistance requires a profound increase in cardiac index in order to sustain oxygen delivery and cellular oxygen uptake. Increased vascular permeability also reduces effective arterial volume and widens capillary-cell diffusion distance, further contributing to the oxygen extraction deficit.

The resulting hypotension represents both the compensatory response, attempting to increase O_2 delivery to tissue, and a pathologic response, vasodilation caused by cascading mediators, procoagulation, and platelet aggregation. The oxygen extraction deficit is initially compensated for by an increase in Dao_2.

As oxygen deficit becomes more severe, continual inflammation at the cellular level and organ dysfunction ensue. Cells increase lactate production from anaerobic metabolism of pyruvate, the ATP ionic gradient fails, and cells begin to lyse, further contributing to the stimulating signal of the SIRS cascade. Hypermetabolic demand coupled with an acute deficit in oxygen extraction and metabolic failure are initiators of MODS.

CELLULAR SIGNALING, SIRS, SEPSIS, AND MODS

Historically infection has been considered the primary cause of SIRS and MODS; however, recent studies indicate that the precipitating inflammatory response may be independent of infection. In fact, any severe insult may stimulate the host-defense mechanisms implicated in the evolution of SIRS and MODS.

Activation of the body's host-defense mechanisms precipitates a widespread inflammatory response that is not organism specific. In fact, the inflammatory response may be independent of infection.[13,14] The innate immune system provides a first-line defense against pathogens and activates a humoral-mediated response. The evolution of an uncontrolled inflammatory response and the concomitant MODS is now recognized as a defect in cellular signaling.[15-17]

CYTOKINES. The first line of defense in resisting bacterial invasion is the macrophage. In addition to their phagocytic and bactericidal functions, macrophages rapidly release cytokines that activate other cells of the immune system and alter the host metabolism after an inflammatory insult. The role of the cytokine is to communicate messages between cells. Cytokines promote proinflammatory effects, pyrogenesis and upregulation of acute phase proteins, and an antiinflammatory response. Through their effect on both the innate and specific (acquired) immune systems, the overlapping stimulatory and inhibitory functions among the various cytokines regulate the host's response to injury, promoting control of the invading insult and tissue repair.[15] Prolonged or exaggerated elaboration of cytokines can have deleterious effects, perpetuating SIRS and contributing to MODS. Tumor necrosis factor (TNF), interleukin 1 (IL-1), and interleukin 6 (IL-6) have received the most attention as mediators of the inflammatory response.

TNF is primarily produced by macrophages, initiating a process that can lead to tissue injury and shock. It elicits a dose-responsive hypotension and can cause acute vasodilation, tachycardia, pyrexia, and hypermetabolism in both animals and human volunteers.[18,19] The primary effect is on the vascular endothelium, promoting adhesion of leukocytes and stimulating further chemokine secretion. In addition, TNF acts on hepatocytes, increasing the synthesis of the acute phase proteins, decreasing expression of albumin, and enhancing the synthesis of triglycerides.[20,21] Infusion of TNF in animals elicits many of the clinical symptoms associated with MODS, including hypotension, tachypnea, metabolite acidosis, hemoconcentration, and hyperglycemia that is superseded by hypoglycemia. At necropsy, severe thickening of the alveolar septum, ischemia of the gastrointestinal tract, renal and pancreatic hemorrhage, and renal tubular necrosis are observed. In addition, chronic exposure to low plasma concentrations of TNF induces the wasting diathesis observed in various disease states. Recent evidence also implicates the contributory role of TNF in accelerating apoptosis, or programmed cell death (PCD).[13,14] Although PCD is a homeostatic process, its acceleration via specific cell signaling accounts for the progression from SIRS to multiple organ dysfunction.

IL-1 is an additional macrophage-derived cytokine with potent biologic effects. In myelohematopoietic tissues, IL-1 is required for optimal cellular activation and proliferation and has been implicated in inducing apoptosis signaling, as well as directly affecting pancreatic cell apoptosis.[13,14] IL-1 is pyrogenic, accelerates the basal metabolic rate, increases oxygen consumption, augments skeletal muscle catabolism and consequently releases amino acids, and reduces vascular smooth muscle reactivity.[22]

IL-6 contributes both proinflammatory and antiinflammatory effects in the cascade, as well as acceleration of apoptosis. IL-6 primarily affects hepatic acute-phase protein production and is a potent pyrogenic.[15] In patients with sepsis, IL-6, IL-8, and TNF may be elevated. However, trauma patients appear to have initial elevation, then inhibition, of TNF and a primary elevation of IL-6.[23,24] Another inflammatory cytokine that has been identified and correlates with survival after severe trauma is IL-10.[23,25]

COMPLEMENT ACTIVATION.   Bacterial infection induces a complex interaction of humoral and cellular responses. The humoral response induces a primary sequence of relatively nonspecific immunologic reactions. The early responding cytokines and the acute-phase proteins such as C-reactive protein and opsonic fibronectin bind to antibody proteins on the cell walls of the offending organisms. Stimulation of the complement system elicits the generation of complement split products, collectively known as anaphylatoxins. Three of the most notable are C3a, C3b, and C5a. Both C5a and C3b possess chemotactic properties for neutrophils, macrophages, and monocytes. They serve to attract these cells to areas of inflammation, enhance their adhesiveness, and promote aggregation.[12,26] All three cell types protect against bacterial invasion by virtue of their ability to engulf bacteria via phagocytosis. Nevertheless, large-scale infiltration and activation of neutrophils, which occur with sepsis and trauma, can be detrimental to tissues rather than protective of them. Activated neutrophils release oxygen free radicals (superoxide, peroxide, and the hydroxyl radical) during phagocytosis. These toxic oxygen products normally serve a protective function by virtue of their bactericidal nature. However, if generated in sizable amounts, oxygen free radicals destroy membrane integrity, which could ultimately lead to widespread tissue injury and impairment of organ function.

This response is followed by complement activation in which C5a enhances leukocyte or macrophage aggregation and opsonization of the organism. C3a induces leukocyte production of oxygen-derived free radicals in the form of superoxides, damaging the microorganism's cell membrane. Like other complement fragments, C3a exhibits chemotaxis. However, it also causes extensive mast cell degranulation, resulting in the liberation of histamine. Histamine relaxes cell-to-cell junctions, permitting the extravasation of fluid into the interstitial spaces. It is for this reason that C3a has been implicated in the genesis of permeability edema, which may contribute to organ dysfunction.[12]

These events facilitate bacterial ingestion by the defending white cells, which promotes changes in the bacterial cell structure as well as the external environment, fostering bacterial death and lysis. Stimulation of the complement cascade has an indirect capability of triggering the activation of other enzyme cascades. These include fibrinolysis and coagulation systems, as well as the generation of prostaglandins and leukotrienes from granulocytes. These substances behave as mediators, which modulate tissue injury during sepsis and MODS. Both IL-1 and IL-2 amplify host-defense responses by stimulation of lymphocyte propagation. Moreover, these immune responses effect blast transformation and proliferation of leukocytes and promote their migration and adherence to the invading organisms and to nonviable or damaged tissues. Consequently the release of leukocyte proteases is increased, which completes the destruction of the bacteria and necrotic tissue, thereby facilitating their removal. Leukotrienes synthesized from white blood cells during this process also stimulate cellular immunity and alter the balance among suppressor, helper, and killer lymphocytes to deal with the secondary organism and tissue-specific aspects of this process.

Although cellular responses are aimed primarily at defense, sepsis may engender an overstimulation of some of these protective mechanisms. Subsequently, certain cells appear to make an abundance of a variety of substances that are postulated to intensify tissue malperfusion and injury. In a process termed "malignant inflammation," neutrophils, macrophages, lymphocytes, and perhaps platelets liberate vasoactive mediators, which may amplify the pathogenesis of the septic process as well as organ failure.

Margination of neutrophils along vascular endothelium likely leads to damage of the cells lining the blood vessels. This injury may be succeeded by exposure of plasma to the underlying collagen. Both are understood to effect activation of the coagulation cascade via Hageman factor (factor XII in the intrinsic pathway). In addition, activated neutrophils release elastase, which may also cause Hageman factor formation. Conversion of biologically inactive precursors, initiated by Hageman factor, catalyzes the synthesis of the vasoactive kinins. The most commonly formed is bradykinin, a potent vasodilator that also increases capillary permeability. Changes in capillary permeability and vasodilation, exacerbated by such substances as bradykinin, have a role in local tissue injury and malperfusion, which may amplify organ dysfunction.

Activated neutrophils extrude a variety of proteases, including elastase, cathepsin G, and collagenase. These proteases have the capability to degrade extracellular matrices if produced in surplus. Excessive free radical production associated with phagocytosis, combined with the release of these proteases, damages surrounding tissues.[27] Neutrophils, macrophages, and monocytes all are known to synthesize metabolic products of arachidonic acid catabolism. The arachidonic acid derivatives, lipid mediators called eicosanoids, include the leukotrienes, prostaglandins, and thromboxane (TX); all have been implicated in modulating the physiologic response to sepsis.

LIPID MEDIATORS

Leukotrienes. Collectively identified as slow-reacting substances of anaphylaxis, leukotrienes (LT) LTC_4, LTD_4, and LTE_4 possess the ability to alter tissue permeability, produce bronchoconstriction, and trigger vasoconstriction in some vascular beds.[28] The exact role of LTC_4, LTD_4, and LTE_4 in sepsis remains unclear; they appear to participate in regional alterations in microvascular perfusion in addition to the exacerbation of tissue edema, particularly in the lung.[28,29] Another leukotriene, LTB_4, is a potent chemotactic agent for leukocytes. Like the stimulus for the other leukotrienes, inflammation and tissue ischemia can induce generation of LTB_4. Once formed, it fosters neutrophil aggregation with release of granular constituents.[28,30] Consequently, more neutrophils are attracted to the area. The aggregation of substantial numbers of cells promotes increased free radical production and perpetuates eicosanoid synthesis. Additionally, leukocyte clumping in the microvasculature can cause mechanical obstruction to blood flow.

Thromboxane. Thromboxane, known to be elevated in trauma and sepsis, is manufactured by white blood cells and platelets, as well as by other vascular and parenchymal tissues.[12] An extremely potent vasoconstrictor, TXA_2 has the additional ability to aggregate both platelets and neutrophils. Frequently, platelet abnormalities are manifested by profound thrombocytopenia, probably as a result of complement system stimulation.[31] Once platelets aggregate, they release TX, which also enhances leukocyte aggregation, thus creating a vicious cycle. Aggregation of white cells and platelets by TX may subsequently aggravate sluggish tissue blood flow. Vasoconstriction resulting from TX synthesis may permit regions of malperfusion, intensifying tissue hypoxia. TX plays a significant role in microvascular thrombosis because it increases vascular resistance and tissue ischemia.[28]

Prostaglandin. The metabolism of arachidonic acid yields prostaglandin (PG). PG is further metabolized into TXA_2, prostaglandin E_2 (PGE_2), or prostaglandin I_2 (PGI_2). PGI_2 regulates the vasomotor tone and inhibits platelet aggregation, whereas PGE_2 contributes more to the antiinflammatory response in sepsis, inhibiting the cytokine response.[28] Prostaglandins decrease afterload and may cause significant hypotension, dilate the coronary arteries, and have antiproteolytic properties.

Free Radicals. Nitric oxide (NO) is a potent and multipurpose free radical. NO is produced by enzymatic conversion of L-arginine to NO and citrulline in the presence of oxygen catalyzed by the enzyme NO synthase (NOS). At normal production levels, NO acts as a messenger and performs as an antioxidant. At higher circulating levels, NO may become cytotoxic.[32,33] NO is one of the compounds implicated as a mediator of the sepsis-induced loss of vascular tone. Its potential involvement stems from its multifactorial role governing interactions among platelets, leukocytes, and vascular endothelium and as an endogenous vasodilator. Besides its affects on vascular tone, NO is involved in other processes considered beneficial to the septic host. These include inactivation of oxygen free radicals, prevention of microvascular thrombi, inhibition of platelet aggregation and leukocyte adhesion, bronchodilation, and protection of myocardium from ischemic damage.[33] Nitrate and nitrite are the inactive and stable end-products of NO production. Plasma concentration of nitrate and nitrite are elevated in septic patients.

Cellular products of both gram-negative (endotoxin) and gram-positive bacteria induce the iNOS form of the enzyme; this induction is cytokine mediated. The induction of iNOS can be prevented by pretreatment with glucocorticoids or inhibitors of protein synthesis. Because protein synthesis is involved in the iNOS response, NO production by this pathway occurs in a longer time frame. NO formed by endothelial NOS is an important regulator of tissue blood flow and plays an essential role in cardiovascular function. Because of its potential to modulate vascular resistance, inhibition of the NOS pathway would be anticipated to raise blood pressure and systemic vascular resistance in septic patients. However, in most studies using an inhibitor of NOS, cardiac index is reduced, heart rate falls, and pulmonary vascular resistance increases. These changes are detrimental to the host in hypodynamic septic shock, in which case the inhibition of NOS may aggravate tissue hypoperfusion.[33] Thus indiscriminate inhibition of NO production may cause more harm than good. Selective inhibition of the iNOS may provide a better therapeutic approach. The rationale is that inhibition of the inducible isoenzyme would limit the deleterious effects of NO without altering the normal actions derived from the expressed isoenzyme.

Patients with persistent inflammation present initially with an overwhelming response cascade. The most common cause of inflammatory stimulation is the local release of bacteria or other toxic mediators. Central to the host's ability to combat a bacterial insult is the immune response. The immune system limits the spread of the pathogen, augments the flux of immune cells, and modulates the host's metabolism to enhance the environment necessary for the destruction of bacteria. These changes are mediated by the factors secreted by cells of the immune system. Complement system fragments are pivotal in the synthesis of cellular and humoral mediators associated with sepsis and MODS. Severe bacterial invasion results in an excessive release of the mediators, which, in their most severe form, elicit a shock state in which inadequate tissue perfusion may lead to organ damage. These toxins stimulate cytokines that increase the inflammatory response, further generating cytokines. The cytokines affect the organs and also act through secondary mediators. The secondary mediators promote both proinflammatory and antiinflammatory responses and adhesion molecules on the endothelial cells, as well as migration of these molecules into the extravascular space, promoting microvascular and tissue injury. The endothelial injury activates the extrinsic pathway and may lead to consumptive coagulopathy and fibrin deposition. White cell and red cell clotting, along with alterations in vascular tone, contribute to the cardiovascular manifestations and systemic deficits noted in inflammatory shock.

CLINICAL EVALUATION OF SEPSIS AND TRAUMATIC SHOCK

Sepsis and hemorrhagic shock with secondary development of MODS continue to be a common cause of death in severely injured patients. The continuum of the inflammatory response and the introduction of a bacterial nidus presents in a significant pattern. Despite advances in therapy and aggressive interventions, mortality from septic shock continues to be high.

PATTERNS OF RESPONSE

HYPERDYNAMIC SEPTIC STATE. Sepsis is characterized by increased oxygen consumption, which must be met with augmented oxygen delivery. Elevated cardiac index and minute ventilation sustain increased oxygen delivery. The primary mechanisms that increase cardiac index are an increase in heart rate and reduced afterload. The diminished afterload is a consequence of reduced arteriolar tone and vasodilation. The combination of an increased cardiac index with decreased vascular resistance characterizes the hyperdynamic cardiovascular state associated with sepsis. This hyperdynamic state is necessary to meet the higher cellular energy demands required to defend against the insult and maintain normal organ function.[34,35] Although management strategies directed toward target "supranormal" values of cardiac index, oxygen delivery, and consumption have not been shown definitively to improve survival, a more critical feature may be the ability of the patient to mount and sustain an increase in cardiac index to support a hyperdynamic state.[1-3,36-41] Patients with hyperdynamic profiles typically have a cardiac index greater than 4.5 L/min/m^2 and a systemic resistance of less than 1000 dyne/sec/cm^{-5}. Although the myocardium has the potential to achieve an increase in cardiac index, this increases cardiac work and myocardial oxygen demands, which must be sustainable for days or even weeks during a septic episode.

The significant and continual demand on the heart can lead to myocardial ischemia and depression in patients with sepsis. Inadequate preload, preexisting cardiac disease, and acquired cardiac dysfunction all contribute to failure to achieve a high-output state. Preexisting cardiac disease such as stenotic valvular lesions, cardiomyopathies, and scarring from previous myocardial infarction limit the ability to increase myocardial contractility. Myocardial dysfunction in sepsis and SIRS arises from a reduction in contractility caused by mediator release (TNF, IL-1, NO) in prolonged inflammation or inadequate resuscitation after a hypovolemic episode.[42] Impaired myocardial function causes a fall

in cardiac index and reduces ejection fraction. In order to compensate for reduced blood flow to the peripheral tissues, cellular extraction of oxygen increases and is associated with widening of the arteriovenous oxygen content gradient. Hypotension and acidosis may occur if the cardiac depression is severe enough to limit oxygen delivery to the tissues or there is a cellular extraction deficit. In the septic state the increased cardiac index appears to support cell function for a time; however, transition from a high to low cardiac output state contributes to the perpetuation of sepsis-related SIRS, maldistribution of flow, and hypoperfusion of tissue beds, and thus progression to MODS.

In addition to myocardial depression, sepsis-related mediator release induces reduced systemic vascular resistance. In a large number of patients, hypotension is unresponsive to treatment with vasopressive agents or fluid resuscitation. There may be a down regulation of alpha-adrenergic receptors secondary to the high circulation of catecholamines. At the macrovascular level, sepsis-induced disturbances unresponsive to treatment are present in a majority of patients. At the microvascular level, disturbances in endothelial function give rise to increased permeability of capillaries and maldistribution of blood flow, reducing tissue perfusion and potentially causing parenchymal cell damage. Subsequent fluid extravasation widens the capillary-cell diffusion difference and further limits cellular oxygen extraction. Both vasodilation, caused by mediators such as histamine, kinins, and prostaglandins, and vasoconstriction (e.g., as a result of thromboxane and TNF release) contribute to inhomogeneous perfusion. The combined result is profound oxygen deficiency and cellular dysfunction.

ANOXIA, HYPOXIA, AND ISCHEMIA. Differentiation of anoxia, hypoxia, and ischemia is important. Although all three conditions result in diminished oxygen delivery to the tissues, the consequences of each condition with regard to energy metabolism are different. In the strictest sense, anoxia is defined as an absence of oxygen where blood flow is either normal or increased. In hypoxia the arterial oxygen content is decreased, but blood flow is maintained at normal values. Primarily, inadequate hemoglobin or Sao$_2$ and Pao$_2$ reduce oxygen transport. Ischemia is caused by decreased blood flow, which results in inadequate oxygen delivery. Ischemia differs from anoxia and hypoxia in that oxygen content is normal but blood flow is curtailed. An ischemic condition may exist when (1) blood flow falls below that required to meet the normal energy needs at rest, (2) blood flow fails to augment oxygen delivery in response to an increased oxidative demand, or (3) capillary perfusion is altered by humoral and chemical substances. Reduced blood flow also results in decreased "wash out" of the hypoperfused capillary beds and leads to accumulation of potentially harmful metabolic products in the surrounding tissues.[4] These metabolic products such as lactate or long-chain fatty acyl esters are themselves toxic to the cell and promote further damage. Therefore, ischemia may be a more detrimental insult than hypoxia or anoxia alone. The toxic metabolic byproducts encourage surrounding cell failure, and when reperfusion through previously shunted capillary beds does occur, these products are "washed out," causing damage even to distant tissues.

PHYSIOLOGIC MONITORING

Monitoring alterations in cardiac function, oxygen delivery, and metabolic response has become a standard by which to evaluate the physiologic response to posttraumatic shock and sepsis and to the management of these. Traditional endpoints for medical management of shock—that is, return of arterial blood pressure, heart rate, and urine output to normal—are inadequate. Hypoperfusion may be masked by normal vital signs in compensated shock states.[36,37,40] Specific methods for monitoring tissue oxygenation may provide a more focused perspective on peripheral perfusion and resolution of oxygen debt.

OXYGEN DELIVERY AND DEBT.

In the initial presentation of traumatic shock, both the delivery of oxygen and the oxygen extraction are affected. Hemorrhagic hypovolemia profoundly decreases DaO_2 and oxygen extraction dramatically increases in an attempt to meet oxidative requirements. Oxygen debt, the difference between cellular oxygen requirement and the actual cellular oxygen consumption, may result and must be "repaid." (Figure 12-7) If it is not, organ function may become unrecoverable. Clinical evidence of oxygen deficit includes a reduction of oxygen consumption, rising serum lactate concentration and base deficit, and derangement of other metabolic indicators. Some evidence supports increasing oxygen delivery to supranormal levels during resuscitation from traumatic shock as a means of repaying the oxygen deficit.[2] Supranormal oxygen delivery is defined as achieving predetermined goals of a cardiac index greater than 4.5 l/min/m², oxygen delivery index greater

than 600 L/min/m², and oxygen consumption index greater than 170 L/min/m². Despite the conceptual appeal of this theory, achievement of supernormal oxygen delivery goals may not improve mortality and morbidity and in fact may increase in-hospital mortality.[1,41,42]

EVALUATION OF OXYGEN UTILIZATION

Monitoring tissue oxygen uptake is an essential aspect of the clinical evaluation and management of critically ill trauma patients and is described in detail in Chapter 13. Clinical parameters used to assess oxygen delivery and utilization, their formulas, and their normal values are summarized in Tables 12-1, 12-2, and 12-3.

GLOBAL OXYGENATION MONITORING

Mixed Venous Blood Gases.   Oxygen availability is the most important determinant of viable oxidative energy metabolism. Cellular oxygen consumption is influenced by the availability of oxygen delivered via the microcirculation and extraction of oxygen from the capillaries in order to meet cellular oxygen requirements. Most organ systems use less than 50% of the available arterial oxygen. The exception is the myocardium, which extracts nearly 80% of the available oxygen in a single pass.

A reduction in oxygen delivery results in several characteristic changes. A decline in blood flow results in a greater extraction of arterial oxygen. Mixed venous blood gases (Svo_2) from the pulmonary artery may be used to evaluate the oxyhemoglobin reservoir after cellular uptake of dissolved oxygen and subsequent release of oxygen from hemoglobin to keep the dissolved oxygen relatively constant. This is a fairly global indicator of oxygen consumption at the cellular level, because Svo_2 changes may not reflect oxygen extraction in underperfused tissue beds, particularly in sepsis.[4]

Lactic Acidosis.   Plasma lactate concentration and lactic acidosis have correlated with the adequacy of resuscitation in shock and trauma patients.[36,43-51] During shock, when tissue oxygenation is reduced, mitochondrial respiration shifts to anaerobic metabolism. The cellular fuel, pyruvate, rather than being converted into acetyl coenzyme A and subsequently entering into the tricarboxylic acid cycle, is metabolized to lactate. The continued hydrolysis of ATP by cellular processes produces excessive protons, yielding a metabolic acid. Increasing oxygen delivery is a means to reverse the anaerobic processes, which is evidenced by normalization of elevated plasma lactate concentrations (>2 mmol/L).

Base Deficit.   Base deficit is an indirect, calculated measure of tissue acidosis. The measurement of base deficit is related to the amount of base in millimoles required to titrate a liter of whole blood to a pH of 7.40. As an indicator of resuscitation, base deficit correlates with the magnitude of oxygen debt accumulation and is a reasonable predictor of survival.[36,45,47,52]

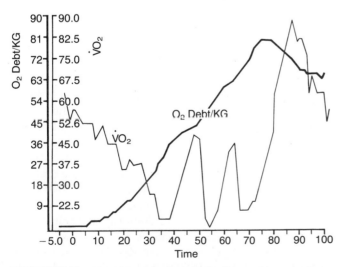

FIGURE 12-7 As oxygen consumption falls, the oxygen debt gradually accumulates. With resuscitation oxygen consumption exceeds the baseline demands, and the oxygen debt is gradually repaid.

REGIONAL OXYGEN MONITORING. As discussed, blood flow and perfusion are not uniformly distributed to all organs. Investigators suggest that it is advantageous to identify and monitor those tissue beds that are significantly at risk for under-perfusion in shock.

Intramucosal pHi. Reduced splanchnic perfusion reflects early signs of hypoperfusion in shock.[53] Tonometry, used to evaluate perfusion of the gastric or intestinal mucosal bed, may allow earlier detection of systemic hypoperfusion. Evaluation of gut perfusion via measurement of gastric mucosal pH (pHi) is based on the assumption that gastric mucosal bicarbonate equals serum bicarbonate. Intramucosal measurement of hydrogen ions via a saline-filled silicone balloon can be used to calculate pHi. Reduced blood flow to the gastrointestinal mucosa causes anaerobic metabolism in these tissue beds and thus a decrease in pHi. Early identification of altered perfusion provides an opportunity to optimize resuscitation efforts and more quickly reverse oxygen debt accumulation.[53,54] Normalization of gastric pH has been shown to be useful as an endpoint for resuscitation in critically ill surgical patients, as well as a predictor of survival.[54,55] However, gastric arterial CO_2 gradient and pHi are more difficult to interpret in sepsis. The anticipated normalization of pHi may not occur in septic patients despite interventions to reverse hypoperfusion.[56-59]

LOCAL OXYGEN MONITORING. Near infrared spectroscopy (NIRS) provides a noninvasive method for the monitoring of oxidized cytochrome aa_3. Oxyhemoglobin absorbs infrared light poorly, and NIRs waves may be passed easily through the skin and tissue. NIRs use in evaluating tissue oxygen saturation, as well as cytochrome aa_3, has been shown to correlate with presently accepted methods for determining resuscitation.[60-63] An early reduction in cytochrome aa_3 despite normal oxygen delivery has been demonstrated in trauma patients.

Peripheral tissues may provide a more complete and preferable indicator of the adequacy of resuscitation in shock. Using fiberoptic probes, skeletal muscle monitoring in recent studies more accurately reflected the level of oxygen delivery required to maximize perfusion. Differences between the evaluation of tissue oxygenation and skeletal muscle oxygenation have been proposed.[61-63]

HEMODYNAMIC MONITORING

The management of multi-injured trauma patients is guided, in part, by parameters measured by a pulmonary artery catheter (PAC), which evaluates left ventricular function and adequacy of intravascular volume and provides intermittent or continuous measurement of mixed venous blood gases and pH. An assumption underlying PAC data interpretation is that changes indicative of left ventricular function will be reflected by the right-sided heart catheter. In a patient in cardiac failure but without preexisting pulmonary disease, this assumption typically is true. However, the information is influenced by changes in the compliance of the right side of the heart, intrathoracic pressures, and the compliance of the pulmonary vasculature, as well as the equal derivatives from the left side of the heart. The PAOP provides an estimation of left ventricular preload; however, it also may be beneficial in evaluating right ventricular ejection fraction and end-diastolic volume to assess the adequacy of preload. In the previously healthy trauma patient, the importance of evaluation of the right side of the heart is at least as significant as assessment of left ventricular function.[64] During and after control of hemorrhage, the major therapeutic effort in trauma is aggressive volume resuscitation. Evaluation of end-diastolic volume as it relates to the Frank-Starling curve (i.e., increasing initial myocardial fiber length to enhance contractile force and stroke volume) is an established principle of resuscitation of the trauma and septic patient population. Careful interpretation of elevated PAOP, RAP, and pulmonary artery pressures is warranted in the presence of a high cardiac index, arterial hypotension, or hypoperfusion as evaluated by tissue metabolic indicators of hypoxia and oxygen debt accumulation. Because PAC-derived parameters are affected by ventricular compliance, pulmonary vascular vasoconstriction, and airway pressure, PAOP and RAP may not be reliable indicators of end-diastolic volume and preload.[64-66] Other traditional indicators for adequate volume resuscitation, such as blood pressure, heart rate, and urine output, are also unreliable as indicators of intravascular and end-diastolic volumes.[37,66,67]

Earlier studies noted a high incidence of right ventricular dysfunction in the trauma and shock population. This is possibly related to increased right ventricular stress and volume overload secondary to acute pulmonary hypertension.[66,67] An associated elevation of PAOP more likely is due to pulmonary hypertension and the inability of the right ventricle to adjust contractile tension to volume and resistance loads, causing a leftward shift of the intraventricular septum and reducing left ventricular compliance. Right ventricular end-diastolic volume index therefore may be a more appropriate indicator of ventricular preload than traditional PAOP.[66-69]

Initially the trauma patient in hemorrhagic hypovolemic shock displays symptoms of tachycardia, hypotension, base deficit, low PAOP and RAP, low stroke index, and systemic shunt. After appropriate volume resuscitation, the patient will generally improve and metabolic indicators of oxygen debt accumulation normalize. Subsets of trauma patients do not improve or have a secondary nidus that triggers SIRS. These patients develop cellular hypoxia and organ dysfunction as a result of humoral mediator and oxygen free radical release, capillary endothelial changes, reduction in ATP production, and mitochondrial dysfunction. Their clinical presentation subsequently includes an increasing cardiac index, reduced systemic vascular resistance, tachycardia, normal to low RAP and PAOP, and metabolic acidosis. As shock or SIRS progresses, cardiac index continues to be elevated; RAP, PA pressures, and PAOP increase; and severe metabolic acidosis ensues.

METABOLIC CHANGES ASSOCIATED WITH IMPAIRED OXYGEN DELIVERY

Reduction in oxygen availability leaves intermediates in the electron-transport chain in a more reduced state. Phosphorylation of ADP via oxidative phosphorylation ceases despite reduced ATP and increased ADP concentrations (Figure 12-8). Creatine phosphate concentrations decline by 80% to 90% within minutes, followed by a slower decline in ATP.[70-72]

This imbalance between energy production and energy utilization results in altered adenine nucleotide metabolism. Initially, high-energy phosphates stored as creatine phosphate are utilized to maintain cellular ATP concentrations near normal. However, the amount of high-energy phosphates the cell can store is limited, and creatine phosphate concentrations are depleted within 5 minutes of the onset of ischemia. After the depletion of creatine phosphate, ATP concentrations begin to fall. The reduction in ATP concentrations is accompanied by a rise in ADP and AMP. As the duration of ischemia is increased, this alteration becomes more pronounced. In addition, there is a fall in the sum of the adenine nucleotides (ATP + ADP + AMP). The concentration of adenine nucleotides may be of importance in maintaining cell viability, as well as in the ability of the cell to recover normal function after restoration of normal blood flow (Figure 12-9).[70-72]

During ischemia the breakdown of ATP for cellular metabolic needs leads to relatively high cellular concentrations of hypoxanthine and xanthine. Reoxygenation of the ischemic area presents oxygen to the large pools of substrate or the enzyme xanthine oxidase, which is felt to be contained in the capillary endothelium, showering the capillary endothelium of the compromised tissues with superoxide free radicals. Once the initial xanthine oxidase-mediated capillary injury has occurred, complement activation can attract leukocytes to the affected area, resulting in cellular death. The monitoring of xanthine oxidase may be used as an indicator of tissue oxygenation in the future.

Simple oxygen deficiency does not itself cause irreversible tissue damage. If the oxygen supply is restored within several minutes, both ATP synthesis and tissue function return to normal. However, if the reduction in oxygen supply is continued, the tissue becomes irreversibly damaged (Figure 12-10). Many hypotheses have been put forward to account for this transition of viable to irreversibly injured cells, and research related to achievement of "supranormal" oxygen delivery has not conclusively demonstrated prevention or preservation of cell function as was anticipated. Because ATP functions as the energy source, much attention has been focused on the role of ATP in reperfusion. Reperfusion and restoration of oxygen delivery to ischemic tissue result in the rapid resynthesis of creatine phosphate, but ATP concentrations remain depressed.

Although a relationship between survival and oxygen deficit has been demonstrated,[73] perhaps a finer relationship can be drawn between oxygen deficit and morphologic and functional injury to cells. It appears that as ischemia worsens cellular perfusion, there is intracellular accumulation of

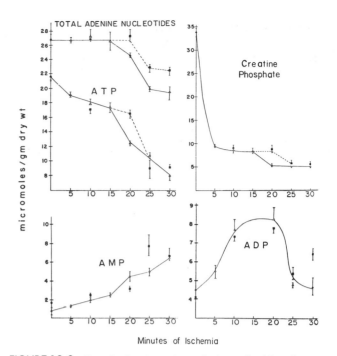

FIGURE 12-8 Effect of ischemia on tissue adenine nucleotide and creatine phosphate concentrations. Hearts were perfused with Krebs-Henseleit solution, supplemented with either glucose *(triangles)* or glucose plus acetate *(squares)* for a 15-minute equilibration period. The hearts were then exposed to a period of severe global ischemia and rapidly frozen. (From Vary TC, Angelakos ET, Schaffer SW: Relationship between adenine nucleotide metabolism and irreversible tissue damage in isolated perfused rat heart, *Circ Res* 45[2]:220, 1979.)

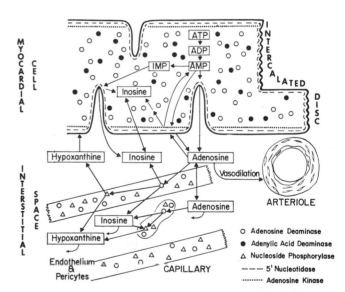

FIGURE 12-9 Formation, fate, and site of action of adenosine. The distribution of the different enzymes involved in the metabolism of adenosine is illustrated by the different symbols defined at the right of the diagram. (From Rubio R, Wiedmeier T, Berne RM: Nucleoside phosphorylase: localization and role in myocardial distribution of purines, *Am J Physiol* 222[3]:554, 1972.)

lactic acid and hydrogen ions. Eventually changes in cell membrane and function occur, followed by influx of sodium and potassium extrusion. This causes increased activity of sodium-potassium ATPase. As discussed earlier, there is a decreased production of ATP during ischemia. Conse-

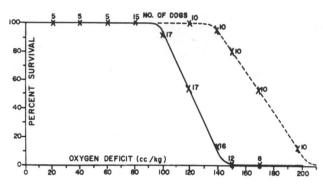

FIGURE 12-10 The total oxygen deficit has been shown to be an excellent quantitative predictor of survival after hemorrhagic shock in the dog model. The *solid line* shows the survival rate for control animals at various oxygen deficits; the *dashed line* shows the survival rate for digitalized animals. (From Crowell JW, Smith EE: Oxygen deficit and irreversible hemorrhagic shock, *Am J Physiol* 206:313, 1964.)

quently the chemiosmotic balance of the intracellular environment is disrupted, leading to intracellular swelling. Mitochondria and cell organelles are disrupted, which ultimately results in cell death.

MODULATION OF NUTRIENT SUBSTRATE FLUX BY SEPSIS

In humans and animals there is a fine balance between anabolism, the building up of energy stores, and catabolism, the breakdown of these energy stores. The adaptive ability of the organism to use alternative fuels instead of glucose is of fundamental importance to the survival of the individual. This is because certain cells such as erythrocytes and cells of the renal medulla and central nervous system have an absolute requirement for glucose, amounting to approximately 180 g/day. Less than half this demand can be supplied simply by the breakdown of glycogen to glucose in the liver. However, the liver and, to a certain extent, the kidneys synthesize glucose from different carbon sources via the process of gluconeogenesis. Glucose is synthesized from glycerol, lactate, pyruvate, and certain amino acids. Glycerol is obtained from adipose tissue after the breakdown of triglycerides. Lactate and pyruvate are derived primarily from skeletal muscle tissue secondary to the breakdown of skeletal muscle glycogen. Amino acids are derived from protein degradation, particularly in skeletal muscle.

When reduced oxygen supply limits oxidative energy production, ATP produced glycolytically via substrate phosphorylation is increased. In cardiac muscle, the maximal rate of glycolytically produced ATP represents only about 25% of the normal energy requirements. In ischemia there is a transient increase in glycolysis that results primarily from the breakdown of glycogen. However, if flow is reduced to a low enough level, the transient increase in glycolysis is succeeded by an inhibition of glycolysis to a rate about 10% the rate observed in anoxia. The mechanism responsible for this difference between ischemia and anoxia appears to be related to the buildup of metabolic products in ischemia. Flux through glycolysis becomes restricted by the accumula-

tion of metabolic products, particularly lactate, which are not removed from the ischemic tissue during poor perfusion.[70-72]

Although oxygen can become rate limiting for energy production, a reduction in blood flow also decreases the delivery of carbon substrates for oxidative metabolism. In anoxia the tissues are oxygen deficient, but flow is fast enough to remove metabolic products and prevent glycolytic inhibition. Under these conditions, glycolysis is maximally stimulated. However, when flow is reduced (<3 ml/g/min), glycolysis becomes inhibited. This suggests that glycolytic inhibition during ischemia is more dependent on flow than on oxygen availability. Oxidation of fatty acids is inhibited in proportion to decreased availability and is not flow dependent other than to the extent that flow affects oxygen delivery.

SEPTIC CATABOLISM

Physiologic monitoring of the septic patient has demonstrated that the normal balance between anabolic and catabolic processes is altered in the direction of catabolic metabolism.[74-76] This results in pathologic alterations in glucose, fatty acid, and amino acid (protein) metabolism, often manifested clinically by mild hyperglycemia, a rise in serum triglycerides, and changes in plasma amino acid and acute-phase protein concentrations. The degree of metabolic dysfunction is ultimately indicative of the extent of organ dysfunction induced by invading organisms or traumatic injury. The pattern of alterations in the plasma concentrations of these fuels is superimposed over changes in the plasma concentration of hormones and cytokines.[74-78] Trauma and sepsis initiate a pattern of physiologic and metabolic adaptation characterized initially by an increase in protein metabolism.[79,80] Severe infection and trauma evoke an interwoven network of responses all designed to limit the extent of damage elicited by the initial insult. Virtually every organ system of the body becomes affected and displays recognizable metabolic alterations.

HORMONAL CHANGES IN SEPSIS

Typically sepsis is characterized by a fall in the thyroid hormone T_3, whereas the other stress hormones (cortisol, epinephrine, and glucagon) are elevated. Glucagon concentrations rise to extraordinarily high levels. Although the rise in glucagon is accompanied by a rise in immunoassayable insulin, the insulin/glucagon ratio is reversed compared with its value in the postabsorptive state. This reversal of the insulin/glucagon ratio may be responsible in part for the accelerated rate of glucose production by the liver in sepsis. Both insulin and glucagon have immediate and delayed effects on hepatic glucose metabolism.

Catecholamines also stimulate both glycogenolysis and gluconeogenesis. The levels of plasma catecholamines epinephrine and norepinephrine have been demonstrated to rise progressively with increasing severity of injury.[75,77-79] Both epinephrine and norepinephrine rise to levels considered high enough to produce metabolic changes. In this regard, plasma epinephrine concentrations are more important for stimulating hyperglycemia than is the severity of the injury itself.

The stimulation of hepatic output of glucose by epinephrine involves the breakdown of glucagon with the release of glucose. However, changes in the hormonal milieu are not solely responsible for enhanced gluconeogenesis in sepsis. Unlike other pathologic conditions such as starvation or diabetes, in sepsis gluconeogenesis is not suppressed by the infusion of glucose.[76,81] This lack of response to glucose has been proposed to occur as a result of enhanced and continual delivery of gluconeogenic precursors, namely lactate, alanine, glycine, serine, and glycerol, from peripheral tissues.[76]

INSULIN RESISTANCE IN SEPSIS.   Abnormal glucose tolerance tests are commonly observed after traumatic injury, burn, shock, or sepsis despite normal or accentuated insulin secretion. The primary sites of insulin resistance are in systemic tissues, particularly skeletal muscle and adipose tissue, where insulin stimulates glucose uptake. This insulin resistance is manifested by either an abnormal glucose tolerance test or simply an elevated plasma glucose concentration for a given insulin concentration. Evidence suggests that the insulin concentration is the same or increased in sepsis; no antiinsulin antibodies have been detected. At the receptor level, alterations in receptor affinity or receptor number also would decrease the biologic response for a given plasma insulin concentration. However, the sensitivity of the receptor to circulating insulin appears to be normal.[81-83] There is a marked decrease in the extent of tyrosine phosphorylation of the insulin-receptor phosphorylation of IRS-1 in response to insulin during sepsis.[83] Thus the septic process affects the initial steps in the signal transduction pathway for insulin.

With regard to the potential mediators responsible for the sepsis-induced insulin resistance, evidence indicates a potential link between TNF and insulin resistance. First, plasma concentrations of TNF-alpha are increased after infection.[84] Second, TNF blocks the action of insulin through its ability to inhibit insulin receptor tyrosine kinase activity.[85-88] Third, obesity-induced insulin resistance is prevented in mice lacking a functional TNF response.[89] Fourth, inhibition of TNF secretion improves insulin action limiting skeletal muscle catabolism and lactate production after infection.[90]

REGULATION OF GLUCOSE METABOLISM IN SEPSIS.   Variations in carbohydrate metabolism after severe trauma and during sepsis include hyperglycemia, increased gluconeogenesis with an increased output of glucose from the liver, elevated blood lactate, and insulin resistance. Hyperglycemia and hyperlactatemia are frequent manifestations of the human metabolic response to sepsis and are implicated in the clinical development of the process.[91]

Sepsis-induced hyperlactatemia with concomitant acidosis is most easily explained when the septic shock episode is associated with tissue ischemia secondary to hypoperfusion.

Under these circumstances, augmenting oxygen delivery through increasing volume resuscitation and cardiac index reduces the lactate production.[45,50,51]

In contrast to the hypodynamic septic state, the hemodynamically stable, hyperdynamic, and hypermetabolic phase of sepsis is characterized by an elevated cardiac index and augmented oxygen consumption, maintenance of normal high-energy phosphate contents in skeletal muscle, and normal lactate/pyruvate ratios.[92] Enhancing oxygen delivery does not decrease plasma lactate concentration in these patients.[43,44] The failure of plasma lactate concentrations to abate after increasing oxygen delivery indicates that metabolic abnormalities other than inadequate oxygen delivery are responsible for the elevation of serum lactate in patients with stable hyperdynamic sepsis.[76] Thus hyperlactatemia results from altered control of glucose metabolic pathways rather than a deficit in oxygen availability in the hyperdynamic septic patient.

LACTATE METABOLISM IN SEPSIS
Interorgan Lactate Metabolism in Sepsis.   The plasma lactate concentration represents a balance between the rate of lactate production and its utilization. The liver and kidney are primarily responsible for uptake and utilization of lactate, whereas systemic tissues such as skeletal muscle represent the major sites of lactate production. The lactate that diffuses into the bloodstream is carried to the liver, where it is taken up and either oxidized or reconverted into glucose. Release of lactate from skeletal muscle, its transport and removal from the blood, and its subsequent resynthesis into glucose by the liver represents an interorgan physiologic pathway. An imbalance in metabolism will lead to changes in the plasma concentration. The increased lactate production by skeletal muscle provides the necessary gluconeogenic precursors for maintenance of sustained rates of gluconeogenesis in sepsis. Lactate production exceeds its use, accounting for elevated plasma lactate concentrations in sepsis.

Role of Pyruvate Dehydrogenase Complex in Controlling Lactate Production.   Impaired glucose oxidation in conjunction with normal or increased lactate, alanine, and/or pyruvate production suggests a specific inhibition of the pyruvate dehydrogenase (PDH) reaction in sepsis. The PDH complex catalyzes the mitochondrial decarboxylation of pyruvate into acetyl CoA, which is a key participant in glucose homeostasis (Figure 12-11). Thus entry of glucose carbon into the tricarboxylic acid cycle may be limiting for glucose oxidation in sepsis. The inhibition of the complex during sepsis provides a biochemical explanation for the shift in skeletal muscle glucose metabolism in sepsis.[92]

The mediators responsible for the inhibition of PDH complex during sepsis remain unclear. A frequent common denominator of organ dysfunction and organ failure during sepsis is the abnormal release of cytokines, particularly by the macrophage. TNF is implicated as playing a pivotal role in mediating some of the metabolic responses to sepsis.

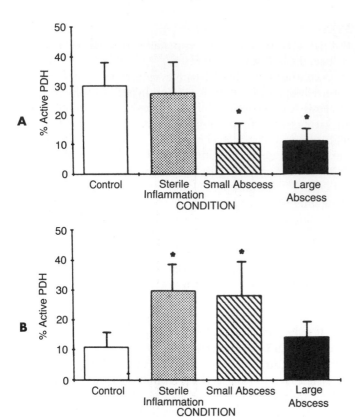

FIGURE 12-11 Effect of sepsis on activity of pyruvate dehydrogenase complex in skeletal muscle (**A**) and liver (**B**). Skeletal muscle and liver samples were frozen in situ 5 days after intraabdominal introduction of a rat fecal agar pellet. Four groups of animals were used: control (no pellet); sterile inflammation (no bacterial inoculation); small septic abscess (*Bacteroides fragilis* 10^8/ml + *Escherichia coli* 10^6/ml; 0.8 ml pellet); and large septic abscess (*B. fragilis* 10^8/ml + *E. coli* 10^2/ml; 1.5 ml pellet). Extracts of frozen tissue were assayed for active and total pyruvate dehydrogenase (PDH) activity in duplicate. Results are presented as a percentage of total PDH complex existing in active form. Values shown are means ± SE for 10 to 14 animals. * P < 0.005 versus control, Scheffe's analysis for all contrasts. (From Vary TC, Siegel JH, Nakatani T et al: Effect of sepsis on activity of pyruvate dehydrogenase complex in skeletal muscle and liver, *Am J Physiol* 250[6 Pt 1]:E636, 1986.)

Attenuation of the TNF response using either a TNF-binding protein[93] or inhibitors of TNF secretion[90] prevent inhibition of PDH complex and attenuate the hyperlactatemia. This observation is consistent with the perspective that altered control of key regulatory enzymes is important in determining the extent of carbohydrate dyshomeostasis in hypermetabolic, hyperdynamic septic states.

Activation of PDH Complex Activity After Hemorrhagic Shock.   Because down-regulation of PDH complex may contribute to hyperlactatemia, the potential role of PDH complex during shock and after resuscitation has been examined. The importance of these studies to human sepsis is that patients whose clinical course is shifted from a stable hemodynamic state to a shock state are more apt to succumb. Dichloroacetate improves survival in a canine model of hemorrhagic shock.[94] Activation of PDH complex with dichloroacetate improves cardiac function in reper-

fused ischemic myocardium,[95] suggesting enhanced cardiac function may be the explanation for improved survival. Dichloroacetate restores diminished ATP contents from endotoxin-treated animals and improves cardiac function and metabolism in the heart after hemorrhagic[95] or endotoxin-induced shock.[96]

Hyperlactatemia in Sepsis.   Altered lactate metabolism plays an important role in the development and clinical complications of sepsis. Hyperlactatemia is a prognostic indictor of organ failure and mortality in critically ill septic patients.[97] Sepsis-induced hyperlactatemia can be easily explained when tissue ischemia exists. In the hyperdynamic, hypermetabolic state of sepsis, oxygen consumption and oxygen delivery are increased, with adequate tissue perfusion and maintenance of normal high-energy phosphate concentrations. The hyperlactatemia is present under conditions in which tissue oxygen delivery is elevated. The ratio of lactate to pyruvate is unchanged, suggesting that the increased plasma lactate does not result from inadequate oxygen delivery.

Increased plasma lactate concentrations in sepsis result from either an increased production or decreased utilization or both. The liver is the major organ responsible for lactate clearance by the body. Lactate taken up by the liver is synthesized to glucose by the pathway of gluconeogenesis. Although the rate of glucose production by the liver is increased in sepsis, the rate of lactate delivery may exceed the capacity for gluconeogenesis. The sepsis-induced increases in plasma lactate probably result from a combination of metabolic abnormalities. Sepsis-induced alterations of skeletal muscle carbohydrate metabolism include increased glucose uptake, accelerated lactate production, and decreased glucose oxidation in muscle.

ALTERED SKELETAL MUSCLE PROTEIN METABOLISM.   In addition to its role in locomotion and respiration, skeletal muscle, by virtue of its mass in relation to body weight, represents the major reservoir of amino acids (Figure 12-12). Some of these amino acids are important substrates for gluconeogenesis in liver and kidney. A hallmark of the septic response is the rapid erosion of lean body mass. The imbalance in protein metabolism leading to loss of lean body mass is manifested by excretion of urea, resulting in a large negative nitrogen balance. The septic condition initiates one of the most severe catabolic responses known. Positive nitrogen balance in septic patients cannot be achieved through aggressive nutritional support alone. Nitrogen losses of 150 to 320 g (or approximately 5% to 17% of body protein) are commonly observed over the course of a septic episode (see Chapter 16). Because skeletal muscle comprises approximately 45% of body weight, the sepsis-induced whole-body negative nitrogen balance reflects increases in net catabolism in this tissue. Mobilization of amino acids from skeletal muscle results from an increase in proteolysis or a decrease in protein synthesis. The relative contribution of protein synthesis and proteolysis to the

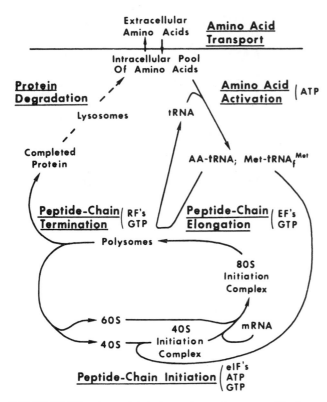

FIGURE 12-12 Pathway of skeletal muscle protein turnover. The figure schematically depicts the major steps involved in protein synthesis and in protein degradation. *ATP*, Adenosine triphosphate; *GTP*, guanosine triphosphate; *tRNA*, transfer RNA; *AA-tRNA*, aminoacyl-transfer RNA; *Met-tRNA$_f^{Met}$*, the initiator methionyl-transfer RNA; *eIF's*, eukaryotic initiation factors; *mRNA*, messenger RNA; *EF's*, elongation factors; *RF's*, releasing factors; *40S* and *60S*, small and large ribosomal subunits, respectively. (From Jefferson LS: Role of insulin in the regulation of protein synthesis, *Diabetes* 29[6]:488, 1980.)

overall net catabolic state in muscle varies depending on the severity of the septic insult. In this regard, protein synthesis is reduced to the same extent regardless of the severity of the septic insult, whereas protein degradation continues to accelerate as the septic episode worsens. The persistent loss of large amounts of protein in sepsis leads to organ system dysfunction and eventually organ failure. Clinical implications of continued loss of skeletal muscle protein in septic patients include poor wound healing, loss of muscle strength, diminished muscle activity, and, if severe enough, death.

Increased net proteolysis results in the release of amino acids from structural protein stores, particularly in skeletal muscle. The rate of release of amino acids across the lower extremities increases two- to fivefold in trauma or septic patients compared with healthy volunteers after an overnight fast. The protein economy of the whole body can be estimated by monitoring the nitrogen balance, and the contribution of muscle tissue can be monitored by measuring the rate of 3-methylhistidine production. 3-Methylhistidine is liberated from muscle in proportion to its concentration in muscle protein.[98] This catabolic phase is an intrinsic response to trauma and sepsis, with the amount of muscle loss exceeding that simply because of bed rest. In trauma

patients the catabolic phase abates within a few days of injury and is followed by the restoration of positive nitrogen balance and lean body mass. In contrast to trauma, the catabolic phase continues in sepsis, even when exogenous nutritional support is provided. Skeletal muscle makes a significant contribution to the rise in whole-body protein breakdown. The rate of muscle protein breakdown increases to a greater degree than that of the whole body, with the contribution of muscle proteolysis to whole-body protein degradation nearly doubling.

Mediators of Proteolysis. A certain amount of muscle catabolism in the trauma patient can be attributed to direct injury to the muscle, with subsequent repair of the damaged tissues. However, enhanced catabolism also occurs in the septic patient with no overt signs of direct tissue trauma. The metabolic milieu of the septic host is complex. The catabolism of muscle is probably the net result of interactions between multiple mediators and regulatory pathways. The potential mediators of muscle catabolism and negative nitrogen balance in sepsis can be broadly divided into two categories: hormones and cytokines. Altered responsiveness to both stress hormones (glucocorticoids, glucagon, and epinephrine) and anabolic hormones (insulin, growth hormone, and insulin-like growth factors) have been implicated in causing the sepsis-induced metabolic derangement in protein turnover. Studies in burn patients have suggested that cortisol is a major determinant of the catabolic response.[99] Some of the effects of cortisol have been confirmed in healthy volunteers subjected to an artificial elevation of cortisol to levels seen in burn patients. However, in the postoperative state, and most probably sepsis, cortisol is of less importance, because the metabolic effects appear to be the net result of an integrated response to hormones and cytokines.

Insulin conserves muscle protein by both stimulating protein synthesis and inhibiting protein degradation.[100,101] However, in sepsis the breakdown of muscle protein, as measured by 3-methylhistidine release, is increased despite increased insulin concentration.[98] Furthermore, animal studies have shown both a decreased sensitivity and maximal response to the inhibitory effects of insulin on protein degradation in sepsis.[76,90,102] These observations also suggest that additional factors resulting from the septic episode accelerate muscle catabolism or that injury renders the muscle resistant to insulin action.

Cytokines are polypeptides released by activated macrophages or lymphocytes in response to infection or trauma. Serum concentrations of the inflammatory cytokines TNF, IL-1, and IL-6 are elevated after infection.[21] Furthermore, administration of TNF or IL-1 to healthy animals mimics many of the cardiovascular and metabolic sequelae observed in septic patients.[21] Cytokines bind to specific receptors on target cells to modulate cellular function. They may circulate in the bloodstream, acting in a endocrine fashion, or exhibit tissue-specific synthesis/activity in a paracrine manner. The association of enhanced plasma cytokine concentrations with derangement in protein metabolism has led to the hypothesis that cytokines are proximal mediators of the septic insult and important regulators of protein metabolism in skeletal muscle. Increased muscle proteolysis induced by incubating muscle strips with serum from septic patients has led to the hypothesis that a serum factor expressed as a result of sepsis is responsible for the accelerated muscle catabolism.[102-105] More recently the evidence indicates that modulation of the cytokine response can prevent or lessen the acceleration of sepsis in both animals[102] and humans.[103] IL-1 and a low-molecular-weight protein, called proteolysis-inducing factor, have been isolated from blood obtained from trauma and septic patients.

Acute-Phase Protein Metabolism.   Trauma and sepsis increase the hepatic synthesis and secretion of a number of proteins referred to as acute-phase proteins. The acute-phase proteins include C-reactive protein, fibrinogen, ceruloplasmin, and alpha-1-antitrypsin. Many of these acute-phase proteins are linked to the host's ability to resist or control infection. These functions include complement activation and opsonization needed for bacterial killing (C-reactive protein); coagulation, surface structure and support lattice formations needed for leukocyte entrapment of foreign material (fibrinogen); superoxide scavenging (ceruloplasmin); and inactivation of excess proteases needed to prevent damage to viable cells (alpha-1-antitrypsin). A differential pattern in the plasma acute-phase protein profile has been demonstrated in trauma and septic patients[106] (Figure 12-13). The presence of sepsis, whether clinically evident or not, modifies the posttraumatic acute-phase protein response to favor the increase of some acute-phase proteins while effecting a decrease in the concentration of other proteins that may not be as critical for survival.

LIPID METABOLISM IN SEPSIS

Dependence on Fatty Acid Metabolism.   The metabolic course of the traumatized or septic patient shows that fatty acids become the preferred fuel for oxidative metabolism. This conclusion is based on analysis of respiratory quotients and indirect calorimetry studies.[107-109] Fatty acids are stored as triglycerides in adipose tissues. Sepsis accelerates the breakdown of triglycerides in adipose tissue with the net result being the release of fatty acids into plasma at a rate far in excess of their oxidation. For tissues that use fatty acids for oxidative fuels, the rate of oxidation of fatty acids is proportional to plasma fatty acid concentrations. Thus large increases in availability of fatty acids leads to a greater reliance on fatty acids as energy sources.[110,111] The accelerated fatty acid oxidation is manifested by a fall in respiratory quotient in septic patients.

. Fatty acids released continually into the bloodstream are delivered to the liver. After removal from the plasma, fatty acids may undergo either oxidation for energy and ketone body production or esterification to triglycerides (Figure 12-14). A significant proportion of fatty acids taken up by the liver are re-esterified, leading to accelerated hepatic

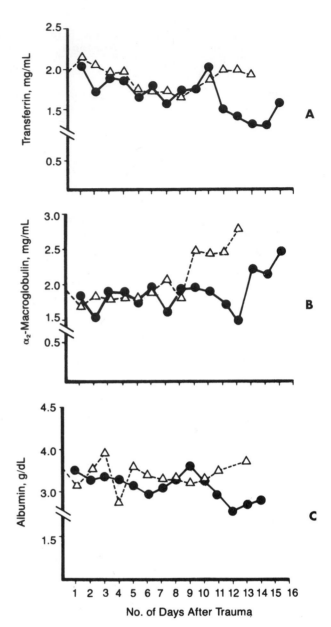

FIGURE 12-13 Plasma acute-phase protein concentrations after trauma in 16 patients *(open triangles)* and trauma complicated by sepsis in 10 patients *(solid circles)*. Mean values for transferrin (**A**), α_2-macroglobulin (**B**), and albumin (**C**) in patients with sepsis developing after trauma are compared with nonseptic trauma patients. Most changes occur only after patients become clinically septic between 5 and 7 days. (From Sganga G, Siegel JH, Brown G et al: Reprioritization of hepatic plasma protein release in trauma and sepsis, *Arch Surg* 120[2]:192, 1985.)

triglyceride formation.[110] Acetyl-CoA synthesis catalyzes the activation of fatty acids to fatty acetyl-CoA esters, which are further metabolized in either anabolic (triglyceride formation) or catabolic (oxidation) pathways. Endotoxin and the proinflammatory cytokines TNF and IL-1 enhance fatty acid synthesis and re-esterification. Lipopolysaccharides (LPS) and cytokines decrease mitochondrial acetyl-CoA synthesis, which may limit oxidation, but increase microsomal mitochondrial acetyl-CoA synthesis, which may support re-esterification of peripherally derived fatty acids for hepatic triglyceride synthesis.[112] A large increase in hepatic

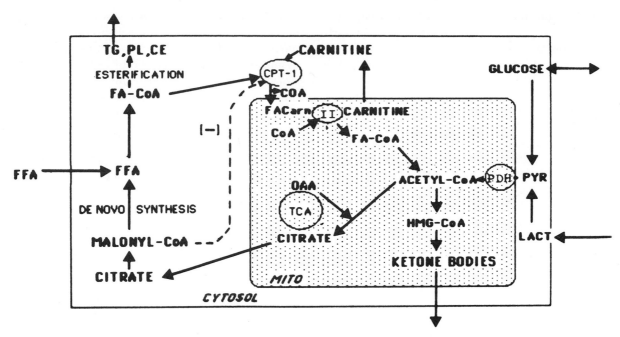

FIGURE 12-14 Relationships of hepatic fatty acid oxidation, ketogenesis, and fatty acid synthesis (---). Malonyl-CoA inhibition of carnitine:acyl-CoA transferase I. Carnitine:acyl-CoA transferases are bound to the inner mitochondrial membrane in vivo, but for clarity the reactions are shown away from membrane. *FFA*, long-chain fatty acids; *FA-CoA*, long-chain fatty acyl-CoA; *FACarn*, long-chain fatty acyl-carnitine; *CoA*, coenzyme A; *OAA*, oxaloacetate; *PYR*, pyruvate; *LACT*, lactate; *TCA*, citric acid cycle; *TG*, triglycerides; *PL*, phospholipids; *CPT-I*, carnitine:acyl-CoA transferase I; *II*, carnitine:acyl-CoA transferase II; *PDH*, pyruvate dehydrogenase complex; *MITO*, mitochondria. (From Vary TC, Siegel JH, Nakatani T et al: A biochemical basis for depressed ketogenesis in sepsis, *J Trauma* 26[5]:420, 1986.)

triglycerides can ensue if the rate of excretion of triglycerides in very low density lipoproteins is not accelerated to the same extent as triglyceride formation. Indeed, elevated hepatic triglyceride levels are a characteristic feature of sepsis.

Virtually all studies of fulminant sepsis have demonstrated increased plasma triglycerides as the septic process worsens. In addition to an increase in hepatic triglyceride synthesis, the systemic triglyceride disposal mechanisms may be impaired. The activity of lipoprotein lipase, the enzyme responsible for clearance of plasma triglycerides, is reduced in both adipose tissue and muscle from septic animals.[113,114] Concomitant with the lowered lipoprotein lipase activity, plasma triglyceride concentrations are increased. TNF is responsible for lowering lipoprotein lipase activity by reducing lipoprotein lipase synthesis in sepsis.

Reduced Ketone Bodies. The normal response of the liver to increased delivery of fatty acids is the synthesis of ketone bodies (3-L-hydroxybutyrate and acetoacetate). In addition, reversal of the insulin/glucagon ratio enhances the ketogenic capacity of the liver. In sepsis there is a rise in the glucagon/insulin ratio, but the hepatic and plasma ketone body concentrations are lower than expected given the hormonal environment. The lack of elevated plasma ketones does not indicate a lack of fatty acid oxidation, because these patients have respiratory quotients of 0.75, indicative of fat oxidation. Sepsis appears to induce changes in hepatic fatty acid metabolism, which prevents or reverses maximal rates of ketogenesis.[115,116]

Failure of hepatic tissue to enhance ketogenesis is important to the clinical outcome of the septic episode, because survival depends on normal liver function. A decrease in the circulating ketone body concentrations would be expected to increase the dependence of systemic tissues on alternative substrates for energy production when cellular metabolism is accelerated by sepsis. The failure to effect similar increases in plasma ketone bodies in nondiabetic septic patients may be an additional factor in the markedly increased rates of proteolysis in septic patients.

Lipogenesis in Sepsis. Ketogenesis may be inhibited during sepsis, but lipogenesis appears to be accelerated. In septic patients receiving only glucose in excess of 800 cal/m², the respiratory quotient rises above 1.0, indicative of net lipogenesis.[107] The capacity to synthesize lipids is increased, suggesting an increased flow of acetyl groups toward fatty acid synthesis and away from ketone body function. These observations support the concept of a reciprocal relationship between lipogenesis and ketogenesis, thus preventing both fatty acids and ketone bodies from being synthesized simultaneously, which would result in an energy-wasting futile cycle.

METABOLIC DYSFUNCTION DURING MODS

Successful resuscitation with repayment of the oxygen debt may improve the patient's well-being in the hours immediately following the trauma episode. However, some combination of inflammatory stimuli, cellular signaling, and ischemia-reperfusion injuries change the stabilized early postresuscitation presentation of many trauma patients. Early stratification of an at-risk group may be essential to treatment and prevention. For example, investigators evaluated trauma patients over 10 years and identified that those with an Injury Severity Score (ISS) of greater or equal to 25 and who had received six or more units of packed cells had a 46% risk of developing MODS and a mortality risk of 30%.[117] Others have defined the MODS score in relationship to number and severity of organ involvement.[118,119] The consistent finding, however, is that significant organ dysfunction is present by 24 hours after injury in the majority of patients who develop multiple organ failure.[120]

MULTIPLE ETIOLOGIC FACTORS

All basic research, as well as clinical practice, supports the hypothesis that the pathogenesis of MODS relates to prolonged systemic inflammatory activation. Immediately after traumatic injury and resuscitation patients progress into a mild, host-beneficial SIRS. The primary factors associated with the development of severe SIRS, MODS, and organ failure have been well documented and include ISS,[117,121] blood transfusions,[122,123] coagulopathy,[124,125] and infectious processes.[10,126,127]

Previously it was commonly accepted that MODS was the expression of an occult septic focus (usually intraabdominal). In operations for intraabdominal sepsis, organ failure developed in 30% to 50% of cases and carried a mortality rate between 30% and 100%, depending on the number of organ systems affected. In the past, two thirds of patients dying of MODS demonstrated an intraabdominal abscess as the bacterial focus.[128] However, as more patients with MODS underwent exploratory laparotomies, it became evident that MODS could exist in the absence of an identifiable bacterial focus. One study reported that only 25% of patients dying of MODS had a major infection at autopsy, only one of which was intraabdominal. Patients dying of MODS and sepsis have enteric bacteremia for which no identifiable focus at autopsy is noted. It is now recognized that bacteria in the gut can lead to infection through translocation or surface spread after the disruption of the intestinal mucosa.[129]

Changes in the intestinal flora coupled with impairment of the normal barrier function of the gastrointestinal tract allow the bowel to serve as a reservoir for pathogens. Bacteria or their products (such as endotoxin) can enter the portal and systemic circulations and initiate a septic process or perpetuate an ongoing septic process. Gut-derived bacteria or endotoxins contribute to the development of MODS in the patient without evidence of infection. In the presence of bacterial translocation, decontamination of the gut with selective suppression of lumina flora would be expected to reduce not only nosocomial infections but also mortality. Although a decline in infection rates has been noted, significant reductions in the incidence and mortality associated with sepsis and MODS have not been achieved.[130-133]

Although the precise mechanisms involved in the failure of organ systems as a consequence of sepsis remains unknown, in those patients who die, the process of organ dysfunction appears metabolic in origin. Sepsis alters the dynamic flux of metabolic substrates between skeletal muscle, gut, kidney, and liver. In the process that culminates in the clinical syndrome of organ failure, instead of the metabolic response to injury abating, hypermetabolism persists. Hypermetabolism represents a phase of altered metabolic regulation that becomes pathologic as the organ failure phase begins. The metabolic dysfunction may be related to either altered hormonal environment, generation of host inflammatory or immunologic mediators, or enhanced substrate fluxes overloading an already damaged organ system. Most likely all three mechanisms are necessary for the manifestation of multiple organ failure in the critically ill patient. This metabolic dysfunction is associated with the development of profound anergy, lymphopenia, inadequate wound healing, and, if left uncorrected, death. The metabolic adaptations in the posttraumatic or septic state are unique and are sometimes different from the physiologic responses in fasting, exercise, starvation, diabetes, and other pathologic conditions. As described, two early manifestations of organ dysfunction in sepsis are a massive excretion of urea and alterations in glucose kinetics resulting in increased rates of glucose appearance. The degree of metabolic dysfunction is indicative of the extent of organ dysfunction induced by the invading organism or inflammatory response to traumatic injury.

ORGAN INTERRELATIONSHIPS IN MODS

Organ and system dysfunction is the sum of individual cellular failures. Thus there most likely exists at any given time a wide spectrum of metabolic and functional abnormalities within any given organ system. Organ dysfunction occurs only when enough cells of that particular organ system fail. The progressive deterioration of two or more organs over a brief period is defined as MODS. Failure of an individual organ affects all organs because of the interdependence of all organ systems and homeostatic mechanisms of the whole individual. For example, hypovolemia or severe myocardial depression also results in hypoperfusion of other organ systems, with the subsequent effects of decreased oxygen delivery to the previously healthy tissues.

After severe trauma, respiratory distress is a common complication necessitating mechanical ventilatory support. In addition, there may be renal, hepatic, gastrointestinal, cardiovascular, and/or metabolic failure. In the absence of severe traumatic injury, individual failure of each of these organ systems is more easily managed and likelihood of effective treatment may be high. However, in the presence of posttraumatic SIRS or whenever two or more of these systems are failing, the mortality from MODS increases. Numerous reports have shown a relationship between the number of organ systems involved and the likelihood of death. One organ system failure is associated with a 40% mortality. The mortality rate increases to 60% with two dysfunctional organs and may be up to 100% as four or more organs fail.[119,134-136] The combination of respiratory failure with renal failure, metabolic failure, or cardiac failure is associated with poor prognosis, particularly in the presence of sepsis.

CLINICAL PROGRESSION

The classic MODS syndrome in trauma patients is described by a pattern of injury, adult respiratory distress syndrome, and hypermetabolism followed by sequential organ failure.[119,137,138] The onset of MODS begins with a low-grade fever, tachycardia, and dyspnea, with appearance of infiltrates on chest radiographs but normal liver and renal function tests. Dyspnea progresses until endotracheal intubation and mechanical ventilatory assistance are required. Initial compensatory mechanisms promote hemodynamic stabilization, often associated with a cardiac index over 5 $L/min/m^2$ and a systemic vascular resistance of less than 600 $dyne/sec/cm^{-5}$. Vo_2 may be greater than 180 $ml/min/m^2$.[139] Hyperglycemia is prevalent in the absence of diabetes mellitus or pancreatitis, and hyperlactatemia and increased urea nitrogen excretion (>15 g/day) are observed, consistent with the hypermetabolic state.

After 7 to 10 days, bilirubin begins to rise progressively, approaches 10 mg/dl, heralding the onset of hepatic dysfunction. Accompanying the increased bilirubin, serum creatinine begins to rise. The hyperdynamic cardiovascular state and hypermetabolism become more pronounced. Bacteremia associated with enteric organisms, positive culture of pathogens, usually gram-negative, from tracheal aspirate, urine, and wounds is not uncommon. Poor peripheral perfusion causes impaired wound healing and development of skin breakdown at pressure points. Positive inotropic support and intravascular volume administration are increasingly required to maintain preload and myocardial contractility, and Dao_2. Between day 14 and 21 compensatory mechanisms begin to fail, and hemodynamic instability ensues despite aggressive intervention. Renal dysfunction worsens and dialysis may be required. By day 21 survivability is doubtful, and death often ensues within 21 to 28 days after the initial insult.[139]

Microbial factors alone do not dictate the host response to traumatic injury. SIRS with progression to MODS can occur without an initial bacterial infection. A number of years ago this observation led to the modification of the definition of sepsis. Consistent definitions of the response to injury and infection were developed by an American College of Chest Physicians and Society of Critical Care Medicine Consensus Conference (Table 12-4).[140] Clinicians previously used the term *sepsis* to refer to the "septic-like" clinical presentation and systemic manifestations of the response to injury even when bacteria could not be cultured. The clinical signs of sepsis such as fever, tachycardia, tachypnea, and leukocytosis were, in fact, those of SIRS.

Simple SIRS/sepsis may progress to severe SIRS/sepsis with the presence of acute organ dysfunction, hypoten-

---

TABLE 12-4 Definitions of Systemic Inflammatory Response Syndrome (SIRS) and Sepsis

SIRS

Response to a variety of severe clinical insults having two or more of the following conditions:

Temperature >38° C or <36° C

Heart rate >90 beats/min

Respiratory rate >20 breaths/min or $Paco_2$ <32 torr

WBC >12,000 cells/mm^3, <4000 cells/mm^3, or >10% immature (band) forms

Infection

Inflammatory response to the presence of microorganisms or the invasion of a normally sterile host by microorganisms.

Sepsis

Systemic response to infection, manifested by two or more of the SIRS criteria as a consequence of infection.

Severe Sepsis

Sepsis associated with organ dysfunction, hypoperfusion, or hypotension; hypoperfusion and perfusion abnormalities may include, but are not limited to, lactic acidosis, oliguria, and an acute alteration in mental status.

Septic Shock

Sepsis with hypotension despite adequate resuscitation with fluids, with the presence of perfusion abnormalities that may include, but are not limited to, lactic acidosis, oliguria, and an acute alteration in mental status; patients receiving inotropic or vasopressor agents may not be hypotensive when perfusion abnormalities are measured.

Hypotension

Systolic blood pressure of less than 90 mm Hg or a reduction of more than 40 mm Hg from baseline in the absence of other causes for hypotension.

MODS

Presence of altered organ function in an acutely ill patient; homeostasis cannot be maintained without intervention.

SIRS, systemic inflammatory response syndrome; *MODS*, multiple organ dysfunction syndrome; *WBC*, white blood cells.

---

sion, or hypoperfusion, and eventually to shock, as hypotension persists despite adequate fluid resuscitation. MODS is the failure of cell and organ function associated with acute illness in which normal homeostasis cannot be maintained. MODS may be a direct result of a well-defined insult or a multiplicity of interreacting pathophysiologic events.

MANAGEMENT

Paramount to the immediate resuscitative effort in the trauma population is the control of hemorrhage. Temporizing and resuscitative efforts are designed to halt oxygen deficit accumulation and repay oxygen debt. Treatment of underlying infections with the correct antibiotic(s) is important for survival (see Chapter 14).

The magnitude of oxygen deficit is directly related to survival and most likely also related to the extent of multiple organ failure that follows a shock episode. Significant oxygen debt accumulation may occur before arrival at the trauma center. The rate and magnitude of accumulation influence the development of cellular dysfunction and lethal metabolic injury. Rapid correction of hypoperfusion is essential (see Chapter13). Although resuscitation endpoints are controversial and definitive evidence supporting use of target endpoints is still lacking, most experts use a combination of base deficit, lactate, and other regional or local tissue perfusion indicators.[36,47,49,139]

Although the mainstay of resuscitation is intravascular volume administration, the types of fluid used and the optimal hemoglobin concentration are not definitive in the literature. Persistent or refractory hypotension may require vasoconstrictive agents to maintain arterial pressure and cardiac index. Catecholamine administration should be evaluated in respect to splanchnic blood flow[57,58] and renal perfusion.[141-143] As catecholamine sensitivity is altered in sepsis, higher doses than usual may be required. However, the requirement for vasopressor support in severe and progressive MODS appears to be associated with nonsurvival.[144]

Despite aggressive management of shock, mortality remains between 40% and 60%. Newer therapies are focused on the metabolic inflammatory processes. Corticosteroid trials and anticytokine therapies have not had the expected positive results in the prevention and treatment of SIRS and sepsis.[136,138,145-148] Studies investigating endotoxin modulation and therapies directed at neutrophil adhesion molecules, among others, are currently underway.

SUMMARY

Severe multiple trauma that overwhelms the numerous compensatory mechanisms designed to stabilize a life-threatening situation results in a complex series of pathophysiologic processes. Subsequent hemorrhagic shock and sepsis result in cellular dysfunction and are reflected in altered hemodynamic and metabolic statuses. The diagnosis and effective treatment of posttrauma shock states is guided by an understanding of these pathophysiologic events and the risk of sequential or multiple organ failure. Although MODS may have many causes in the patient with traumatic injuries, two of the most common are hypovolemia and sepsis. Of the two, the pathophysiology of hypovolemia is best understood and, as a consequence, more readily managed. Because of its more complex nature, sepsis is more difficult to manage in the trauma patient and is associated with higher mortality.[149] Significant advances have been made in the understanding of the pathophysiology of SIRS and MODS; however, much remains to be elucidated. Laboratory and clinical investigations will continue to broaden our knowledge of the complex processes involved in inflammation, sepsis, and MODS and contribute to exploration of more effective prevention and management strategies.

REFERENCES

1. Durham RN, Neunaber K, Mazuski J et al: The relationship of oxygen consumption and delivery as end points for resuscitation in critically ill patients, *J Trauma* 41(1):32-40, 1996.
2. Bishop MH, Shoemaker WC, Appel PL et al: Relationship between supranormal circulatory values, time delays, and outcomes in severely traumatized patients, *Crit Care Med* 21(1):56-63, 1993.
3. Ronco JJ, Fenwick JC, Tweeddale MG et al: Identification of the critical oxygen delivery for anaerobic metabolism in critically ill septic and nonseptic humans, *JAMA* 270(14):1724-1730, 1994.
4. Kearney ML: Imbalance of oxygen supply and demand. In Secor VH, editor: *Multiple organ dysfunction and failure*, St. Louis, 1996, Mosby, 135-147.
5. Siegel JH: Pattern and process in the evolution of and recovery from shock. In Siegel JH, Chodoff PD, editors: *The aged and high risk surgical patient*, New York, 1976, Grune & Stratton, 381-455.
6. Cuthbertson DP: Post-shock metabolic response, *Lancet* 1:433-436, 1942.
7. Shoemaker WC, Lim L, Boyd DR: Sequential hemodynamic events after trauma to the unanesthetized patient, *Surg Gynecol Obstet* 132:1033-1038, 1971.
8. Shoemaker WC: Pathophysiologic basis of therapy for shock and trauma syndromes, *Semin Drug Treat* 3(3):211-229, 1973.
9. Komatsu T, Shibutani K, Okamoto K: Critical level of oxygen delivery of cardiopulmonary bypass, *Crit Care Med* 15(3):194-197, 1987.
10. Waydhas C, Nast-Kolb D, Jochum M et al: Inflammatory mediators, infection, sepsis, and multiple organ failure after severe trauma, *Arch Surg* 127(4):460-467, 1992.
11. Papathanassoglou ED, Moynihan JA, Ackerman MH: Does programmed cell death (apoptosis) play a role in the development of multiple organ dysfunction in critically ill patients? A review and theoretical framework, *Crit Care Med* 28(2):537-549, 2000.
12. Secor VH: The systemic inflammatory response syndrome: role of mediators in multiple organ dysfunction syndrome. In Secor VH, editor: *Multiple organ dysfunction and failure*, St. Louis, 1996, Mosby, 19-45.
13. Haslett C: Granulocyte apoptosis and inflammatory disease, *Br Med Bull* 53(3):669-683, 1997.
14. Savill J: Apoptosis in resolution of inflammation, *J Leukoc Biol* 61(4):375-380, 1997.
15. Oberholzer A, Oberholzer C, Moldawer LL: Cytokine signaling: regulation of the immune response in normal and critically ill states, *Crit Care Med* 28(4):3-12, 2000.
16. Trinchieri G: Interleukin-12: a pro-inflammatory cytokine with immunoregulatory functions that bridge innate resistance and antigen-specific adaptive immunity, *Annu Rev Immunol* 13:251-276, 1995.
17. Gabay C, Kushner I: Acute phase proteins and other systemic responses to inflammation, *N Engl J Med* 340(6):448-454, 1999.

18. Tilg H, Trehu E, Atkins MB et al: Interleukin-6 as an anti-inflammatory cytokine: induction of IL-1 receptor antagonist and soluble tumor necrosis factor, *Blood* 83(1): 113-118, 1994.

19. Evans DA, Jacobs DO, Revhaug A et al: The effects of TNF and their selective inhibition by ibuprofen, *Ann Surg* 209(3): 312-321, 1989.

20. Tracey KJ, Lowry SF, Fahey TJ 3d et al: Cachectin/tumor necrosis factor induces lethal shock and stress hormone responses in the dog, *Surg Gynecol Obstet* 164(5):415-422, 1987.

21. Martin C, Boisson C, Haccoun M et al: Patterns of cytokine evolution (tumor necrosis factor-alpha and interleukin-6) after septic shock, hemorrhagic shock and severe trauma, *Crit Care Med* 25:1813-1819, 1997.

22. Giannoudis PV, Smith RM, Banks RE et al: Stimulation of inflammatory markers after blunt trauma, *Br J Surg* 85(7): 986-990, 1998.

23. Majetschak M, Borgermann J, Waydhas C et al: Whole blood tumor necrosis factor-alpha and its relation to systemic concentrations of interleukin 4, interluekin 10, and transforming growth factor-beta-1 in multiply injured blunt trauma victims, *Crit Care Med* 28(6):1847-1853, 2000.

24. Tschaikowsky K, Sagner S, Lehnert N, et al: Endothelin in septic patients: effects on cardiovascular and renal function and its relationship to proinflammatory cytokines, *Crit Care Med* 28(6):1854-1860, 2000.

25. Keel M, Ungethum U, Steckholzer U et al: Interleukin-10 counterregulates proinflammatory cytokine-induced inhibition of neutrophil apoptosis during severe sepsis, *Blood* 90(9):3356-3363, 1997.

26. Astiz M, Saha D, Lustbader D et al: Monocyte response to bacterial toxins, expression of cell surface antigens, and the release of anti-inflammatory antigens during sepsis, *J Lab Clin Med* 128(6):594-600, 1996.

27. Petrak RA, Balk RA, Bone RC: Prostaglandins, cyclooxygenase inhibitors and thromboxane synthetase inhibitors in the pathogenesis of multiple system organ failure, *Crit Care Clin* 5(2):303-314, 1989.

28. Bugler EM, Maier RV: Lipid mediators in the pathophysiology of critical illness, *Crit Care Med* 28(4 Suppl): N27-N36, 2000.

29. Knoller J, Schoenfeld W, Joka T et al: Generation of leukotrienes in polytraumatic patients with adult respiratory distress syndrome, *Prog Clin Biol Res* 236:311-316, 1987.

30. Smith MJH, Ford-Hutchinson AW, Bray MA: Leukotriene B: a potential mediator of inflammation, *J Pharm Pharmacol* 32(7):517-518, 1980.

31. Dries DJ: Activation of the clotting system and complement after trauma, *New Horiz* 4(2):276-288, 1996.

32. Ancarcrona M, Dypbukt JM, Brune B et al: Interleukin-1 beta-induced nitric oxide production activates apoptosis in pancreatic RIN m5F cells, *Exp Cell Res* 213(1):172-177, 1994.

33. Liaudet L, Soriano FG, Szabo C: Biology of nitric oxide signaling, *Crit Care Med* 28[4 Suppl]: N37-N52, 2000.

34. Siegel JH: Cardiorespiratory manifestations of metabolic failure in sepsis and the multiple organ failure syndrome, *Surg Clin North Am* 63(2):379-399, 1983.

35. Siegel JH, Cerra FB, Coleman B et al: Physiological and metabolic correlations in human sepsis, *Surgery* 86(2): 163-193, 1979.

36. Third European Consensus Conference in Intensive Care Medicine: Tissue hypoxia: how to detect, how to correct, how to prevent, *Am J Respir Crit Care Med* 154(5):1573-1578, 1996.

37. Abou-Khalil B, Scalea TM, Trooskin SZ et al: Hemodynamic responses to shock in young trauma patients: need for invasive monitoring, *Crit Care Med* 22(4):633-639, 1994.

38. Shoemaker WC, Appel P, Kram HB: Tissue oxygen debt as a determinant of lethal and nonlethal postoperative organ failure, *Crit Care Med* 16(11):1117-1120, 1988.

39. Shoemaker WC, Montgomery ES, Kaplan E et al: Physiologic patterns in surviving and nonsurviving shock patients, *Arch Surg* 106(5):630-636, 1973.

40. Shoemaker WC, Appel P, Bland R: Use of physiologic monitoring to predict outcome and to assist clinical decisions in the critically ill postoperative patients, *Am J Surg* 146(1): 43-50, 1983.

41. Gattinoni L, Brazzi L, Pelosi P et al: A trial of goal-oriented hemodynamic therapy in critically ill patients, *N Engl J Med* 333(16):1025-1032, 1995.

42. Gates DM: Myocardial dysfunction in sepsis and multiple organ dysfunction syndrome. In Secor VH, editor: *Multiple organ dysfunction and failure*, St. Louis, 1996, Mosby, 252-275.

43. Yu M, Burchell S, Takiguchi S et al: The relationship of oxygen consumption measured by indirect calorimetry to oxygen delivery in critically ill patients, *J Trauma* 41(1):32-40, 1996.

44. Weil MH, Afifi AA: Experimental and clinical studies on lactate and pyruvate as indicators of the severity of acute circulatory failure, *Circulation* 41(6):989-1001, 1970.

45. Mizock BA: Lactic acidosis in critical illness, *Crit Care Med* 20(6):80-93, 1992.

46. Dunham CM, Frankenfield D, Belzberg H et al: Inflammatory markers: superior predictors of adverse outcome in blunt trauma patients? *Crit Care Med* 22(4):667-672, 1994.

47. Bakker J, Gris P, Coffernils M et al: Serial blood lactate levels can predict the development of multiple organ failure following septic shock, *Am J Surg* 171(2):221-226, 1996.

48. Maniskis P, Jankowski S, Zhang H et al: Correlation of serial blood lactate levels to organ failure and mortality after trauma, *Am J Emerg Med* 13(6):619-622, 1995.

49. Friedman G, Berlot G, Kahn RJ et al: Combined measurements of blood lactate concentrations and gastric intramucosal pH in patients with severe sepsis, *Crit Care Med* 23(7):1184-1193, 1995.

50. Dunham CM, Siegel JH, Weireter L et al: Oxygen debt and metabolic acidemia as quantitative predictors of mortality and the severity of the ischemic insult in hemorrhagic shock, *Crit Care Med* 19(2):231-243, 1991.

51. Vincent JL, Dufaye P, Berre J et al: Serial lactate determinations during circulatory shock, *Crit Care Med* 11(6):449-451, 1983.

52. Rutherford EJ, Morris JA Jr, Reed GW et al: Base deficit stratifies mortality and determines therapy, *J Trauma* 33(3): 417-422, 1992.

53. Gutierrez G, Brown SD: Gastrointestinal tonometry: a monitor of regional dysoxia, *New Horiz* 4(4):413-419, 1996.

54. Barquist E, Kirton O, Windsor J et al: The impact of antioxidant and splanchnic-directed therapy on persistent uncorrected gastric mucosal pH in the critically injured trauma patient, *J Trauma* 44(2):355-359, 1998.

55. Ivatury RR, Simon RJ, Islam S et al: A prospective randomized study of end points of resuscitation after major trauma: global oxygen transport indices versus organ-specific gastric mucosal pH, *J Am Coll Surg* 183(2):145-154, 1996.

56. Lorente J, Ezpeleta A, Esteban A et al: Sytemic hemodynamics, gastric mucosal PCO_2 changes, and outcome in critically ill burn patients, *Crit Care Med* 28(6):1728-1735, 2000.

57. Silverman MJ, Tuna P: Gastric tonometry in patients with sepsis: effects of dobutamine and packed red blood cell transfusion, *Chest* 102(1):184-188, 1992.

58. Marik PE, Mohedin M: Contrasting effects of dopamine and norepinephrine on systemic and splanchnic oxygen utilization in hyperdynamic sepsis, *JAMA* 272(17):1354-1357, 1994.

59. Forrest D, Baigorri F, Chittock D: Volume expansion using pentastarch does not change gastric arterial CO_2 gradient or gastric mucosal pH in patients who have septic syndrome, *Crit Care Med* 28(7):2254-2258, 2000.

60. Beilman GJ, Groehler KE, Lazaron V et al: Near-infrared spectroscopy measurement of regional tissue oxyhemoglobin saturation during hemorrhagic shock, *Shock* 12(3):196-200, 1999.

61. Piantodosi CA, Jobsis-Vander Vliet FF: Near infrared optical monitoring of intact skeletal muscle during hypoxia and hemorrhagic hypotension in cats, *Adv Exp Med Biol* 191:855–862, 1985.

62. McKinley BA, Marvin RG, Cocanour CS et al: Tissue hemoglobin O_2 saturation during resuscitation of traumatic shock monitored using near infrared spectrometry, *J Trauma* 48(4):637-642, 2000.

63. McKinley BA, Ware DN, Marvin RG et al: Skeletal muscle pH, PCO_2, and PO_2 during resuscitation of severe hemorrhagic shock, *J Trauma* 45(3):633-636, 1998.

64. Chang MC, Mondy JS III, Meredith JW et al: Redefining cardiovascular performance during shock resuscitation: ventricular stroke work, power, and the pressure-volume diagram, *J Trauma* 45(3):470-478, 1998.

65. Calvin JE, Driedger AA, Sibbald WJ: Does the pulmonary capillary wedge pressure predict left ventricular preload in critically ill patients, *Crit Care Med* 9(6):437-443, 1981.

66. Chang MC, Meredith JW: Cardiac preload, splanchnic perfusion, and their relationship during resuscitation in trauma patients, *J Trauma* 42(4):577-584, 1997.

67. Diebel LN, Wilson RF, Tagett MG et al: End-diastolic volume: a better indicator of preload in the critically ill, *Arch Surg* 127(7):817-821, 1992.

68. Chang MC, Mondy JS III, Meredith JW et al: Clinical application of ventricular end-systolic elastance and the ventricular pressure-volume diagram, *Shock* 7(6):413-419, 1997.

69. Chang MC, Blinman TA, Rutherford EJ et al: Preload assessment in trauma patients during large-volume shock resuscitation, *Arch Surg* 131(7):728-731, 1996.

70. Neely JR, Vary TC, Liedtke AJ: Substrate delivery in ischemic myocardium. In Tillsmanns H, Kubler W, Zebe H, editors: *Microcirculation of the heart,* Berlin, 1982, Springer-Verlag.

71. Vary TC, Angelakos ET, Schaffer SW: Relationship between adenine nucleotide metabolism and irreversible tissue damage in isolated perfused rat heart, *Circ Res* 45(2):218-225, 1979.

72. Reibel DK, Rovetto MJ: Myocardial ATP synthesis and mechanical function following oxygen deficiency, *Am J Physiol* 234(5):H620-H624, 1978.

73. Crowell JW, Smith EE: Oxygen deficit and irreversible hemorrhagic shock, *Am J Physiol* 206:313-316, 1964.

74. Liddell MJ, Daniel AM, McClean LD et al: Role of stress hormones in the catabolic metabolism of shock, *Surg Gynecol Obstet* 149(6):822, 1979.

75. Marchuk JB, Finley RJ, Groves AC et al: Catabolic hormones and substrate pattern in septic patients, *J Surg Res* 23(3):117, 1977.

76. Vary TC: Inter-organ protein a carbohydrate relationships during sepsis: necessary evils or uncanny coincidences, *Curr Opin Clin Nutr Metab Care* 2(3):235-242, 1999.

77. Frayn KN, Little RA, Maycock PF et al: The relationship of plasma catecholamines to acute metabolic and hormonal responses to injury in man, *Circ Shock* 16(3):229-240, 1985.

78. Davies CL, Newman CJ, Molyneaux SG et al: The relationship between plasma catecholamines and severity of injury in man, *J Trauma* 24(2):99-105, 1984.

79. Vary TC, Siegel JH: Sepsis, abnormal metabolic control and multiple organ failure syndrome. In Siegel JH, editor: *Trauma: emergency surgery and critical care,* New York, 1987, Churchill Livingstone, 411-501.

80. Vary TC: Regulation of skeletal muscle protein turnover during sepsis, *Curr Opin Clin Nutr Metab Care* 1(2):217-224, 1998.

81. Black PR, Brooks DC, Bessey PQ et al: Mechanism of insulin resistance following injury, *Ann Surg* 196(4):420-425, 1982.

82. Vary TC, Drnevich D, Jurasinski CV et al: Mechanisms regulating skeletal muscle glucose metabolism in sepsis, *Shock* 3(6):403-410, 1995.

83. Fan J, Li Y, Wojnar M, et al: Endotoxin-induces alterations in insulin-stimulated phosphorylation of insulin receptor, 1RS-1, and MAP kinase in skeletal muscle, *Shock* 3(6):164-170, 1996.

84. Chang H, Bristian B: The role of cytokines in the catabolic consequences of infection and injury, *J Parenter Enteral Nutr* 22(3):156-166, 1998.

85. Feinstein R, Kanety H, Papa M et al: Tumor necrosis factor-alpha suppresses insulin-induced tyrosine phosphorylation of insulin receptor and its substrates, *J Biolog Chem* 268(35):26055-26058, 1993.

86. Kroder G, Bossenmaier B, Kellerer M et al: Tumor necrosis factor-alpha and hyperglycemia-induced insulin resistance: evidence for different mechanisms and different effects on insulin signaling, *J Clin Invest* 97(6):1471-1477, 1996.

87. Peraldi P, Hotamisligil G, Buurman W et al: Tumor necrosis factor (TNF)-alpha inhibits insulin signaling through stimulation of the p55 receptor and activation of sphingomyelinase, *J Biol Chem* 271(22):13018-13022, 1996.

88. Peraldi P, Spiegelman B: TNF-alpha and insulin resistance: summary and future prospects, *Mol Cell Biochem* 182(1-2):169-175, 1998.

89. Uysal T, Wiesbrock S, Marino M et al: Protection from obesity-induced insulin resistance in mice lacking TNF-alpha function, *Nature* 389(6651):610-614, 1997.

90. Vary TC, Dardevet D, Obled C et al: Modulation of skeletal muscle lactate metabolism during epsis by insulin or insulin-like growth factor-I: effects of pentoxifylline, *Shock* 7(6):432-438, 1997.

91. Vincent JL, Dufaye P, Berre J et al: Serial lactate determinations during circulatory shock, *Crit Care Med* 11(6):449-451, 1983.

92. Vary TC: Down regulation of pyruvate dehydrogenase complex in skeletal muscle during sepsis: Implications for sepsis-induced hyperlactatemia, *Sepsis* 2:303-312, 1998.

93. Vary TC, Hazen SA, Maish III G et al: TNF binding protein prevents hyperlactatemia and inactivation of PDH complex in skeletal muscle during sepsis, *J Surg Res* 80(1):44-51, 1998.

94. Curtis SE, Cain SM: Regional and systemic oxygen delivery/uptake relations and lactate flux in hyperdynamic endotoxin-treated dogs, *Ann Rev Respir Dis* 145(2 Pt 1):348-354, 1992.

95. Kline JA, Maiorano PC, Schroeder JD et al: Activation of pyruvate dehydrogenase improves heart function and metabolism after hemorrhagic shock, *J Mol Cell Cardiol* 29(9)2465-2474, 1997.

96. Burns AH, Giamo, Summer WR: Dichloroacetate improves in vitro myocardial function following in vivo endotoxin administration, *J Crit Care* 1:11-17, 1986.

97. Vary TC, Siegel JH, Rivkind A: Clinical and therapeutic significance of metabolic patterns of lactic acidosis, *Perspect Crit Care* 1:85-132, 1988.

98. Long CL, Birkhahn RH, Geiger JW et al: Urinary excretion of 3-methylhistidine: an assessment of muscle protein catabolism in adult normal subject and during malnutrition, sepsis and skeletal muscle trauma, *Metabolism* 30(8):765-776, 1981.

99. Wilmore DW, Aulick LH, Mason AP et al: Influence of burn wound on local and systemic response to injury, *Ann Surg* 186(4):444-458, 1977.

100. Jefferson LS: Role of insulin in the regulation of protein synthesis, *Diabetes* 29(6):487-490, 1980.

101. Morgan HE, Chua B, Beinlich CJ: Regulation of protein degradation in heart. In Wildenthal K, editor: *Degradative processes in heart and skeletal muscle*, Amsterdam, 1980, Elsevier-North Holland, 87-112.

102. Vary TC, Dardevet D, Grizard J et al: Pentoxifylline improves insulin action limiting skeletal muscle catabolism after infection, *J Endocrinol* 163(1):15-24, 1999.

103. Cooney RA, Pantaloni A, Sarson Y et al: *A pilot study on the metabolic effects of IL-1ra in patients with severe sepsis.* 4th International Congress on Immune Consequences of Trauma, Shock and Sepsis, Bologne, Italy, 1997, Mondozzi Editore S.P.A., 909-912.

104. Clowes GHA Jr, George BC, Villee CA Jr et al: Muscle proteolysis induced by a circulating peptide in patients with sepsis and trauma, *N Engl J Med* 308(10):545-552, 1983.

105. Loda M, Clowes GHA Jr, Dinarello CA et al: Induction of hepatic protein synthesis by a peptide in blood plasma of patients with sepsis and trauma, *Surgery* 96(2):204-213, 1984.

106. Sganga G, Siegel JH, Brown G et al: Reprioritization of hepatic plasma protein release in trauma and sepsis, *Arch Surg* 120(2):187-199, 1985.

107. Nanni G, Siegel JH, Coleman B et al: Increased lipid fuel dependence on critically ill septic patients, *J Trauma* 24(1):14-30, 1984.

108. Sganga G, Siegel JH, Coleman B et al: The physiologic meaning of respiratory index in various types of critical illness, *Circ Shock* 17(3):179-193, 1985.

109. Stoner HB, Little RA, Frayn KN et al: The effect of sepsis on the oxidation of carbohydrate and fat, *Br J Surg* 70(1):32-35, 1983.

110. Wolfe RR: Substrate utilization/insulin resistance in sepsis/trauma, *Baillieres Clin Endocrinol Metab* 11(4):645-657, 1997.

111. Wolfe RR, Martini WZ: Changes in intermediary metabolism in severe surgical illness, *World J Surg* 24(6):639-647, 2000.

112. Mennon RA, Fuller J, Moser AH et al: In vivo regulation of acytl-CoA synthetase mRNA and activity by endotoxin and cytokines, *Amer J Physiol* 275(1 Pt 1):E64-72, 1998.

113. Pekala PH, Kawakami M, Angus CW et al: Selective inhibition of synthesis of enzymes for de novo fatty acid biosynthesis by an endotoxin-induced mediator from exudate cells, *Proc Natl Acad Sci U S A* 80(9):2743-2747, 1983.

114. Scholl RA, Lang CH, Bagby GJ: Hypertriglyceridemia and its relation to tissue lipoprotein lipase activity in endotoxemic *Escherichia coli* bacteremic, and polymicrobial septic rats, *J Surg Res* 37(5):394-401, 1984.

115. Wannemacher RW, Pace JG, Beall FA et al: Role of liver in regulation of ketone body production during sepsis, *J Clin Invest* 64(6):1565-1572, 1979.

116. Pailla K, Lim SK, De Bandt JP et al: TNF-alpha and IL-6 synergistically inhibit ketogenesis from fatty acids and alpha-ketoisocaproate in isolated rat hepatocytes, *J Parenter Enteral Nutr* 22(5):286-290, 1998.

117. Sauaia A, Moore FA, Moore EE et al: Early predictors of postinjury multiple organ failure, *Arch Surg* 129(1):39-45, 1994.

118. Marshall JC, Cook DJ, Christou NV et al: Multiple organ dysfunction score: a reliable descriptor of a complex clinical outcome, *Crit Care Med* 23(10):1638-1652, 1995.

119. Vincent JL, de Mendonca A, Cantraine F et al: Use of SOFA score to assess the incidence of organ dysfunction/failure in intensive care units: results of a multicenter, prospective study, *Crit Care Med* 26(11):1793-1800, 1998.

120. Cryer HG, Leong K, McArthur DL et al: Multiple organ failure: by the time you predict it, it's already there, *J Trauma* 46(4):597-606, 1999.

121. Tran DD, Cuesta MA, van Leeuwen PAM et al: Risk factors for multiple organ failure and death in critically injured patients, *Surgery* 114(1):21-30, 1993.

122. Maetani S, Nishikawa T, Tobe T et al: Role of blood transfusion in organ system failure following major abdominal surgery, *Ann Surg* 203(3):275-281, 1986.

123. Cue JI, Peyton JC, Malangoni MA: Does blood transfusion or hemorrhagic shock induce immunosuppression? *J Trauma* 32(5):613-617, 1992.

124. Cosgriff N, Moore EE, Sauaia A et al: Predicting life-threatening coagulopathy in the massively transfused trauma patient: hypothermia and acidosis revisited, *J Trauma* 42(5):857-861, 1997.

125. Moore EE: Staged laparotomy for the hypothermia, acidosis, coagulopathy syndrome, *Am J Surg* 172(5):405-410, 1996.

126. Sauaia A, Moore FA, Moore EE et al: Pneumonia: cause or symptom of postinjury multiple organ failure? *Am J Surg* 166(6):606-611, 1999.

127. Moore FA, Sauaia A, Moore EE et al: Postinjury multiple organ failure: a bimodal phenomenon, *J Trauma* 40(4):501-512, 1996.

128. Meakins JL, Wicklund B, Forse RA et al: The surgical intensive care unit: current concepts in infection, *Surg Clin North Am* 60(1):117-132, 1980.

129. Dietch EA: Gut failure: its role in the multiple organ failure syndrome. In Dietch EA, editor: *Multiple organ failure: pathophysiology and basic concepts of therapy,* New York, 1990, Thieme, 40-60.

130. Cerra FB, Abrams J, Negro F et al: Multiple organ failure syndrome: clinical epidemiology and effect of current therapy. In Vincent JL, editor: *Update in intensive care and emergency medicine,* Berlin, 1990, Springer-Verlag, 22-31.

131. Ramsey G, Ledingham I: Management of multiple organs: control of the microbial environment, *New Horiz* 2:327-337, 1989.

132. Wichmann MW, Inthorn D, Andress HJ et al: Incidence and mortality of severe sepsis in surgical intensive care patients: the influence of gender on disease process and outcome, *Intensive Care Med* 26(2):167-172, 2000.

133. Hardaway RM: A review of septic shock, *Am Surg* 66(1): 22-29, 2000.

134. Fry DE: Diagnosis and epidemiology of multiple organ failure. In Deitch EA, editor: *Multiple organ failure: pathophysiology and basic concepts of therapy,* New York, 1990, Thieme, 13-25.

135. Balk RA: Pathogenesis and management of multiple organ dysfunction or failure in severe sepsis and septic shock, *Crit Care Clin* 16(2):337-352, 2000.

136. Baue AE: Multiple organ failure, multiple organ dysfunction syndrome, and systemic inflammatory response syndrome: why no magic bullet? *Arch Surg* 132(7):703-707, 1997.

137. Cerra FB: Hypermetabolism-organ failure syndrome: a metabolic response to injury, *Crit Care Clin* 5(2):289-302, 1989.

138. Jarrar D, Chaudry IH, Wang P: Organ dysfunction following hemorrhage and sepsis: mechanisms and therapeutic approaches, *Int J Mol Med* 4(6):575-583, 1999.

139. Von Rueden KT, Dunham CM: Evaluation and management of oxygen delivery and consumption in multiple organ dysfunction syndrome. In Secor V, editor: *Multiple organ dysfunction and failure: pathophysiology and clinical implications,* ed 2, St Louis, 1996, Mosby, 384-401.

140. ACCP/SCCM Consensus Conference Committee, American College of Chest Physicians/Society of Critical Care Medicine Consensus Conference: Definitions for sepsis and organ failure and guidelines for the use of innovative therapies in sepsis, *Crit Care Med* 20(6):864-874, 1992.

141. Rudis M, Basha M, Zarowitz B: Is it time to reposition vasopressors and inotropes in sepsis? *Crit Care Med* 24(3): 525-37, 1996.

142. Neviere R, Mathieu D, Chagnon JC et al: The contrasting effects of dobutamine and dopamine on gastric mucosal perfusion in septic patients, *Am J Respir Crit Care Med* 154(6 Pt 1):1684-1688, 1996.

143. Levy B, Bollaert PE, Lucchelli JP et al: Dobutamine improves the adequacy of gastric mucosal perfusion in epinephrine-treated septic shock, *Crit Care Med* 25(10): 1649-1654, 1997.

144. Abid O, Akca S, Haji-Michael P et al: Strong vasopressor support may be futile in the intensive care unit patient with multiple organ failure, *Crit Care Med* 28(4):947-949, 2000.

145. Lynn W, Cohen J: Adjunctive therapy for septic shock: a review of experimental approaches, *Clin Infect Dis* 20(1): 143-158, 1995.

146. Zeni F, Freeman B, Natanson C: Anti-inflammatory therapies to treat sepsis and septic shock: a reassessment, *Crit Care Med* 25(7):1095-1100, 1997.

147. Bone RC: Why sepsis trials fail, *JAMA* 276(7):565-566, 1996.

148. Liu M, Slutsky A: Anti-inflammatory therapies: application of molecular biology techniques in intensive care medicine, *Intensive Care Med* 23(7):718-731, 1997.

149. Deitch EA, Livingston DH, Hauser CJ: Septic complications in the trauma patient, *New Horiz* 7:158-172, 1999.

INITIAL MANAGEMENT OF TRAUMATIC SHOCK

Thomas M. Scalea • Sharon A. Boswell

The rapid recognition and therapy of shock is at the cornerstone of the early evaluation and treatment phase of badly injured patients. Sometimes shock is obvious, and even the unsophisticated clearly recognize the patient in extremis from blood loss. However, much more frequently the findings are substantially more subtle and increasing levels of clinical sophistication and experience are necessary to recognize shock, particularly when the victim is able to compensate for the disruption. Shock represents an uncoupling of the normal physiologic functions. Compensatory mechanisms initially strive to maintain homeostasis. This compensation can be quite profound, particularly in young patients, and patients with substantial blood loss or severe injuries can appear relatively stable initially.

The importance of early recognition of shock cannot be overemphasized. When untreated or treated very late, shock produces acute organ dysfunction that almost always leads to death—often within 24 hours.[1] However, late recognition of shock, even if not accompanied by classic signs, produces a profound hypoperfusion insult, with the accumulation of a significant oxygen debt. Patients may survive for the short term but then develop sequential organ failure several days later.[2] Despite an increased understanding of injury and resuscitation, we have yet to significantly alter the mortality associated with multiple organ failure.

Although the term *traumatic shock* may seem redundant, it actually describes a distinct clinical entity. Shock following injury is multifactorial. Hemodynamic alteration from blood loss can be compounded by mediator release from injured soft tissue. Both of these can be further compounded by cardiovascular dysfunction resulting from blunt cardiac injury or cardiac tamponade. Hypoxia from pulmonary contusion may limit oxygen delivery and worsen cardiac function. Thus traumatic shock can include aspects of many other types of shock.

OXYGEN TRANSPORT

Central to the understanding of the concept of shock is the principle of oxygen transport (Table 13-1). The vast majority of oxygen (98% to 99%) exists in the body bound to hemoglobin. A small portion is freely dissolved in plasma. Thus oxygen content is a function of hemoglobin and oxygen saturation. Cardiac output delivers oxygen to the periphery. The cells then unload the amount of oxygen they need, and the unneeded portion is returned back to the heart via the venous circulation. The oxygen extraction ratio is approximately 25%.

A number of physiologic variables can alter this relationship. After injury, loss of circulating blood volume (via hemorrhage or loss of serum into the soft tissue) decreases cardiac preload impeding cardiac output. Increased needs in the periphery create a state in which the body must compensate by increasing oxygen delivery. This can be accomplished in a number of ways. Cardiac output, a function of the stroke volume of the heart and the heart rate, can increase. The stroke volume is a function of preload, afterload, and contractility. Thus an increase in myocardial contractility or heart rate can increase cardiac output. An increase in vascular resistance, which initially maintains blood pressure, also limits cardiovascular performance. Alternatively, the cells can unload more oxygen in the periphery, thus maintaining oxygen consumption. Both methods can be used simultaneously.

The ability of the cell to unload oxygen can be affected by a number of factors. The oxyhemoglobin dissociation curve governs the principles of oxygen affinity to the hemoglobin molecule (Figure 13-1). Some conditions such as alkalosis, hypothermia, or a loss of 2,3-diphosphoglycerate (2,3-DPG) increase oxygen's affinity for hemoglobin, thus impeding the body's ability to unload oxygen at the cellular level. Conversely, acidosis, hyperthermia, and increases in 2,3-DPG, shift the curve in the opposite direction, allowing for increased peripheral oxygen unloading. These relationships can be quite dynamic, particularly in a patient with complicated diagnoses.

At some point, oxygen demand can exceed oxygen supply. As compensation fails, the cells must shift to anaerobic metabolism to generate the high-energy phosphate compounds needed for cellular metabolism.[3] Anaero-bic metabolism is an extremely inefficient means of generating adenosine triphosphate (ATP)—approximately 5% as efficient as aerobic metabolism using the Krebs cycle (Figure 13-2).[4] In addition, lactate is a byproduct of anaerobic metabolism. Lactate may depress cardiac function and limit oxygen delivery. As acidosis worsens, so does cardiac performance, and ultimately death ensues.

Shock then can be defined as any state in which oxygen demand exceeds oxygen supply or oxygen utilization regard-

TABLE 13-1   Oxygen Transport

Variables	Abbreviation	Units	Calculation	Normal Value
Hb saturation	Sao_2	%	Direct measurement	95-99
Arterial oxygen content	Cao_2	ml O_2/dl	$Cao_2 = (Hb \times 1.39 \times Sao_2) + (.003 \times Pao_2)$	16-22
Venous oxygen content	Cvo_2	ml O_2/dl	$Cvo_2 = (Hb \times 1.39 \times Svo_2) + (.003 \times Pvo_2)$	12-17
Oxygen delivery	Do_2 I	ml/min/m^2	$Do_2 = Cao_2 \times CI \times 10$	520-720
Oxygen consumption	Vo_2 I	ml/min/m^2	$Vo_2 = C(a-v)O_2 \times CI \times 10$	100-180

Modified from Shoemaker WC: Relation of oxygen transport patterns to the pathophysiology and therapy of shock states, *Intensive Care Med* 13:234, 1987.
CI, Cardiac index; *Hb,* Hemoglobin.

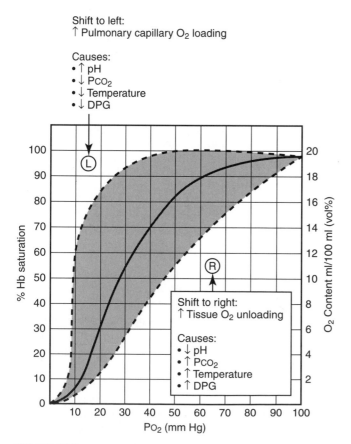

FIGURE 13-1 Oxyhemoglobin dissociation curve. (From Moms MT: *Adult respiratory distress syndrome.* In Secour VH, editor: *Multiple organ dysfunction & failure,* ed 2, St. Louis, 1996, Mosby, 174.)

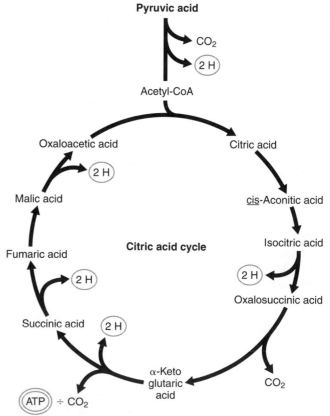

FIGURE 13-2 Diagram of Krebs cycle. (From Porth CM, Curtis RL: Cell and tissue characteristics. In Porth CM, editor: *Pathophysiology concepts and altered states,* ed 4, Philadelphia, 1994, JB Lippincott, 16.)

less of the underlying cause. Thus all shock can be defined as a type of cardiogenic shock or inadequate cardiovascular performance. Given the nature of injury, we attempt to estimate peripheral oxygen delivery through the use of blood pressure or target organ function. Although this practice has the advantage of being quick and readily available in the clinical arena, these parameters are at best nonspecific and in some cases can lead to faulty decision making. Some patients who are hypotensive may not be in shock. Conversely, many patients who are not hypotensive may be in shock. Recognizing this concept and knowing when it is necessary to obtain more data is key to optimizing care, particularly in patients with complex diagnoses.

PATHOPHYSIOLOGY OF SHOCK

PHYSIOLOGY OF BLOOD LOSS

Blood loss is the most common cause of inadequate cardiac performance after injury.[5] It can be accompanied by other volume losses such as fluid losses from soft tissue or bony injury, further depressing cardiovascular performance. Initial attempts to compensate for blood loss are multifactorial. Catecholamine-mediated systemic vasoconstriction is primarily responsible for the increase in systemic vascular resistance seen in many shock states. This allows for the shunting of blood flow away from nonessential organs. Blood is initially directed away from the skin and skeletal muscle, maintaining flow to the more central vascular beds. Ultimately, as blood loss continues, the only core organs protected are the most essential—the heart and the brain. Under normal conditions the perfusion pressure and degree of smooth muscle tone in the supplying vessels determine regional blood flow to any individual organ. As organisms bleed, autoregulatory mechanisms attempt to maintain a steady-state pressure flow to these vital organs. Thus tissue

hypoxia will initially be more marked in tissues and organs in which autoregulatory compensation fails.

Clinically measurable parameters that are thought to change first include heart rate, pulse pressure, and skin temperature (Table 13-2). Tachycardia, a narrowing of pulse pressure, and loss of capillary refill are thought to be the first measurable signs after hemorrhage. As blood loss continues, there may be a stepwise change in these and other parameters. When blood loss approximates 40% to 50% of total circulating blood volume (>2 L in a 70-kg man), compensation fails and patients develop bradycardia, obtundation, and cardiac arrest.[6] The stepwise change in vital signs allows for estimation of the amount of blood loss and thus can be used to direct care. For instance, patients who are stable (i.e., normotensive and not tachycardic) could be presumed to have a minor injury and have suffered less than a 15% loss in circulating blood volume. Those who are initially somewhat hypotensive or tachycardic and who respond to initial resuscitation may then be classified as "stabilizable." Although they must be presumed to have suffered a significant blood loss, most often they are able to undergo diagnostic evaluation to precisely identify the source of blood loss. Some of these patients may even be managed nonoperatively. Conversely, patients who present in extremis and do not respond to initial resuscitation must be presumed to have serious ongoing blood loss. Their initial evaluation should be tailored to minimize time, and hemorrhage must be arrested immediately.

Unfortunately, vital signs are often imprecise and may incorrectly classify patients with marginally compensated shock as stable. Tissue oxygen extraction, as measured by either mixed venous or central venous oxygen saturation, is much more specific and correlates reliably with blood loss (Figure 13-3). This has been demonstrated in controlled laboratory models of both anesthetized and unanesthetized

TABLE 13-2 Estimated Fluids and Blood Losses Based on Patient's Initial Presentation

	Class I	Class II	Class III	Class IV
Blood Loss (mL)	Up to 750	750-1500	1500-2000	>2000
Blood Loss (% Blood Volume)	Up to 15%	15%-30%	30%-40%	>40%
Pulse Rate	<100	>100	>120	>140
Blood Pressure	Normal	Normal	Decreased	Decreased
Pulse Pressure (mm Hg)	Normal or increased	Decreased	Decreased	Decreased
Respiratory Rate	14-20	20-30	30-40	>35
Urine Output (mL/hr)	>30	20-30	5-15	Negligible
CNS/Mental Status	Slightly anxious	Mildly anxious	Anxious, confused	Confused, lethargic
Fluid Replacement (3:1 Rule)	Crystalloid	Crystalloid	Crystalloid and blood	Crystalloid and blood

Modified with permission from American College of Surgeons, Committee on Trauma: *Advanced trauma life support for doctors, student course manual,* ed 6, Chicago, 1997, American College of Surgeons, p. 98.

For a 70-kg man.

The guidelines in Table 13-2 are based on the "3-for-1" rule. This rule derives from the empiric observation that most patients in hemorrhagic shock require as much as 300 mL of electrolyte solution for each 100 mL of blood loss. Applied blindly, these guidelines can result in excessive or inadequate fluid administration. For example, a patient with a crush injury to the extremity may have hypotension out of proportion to his or her blood loss and requires fluids in excess of the 3:1 guidelines. In contrast, a patient whose ongoing blood loss is being replaced by blood transfusion requires less than 3:1. The use of bolus therapy with careful monitoring of the patient's response can moderate these extremes.

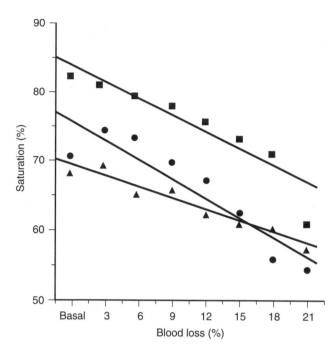

FIGURE 13-3 Relationship between venous oxygen saturation and blood loss in awake and anesthetized dogs. Squares represent mixed venous oxygen saturation (anesthetized); circles represent central venous oxygen saturation (awake); and triangles represent mixed venous oxygen saturation (awake). (Modified from Scalea TM, Holman M, Fuortes M et al: Central venous blood oxygen saturation: an early, accurate measurement of volume during hemorrhage, *J Trauma* 28:728, 1988.)

canine hemorrhage.[7] More recently it has been investigated in humans who presented to an emergency department with mechanisms of injury suggestive of acute blood loss but who initially seemed to be hemodynamically stable.[8] Fully 40% of these stable patients had central venous oxygen desaturation, though their blood pressure and pulse rate were similar to those of patients with normal central venous oxygen saturations. Central venous oxygen desaturation was used to reliably predict patients with injuries causing major blood loss, such as large hemothoraces or hemorrhage from pelvic fractures.

Urine output has been reported to be a reliable indicator of the depth of shock.[6] Thus patients who are oliguric should be presumed to be underresuscitated. More importantly, patients who are nonoliguric are deemed stable. However, work from the authors' laboratory seems to refute those conclusions.[9] In a porcine model of nonhypotensive shock, animals that lost 15% of their total circulating volume behaved as expected by becoming oliguric. They held on to both salt and water, as evidenced by low urine sodium concentrations. In contrast, animals bled more severely—losing 21%, 27%, and 35% of the total circulating blood volume—all developed an acute salt-wasting nephropathy and acute tubular insufficiency. These animals had high urine-sodium concentrations, and their urine output was not different from that of control animals.

Other factors may alter cardiac performance and perfusion parameters after blood loss. One is mechanism of injury. Patients who have sustained blunt trauma respond differently than patients with penetrating injuries. Penetrat-

ing trauma approximates a pure blood loss situation with acute cardiac insufficiency. A tissue crush injury that accompanies blunt trauma, however, can stimulate a cascade that even acutely liberates vasoactive mediators, which can affect hemodynamic performance. Patients with this type of injury may develop a high cardiac output/low vascular resistance state similar to sepsis. Ethanol use, which is commonly associated with trauma, has been shown to modulate plasma norepinephrine concentrations after injury, blunting the vascular response and moderating the affect of adrenergic stimuli.[10] Street drugs such as cocaine may also affect cardiovascular performance. In a recent study animals pretreated with cocaine and then subjected to blood loss had a blunted response to hemorrhage compared with control animals.[11]

Some vascular beds may respond differently than others. Global parameters such as mixed venous oxygen saturation reflect a mixing of blood from all vascular beds. Identification of the most responsive vascular beds could allow earlier diagnosis of blood loss. The mesenteric circulation is exquisitely sensitive to falls in preload.[12] Blood flow to the gut is reduced primarily via vasoconstriction caused by elevated renin angiotensin activity. This is opposed to the renal circulation, in which hemorrhagic hypotension may activate renal vasodilatory signals via local release of prostaglandins and nitric oxide. Monitoring of mesenteric circulation could potentially provide early warning signals to critical but non-hemodynamically significant hemorrhage. The adequacy of flow can be measured via intracellular pH. Indirect measurement of this parameter via gastric tonometry catheters has been demonstrated to predict adequacy of resuscitation in the general class of intensive care unit (ICU) patients.[13] Unpublished work from the authors' laboratory has demonstrated that gastric tonometry is an extremely sensitive indicator of blood loss that changes before other vital signs. In addition, the authors have demonstrated that reduction in gastrointestinal oxygen delivery is accompanied by oxygen supply dependency.

NEUROGENIC SHOCK

Efferent sympathetic neurons in the thoracic and cervical spinal cord are dependent on descending input from the hypothalmus and brainstem for vasomotor control. Brainstem damage or spinal cord injury may then produce neurogenic shock. In this type of shock, loss of vasoconstrictor-sympathetic activity leads to vascular collapse. With loss of vasomotor control, even previously adequate blood volume becomes incapable of filling the now dilated capacitance vessels. Bradycardia and hypotension are common. However, unlike hemorrhagic shock, neurogenic shock is characterized by a slow pulse rate and warm, dry skin. This is a relative hypovolemia resulting from decreases in peripheral vascular and cardiac sympathetic activity. Hemodynamic patterns can be variable. Decreases in systemic vascular resistance, central venous pressure, and pulmonary capillary wedge pressure are nearly universal. Cardiac output, on the other hand, may be low, normal, or elevated. The loss of vascular resistance allows unimpeded forward flow from the heart. These salutory effects on cardiac performance may be counterbalanced, however, by the negative effect of inadequate preload from the vasodilation. Refer to Chapter 22 for information on management of neurogenic shock.

The hemodynamics of neurogenic shock may be further complicated by differences in mechanism of injury. A spinal cord injury may be accompanied by blood loss, which can exacerbate any of the hemodynamic consequences. The lack of sympathetic response may also mask the signs of acute blood loss. Soderstrom et al demonstrated that nearly 70% of patients with cervical spine injury and blunt trauma are hypotensive from their spinal cord injury, not concomitant blood loss.[14] In contradistinction, a recent series of patients with penetrating spinal cord injuries found that neurogenic shock explained hypotension in approximately 20% of patients.[15] This underscores the need to completely evaluate all patients regardless of the obvious nature of one particular injury.

Cardiogenic Shock

The most frequent cause of cardiogenic shock is acute myocardial infarction.[5] This can accompany injury, particularly in elderly patients. Cardiogenic shock occurs when 35% to 40% of the left ventricular muscle mass is damaged.[16] The resulting impairment in left ventricular function produces elevated end-systolic volumes and filling pressures. This in turn limits diastolic filling. Cardiac output falls and produces often profound hypotension. Coronary perfusion is thereby decreased, potentially extending the area of ischemia. This ischemia further drops cardiac output and creates an ever-widening cyclic process, which will result in patient death unless truncated early.

Patients with acute cardiac failure after injury are a special subset of patients and present many challenges. Peripheral oxygen delivery needs must be met to maintain aerobic metabolism. Cardiovascular support often involves "supranormal" levels of circulating blood volume in order to achieve adequate cardiac output. Inotropic support may be necessary to support the failing heart. All these changes, however, further increase myocardial work and myocardial oxygen demand.

Cardiac protection with beta blockade afterload reduction and conservative fluid administration will help preserve myocardium but will limit forward flow. Despite all interventions, cardiogenic shock in this setting is often a lethal state.[17]

Septic Shock

Pure septic shock resulting from infection is unusual immediately after acute trauma. The only exception may occur in patients with grossly contaminated wounds. Significant soft tissue infection is seen in patients with multiple long-bone fractures, and these patients occasionally present with septic shock several hours after injury. The mediator release stimulated by significant soft tissue injury, especially when accompanied by gross contamination or dead muscle, often presents in a manner similar to septic shock.

Septic shock is most commonly characterized by vasodilation, and the resulting hemodynamics are generally related to unopposed forward cardiac flow. Septic shock is not a pure hypovolemic state. It is better described as maldistribution of blood flow. The vasodilation, with resultant arteriolar and venous dilation, lowers cardiac preload as well as afterload. Although many patients present with warm, seemingly well-perfused extremities and high cardiac output, those with septic shock may actually exhibit high, normal, or low cardiac output states. Relative myocardial failure can come as a result of inadequate cardiac preload or direct myocardial depression from circulating mediators. A subset of patients, usually the elderly, who are septic in fact can present with high systemic vascular resistances and low cardiac outputs in a manner similar to that of cardiogenic shock. This form of septic shock carries an extremely poor prognosis.

The initial decrease in blood pressure seen with all forms of septic shock is multifactorial. An infectious process leads to the release of vasoactive mediators such as histamine and bradykinin. These vasoactive agents ultimately cause pooling of peripheral blood and occasionally extravasation of plasma into the interstitium. The acute capillary leak and peripheral pooling decrease venous return, with resultant falling cardiac output and blood pressure. Compensation for this decrease in ventricular filling is mediated initially through increases in sympathoadrenal stimulae. Ultimately, however, myocardial dysfunction will override this attempt at compensation.

Initially the availability of substrates (particularly oxygen and glucose) is increased to support metabolic need as demands rise. However, as peripheral perfusion decreases, substrate delivery may be inadequate and anaerobic metabolism ensues. In addition, visceral redistribution of flow creates a state of relative mitochondrial failure. Even with increased peripheral oxygen delivery, the ability of the cell and the mitochondria to unload and use oxygen decreases.

Diagnosis and Treatment of Shock

The diagnosis of shock is based on the ability to identify problems with peripheral perfusion. As the patient traverses the trauma care system, the ability to diagnose shock increases with the sophistication of the tools available.

Prehospital care providers have only rudimentary tools, in addition to their clinical acumen, to use in the identification of blood loss. Thus it can be reasonably assumed that they will not be as accurate or specific in diagnosing shock as clinicians in an ICU, whose arsenal includes invasive hemodynamic monitoring devices as well as knowledge of the patient's clinical course up to that point.

Prehospital Care

The goal in caring for any trauma patient is to identify those most severely injured as early as possible and then to minimize the time from injury to definitive therapy. Unfortunately, diagnosis of shock in the field can be quite difficult. Blood pressure and pulse rate are crude measures of the adequacy of peripheral perfusion,[7] yet little else is available to the prehospital care provider. These individuals must make rapid decisions based on a paucity of information. Thus in most emergency medical services (EMS) systems the tendency has been to overtriage as opposed to undertriage in order to avoid delivering a patient to an institution not capable of providing adequate care.

Skin temperature, capillary refill, and the initial response of blood pressure and pulse rate to a fluid bolus are the primary assessment parameters available in the prehospital arena. A gauge of anatomic severity may also provide some clue as to the likelihood of blood loss. For instance, patients with multiple long-bone fractures must be presumed to have substantial blood loss and should be treated accordingly despite normal vital signs. Large scalp lacerations are notorious for producing exsanguinating hemorrhage, and patients with this type of injury must be presumed to have lost a substantial amount of blood regardless of their blood pressure or pulse rate. Patients with pelvic instability or a tense, distended abdomen must likewise be presumed to have bled into their retroperitoneum or abdominal cavity. Physical examination of the chest provides some clue, though relatively crude, as to blood loss into the thoracic cavity. Lastly, the patient's own medical history, such as presence or absence of cardiac disease and medication use, may help determine his or her ability to withstand blood loss and respond hemodynamically. Patients on beta blockers will not be able to use tachycardia to augment forward flow.

Several philosophies exist regarding the care of patients who are confirmed or suspected to be in shock (Table 13-3). The first is to attempt to stabilize these patients in the field. This "stay and play" philosophy is based on an assumption that time in the field can be well spent stabilizing the patient's physiologic status.[18] Correction of oxygenation or ventilatory problems can be lifesaving. The insertion of

intravenous (IV) catheters for fluid resuscitation can help correct cardiovascular instability. A brief neurologic assessment can identify patients at high risk for severe brain injury, particularly those with impending herniation. Therapy can then be directed and triage possibly improved. Unfortunately, the time involved in even rapid evaluation and temporary stabilization often causes concern.

Excessive time in the field can prolong the interval from injury to definitive therapy. Proponents of the "scoop and run" philosophy believe that only immediately life-threatening problems such as airway issues should be addressed in the field.[19] Patients should be immobilized on spine boards and external hemorrhage controlled with direct pressure. All other therapies should be attempted only en route. Prolonging field time even long enough to insert an IV catheter may negatively alter ultimate outcome.

In 1983 Smith et al reviewed the prehospital care of 52 trauma victims who underwent attempts at in-field stabilization.[20] In all cases the IV insertion time was longer than the transport time. Failure of line placement occurred 28% of the time and occurred most often in those patients most severely injured. The average IV insertion time in the field was between 10 and 12 minutes. Border et al estimated that blood loss during this time may be in excess of 1500 ml in badly injured patients.[21]

This issue was further investigated by clinicians at Los Angeles County Hospital.[22] In this study nearly 6000 trauma patients admitted via the emergency department were evaluated for field time and mode of transportation. Patients who were transported by private vehicle as opposed to the city EMS system got to the hospital statistically significantly faster. The main reason for this appeared to be the amount of time the prehospital personnel spent in the field attempting to stabilize the patient. The moderate to severely injured patients (Injury Severity Score [ISS] 15-25)

TABLE 13-3	**Field Resuscitation Time**		
	Stay and Play		**Load and Go**
Time at scene	Longer (20-30 min)		Shorter (<10 min)
Interventions	Airway stabilization		Airway stabilization
	Spinal stabilization		Spinal stabilization
	• IV access		
	• Fluid therapy		
	• Wound/fracture stabilization		
Appropriate Locale	Rural		Urban
Advantages	• Earlier fluid therapy		• Shorter time to definitive care
	• Earlier administration of pain control therapy		
	• Earlier administration of effective measures for cardiac arrhythmias		
	• Broader assessment with possible better triage		
Disadvantages	• Longer time to definitive care		• Delay in beginning fluid therapy
	• Potential for increased bleeding with increased fluid volume		• Possible increase in mistriage

Modified from Border JR, Lewis FR, Aprahamian C et al: Panel: prehospital trauma care—stabilize or scoop and run, *J Trauma* 23: 708-711, 1983; and Gold CR: Prehospital advanced life support vs "scoop and run" in trauma management, *Ann Emerg Med* 16: 797-801, 1987.

arriving at the hospital without the benefit of ambulance transport had a lower mortality than their EMS-transported counterparts. This compelling data argues strongly in favor of "scoop and run."

Some middle ground would presumably be the wisest. In dense urban areas where prehospital transport times are shorter, it is hard to imagine that spending a prolonged amount of time in the field is wise. This would be particularly true for patients with penetrating trauma, primarily penetrating torso trauma. Attempts to stabilize these patients in the field will almost certainly result in longer than necessary prehospital care. Survival of these patients is a function of rapid transport and definitive control of life-threatening blood loss. Patients with vascular injuries can bleed faster than they can be resuscitated.

On the other hand, patients in rural areas with blunt trauma may be best served by an attempt at stabilization. An additional 10 minutes of prehospital time may not substantially increase total time in areas where long transport times are the norm. Airway control and some attempt at cardiovascular stability may be lifesaving, particularly in patients with traumatic brain injury. Each EMS system should address these issues individually. It is important to understand the local climate in order to stratify policies by level of sophistication of the prehospital care provider as well as transport time.

Fluid administration in the prehospital arena has evolved considerably in the past several years. Original treatment algorithms called for establishment of large-bore IV access and instillation of 2 L of crystalloid fluid as rapidly as possible, with the goal of normalizing both blood pressure and pulse rate. Early in the twentieth century, however, Cannon suggested that IV fluids administered in the field to patients with hypotension could be injurious.[23] He theorized that crystalloid fluid would serve only to displace a hemostatic clot that may have formed on injured blood vessels as blood pressure fell. In addition, he felt that if bleeding persisted despite hypotension, administration of IV fluids would not positively influence outcome.

This thought was corroborated scientifically in 1965, when Shaftan et al investigated this theory in a canine hemorrhagic shock model.[24] They investigated various resuscitation regimens to elucidate the relative effects of pressure and volume on the hemodynamic response to crystalloid fluid resuscitation. They demonstrated that the time to hemostasis was longest and blood loss greatest in animals resuscitated to normal volume status and blood pressure. Subsequently, numerous animal models have been used, most often a porcine aortotomy model of hemorrhagic shock.[25-27] All these investigations demonstrated that intraperitoneal blood loss is greatest when animals are resuscitated to normal blood pressure. The excessive amount of crystalloid fluid required to maintain normal blood pressure seems to hemodilute the available hemoglobin and increase intraperitoneal blood loss, presumably by displacing the clot that forms on top of the injured aorta at the time of hypotension. In 1994 Bickell et al. randomized patients with

penetrating torso trauma and hypotension in the field to receive no fluid or standard crystalloid fluid, with a target systolic blood pressure of 100 mm Hg.[28] Patients in the fluid-restricted group received fluids only at the time of anesthetic induction for surgical control of their hemorrhagic shock. In this study there was a statistically significant survival advantage to fluid restriction.

Thus it seems that moderate hypotension, although potentially detrimental, is in fact relatively well tolerated, at least for short periods. This may be better than the alternative of increased blood loss and hemodilution with crystalloid resuscitation to attain normal blood pressure. It is important to remember that this has been investigated only in humans with penetrating torso trauma. Other subsets of patients who are badly injured may be significantly harmed by hypotension. There is no human data to suggest the same treatment strategy is wise after blunt trauma, though it is possible. In addition, in patients with traumatic brain injury, hypotension has been shown to double mortality.[29] Thus fluid restriction is probably not wise in these patients. Alternatively, geriatric patients with limited cardiovascular reserve may require different treatment algorithms to avoid development of acute cardiac ischemia, which almost certainly will lead to death.

The type of fluid used in the prehospital environment has likewise been called into question (Table 13-4). In most EMS systems, crystalloid fluid is the preferred volume expander. There is, however, some evidence that hypertonic saline may have the advantages of more rapid restoration of cardiovascular function with a smaller volume of fluid. As little as 4 ml/kg, if given rapidly, may have the same hemodynamic effect as several liters of crystalloid.[30] The increase in cardiac output and mean arterial pressure with hypertonic saline results from an osmotic shift of fluid from the interstitial and intracellular spaces into the intravascular space. This is mediated by rapid increases in serum osmolarity that accompany the infusion of 7.5% sodium chloride, which has a milliosmolarity of 2400. The addition of dextran prolongs this plasma expansion.[31] In several animal models of hemorrhage, hypertonic saline/dextran improved stroke volume and decreased both heart rate and systemic vascular resistance.[32,33] Enthusiasm for use of hypertonic solutions has been counterbalanced by several small studies suggesting that re-bleeding and hemodynamic instability may occur after the infusion of hypertonic saline when blood loss is not fully controlled.[34,35]

Hypertonic saline and hypertonic saline/dextran have been investigated in several randomized prospective trials in humans. Mattox et al demonstrated increases in blood pressure in a multiinstitutional study on the use of hypertonic saline in the prehospital arena.[36] In the subset of patients requiring emergency life-saving surgery to control hemorrhage, survival was statistically significantly better in patients who were treated with hypertonic saline compared with those treated with dextran or crystalloid fluid. Vassar et al investigated this issue in four separate randomized trials during the early 1990s.[37-40] They were unable to demon-

TABLE 13-4	**Fluid Therapy**		
	Crystalloids	Hypertonic Saline	Hypertonic Saline/Dextran
Amount required	Two L	4 ml/kg	4 ml/kg
Osmolarity	273-308 mOsm/L	1026 mOsm/L for 3% 2565 mOsm/L for 7.5% 8008 mOsm/L for 23.4%	2400 mOsm/L for 7.5% HTS in 6% dextran 70 (will vary depending on HTS and dextran concentrations used)
Longevity	Minutes	15-30 min	3-4 hr
Advantages	• No side effects	• Faster increase in BP than with crystalloids • Requires less volume • Requires less time for infusion • May increase survival in patients with GCS ≤ 8 by decreasing intracranial pressure	• Faster increase in BP than with crystalloids • Requires less volume • Requires less time for infusion • May increase survival in patients with GCS ≤ 8 by decreasing intracranial pressure
Disadvantages	• May exacerbate bleeding in large volumes • May worsen head injury in large volumes	• No increase in survival over crystalloids in the general trauma population • Potential for adverse reactions such as seizures or coagulopathies	• No increase in survival over crystalloids in the general trauma population • Potential for adverse reactions such as seizures, coagulopathies, or anaphylaxis

Modified from Mattox KL, Maningas PA, Moore EE et al: Prehospital hypertonic saline/dextran infusion for post-traumatic hypotension, *Ann Surg* 213:482-491, 1991; and Vassar MJ, Fischer RP, O'Brien PE et al: A multicenter trial for resuscitation of injured patients with 7.5% sodium chloride, *Arch Surg* 128:1003-1013, 1993.

strate any survival advantage in the broad group of patients randomized to hypertonic saline compared with crystalloid fluid. However, in the subset of patients with severe traumatic brain injury, there appeared to be a survival advantage to using hyperosmotic resuscitation. This may have been due to a decrease in secondary brain injury from the more rapid restoration of cardiovascular function or decreases in intracranial pressure, as seen with the administration of hypertonic saline. The cerebral osmotic effects of hypertonic saline are similar to those of mannitol. In a metaanalysis Wade et al demonstrated a distinct survival advantage for patients with serious traumatic brain injury treated with hypertonic saline.[31]

There are some distinct disadvantages to the use of hypertonic saline as well. Although the hemodynamic effects are rapid and profound, they are relatively short lived. At some point, the intracellular hypernatremia can become problematic and sufficient free water must be administered to repay the intracellular debt. Rapid instillation of hyperosmotic saline may be unsafe in patients with limited cardiac reserve (e.g., elderly patients), as it may precipitate heart failure. The lack of convincing randomized prospective data and the concerns about potential disadvantages of hypertonic saline have combined to limit its widespread use in the prehospital arena.

In the late 1980s military antishock trousers (MAST) were thought to be useful in the resuscitation scheme after trauma. MAST were thought to autotransfuse volume by applying pressure to the capacitance vessels in the lower extremities. Added advantages included the potential stabilization of long-bone fractures and reduction of pelvic fractures. More recent data, however, has failed to demonstrate any real utility to MAST. In fact, increases in blood pressure seen with the use of MAST seem to be secondary to increases in systemic vascular resistance, and MAST do not augment cardiac preload. In a randomized trial of 911 patients, Mattox et al demonstrated no survival advantage with use of MAST.[41] Wangensteen et al reported that pneumatic external compression without concomitant intervascular volume replacement accelerated the development of lactic acidosis and decreased the survival rate in animal models.[42] In general, the widespread use of MAST has fallen out of favor and many EMS systems have abandoned their use in the prehospital arena. However, there may be some uses for MAST. They can be helpful as a temporary splint in patients with extensive long-bone fractures. In addition, they can be helpful in patients with complex pelvic fractures by reducing the fracture, limiting pelvic volume, and potentially reducing blood loss. They do, however, introduce the possibility of cardiovascular effects resulting from increased intraabdominal pressure. In addition, MAST may be useful during long transports to help support at least some blood pressure when no other mode of therapy is available.

TRANSPORT DECISIONS

Transport decisions are as important as any other prehospital decisions. The concept of triage is designed around delivering the patient to the most appropriate facility as quickly as possible. Rapid transport to an emergency department or hospital that does not have the capability of providing the appropriate level of care to the patient may only jeopardize long-term outcome. All emergency departments should be able to provide immediately life-saving therapies such as establishing an airway and shock resuscitation. However, more sophisticated diagnostics and therapeutics are available in only a few facilities. For instance, access to a computed tomography (CT) scanner and the ready availability of a neurosurgeon may be lifesaving in a

TABLE 13-5	**Trauma Center Descriptors**			
	Level I	Level II	Level III	Level IV
Admission requirements	1200 trauma patients per year; 20% must have an ISS ≥15 or 35 patients per surgeon with ISS ≥15	Depends on geographic area served, population density, resources available, and maturity of system	No requirement	No requirement
Surgeon availability	24-hour in-house attending surgeon required	Surgeon must be rapidly available on short notice	A general surgeon must be promptly available	24-hour emergency coverage by a physician
Research center	Required	Not required	Not required	Not required
Education, prevention, and outreach	Required	Required	Required	Required

Modified from Committee on Trauma, American College of Surgeons: *Resources for optimal care of the injured patient: 1999*, Chicago, 1998, The College.

patient with operable traumatic brain injury. The ready availability of a general surgeon and an operating room likewise can be the only method of salvaging a patient who is in hemorrhagic shock from blunt or penetrating torso trauma.

In the United States there has been an attempt to classify hospitals in order to rank the degree of care they may reasonably be expected to provide 24 hours a day, 365 days a year. Various agencies (e.g., local EMS systems or state governmental agencies) are responsible for this designation and verification process. Decisions regarding criteria for the various levels of trauma centers and the number of centers necessary in any given locale vary among municipalities. In some locations any center that meets the criteria is designated. This makes the highest number of centers available but dilutes each center's experience. In other areas the issue of capacity is more important and there is a limit on the number of centers that can be designated within each geographic location. This may increase transport times slightly but concentrates experience in a smaller number of hospitals.

The American College of Surgeons (ACS) has a verification process that provides a national standard (Table 13-5).[43] In order to be verified as a Level I trauma center by the ACS, a hospital must have continuous coverage by an attending trauma surgeon and must provide care for at least 1200 patients each year, at least 20% of whom have an ISS greater than 15. Level I centers must also be leaders in education, prevention, and trauma research. A Level II designation allows for consultation specialties, such as orthopedics and neurosurgery, to be available on an on-call basis. Level II centers are generally not teaching or research facilities. Level III centers are equipped to deal with life-threatening injuries only on a short-term basis.

The issue of the triage of severely injured patients remains somewhat controversial. Should a badly injured patient be transported directly to a Level I trauma center, bypassing a Level II or Level III center? Alternatively, is that patient best seen at the nearest trauma center for stabilization and then transferred to a Level I trauma center if deemed necessary? Unfortunately, this debate is often fueled more by economic agendas than a real concern about the patient's welfare. There is a relative paucity of data to guide system decisions. In addition, triage criteria are often vague, which has the advantage of allowing prehospital care personnel the latitude to make triage decisions in the field but also opens them to criticism should they bypass any center.

In a study of 4364 significantly injured patients (mean ISS of 14), Sampalis et al demonstrated that patients who were transferred from the initial receiving hospital had an adjusted increase in odds of dying of 57% compared with equally injured patients taken directly to a Level I trauma center.[44] However, this study included only urban hospital transfers. Young et al demonstrated that patients with traumatic brain injury have a statistically significant increase in survival when transported directly to trauma centers in Virginia, a state that has a much more rural appearance.[45] In another study conducted in a rural setting, Rogers et al[46] found that patients transferred to a Level I trauma center from outlying hospitals had the same mortality as those admitted directly to a Level I center. This was true of even more severely injured patients. However, twice as many patients died at the scene in rural environments than in more urban environments (72% versus 40%). The authors postulated that this difference was due to delay in discovery of patients and to prolonged EMS arrival and transport times even to the regional hospitals.

INJURY DEMOGRAPHICS

This year nearly 40,000,000 people will be seen in our nation's emergency departments as a result of unintentional injury. More than 2.5 million of them will require hospitalization. In 1996 the number of deaths from unintentional injury increased for the fourth consecutive year, to 93,874.[47] Experts expect this trend to continue.

Patients die in a trimodal distribution after injury. The vast majority of deaths occur at the scene from immediately life-threatening airway compromise, brain injury, and exsanguinating hemorrhage. In fact, there is little that trauma care can do to improve these patients' survival other than trauma prevention strategies. An additional 20% of trauma deaths occur in the early phase, generally from exsanguinating hemorrhage.[48] It is this group of patients in whom prehospital and emergency department decision making can potentially have an effect. The last group of patients die later from multiple organ failure, usually septic in origin. This group represents approximately 10% of trauma deaths.[48] Some of these deaths may be prevented by limiting shock and using optimal resuscitation strategies. The exact percentage of lives that can be saved by altering trauma care, although not insignificant, remains unknown.

BLUNT TRAUMA. Blunt trauma is the most common mechanism of injury in the United States.[49] The mechanics of blunt injury involve a compression or crushing mechanism via energy transmission and direct injury. If compressive, shearing, or stretching forces exceed the tolerance limit of a tissue or an organ, the tissues are disrupted. This may result in injury to the solid viscera, such as the liver or spleen, or rupture of the hollow viscera, such as the gastrointestinal tract.

Injury can also result from movement of the organs within the body. Some organs are rigidly fixed, whereas others are more mobile. Injuries are particularly common in areas of transition from mobile to immobile organ because the part not rigidly fixed is free to move with a great degree of velocity.

The most common cause of death and disability from unintentional injuries worldwide is the motor vehicle crash. In 1996 the number of deaths from motor vehicle-related incidences in the United States alone rose to more than 43,000, and nearly 21,000,000 people suffered some disabling injury.[47] The injury patterns seen with motor vehicle crashes are difficult to predict because a number of factors contribute to them. Certainly the speed of the vehicle and the surface that it strikes are important in determining the vectors of energy. The use of restraint systems such as seat belts and air bags also influence not only the severity of injury but also the type of injury seen. A high-speed, head-on collision into a bridge abutment with an unrestrained driver at the wheel is far different than the car traveling at 20 mph that strikes a tree with a glancing blow with a driver protected by a seat belt and an air bag. Both are motor vehicle crashes, but the injury patterns will be substantially different.

Falls are the second leading cause of unintentional death in the United States and were responsible for more than 8,000,000 emergency department visits in 1994. They continue to account for more than 20% of all injury-related hospital admissions.[47] Falls from a height can produce a unique pattern of injury. The degree of injury is a function of the distance of the fall, the surface on which the victim lands, and whether the fall is broken by objects during flight. The center of gravity in adults resides in the pelvis, whereas in young children the center of gravity is in the head. Therefore children who fall a great distance often land on their head and thus are likely to suffer severe traumatic brain injury. Adults, on the other hand, often right themselves as they fall and land on their feet. The force is then transmitted up the axial skeleton into the spine. Lower extremity, pelvic, and thoracolumbar spinal fractures are common, as well as injuries to the retroperitoneal viscera. Brain injury and intraabdominal injury, however, are relatively rare.

Pedestrians struck by cars may likewise have unique patterns of injury. Pedestrians are completely unprotected, so all the force is applied directly to the portion of the body that is struck. Additional injury can be caused if victims are thrown through the air and strike a second object. Motorcyclists or bicyclists are also poorly protected, except for the protection afforded by helmets. Their injuries are also compounded by the fact that vehicles such as motorcycles can travel at great rates of speed.

PENETRATING TRAUMA. Penetrating trauma differs from blunt trauma in that it does not cause a diffuse pattern of injury. In the case of stabbings the wounding blade directly injures tissues as it passes through the body. Because the penetrating object produces a hole in the skin no larger than the blade, external examination of the size of the wound may grossly underestimate the degree of internal damage. In addition, the trajectory of the blade is not apparent by external examination. Any stab wound located in the lower chest, pelvis, flank, or back must be presumed to have a transabdominal trajectory and accompanying injury until proven otherwise.

Gunshots injure in several ways. Bullets may injure organs directly. Secondary missiles can be formed as bullets shatter bone and the bony fragments then disperse. In addition, the bullet produces a concussive zone of injury from energy transmission as it travels through the body. High-energy missiles can cause a significant amount of injury somewhat distant from their direct path. Some bullets are designed to expand or break apart as they enter the victim. These tend to cause more tissue destruction.

Entrance and exit wounds can approximate missile trajectory. Plain radiographs help to localize the foreign body, allowing prediction of vascular structures at risk for injury. Unfortunately, however, bullets often do not travel in a straight line. Thus all structures in any proximity to the presumed trajectory must be considered injured until proven otherwise.

THE EVALUATION PROCESS

The evaluation of patients after trauma must be rapid, systematic, and organized (Table 13-6). Injuries must be identified in the order in which they are likely to produce death or serious disability. These must then be dealt with in the same order in which they are identified. It is also important to remember that injury is a tremendously

TABLE 13-6	**Initial Evaluation**
Phase	**Evaluation/Intervention**
Primary survey	Airway
	Breathing
	Circulation
	Disability
	Exposure
	Identify and immediately treat life-threatening injuries
Resuscitation	Electrocardiogram
	Pulse oximetry
	Foley catheter
	Nasogastric tube
	End-tidal CO_2 monitoring
	Two large-bore peripheral IV lines (cutdown and central access as necessary)
	Routine lab work
	Blood for type and crossmatch
	ABG (with high index of suspicion)
	Initial IV fluid therapy
Secondary survey	Rapid head-to-toe evaluation
Diagnostic studies	Initial surveillance radiographs:
	• Lateral cervical spine
	• Chest x-ray
	• A/P pelvis
	Thoracic and lumbar spine films if needed
	Extremity x-ray studies as indicated
	Ultrasound, CT, angiography as necessary

Modified from Border JR, Lewis FR, Aprahamian C et al: Panel: prehospital trauma care—stabilize or scoop and run, *J Trauma* 23:708-711, 1983; and Gold CR: Prehospital advanced life support vs "scoop and run" in trauma management, *Ann Emerg Med* 16:797-801, 1987.
ABG, Arterial blood gases; *A/P,* anterior to posterior.

dynamic process, particularly immediately on patient arrival to the hospital. A stable patient can almost immediately become grossly unstable, and injuries that seem minor initially can evolve into life-threatening ones in a very short time. Thus the evaluation process must be repetitive to avoid missing this progression. A primary survey usually is conducted first; it is designed to identify immediately life-threatening injury. The survey should be followed by a resuscitation period, during which patients are reevaluated and monitored. The secondary survey—a head-to-toe physical examination—follows the resuscitation phase. At the end of the secondary survey, radiographic evaluation and other diagnostic tests should be performed. Results of these should be compiled to plan definitive care.

PRIMARY SURVEY. A primary survey is done specifically to identify and treat immediately life-threatening injury. Airway issues always assume the highest priority. In any badly injured patient, airway control must be accomplished immediately. Consideration should be given to definitive airway management in patients who present in shock and those who have significant traumatic brain injury (a Glasgow Coma Scale [GCS] score < 8), neck injuries, significant maxillofacial injury, or any other injury that potentially compromises airway integrity. Airway control in the field is generally accomplished by the orotracheal route, though nasal intubation is a viable alternative as well. Disposable end-tidal CO_2 detectors, if available, are extremely useful to confirm endotracheal tube position. However, CO_2 may be impossible to detect because of lack of cellular respiration from profound shock. Breath sounds may be difficult to interpret as well. In these cases further attempts at airway control in the field should be abandoned and the patient should be transferred to the hospital as quickly as possible.

In the resuscitation unit, airway control is most often obtained via the orotracheal route using a rapid-sequence technique with strict in-line stabilization of the cervical spine. Once the patient has been intubated, the endotracheal tube must be properly secured. Tube position should be confirmed, documented, and periodically rechecked.

Once the patient's airway has been controlled, rapid assessment of the adequacy of oxygenation and ventilation is the next highest priority. Supplemental oxygen should be administered to all patients in order to maximize peripheral oxygen delivery. The assessment of breathing includes evaluating for the six most life-threatening injuries: tension pneumothorax, open pneumothorax, massive hemothorax, pericardial tamponade, airway obstruction, and flail chest.

Tension pneumothorax or massive hemothorax should be diagnosed and treated on clinical grounds. Relying on breath sounds to make the diagnosis is unwise and could prove to be fatal. Chest decompression with tube thoracostomy is ideal therapy. However, a tension pneumothorax may be temporized by placing a 14-gauge IV catheter in the chest anteriorly through the second intercostal space. An open pneumothorax should be treated with an occlusive dressing such as Vasoline gauze followed by a chest tube. Flail chest is a clinical diagnosis in which a portion of the chest wall moves paradoxically from the remainder of the thoracic cage. This is caused by at least two or three ribs broken in two places. Endotracheal intubation should be considered for all patients with flail chest. However, most of the pulmonary dysfunction is from underlying pulmonary contusions and lacerations, not from the mechanical problems of the injured bony segment. Some patients can be managed without endotracheal intubation using good pain control techniques and directed pulmonary therapy. Intravenous or epidural patient-controlled analgesia (PCA) or an intrathoracic anesthetic block can be efficacious.

The physical findings often associated with the most life threatening of these conditions are depicted in Table 13-7. Unfortunately, these conditions often occur simultaneously, and the physical findings can be confusing. For instance, the patient who has exsanguinated from concomitant pulmonary hilar injury and has cardiac tamponade will not have jugular venous distention until very late. Therefore these conditions should be treated aggressively based on clinical suspicion.

TABLE 13-7 **Physical Findings in Thoracic Trauma Patients**				
	JVD	**Resonance**	**Breath Sounds**	**Tracheal Position**
Cardiac tamponade	Yes	Normal	Normal	Normal
Tension pneumothorax	Yes	Hyper	Decreased	Deviated airway
Massive hemothorax	No	Hypo	Decreased	Normal

JVD, Jugular vein distention.

Circulation, or the adequacy of peripheral oxygen delivery, is the next highest priority. Adequate perfusion depends on oxygen delivery meeting oxygen demand. The body cannot store oxygen; therefore an oxygen debt can be incurred rapidly. As previously noted, clinical signs often occur late in the trauma cycle, after oxygen debt is well established.

The degree of hemodynamic instability will be a function of the rapidity of ongoing blood loss and the degree or efficacy of compensation. Vasoconstriction may mask clinical signs until very late in the clinical course.[6] This is particularly true in young patients, most of whom have extremely compliant capacitance vessels. More than 50% of total circulating blood volume can be lost before patients show clinical signs. These patients often develop relatively sudden cardiovascular collapse. Commonly used parameters such as heart rate, blood pressure, pulse pressure, and urine output grossly underestimate the degree of blood loss. Calculation of base deficit via arterial blood gas analysis can be extremely useful in estimating blood loss and should be routine in any patient suspected of having significant blood loss.[50]

Large-bore IV access should be established and blood obtained for laboratory values. Two peripheral IV lines usually are sufficient. However, in patients who are in shock, vasoconstriction may make placement of large-bore peripheral IV lines problematic or impossible. In this case central access must be obtained. Percutaneous placement of pulmonary artery catheter introducers for infusion of volume is favored. Peripheral cutdown can take an excessive amount of time. The saphenous vein at the ankle is unlikely to be suitable for large-bore access. Saphenous cutdown in the groin risks iatrogenic injury to the femoral artery or femoral vein. Percutaneous access has been shown to be safe if done by experienced practitioners or residents with adequate supervision.[51] Flow characteristics of the fluid infused are a function of the length and diameter of the catheter. Short, wide catheters impede flow the least. Therefore long central venous pressure lines are not the best idea because flow through this type of catheter will be much slower than via an introducer.

A brief neurologic assessment (D for disability) is the next highest priority. Usually patients are asked to wiggle their toes, which assesses mentation and the ability to process information. In addition, it allows early identification of complete spinal cord injuries. In patients with some degree of mental obtundation, a GCS score should be calculated (see Chapter 19). This should be compared with the neurologic assessment obtained by the prehospital care providers in the field. Focal signs on physical examination, such as a unilaterally dilated pupil or a decrease of 2 in the GCS score, particularly if that decrease is in the motor component, are strong predictors of an intracranial lesion requiring evacuation.[52] This is an emergency situation that demands immediate CT examination, if the patient is hemodynamically stable, to plan operative decompression. Performing blind burr holes in the emergency department is useful only in very remote locations when patients are dying and transfer is not possible.

Any patient with a significant decrease in mental status should have airway control before leaving the emergency department. Suspected increases in intracranial pressure can be controlled temporarily with hyperventilation and the use of intravenous mannitol. It is important to remember that the diuretic effect of mannitol may make patients hypovolemic in 15 to 20 minutes. These patients may require additional intravenous fluid or blood transfusion to maintain circulating blood volume.

Complete exposure of the patient, with environmental precautions, is the next essential step in completing the primary survey. Many patients present with obvious injury, and the natural tendency is to focus on that injury. It is important to totally examine the patient to avoid missing a subtle but potentially life-threatening injury. Patients must be log rolled and their back examined, as well as the perineum and axillae. Despite the need for complete exposure, the patient must be kept warm and dry. Hypothermia depresses cardiac performance, impedes pulmonary function, and worsens any coagulopathy. Hypothermia often begins either in the field or in the emergency department. Warming fluids and autotransfusing any blood collected from the thoracic cavity can be helpful in preventing hypothermia. In addition, the ambient temperature in the resuscitation area should be kept above 70° F and patients should be covered after thorough examination.

RESUSCITATION. The primary survey should have identified all immediately life-threatening injuries, and those injuries should be dealt with as they are discovered. Resuscitation often occurs in concert with the primary survey because resuscitation accompanies therapy for life-threatening injuries. If the patient has been deemed stable after the primary survey, the resuscitation phase is the period in which the patient is monitored and cardiovascular stability issues are readdressed. If large-bore peripheral access was not established during the primary survey, it is important to obtain it at this point. Patients should be connected to a cardiac monitor and a pulse oximeter. End-tidal CO_2 monitors should be used in patients who have undergone intubation. A Foley catheter and gastric tube should be inserted if there are no contraindications. Contraindications to nasal insertion of a gastric tube include any significant midface fracture. In patients with a cribriform plate fracture, a nasogastric tube may inadvertently be placed within the cranium. Evidence of a urethral injury is a contraindication to bladder catheterization. Physical findings such as a high-riding prostate on rectal exam, blood at the urethral meatus, or a scrotal hematoma are absolute contraindications to placement of a Foley catheter. In male patients with clinical evidence of a pelvic fracture, Foley catheterization can be deferred until imaging studies are completed if the patient remains stable. It may be wise to obtain a urethrogram to document the integrity of the urethra in men with complex pelvic fractures before inserting a Foley catheter, even in the absence of clinical signs.

The initial fluid bolus given is generally 2 L of isotonic crystalloid. Patients who present with some degree of shock can be stratified over several response groups. The immediate responders are those who have a complete response to the initial crystalloid fluid bolus and show no evidence of ongoing blood loss or perfusion deficits. These patients in general have Class I or Class II shock (see Table 13-2). Transient responders are those who initially respond but then show signs of ongoing blood loss or perfusion deficit. These patients generally have Class II or Class III hemorrhage or have bled once and then re-bled. Fluid should be continued and a rapid search for occult traces of blood loss undertaken. Real consideration should be given to early transfusion in these patients. Patients who do not respond have life-threatening hemorrhage. The highest priority must be given to ascertaining the site of blood loss and stopping it immediately. These patients all require blood transfusion; uncrossmatched blood is a perfectly acceptable choice.

The transition between primary survey and resuscitation into the secondary survey is a useful time to obtain initial radiographs. It is also important to ensure that appropriate laboratory tests have been ordered and that blood has been sent to be typed and crossmatched.

SECONDARY SURVEY.   The secondary survey consists of a careful examination of the entire patient to elucidate injury and areas of potential injury. It is generally done in a head-to-toe fashion. It is important to remember to examine the pupils for reactivity and the tympanic membrane for evidence of membrane rupture and cerebral spinal fluid leak. Battle's sign, ecchymosis over the mastoid area, may be the only presenting indication of a basilar skull fracture. The midface area should be examined for swelling, tenderness, and stability. The neck should be kept immobilized until a cervical spine injury has been ruled out. However, it is possible to remove the collar carefully and elucidate the presence or absence of cervical spine tenderness. The neck should also be examined for the presence of subcutaneous

air, as well as ecchymoses or abrasions. The chest wall should be palpated for evidence of subcutaneous air, instability, or tenderness. The lungs and heart should be carefully auscultated. The presence or absence of hyperresonance or dullness on percussion of the chest wall along with characteristic breath sounds can raise suspicion of pneumothorax or hemothorax. The abdomen should be auscultated, inspected, and palpated. The presence or absence of tenderness will help determine the need for further investigation. The pelvis should be examined gently for evidence of tenderness and stability. It is important to avoid rocking the pelvis because unstable pelvic fractures have a tendency to bleed with any motion. The patient should be log rolled and the back examined. It is necessary to carefully palpate all bony prominences over the spine and examine any tender areas of the flank. Bruising and soft tissue injury should be noted. All four extremities should be examined for pain, tenderness, ligamentous stability, and adequacy of pulses. Finally the patient should undergo a complete neurologic evaluation.

CLINICAL DECISION MAKING

At this point the clinician should have identified all areas of defined and potential injury. It is now time for further diagnostics and definitive care. A priority must be assigned to each injury. Several principles apply.

Injuries should be investigated in the order in which they are likely to cause death or permanent disability. Most badly injured trauma patients require a multiplicity of diagnostic images, particularly radiographs and scans. The plan should maximize efficiency. Transporting patients can divert precious resources. When nurses transport patients for diagnostic testing, they are unable to care for other patients. Therefore it is important to realistically approximate the time needed for a diagnostic examination. An urgent CT scan of the head should not be delayed to obtain all the plain films simply for convenience.

The initial films generally obtained are of the lateral cervical spine, the chest, and the pelvis. These are good screening examinations to detect potentially life-threatening injuries and areas of possible blood loss. They can be obtained rapidly without transporting the patient from the resuscitation area.

Patients can lose blood into one or more body cavities—chest, abdomen, pelvis and retroperitoneum, and muscle compartments—and outside the body (e.g., on the street). Intrathoracic injury can be diagnosed with a combination of clinical suspicion, physical examination, and a plain chest x-ray examination. Pelvic bleeding can be extremely substantial and produce life-threatening hemorrhage. Virtually every patient who has significant retroperitoneal bleeding has a pelvic fracture. This diagnosis can be made with a combination of physical examination and a pelvic x-ray examination. Muscle compartment bleeding, if significant, will be obvious on physical examination.

External blood loss can be life threatening and may occur from injuries that appear innocuous at the time of initial presentation, such as scalp lacerations. It is difficult to quantitate blood at the scene, but the prehospital care providers will be the best gauge as to whether there was substantial external blood loss in the field. It is important to remember that even major vascular injury or significant scalp bleeding may stop, particularly if the patient develops hypotension at some point. These injuries may re-bleed once the patient's blood pressure is normalized.

Intraabdominal bleeding can be more difficult to detect. A plain film of the abdomen is not helpful in diagnosing intraabdominal bleeding, and physical examination is not at all specific or sensitive. Bedside ultrasonographic examination can be helpful in determining the presence or absence of intraabdominal bleeding, particularly in a patient in shock (Figure 13-4).[53] Diagnostic peritoneal lavage is also rapid and can be performed at the bedside. Although CT scanning is the most precise method of diagnosing abdominal blood loss, it is time consuming and usually takes the patient out of the resuscitation area. This technique should be reserved for patients who are hemodynamically stable.

RESUSCITATION FLUIDS. The goal of fluid administration in the trauma patient is to support cardiovascular function and maintain adequate peripheral oxygen delivery. Volume increases cardiac preload, thus supporting cardiac output. The standard initial fluid is isotonic crystalloid, though advocates of colloids and hypertonic saline do exist.[31,36-40] Both hypertonic saline and colloid infusion have the advantage of supporting cardiac function with a limited amount of fluid. Both rely partially on recruitment of interstitial volume to achieve this. Crystalloid fluid in adequate volume is as capable of cardiac augmentation as either of the other two choices. None of these fluids increase oxygen-carrying capacity. Overzealous administration of any of them can limit oxygen delivery in several ways. Fluid infusion will dilute hemoglobin levels, thus limiting oxygen

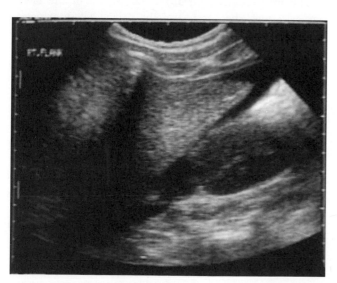

FIGURE 13-4 Focused assessment with sonography for trauma (FAST) demonstrates free intraperitoneal blood.

delivery. If hemoglobin falls dangerously low and myocardial oxygen delivery become insufficient, cardiovascular function may be compromised. If the heart is unable to accept a large volume load, be it colloid, crystalloid, or hypertonic saline, the heart can fail as it is pushed over the peak of its myocardial performance curve.

The only readily available fluid that increases oxygen-carrying capacity and preload is blood. Although clinicians are aware of bloodborne pathogens and transfusion reactions, equal concern must be raised regarding the consequence of delaying transfusion when blood is needed. The exact indication for transfusing blood remains controversial.[54-56] However, several principles seem reasonable.

Patients who are hemodynamically unstable and those with evidence of persistent tissue hypoxia despite fluid resuscitation should be given blood transfusions. Cross-matched blood is preferable, but the patient's clinical condition must dictate whether delaying transfusion is prudent. Major transfusion reactions are uncommon given today's level of sophistication in blood banking. Even transfusion with type O blood is relatively safe and is necessary in major blood loss situations.

Some patients may have a dangerous tissue hypoxia despite relatively normal vital signs. Patients with sufficient metabolic acidosis, as indicated by arterial blood gas values, must be presumed to be in shock. Clinicians should give strong consideration to transfusing these patients even if they are not significantly hypotensive. All patients whose metabolic acidosis persists after initial fluid resuscitation should likewise be given blood transfusions. Insertion of central monitoring devices and measurement of central venous oxygen saturation can be helpful. Patients with central venous oxygen saturations lower than 55% should be presumed to be in shock and bleeding. Consideration should be given to empiric blood transfusion.

Hematocrit, expressed in percent, is a ratio of red blood cells to circulating intravascular volume. If patients bleed acutely, they lose cells and volume equally. Thus patients who are bleeding acutely will maintain a normal hematocrit during the initial resuscitation. Hematocrit falls when patients receive exogenous fluids that dilute the red blood cells and the kidney compensates for blood loss by retaining salt and water. Initial hematocrit should not be used as the trigger for transfusion. Serial hematocrits may be better, but the time required to obtain laboratory results makes this impractical as a minute-to-minute guide during the initial phase of care.

In addition to red blood cell transfusions and use of hemoglobin substitutes, it is necessary to remember the important role that fresh frozen plasma (FFP) and platelets play in the care of the patient that requires massive blood transfusion. Standard blood transfusions replace only red blood cells, not coagulation factors or platelets. Coagulopathy after significant injury is quite common.

Thrombocytopenia is the most common disorder after massive transfusion. Although platelet counts of

$20,000/mm^3$ are generally sufficient to prevent spontaneous bleeding, patients in shock who are being resuscitated with large volumes of fluid and blood have much less predictable platelet function. Platelet counts must be monitored closely. In general, platelets should be given if the platelet count is less than $100,000/mm^3$ or if there is clinical evidence of ongoing bleeding. Alternatively, platelets can simply be given empirically as part of the massive resuscitation. Many patients take nonsteroidal antiinflammatory drugs on a regular basis. These drugs, as well as aspirin, inhibit platelet function, increasing bleeding after injury.

Likewise, massive transfusion rapidly depletes coagulation factors. Hepatic function may be impaired in the patient who is in shock, thus limiting the ability to rapidly mobilize additional coagulation factors. FFP can be lifesaving when given. It is easy to underestimate the need for plasma, and delays will certainly impede hemostasis. Prothrombin and partial thromboplastin times should be carefully monitored and kept normal.

Coagulopathy becomes clinically important when more than 10 units of red blood cells are rapidly administered. Prophylactic administration of FFP or platelets, based on the number of red cells administered, makes intuitive sense but has never been proven to have demonstrable benefits. However, taking time during massive transfusion to obtain coagulation profile laboratory results and then waiting for the FFP or platelets to be processed can delay necessary transfusion of these blood products, thereby worsening coagulopathy.

BLOOD SUBSTITUTES. The blood supply today is the safest it has ever been. However, the risks of hepatitis and human immunodeficiency virus (HIV) transmission via blood are real. In addition, the availability of blood for transfusion is at risk and the available allogenic blood product pool is shrinking. A shortage of 4 million units of packed red blood cells per year is projected by the year 2030.[57]

The storage of red blood cells has distinct limitations. Ideally, red blood cell storage maximizes the number of available viable red cells. The lower limit for successful transfusion is 70% red blood cell survival 24 hours after transfusion.[58] As storage time increases, red cell viability decreases as a result of a myriad of biochemical changes such as depletion of ATP 2,3-DPG. Stored blood becomes depleted of 2,3-DPG within 3 weeks. These cells do regain the ability to synthesize DPG once they are infused, but this does not occur for approximately 24 hours.[58] Animal studies have shown a significant increase in mortality and development of multiple organ failure when blood low in 2,3-DPG is transfused.[59]

Blood substitutes are an extremely attractive alternative. Unlike blood, hemoglobin substitutes do not require crossmatching and should carry no risk of bloodborne viral pathogens. Hemoglobin-based red cell substitutes are readily available, have a long shelf life, and are not immunosuppressive. In general, they have a lower viscosity than blood, which enhances flow through smaller capillaries and potentially increases peripheral oxygen delivery.

In initial trials hemoglobin substitutes produced toxicities of great concern, particularly renal toxicity. However, the methods for polymerization and tetrameric formation of free hemoglobin have vastly improved. Therefore toxicity occurs less often and circulation times, a problem in earlier trials, have been prolonged. In addition, oxygen-loading properties have been improved.

Hemoglobin-based red cell substitutes come from various sources of hemoglobin. Human hemoglobin-based preparations are naturally occurring; however, there is limited availability of outdated units of blood, which are the sources of this hemoglobin substitute. Elderly people, constituting an increasing percentage of society, are undergoing emergency and elective surgery more often, increasing the need for blood products. There has also been a decrease in the donor population in proportion to the population using allogenic blood products.[60] Bovine hemoglobin-based products offer the advantages of near limitless supply and lower cost. The last option is recombinant therapy to produce synthetic hemoglobin substitutes.

The various hemoglobin substitutes currently available are depicted in Table 13-8. Human polymerized hemoglobin has been administered safely in Phase II trials during both

TABLE 13-8 Hemoglobin Substitutes

Company	Corporate Sponsor	Product	Type	Clinical Trial Status
Baxter	None	Hem-Assist diaspirin crosslinked	Human	Patient efficacy: trauma, surgical, cardiac
Northfield	Pharmacia	PolyHeme glutaralde hydepolymerized	Human	Late patient safety: trauma, surgical
Hemosol	Fresenius	Hemo-Link o-raffinose polymerized	Human	Early patient safety: surgical
Biopure	B. Braum Melsungen	Hemopure glutaraldehyde polymerized	Bovine	Late patient safety: surgical, trauma, cardiac
Somatogen	Eli Lilly & Co.	Optro recombinantly crosslinked	Recombinant	Late patient safety: surgical
Perflubron	Alliance Pharmaceuticals	Perfluorocarbons	Organic	Phase II clinical trials

elective and urgent surgery, as well as to trauma patients requiring up to six units of transfusion in 24 hours.[61] Diaspirin crosslinked hemoglobin originally showed promise in animal trials. Phase II trials in trauma patients, however, demonstrated excessive mortality in the patients resuscitated with hemoglobin substitutes versus standard crystalloid fluid. That trial was truncated after 100 patients were enrolled.[62] Currently the use of Hemapure is being studied in elective orthopedic surgery patients.[61]

Perfluorochemical emulsions are another alternative to human blood. Perfluorochemicals are organic liquids derived from hydrocarbons, which are able to carry large amounts of dissolved oxygen. However, they require a high partial pressure of oxygen, thus potentially limiting their clinical use. One of their greatest advantages is that the purity of perfluorocarbons can be more easily controlled. Certainly one of the potential uses for these compounds is in patients whose religion does not allow them to accept donated blood or products prepared from blood. Perfluorocarbons are currently in Phase II trials.[10]

HYPOTHERMIA.   Hypothermia is a common problem in patients with serious injury and shock. Hypothermia can be classified as moderate or severe. In general, core body temperature is regulated and even relatively small changes in body temperature trigger a compensatory mechanism. This generally involves vasoconstriction at the level of the skin, which reduces heat loss, and shivering, which increases heat production. Unfortunately, many injured patients are subjected to environmental factors that predispose them to hypothermia. Shock, particularly if profound, is almost always accompanied by hypothermia. Patients who are injured and lie at ambient temperature on the street often become hypothermic even before they are discovered, particularly if they lie in wet clothes or are exposed to ambient temperatures significantly less than core body temperature. Decisions made by health care providers can significantly exacerbate hypothermia. Infusion of room-temperature intravenous fluids or cold blood can drop core body temperature. If patients are exposed and examined for potential injuries, care might not be taken to cover them or to warm the ambient temperature of the resuscitation area. Thus hypothermia begins in the field and can be exacerbated during resuscitation. In a series of patients requiring operation, Gregory et al demonstrated that most patients are hypothermic at the time of anesthetic induction.[63] These problems can be compounded by heat loss in the operating room from open body cavities, ongoing resuscitation, and cool irrigation fluids. In addition, anesthetic agents and narcotics suppress compensatory mechanisms.

Hypothermia affects all body systems. The extent to which each system is affected depends on the severity of the hypothermia and its duration. Initial cardiovascular response includes increases in heart rate, cardiac output, and mean arterial pressure secondary to increases in circulating catecholamines, peripheral vasoconstriction, and the resultant increase in central blood volume. Ultimately, however,

cardiac output, heart rate, and blood pressure fall. There is a generalized slowing of conduction, often accompanied by T-wave inversion and increases in the QT interval. A J wave may be seen as hypothermia worsens. Both atrial and ventricular arrhythmias such as atrial fibrillation can occur. Ventricular fibrillation can be seen as temperature falls below 30° C.

Hypothermia produces central stimulation of the respiratory system initially with an increased respiratory rate. However, as cooling progresses, respiratory depression ensues with decreased respiratory rate and tidal volume. This is often accompanied by marked increases in dead space. Epithelial mucosa may become swollen and the ability to clear secretions is depressed.

Decreased tubular enzymatic activity in the kidneys secondary to increased circulating blood volume from vasoconstriction produces a cold diuresis. This may be seen relatively early after a drop in core temperature of only 2° to 3° C.[64] This can give the false impression of an adequately resuscitated patient as vasoconstriction maintains blood pressure at normal despite a drop in cardiac output and urine output remains normal or even above normal. Oliguria and vasotemia occur quite late. Cerebral blood flow decreases as temperature decreases and may be accompanied by impaired mentation, agitation, drowsiness, or seizure.

The diagnosis of hypothermia depends on accurate measurement of temperature. Peripheral determinations of temperature such as oral or tympanic membrane temperature may not accurately reflect core temperature, particularly as vasoconstriction and other cardiovascular compensatory mechanisms increase. In addition, some methods of measuring body temperature are not designed to measure temperatures below 35° C. Core body temperature can best be measured by the thermistor on a pulmonary artery catheter. In addition, thermistors have been incorporated into Foley catheters and provide continuous readout of core body temperature in the bladder. Nierman demonstrated good correlation between pulmonary artery temperature and bladder temperature as long as the bladder is not being irrigated.[65] This included temperatures of approximately 35° C.

Clearly the best treatment of hypothermia is to limit heat loss and prevent it if at all possible. Treatment of mild to moderate hypothermia can be passive. This involves preventing additional heat loss and allowing the body to compensate by covering the patient with a blanket, increasing the ambient temperature, or using devices such as aluminum caps to prevent heat loss from the head. Convective air blankets can be beneficial as well.

When patients have developed severe hypothermia, active rewarming is generally used. Heat can be exchanged across any membrane such as the lungs, pleural cavity, or peritoneal cavity. The efficacy of rewarming is a function of the surface area across which heat can be exchanged. Thus peritoneal dialysis or irrigation of a chest tube with warmed, sterile fluid can increase body temperature. Warming inspired gases via the ventilator is another option. Intravenous fluids, including blood, should be warmed to at least to body temperature. There is some evidence that hot fluids can be used without concern for safety.[66] Convective warming units can be used, but they are not as efficient as the above-mentioned methods. Finally, extracorporeal rewarming techniques can be used in some cases. Gentilello et al described continuous arterial venous rewarming via modification of the commercially available warmers used to warm IV fluids.[67] Impressive rates of rewarming can be achieved using this or some other circuit.

Hypothermia may be a marker of the severity of injury as opposed to an independent predictor of mortality. In addition, some patients, such as those with brain injury, may actually benefit from hypothermia. Marion et al demonstrated improved survival among patients with traumatic brain injury who were randomized to sustained core body temperatures of 32° C for 24 hours.[68] In addition, there are case reports of patient survival when usually fatal injuries were repaired while the patient was in hypothermic circulatory arrest. Finally, Tisherman et al demonstrated the cerebral protective effects of deep hypothermia, up to 60 minutes in dogs, even in the face of cardiac arrest.[69] The potential applications in humans involve inducing a state of suspended animation accompanied by deep hypothermia to allow repair of injuries during heroic resuscitation.

HEMODYNAMIC MONITORING.   Evidence of inadequate perfusion should prompt simultaneous investigation and therapy. Patients who demonstrate inadequate resuscitation despite seemingly adequate treatment for the injuries identified may well have a missed injury. Untreated, these often are fatal. This should prompt a rapid but comprehensive search for injuries that were missed at the time of initial investigation or that were thought to be minor but have now become more profoundly symptomatic. In addition, resuscitation efforts should be continued.

Virtually every patient who has been inadequately resuscitated is volume depleted and can benefit from increased cardiac preload. Thus a reasonable response would be to augment cardiac preload with increased intravenous fluid. Blood is an excellent choice because it has the ability to increase cardiac output by increasing preload and to increase oxygen delivery by increasing hemoglobin. Serial measurements of serum lactate levels can be used to demonstrate the return of aerobic metabolism. Patients who undergo further resuscitation efforts and then have their lactate cleared to normal can reasonably be assumed to be more fully resuscitated.[70] It is important to remember that serum lactates can be misleading, especially when followed over a short period. There is often a washout phenomenon, particularly in badly injured patients. Thus serum lactate is high initially and either fails to fall or actually increases after resuscitation. This usually represents washout as resuscitation reperfuses beds that were previously underperfused. The next serum lactate measurement then begins to show normalization.

Patients who are not fully resuscitated often benefit from more sophisticated monitoring. Occult cardiovascular dysfunction is quite common after injury. An 80% incidence of inadequate resuscitation has been demonstrated in seriously injured patients with traumatic brain injury despite normal vital signs.[71] In addition, patients with significant penetrating torso trauma often have substantial perfusion abnormalities despite normal vital signs. In patients such as these, insertion of a pulmonary artery catheter can help define the problematic cardiovascular parameters. A more sophisticated understanding of vascular resistance and preload issues allows the resuscitation to be guided more precisely.

SPECIAL CONSIDERATIONS

PEDIATRIC TRAUMA

Although the pathophysiology of shock does not differ remarkably between children and adults, the manifestation does. Pediatric patients develop system dysfunction and organ failure in a consuming manner rather than the slower, progressive organ failure seen in adults. Children normally have a higher metabolic rate than adults, and trauma and sepsis only increase their metabolic needs. This hypermetabolic state quickly depletes the limited energy stores available to a child, and anaerobic metabolism occurs earlier. Liver failure can rapidly ensue, and the hypermetabolic state cannot be sustained. Cellular energy production becomes further decreased, thus limiting oxygen supply and ultimately producing cellular death.

The most frequent cause of shock in children, as well as adults, is hypovolemia.[72] Although the circulating blood volume in a child is relatively larger than in an adult, absolute blood volume is small. Most of the total fluid volume in children is extracellular and can be lost even without extensive hemorrhage. The early symptoms of hypovolemia in children are decreased peripheral perfusion, oliguria, and tachycardia. As with adults, blood pressure is not an accurate indicator of shock in children. As cardiac output decreases, vasoconstriction increases, artificially maintaining blood pressure. Cardiac failure follows hypotension relatively quickly. Stroke volume is relatively fixed in children and thus responds to shock by increasing heart rate. Thus in order to maintain adequate output in critically ill children, heart rates should be maintained within the high normal range.

Respiratory failure also occurs relatively quickly in pediatric patients. Children have little respiratory reserve because their chest wall is more compliant and their abdomen is larger, decreasing the ability to raise intrathoracic pressure. Children's thoracic musculature tires more easily than adults, predisposing them to respiratory failure.

There are also differences in the immune system in children relative to adults. Young children have few neutrophils and are not able to produce white blood cells in the face of stress as well as an older child. Complement levels do not reach adult normal ranges until the age of 3 to 6 months.[73] In addition, because immunoglobulin levels are transferred from mother to child, they wane at 4 to 5 months of age at which point infants become extremely susceptible to viruses, *Candida* infections, and bacteria. The child does not have the ability to launch an immune response to these contagions and may develop acute organ dysfunction as a result of infection after injury.

TRAUMA IN THE ELDERLY

During the past 10 years geriatric trauma has become an increasingly important segment of injury care. Several principles are important to maximize functional outcome and survival of this special subset of patients. The presentation of injured geriatric patients differs from that of their younger counterparts. As with everyone, the triage and initial care of geriatric patients must be based on a stepwise evaluation of anatomy, injury, and stability. Undertriage in the field can be particularly lethal in geriatric trauma patients. Their injuries are often occult. Symptoms such as confusion or pain may be ascribed to preexisiting disease. Unfortunately, the margin of error that a geriatric patient will tolerate is small. In fact, Osler et al found that, when controlled for degree of injury (using the Trauma and Injury Severity Score), six times as many elderly die as younger victims.[74] Despite this, most trauma systems currently do not have specialty centers for geriatric injury or different triage protocols for the elderly. Yet these same systems often subsegment the pediatric population because of its special needs.

The care of the elderly patient in the prehospital phase should be modified. Conditions as simple as isolated fractures can be life threatening. The loss of tissue turgor and the atherosclerosis that affect virtually every elderly person may limit tamponade and increase blood loss into muscle compartments.[75] The lack of cardiovascular reserve limits the heart's ability to rapidly accept the volume load. Cerebral atrophy makes potentially life-threatening, traumatic brain injury relatively asymptomatic initially. Elderly patients can then become suddenly and profoundly symptomatic up to hours after injury. Outcome at that point is likely to be poor, particularly if the patient has been undertriaged to a local emergency department. Paramedics should be advised to recognize that occult injuries can kill elderly patients. Intravenous fluids are best given in small boluses such as 250 ml aliquots to avoid precipitating heart failure. Fractures should be splinted and patients transported rapidly. The suspicion of traumatic brain injury should prompt transport to a trauma center.

The physiology of aging limits the elderly patient's ability to respond to the stresses of injury. This is perhaps most important in the cardiovascular system. Cardiac output remains relatively stable as the patient ages, but the ability to augment cardiovascular performance is blunted. The same is true for heart rate, a compensatory mechanism used to maintain peripheral oxygen delivery. Autoregulation attempts to hold coronary perfusion stable over a wide range of physiologic states. This becomes particularly problematic when fixed coronary artery lesions begin to limit flow. The coronary circulation is significantly venous extracted even at rest.

Increased peripheral oxygen demands after injury can precipitate a dangerous set of circumstances. As oxygen demand increases, cardiac output must likewise increase. Blood loss limits peripheral oxygen delivery and myocardial oxygen demands increase as the heart attempts to compensate and increase cardiac output. Coronary ischemia can occur, which itself limits cardiac output. This can quickly lead to irreversible shock.

Other organ systems, such as the lungs and kidneys, behave similarly. Ventilation/perfusion mismatch can approach 15% to 20% in the elderly.[75] A drop in cardiac output may itself be sufficient to precipitate hypoxia. Nephron mass decreases as people age, and creatinine clearance follows. However, the loss of circulating muscle mass generally means that blood urea nitrogen and creatinine levels remain normal. Even dehydrated elderly patients may produce large volumes of relatively dilute urine secondary to a loss in the reabsorptive capacity of the distal tubule. Finally, diuretic medications, which are used by many elderly people, may make the average person dehydrated at rest. Thus these patients may have significant renal impairment even though at first glance renal function is normal.

The role of occult hypoperfusion and its impact on outcome have recently been recognized. Cardiovascular insufficiency is common in elderly people, even in those who appear relatively stable.[76] Early recognition of this condition is extremely important because delays in therapy can be lethal. High-risk patients include those with traumatic brain injury or multiple long-bone fractures, those who were struck by an automobile, and those who present with initial hypotension. Invasive hemodynamic monitoring can be lifesaving in these patients.[1] In a prospective study of elderly patients at high risk, Scalea et al demonstrated that half these patients were in cardiogenic shock.[76] Survival was no different than when monitoring was initiated late in the patient's course of treatment. However, when the initial evaluation process was truncated, mean time to monitoring fell from 5.5 to 2.5 hours. Mortality was reduced by approximately 50% when important cardiovascular issues were identified and treated early. Thus it seems that the degree of physiologic alteration at the time of admission is not as important as early recognition and treatment.

The cause of this cardiovascular dysfunction has been thought to be pump failure secondary to a combination of chronic illness and acute cardiovascular need. More recently, however, the possibility of occult acute cardiac ischemia precipitating pump failure has been raised. This unstable angina may go unrecognized by both the patient and the physician. Chest pain may be masked by pain from other injuries. If the patient has not had angina previously, this may be dismissed as indigestion or thought to be secondary to the injury. Patients who are critically ill may be intubated and sedated and thus be unable to complain of chest pain even if it is present. If acute cardiac ischemia does occur, a different strategy is mandated. Cardiac support for the failing pump involves volume loading and inotropic support to maximize peripheral oxygen delivery. Acute cardiac ischemia, however, requires a strategy of myocardial protection involving beta blockade, judicious fluid administration, and nitrates. A 12-lead electrocardiogram and a single set of cardiac enzymes may be insufficient to detect cardiac ischemia. More work is needed to determine the exact incidence of cardiac ischemia and whether a different algorithm alters outcome in these high-risk patients.

CONCLUSION

The evaluation process and initial resuscitation of patients after significant injury is a tremendously dynamic process. It is important to identify injuries in the order in which they are likely to produce death or disability. Vital signs are imprecise, and although they can identify patients in extremis, they often underestimate the magnitude of physiologic derangement. Resuscitation schemes must be tailored to the population being treated. Some groups, such as pediatric and elderly patients, may well require specialized evaluation and resuscitation schemes.

Far and away the most important principle is for clinicians to remain suspicious. Nothing should be taken for granted; the trauma team should assume patients are badly injured with significant physiologic derangement until proven otherwise. A healthy skepticism and real clinical suspicion may prove to be the difference between survival and death.

REFERENCES

1. Scalea TM, Duncan AO: Initial management of the critically ill trauma patient in extremis. *Trauma Q* 10:3-11, 1993.
2. Abou-Khalil B, Scalea TM, Trooskin SZ et al: Hemodynamic responses to shock in young trauma patients: need for invasive monitoring, *Crit Care Med* 22:633-639, 1994.
3. Kearney ML: Imbalance of oxygen supply and demand. In Secour VH, editor: *Multiple organ dysfunction & failure*, ed 2, St. Louis, 1996, Mosby, 135-147.
4. Ozawa K: Energy metabolism. In Cowley RA, Trump BF, editors: *Pathophysiology of shock, anoxia and ischemia*, Baltimore, 1982, Williams & Wilkins, 74-83.
5. Gann DS, Amaral JF: Pathophysiology of trauma and shock. In Zuidema GD, Rutherford RB, Ballinger WR, editors: *The management of trauma*, ed 4, Philadelphia, 1985, WB Saunders, 37-103.
6. American College of Surgeons' Committee on Trauma: *Advanced trauma life support. Program for physicians.* Chicago, 1993, The College.
7. Scalea TM, Holman M, Fuortes M et al: Central venous blood oxygen saturation: an early, accurate measurement of volume during hemorrhage, *J Trauma* 28:725-732, 1988.
8. Scalea TM, Hartnett R, Duncan AO: Central venous oxygen saturation: a useful clinical tool in trauma patients, *J Trauma* 30:1539-1543, 1989.
9. Sinert RH, Baron BJ, Low RB et al: Is urine output a reliable index of blood volume in hemorrhagic shock? *Acad Emerg Med* 3:448, 1996.
10. Baron BJ, Scalea TM: Acute blood loss, *Emerg Med Clin North Am* 14:35-55, 1996.
11. Bania TC, Baron BJ, Almond GL et al: The hemodynamic effects of cocaine during acute controlled hemorrhage in conscious rats, *J Toxicol* 38:1-6, 2000.
12. Dutton RP: Shock and trauma anesthesia, *Anesth Clin North Am* 17:83-95, 1999
13. Gomersall CD, Joynt GM, Freebairn RC et al: Resuscitation of critically ill patients based on the results of gastric tonometry: a prospective, randomized, controlled trial, *Crit Care Med* 28:607-614, 2000.
14. Soderstrom CA, McArdle DQ, Ducher TB et al: The diagnosis of intra-abdominal injury in patients with cervical cord trauma, *J Trauma* 23:1061-1065, 1983.
15. Zipnick RI, Scalea TM, Trooskin SZ et al: Hemodynamic responses to penetrating spinal cord injuries, *J Trauma* 35:578-583, 1993.
16. Downing SE: The heart in shock. In Altura BM, Lefer AM, Schumer W, editors: *Handbook of shock and trauma*, New York, 1983, Raven, 5-28.
17. Muller JE: Treatment of myocardial infarction. In Cowley RA, Trump BF, editors: *Pathophysiology of shock, anoxia, and ischemia*, Baltimore, 1982, Williams & Wilkins, 684-701.
18. Reines HD, Bartlett RL, Chudy NE et al: Is advanced life support appropriate for victims of motor vehicle accidents: the South Carolina Highway Trauma Project, *J Trauma* 28: 563-570, 1988.
19. Sampalis JS, Lavoie A, Williams JI et al: Impact of on-site care, prehospital time, and level of in-hospital care on survival in severely injured patients, *J Trauma* 34:252-261, 1993.
20. Smith JP, Boda BI, Hill AS et al: Prehospital stabilization of critically injured patients: a failed concept, *J Trauma* 25:65-70, 1985.
21. Border JR, Lewis RF, Aprahamian C et al: Panel: prehospital trauma care—stabilize or scoop and run, *J Trauma* 23:708-711, 1983.
22. Cornwell EE, Belzberg H, Hennigan K et al: Paramedic vs private transportation of trauma patients: effect on outcome, *Arch Surg* 135:315-319, 2000.
23. Cannon WB, Fraser J, Cowell EM: The preventive treatment of wound shock, *JAMA* 70:618-621, 1918.
24. Ryzoff RI, Shaftan GW, Herbsman H: Selective conservatism in penetrating abdominal trauma, *Surgery* 59:650-653, 1966.
25. Marshall HP, Capone A, Courcoulas AP et al: Effects of hemodilution on long-term survival in an uncontrolled hemorrhagic shock model in rats, *J Trauma* 43:673-679, 1997.
26. Bickell WH, Bruttig SP, Millnamow GA et al: The detrimental effects of intravenous crystalloid after aortotomy in swine, *Surgery* 110:529-536, 1991.
27. Kowalenko T, Stern S, Dronen SC et al: Improved outcome with hypotensive resuscitation of uncontrolled hemorrhagic shock in a swine model, *J Trauma* 33:349-362, 1992.
28. Bickell WH, Wall MJ Jr, Pepe PE et al: Immediate versus delayed fluid resuscitation for hypotensive patients with penetrating torso injuries, *N Engl J Med* 331:1105-1109, 1994.
29. Chesnut RM, Gautelle T, Blunt BA et al: Neurogenic hypotension in patients with severe head injuries, *J Trauma* 44: 958-963, 1998.

30. Younes RN, Aun F, Accioly CQ et al: Hypertonic solutions in the treatment of hypovolemic shock: a prospective, randomized study in patients admitted to the emergency room, *Surgery* 111:380-384, 1992.

31. Wade CE, Kramer GC, Grady JJ et al: Efficacy of hypertonic 7.5% NaCl/6% dextran-70 in treating trauma: a meta-analysis of controlled clinical studies, *Surgery* 122:609-616, 1997.

32. Maningas PA, Volk K, DeGuzman L: Resuscitation with 7.5% NaCl/6% dextran-70 for the treatment of severe hemorrhagic shock in swine, *Crit Care Med* 15:1121-1126, 1987.

33. Velasco IT, Rocha-e-Silva M, Oliveira MA et al: Hypertonic and hyperoncotic resuscitation from severe hemorrhagic shock in dogs: a comparative study, *Crit Care Med* 17:261-264, 1989.

34. Krausz MM, Landau EH, Klin B et al: Hypertonic saline treatment of uncontrolled hemorrhagic shock at different periods from bleeding, *Arch Surg* 127:93-96, 1992.

35. Bickell WH, Bruttig SP, Millnamow GA et al: Use of hypertonic saline/dextran versus lactated Ringers solution as a resuscitation fluid after uncontrolled aortic hemorrhage in anesthetized swine, *Ann Emerg Med* 21:1077-1085, 1992.

36. Mattox KL, Maningas PA, Moore EE et al: Prehospital hypertonic saline/dextran infusion for post-traumatic hypotension: the U.S.A. multicenter trial, *Ann Surg* 213:482-491, 1991.

37. Vassar MJ, Fischer RP, O'Brien PE et al: A multicenter trial for resuscitation of injured patients with 7.5% sodium chloride: the effect of added dextran 70: the multicenter group for the study of hypertonic saline in trauma patients, *Arch Surg* 128:1003-1013, 1993.

38. Vassar MJ, Perry CA, Holcroft JW: Prehospital resuscitation of hypotensive trauma patients with 7.5% NaCl versus 7.5% NaCl with added dextran: a controlled trial, *J Trauma* 34:622-632, 1993.

39. Vassar MJ, Perry CA, Gannaway WL et al: 7.5% sodium chloride/dextran for resuscitation of trauma patients undergoing helicopter transport, *Arch Surg* 126:1065-1072, 1991.

40. Vassar MJ, Perry CA, Holcroft JW: Analysis of potential risks associated with 7.5% sodium chloride resuscitation of traumatic shock, *Arch Surg* 125:1309-1315, 1990.

41. Mattox KL, Bickell W, Pepe PE et al: Prospective MAST study in 911 patients, *J Trauma* 29:1104-1112, 1989.

42. Wangensteen SL, Deoll JD, Ludwig RM et al: The detrimental effect of the G-suit in hemorrhagic shock, *Ann Surg* 170:187-192, 1969.

43. Committee on Trauma, American College of Surgeons: *Resources for optimal care of the injured patient: 1999,* Chicago, 1998, American College of Surgeons.

44. Sampalis JS, Denis R, Frechette P et al: Direct transport to tertiary trauma centers versus transfer from lower level facilities: impact on mortality and morbidity among patients with major trauma, *J Trauma* 43:288-295, 1997.

45. Young JS, Bassam D, Cephas GA et al: Interhospital versus direct scene transfer of major trauma patients in a rural trauma system, *Am Surg* 64:88-92, 1998.

46. Rogers FB, Osler TM, Shackford SR et al: Study of the outcome of patients transferred to a level I hospital after stabilization at an outlying hospital in a rural setting, *J Trauma* 46:328-333, 1998.

47. Scalea TM, Boswell SA. Abdominal injuries. In Tintinalli JE, Kelen GD, Stapczynski, editors: *Emergency medicine: a comprehensive study guide,* ed 5, New York, 2000, McGraw-Hill, 1699-1708.

48. Rivera FP, Grossman DC, Cummings P: Injury prevention: first of two parts, *N Engl J Med* 337:543-548, 1997.

49. Scalea TM, Low RB: Approach to multiple trauma. In Howell JM, editor: *Emergency medicine,* vol 2, Philadelphia, 1998, WB Saunders, 975-984.

50. Mikulaschek A, Henry SM, Donovan R et al: Serum lactate is not predicted by anion gap or base excess after trauma resuscitation, *J Trauma* 40:218-224, 1996.

51. Scalea TM, Sinert R, Duncan AO et al: Percutaneous central access for resuscitation in trauma, *Acad Emerg Med* 1:525-531, 1994.

52. Gallbraith S, Teasdale G: Predicting the need for operation in the patient with an occult traumatic intracranial hematoma, *J Neurosurg* 55:75-81, 1981.

53. Scalea TM, Rodriguez A, Chiu WC et al: Focused assessment with sonography for trauma (FAST): results from an international consensus conference, *J Trauma* 46:466-472, 1999.

54. Consensus conference: Perioperative red blood cell transfusion, *JAMA* 260:2700-2703, 1988.

55. Practice guidelines for blood component therapy: a report by the American Society of Anesthesiologists Task Force on Blood Component Therapy, *Anesthesiology* 84:732-747, 1996

56. Farion KJ, McLellan BA, Boulanger BR et al: Changes in red cell transfusion practice among adult trauma victims, *J Trauma* 44:583-587, 1998.

57. Scott MG, Kucik DF, Goodnough LT et al: Blood substitutes: evolution and future applications, *Clin Chem* 43:1724-1731, 1997.

58. Ketcham EM, Cairns CB: Hemoglobin-based oxygen carriers: development and clinical potential, *Ann Emerg Med* 33:326-337, 1999.

59. Harmening DM: *Modern blood banking and transfusion practices,* ed 3, Philadelphia, 1994, FA Davis.

60. Chang TM: Future prospects for artificial blood, *Trends Biotech* 17:61-67, 1999.

61. Cohn SM: The current status of hemoglobin-based blood substitutes, *Ann Med* 29:371-376, 1997.

62. Slone EP, Koenigsberg M, Gens D: Diaspirin cross-linked hemoglobin (DCLHb) in the treatment of severe hemorrhagic shock: a randomized controlled efficacy trial, *JAMA* 282:1857-1864, 1999.

63. Gregory JS, Flancbaum L, Townsend MC et al: Incidence and timing of hypothermia in trauma patients undergoing operations, *J Trauma* 31:795-800, 1991.

64. Fisher DA: Cold diuresis in the newborn, *Pediatrics* 40:636-641, 1967.

65. Nierman DM: Core temperature measurement in the intensive care unit, *Crit Care Med* 19:818-823, 1991.

66. Werwath DL, Schwab CW, Scholten JR et al: Microwave ovens: a safe new method for warming crystalloids, *Am Surg* 50:656-659, 1984.

67. Gentilello LM, Cobean RA, Offner PJ et al: Continuous arteriovenous rewarming: rapid reversal of hypothermia in critically ill patients, *J Trauma* 32:316-327, 1992.

68. Marion DW, Obrist WD, Carlier PM et al: The use of moderate therapeutic hypothermia for patients with severe head injuries: a preliminary report, *J Neurosurg* 79:354-362, 1993.

69. Tisherman SA, Rodriguez A, Safar P: Therapeutic hypothermia in traumatology, *Surg Clin North Am* 79:1269-1289, 1999.

70. Abramson D, Scalea TM, Hitchcock R et al: Lactate clearance and survival following injury, *J Trauma* 35:581-589, 1993.

71. Scalea TM, Maltz S, Yelon J et al: Resuscitation of multiple trauma and head injuries: role of crystalloid fluid and inotropes, *Crit Care Med* 22:1610-1615, 1994.

72. Hauda WE II: Pediatric trauma. In Tintinalli JE, Kelen GD, Stapczynski JS: *Emergency medicine: a comprehensive study guide,* ed 5, New York, 2000, McGraw-Hill, 1614-1623.

73. Moloney-Harmon PA, Czerwinski SJ: The pediatric patient with multiple organ dysfunction syndrome. In Secor VH, editor: *Multiple organ dysfunction & failure,* ed 2, St. Louis, 1996, Mosby, 327-356.

74. Osler T, Hales K, Baack B et al: Trauma in the elderly, *Am J Surg* 156:537-543, 1988.

75. Scalea TM, Kohl L: Geriatric trauma. In Feliciano D, Moore EE, Mattox K, editors: *Trauma,* ed 3, Stamford, 1996, Appleton & Lange, 899-912.

76. Scalea TM, Simon HM, Duncan AO et al: Geriatric blunt multiple trauma: improved survival with early invasive monitoring, *J Trauma* 30:129-136, 1990.

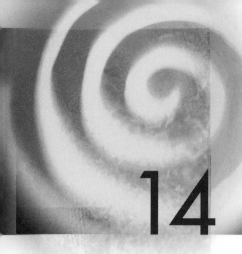

INFECTION AND INFECTION CONTROL

14

Patricia B. Casper • Manjari Joshi

Trauma and infectious diseases have been the leading causes of death, serious morbidity, and debilitating physical handicaps since the dawn of recorded history. However, both trauma and infection control are viewed as newly defined subspecialties of modern health care delivery. Only since World War II has technology provided a means to treat these diseases and ameliorate the outcomes. For example, rapid transport vehicles such as Med-Evac helicopters did not exist, so most trauma victims died either at the incident scene or during the transport to the hospital. The evolution of sophisticated, invasive medical technology has made emergent resuscitation and life support possible, thereby saving the lives of critically injured trauma patients. Similarly, with the discovery of antibiotics and vaccines, many of the predominantly fatal and debilitating infectious diseases became treatable and preventable. One would expect that new technologic advances would prevent development of infection. However, infection is the predominant complication that jeopardizes the recovery and life of severely traumatized patients surviving more than 5 days. Twenty-two percent to 63% of surviving trauma patients develop infection.[1,2,3] Studies of patients with blunt or penetrating traumas document that infection is responsible for 30% to 88% of posttrauma deaths.[1,2] Infection is ranked second only to severe head and high cervical spinal injury as the leading cause of death in this population.[1] It is a medical paradox that the many invasive therapies necessary to resuscitate and sustain these trauma patients can increase the risk of life-threatening infections.

The purpose of this chapter is to provide an understanding of the relationships that exist among factors influencing the development of infection in severely traumatized patients. These factors include the following:

- The nature of the underlying injuries
- Invasive therapies
- Mechanical support devices
- Loss of host-defense mechanisms
- The body's resident microbial flora
- The hospital environment

- Antibiotic use
- Clinical scenarios of resuscitation and patient care delivery
- Attention to infection-control guidelines

Only by understanding these relationships and the dynamic changes that occur during the patient's cycle from the initial injury through recovery can nurses, through the care that they provide, directly affect the ultimate outcome.

HOST-DEFENSE MECHANISMS

Compromise of host-defense mechanisms after trauma is the major determinant of subsequent infection. Therefore the primary goal of nursing care throughout the trauma cycle is to promote and safeguard the patient's ability to resist infection by carefully evaluating the host-defense mechanisms. Nurses must recognize and understand the relationship between the defense mechanisms and infection if they are to maximize the quality of their patient care.

Natural host defenses against infection consist of the external mechanisms of the anatomic barriers, the internal mechanisms of the humoral and cell-mediated immune responses, and the interactions that mediate between the external and internal defenses.[4] These protective defense mechanisms can be impeded or in some cases completely obliterated as the consequence of injury, disease, invasive therapy, chemotherapy, nutrition, or age.

Severely traumatized patients are frequently included in discussions of infection in immunosuppressed patients.[1,5,6] Although immunosuppression has been described most often in trauma patients sustaining thermal injury,[7] it also occurs in the multisystem trauma patient.[6,8,9] However, suppression of the immune responses in these patients does not appear to be a sustained phenomenon.

It is important to realize that trauma patients are not immunosuppressed like cancer patients, who are compromised by direct immunosuppressive therapy, cytotoxic drugs, cellular immune dysfunction, or granulocytopenia.[10,11] Trauma patients have functioning immune systems and can respond to invasion by exogenous antigens.

The natural host defense against infection consists of both external and internal mechanisms. Pathogens bypass the external, first-line defense, when broken skin and mucosal surfaces are contaminated during injury and later by surgery and debridement. Surgical interventions increase the risk of infection with placement of surgical drains or external fixation devices and compromise local tissue perfusion with hematoma formation, aggressive tissue handling, and the creation of dead space. The integumentary system is further compromised by microbes entering via intravenous catheters, central nervous system pressure monitors, rectal tubes, urinary catheters and endotracheal tubes. Breaks in the anatomic barriers and the patient's exposure to the intensive care environment are the primary causes of defense compromise (immunocompromise) in the trauma population. Virulent, highly resistant bacteria within the critical care unit may be spread among patients by personnel or shared equipment.[2,3,12,13] Trauma is primarily an event of the young; the mean patient age is between 29 and 31 years. Most trauma patients do not have premorbid conditions, such as diabetes mellitus, chronic renal failure, cirrhosis, or cancer, which jeopardize their defense mechanisms.

EXTERNAL DEFENSE MECHANISMS

SKIN. The skin acts as the major mechanical barrier blocking invasion by pathogenic microorganisms. The skin's protective ability is enhanced by its normally acidic pH, which inhibits the growth of some organisms.[14] Sebum, the oily secretion of the sebaceous glands, has long-chain fatty acids that act as germicidal agents. The biochemical characteristics of skin are regulated by the resident microbes of the normal flora. The major inhabitants include coagulase-positive and coagulase-negative staphylococci, streptococci, and diphtheroids.Extensive tissue destruction from burns, degloving and avulsion injuries, traumatic amputations, and high-energy open fracture injuries destroys the skin's protective barrier and sensing mechanisms. Destruction of tissue prevents delivery of cellular components of the immune system to the site of injury.

Compromise of perfusion to the skin from pressure on bony prominences, retraction by surgical instruments, or the presence of a hematoma or indwelling device can cause ischemia and subsequent necrosis, which provide the bacteria an enriched environment. Chemical irritation from degerming and defatting agents, adhesive tape, or excoriating exudates, as well as mechanical irritations created from sheet burns or restraint friction abrasions, also contribute to loss of the skin's defense mechanisms.

Elderly patients have the added burden of the age-related changes that affect the skin's normal function. Their skin has less oil, blood flow, innervation, and subcutaneous fat. Thus elderly patients are more prone to skin breakdown and wound infection than younger patients. Similarly, obese patients have reduced perfusion of tissues because of a large amount of subcutaneous fat. These patients have an increased risk of wound infection and skin breakdown.

Infection control guidelines relative to the defense mechanisms of the skin include meticulous aseptic technique, gentle tissue handling, alleviation of pressure, selection of the least irritating but most effective antiseptic solutions, and diligent handwashing.

RESPIRATORY TRACT. The respiratory tract has a complex system of host-defense mechanisms. Mucociliated epithelium cleans and protects airways and coughing, sneezing, and deep breathing provide mechanical clearing actions. Other pulmonary defense mechanisms include: secretory antibody immunoglobulin A (IgA), lysozymes, and phagocytes.[15]

Although respiratory defenses may be affected by chronic obstructive pulmonary disease, tobacco smoking, and immunosuppressive therapy, the primary loss of defenses in trauma patients occurs when the patient is intubated. All the natural defense mechanisms are circumvented, and microorganisms from the environment can be afforded unobstructed entry into the lungs. The risk for the development of nosocomial infection is greatly increased if respiratory equipment is not scrupulously maintained. Inadvertent contamination of the inspiratory circuits with an organism such as *Pseudomonas* spp. can be fatal because the rapidly replicating bacteria is aerosolized into the lungs.

The patient can be further compromised if chest wall integrity is disrupted or ventilation impaired. For example, flail chest injury, rib fractures, thoracic or abdominal surgical incisions, chest tubes, decreased level of consciousness, central nervous system dysfunction, and paralyzing agents limit normal clearing of secretions. Furthermore, immobility as a result of coma, traction and fixation devices, or spinal injury leads to retention or pooling of secretions because normal clearing actions are compromised. Elderly patients are prone to pneumonia secondary to the age-related changes that hinder their ability to cough and expectorate sputum. These changes include decreased elasticity of the alveoli, decreased tonicity of the intercostal muscles and diaphragm, and poor vital capacity and blood flow.

Damage from inhalation burn injuries secondary to heat, carbon monoxide, vaporization of toxic chemicals, and smoke can produce both temporary and permanent destruction of lung defense mechanisms. In addition, the restriction from unreleased circumferential thoracic eschars can impede breathing and contribute to hypoxemia.

Aspiration can cause pneumonia, lung abscess, or empyema and is a major concern in unconscious, immobile, or intubated patients. Normal respiratory flora can be altered by coma, hypotension, leukocytosis, azotemia, intubation, or antibiotic therapy.[16]

In community-acquired aspiration pneumonia, *Streptococcus* species are the most common isolates. In contrast, gram-negative bacilli and *Staphylococcus aureus* are the organisms most commonly isolated from nosocomial aspiration pneumonia.[16]

Nasal and tracheal tubes also increase the risk of upper respiratory infection. Indwelling nasogastric and nasoendotracheal tubes can obstruct the drainage of the sinuses and result in nosocomial sinusitis or can obstruct the eustachian tubes, causing otitis media. The presence of chest tubes has been shown to be a highly significant factor in the development of nosocomial empyema.[12]

Nurses can assist respiratory tract defense mechanisms by frequently repositioning unconscious or immobile patients, preventing the retention of pulmonary secretions by chest physiotherapy, and encouraging use of incentive spirometry coughing and deep breathing. The American Thoracic Society Consensus Statement documents the reduction of pneumonia with the use of lateral rotation beds by mobilization of tracheobronchial secretions.[17] Joshi et al demonstrated the importance of chest physiotherapy in 39 ventilated critically ill patients with a new pulmonary infiltrate, fever, leukocytosis, and purulent sputum. Within 4 to 8 hours after receiving vigorous chest percussion, 80% of the patients had partial or complete resolution of the pulmonary infiltrates.[18]

GASTROINTESTINAL TRACT.   The heavily colonized gastrointestinal tract serves as a major reservoir for microorganisms that can cause nosocomial infection. External defenses of the gastrointestinal tract include an intact mucosal epithelium, acid barrier of the stomach, and peristalsis to continually evacuate the tract. The lytic enzymes in saliva, secretory antibody IgA, lysozyme, and phagocytic cells work in concert to destroy bacteria that are ingested. Normal stomach, duodenum, and jejunum are colonized with low concentrations of mouth flora. The trauma patient soon loses the protection provided by the normal gut flora as the microenvironment is disrupted by injury, ischemia, impaired motility, pH changes, fasting, and antibiotics.

Drug therapy can have a negative influence on the defense mechanisms of the gastrointestinal tract. Antacids and H_2-blocking agents affecting gastric acid secretions can elevate the normal pH of the stomach and eliminate the protective acid barrier.[19] Gastric motility can be reduced by muscle relaxants, sedatives, and analgesia. Antibiotics shift the normal composition of the microbes colonizing gut flora. Despite the use of prophylactic antibiotics, peritonitis and deep-seated abscesses can develop when the integrity of the gastrointestinal mucosa has been broken.

GENITOURINARY TRACT.   The external defense mechanisms of the genitourinary tract include the ciliated mucosa that blocks bacterial adherence and the flushing actions of a distensible bladder. The bacteriostatic characteristic of urine is produced by a low pH and the hyperosmolar composition. Therefore urine is sterile because the environment of the bladder is not conducive to the growth of bacteria.[20]

The major predisposing infection risk factor in the genitourinary tract is the use of an indwelling urinary catheter, which creates an easy portal of entry for the microorganisms colonizing the perineum. Infection risks are higher in females because they have a short urethra and the added reservoir of the organisms colonizing the vagina. Other clinical conditions that increase susceptibility to infection include obstructions in the urinary system, changes in the chemical composition of the urine, renal failure, and frequent manipulations of the indwelling drainage system.

INTERNAL DEFENSE MECHANISMS

Compromise of internal host mechanisms after trauma can contribute to subsequent infection. The primary goal of nursing care throughout the trauma cycle is to promote and safeguard the patient's ability to resist infection.

The internal defense mechanisms include the humoral (e.g., B lymphocytes, leukocytes) and complex cell-mediated (e.g., macrophages, T lymphocytes) immune responses that support the patient's resistance to infection.[2]

Polymorphonuclear neutrophils are the first of the phagocytic leukocytes to arrive at the site of inflammation, usually within 6 to 12 hours after initial injury. Their role is to ingest bacteria, dead cells, and cellular debris. The number of circulating neutrophils increases during infection and usually is accompanied by an increase in the ratio of immature (bands, metamyelocytes, myelocytes) to mature neutrophils, known as a left shift.

Macrophages are similar to neutrophils in characteristics and functions. Produced within the bone marrow, monocytes circulate in the bloodstream and become macrophages when they infiltrate the tissues. Macrophages process and present antigens to the lymphocytes. They also have receptors for complement, antibodies, and lymphokines. Plasma proteins activated by inflammation include the complement, clotting, and kinin systems. When activated, a specific sequence of complement components leads to fluid accumulation within the cell, causing the membranes to rupture. The clotting system forms a fibrous meshwork trapping exudate, microorganisms, and foreign bodies to prevent the spread of infection, stop bleeding, and provide a framework for repair. Kinin system proteins dilate vessels, increase vascular permeability, and can increase leukocyte chemotaxis.

Lymphocytes migrate through lymphoid tissues and become either B lymphocytes, responsible for humoral immunity, or T lymphocytes, responsible for cell-mediated immunity. Each individual B or T cell recognizes a specific antigen. B cells produce antibodies that attack antigens; T cells directly attack antigens. B-cell lymphocytes are responsible for immunoglobulin production. Specific antibody production may be decreased after blunt trauma.[21]

T lymphocytes of the cell-mediated system have a variety of roles and are further divided into subclasses: the helper cells (T helper-inducer, CD4) and suppressor T cells (T suppressor-cytotoxic, CD8). Trauma can decrease total T cells within 24 hours of injury, with effects lasting 10 days. In addition to T cell dysfunction, alteration in cytokine production also occurs. Patients receiving high-volume transfusions may have lowered T cell counts.

The reticuloendothelial system of the liver and spleen removes as much as 80% to 90% of the particulate matter in the blood. The digestive capacity of Kupffer's cells of the liver is decreased after trauma.

SPLEEN.   The immune responses mediated by the spleen include filtration of aging or deformed blood cells, antibody synthesis, promotion of phagocytosis, and complement and T-cell amplification. Asplenic patients have significantly decreased levels of immunoglobulin M (IgM), lack the ability to switch from IgM to IgG antibody production,[22] and have diminished properdin activity (an alternative complement pathway factor).[23] The net effect of impaired antibody formation and diminished complement activity is a reduction in opsonic activity.[24] Opsonization facilitates the preliminary adherence of a phagocyte to a bacterium. This is especially important for the phagocytosis of encapsulated bacteria such as pneumococci, salmonellae, haemophilus, meningococci, and *S. aureus.*

Because the spleen is a solid, highly vascularized organ, blunt abdominal trauma can produce splenic rupture and massive hemorrhage. In the past emergent splenectomy was commonly performed. However, with the awareness of the spleen's role in immunity and reports of postsplenectomy sepsis, splenic salvage or splenorrhaphy is now the treatment of choice.[25]

Overwhelming postsplenectomy sepsis has been well described in children and is being increasingly reported in splenectomized adults.[24,26] Postsplenectomy sepsis is fulminant and usually fatal. Therapy must be aggressive, with early initiation of antibiotics and vigorous hemodynamic support. The incidence of postsplenectomy sepsis after trauma is relatively low, occurring in approximately 1.4% of patients.[27] However, because the associated mortality rate is high, prevention is imperative. Patients undergoing splenectomy secondary to trauma should receive the pneumococcal vaccine (Pneumovax 23), a polyvalent vaccine directed against 23 of the pneumococcal capsular antigens. One study has shown that the antibody response to a polyvalent pneumococcal vaccine among splenectomized trauma patients is similar to that in normal, healthy control patients.[28] Although this study could not determine whether these patients were adequately protected from pneumococcal disease, the investigators recommended vaccination within 72 hours of splenectomy. Revaccination in 5 years has been suggested, but further research is needed to determine the duration of response to the vaccination.[29]

Throughout the trauma cycle, nurses can aid the prevention and outcome of postsplenectomy sepsis by ensuring that the pneumococcal vaccination has been given and educating the patient about infection risks and disease symptoms. Formal recommendation as to the benefits of the *Haemophilus influenzae* B, or meningococcal, vaccine have not been made. Patients should also be counseled to discuss the immunizations with their private physicians.

INFLAMMATORY RESPONSE.   Inflammation is a nonspecific response to tissue damage that can be caused by direct trauma or induced by a variety of mechanical, chemical, and biologic stimuli. A complex pathologic process consisting of cellular and histologic reactions occurs in the affected blood vessels and adjacent tissues. The fundamental process includes local reactions and resulting morphologic changes, destruction and removal of the injurious material, and responses that lead to repair and healing.[30] The systemic response to inflammation is characterized by a hyperdynamic state and increased permeability of vascular endothelium.

When damage occurs, local blood flow, vasodilation, and capillary permeability are increased. Edema and the increased volume of bound water results in a swelling of the inflamed area. The inflamed tissue induces leukocyte-promoting factor that attracts the circulating white cells and causes the reticuloendothelial system to release granulocytes, particularly neutrophils. Granulocytes and monocytes cross the walls of venules and capillaries via ameboid movement and invade the affected area. Inflammatory responses induced by infection can be brought under control by these phagocytic cells as they invade the inflamed tissue and engulf and kill the pathogenic organisms. This response is amplified by the release and elaboration of several humoral mediators from the killed or injured cells. These substances include histamine, serotonin, leukotrienes, kinins, prostaglandins, and the early components of complement.[31] Other factors released from the inflamed tissue stimulate the liver to produce a number of proteins, including fibrinogen. The beneficial effects of the inflammatory response include the following:

- Presence of leukocytosis
- Interaction of plasma proteins (i.e., specific and nonspecific humoral agents)
- Production of fibrinogen, which is converted to fibrin, aiding the localization of the infectious process by providing a matrix for phagocytosis
- Increased blood and lymph flow, which dilutes and flushes the toxic material

Neutrophils (polymorphonuclear leukocytes) and macrophages (reticuloendothelial system cells) are the primary cells involved in phagocytosis. In the early stages of inflammation the exudate is primarily alkaline and polymorphonuclear leukocytes predominate. As the reactions persist, congestion of the capillaries leads to anoxia in the inflamed area and induces anaerobic respiration. Glycolysis creates lactic acid production and accumulation and decreases the pH of the exudate. If the inflammation is caused by bacteria, the lymphocytes produce antibodies against the invading microorganisms. In bacterial infections macrophages become the predominant cells of inflammatory exudate. Although the acidic pH and the antibodies of the exudate may inhibit bacterial growth, the major defense against infection is attributable to the actions of the phagocytic cells. These cells interact to engulf the cell remnants and fibers altered by the tissue damage and the inflammatory response.

When tissue damage is severe or inflammation persists, large numbers of neutrophils migrate to the site. Many of these cells are killed by the inflammatory agent, and others die because of the acid pH of the exudate. Enzymes released from the stimulated, injured, or dead leukocytes can degrade local connective tissue, causing further destruction, necrosis, and tissue liquefaction. The resulting inflammatory exudative fluid material is called *pus*. Pus consists of dead and dying leukocytes, blood, plasma, fibrin, cellular debris, and living and dead microorganisms. Resolution of the inflammatory response is impeded when extensive tissue damage and necrosis have occurred. Surgical debridement is then required.

Clinical manifestations of the inflammatory response include redness, heat, swelling, pain, and loss of or inhibited function. The redness and warmth result from the increased blood flow to the affected area. Swelling results from the congestion and exudation from the capillaries. Pain is caused by changes in osmotic pressure and pH of the exudate and the pressure and stretching of nerve endings. Loss of function may be secondary to injury or the destructive mechanisms of the inflammatory response.

Systemic pathologic manifestations include peripheral leukocytosis, increased sedimentation rate, and fever. When tissue is overwhelmed by invasive infection or tissue necrosis, the usual inflammatory response mechanisms cannot compensate for the insult and bacteremia ensues. In this condition bacteria or the toxins of tissue necrosis invade the bloodstream, producing a constellation of symptoms including fever, shaking chills, and confusion, as well as signs and symptoms of shock (i.e., hypotension, tachycardia, tachypnea, and oliguria).

Infection from a variety of bacteria, viruses, fungi, and rickettsiae can cause septic shock. Toxins from gram-negative enteric bacilli, gram-positive organisms such as *S. aureus*, group A β-hemolytic streptococci, pneumococci, and histotoxic strains of anaerobic *Clostridium* most commonly induce septic shock in trauma patients.[32,33] Toxins such as lecithinase (α-toxin), hemolysins, enterotoxins, coagulases, and hyaluronidases destroy cellular membranes, alter vascular endothelial permeability, and induce tissue necrosis. Bacterial toxins increase vascular permeability, which may result in significant losses of plasma fluid into the interstitial spaces.[34] This is commonly referred to as "third spacing" and results in inadequate circulatory volume, circulatory collapse, and potentially profound hypotension. Release of exotoxins is directly responsible for the progression of disease.[34] Furthermore, when inflammatory response results from tissue necrosis, the progression of disease is rapid and blood cultures are often negative.

Hypovolemia decreases perfusion of nonvital tissues, producing anaerobic cellular metabolism with increased production of lactate. This is the primary cause of metabolic acidosis in septic shock. The alteration in cellular metabolism, especially when coupled with the destructive effects of bacterial toxins, causes the lungs to compensate for the resultant hypoxia and acidosis. The patient's respirations become more rapid and shallow, because of acidosis, as the shock state progresses. This respiratory insufficiency can ultimately lead to acute respiratory failure. If hypovolemic shock is not corrected within 1 hour of injury or insult, the patient's survival is jeopardized.[35]

The inflammatory response results from a number of events and stimuli in the trauma population. Inflammation can occur directly from the injury. The more extensive the tissue destruction, the greater the inflammatory response.[36] It is not uncommon to have very high white blood cell counts (i.e., 20,000 to 40,000 cells/mm^3) immediately after severe traumatic injury. In addition to the trauma, inflammation can be induced by a variety of stimuli, including the presence of foreign objects such as bullets, stones, sutures, catheters, and orthopedic hardware; exposure to toxic agents such as extremes of temperature, ionizing radiation, and chemicals; and the presence of biologic agents such as microorganisms, bacterial toxins, antigen-antibody complexes, and devitalized and necrotic tissue.

It is important to determine the source of the inflammation so that appropriate therapy can be initiated. It may be virtually impossible to distinguish an inflammatory response that is induced by infection from one that is not. In such cases the diagnosis of infection must be determined by the overall trend of the patient's clinical condition. Strategies to facilitate this diagnosis are outlined later in this chapter.

Cellular immunologic responses can be altered by the inflammatory response, hematoma formation, edema, and the extent and characteristics of tissue destruction. The multifactorial effects of trauma on the complex interactions of the humoral and cell-mediated immune responses are often difficult to elucidate. Whether an overall depression of the immunologic response occurs remains unclear.[2] Various defects of immunity after trauma have been identified. These include (1) responses and interactions of neutrophils,[37-39] lymphocytes,[10,22,23] monocytes, and macrophages[23,40]; (2) delayed hypersensitivity reactions[41]; (3) the function of the reticuloendothelial system; (4) opsonization[42]; and (5) the activation of complement.[43] Although there is some disagreement regarding the function of specific elements of these responses, it is generally agreed that the key determinants of immunologic dysfunction emerge from the overall severity and characteristics of the injury, the presence of shock, the obliteration of anatomic barriers, and the dilutional effects of massive fluid replacement.[2,39]

As the patient progresses through the trauma cycle, the precipitating events of inflammation resolve, cell function is restored, and fewer invasive interventions and mechanical support devices are required. Therefore new onset of inflammation developing during later phases of recovery may be more easily attributed to infection than to the systemic inflammatory response.

FEVER. Under normal conditions, body temperature is determined by the "set point" of the hypothalamic thermoregulatory system and a delicate balance between heat production and heat loss. Heat production is derived from the metabolism of food and body activity. Heat loss occurs via radiation, convection, and vaporization and is regulated by peripheral blood flow to the skin, sweating, and heat loss with vapor from the lungs. The normal body temperature has a set point of 98.6° F (37° C), but variations of ±0.6° F can be observed. Therefore the normal temperature range can vary from 98° to 99.2° F (36.6° to 37.5° C). Fever results from any disturbance in the hypothalamic thermoregulatory activity that leads to an increase of the thermal set point. Clinically, fever is defined as any temperature above 100.5° F (37.8° C) if taken orally or above 101.5° F (38.4° C) if taken rectally. Axillary temperature measurement is the least desirable method; core or oral temperatures are preferable.

In healthy individuals a fever is most frequently triggered by an infection from microorganisms, bacterial toxins, or antigens; an allergic reaction caused by the invasion of antigens; or the formation of antigen-antibody complexes.[44] These external agents, or exogenous pyrogens, stimulate the inflammatory response. Activation of the polymorphonuclear leukocytes, monocytes, and macrophages, which mediate the inflammatory response, releases an endogenous pyrogen.[45] When the fever pathway is triggered by antigenic stimulation, activation of the lymphocytes precedes activation of the phagocytic cells. In this case the lymphocytes produce a "lymphokine" that then activates phagocytic cell populations. The exact mechanisms for the release of endogenous pyrogens are not known, but recent studies suggest the operation of more than one mechanism, as well as the existence of more than one type of pyrogen.[46]

Endogenous pyrogen is released into the circulation, travels to the thermosensitive neurons in the anterior hypothalamus, and reduces the inhibitory effect of thermosensitive neurons on the "thermal-blind" neurons of the posterior hypothalamus. Peripheral vasoconstriction results, accompanied by a drop in body surface temperature. Thermal receptors in the skin activate somatic motor nerves innervating the skeletal muscles. Muscle contractions increase and are expressed as shivering or shaking chills. A new thermal set point is established with an increase in body heat and a rise in body temperature (i.e., fever).

Fever is often described as one of the classic manifestations of infection. In trauma patients the significance of the febrile response and the pattern of the temperature must be evaluated carefully. Many of the thermoregulatory mechanisms can be compromised by the nature of the injury. Patients sustaining massive burns, extensive soft tissue injury, and severe spinal cord injury lose the skin's thermoregulatory functions. These patients may have a hypothermic set point—that is, a set point below 96° F (35.5° C). Therefore a sudden increase of temperature to 99° F (37.2° C) may be indicative of fever in these patients. Elderly patients also can have a lower thermal set point, which is attributed to the deterioration of the skin's normal function. On the other hand, activation and chronic stimulation of the inflammatory response may cause some patients to establish a higher than normal set point. These patients appear to have a persistent fever. Patients sustaining severe brain injury resulting in compromise or injury of the hypothalamus may have irregular, widely variant temperature patterns. This condition is known as central fever.

Because fever is a manifestation of both infectious and noninfectious inflammatory responses, its utility for the diagnosis of infection is limited. Therefore continuous evaluation of the overall clinical condition compared with the temperature pattern trend is essential. This is crucial during the early phases of the trauma cycle, when the inflammatory responses are complex and acute.

THE MICROBIOLOGIC RESERVOIR

As the patient progresses through the phases of the trauma cycle, the reservoirs of the microorganisms that can induce infection continually change. Contributory factors include the events of the initial trauma, the different locations of the patient in the health care delivery system, antibiotic use, and the characteristics of the injuries and clinical course.

There are both endogenous and exogenous sources of microorganisms.[47] The primary reservoir is the patient's own endogenous flora.[48] These organisms are generally nonpathogenic and colonize the skin, respiratory tract, gastrointestinal tract, and genitourinary tract. The predominant pathogens recovered from infections occurring in trauma patients are coagulase-positive and coagulase-negative staphylococci, which colonize all four body systems. However, the organisms of the normal flora act as pathogens when they are provided access into normally sterile body sites. These avenues are created by disruptions of the natural barriers. The composition of the normal flora and their usual patterns of antibiotic susceptibility can be altered by antibiotic therapy, changes in the patient's clinical condition, and exposure to the intensive care unit (ICU) setting. The emergence of highly resistant strains results, creating complex dilemmas for therapy because more toxic antimicrobial agents must be employed when a serious infection develops. A summary of the normal flora is shown in Table 14-1.

Exogenous sources of microorganisms arise from the conditions at the incident scene and the hospital setting. Although relatively rare, organisms encountered at the incident scene can later cause serious, even fatal infection. These microorganisms become pathogenic and gain entry into normally protected tissues or are aspirated into the lung if they are not debrided from open wounds.

On the other hand, nosocomial organisms are frequently the causative agents of infection.[49,50] Unwashed hands of personnel, contaminated equipment, and sharing of supplies and equipment provide vehicles for pathogens to cross-contaminate patients. The primary objectives of infection control are to prevent these organisms from gaining access to sterile body sites, eliminate the modes of transmission or cross-contamination, and minimize alterations of the patient's normal flora.

TABLE 14-1   The Microbiologic Reservoir: The Normal Flora

Skin
Coagulase-positive staphylococci
Coagulase-negative staphylococci
Aerobic and anaerobic streptococci
Bacillus species
Diphtheroids

Respiratory Tract
Coagulase-positive staphylococci
Aerobic and anaerobic streptococci
Neisseria species
Bacteroides species
Fusobacterium species
E. coli
Hemophilus species
Diphtheroids
Lactobacilli
Actinomyces species

Gastrointestinal Tract
Aerobic and anaerobic streptococci
Diphtheroids
Bacteroides species
Lactobacilli
Clostridium species
Veillonella species
E. coli
Proteus species
Candida species
Fusobacterium species
Klebsiella species
Actinomyces species
Enterococcus species

Genitourinary Tract
Coagulase-positive staphylococci
Diphtheroids
Aerobic and anaerobic streptococci
Hemophilus species
Coagulase-negative staphylococci
Fusobacterium species
Lactobacilli
Clostridium species
Actinomyces species
Bacteroides species
Candida species

The presence of a microorganism in and of itself does not necessarily mean that an infection is evident. Nor does a positive culture necessarily mean that the patient is infected. A positive culture merely means that an organism is growing in the culture medium. Positive culture results must be evaluated from the perspective of the patient's clinical picture. In other words, there must be a specific host-parasite relationship in order for infection to occur.

Colonization occurs when microorganisms exist in or on a body system and no detrimental effects result. In some instances this may be a symbiotic relationship where both host and microorganism benefit. For example, the organisms colonizing the skin help to regulate the skin's pH and prevent establishment of pathogenic organisms. Similarly, the gut flora provide the body with a natural source of vitamin K and add bulk to fecal material to promote peristalsis. Open wounds and the respiratory secretions of ventilator-dependent patients may be abundantly colonized, but the presence of microorganisms does not necessarily mean that an infection has developed. Infection occurs when the organisms cause injury or damage to the tissues.

The relationship between the microorganisms and the patient and the development of infection is illustrated by the following formula[47]:

Possibility of infection = number of organisms × virulence/patient's resistance

The number of organisms is the dose or inoculum of microorganisms. The inoculum can stem from endogenous flora, the hands of personnel, the environment of the hospital setting, and occasionally the incident scene. It can be reduced by the use of meticulous aseptic technique, adequate debridement of the wounds, proper cleaning and maintenance of equipment, strict compliance with infection control guidelines, and handwashing.

The virulence of the organism is its ability to cause disease. For example, *S. aureus,* which produces the enzyme coagulase, is more capable of inducing infection than *Staphylococcus epidermidis,* which does not produce coagulase. However, among critically ill patients, organisms such as coagulase-negative staphylococci and fungi previously thought to be nonpathogenic organisms are now considered the pathogens of serious and fatal infections.[51,52]

Two factors contribute to this trend in nosocomial pathogens:

- Increased use of invasive devices
- Availability of potent new antibiotics

Therefore, in the critically ill trauma population, any microorganism has the potential to cause serious and even fatal disease.

INFECTION RISK FACTORS

Infection risks factors constantly change as the patient proceeds through the cycle from initial injury to recovery. The risk of infection is influenced by the following factors: clinical setting; therapeutic interventions (e.g., antibiotics, surgery, invasive devices, infusates, medications); the amount of attention given to infection control guidelines; and, most importantly, the nature and extent of the injuries and compromise of the host-defense mechanisms. Prevention of infection depends on not only identifying these factors but also recognizing the influences that each has on the others.

CLINICAL SETTING

Adherence to infection control guidelines influences the environmental infection risks. Emergent procedures are often crucial to survival. During initial resuscitation, there may be little time to comply with rigorous infection control practices (e.g., meticulous skin preparation of operative and procedure sites, scrupulous aseptic technique, gentle tissue handling, adherence to proper dress codes, or even handwashing). Sterile trays and fields can be easily contaminated as the attention of the staff focuses on the needs of the patient rather than the equipment in the environment. As more people become involved in the resuscitation, the less space there is for the staff to function, and the environment becomes more chaotic and cluttered. These factors increase the probability of contamination.

In nonemergent settings the lack of attention to handwashing by hospital staff continues to be the primary cause of cross-contamination among patients. The frequency with which handwashing should be performed—before and after each patient contact—can be time consuming. In addition, the nurse/patient ratio can influence handwashing practices and overall compliance with infection control guidelines.[53,54] The trauma team comprises many members including: physicians, nurses, allied health professionals, and ancillary personnel. Therefore it is not uncommon for one person to have multiple patient contacts during the course of his or her shift. Each time a health team member fails to wash hands, the chances of cross-contamination increase. This is a particular hazard in the intensive care unit, where nurses and others frequently manipulate vascular lines and other invasive devices. Equipment becomes inoculated by bacteria from their hands, and these bacteria can then gain direct access to the patient. Unfortunately, the practice of handwashing is too often forgotten. In addition, the hands of the patient, especially the fingernails, require care because confused or stuporous patients may scratch off dressings or scratch suture lines. Other actions that increase the risk of infection hazards include uncapping needles with teeth, contaminating sterile fields with clothing or bare hands, allowing fluid to reflux from drainage vessels back into the patient's body cavity, and dress code infractions.[55]

The care of trauma patients often requires a vast array of equipment and supplies. Improper and inadequate cleaning of equipment, use of supplies and equipment beyond recommended sterility intervals, and sharing supplies among patients promote the risk of infection, create reservoirs of microorganisms, and potentiate infectious outbreaks and epidemic situations. Tape and scissors are common vehicles of cross-contamination. For example, the practice of placing strips of tape on objects such as bed rails, countertops, and IV poles before application to the dressings may result in tape contamination. If surfaces of the equipment are contaminated with bacteria, microorganisms adhere to the tape and thus inoculate the dressing. Scissors become a vehicle for cross-contamination when they are used to remove wound dressings. The grooves and notches of the scissor blades can become contaminated with wound drainage and exudates. This material is often teeming with bacteria, which can then be introduced into another patient's wounds at the next dressing change. Disposable scissors may be best used for dressing changes on open wounds.

Nurses have a vital role in counteracting the environmental infection risks. The most important action is to increase their awareness and practice of infection control guidelines. This must be emphasized in all phases of the trauma cycle.

NATURE OF THE INJURIES

It is well documented that critically ill patients are predisposed to infection by the very nature of their underlying illnesses.[11,56,57] In the trauma population those sustaining severe and multisystem injuries are at greatest risk.[3,5,12,13] Specific characteristics of different injuries (e.g., open injuries, aspiration of fluids and objects into the lungs, extensive soft-tissue injuries and burns, crushing injuries, and penetrating injuries) create specific infection risks. Open injuries, such as open bone fractures, traumatic amputations, degloving and avulsion injuries, and gunshot and stab wounds, annihilate external barriers. These wounds can be heavily contaminated with microorganisms from a variety of foreign objects such as bullets, glass, leaves, and sticks. As previously described, hypoperfusion and hematoma formation can hinder inflammatory responses, lead to tissue necrosis, and create environments in which bacteria can thrive. The physiologic aspects of the underlying injury, coupled with the consequences of invasive procedures and devices, reduce the patient's resistance to infection.

Management of traumatic injuries often requires complex drug therapy that may contribute to the patient's susceptibility to infection. Antibiotics alter the composition of the normal flora, and their toxic side effects can cause the failure of many body organs.[58] Anesthetic agents, corticosteroids, antacids, and H_2-blocking agents are but a few of many medications that alter normal system functions and hinder both internal and external defense mechanisms.[10,59,60] Therefore understanding and recognizing the dual-edged nature of medication relative to infection risks is important.

After the resuscitative phase a number of pathologic events can occur, confusing the overall clinical picture and hampering the diagnosis of infection. Examples of such events include coma, fever, hypotension, shock, atelectasis, respiratory distress syndrome, hyperglycemia, and renal failure. The severely injured patient may have one or many of these events occurring at the same time. Understanding the characteristics and manifestations of these clinical conditions, as well as their similarities and relationships to the diagnostic parameters delineating infection, is important. Effective infection control practices for the trauma population must arise from the recognition of the patient's predisposing risks relative to the underlying nature of injuries and the consequences of therapy.

INVASIVE THERAPY

A paradox of modern medical care is the use of invasive interventions to resuscitate and sustain the patient's life and the effect of these interventions in the breakdown of natural defenses and the subsequent development of infection.[2,3,47,57,61] A majority of trauma patients undergo at least one operative procedure, have several intravenous (IV) catheters, an arterial catheter, an endotracheal tube, a nasogastric tube, a urinary catheter, various types of surgical drainage devices, orthopedic hardware, cerebral pressure-sensing devices, and chest tubes. Each of these creates a portal of entry for microorganisms. Once the microbes are established at a new site, the probability that infection will later develop is greatly increased.

Patients in the intensive care unit are placed at risk of infection because of the various indwelling devices commonly in use. The need to frequently handle and manipulate these devices, failure to practice handwashing, and failure to maintain the systems as closed systems can inoculate the patient with the exogenous bacteria of the intensive care unit.

These devices may also be contaminated with substances that enhance bacterial colonization, such as dried blood, providing bacteria with essential nutrients. In addition, the tacky residue left by some antiseptic solutions may actually facilitate bacterial adherence and lead to the cracking and staining of some plastic or rubber materials.[62] Similarly, adhesive tape residue aids both bacterial adherence and nutrition. Respiratory secretions provide nutrients, as well as their own source of intrinsic microorganisms. Therefore nursing care includes keeping these devices clean and properly maintained. Dried blood can be easily removed with hydrogen peroxide, and lines used for frequent blood sampling should be thoroughly flushed.

The patient with multiple invasive devices is at risk for autoinfection. This can be a direct or secondary event. An example of direct autoinfection is the development of septic phlebitis at a catheter insertion site. If this infection is serious, a secondary bacteremia can develop. If the bacteremia persists, this secondary event can cause infection at yet another site. The bacteremia can seed implanted devices such as orthopedic hardware and induce later bone infection, or it directly infects another tissue such as the brain and induces a brain abscess.

Although the infection risk associated with the use of invasive devices is greatest during the initial phases of resuscitation and in the intensive care unit setting, the risk remains as long as an invasive or implanted device is present. Therefore it is absolutely essential that nurses search for methods to keep microorganisms in their normal habitats, eliminate the modes of transmission of organisms, and be ever attentive to infection control guidelines.

To promote understanding of infections and pathogens within the trauma experience, the stages of the trauma cycle have been arbitrarily defined in this chapter as early (1 to 5 days of ICU stay), mid (ICU stay greater than 6 days), late (after the ICU stay), and chronic (after discharge or rehabilitation). During hospitalization the

pathogenic flora supercedes the patients' normal endogenous flora. The pathogens and infections common during different phases of the trauma cycle are summarized in Tables 14-2 and 14-3.

ANTIBIOTIC USE

Although modern antibiotic therapy has dramatically reduced the morbidity and mortality of infectious disease, antibiotic use is a complex issue in patient care. Antibiotics are powerful drugs with dual-edged consequences. They can prevent and cure infection, but they also can alter the composition of the body's resident flora, promote "superinfections," and induce the emergence of antibiotic-resistant flora. Therefore antibiotics must be used judiciously.

TABLE 14-2   Occurrence of Pathogens in the Trauma Cycle*

Early (1-5 Days)
- *S. aureus*
- *H. influenzae*
- Streptococci
- Anaerobes
- *E. coli*
- *Klebsiella* sp.
- *Proteus* sp.
- Enterobacteriaceae
- Mycoplasma
- Chlamydia
- Legionella

Mid (ICU Stay More Than 6 Days)
- Methicillin-sensitive *S. aureus* (MSSA)
- Methicillin-resistant *S. aureus*
- Coagulase-negative staphlococci
- *Pseudomonas* sp.
- Acinetobacter sp.
- Enterobacter sp.
- Other resistant negative rods
- *Clostridium difficile*
- Fungi
- Vancomycin-sensitive enterococci (VSE)
- Vancomycin-resistant enterococci (VRE)

Late (After ICU)
- Patient off antibiotics (>10 days)
  → early pathogens
- Patient on antibiotics
  → midcycle pathogens

Chronic (After Discharge/Rehabilitation)
- No lines or invasive devices
  → early pathogens
  → occasionally midcycle pathogens
- Invasive devices
  → midcycle pathogens

*The presence of resistant pathogens is dependent on premorbid risk factors, severity of illness, prior antibiotic use, among other factors.

TABLE 14-3   Sites of Infection* During the Trauma Cycle

Early (1-5 Days)
- Community-acquired pneumonia
- Aspiration pneumonia
- Cellulitis/wound infection
- Line-related infection

Late (After ICU)
- Urinary tract infection
- Line sepsis
- Pneumonia
- *Clostridium difficile* colitis
- Osteomyelitis
- Skin/soft tissue infection

Mid (ICU Stay More Than 6 Days)
- Urinary tract infection
- Pneumonia
- Line-related infection
- Skin/soft tissue infection
- Meningitis (violation of dura)
- Intraabdominal abscess
- Sinusitis
- *Clostridium difficile* colitis
- Fungal infection

Chronic (After Discharge/Rehabilitation)
- Urinary tract infection
- *Clostridium difficile* colitis
- Skin/soft tissue infection (decubitus ulcers)
- Osteomyelitis
- Line sepsis

*In order of frequency of occurrence.

SELECTION.   Factors guiding the selection of appropriate antibiotics for the treatment of infection[58] include the following:

1. Site of infection (effectiveness of antibiotics varies for different tissues)
2. Severity of infection
3. Identity of the organism
4. Antibiotic susceptibility of the organism
5. Clinical condition of patient (selection influenced by presence of renal or liver failure or septic shock, which requires more aggressive broad-spectrum therapy)
6. Basic knowledge of what organisms usually cause infection in a specific hospital unit

When a patient develops a severe infection, there is often no time to wait for culture results before initiating treatment. It takes approximately 72 hours to identify the organism and determine sensitivity patterns. Initial antibiotic selection can be aided by the use of a Gram stain, which can be performed in a matter of minutes. It is important to remember that this does not identify a specific organism; it qualitatively characterizes the nature of the specimen by demonstrating the presence and morphology of cells and organisms. Once the culture and sensitivity results are known, the antibiotics can be adjusted accordingly. The goal is to select a drug that maximizes effectiveness without inducing toxic side effects in the patient.

For severely traumatized patients, antibiotic use becomes more complex. Because of the nature of their injuries, the major compromise of their defense mechanisms, and their exposure to the flora of the ICU, it is highly probable that the overall composition of their normal flora will change. It is not at all uncommon for these patients to be subjected to repeated courses of antibiotics. These drugs can be given both as prophylaxis for injury or surgery and as therapy for infection. Each time an antibiotic is used, the possibility of the emergence of resistant organisms increases. Thus while the antibiotic is treating one infection, it may very well be inducing colonization at another site in the patient. This other site may then become the focus of a subsequent infection. It is important to remember which antibiotics an individual patient has received so that the organism of an ensuing infection can be more readily determined.

PROPHYLAXIS.   Although the prophylactic use of antibiotics is beneficial before some elective surgeries,[63] the benefits of prophylaxis for certain open injuries remains unclear.[64,65] Supporting the argument is the premise that administration of antibiotics after open injury is never prophylactic because of the extensive presence of bacterial contamination. It has been shown in animal models that there is a critical period within 3 to 4 hours of injury when antibiotic administration appears to be effective in reducing the incidence of wound infection.[66,67] Real-life situations may prevent early administration of prophylactic antibiotics. In addition, antibiotics are ineffective in the presence of devitalized tissue and indwelling contamination by foreign objects such as bullets.

Because of the complex dilemmas that antibiotic utilization presents, prophylactic use must be considered carefully. Unfortunately, there is no one "wonder antibiotic" that can effectively eradicate all the microorganisms that can cause infection. No matter what antibiotic is selected, an advantage to proliferate will always be given to another organism. For example, if a first-generation cephalosporin is administered to minimize infection from staphylococci, the composition of the patient's normal microbial flora may be shifted to favor *Pseudomonas* organisms.

Prolonged administration of antibiotics changes the normal flora and creates antibiotic-resistant organisms. When prolonged antibiotic administration is coupled with the use of invasive support devices that provide access to normally sterile body sites, a "superinfection" may develop. Therefore the duration of prophylaxis should be kept short. Efficacy has been confirmed using a single preoperative dose and a repeat dose at an interval of 12 hours or less after the procedure. In addition, in comparison studies, short courses (≤24 hours), versus long courses (3 to 5 days), have had equivalent outcomes in injuries. For example, with short-course antibiotics for penetrating abdominal trauma, 1-day therapy has been shown to be as effective as 5-day therapy.[66,68,69]

Benefits versus risks of antibiotic administration must always be considered. Many prophylactic antibiotic uses once believed to be effective are now subject to controversy and debate. For example, previously standard practice dictated use of prophylactic antibiotic for any patient sustaining a cerebrospinal fluid leak in order to minimize the possibility of meningitis. However, studies show that prophylactic antimicrobial therapy does not prevent meningitis and may promote the development of gram-negative meningitis.[65] Current recommendations for antibiotic prophylaxis in trauma patients include only those injuries producing open bone fractures, disruption of the intraoral mucosa, or penetrating injury of the colon. Courses of therapy should be short (e.g., 48 to 72 hours).[2,3,12,13,70]

RESISTANCE.   Although some microorganisms are naturally resistant to certain antibiotics, many gram-negative bacilli can acquire drug resistance by extrachromosomal fragments of deoxyribonucleic acid (DNA) known as plasmids, or R-factors.[71] Plasmids allow the organisms to synthesize enzymes that can inactivate the antibiotic, change the structure of the bacterial cell wall, or produce metabolic enzymes that make the cell resistant to inhibition by the antibiotic. The β-lactamases, penicillinase and cephalosporinase, which hydrolyze the peptide bond of the β-lactam antibiotics, are good examples of enzymes that can inactivate an antibiotic. Expression of these enzymes is induced by exposure of the bacteria to the respective antibiotics.[71-73] Similarly, the emergence of aminoglycoside resistance also has been demonstrated to occur in patients exposed to repeated courses of aminoglycoside antibiotics.[74] Expression of these enzymes increases organisms' survival advantage.

The greatest impact of an antibiotic-resistance emergency occurs in the intensive care unit. Because of the many different procedures necessary to care for these patients, the opportunity for transmission of an antibiotic-resistant organism from one patient to another is always present. In addition, it has been demonstrated that the intensive care unit environment itself can promote this phenomenon.[75-77] It is important to monitor the antibiotic history of the patient, as well as the overall antibiotic use of the unit and the antibiograms of the recovered pathogens.

IMPACT OF ANTIBIOTIC USE.   Medical management of critically ill patients infected with resistant organisms is complex. The toxic side effects attributed to the use of antibiotics may in some instances be as devastating as the infection itself. Sensitive monitoring procedures demonstrating the effectiveness of therapy are required; these include pharmacokinetic evaluation, synergy studies, and determination of minimum inhibitory concentrations or serum bactericidal levels of the antibiotics. Clinical parameters that may indicate the deleterious effects of therapy should be monitored daily. Moreover, because more than one infectious process may be occurring simultaneously, antibiotic selection must be reevaluated daily. The indication for and length of antibiotic therapy should be well defined. When the patient has received what is considered appropriate therapy, antibiotics should be discontinued.

Courses of therapy should be site- and organism-directed. Long-term use of antibiotics, which could lead to increased colonization and subsequent infection with resistant and more opportunistic organisms, is not appropriate. Patients who are continuously febrile while on antibiotic therapy should be reevaluated for noninfectious causes.

The problem of antibiotic resistance emergencies has promoted the search for new antimicrobial agents. During the middle to late 1980s, many new antibiotics became available; these included the newer cephalosporins, penicillins, macrolides, and quinolones.[78,79] These newer antibiotics are more stable against attack by the bacterial enzymes, so the induction of resistance is impeded. In addition, these drugs have an expanded spectrum of activity against a variety of microorganisms. The expanded spectrum may eliminate the need to give several antibiotics when treating infections caused by more than one organism. Many have longer half-lives and can be given less frequently. These advantages can be offset by an increased risk of superinfection, toxic side effects, and misuse in which a less expensive but therapeutically equivalent drug can adequately treat an infection.

Because of the complexities of antibiotic therapy, the need to avoid the emergence of antibiotic-resistant microorganisms, and the demand for cost-containment measures for these very expensive drugs, overall antibiotic use must be continuously monitored.[80] Mechanisms to enforce recommended prescription guidelines must be sought. In fact, the Joint Commission on Accreditation of Hospitals has required health care facilities to define prescribing guidelines and audit antibiotic utilization.[81] An example of guidelines for antibiotic use in the trauma patient is presented in Table 14-4.

TABLE 14-4　Guidelines for Antimicrobial Use

1. Restrict the prophylactic use of antibiotics to situations in which effectiveness has been demonstrated.
2. Use narrow-spectrum rather than expanded-spectrum antibiotics.
3. Prescribe adequate dosages to ensure eradication of the organisms and minimal toxicity to the patient.
4. Use short therapeutic courses, such as 7 to 10 days, whenever possible.
5. Reserve the more potent agents for use against resistant organisms.
6. Closely monitor patients for adverse effects of antibiotics.
7. Conduct general audits of antibiotic use to evaluate the effectiveness of therapy and utilization abuses.

SURVEILLANCE AND IDENTIFICATION OF INFECTION

Routine surveillance for infection is essential in the critically ill trauma population. Evaluation of infection among the critically ill trauma population can be difficult and complex. The patients are usually unable to communicate or sense their symptoms as a result of a decreased level of consciousness, disorientation, sedation, endotracheal intubation, or central nervous system injury. Usual physical examination findings may be hampered by bandages, multiple indwelling devices, casts, traction or fixation devices, the patient's immobility, and the use of isolation precautions. Some diagnostic tests may be difficult to obtain because it is cumbersome or risky to transport the patient or because it is impossible to place the patient in the optimal position for the study that yields definitive results.

Classic indicators of infection such as leukocytosis and fever may not be specific in the critically ill trauma patient. For example, fever may be the result of atelectasis, drug or transfusion reactions, central nervous system dysfunction, hematoma formation, the presence of necrotic tissue, or inflammation. Trauma patients can be hemodynamically unstable as a result of hemorrhage, cardiac and pulmonary dysfunction, neurologic dysfunction, or sepsis. These multiple aspects of the patient's clinical status must be differentiated from infection.

Because the evaluation of infection is complex in the critically ill trauma population, one of the most effective infection surveillance systems is an infectious disease team, whose primary responsibility is to evaluate all high-risk patients.[70] However, whether the trauma center utilizes the infectious disease team approach or not, prospective trend analysis of individual patients is essential. Clinical parameters such as the pattern of the fever curve, white blood cell count, platelet count, creatinine level, use of corticosteroids and antibiotics, roentgenograms, Gram stain and culture results, and placement of indwelling devices should be documented and monitored daily by the team. Prospective surveillance facilitates trend analysis and early diagnosis of infection and directs appropriate antibiotic therapy. It also establishes endemic infection rates, identifies infection hazards, monitors effectiveness of infection control practices, and establishes baselines. Early diagnosis of infection may be enhanced by surveillance cultures of the sputum of patients on mechanical ventilators and of the urine of patients with indwelling urinary catheters, since colonization patterns, as well as the impact of antibiotic therapy, can be determined. The use of a "fever protocol" may be beneficial. For example, with each temperature spike of 102.2° F (39° C) or change of 1.8° F (1° C), the following fever protocol could be automatically obtained: two sets of percutaneously drawn blood cultures, white blood cell count with differential, urine culture and urinalysis, sputum Gram stain and culture, and chest x-ray examination. Sites of wounds and indwelling catheters should be examined, suspect lines removed and cultured via semiquantitative technique, and any purulent drainage sent for culture and Gram stain. Sinus radiographs should be obtained on patients with indwelling nasal tubes. If a central nervous system infection is suspected in a patient with head and spinal cord injuries, the neurosurgeon should be consulted so that the safety of performing a lumbar puncture can be determined.

Although infection surveillance should be comprehensive and aggressive during the initial and intensive phases of the trauma cycle, it is a continuous process across the entire cycle. The infection risks are always in a dynamic state, and they must be constantly reevaluated as the status of the patient changes. As the patient recovers, the infection risks tend to decrease. However, eradication of many infections may be difficult during these later phases. These infections may be caused by the more resistant microorganisms or develop chronic patterns that are difficult to manage. Infection developing during any phase of the cycle always jeopardizes the final outcome; it prolongs the recovery and may even prevent saving the patient's life.

INFECTION RELATED TO DISRUPTION OF THE SKIN

Wound infection has been described extensively in literature and is one of the most frequently cited infectious complications after trauma.[5,82-84] However, these infections constitute only 8% to 20% of overall infections, and the majority of serious bacteremic illnesses in the severely traumatized patient are actually related to vascular and pulmonary infections.[2,3,12,13]

Any disruption or compromise of skin integrity can result in infection. These events include physical trauma, operative and invasive procedures, and inadequate tissue perfusion secondary to prolonged pressure, avascular necrosis, ischemia, hematoma, edema, or inflammation. At highest risk are massive, open soft-tissue injuries such as traumatic amputations, degloving and avulsion injuries, burns, and high-energy open fractures. Stratification of the infection risks for operative wounds are defined by the class of surgery. These classes are outlined in Table 14-5 and are

TABLE 14-5	**Classification of Surgical Procedures**

Class I: Clean Surgical Procedures

Definition: Nontraumatic, uninfected operative wounds in which no inflammation is encountered, there is no break in technique, and neither the respiratory, alimentary, or genitourinary tracts nor the oropharyngeal cavities are entered.

Expected infection rate: 1% to 5%

Class II: Clean-Contaminated Surgical Procedures

Definition: Operations in which the respiratory, alimentary, or genitourinary tracts are entered under controlled conditions and without unusual contamination.

Expected infection rate: 8% to 11%

Class III: Contaminated Surgical Procedures

Definition: Operations associated with open, fresh accidental wounds; major breaks in sterile technique or gross spillage from the gastrointestinal tract occur; or acute, nonpurulent inflammation is encountered.

Expected infection rate: 15% to 20%

Class IV: Dirty and Infected Procedures

Definition: Operations involving old traumatic wounds with devitalized tissue and those that involve existing clinical infection.

Expected infection rate: more than 25%

---

determined according to the degree of expected bacterial contamination relative to the surgical procedure.[85]

Management of the wound must address three factors if wound infection is to be prevented.[82] First, bacteria can contaminate any wound, whether it results from trauma or an operative procedure. Second, the risk of infection increases proportionately with the extent of contamination. Third, devitalized tissue creates an environment supportive of bacterial growth. Therefore the importance of meticulous aseptic and surgical technique cannot be overemphasized. Gentle tissue handling, hemostasis, adequate blood supply, debridement of dead tissue, obliteration of dead space, avoidance of hematoma, and wound closure without tension significantly reduce the incidence of postoperative wound infections.[83,84,86] Practices that do not reduce wound infection rates include preoperative shaving,[87] adhesive plastic drapes,[84] drains other than closed-suction systems,[84,88] ultraviolet lights,[89] and topical antibiotic and antiseptic irrigation solutions.[90]

Wound infections are divided into superficial (above the fascial planes) and deep seated (below the fascial planes).[84,91] Deep-seated infections are discussed elsewhere in this chapter.

Superficial infections range from mild conditions such as cellulitis to serious, fulminant conditions such as necrotizing fasciitis.[91] Clear definitions for some of these infections remain obscure because many underlying conditions, infectious or noninfectious, present the same signs and symp-

toms. For example, pain, swelling, tenderness, redness, fever, and elevated white blood cell count are common signs and symptoms of inflammatory response. It is equally impossible to identify a causative organism by the color, odor, or consistency of drainage material.

Cellulitis is a superficial inflammatory reaction without any specific characteristics or purulent discharge. Suppurative wound infections or abscesses are defined by inflammation, induration, and the presence of purulent material. Surgical excision and debridement of the abscess and initiation of antibiotics are usually required. The most frequently isolated organism is *S. aureus*. However, if these infections develop after antibiotic therapy or prolonged hospitalization, gram-negative bacilli such as *Escherichia coli, Pseudomonas aeruginosa, Enterobacter* species, or other gram-positive cocci such as coagulase-negative staphylococci may be recovered from the exudate.

Gram stain, culture, and sensitivity testing of isolated organisms are key diagnostic tools for the evaluation of infection. The results of a Gram stain can be known in a matter of minutes. The relative proportion of white blood cells and epithelial cells, as well as the morphology and staining properties of any organisms (e.g., gram-positive cocci, gram-negative bacilli), provide the basis for empiric antibiotic selection. Treatment is modified in the next 72 hours when specific bacteria are identified by culture and antibiotic susceptibility is known.

NECROTIZING SOFT TISSUE INFECTIONS

Necrotizing soft tissue infections (NSTIs) classically present as rapidly progressing conditions of the skin, subcutaneous fat, and fascia. They are difficult to diagnose, their treatment is complicated and expensive, and they have a high mortality. Survivors tend to require lengthy hospitalization, undergo prolonged courses of rehabilitation, and then have residual physical limitations that, in many cases, prevent independent living.

NSTIs are severe, fulminant infections that usually have a rapidly progressive course (occasionally hours); in rare cases, the process is insidious and subacute. The early local clinical manifestation of NSTI is an exquisitely tender, edematous, hot area of shiny skin that cannot be differentiated readily from cellulitis.[33,92,93] As the infection spreads, the skin color changes to bronze and blue-gray and bullae eventually form. The skin may become gangrenous and anesthetic. Sloughing occurs from destruction of the underlying subcutaneous tissue and thrombosis of nutrient-carrying vessels.[94] When the infection is well established, necrosis of superficial fascia and fat results in exudation of thin, watery, foul-smelling fluid.

Systemic manifestations include tachycardia, hypotension, tachypnea, fever/chills, oliguria, and altered sensorium.[33,93,94] The patient can also manifest leukocytosis, metabolic acidosis, hypoalbuminemia, electrolyte imbalance, hyperglycemia, and dehydration.[33,93,94] In the absence of medical intervention most necrotizing infections will progress to multiple organ dysfunction syndrome (MODS)

| TABLE 14-6 | **Bacteriology of Necrotizing Soft Tissue Infection** |

Gram-Negative Rods	**Gram-Positive Cocci**
Escherichia coli	β-Hemolytic *streptococci* (Group A, B, other)
Klebsiella sp.	α-Hemolytic *streptococci*
Enterobacter sp.	Group D *enterococci*
Proteus sp.	*Staphylococcus aureus*
Acinetobacter sp.	*Staphylococcus* coagulase-negative
Citrobacter sp.	
Serratia sp.	
Anaerobes	**Fungus**
Bacteroides sp.	*Candida* sp.
Clostridium perfringens	Others
Peptococcus	
Peptostreptococcus	

and death. Causative agents of NSTIs are presented in Table 14-6.

A variety of conditions can predispose a patient to necrotizing infection. By far the most important are diabetes mellitus (with an incidence of 30% to 55%)[95] and morbid obesity (in about one third of patients).[95] Other factors include trauma, the presence of a foreign body, surgical procedures, burns, parenteral drug abuse, insect bites, odontogenic infections, decubitus ulcers,[96] and systemic diseases states such as peripheral vascular disease, alcoholism, malignancy, and acquired immunodeficiency syndrome (AIDS).[96] The immunocompromised state induced by chemotherapy or corticosteroid therapy can also predispose patients to NSTIs.[91,92,96]

A number of studies have documented that rapid diagnosis and early surgical debridement of NSTIs improve patients' outcomes.[97] A definitive diagnosis can be made only by direct visualization of the skin, subcutaneous tissue, muscle, and fascia, followed by bacterial culture. Evaluation of frozen sections of soft-tissue biopsies for characteristic histopathologic findings may also be useful in early diagnosis. Plain radiographic studies may reveal gas in the soft tissue. Demonstration of soft tissue gas and asymmetric edema within different soft tissue planes on computed tomography or magnetic resonance imaging strongly suggests necrotizing infection. The immediate goal in the treatment of NSTIs is prevention of death. This entails early, aggressive resuscitation; close monitoring of hemodynamic and respiratory status; correction of metabolic derangements; and institution of supportive measures.

Repeated surgical debridement is essential to excise infected tissue. This is accompanied by administration of broad-spectrum antibiotics modulated as culture results accumulate. Hyperbaric oxygen (HBO) therapy is often added as adjunct treatment, but the use of this costly and complex therapy in cases of necrotizing infection has not been evaluated scientifically. Anecdotal accounts describe its apparent benefits: reduction in the progress of infection and enhancement of wound healing. Although it may offer clinical benefit, the integration with other therapies is logistically challenging and limited to a few centers throughout the country with hyperbaric oxygen chambers.

CLOSTRIDIAL INFECTIONS

Fortunately, infections caused by *Clostridium* species are relatively rare. However, because they are rapidly progressive infections, when they occur they are almost always fatal. Because clostridia are widely distributed in nature, wound contamination of open traumatic injuries is quite common. The pathogenic clostridia can be divided into three major groups according to the diseases they produce: (1) histotoxic clostridia, *C. perfringens, C. novyi, C. septicum, C. histolyticum, C. bifermentans,* and *C. fallax,* which cause a variety of tissue infections, the most common being myonecrotic gas gangrene; (2) *C. tetani,* the causative agent of tetanus; and (3) *C. botulinum* type A, the cause of wound botulism. In all these infections the production of potent exotoxins is primarily responsible for the rapid progression of disease and the extent of damage to the involved tissues.

GAS GANGRENE

Gas gangrene is a rapidly progressive, life-threatening toxemic infection of the skeletal muscle. It is most frequently associated with open bone fractures, but it can develop secondary to biliary and bowel surgery. Clostridial myonecrosis results when the wound is inoculated by clostridial spores or by the vegetative forms of the organism. Symptoms begin suddenly with severe local pain and tense swelling around the wound site. Accompanying systemic signs include tachycardia, hypotension, fever, agitation, and disorientation. Muscle necrosis is marked by distinct, advancing margins, and crepitance is usually evident. Serous hemorrhagic bullae can develop. A Gram stain of the exudate will show gram-positive rods and an absence of polymorphonuclear leukocytes.[98]

Treatment necessitates immediate and extensive surgical exploration, with excision of all necrotic tissue and emergent institution of large doses of penicillin. Hyperbaric oxygen enhances the rate of wound healing in devascularized hypoxic wounds by increasing the partial pressure of oxygen (Po_2) in the damaged tissues.[99] It also inhibits toxin production by the bacteria.[99] However, bactericidal effects of hyperbaric oxygen therapy have not been clearly established.

TETANUS

The spores of *C. tetani* are ubiquitous. Simple puncture wounds from nails, splinters, thorns, or contaminated syringes and IV needles can provide conditions conducive to the development of tetanus. Open fractures, punctures by dirty metal objects, and injuries from farm cultivation equipment offer the same environment. However, tetanus is a preventable disease with proper immunization. Key determinants of infection are the characterization of the wound and the patient's immunization history. Table 14-7 summarizes tetanus prophylaxis based on these two variables.

TABLE 14-7	Guide to Tetanus Prophylaxis in Routine Wound Management in Adults			
Number of Doses of Tetanus Toxoid	Clean, Minor Wounds Td	TIG	All Other Wounds Td	TIG
Unknown or <3	Yes	No	Yes	Yes
3	No*	No	No†	No

Td, Tetanus toxoid; *TIG*, tetanus immune globulin.
*Yes, if more than 10 years since last dose.
†Yes, if more than 5 years since last dose.

Tetanus should be suspected in patients who have risk factors and show symptoms of neuromuscular dysfunction. Symptoms include profound neuromuscular rigidity in the injured region followed by progressive central nervous system dysfunction: tremors and spasms of facial, pharyngeal, and laryngeal muscles (lockjaw); nuchal rigidity; and opisthotonos (hyperextension spasms of the paraspinous muscles). Seizures and autonomic nervous system involvement are common. Treatment involves sedation, paralytic agents, mechanical ventilation, high doses of penicillin, and large doses of tetanus immune globulin (TIG). Mortality has been reported at 50%.[100]

BURN WOUND INFECTIONS

The disruption of homeostasis associated with severe burns exceeds that of any other injury. Current techniques of burn wound care have reduced the incidence and mortality associated with infection.[101] However, increased mortality after burns of more than 40% of body surface area is still primarily attributable to infection.

Burns have unique wound infection risks relative to the depressed immunity in the host and the nature of the injury.[102] Contributory factors include loss of the skin's mechanical barrier; an impeded ability to sense toxic stimuli; the inability to control heat and water loss; the agent inducing the burn; the size and degree of the burn; and injury of other organ systems.

A full-thickness burn results in residual avascular and nonviable cutaneous tissue that is dead protein, called eschar. This devitalized tissue becomes contaminated and colonized with bacteria. This is true even in the early stages of injury. Infection develops when the colonization becomes dense and subsequently invades adjacent viable tissue.

A variety of microorganisms—bacteria, mycobacteria, yeast, fungi, and viruses—have been cited as the causative agents of burn infections. The pattern of infecting organisms tends to be cyclical. The first organisms are generally the invasive gram-positive cocci, such as coagulase-positive staphylococci and group A β-hemolytic streptococci, followed by gram-negative bacteria, especially *P. aeruginosa*, and then yeast. The emergence of multiple-antibiotic-resistant organisms is not uncommon, and antibiotic selection pressures can evolve from both topical antiseptic agents and parenterally administered drugs. Organisms that predominate as problem agents of infection may change with time, and more resistant flora may produce "mini-epidemics."[103]

The diagnosis of infection in burn patients is often difficult. Purulence may be evident below the eschar, but wounds may appear clean even when they are infected. Although the utility of quantitative tissue cultures remains controversial, it is the primary tool used to identify the predominant organism in the wound. Histologic examination of a biopsy specimen is the only reliable means of differentiating wound colonization from invasive infection.[104]

Prevention of infection in burn wounds is achieved by the following methods:

1. Frequent evaluation of the wound and surrounding tissue for evidence of infection
2. Application of topical antimicrobial agents such as silver sulfadiazine on a daily basis[105]
3. Alternation of topical agents to decrease or delay the emergence of resistant wound organisms and minimize side effects[106]
4. Administration of combinations of topical agents with systemic antibiotics to provide synergy against resistant organisms[107]
5. Administration of antibiotic before and during burn wound excision to prevent bacteremia[101]
6. Early excision of the burn wound to the level of viable tissue, followed by application of skin grafts to the wound surface[108]
7. Minimization of cross-contamination of patient's wounds (gowns, gloves, and masks used by medical staff and visitors; frequent handwashing; not sharing supplies and equipment among patients; cohorting patients also shown to be effective)

Prevention of immune dysfunction after burn injury with certain immune modulators has been demonstrated in animal experiments. Most of these modalities have not proven to be clearly useful in humans. The importance of aggressive nutritional replenishment is also vital to maintaining immune functions.[109]

Upon suspicion or confirmation of burn wound sepsis, plans are made for surgical excision of residual nonviable, infected tissue. Systemic antibiotic coverage is also instituted based on the known or likely identification of wound organisms. Routine surveillance cultures of the wounds aids in making the choice of antibiotics. Intensive care management of severely burned patients includes airway management, fluid resuscitation, support of the hypermetabolic response, and treatment of smoke inhalation injury. After initial surgery, plastic reconstruction and long-term rehabilitation are also essential.[104,110]

WOUND CARE THROUGH THE TRAUMA CYCLE

The primary objective of wound care throughout the trauma cycle is the prevention of infection. Nursing actions

TABLE 14-8	**Infection Control Guidelines for the Care of Wounds**

1. Wash hands before and after patient care.
2. Use aseptic technique for dressing changes of open wounds.
3. Change dressings that become saturated with drainage fluid and notify the physician of changes in its character, such as amount, color, odor, viscosity. Document all changes.
4. Maintain the patency and function of wound drains.
5. Notify the physician of any signs of increasing inflammation, purulent drainage, or breakdown in the integrity of suture lines.
6. Perform wound cultures correctly.
7. Clean and disinfect scissor blades after each use.

should minimize cross-contamination and promote wound healing. The most effective measures are meticulous aseptic technique and handwashing. Scissors and tape used for multiple patients must be handled properly to prevent cross-contamination.

Careful nursing assessment can detect the early development of infection. Assessment in such situations involves a trend analysis. Increasing signs of inflammation, increased drainage or purulence, breakdown of the integrity of suture margins, and systemic signs of deterioration should be reported immediately. Nursing care must minimize patient immobility and stimulate tissue perfusion. Frequent turning and repositioning of the patient can prevent the development of decubitus ulcers. Nurses can promote wound healing and enhance the patient's resistance to infection by ensuring adequate nutrition. Environmental and iatrogenic factors can contribute to emergence of multiple-antibiotic-resistant organisms (MARO) in patients with burns and large wounds. These include methicillin-resistant *S. aureus,* also known as oxacillin-resistant *S. aureus,* and vancomycin-resistant enterococci. Isolation precautions are required for patients with infections attributed to MARO.[111] Specific institutional requirements may also isolate for *Clostridium difficile* or imipenem-resistant *P. aeruginosa.*

Throughout the trauma cycle, wound care must reflect the underlying nature of the patient's injuries. Guidelines for the care of wounds are found in Table 14-8.

INFECTION RELATED TO ORTHOPEDIC INJURY

Infections after orthopedic injuries cause substantial morbidity worldwide despite continued progress toward understanding its pathophysiology and optimal management. The pathogenesis of such infections is related to the nature and extent of the underlying injury, management of the wound, use of fixation devices, and antibiotic therapy.

NATURE OF THE INJURY

Patients sustaining multisystem trauma including orthopedic injury are at highest risk for infection. Hemodynamic instability of these patients can create a therapeutic dilemma

for the trauma team. Immediate fracture fixation and stabilization are often the primary goals. To do so lessens the degree of avascular necrosis at the fracture site and promotes early mobilization of the patient in order to minimize or prevent pulmonary complications. However, fixation and stabilization may have to be delayed as indicated by the extent of the injuries and the priorities of resuscitation. Delay can contribute to the amount of ischemia at the fracture site and increase the amount of soft tissue damage and bone loss. Not only does this promote the chance of infection, but it also can jeopardize the ultimate salvage of a limb or necessitate later skin- and bone-graft procedures.

The primary index for fracture site infection is the severity of injury. Contributory factors include the amount of bone loss, comminution, displacement, and periosteal stripping; the extent of soft tissue injury; wound contamination; compromise to tissue perfusion; and vascular injury. The presence of foreign bodies, coupled with conditions producing ischemia, hypovolemia, and avascular necrosis, creates an environment in which any bacterial inoculum can thrive.[83,84] Long bone fractures tend to have greater infection risks than flat bone fractures. Traumatic amputations; open fractures with vascular injury resulting from high-energy impact, such as pedestrian road traffic crashes and gunshots; and fractures inducing compartmental syndromes have the greatest infection risks. All these injuries have extensive tissue damage and massive wound contamination.

MANAGEMENT OF FRACTURES

Fracture management must minimize the consequences of bacterial contamination and the devitalization of tissues that occur secondary to the fracture itself.[82] Interventions generally accepted as preventative measures include early fixation and stabilization, adequate debridement, meticulous surgical technique, and antibiotic use.

Meticulous surgical technique cannot be overemphasized, and adherence to these principles significantly reduces the incidence of postoperative wound infection.[83,84] However, extensive surgical dissection with loss of vital tissue attachments, failure to remove freed fracture fragments, and prolonged duration of operative time tend to induce later infectious complications.

Ideally, fixation of the fracture should occur as close to the initial time of injury as possible. A long bone fracture causes tearing of the periosteum and disruption of the longitudinally lying haversian system, resulting in devitalization and avascular necrosis. This creates an environment conducive to the growth of bacteria, which can be introduced either by trauma or surgical intervention. Therefore early and adequate debridement of injury tends to reduce the infection risks.

Immobilization is an important adjunct to the healing of soft tissue injury.[112] Stabilization helps to restore the fracture to a near approximation of the bone's normal anatomic position. The stability realigns vital neurovascular structures, strengthens soft tissue planes, and promotes reestablishment of the microcirculation. Early revascularization of devitalized structures improves the local immune responses of the tissues and enhances resistance to infection. However, for some open fractures with accompanying soft tissue injury and a high level of contamination, the method of wound closure and stabilization is still controversial. Most agree that infection risk is reduced when open wounds are not closed primarily. A recent study demonstrated that the immediate primary closure of open fracture wounds seemed to cause no significant increase in infection or delayed union.[113]

At the crux of the controversy surrounding open fracture management is the type of fixation—internal versus external. Some argue that the presence of a foreign body in an already heavily contaminated wound provides bacteria with a convenient surface on which to establish a habitat in an environment already conducive to their growth. Therefore the risk of infection outweighs the benefits of closure. There is also clinical support for immediate internal fixation of open proximal long bone fractures, particularly to decrease pulmonary complications by early mobilization. These situations include open fractures in patients with multiple traumas, type I and some type II open fractures, intraarticular fractures, open fractures with associated vascular injury, and open femur fractures in the elderly.[112,114,115] In these cases the benefits of stabilization outweigh the risks of infection.

The use of external fixation devices can both facilitate and reduce infection risks.[114] Advantages include the relative ease and speed of application, achievement of reasonable anatomic reduction and stabilization, and the occurrence of minimal additional soft tissue trauma. The disadvantages include intricate and time-consuming application in large, complex open wounds; malunion; delayed union; interference with soft tissue reconstructive surgery; and development of pin tract infections.[112]

Orthopedic appliances are foreign bodies that can lead to necrosis and provide surfaces for bacterial adherence.[116] Technical placement also can be a contributory factor. Technical factors that promote infectious complications include the use of dull and worn drill bits, failure to control the direction of a cutting tool, and heat generated by drilling.[117] After insertion, any adverse stress and strain on the hardware or a loosening of the hardware can amplify the devitalization of the surrounding tissue and aid the development of infection.[116,118]

ANTIBIOTIC USE

The prophylactic use of antibiotics has been proven beneficial to the management of open fractures.[64,66,68] Most antibiotic prophylaxis is directed against *S. aureus*. First-generation cephalosporins, such as cephalothin (Keflin) or cefazolin (Ancef, Kefzol), and semisynthetic penicillins such as nafcillin are acceptable choices. Because of the previously described consequences of antibiotic therapy, the duration of prophylaxis should be kept short, and risk/benefit ratios must be evaluated for each patient.

The local use of antibiotics in the form of antibiotic-impregnated cement and beads for orthopedic infections and prevention of infection has been advocated. Despite high initial interest, controversies remain regarding their indications, and some express concerns regarding their safety.[119]

ORTHOPEDIC HARDWARE-ASSOCIATED INFECTIONS

Indwelling orthopedic hardware can be associated with both superficial and deep-seated infections. Four percent to 30% of patients in whom external fixation devices have been placed develop associated infections.[120] The associated infections include small areas of cellulitis and local abscess surrounding the pin insertion sites, muscle infections of the surrounding tract, and bone infections. An indication that a superficial infection has disseminated into the underlying tissues is the loosening of an implanted orthopedic bone pin. Pin or bone infection may necessitate pin removal for resolution of disease. It is a difficult decision because removal may decrease stability and further jeopardize the outcome.

Because of the local tissue responses to the presence of a pin, it is important to continually observe the pin-skin interface. Serous drainage is produced when tissues slide over the pin, and it may form a crust at the pin-skin interface. As long as this fluid can drain freely, infection risks are reduced. Consequently, crust formations must be gently removed. For newly placed pins, pin-site care may be necessary several times a day. Special care should be taken during cleansing so that additional trauma or cavitation around the pin-skin junction is not induced, since this can produce localized suppuration and necrosis. On the other hand, skin tension can impede the flow of fluid and promote inflammation, necrosis, and infection. Increased frequency of cleansing and surgical debridement may be required to alleviate the tension. The primary goals of pin-site care should be to promote the free drainage of fluid and minimize local tissue damage.

Internal fixation devices (e.g., plates, nails, screws, pins, and prostheses) also can foster the development of infection. They cause a local tissue response and provide surfaces on which bacteria can adhere and establish new habitats. Bacterial seeding can occur either at the time of insertion or by hematogenous spread from another site. Infection can then develop in poorly vascularized crevices where the internal fixation devices adjoin the bone. Clinical manifestations can include pain, inflammation, fever, purulent drainage, and leukocytosis. Resolution of infection cannot occur until the hardware is removed. These infections can range from low-grade infection around the hardware to deep-seated bone infections. Infection control guidelines for the care of external fixation devices are outlined in Table 14-9.

TABLE 14-9   Infection Control Guidelines for the Care of External Fixation Devices

1. Do not impede the flow of serous drainage fluid.
2. Do not use occlusive dressings or a thick coating of antimicrobial ointment at the skin-pin junction.
2. Notify the physician if skin tension develops at the skin-pin junction.
4. Gently remove any crust formation at the skin-pin junction.
5. Avoid inducing local tissue trauma or cavitation at the skin-pin junction.
6. Use a combination of antiseptic solutions determined by the needs of the patient.
7. Minimize any unnecessary stress and strain on the fixator; lubricate any pin-traction junctions.

BONE INFECTIONS

Osteomyelitis is an infection involving both the bone and its marrow. It can be caused by (1) hematogenous spread from another site of infection, (2) extension from a contiguous infection, or (3) direct introduction from trauma or a surgical procedure.[121,122] Acute hematogenous osteomyelitis infects previously normal bone and develops as a sequela to systemic diseases or prior infection at another site; it can also develop from vascular insufficiencies. Posttraumatic osteomyelitis, or fracture infection, is an infection that develops as a result of injury, impedance of the microcirculation, failure to debride necrotic tissue or evacuate hematomas, or the presence of indwelling fixation devices. It develops in bone that is devitalized and necrotic from the onset. Therefore aggressive debridement with removal of sequestra and appropriate antibiotic therapy often can prevent acute infections from becoming chronic problems. Chronicity tends to be more commonly associated with nontraumatic osteomyelitis.[121,122]

Posttraumatic bone infections are not clearly defined in the medical literature. They can be caused by hematogenous seeding of implanted orthopedic hardware from a nosocomial bacteremia, dissection from an overlying superficial wound infection, or inadequate debridement or evacuation of a hematoma at the time of initial fixation. These infections may appear weeks, months, and even years after the initial injury. The clinical manifestations can include any combination of local pain, erythema, heat, tenderness, and draining sinuses over the involved site of bone infection. Elevated white blood cell count, rising sedimentation rates, and fever are not usually present. Treatment includes surgical debridement, removal of associated hardware, and appropriate parenteral antibiotic therapy for a minimum of 4 weeks.[123]

Prevention of infection in patients sustaining orthopedic injury is a challenge throughout the trauma cycle. Nursing interventions should be directed toward minimizing infectious complications attributed to immobility. Most important are actions that promote pulmonary function and maintain adequate perfusion of the skin. Meticulous care and evaluation of fixation devices and maintenance of proper alignment can reduce infection risks. During the later phase of the cycle, nurses should be alert to the development of bone infection.

SYSTEMIC INFLAMMATORY RESPONSE SYNDROME

The introduction of the term *systemic inflammatory response syndrome* (SIRS) by the American College of Chest Physicians and Society of Critical Care Medicine[124] recognized the role that endogenous mediators of systemic inflammation play in "sepsis syndrome" (which is no longer regarded as being caused by microbial pathogens alone). SIRS is an overall inflammatory response that affects multiple organs with or without infection. SIRS can be precipitated by events such as infection, trauma, pancreatitis, and surgery. The similar features of sepsis syndrome and SIRS indicate a change of perspective rather than a new clinical entity. Sepsis syndrome/SIRS is viewed as a trigger-mediator-response sequence, whereas SIRS is the response to the action of intrinsic mediators. At times SIRS can compromise the function of various organ systems resulting in multiple organ dysfunction syndrome (MODS) (see Chapter 12).[125,126]

The clinical signs of infection, such as fever, tachycardia, tachypnea, and leukocytosis, are common responses to systemic insults. It is now recognized that events such as trauma, infections, and burns are the triggers and produce identical clinical and inflammatory responses independent of the precipitating process.[127] Early recognition, determination of the underlying cause, and aggressive treatment can curtail the progression to severe forms of SIRS. Table 14-10 defines the currently accepted definitions of SIRS.

CARDIOVASCULAR SYSTEM INFECTIONS

Infections related to the cardiovascular system include bacteremia, phlebitis, arterial abscess, infusate-associated sepsis, endocarditis, and intravascular catheter-related sepsis.

Bacteremia is the presence of bacteria in the bloodstream.[128,129] It can be a transient phenomenon following the instrumentation of tissues abundant with microorganisms, such as cystoscopic procedures, endotracheal suctioning, and debridement of a local abscess. Generally this is a short, self-limiting condition, and the organisms are eradicated by cellular immune responses. However, it is important to be aware of this phenomenon because blood cultures drawn immediately after such procedures can be positive. Accurate clinical diagnosis may be obscured by the positivity of these blood cultures, and inappropriate therapy subsequently may be initiated.

Bacteremia originates from an underlying infection or reservoir at another site. Determining the origin of and the

TABLE 14-10	Systemic Inflammatory Response Syndrome Definitions Given by the ACCP/SCCM Consensus Conference	
Term	**Definition**	
SIRS	The systemic inflammatory response to a variety of severe clinical insults. Manifested by two or more of the following conditions: temperature >38° C or <36° C; heart rate >90 beats/min; respiratory rate >20 breaths/min or $Paco_2$ <32 torr (<4.3 kPa); WBC >12,000 cells/mm^3, <4000 cells/mm^3, or >10% immature (band) forms.	
Infection	A microbial phenomenon characterized by an inflammatory response to the presence of microorganisms or the invasion of normally sterile host tissue by those organisms.	
Sepsis	The systemic response to infection. Manifested by two or more of the SIRS criteria as a result of infection.	
Bacteremia	The presence of viable bacteria in the blood.	
Severe sepsis	Sepsis associated with organ dysfunction, hypoperfusion, or hypotension; hypoperfusion and perfusion abnormalities may include, but are not limited to, lactic acidosis, oliguria, or an acute alteration in mental status.	
Septic shock	Sepsis with hypotension despite adequate resuscitation with fluids, along with the presence of perfusion abnormalities that may include, but are not limited to, lactic acidosis, oliguria, or an acute alteration in mental status. Patients who are on inotropic or vasopressive agents may not be hypotensive when perfusion abnormalities are measured.	
Hypotension	A systolic blood pressure of <90 mm Hg or a reduction of >40 mm Hg from baseline in the absence of other causes of hypotension.	
MODS	The presence of altered organ function in an acutely ill patient such that homeostasis cannot be maintained without intervention.	

Modified from Bone RC, Balk RA, Cerra FB et al: Definitions for sepsis and organ failure and guidelines for the use of innovative therapies in sepsis. ACCP/SCCM consensus conference committee, *Chest* 101:1644-1655, 1992.
SIRS, Systemic inflammatory response syndrome; *MODS,* multiple organ dysfunction syndrome.

microorganism causing the infection is important so that appropriate antimicrobial and supportive therapy can be initiated.

Primary, or unexplained, bacteremia is defined as the presence of organisms recovered from blood cultures that are not recovered from cultures taken from other possible sites. Most organisms responsible for primary bacteremia are similar to those causing intravascular catheter-related infections. Vascular catheters offer many opportunities for microorganisms to gain access to the bloodstream and provide sites for the organisms to colonize. Some of these infections are related to contaminated fluids, or the catheters themselves may become colonized and result in bacteremia. However, the vascular catheters may have been removed before identification of the bacteremia, and subsequently determination of the source of infection may be difficult.

Approximately 20% to 25% of serious bacteremic infections are related to the use of intravascular catheters.[2,3,12,13] The major infection risks for cardiovascular infection stem from the urgent conditions under which the catheters were placed and the need to frequently manipulate the lines to obtain hemodynamic pressures or blood samples or to administer medications, fluids, blood, and blood products.[130-131]

PHLEBITIS

Phlebitis is an inflammation of a vein. It can develop from irritation produced by either mechanical trauma from the catheter or the chemical nature of the infusate and medications. Chemical phlebitis is generally not classified as an infection. Septic phlebitis may be defined as suppurative or septic nonsuppurative. Chemical and suppurative phlebitis

may both present with signs of erythema, heat, tenderness, and a palpable cord. However, suppurative phlebitis is usually differentiated when purulent, culture-positive material can be expressed from the catheter insertion site. The causative organism is usually coagulase-positive staphylococci. When a systemic reaction (e.g., fever, elevated white blood cell count, or associated bacteremia) does not occur, heat and elevation of the afflicted body part may be adequate treatment. Management of systemic infection includes parenteral antibiotics directed toward staphylococci. However, if there is no improvement within 24 hours, surgical excision of the vein may be necessary.

Septic nonsuppurative thrombophlebitis should be suspected when a patient presents with a persistent gram-negative bacillary bacteremia with a member of the Klebsielleae tribe (*Enterobacter, Klebsiella,* and *Serratia*) and no site of infection can be identified.[132] This diagnosis can be further supported when appropriate antimicrobial therapy is initiated and subsequent blood cultures continue to be positive. Excision of the infected vein is necessary. It may be difficult to determine exactly which vein is involved, since there may be no evidence of purulence at an insertion site and a palpable cord cannot be detected. Veins through which the IV solutions are being administered are usually implicated.

ARTERIAL ABSCESSES

Arterial lines are occasionally the source of serious infection.[133] Arterial abscess may result when a local stitch abscess at the catheter-skin interface disseminates into the arterial wall or the tip of the indwelling catheter produces trauma to the arterial wall. Frequently there is an associated secondary bacteremia and the presence of septic emboli distal to the insertion site. The emboli will be evident on the palm of the hand if a radial or brachial artery is involved or on the sole of the foot if a femoral artery is involved. Septic emboli appear as small hemorrhagic areas that may have necrotic centers. If emboli are observed, the line must be removed immediately and antibiotics begun. Careful observation for pseudoaneurysm is indicated, and if found, the artery must be resected. In one study cannulation of the femoral artery resulted in fewer infectious complications than use of the radial artery.[134]

INFUSATE-ASSOCIATED SEPSIS

Hyperalimentation solutions are documented as being a source of catheter- and infusate-associated sepsis.[135] Fat-emulsion solutions pose an infectious threat because they provide a rich medium for luxuriant microbial growth.[136]

Although relatively rare, septicemia associated with contaminated infusion fluids has been documented.[137] *Enterobacter* bacteremia has been associated with contaminated dextrose solutions, *Pseudomonas cepacia* attributed to normal serum albumin, and *Salmonella* bacteremia related to contaminated platelet transfusions.

ENDOCARDITIS

Infective endocarditis (IE) is caused by the invasion of microorganisms into the endocardial surface of the heart.[138] Although infection may occur at any site on the endocardial surface, heart valves are the most frequently affected. IE has been caused by a variety of microorganisms and associated with many different predisposing illnesses, cardiac anomalies, and parenteral drug abuse. In severely traumatized patients another form of this infection has emerged as nosocomial infective endocarditis (NIE).[139] Development of NIE is directly related to the prolonged use of pulmonary artery catheters, central venous catheters, hemodialysis shunts, intracardiac prostheses, vascular grafts, and intracardiac pacemaker wires. NIE may also develop as a complication of a serious bacteremic infection. Identification of NIE may be obscure and should be considered in patients who have persistent bacteremia with the same organism and predisposing risk factors. Treatment requires prolonged parenteral antibiotic therapy for 4 to 6 weeks.

INTRAVASCULAR CATHETER-RELATED INFECTIONS

Intravascular devices are indispensable in critically ill patients and are used to administer IV fluids, medications, blood products, and parenteral nutrition and to monitor hemodynamic status. The use of IV devices can be complicated by a variety of infectious complications, including bloodstream infection, endocarditis, septic thrombophlebitis, and metastatic infections.[140] Catheter-related infections can be associated with increased morbidity and mortality and prolonged hospitalization.[141] The incidence of and potential risk factors for intravascular device-related infec-

---

TABLE 14-11   Current CDC Guidelines for Prevention of Nosocomial Intravascular Device-Related Infections

1. Educate and train health care workers in appropriate infection control measures to prevent intravascular device-related infection.
2. Implement surveillance for catheter-related infection:
   - Inspect the catheter-skin interface and report any signs of inflammation or purulent drainage to the physician immediately.
   - Remove lines immediately if they are suspected of being infected, and obtain a culture and Gram stain of any drainage from the insertion site.
   - Obtain a line culture using semiquantitative technique.
3. Wash hands before and after inserting or maintaining IV catheter.
4. Use barrier precautions during catheter insertion and care.
5. Do not use cutdown procedures.
6. Provide appropriate catheter site care:
   - Cleanse the skin with appropriate antiseptic before catheter insertion.
   - Use sterile gauze or transparent dressing to cover the catheter site.
7. Select or replace an IV device with lowest risk of complication and the lowest cost.
8. Replace IV tubing at 72-hour intervals. If administering blood or lipid emulsion, replace tubing within 24 hours.
9. Clean injection ports with antiseptic agents.
10. Prepare all parenteral fluids using aseptic technique.

---

tions can vary with the type of device and the therapy it is used to render. Comparison of research may be difficult because studies have been conducted on variable patient populations.

Coagulase negative staphylococci have become the most frequently isolated pathogens in catheter-related infections. Other pathogens often isolated are *S. aureus,* enterococci, gram-negative bacilli, and fungal pathogens.[142,143] Diagnosis is based on clinical and laboratory criteria. The semiquantitative methods for obtaining cultures of catheters has enhanced the ability to diagnose catheter-related infections.[144] Table 14-11 demonstrates the current Centers for Disease Control and Prevention (CDC) guidelines for prevention of nosocomial intravascular device-related infections.[145]

CENTRAL NERVOUS SYSTEM INFECTION

RISK FACTORS

The major risk factor for development of a central nervous system (CNS) infection after CNS trauma is violation of the dural membrane.[146-148] Disruption of the dura can result from direct penetrating injury, cranial fractures such as Le Fort II and III, nasal and basilar skull fractures, placement of intraventricular catheters, and extensive neurosurgical procedures. Prophylactic antibiotics after open CNS injuries, unless administered for a penetrating wound, are not recommended because they are not effective in preventing infection and may shift the normal flora toward a predominance of gram-negative bacillary organisms.[65] Nor are antibiotics effective on bullets, foreign objects, or devascularized and necrotic tissues. The best preventive measures remain adequate debridement and meticulous surgical technique.

Use of certain medical devices increases the risk of CNS infections. Nasal tubes such as nasogastric and nasotracheal tubes should not be placed in patients with known or suspected CSF leaks, and nasopharyngeal suctioning should not be performed. These procedures can significantly increase the risk of sinusitis and subsequent meningitis.[149] Many patients with CNS injuries receive antacids or H_2-blocking agents to help minimize gastrointestinal stress. These drugs raise the gastric pH and cause the acidic barrier of the stomach to be lost, creating a reservoir for microorganisms. If a vented gastric tube is used, special attention must be given to preventing reflux of the microbiologically abundant gastric fluids on to neurosurgical drains or intracranial pressure (ICP) monitoring devices. The consequence could be development of meningitis or ventriculitis.

INTRACRANIAL PRESSURE MONITORING DEVICES

Meningitis and ventriculitis can be associated with the use of intraventricular catheters.[150,151] The infection risks are related to the length of time these catheters are in place, the ability to maintain a "closed system," the monitoring and drainage systems, and the need to vent CSF. Only drainage systems manufactured specifically for use as intraventricular monitoring and drainage devices should be used. When intraventricular catheters are used, culture and Gram stain, complete cell count with differential, and protein and glucose determinations should be obtained from a CSF sample withdrawn from the catheter if intracranial infection is a possibility. A CSF sample is obtained whenever the patient becomes febrile, has a mental status change, or has an unexplained increase in serum white blood cells. The results and trends of the cell count and glucose determination afford early detection of infection and aid in the evaluation of positive culture and Gram stain results. For example, if the glucose level is low or less than two thirds the serum value and the white blood cell count is high with a predominance of polymorphonuclear leukocytes, the patient may have meningitis. Because culture results require a minimum of 72 hours before identification and antibiotic susceptibility patterns can be determined, antibiotic therapy should be initiated before culture results are complete and then adjusted accordingly. Catheters should be inserted using strict sterile technique and changed with a consistent protocol. When the catheter is discontinued, it should be removed using aseptic technique. The infectious hazards related to ICP monitoring can be reduced if subarachnoid/subdural or parenchymal devices are used instead of the more invasive intraventricular catheter.[151,152] Infection rates with the fiberoptic ICP monitoring devices are also low.[153]

CEREBROSPINAL FLUID SHUNTS

Posttraumatic hydrocephalus can be a complication of head injury and often necessitates the use of CSF shunts. These include ventriculoatrial, ventriculoperitoneal, lumbar-peritoneal, and ventriculopleural varieties.

Complications of infection secondary to the placement of CSF shunts can lead to impaired intellectual and neurologic function and, in some cases, death.[154] These infections can include meningitis, brain abscess, wound infection, and peritonitis (for peritoneal shunts). The clinical manifestations of such an infection may be fever alone or any combination of the systemic signs of infection. The predisposing infection risks are related to technical placement, operative time, intracerebral hemorrhage, intracranial pressure of 20 mm Hg or more, irrigation of system, and ventricular catheterization for more than 5 days.[150] The role of prophylactic antibiotics remains unclear. Positive cultures of the CSF, blood, shunt apparatus, incisions, or peritoneal fluid may be obtained. Treatment involves appropriate antimicrobial therapy or shunt removal, replacement, or revision.

Although S. aureus and gram-negative bacillary organisms have been identified as the causative agents, most report strains of coagulase-negative staphylococci as the predominant pathogen. This organism produces an excess of a mucoid substance that appears to promote adherence to smooth surfaces and may be protective against the lytic actions of lysozyme.[155] The major reservoir of coagulase-negative staphylococci is the patient's skin.

MENINGITIS

Classic signs of meningitis may be obscure in patients sustaining severe brain injury. Decreasing level of consciousness and nuchal rigidity may sometimes be absent or difficult to evaluate. Fever may be absent, demonstrate erratic patterns, or be the result of blood in the CSF. Leukocytosis can be influenced by the underlying injury or by the presence of blood. If intracranial pressure is elevated, it may be impossible to perform a lumbar puncture to obtain CSF for culture because of the risk of inducing brain herniation.

When a sample of the CSF can be obtained, diagnosis of meningitis is based on the presence of pleocytosis, hypoglycorrhachia, elevation of CSF protein not attributable to a noninfectious cause, and the isolation of an organism. Gram-negative meningitis is more common if the patient has received prior antibiotic therapy. When CSF culture is not obtainable, the diagnosis of infection is more difficult. In these patients antibiotic therapy should be initiated when the patient shows signs of mental and clinical deterioration in conjunction with the suspicion of infection. An effective antibiotic regimen for the empirical treatment of meningitis when the causative organism is not known should

TABLE 14-12	**Infection Control Guidelines for Preventing Central Nervous System Infection**

1. Do not use prophylactic antibiotics in patients with CSF leaks.
2. Do not place nasal tubes or perform nasopharyngeal suctioning in patients with CSF leaks.
3. Avoid reflux of fluid into drainage tract of intracranial drains.
4. Use subarachnoid/subdural or parenchymal devices instead of intraventricular catheters whenever possible.
5. Remove monitoring devices and drains as soon as possible.
6. Use strict aseptic technique for insertion of monitoring systems.
7. Use strict aseptic technique to manipulate and calibrate monitoring systems.
8. Obtain CSF samples for culture, Gram stain, complete cell count, and glucose determination on patients with intraventricular catheters when indicated.
9. Use aseptic technique when manipulating any neurosurgical drain.

provide coverage against both gram-positive cocci and gram-negative bacillary organisms.[156]

Brain abscess, epidural abscess, meningitis, and osteomyelitis of the cranium or spine may develop from a dissecting wound infection. In addition, these infections can result from inadequate debridement of the initial injury, failure to comply with the principles of meticulous surgical technique, or hematogenous seeding from a bacteremia. Eradication of infection may be difficult and requires prolonged antibiotic therapy (i.e., 6 to 8 weeks). Surgical intervention also may be necessary.

INFECTION CONTROL MEASURES THROUGHOUT THE TRAUMA CYCLE

The primary infection risks for CNS infection occur during the initial phase of the trauma cycle when the dura is broken. CSF infection is more likely to occur in the acute stages, whereas the deep-seated infections often develop much later. Trauma patients sustaining CNS injury have the highest infection risks because they often require prolonged mechanical support of many organ systems.[157,158] Throughout the trauma cycle, nurses must be alert to subtle changes in the patient's clinical condition that signal the presence of an incubating infection. This vigilance will promote earlier recognition of infection and initiation of appropriate therapy. Infection control guidelines for preventing CNS infection are found in Table 14-12.

RESPIRATORY TRACT INFECTION

Despite recent progress in the diagnosis, prevention, and treatment of hospital-acquired infections, nosocomial pneumonia remains an important problem, particularly among the critically ill. According to data from the National Nosocomial Infections Surveillance System, nosocomial pneumonia is now the second most frequent cause[159] of hospital-acquired infections in the United States, occurring in 5 to 10 patients per 1000 hospital admissions,[160] or about 300,000 patients each year.[161] These patients are often in medical or surgical intensive care units, where reports of the incidence of nosocomial pneumonia have ranged from 9% to 40%, or 15 cases per 1000 ventilator days.[162] Pneumonia remains the leading cause of death from nosocomial infection.[163] Reviewing 200 consecutive deaths at a university hospital and a community hospital, Gross et al found nosocomial pneumonia either directly caused or contributed to 16% of all deaths.[163] Although mortality rates as high as 72% have been reported for bacteremic nosocomial pneumonia caused by *P. aeruginosa*,[164] the overall mortality rate of this hospital-acquired infection is felt to be in the range of 33% to 50%. In addition, the associated morbidity of nosocomial pneumonia is considerable, adding an estimated 5 days to the hospital stay of surviving patients and increasing health care costs by billions of dollars.

UPPER RESPIRATORY TRACT INFECTION

SINUSITIS/OTITIS. Upper respiratory tract infections are usually related to intubation and most are of nosocomial etiology.[165,166] Nosocomial sinusitis usually presents as cryptic fever in patients with indwelling nasal tubes and a decreased level of consciousness.[165] The presence of a large-bore tube in the nose can cause inflammation and edema of the nasopharyngeal mucosa with blocked ventilation of the sinuses. In addition, supine positioning of critically ill patients prevents gravity-induced drainage of sinuses. Blood in sinus cavities secondary to facial trauma presents an excellent bacterial culture medium. The end result is the colonization of sinus cavities with pathogenic oropharyngeal flora.

Diagnosis is based on positive roentgenograms consistent with sinusitis and either purulent material aspirated from the sinuses or the presence of purulent nasal discharge. However, less than one third of patients described as having this disease have purulent nasal discharge. Most infections are polymicrobial, with a predominance of gram-negative bacilli. Similarly, otitis can develop secondary to indwelling nasal tubes or implanted myringotomy tubes. Purulent drainage may not be evident, and the diagnosis may be overlooked. Careful examination and assessment of the patient are key to the diagnosis. Failure to identify sinusitis or otitis can result in the institution of inappropriate therapy if the source of the fever is attributed to other factors. Resolution of infection requires the removal of the tubes and administration of appropriate antibiotics. Surgical drainage of an abscess or aspiration of the sinus also may be necessary.

TRACHEITIS. Tracheitis may be associated with endotracheal intubation. Prolonged hyperinflation of endotracheal cuffs causes localized tracheal ischemia, creating

TABLE 14-13   Risk Factors Associated with Colonization and Development of Nosocomial Pneumonia

Host Factors	Surgery	Medications	Invasive Devices

• Age >70 years
• Underlying medical conditions:
  -coma
  -COPD
  -diabetes mellitus
  -alcoholism
  -smoking
  -immunosuppresion
  -malnourishment
• Delayed gastrointestinal motility
• Immobility
	• Thoracic
	• Abdominal
	• ENT
		• Antibiotics
		• Steroids
		• Cytotoxic drugs
		• Antacids
		• H_2-blockers
		• CNS depressants
			• NG tube
			• Endotracheal tube
			• Tracheostomy
			• Intracranial pressure monitor
			• Gastric feeding

COPD, Chronic obstructive pulmonary disease; ENT, ear, nose, and throat; CNS, central nervous system; NG, nasogastric.

an environment that facilitates the growth of oral anaerobes. Purulent tracheitis that may have secondary cellulitis is generally attributed to anaerobes. Patients with tracheostomy tubes should be monitored for the development of purulent tracheitis. Discharges usually are copious, thin in viscosity, dirty brown in color, and foul smelling. Most patients do well with appropriate antibiotic therapy, which is usually directed against the oral anaerobes.

LOWER RESPIRATORY TRACT INFECTION

PNEUMONIA.   In hospitalized patients the occurrence of nosocomial pneumonia is related to circumvented pulmonary defenses, altered upper respiratory physical barriers, and colonization. Table 14-13 summarizes the risks factors associated with nosocomial pneumonia.

The etiologic agents of nosocomial pneumonia include a diverse group of pathogens. Gram-negative bacilli and staphylococci are the most frequent isolates in most studies.[167] P. aeruginosa is the most frequently isolated gram-negative bacillus. In some centers and in patients previously treated with antibiotics, Acinetobacter and Enterobacter species are becoming an increasing problem.[168] S. aureus is the most common gram-positive organism associated with nosocomial pneumonia and, given the growing incidence of methicillin-resistant strains, has important implications in the design of treatment regimens.

Although their role in hospital-acquired pneumonia is not clear, anaerobes are identified in 35% of specimens appropriately obtained and cultured.[169] H. influenzae and Streptococcus pneumoniae, when present, are usually identified in patients with chronic obstructive pulmonary disease (COPD) or early in the course of hospitalization in patients who have not received prior antibiotics.[170]

The diagnosis of hospital-acquired pneumonia is fraught with problems, particularly among critically ill and mechanically ventilated patients. Largely as a result of the accessibility of the lower airway, most studies have addressed the problem of diagnosis only in ventilated patients. The clinician is faced with the decision of whether to make the diagnosis on clinical grounds alone[171] and treat empirically versus pursuing a more invasive approach in the hopes of obtaining a specific diagnosis. The criteria used most often for the clinical diagnosis of nosocomial pneumonia include the following:

- Fever with a temperature higher than 38.5° C or lower than 35° C
- Leukocytosis or leukopenia
- New or increasing pulmonary infiltrate persistent for 48 hours on chest radiographs
- Purulent tracheobronchial secretions
- Isolation of pathogenic bacteria from an endotracheal aspirate

The clinical picture, however, can often be confused with a variety of other infectious and noninfectious pulmonary processes in the mechanically ventilated patient.

Over the past decade, several studies have specifically evaluated the incidence and risk factors associated with pneumonia in trauma patients. In 1992 Rello et al concluded that nosocomial respiratory tract infections were a frequent problem (26% incidence) in multiple trauma patients, especially those with Glasgow Coma Scale (GCS) scores less than 9. *S. aureus* was a frequent isolate among such patients.[168] In 1997 Montgomerie reviewed the incidence of various infections in spinal cord-injured patients. Pneumonia occurred in 5% to 20% of all patients with spinal cord injuries.[172] Ewig et al in 1999 evaluated the bacterial colonization patterns in mechanically ventilated patients with traumatic head injury.[171] They concluded that patients with head injury are colonized in the airways by group I pathogens (*S. pneumoniae, S. aureus, H. influenzae*) early in the evolution of illness. After 4 days, group II pathogens (gram-negative rods) colonize the airways. Previous antibiotic treatment was protective against colonization with group I pathogens but increased the subsequent colonization with group II pathogens. Campbell et al in 1999 demonstrated that nasal colonization with *S. aureus* at the time of severe head injury increased the risk of *S. aureus* pneumonia.[173] Finally Berrouane et al conducted a study in a neurosurgical intensive care unit[174] and confirmed the high incidence of early-onset pneumonia in trauma patients.

Nosocomial pneumonia is a serious disease. It is often complicated by bacteremia and has a high mortality rate. Pneumonia and aspiration can induce lung abscess and empyema. Therefore all efforts to prevent it must be undertaken.

EMPYEMA.   Thoracic empyema has been described as a sequela of prior pneumonia, aspiration, or pleural effusion.[175] Predisposing risk factors appear to be related to chest tube insertion for evacuation of blood after chest trauma or emergency intervention for internal cardiac massage and after barotrauma in patients requiring high levels of positive end-expiratory pressure or controlled mechanical ventilation.[176,177] The primary pathogen is usually coagulase-positive staphylococci.[176] Empyema that follows barotrauma and chest tube insertion generally develops late in the hospitalization, and therefore patients may have a colonized lower respiratory tract. Organisms recovered from empyema via this mechanism are usually gram-negative bacilli and anaerobes.[176] Empyema may be a consequence of surgical misadventure during the placement of subclavian and jugular central venous catheters.[178] These incidents can cause pneumothorax, hemothorax, and hydrothorax, which contaminate the lungs and pleural space and may warrant the emergent insertion of chest tubes.

Diagnosis of nosocomial empyema is based on purulent drainage from the pleural space and increasing trends in temperature and white blood cell count. Culture and Gram stain, complete cell count with differential, and pH and protein determinations of the drainage fluid can support the diagnosis. Pleural fluid cultures should not be obtained from the collection chambers, since this fluid may be contaminated and may not reflect the clinical picture. Samples are drawn from a site on the latex tubing that is as close as possible to the thoracotomy tube. The tubing should be washed with an antiseptic soap and then disinfected with alcohol. A 25-gauge needle is used to aspirate a small amount of pleural fluid. Specimens should be sent to the laboratory in the syringe, not in blood culture bottles. Treatment may require decortication and rib resection.[179] Appropriate parenteral antibiotics are given until the chest tube is converted to a treatment port.

Infection control measures that may minimize the development of nosocomial empyema include strict aseptic chest tube insertion technique and maintenance of occlusive dressings at the insertion site that should be changed routinely. Gentle milking of the latex tubings of the drainage system prevents local trauma at the skin-tube interface and catapulting of organisms back into the pleural space.

INFECTION CONTROL MEASURES THROUGHOUT THE TRAUMA CYCLE

Respiratory infections can develop in any phase of the trauma cycle subsequent to initial resuscitation. The greatest chance for pneumonia is when the patient is in the intensive care unit and is ventilator dependent, unconscious, or immobilized. However, infection hazards are present throughout the cycle and may exist in the prehospital phase. Nursing actions promote pulmonary function and prevent the retention of secretions. These actions include chest physiotherapy, frequent repositioning and turning, incentive spirometry, encouraging cough and deep breathing exercises in nonventilated patients, and providing frequent pulmonary toilet to ventilator-dependent patients. Infection control guidelines for prevention of nosocomial pneumonia are outlined in Table 14-14.[180,181]

GASTROINTESTINAL TRACT INFECTION

The risks of intraabdominal infection after operative procedures are well documented.[1,5,47,84,86] The risk of developing an infection is influenced by the following:

- Type and classification of surgery performed
- Duration of surgery
- Skill of the surgeon
- Manner in which the skin is prepared before incision
- Hollow viscus injury

Compromised tissue perfusion causes devitalized tissue, providing a medium in which microorganisms thrive. Other predisposing factors are hematoma formation, dead spaces, abrasive tissue handling, surgical misadventures, placement of drains, peritoneal dialysis, CNS dysfunction, and use of enteral feeding tubes. Often, despite prophylactic antibiotic therapy, peritonitis and deep-seated abscesses can develop

TABLE 14-14   Infection Control Guidelines for Prevention of Lower Respiratory Tract Infections

1. Conduct surveillance for bacterial pneumonia in ICU patients to determine trends, causative organisms, and their antimicrobial susceptibility patterns.
2. Perform procedures to interrupt transmission of microorganisms:
   - Sterilize or disinfect and maintain equipment and devices. For example, change ventilator circuits every 48 hours; discard unused portion of fluid in nebulizer or humidifier; dedicate one bag-mask resuscitator to each patient; and periodically drain and discard any condensation that collects in the tubing of a breathing circuit.
   - Interrupt person-to-person transmission of bacteria using handwashing, barrier precautions such as gloves, and suctioning of respiratory secretions.
3. Modifying host risk for infection:
   - Discontinue endotracheal, tracheostomy, and enteral tubes as soon as possible.
   - Prevent aspiration associated with enteral feeding by verifying placement of tubes, elevating head end of patients' beds, and assessing intestinal motility.
   - Prevent gastric colonization by use of an agent that does not raise the patient's gastric pH (for stress ulcer prophylaxis).
   - Postoperative pneumonia can be prevented by frequent coughing, deep breathing, and ambulating as soon as possible; adequate control of pain; and use of incentive spirometer or intermittent positive pressure breathing.
4. Vaccinate high-risk patients with pneumococcal vaccine.

when the integrity of the gastrointestinal (GI) mucosa has been broken.[2,3,12,13] Mortality from these infections has been reported to approach 30%, and the prognosis worsens with increasing age, organ failure, bacteremia, and persistent abscess.[2]

Penetrating trauma can disrupt the colonic mucosa, causing fecal contamination of the peritoneal cavity, and can sever the major deep vessels. Blunt trauma causes rupture of the solid, highly perfused organs such as liver and spleen, which may cause massive hemorrhage necessitating emergent surgery with inadequate time for meticulous skin preparation or gentle tissue handling. In addition, trauma patients are prone to development of infection as a result of altered GI function caused by CNS injury, anesthetic agents, and antibiotic use.[58] The most common sites for intraabdominal abscess after trauma are within the subphrenic and subhepatic spaces.

Contusion of the gallbladder secondary to trauma or a hepatobiliary procedure is one cause of acute acalculous cholecystitis.[182] The contusion impedes perfusion, which may cause necrosis and provide a medium for bacterial growth and an access route for entry into the bloodstream. The development of acute acalculous cholecystitis can be a serious, life-threatening disease.

Diagnosis of intraabdominal infection can be hindered by the patient's clinical condition. Physical examination may be difficult due to the presence of drainage tubes and bandages or the patient's immobility. Diagnostic tests such as ultrasound, computed tomography scan, and x-ray films may be unobtainable because the patient is too critically ill to be moved or the extent of the injury prevents the proper positioning of the patient for performance of the test.

Assessment of intraabdominal infection depends on evaluation of bowel function, the integrity of suture lines, the character of any drainage fluid, and trending fever pattern and white blood cell count. Purulent material from incisions or drainage tubes should be sent for Gram stain and culture.

Diarrhea in severely compromised patients is usually caused by the hyperosmolarity of the feeding solution. However, infectious causes such as pseudomembranous colitis and antibiotic-associated colitis must be considered. In critically ill patients the incidence of *Salmonella*, *Shigella*, and *Campylobacter* enterocolitis is extremely rare. Therefore stool cultures for these pathogens should not be a routine diagnostic test. Persistent diarrhea, defined as three or more large, loose stools a day, in patients on or completing antibiotic therapy may be an indication of the presence of *C. difficile* colitis.[183] Characteristically the diarrhea is watery and large in volume, but evidence of blood and mucus may be absent. Fever, leukocytosis, and abdominal cramping are present in most cases. Antibiotic-related pseudomembranous colitis has been associated with almost every antimicrobial agent.[183] Diagnosis is based on onset of diarrhea during or after antibiotic therapy, presence of *C. difficile* toxin in stool specimens, and observation of pseudomembranes during endoscopic examination. Most patients do well with administration of oral metronidazole.[183,184] Cross-contamination is likely if patients are placed in close proximity. Body fluid precautions are necessary for patients with diarrhea associated with gastrointestinal infections.[185]

Indwelling nasogastric tubes and gastrostomy tubes can result in staphylococcal enterocolitis. The staphylococci invade the GI tract from the skin's reservoir via either the nares or the gastrostomy tube-skin interface or, in some cases, as a result of contamination of the feeding solution and apparatus. Needle jejunostomy tubes can produce localized ischemia, which can later lead to necrosis, intestinal perforation, peritonitis, and intraabdominal abscess.

Special consideration must be given to trauma patients receiving enteral feeding and who have dysfunctional GI tracts or increased gastric pH.[186] The primary infection risk is related to bacterial growth in residual solutions that accumulate within the administration sets.[187] Some studies suggest that contaminated enteral nutrition represents a significant cause of bacteremic infection.[188] Infection risks for these patients can be reduced by thoroughly cleaning or changing the administration sets a minimum of every 24 hours.[189]

Although many gastrointestinal infections tend to manifest later in the trauma cycle, infection risks throughout the

TABLE 14-15 Infection Control Guidelines for the Gastrointestinal Tract

1. Use sterile technique for wound and drain care.
2. Use sterile measuring devices when emptying drainage vessels.
3. Maintain the patency and function of all drainage tubes to ensure proper evacuation.
4. Document the characteristics of all drainage fluids, such as amount, color, viscosity, and odor.
5. Document the appearance of surgical sites, and notify the physician of any leakage through the incision.
6. Obtain culture and Gram stain of any purulent material from wounds or drainage tubes.
7. Assess bowel sounds and function at the beginning of every shift.
8. Obtain *C. difficile* culture for persistent diarrhea.
9. Use blood-warming apparatus for warming peritoneal solutions rather than water baths.
10. Change enteral feeding apparatus daily.

cycle are ever present. Frequent assessment of GI function facilitates early diagnosis and treatment of disease. Therefore any deviation from the patient's normal baseline may signal the presence of an incubating infection. Infection control guidelines are shown in Table 14-15.

GENITOURINARY TRACT INFECTION

Catheter-associated urinary tract infection (UTI) is the most frequently cited nosocomial infection developing among hospitalized patient populations.[159,190] Approximately 20% of the infections developed in severely traumatized patients have been reported to be UTIs.[1-3,12,13,191] Underlying illness, advanced age, female sex, burns, CNS injury, genitourinary (GU) injury, metabolic imbalances, and renal failure contribute to the infection risks.[190]

The major cause of UTI is an indwelling catheter, which affords bacteria a direct portal of entry into the bladder. Bacteria may be inoculated into the system during catheter insertion, by traveling the mucous coating that forms along the catheter,[192] from contamination of the drainage bag if urine refluxes into the bladder, and by frequent manipulations of the drainage system.[193] The probability of developing bacteriuria and UTI increases proportionately as the duration of catheter indwelling time increases.[194]

Because of the high frequency of bacterial colonization in the urinary drainage system, the criteria for diagnosis of UTI may require refinement. A useful definition for UTI in the catheterized patient is two or more consecutive positive urine cultures with more than 100,000 colony-forming units per milliliter, pyuria of at least 10 white blood cells per high-power field of unspun fresh urine, and clinical signs of infection.[2,3,12,13] Treatment of colonization rather than infection can encourage the emergence of antibiotic-resistant bacteria or mask the development of a more serious infection.

In patients sustaining spinal cord injury with neurogenic bladder, regimens for bladder training should be initiated as soon as possible. There seems to be less of an associated risk for UTI from intermittent catheterizations than with indwelling catheters.[195,196] However, in male patients, epididymitis and prostate gland infection may be induced by repetitive instrumentations or intermittent catheterizations.

Although reports cite UTI as one of the predominant types of nosocomial infection, UTIs have a comparatively low incidence of associated bacteremia. The vast majority of UTIs are caused by *E. coli* and other gram-negative bacillary bacteria. An indwelling catheter should not be changed during a fever spike or an acute infectious crisis. If the patient has colonized or infected urine, the bacteria may gain access to the bloodstream as the catheter is being changed. Catheter tip cultures are unnecessary because the tip becomes contaminated when withdrawn from the urethral mucosa. Urine culture and urinalysis obtained by needle aspiration of the catheter system are more appropriate.

Infection control practices and preventive efforts in the development of UTI have been widely examined.[197] Certain measures are ineffective, such as routine bladder irrigation, suppressive antibiotic therapy, povidone-iodine solutions for meatal care, and instillation of hydrogen peroxide into the drainage bag. In the intensive care unit the sharing of collection vessels used to empty the drainage bags has been associated with outbreaks of gram-negative UTIs.[198]

Bladder injury can promote UTI secondary to dysfunction of the bladder, as well as increase the necessity for prolonged instrumentation. Indwelling suprapubic tubes may induce infection at the skin-tube junction. Patency of these tubes is important. Leakage around the catheter and signs of inflammation or purulent drainage need to be reported to the physician.

UTIs occur in any phase of the trauma cycle, even at the time of admission. As the patient progresses through the trauma cycle, recurrence of UTI may occur in patients requiring prolonged instrumentation. Concomitantly, repeated courses of antibiotic therapy increase the reservoir of antibiotic-resistant microorganisms. Because of the high risk for UTI, the use of indwelling catheters for the management of urinary incontinence should be considered carefully. Promoting noninvasive management, such as condom catheters in males and disposable diapers in females whenever possible, is necessary.

OCCUPATIONAL EXPOSURE TO BLOODBORNE DISEASES

Occupational concern about acquisition of an infectious disease while performing emergency medical services (EMS) has intensified largely as a result of AIDS.[199] Although needle-stick injuries are the most common method of exposure to dangerous viruses, bloodborne pathogens can also be transmitted through contact with mucous membranes or nonintact skin of the health care provider. In 1987 the CDC called for the institution of universal precautions for infection control to prevent occupational acquisition of the bloodborne infections hepatitis B virus (HBV) and human immunodeficiency virus (HIV).[200] These guidelines recommend the following:

- Consider all blood, bloody body fluids, and other body fluids to be infectious.
- Wear appropriate protective attire (gloves, gowns, eyewear, and masks) for tasks that could cause bloody fluid contamination of personnel.
- Define the circumstances of exposures to blood and body fluids.
- Outline employee health guidelines for follow-up medical care for personnel sustaining an exposure.

The CDC has no power of enforcement for their guidelines. The U.S. Department of Labor, through the Occupational Safety and Health Administration (OSHA), codified the CDC guidelines into federal regulations that became effective in 1992.[201] The OSHA regulations are much more explicit with regard to definitions of infectious body fluids, requirements for education and training, mandating hepatitis B vaccine programs at the expense of the employer, guidelines for employee health programs, environmental controls, and documenting compliance with the regulations. OSHA standards extend to all private sector employers with one or more employees.

In 1996 the CDC discontinued use of the term *universal precautions,* replacing it with *standard precautions.* This term change reflected the need to protect medical personnel not only from bloodborne infections but also from an array of other infectious organisms.

HIV AND THE TRAUMA PATIENT

Most trauma patients admitted with HIV infection are in the asymptomatic carrier phase of the illness. Common demographic features among trauma and HIV patients have been documented.[202] More than 90% of AIDS cases occur in people between 20 and 49 years; more than 90% of these are male; and approximately 15% use IV drugs. Similarly, trauma is the leading killer of U.S. residents under the age of 38, most victims are male, and drug and alcohol abusers seem to have higher trauma rates. Patients sustaining gunshot wounds resulting from situations related to IV drug abuse or dealing are seen more frequently within large metropolitan areas and surrounding communities than in rural settings. Studies describing the incidence rates of HIV among trauma patients reflect the demographic patterns of HIV infection, with significantly greater numbers concentrated in larger cities.[203-205] Sloan et al found that out of 994 patients admitted to an urban level I trauma center, 43 patients (4.3%) tested HIV positive. Infection was related to age (20-49 years), IV drug use, history of hepatitis or sexually transmitted disease, prior HIV testing, shock, and death. Young urban trauma patients were 15 to 17 times more likely to be HIV infected than the overall trauma population.[203] A study by Tardiff et al of 1242 trauma patients from New York City concluded that the rate of HIV infection (7.2% overall) was significant especially in those with cocaine use.[205] By contrast, a hospital whose trauma population was mostly referred from outside the city limits, reported a much lower seropositivity rate of 1.7% of admissions.[204]

The total number of HIV cases has steadily increased since 1986, with the northeastern United States and the Atlantic Coast having the highest rates. HIV has been isolated in many body fluids, but only contact with blood, semen, genital secretions, and breast milk has been documented as a source of transmission. Contact with nonintact skin in the trauma patient has rarely resulted in HIV infection.[206,207]

Identification of HIV-infected patients who may pose an occupational risk to emergency health care workers cannot be guaranteed. Two types of HIV antibody tests are widely used at present: enzyme-linked immunosorbent assay (ELISA) and Western blot electrophoresis. Both have intrinsic flaws.[208] ELISA is a highly sensitive test (>99%) for antibody response; however, it is not as specific (95% to 99%) because reactivity with similar antibodies can give false positive results. Many conditions, including collagen-vascular diseases, chronic hepatitis, and malaria, have been associated with false positive results on ELISA. Western blot electrophoresis is a highly specific test for HIV antibody proteins; however, it is not an extremely sensitive test, and results can be inconclusive. Therefore the most widely accepted criteria for HIV antibody positivity require that both tests be performed and both tests be positive. Within 2 weeks of exposure, a period of viremia and P24 antigenemia occurs. During this phase, ELISA and Western blot tests remain negative. P24 testing is useful in evaluating patients with suspected acute retroviral syndrome.[209] In the early 1990s new technologies, including quantitative reverse transcriptase polymerase chain reaction (PCR), branched DNA, and nucleic acid sequence-based assay (NASBA) techniques, allowed accurate measurement of viral-associated circulating HIV RNA in plasma.[210]

Massive fluid replacement in trauma patients may influence HIV antibody positivity. The antibodies are diluted, and the patient's HIV antibody test could be falsely negative. Newly infected individuals may test negative because their body has not had adequate time to mount an antibody response, yet they may have viral particles in their blood that can infect a health care worker who sustains percutaneous or mucocutaneous exposure. Knowledge of the patient's HIV antibody status could give the care provider a false sense of security, and thus infection control precautions might be relaxed at a time when the patient's blood is most infectious. Accurate detection of those patients who have the virus is impossible without serologic testing, even with a detailed history. This fact reinforces the need for consistent use of standard precautions in the care of all trauma patients. If one of the bloodborne diseases or any communicable disease is diagnosed while the patient is hospitalized, prehospital EMS providers must be notified of their exposure. Notification mechanisms must ensure both accurate information and protection of the patient's and provider's legal rights.

Informed consent is mandatory for HIV testing in most states and a requirement by OSHA for serotesting a patient in cases of occupational exposure.[201] Informed consent is particularly important for trauma patients because the circumstance of their admission is not HIV infection. For this reason, substitute consent of unconscious or cognitively impaired patients may not be legal unless formal legal guardianship has been established.

Public health measures for HIV prevention have focused on limiting exposure through condom use, needle exchange programs, education, and safety protocols. Still, HIV transmission continues at epidemic levels and additional strategies are needed. Data reported from the CDC suggest that the vast majority of documented occupational transmissions are a result of percutaneous exposure. The average risk for acquisition of HIV through percutaneous exposure to infected blood is approximately 0.3%. Postexposure prophylaxis is an exciting advance in the management of HIV exposure in the workplace. The success of this prophylaxis led the CDC to recommend a more aggressive, multidrug antiviral regimen.[211,212] Rapid HIV testing allows same-day results. In some instances results may be available within 1 to 2 hours. Kelen found the sensitivity and specificity of the rapid test were 100% and 98.9%, respectively. Rapid-result HIV testing facilitates prompt initiation of post-HIV exposure prophylaxis in the health care worker.[213]

HEPATITIS B AND HEPATITIS B VACCINE

Unlike HIV, hepatitis B virus can be easily and reliably detected in patients with a chronic carrier state or active state of infection. Serotesting for HBV is done by radioimmunoassay (RIA), which detects the presence of hepatitis B surface antigen (HBsAg), and positivity is an indication of existing HBV. However, HBsAg testing is not routinely performed by the majority of health care facilities for several reasons:

1. Chronic HBV infection afflicts 1.25 million people in the United States; routine screening of all patients may be prohibitively expensive for many hospitals.
2. An HBsAg test may be irrelevant to the reason for the patient's admission to the hospital.
3. Many hospitals are not equipped to perform these tests on site.
4. Employees can be vaccinated against HBV infection.

Therefore it is estimated that approximately 90% of HBsAg carriers who are hospitalized are not detected as carriers of the virus during admission.[214]

Although prophylactic treatment is available, in 1993 the CDC estimated that 1450 health care workers became infected with hepatitis B virus after occupational exposure. Of these, 100 to 200 eventually died from the lethal sequelae of this disease. A recent study in a level I trauma center

reported the following incidence of bloodborne pathogens: HBV 1.5%, HCV 13.8%, and HIV 0.52%.[202] Six percent to 30% of health care workers not vaccinated or receiving prophylaxis who incur blood or body fluid exposure involving patients with hepatitis B will develop disease[202,214]; fewer than 1% of those incurring similar misadventures involving people with AIDS will become HIV antibody positive.[212] Reports of health care workers who have died from documented or suspected occupational acquisition of HIV infection are rare.

The occupational risk of HBV infection among health care workers is high. Health care workers have a seroincidence 2 to 4 times higher (6% to 15%) than that of the general U.S. population. Among health care workers, dentists, laboratory workers, dialysis workers, cleaning service employees, and nurses have the highest rate of occupationally acquired HBV.[215]

Despite these statistics and the CDC's recommendation that health care workers in high-risk settings be vaccinated with hepatitis B vaccine, vaccination programs have met with little success, resulting in the decline but not the elimination of hepatitis.[215,216] Concern over safety, efficacy, lack of education regarding the vaccine, and fear of needles have been identified as factors related to vaccine nonacceptance.[217] However, the OSHA regulations[201] mandate that employers make hepatitis B vaccine available at no charge to employees and require employers to document proof of vaccination refusal by employees. Indications for HBV vaccination in the United States include individuals with a high risk of exposure to HBV who have not been previously infected. Universal vaccination of children in the United States was recommended in 1991.[218]

OCCUPATIONAL PROTECTIVE ATTIRE AND PROCEDURES

OSHA estimates that more than 5.6 million health care and public safety workers are potentially exposed to infectious material and other body fluids that may contain HIV and HBV.[219] Most commonly, exposure is secondary to needle-stick injury; however, contact with mucous membranes and nonintact skin of workers are also means of exposure.

OSHA regulations to reduce the risk of occupational exposure by bloodborne pathogens are outlined in Table 14-16. The guidelines apply to all persons exposed to blood, blood products, or other potentially infectious materials, including all body fluids (semen, vaginal secretions, cerebrospinal fluid), body tissue, and organs (living or dead) or HIV-containing cell or tissue cultures.

When the CDC recommended the implementation of standard precautions for the prevention of occupational acquisition of bloodborne diseases, glove use both inside and outside hospitals dramatically increased.[220] Gloves should be worn only when a task involves direct contact with blood or body fluids. They should be removed as soon as the task is completed, and handwashing should be performed. Wearing gloves should never be viewed as a substitute for

TABLE 14-16   Infection Control Guidelines for Prevention of Bloodborne Infections in the Healthcare Environment

1. Treat the blood and body fluids of all patients as if they were infectious.
2. Wear gloves when handling any blood or body fluid or performing invasive procedures (e.g., IV insertions, percutaneous venous or arterial punctures, and dressing changes).
3. Wear masks and eye protection when the chance of blood or body fluids being splashed is high.
4. Avoid needle-stick injuries and do not recap needles. All needles and sharps must be disposed of in impervious, puncture-resistant containers.
5. Protect broken skin with Band-Aids or small dressings.
6. Wash hands after all patient care procedures.
7. Use respiratory assist devices when performing mouth-to-mouth resuscitation.
8. Change clothing or scrub attire contaminated with blood or body fluids as soon as possible.
9. Report all percutaneous and mucocutaneous exposures to a patient's blood or body fluid and provide appropriate follow-up care.
10. Prehospital providers should wear heavy-weight gloves, such as leather ones, during extrication procedures to prevent hand injury.
11. Use chemical disinfectants responsibly and according to manufacturers' guidelines for both equipment and disinfecting agent.
12. Establish vaccination programs for HBV.

handwashing. In addition, the failure to remove gloves promptly can facilitate cross-infection among hospitalized patients and increase nosocomial infection rates. Failure to remove gloves also can promote occupational acquisition of bloodborne infection because personnel can inoculate themselves with the blood or secretions on the outside of the gloves by unconscious habits such as wiping their eyes or placing contaminated pens in their mouth.

Glove strength, not sterility, and proper fit of the gloves are the key factors for preventing occupational exposure. There is no single type or thickness of glove that is appropriate in all situations.[221] Sterile gloves should be worn only for procedures in which the patient needs protection from nosocomial infection. These include invasive and operative procedures. Sized nonsterile disposable gloves should be used for any other procedures or tasks in which finger dexterity is important and that involve manipulation of blood samples, IV monitoring lines, or the performance of a variety of laboratory tasks. Midweight plastic or rubber gloves should be worn for cleaning procedures, and heavy gloves (e.g., leather) should be worn for prehospital extrication procedures or trash removal. Gloves, which should be readily available, must be task specific and ensure the safety of both patients and personnel.

Proper eye protection facilitates safety and maintains vision. Visors, face shields, or goggles are most appropriate for procedures that involve cutting or drilling bone, when using pulsatile-jet lavage irrigation systems, when controlling hemorrhage, and while performing vascular surgery or dental procedures.[222]

All patient care procedures should be evaluated for safety; when appropriate, alternatives should be sought to minimize risks. Recapping needles is an unsafe practice. Technical proficiency should be monitored, and procedures identified as resulting in needle-stick injuries must be improved. The best mechanism to accomplish this is to document all needle sticks. This allows monitoring of the acquisition of disease and the safety of patient care practices.

The CDC states that handwashing "is the single most important procedure for preventing nosocomial infections." Handwashing, according to the Association of Professionals in Infection Control (APIC) guidelines, is the use of a broad-spectrum antimicrobial soap that is nonirritating, fast-acting, and designed to reduce the number of transient flora by suspending microorganisms and allowing them to be rinsed off. It facilitates protection of the patient from acquisition of nosocomial infection and the provider from occupational acquisition of an infectious disease. Waterless hand-cleaning products, especially in the prehospital setting, can be useful when there is no easy access to water sources and sinks. However, such products should not be considered a substitute for handwashing. Hands should be washed thoroughly as soon as patient care allows. Personnel should wash hands after contact with blood or body fluids regardless of whether gloves are worn. Hands should also be washed immediately after gloves are removed between patient contacts. It may also be necessary to wash hands between tasks or procedures on the same patient to prevent cross-contamination of different body sites. The CDC recommends a vigorous rubbing together of lathered hands for at least 10 seconds, followed by rinsing in running water.[223-225] More time may be necessary if the hands are visibly soiled. There are no well-controlled studies comparing soaps, detergents, and antimicrobial-containing products. Handwashing with plain soap appears to be sufficient.[225]

Failure to perform handwashing can be implicated in the acquisition of viral disease and may be an important factor in HBV transmission. Although it is clear that HBV transmission occurs by direct percutaneous or mucocutaneous exposure in the workplace, a significant number of those infected disclaim any knowledge of previous misadventure. Although acquisition of infection could have resulted from an exposure in the community, the mode of transmission in most of these cases may be the unconscious habits of personnel and failure to comply with infection control policies.

CLEANING, DISINFECTION, AND STERILIZATION

No other infection control guidelines create more confusion than those outlining cleaning, disinfection, and sterilization recommendations. These terms are often misused or inappropriately interchanged by supervisory personnel or even authorities on the subject. Decontamination is a process that removes disease-producing microorganisms and renders the object or the environment safe (e.g., washing a surface with hot soapy water). Disinfection is a process that kills or destroys most disease-producing microorganisms except the resistant bacterial endospores. The process can vary from low level (which kills bacteria, fungi, and viruses) to high level (which kills bacteria, tubercle bacilli, some spores, and viruses). Sterilization is a chemical or physical process that results in the total destruction of all microorganisms, including highly resistant bacterial spores or prions. Prions are infectious agents smaller than viruses that can initiate infection without the inflammatory response.

Application of these procedures is determined by the specific use of the equipment or instrument.[226] Sterilization is required for critical items; these include surgical instruments, cardiac catheters, orthopedic implants, and other devices placed into normally sterile body environments. Disinfection is required for semicritical items such as those that touch or invade mucous membranes. High-level disinfection is recommended for respiratory equipment to ensure eradication of mycobacteria. All other items and surfaces that contact intact skin but not mucous membranes are considered noncritical and require cleaning, decontamination, sanitizing, or low-level disinfection.

Disinfection and sterilization procedures must be performed on precleaned surfaces, as disinfectants are inactivated in the presence of organic matter. Concentrations of disinfectants and sterilants must be exact and in accordance with label instructions. Most disinfectants can be toxic, requiring personnel who use them to wear appropriate protective attire. Toxicity of products can be assessed from a material safety data sheet. In addition, it is federal law that all employees using disinfectants be educated about and protected against associated hazards.

A major disinfectant dilemma of recent years has centered on the eradication of HIV and HBV in the environment. Early in the AIDS epidemic, most infection guidelines recommended the use of household bleach in 1:10 dilution for environmental cleaning. This recommendation was largely derived from those developed in the 1970s for HBV and the fact that bleach is inexpensive and widely available to the medical and general community. However, as our knowledge of HIV has advanced, no environmental mechanisms of HIV infection have been documented, and a variety of disinfectants have been proved to be effective against this virus.[227] Subsequently the CDC changed its recommendation to detergent disinfectants for environmental cleaning.[200] Therefore standard recommendations for cleaning, disinfection, and sterilization are adequate measures to control this virus in health care settings.

HBV has often been considered some sort of "supervirus" because of its ability to survive under a variety of environmental conditions.[228] Studies demonstrated that undiluted serum from HBsAg carriers could be inactivated in 30 minutes by a 1:10 dilution of household bleach. However, even at much smaller concentrations, bleach solutions still can be corrosive to metals.

Detergent disinfectants were recommended for environmental cleaning even when the area was visibly contaminated with the blood or feces of a patient with hepatitis. However, bleach solutions were still recommended for surfaces such as curled or grooved instrument knobs that could not be cleaned easily. Environmental disinfection with bleach solutions was recommended for hemodialysis units to reduce the nosocomial transmission of HBV. In this setting it was theorized that critical and semicritical items used during dialysis could be contaminated by environmental HBV even if the person wore gloves.[229]

A mucocutaneous or percutaneous exposure to HBV is still necessary to cause disease. The best means of protection is wearing appropriate gloves, face masks, and gowns while performing cleaning, decontamination, and disinfection procedures and to meticulously clean the environment.

PREHOSPITAL PHASE

Prehospital EMS providers deal with unique and complex infection control issues. Nowhere within the trauma cycle is the application of infection control guidelines a greater challenge. Nurses can positively influence the infection control guidelines and educational programs of EMS systems.

At the time of initial resuscitation of a patient, the presence of bloodborne viruses is generally unknown because emergency care providers usually do not know the patient's medical history or lifestyle. This information may be difficult to obtain if the patient dies at the injury scene or shortly after admission or if the patient sustained an injury or complication of disease that results in permanent cognitive impairment. Infection risks may never be subsequently determined. Prehospital providers can be in situations where the blood of more than one patient contaminates the same environment. Any patient's blood or body fluids must be considered infectious. Needle sticks or cuts causing percutaneous or mucocutaneous exposure should be treated at this time, and the provider should be reminded to report these exposures and receive follow-up care according to the individual EMS system's policy.

The physical environment can be unstable and adverse, and the EMS provider's life itself may be in jeopardy. There are no truly aseptic conditions in the field. EMS must often be performed under conditions of inclement weather, within very confined spaces, with limited supplies and equipment, and without adequate lighting or water sources. These situations underscore the importance of wearing appropriate protective attire.

Prehospital infection control programs have been developed to help ensure patient and practitioner safety during delivery of EMS.[230] Prehospital care providers must be protected from both biologic and physical hazards. Heavy-duty hand protection such as leather gloves or gauntlets should be available for extrication procedures in order to prevent hand injury. Because water sources are unavailable, handwashing should be performed as soon as patient care allows once the providers have arrived at the hospital. Gowns are not recommended because they can be dangerous and cumbersome in rescue operations and are generally inadequate in the field. Turnout coats may offer a better alternative.

Formulation of infection control guidelines must be based on a clear understanding of a specific EMS system, that is, how the system works, the kind of care provided, and the limitation of personnel, supplies, and financing. In addition, notification of prehospital care providers of the diagnosis of an infectious disease in persons transported by them is a federal law.[210]

INFECTION CONTROL PROGRAM IN A TRAUMA UNIT

Infection control throughout the trauma cycle is a multifactorial problem. Trauma patients can have injuries that involve every organ system, and the severity of injuries can be highly varied. The infection risks and the reservoir of microorganisms are continually changing. Infection control guidelines must offer dual protection; that is, both the patients and staff must be protected from infection hazards. The overall infection control program must be monitored constantly. The incidence and prevalence of the infections, the infection rates, the safety and efficacy of patient care practices, the colonization and antibiotic susceptibility patterns of the organisms, antibiotic utilization, and acquisition of infection among the staff must be evaluated prospectively and comprehensively on a daily, monthly, and yearly basis. All the members of the trauma team—physicians, nurses, allied health professionals, and ancillary personnel—must be adequately educated about infection control principles and guidelines to ensure consistency of patient care and compliance with control measures. Therefore the primary objectives of the infection control program are (1) to identify the infection risks, (2) to determine the reservoirs of the microorganisms, (3) to provide dual protection of both patients and staff, (4) to have comprehensive and prospective surveillance, (5) to determine the efficacy and cost-effectiveness of patient care practices, and (6) to provide adequate education to all staff.

DRESS CODES

Recommendations for dress codes must address both the occupational protection of personnel and the protection of patients from nosocomial infection. Although the use of scrub clothes and cover gowns is generally thought not to be effective for reducing nosocomial infection risks in these areas, there may still be benefits. The requirement for wearing scrub clothes can regulate traffic of personnel and serve as a physical reminder to the personnel that they are caring for a special patient population.

The efficacy of wearing hats is not known. Although hair can be a reservoir for many microorganisms,[231] the risk to the patient results when personnel unconsciously handle their hair and then fail to wash their hands before patient contact. The Association of Operating Room Nurses' (AORN) standards require that all scalp and facial hair be covered when performing invasive procedures. Bouffant and hood-style covers are preferable.

One approach that may be beneficial in the prevention of nosocomial infection is the use of a procedural dress code. For example, insertion of a pulmonary artery catheter should require sterile gowns, hats covering all hair, masks, and sterile gloves, whereas obtaining blood cultures would require sterile gloves only. In other words, each procedure would be assigned a specific dress code category.[93] For example:

Category I: Sterile gown, hat, mask, and sterile gloves
Category II: Clean scrub attire or cover gown, hat, mask, and sterile gloves
Category III: Hat, mask, and sterile gloves
Category IV: Sterile gloves only
Category V: Good handwashing

NEW PRODUCT EVALUATION

Another important aspect of infection control in a trauma center is new product evaluation. It is important to remember that new or innovative is not necessarily better and that the use of a new product in or on a patient requires special evaluation. The use and effectiveness of hospital devices have not been as carefully regulated as drugs and medications. Benefits to patient care may only be speculative, and apparent cost benefits may be obscure. For example, a change to a less expensive arterial catheter may appear to reduce costs. However, if the catheter cannot be inserted easily via percutaneous placement, a cutdown procedure may be necessary; both cost and infection risk are substantially increased. Similarly, changes in procedure or policy should be examined carefully. Therefore an ongoing infection surveillance baseline is mandatory for judicious decisions regarding changes in product and procedural policy.[224]

DESIGN OF THE TRAUMA CENTER

The design of a trauma center should provide an environment that minimizes infection hazards. The primary objective is to reduce mechanisms of cross-infection among the patients. An important factor is the separation of patients by either physical barriers or spatial arrangements. An effective design involves the use of individual patient rooms.

Patient care supplies must be adequate, but areas should not be overstocked. Supplies must be continually checked to ensure the sterility of the products (e.g., integrity of packaging, expiration dates). Overstocking risks the use of nonsterile supplies and jeopardizes patient safety. The arrangement must allow rapid access during emergency situations, as well as promote infection control measures. Whenever possible, supplies and equipment should not be shared among patients. In addition, adequate space should be allocated for the proper cleaning and maintenance of equipment. Cross-contamination from dirty supplies to clean supplies must be avoided.

Because failure to comply with handwashing recommendations has been identified as the major cause of cross-contamination among patients,[75] it is essential that sinks are conventionally placed. Government standards recommend that the ratio of beds to sinks be no more than 6:1 in a multibed unit.[232] Ideally, there should be a sink next to every patient bed, and these sinks should operate via foot pedal or knee mechanisms. Because sinks can be a reservoir for gram-negative organisms,[233] special attention must be given to the proper maintenance of sinks and aerators on faucets should be removed.

SUMMARY

Infection control throughout the trauma cycle is a challenge. Infection will always be a potential complication of traumatic injuries, resuscitation, and invasive procedures. No matter the causative factor, infection can increase morbidity, prolong hospitalization, increase the cost of care, and jeopardize the final outcome. Therefore every effort must be undertaken to prevent and minimize the infection risks.

Despite all the advances in the care of trauma patients, early lessons on the importance of handwashing,[234] meticulous aseptic technique, and careful attention to and awareness of infection threats continue to be the most effective measures to prevent cross-contamination and infection in this population. Valuable lessons of nosocomial infection control learned from trauma patients can be applied to all patient populations, especially those whose survival is dependent on mechanical and invasive support devices.

REFERENCES

1. Allgower M, Durig M, Wolff G: Infection and trauma, *Surg Clin North Am* 60:133-144, 1980.
2. Stillwell M, Caplan ES: The septic multiple-trauma patient, *Infect Dis Clin North Am* 3:155-183, 1989.
3. Caplan ES, Joshi M, Hoyt NJ et al: *Changing patterns of infection and infection-related mortality in 10,308 multiply traumatized patients over a seven-year period.* Presented before the American Association for the Surgery of Trauma, Honolulu, Hawaii, September 17, 1986.
4. Youmans GP, Paterson PY, Sonmers HM: *The biological and clinical basis of infectious diseases,* Philadelphia, 1985, WB Saunders, 9-18.
5. Fry DE: Infection in the trauma patient: the major deterrent to good recovery, *Heart Lung* 7:257-261, 1978.
6. McRitchie DI, Girotti MJ, Rotstein OD et al: Impaired antibody production in blunt trauma: possible role for T cell dysfunction, *Arch Surg* 125:91, 1990.
7. Dobke M, Sztaba-Kania M: The occurrence of immune complexes in patients with thermal injuries. In Ninnemann JL, editor: *Traumatic injury, infection, and other immunologic sequelae,* Baltimore, 1983, University Park, 153-161.

8. Abraham E: Immunologic mechanisms underlying sepsis in the critically ill surgical patient, *Surg Clin North Am* 65(4): 991-1003, 1985.
9. Border JR: Hypothesis: sepsis, multiple system organ failure, and the macrophage, *Arch Surg* 123(3):285-286, 1988.
10. Craddock CG: Corticosteroid-induced lymphopenia, immunosuppression, and body defense, *Ann Intern Med* 88: 564-566, 1978.
11. Eickhoff TC: Infections in immunosuppressed patients, *Drug Ther,* 2(11):19-23, 27-30, 1972.
12. Caplan ES, Hoyt NJ: Infection surveillance and control in the severely traumatized patient, *Am J Med* 70:638-640, 1981.
13. Caplan ES, Hoyt NJ: Identification and treatment of infection in multiply traumatized patients, *Am J Med* 79(A):68-76, 1985.
14. Tramont EC, Hoover DL: General or nonspecific host defense mechanisms. In Mandell GL, Bennet JE, Dolin R, editors: *Principles and practice of infectious diseases,* ed 5, Philadelphia, 2000, Churchill Livingstone, 31-38.
15. Reynolds HY: Pulmonary host defenses, *Chest* 95(suppl): 223S-230S, 1989.
16. Lober B, Swenson RM: Bacteriology of aspiration pneumonia: a prospective study of community and hospital-acquired cases, *Ann Intern Med* 81:329-331, 1974.
17. Sahn SA: Continuous lateral rotational therapy and nosocomial pneumonia, *Chest* 99(5):1263-1267, 1991.
18. Joshi M, Ciesla N, Caplan E: Diagnosis of pneumonia in critically ill patients, *Chest* 94:4S, 1988.
19. Donowitz LG, Page C, Mileur BL et al: Alteration of normal gastric flora in critical care patients receiving antacid and cimetidine therapy, *Infect Control* 7:23-26, 1986.
20. Kaye D: Host defense mechanisms in the urinary tract, *Urol Clin North Am* 2:407-422, 1975.
21. Faist E, Ertel W, Baker C et al: Terminal B-cell maturation and immunoglobulin: Ig synthesis in vitro in patients with major injury, *J Trauma* 29:2-9, 1989.
22. Sullivan JL, Ochs HD, Schiffman G et al: Immune response after splenectomy, *Lancet* 1:178-181, 1978.
23. Constantopoulos A, Najjar A, Wish JB: Defective phagocytosis due to tuftsin deficiency in splenectomized patients, *Am J Dis Child* 125:663-665, 1973.
24. Krivit W, Giebink GD, Leonard A: Overwhelming postsplenectomy infection, *Surg Clin N Am* 59(2):223-233, 1979.
25. Scher KS, Scott-Conner C, Jones CW et al: Methods of splenic preservation and their effect on clearance of pneumococcal bacteremia, *Ann Surg* 202:595-599, 1985.
26. Waldron DJ, Harding B, Duignan J: Overwhelming infection occurring in the immediate post-splenectomy period, *Br J Clin Practice* 43(11):421-422, 1989.
27. Cullingford GL, Watkins DN, Watts AD et al: Severe late postsplenectomy infection, *Br J Surg* 78(6):716-721, 1991.
28. Caplan ES, Boltansky H, Synder MJ et al: Response of traumatized splenectomized patients to immediate vaccination with polyvalent pneumococcal vaccine, *J Trauma* 23:801-805, 1983.
29. Centers for Disease Control and Prevention: Recommendation of the Immunization Practices Advisory Committee (ACIP): pneumococcal polysaccharide vaccine, *MMWR* 64(8):73-76, 1989.
30. Youmans GB: *The biological and clinical basis of infectious diseases,* Philadelphia, 1985, WB Saunders, 97-112.

31. Mims C: *The pathogenesis of infectious disease,* Orlando, Fla, 1987, Academic, 55-62.

32. Davis JP, Chesney PJ, Wand PJ et al: Toxic-shock syndrome: epidemiologic features, recurrence, risk factors, and prevention, *N Engl J Med* 303:1429-1439, 1980.

33. Stevens DL. Tanner MH, Winship J et al: Severe group A streptococcal infection associated with a toxic shock-like syndrome and scarlet fever toxin, *N Engl J Med* 321:1-7, 1989.

34. Schumer W: Septic shock, *JAMA* 242:1906-1907, 1979.

35. Cowley RA: The resuscitation and stabilization of major multiple trauma patients in a trauma center environment, *Clin Med* 83(1):14-22, 1976.

36. Baue AE, Durham R, Faist E: Systemic inflammatory syndrome (SIRS), multiple organ dysfunction syndrome (MODS), multiple organ failure: are we winning the battle? *Shock* 10(2):79-89, 1998.

37. Nakagawa M, Terashima T, D'yachkova Y et al: Glucocorticoid-induced granulocytosis: contribution of marrow release and demargination of intravascular granulocytes, *Circulation* 21:2307-2313, 1998.

38. Heck E, Edgar M, Hunt J et al: A comparison of leukocyte function and burn mortality, *J Trauma* 20:75-77, 1980.

39. Polk H, Wellhausen S, Regan M et al: A systematic study of host defense processes in badly injured patients, *Ann Surg* 204:282-299, 1986.

40. Kane R, Munster A, Birmingham W et al: Suppressor cell activity after major injury: indirect and direct functional assays, *J Trauma* 22:770-773, 1982.

41. Meakins J, Pietsch J, Rubenick O et al: Delayed hypersensitivity: indicator of acquired failure of host defenses in sepsis and trauma, *Ann Surg* 186:241-250, 1977.

42. Scovill W, Saba T, Kaplan J et al: Disturbances in circulating opsonic activity in man after operative and blunt trauma, *J Surg Res* 22:709-716, 1977.

43. Alexander J, Stinnett J, Ogle C et al: A comparison of immunologic profiles and their influence on bacteremia in surgical patients with high risk of infection, *Surgery* 86:94-104, 1979.

44. Dinarello CA, Wolff SM: Pathogenesis of fever in man, *N Engl J Med* 298:607-611, 1978.

45. Dinarello CA: Endogenous pyrogens. In Lipton JM, editor: *Fever,* New York, 1979, Raven, 1-10.

46. Bodel P: Studies on the mechanism of endogenous pyrogen production: II. Role of cell products in the regulation of pyrogen release from blood leukocytes, *Infect Immun* 10:451-457, 1974.

47. Altmeier WA, Culbertson WR: Surgical infections. In Moyer C, Rhoads JE, Allen JG et al, editors: *Surgery: principles and practice,* ed 3, Philadelphia, 1965, JB Lippincott.

48. Mackowiak PA: The normal microbial flora, *N Engl J Med* 307:83-93, 1982.

49. Petras GY, Bognar SZ: Origin and spread of *Pseudomonas aeruginosa, Proteus,* and *Klebsiella* during twenty years in an infectious disease hospital, *Acta Microbiol Acad Sci Hung* 28:367-380, 1981.

50. Teres D, Schweers P, Bushnell LS et al: Sources of *Pseudomonas aeruginosa* infections in a respiratory-surgical intensive therapy unit, *Lancet* 1:415-417, 1973.

51. Kirchhoff LV, Sheagren JN: Epidemiology and clinical significance of blood cultures positive for coagulase-negative staphylococcus, *Infect Control* 6:479-486, 1985.

52. Walsh TJ, Bustamente C, Vlahov D et al: Candidal suppurative peripheral thrombophlebitis: recognition, prevention, and management, *Infect Control* 7:16-22, 1986.

53. Garner JS, Favero MS: CDC guideline for handwashing and hospital environmental control, *Infect Control* 7:231-235, 1986.

54. Larson E: APIC Guidelines Committee: APIC guideline for handwashing and hand antisepsis in health care settings, *Am J Infect Control* 23(4):251-269, 1995.

55. Caplan ES, Hoyt NJ: Infection control for adult and neonatal intensive care patients. In Gurevich I, Tafuro P, Cunha B et al, editors: *Practical aspects of infection control,* New York, 1984, Praeger, 130-155.

56. Britt MR, Schleupner CJ, Matsumiya S: Severity of underlying disease as a predictor of nosocomial infection: utility in the control of nosocomial infection, *JAMA* 239:1047-1051, 1978.

57. Goris RJA, Draaisma J: Causes of death after blunt trauma, *J Trauma* 22(2):141-146, 1982.

58. Moellering RC Jr: Principles of anti-infective therapy. In Mandell GL, Bennett JE, Dolin R, editors: *Principles and practice of infectious diseases,* ed 5, Philadelphia, 2000, Churchill Livingstone, 223-235.

59. Fuenfer MM, Olson GE, Polk HC: Effect of various corticosteroids upon the phagocytic bactericidal activity of neutrophils, *Surgery* 78:27-33, 1975.

60. Driks MR, Craven DE, Celli BR et al: Nosocomial pneumonia in intubated patients given sucralfate as compared with antacids or histamine type-2 blockers. The role of gastric colonization, *N Engl J Med* 317:1376-1382, 1987.

61. Maki DG: Risk factors for nosocomial infection in intensive care: "devices vs. nature" and goals for the next decade, *Arch Intern Med* 149:30-33, 1989.

62. Rutala, WA: APIC Guidelines for selection and use of disinfectants. In Abrutyn E, Goldmann DA, Scheckler WE: *Saunders' infection control reference service,* Philadelphia, 1998, WB Saunders, 1242-1261.

63. Boyd R, Burke J, Cloton T: A double blind clinical trial of prophylactic antibiotics in hip fractures, *J Bone Joint Surg* 58A:1251-1254, 1973.

64. Edlich RF, Smith QT, Edgerton MT: Resistance of the surgical wound to antimicrobial prophylaxis and its mechanism of development, *Am J Surg* 126:583-591, 1973.

65. Haines SJ: Systemic antibiotic prophylaxis in neurological surgery, *Neurosurgery* 6:355-356, 1980.

66. Burke JF: The effective period of preventive antibiotic action in experimental incisions and dermal lesions, *Surgery* 50:161-168, 1961.

67. Classen DC, Evans RS, Pestotnik SL et al: The timing of prophylactic administration of antibiotics and the risk of surgical-wound infection, *N Engl J Med* 326:282-286, 1997.

68. Gustilio RB, Mendoza RM, Williams DN: Problems in the management of type III (severe) open fracture: a new classification of type III open fractures, *J Trauma* 24(8):742-746, 1984.

69. Oreskovich MR, Dellinger EP, Lennard ES et al: Duration of preventive antibiotic administration for penetrating trauma, *Arch Surg* 117:200-205, 1982.

70. Dunham CM, Cowley RA, editors: Infection control. In *Shock trauma/critical care manual: initial assessment and management,* Baltimore, 1991, University Park, 401-430.

71. Mayer KH, Opal SM, Medeiros AA: Mechanisms of antibiotic resistance. In Mandell GL, Bennett JE, Dolin R, editors: *Principles and practice of infectious disease,* ed 5 Philadelphia, 2000, Churchill Livingstone, 236-253.

72. Banerjee SN, Emori TG, Culver DH et al: Secular trends in nosocomial primary bloodstream infections in the United States, 1980-1989, *Am J Med* 3B:86S-89S, 1991.

73. Holmberg SD, Solomon SL, Blake PA: Health and economic impacts of antimicrobial resistance, *Rev Infect Dis* 6:1065-1078, 1987.

74. Mayer KH: Review of epidemic aminoglycoside resistance world-wide, *Am J Med* 80(suppl 6B):56-64, 1986.

75. Morse LJ, Williams HL, Grenn FP et al: Septicemia due to *Klebsiella* pneumoniae originating from a hand cream dispenser, *N Engl J Med* 279:472-474, 1967.

76. Salzman MB, Isenberg HD, Shapiro JF et al: A prospective study of the catheter hub as the portal of entry for microorganisms causing catheter-related sepsis in neonates, *J Infect Dis* 167:487-490, 1993.

77. Inglis TJ, Millar MR, Jones G: Trachael tube biofilm as a source of bacterial colonization of the lung, *J Clin Microbiol* 27:2014-2018, 1989.

78. Sanders CC: Cefepime, *Clin Infect Dis* 17:369-379, 1993.

79. Hendershot EF: Fluoro quinolones, *Infect Dis Clin N Am* 9:715-730. 1995.

80. Weinstein RA, Kabins SA: Strategies for prevention and control of multiple drug resistant nosocomial infections, *Am J Med* 70:449-454, 1981.

81. Joint Commission on Accreditation of Hospitals: *The comprehensive accreditation manual of hospitals,* Oakbrook Terrace, Ill, 2000, The Commission.

82. Burke JF: Infection. In Hunt TK, Dunphy JE, editors: *Fundamentals of wound management,* New York, 1979, Appleton-Century-Crofts, 513-527.

83. Culver DH, Horan TC, Gaynes RP et al: Surgical wound infection rates by wound class, operative procedure, and patient risk index, *Am J Med* 91(suppl 3B):152S-157S, 1991.

84. Cruse PJE, Foord R: The epidemiology of wound infections: a ten-year prospective study of 62,939 wounds, *Surg Clin North Am* 60(1):27-40, 1980.

85. Centers for Disease Control and Prevention: *Guidelines for prevention of surgical wound infections,* Atlanta, 1982, U.S. Department of Health and Human Services.

86. Nagachinta T, Stephens M, Reitz B: Risk factors for surgical-wound infection following cardiac surgery, *J Infect Dis* 156:967-973, 1987.

87. Seropian Reynolds BM: Wound infections after preoperative depilatory versus razor preparation, *Am J Surg* 121:251-254, 1971.

88. Nora PF, Vanecko RM, Branfield JJ: Prophylactic abdominal drains, *Arch Surg* 105:173-179, 1982.

89. Howard JM, Barker WF, Culbertson WR et al: Postoperative wound infections: the influence of ultraviolet irradiation of the operating room and various other factors, *Arch Surg* 160(suppl):1-92, 1964.

90. Galle PC, Homesley HD, Phyne AL: Reassessment of the surgical scrub, *Surg Gynecol Obstet* 147:215-218, 1978.

91. Swartz MN: Cellulitis and subcutaneous tissue infections. In Mandell GL, Bennett JE, Dolin R, editors: *Principles and practice of infectious diseases,* ed 5, Philadelphia, 2000, Churchill Livingstone, 1037-1057.

92. Wang K, Shin C: Necrotizing fasciitis of the extremities, *J Trauma* 32:179-182, 1992.

93. Forni AL, Kaplan EL, Schlievert PM, Roberts RB: Clinical and microbiological characteristics of severe group A streptococcus infections and streptococcal toxic shock syndrome, *Clin Infec Dis* 21(2):33-40, 1995.

94. Stone HH, Martin JD: Synergistic necrotizing cellulitis, *Ann Surg* 175:702-711, 1972.

95. Elliott DC, Kufera JA, Myers RAM: Necrotizing soft tissue infections: risk factors for mortality and strategies for management, *Ann Surg* 224:672-683, 1996.

96. Asfar SK: Necrotizing fasciitis, *Br J Surg* 7(8):828-840, 1991.

97. Sudarsky LA, Laschigan JC, Coppa F et al: Improved results from a standardized approach in treating patients with necrotizing fasciitis, *Ann Surg* 206:661-665, 1987.

98. Caplan ES, Kluge RM: Gas gangrene: review of 34 cases, *Arch Intern Med* 136:788-791, 1976.

99. Park MK, Muhvick KH, Myers RA et al: Effects of hyperbaric oxygen in infectious diseases: basic mechanisms. In Kindall EP, editor: *Hyperbaric medicine practice,* Flagstaff, Ariz, 1994, Best, 169-204.

100. Bardenheier B, Prevots DR, Khetsuriani et al: Tetanus surveillance—United States, 1995-1997, *MMWR* 3:47(2):1-13, 1998.

101. Sasaki TM, Welch UW, Herndon DN et al: Burn wound manipulation induced bacteremia, *J Trauma* 19:46-48, 1979.

102. Bang, RL, Gang RK, Sanyul SC et al: Burn septicemia: an analysis of 78 patients, *Burns* 24(4):354-361, 1998.

103. Wisplinghoff H, Perbix W, Seifert H: Risk factors for nosocomial bloodstream infections due to *Acinetobacter baumannii:* a case-control study of adult burn patients, *Clin Infect Dis* 28(1):59-66, 1999.

104. Pruitt BA Jr, McManus AT, Kim SH et al: Burn wound infections: current status, *World J Surg* 22(2):135-145, 1998.

105. Hansbrough JF: Burn wound sepsis, *J Intensive Care Med* 2:313-327, 1987.

106. McCauley RL, Robson MC, Heggers JP: Alternating therapy in major burns silver sulfadiazine vs. silver sulfadiazine-nitrofurazone, *J Burn Care Rehab* 5:384-387, 1984.

107. Modak SM, Fox CL: Synergistic action of silver sulfadiazine and sodium piperacillin on resistant *Pseudomonas aeruymosa* in vitro and in experimental burn wound infection, *J Trauma* 25:27-31, 1985.

108. Demling RH: Improved survival after massive burns, *J Trauma* 23:179-184, 1983.

109. Alexander JW, MacMillan BG, Stinnett JD et al: Beneficial effects of aggressive protein feeding in severely burned children, *Ann Surg* 192:505-517, 1980.

110. Ramzy PI, Barret JP, Herndon DN: Thermal injury, *Crit Care Clin* 15(2):333-352, 1999.

111. U.S. Department of Health, Education and Welfare: *Isolation techniques for use in hospitals,* HEW Pub No (CDC) 78-8314, Atlanta, 1985, Centers for Disease Control and Prevention, U.S. Public Health Service.

112. O'Meara PM: Management of open fractures, *Orthop Rev* 21(10):1177-1185, 1992.

113. DeLong WJ Jr, Born CT, Wei SY et al: Aggressive treatment of 119 open fracture wounds, *J Trauma* 46(6):1049-1054, 1999.

114. Chapman MW, Mahoney M: The role of early internal fixation in management of open fractures, *Clin Orthop* 138:120-131, 1979.

115. Chapman MW, Hansen ST: Current concepts in the management of open fracture. In Rockwood CA, Green DP, editors: *Fractures in adults,* ed 4, vol 1, Philadelphia, 1996, JB Lippincott, 169-207.

116. Turek SL, editor: *Orthopaedics—principles and their application,* Philadelphia, 1977, JB Lippincott, 48-82.

117. Harkess JW, Ramsey WC, Admadi B: Definitive treatment of fractures and dislocations. In Rockwood CA, Green DP, editors: *Fractures in adults,* ed 4, vol 1, Philadelphia, 1996, JB Lippincott, 1-139.

118. Trafton PG: Infected fractures. In *Complications of fracture management,* New York, 1982, JB Lippincott, 51-78.

119. Winniger DA, Fass RJ: Antibiotic-impregnated cement and beads for orthopedic infections, *Antimicrob Agents Chemother* 1996 40(12):2675-2679, 1996.

120. Anderson LD, Hutchins WC: Fractures of the tibia and fibula treated by casts and fixation devices, *Clin Orthop* 105:179-192, 1974.

121. Waldvogel FA, Vasey H: Osteomyelitis: the past decade, *N Engl J Med* 303:360-370, 1980.

122. Lew DP, Waldvogel FA: Osteomyelitis, *N Engl J Med* 336(14):999-1007, 1997.

123. Haas DW, McAndrew MP: Bacterial osteomyelitis in adults: evolving considerations in diagnosis and treatment, *Am J Med* 101:550-561, 1996.

124. Bone RC, Balk RA, Cerra FB et al: Definitions for sepsis and organ failure and guidelines for the use of innovative therapies in sepsis. ACCP/SCCM consensus conference committee, *Chest* 101:1644-1655, 1992.

125. Zimmerman JE, Knaus WA, Wagner DP: A comparison of risks and outcomes for patients with organ system failure: 1982-1990, *Crit Care Med* 24:1633-1641, 1996.

126. Goris RJ, te Boekhorst TP, Nuytinck JK et al: Multiple-organ failure: generalized autodestructive inflammation? *Arch Surg* 120:1109-1115, 1985.

127. Rangel-Frausto MS, Pittet D, Costigan M et al: The natural history of the systemic inflammatory response syndrome (SIRS): a prospective study, *JAMA* 273:117-123, 1995.

128. Kreger BE, Craven DE, McCabe WR: Gram-negative bacteremia: IV. Reevaluation of clinical features and treatment in 621 patients, *Am J Med* 68:344-355, 1980.

129. Martin MA: Epidemiology and clinical impact of gram-negative sepsis, *Infect Dis Clin North Am* 5:739-752, 1991.

130. Berkowitz FE, Argent AC, Baise T: Suppurative thrombophlebitis: a serious nosocomial infection, *Pediatr Infect Dis J* 6:64-67, 1987.

131. Kopman EA, Sandza JG: Pulmonary-artery catheter after placement: maintenance of sterility, *Anesthesiology* 48:373-374, 1978.

132. Zinner MJ, Zuidema GD, Lowery RD: Septic nonsuppurative thrombophlebitis, *Arch Surg* 111:122-125, 1976.

133. Band JD, Maki DG: Infections caused by arterial catheters used for hemodynamic monitoring, *Am J Med* 67:735-741, 1979.

134. Soderstrom CA, Wasserman DH, Dunham MC et al: Superiority of the femoral artery for monitoring: a prospective study, *Am J Surg* 144:309-313, 1982.

135. Josephson A, Gombert ME, Sierra MF et al: The relationship between intravenous fluid contamination and the frequency of tubing replacement, *Infect Control* 6:367-370, 1985.

136. Maki DG: Growth properties of microorganisms in lipid for infusion and implications for infection control (abstract), *Am J Infect Control* 8(3):89, 1980.

137. Maki DG, Martin WT: Nationwide epidemic of septicemia caused by contaminated infusion products: IV. Growth of microbial pathogens, *J Infect Dis* 131:276, 1975.

138. Scheld WM, Sande MA: Endocarditis and intravascular infections. In Mandell GL, Dolin R, Bennett JE, editors: *Principles and practice of infectious diseases,* New York, 1995, Wiley Medical, 740-783.

139. Terpenning MS, Buggy BP, Kaufmann CA: Hospital-acquired infective endocarditis, *Arch Intern Med* 148:1601-1603, 1988.

140. Arnow PM, Quimosing EM, Brech M: Consequences of intravascular catheter sepsis, *Clin Infec Dis* 16:778-784, 1993.

141. Haley RW, Schaberg DR, Von Allmen SD et al: Estimating the extra charges and prolongation of hospitalization due to nosocomial infections. A comparison of methods, *J Infec Dis* 141:248-257, 1980.

142. Rello J, Coll P, Net A et al: Infection of pulmonary artery catheters. Epidemiologic characteristics and multivariate analysis of risk factors, *Chest* 103:132-136, 1993.

143. Martin MA, Pfaller MA, Wenzel RP: Coagulase-negative staphylococcal bacteremia, *Ann Intern Med* 110:9-16, 1989.

144. Burn-Buisson C, Abrouk F, Legrand P et al: Diagnosis of central venous catheter related sepsis. Critical level of quantitative tip cultures, *Arch Intern Med* 147:873-877, 1987.

145. Abrutyn E, Goldmann DA, Scheckler WE: *Saunders' infection control reference service,* Philadelphia, 1998, WB Saunders, 924-934.

146. Kaufman BA, Tunkel AR, Pryor JC et al: Meningitis in the neurosurgical patient, *Infect Dis Clin North Am* 4:677-701, 1990.

147. Buckwold FJ, Hand R, Hansebout RR: Hospital-acquired bacterial meningitis in neurosurgical patients, *J Neurosurg* 45:494-500, 1977.

148. Stillwell M, Hogue C, Hoyt NJ et al: Post-traumatic meningococcal meningitis, *J Trauma* 31:1693-1695, 1991.

149. Marion DW: Complications of head injury and their therapy, *Neurosurg Clin N Am* 2(2):411-424, 1991.

150. Mayhall CG, Archer NH, Lamb VA et al: Ventriculostomy-related infections. A prospective epidemiologic study, *N Engl J Med* 310(9):553-559, 1984.

151. Hickman KM, Mayer BL, Muwaswes M: Intracranial pressure monitoring: review of risk factors associated with infection, *Heart Lung* 19(1):84-90, 1990.

152. Winn HR, Dacey RG, Jane JA: Intracranial subarachnoid pressure recording: experience with 650 patients, *Surg Neurol* 8:41-47, 1977.

153. Bekar A, Goren S., Korfali E et al: Complications of brain tissue pressure monitoring with a fiberoptic device, *Neurosurg Rev* 21(4):254-259, 1998.

154. Walters BC, Hoffman HJ, Hendrick EB et al: Cerebrospinal fluid shunt infection: Influences on initial management and subsequent outcome, *J Neurosurg* 60:1014-1021, 1984.

155. Holt RJ: The colonization of ventriculo-atrial shunts by coagulase-negative staphylococci. In Finland M, Marget W, Bartman K, editors: *Bacterial infections: changes in their causative agents, trends, and possible bases*, New York, 1971, Springer-Verlag, 81- 87.

156. Trunkel AR, Scheld WM: Acute meningitis. In Mandell GL, Bennett JE, Dolin R, editors: *Principles and practice of infectious diseases*, ed 5, Philadelphia, 2000, Churchill Livingstone, 959-997.

157. Neiderman MS, Craven DE, Fein AF et al: Pneumonia in the critically ill hospitalized patient, *Chest* 97:170-181, 1990.

158. Piek J: Medical complications in severe head injury, *New Horiz* 3(3):534-538, 1995.

159. Emori TG, Gaynes RP: An overview of nosocomial infections, including the role of the microbiology laboratory, *Clin Microbiol Rev* 6(4):428-442, 1993.

160. Hospital-acquired pneumonia in adults: diagnosis, assessment of severity, initial antimicrobial therapy, and preventive strategies: a consensus statement, *Am J Respir Crit Care Med* 153:1711-1725, 1995.

161. Dal Nogare AR: Nosocomial pneumonia in the medical and surgical patient, *Med Clin North Am* 78:1081-1090, 1994.

162. Cook DJ, Walter SD, Cook RJ et al: Incidence of and risk factors for ventilator-associated pneumonia in critically ill patients, *Ann Intern Med* 129(6):433-440, 1998.

163. Gross PA, Neu HC, Aswapokee P et al: Deaths from nosocomial infections: experience in a university hospital and a community hospital, *Am J Med* 68:219-223, 1980.

164. Bryan CS, Reynolds KL: Bacteremic nosocomial pneumonia: analysis of 172 episodes from a single metropolitan area, *Am Rev Respir Dis* 129:668-671, 1984.

165. Caplan ES, Hoyt NJ: Nosocomial sinusitis, *JAMA* 247(5):639, 1982.

166. Carter BL, Ankoff MS, Fisk JD: Computed tomographic detection of sinusitis responsible for intracranial and extracranial infections, *Radiology* 147:739-742, 1983.

167. Horan T, Culver D, Jarvis W: Pathogens causing nosocomial infections, *Antimicrob Newslet* 5:65-67, 1988.

168. Rello J, Ausina V, Castella J et al: Nosocomial respiratory tract infections in multiple trauma patients. Influence of level of consciousness with implications for therapy, *Chest* 102(2):525-529, 1992.

169. Barlett JG, O'Keefe P, Tally FP et al: Bacteriology of hospital-acquired pneumonia, *Arch Intern Med* 146:868 871, 1986.

170. Schleupner CJ, Cobb DK: A study of the etiologies and treatment of nosocomial pneumonia in a community-based teaching hospital, *Infect Control Hosp Epidemiol* 13:515-528, 1992.

171. Ewig S, Torres A, El-Ebiary M et al: Bacterial colonization patterns in mechanically ventilated patients with traumatic and medical head injury. Incidence, risk factors, and association with ventilator-associated pneumonia, *Am J Respir Crit Care Med* 159:188-198, 1999.

172. Montgomerie JZ: Infections in patients with spinal cord injuries, *Clin Infect Dis* 25(6):1285-1290, 1997.

173. Campbell W, Hendrix E, Schwalbe R et al: Head-injured patients who are nasal carriers of *Straphylococcus aureus* are at high risk for *Staphylococcus aureus* pneumonia, *Crit Care Med* 27(4):798-801, 1999.

174. Berrouane Y, Daudenthun I, Riegel B et al: Early onset pneumonia in neurosurgical intensive care unit patients, *J Hosp Infect* 40(4):275-280, 1998.

175. Weese WC, Shindler ER, Smith IM et al: Empyema of the thorax then and now—a study of 122 cases over 4 decades, *Arch Intern Med* 131:516-520, 1973.

176. Caplan ES, Hoyt NJ, Rodriguez A et al: Empyema in the multiply traumatized patient, *J Trauma* 24:785-789, 1984.

177. Cullen DJ, Calders DL: The incidence of ventilator-induced pulmonary barotrauma in critically ill patients, *Anesthesiology* 50:185-190, 1979.

178. Arnold S, Feathers RS, Gibbs E: Bilateral pneumothoraces and subcutaneous emphysema: a complication of internal jugular puncture, *Br Med J* 1:211-212, 1973.

179. Coon JL, Shuck JM: Failure of tube thoracostomy for post-traumatic empyema: an indication for early decortication, *J Trauma* 15(7):588-594, 1975.

180. Centers for Disease Control and Prevention: Guidelines for prevention of nosocomial pneumonia, *MMWR* 3(46 RR-1): 1-79, 1997.

181. Bergogne-Berezin E: Treatment and prevention of nosocomial pneumonia, *Chest* 108(suppl 2):26S-34S, 1995.

182. DuPriest RW, Khaneja SC, Cowley RA: Acute cholecystitis complicating trauma, *Ann Surg* 189:84-89, 1979.

183. Cleary RK: *Clostridium difficile*-associated diarrhea and colitis: clinical manifestations, diagnosis, and treatment, *Dis Colon Rectum* 41(11):1435-49, 1998.

184. FeKety R, Shah AB: Diagnosis & treatment of *C. difficile* colitis, *JAMA* 269:71-75, 1993.

185. Worsley MA: Infection control and prevention of *Clostridium difficile* infection, *J Antimicrob Chemother* 41(suppl C):59-66, 1998.

186. Cunha BA: Nosocomial diarrhea, *Crit Care Clin* 14(2):329-38, 1998.

187. White WT III, Acuff TE, Sykes TR et al: Bacterial contamination of enteral nutrient solution: a preliminary report, *J Parenter Enteral Nutr* 3:459, 1979.

188. Levy J: Enteral nutrition: an increasingly recognized cause of nosocomial bloodstream infection, *Infect Control Hosp Epidemiol* 10:395-397, 1989.

189. Anderton A, Aidov KE: The effect of handling procedures on microbial contamination of enteral feeds, *J Hosp Infect* 11:364-372, 1988.

190. Turck M, Stamm WE: Nosocomial infection of the urinary tract, *Am J Med* 70:651, 1981.

191. Wallace WC, Cinat M, Gornick WB et al: Nosocomial infections in the surgical intensive care unit: a difference between trauma and surgical patients, *Am Surg* 65(10):987-990, 1999.

192. Kass EH, Schneiderman JL: Entry of bacteria into the urinary tracts of patients with inlying catheters, *N Engl J Med* 264:556, 1957.

193. Classen DC, Larsen RA, Burke JP et al: Prevention of catheter-associated bacteriuria: Clinical trial of methods to block three known pathways, *Am J Infect Control* 19:136-142, 1991.

194. Garibaldi RA, Burke JP, Britt MR et al: Meatal colonization and catheter-associated bacteriuria, *N Engl J Med* 303: 315-318, 1980.

195. Warren JW: Catheter-associated urinary tract infections, *Infect Dis Clin N Am* 11(3):609-622, 1997.

196. National Institute on Disability and Rehabilitation Research: The prevention and management of urinary tract infections among people with spinal cord injuries. National Institute on Disability and Rehabilitation Research consensus statement, January 27-29, 1992, *Sci Nurs* 10(2):49-61, 1993.

197. Centers for Disease Control and Prevention: *Guideline for the prevention of catheter-associated urinary tract infections,* Atlanta, 1982, U.S. Department of Health and Human Services.

198. Rutula WA, Kennedy VA, Loflin HB et al: *Serratia marcescens* nosocomial infections of the urinary tract associated with urine measuring containers and urinometers, *Am J Med* 70:699, 1981.

199. Hoyt NJ: Infection control and emergency medical services: Facts and myths, *Md Med J* 37:551-557, 1988.

200. Centers for Disease Control and Prevention: Recommendations for prevention of HIV transmission in health care settings, *MMWR* 36(suppl):1S-16S, 1987.

201. Occupational exposure to bloodborne pathogens, *Fed Reg* 58(235):64174-64182, 1991.

202. Henein MN, Hoyd L: HIV, hepatitis B and hepatitis C in the code one trauma population, *Am Surg* 63(7):657-659, 1997.

203. Sloan EP, McGill BA, Zalenski R et al: Human immunodeficiency virus and hepatitis B virus seroprevalence in an urban trauma population, *J Trauma* 38(5):736-741, 1995.

204. Soderstrom CA, Furth PA, Glasser D et al: HIV infection rates in a center treating predominantly rural blunt trauma victims, *J Trauma* 29:1526-1530, 1989.

205. Tardiff K, Marzuk PM, Leon AC et al: Human immunodeficiency virus among trauma patients in New York City, *Ann Emerg Med* 32(20):151-154, 1998.

206. McEvoy M, Porter K, Mortimer P et al: Prospective study of clinical, laboratory and ancillary staff with accidental exposures to blood or other body fluids from patients infected with HIV, *Br Med J* 294:1595-7, 1987.

207. Mason JO, Murphy FA, Hughes JM et al: Recommendations for prevention of HIV transmission in health care settings. In Abrutyn E, Goldmann DA, Scheckler WE, editors: *Saunders' infection control reference service,* Philadelphia, 1998, WB Saunders, 877-884.

208. Council on Scientific Affairs: Status report on the acquired immune deficiency syndrome: human T-cell lymphotrophic virus type III testing, *JAMA* 254:1342-1345, 1985.

209. Miles SA, Balden E, Magpantry L et al: Rapid serologic testing with immune-complex associated HIV p24 antigen for early detection of HIV infection in neonates, *N Engl J Med* 328:297-302, 1993.

210. Strathdee SA, O'Shaughnessy MV, Montaner JS et al: A decade of research on the natural history of HIV infection: Part I. Markers, *Clin Invest Med* 19(2):112-120, 1996.

211. Lane TW, Ivey FD, Falk PS et al: False-negative human immunodeficiency virus (HIV) testing in an organ donor (abstract), *Am J Infect Control* 15(2):87, 1987.

212. Centers for Disease Control and Prevention: Recommendations for postexposure prophylaxis after occupational exposure to HIV, *MMWR* 45(22):471, 1996.

213. Kelen GD, Shahan JB, Quinn TC: Emergency department-based HIV screening and counseling: experience with rapid and standard serologic testing, *Ann Emerg Med* 33(2): 147-155, 1999.

214. Dienstag JL, Ryan DM: Occupational exposure to hepatitis B virus in hospital personnel: infection or immunization? *Am J Epidemiol* 115:26-39, 1982.

215. Sepkowitz KA: Nosocomial hepatitis and other infection transmitted by blood and blood products. In Mandell GL, Bennett JE, Dolin R, editors: *Principles and practice of infectious diseases,* ed 5, Philadelphia, 2000, Churchill Livingstone, 3039-3052.

216. Mahoney FJ, Stewart K, Hu H et al: Progress toward the elimination of hepatitis B virus transmission among health care workers in the United States, *Arch Intern Med* 157: 2601-2605, 1997.

217. Christian MA: Influenza and hepatitis B vaccine acceptance: a survey of health care workers, *Am J Infect Control* 19:177-184, 1991.

218. Advisory Committee for Immunization Practices: Hepatitis B virus: a comprehensive strategy for eliminating transmission in the United States through universal childhood vaccination, *MMWR* 40(RR-13):1-25, 1991.

219. US Department of Labor, Occupational Safety and Health Administration: Occupational exposure to bloodborne pathogens. In Abrutyn E, Goldmann DA, Scheckler WE, editors: *Saunders' infection control reference service,* Philadelphia, 1998, WB Saunders, 1109-1113.

220. Kaczmarek RG, Moore RM, McCrohan J et al: Glove use by health care workers: results of a tristate investigation, *Am J Infect Control* 19:228-32, 1991.

221. US Department of Health and Human Services/Public Health: Update: universal precautions for prevention of transmission of human immunodeficiency virus, hepatitis B virus, and other bloodborne pathogens in health-care settings. In Abrutyn E, Goldmann DA, Scheckler NE, editors: *Saunders' infection control reference service,* Philadelphia, 1998, WB Saunders, 1072-1074.

222. Department of Labor, Occupational Safety and Health Administration: Occupational exposure to bloodborne pathogens: final rule. *Fed Reg* 56(235):64175-64182, 1991.

223. Graham M: Frequency and duration of handwashing in an intensive care unit, *Am J Infect Control* 18(2):77-81, 1990.

224. Ahrens T: Outlier management: influencing the highest resource-consuming areas in acute and critical care, *Crit Care Nurs Clin N Am* 11(1):107-116, 1999.

225. Larson E: Guidelines for infection control practice: APIC guidelines for handwashing and hand antisepsis in health-care settings. In Abrutyn E, Goldmann DA, Scheckler NE, editors: *Saunders' infection control reference service,* Philadelphia, 1998, WB Saunders, 1230-1242.

226. Rutala WA: APIC guidelines for selection and use of disinfectants. In Abrutyn E, Goldmann DA, Scheckler NE, editors: *Saunders' infection control reference service,* Philadelphia, 1998, WB Saunders, 1242-1260.

227. Spire B, Barre-Sinoussi F, Montagnier L et al: Inactivation of lymphadenopathy-associated virus by chemical disinfectants, *Lancet* 1:899-901, 1984.

228. Bond WW, Peterson JJ, Favero MS: *Viral hepatitis B.* Aspects of environmental control series, Washington, DC, 1977, U.S. Department of Health, Education and Welfare, 2-19.

229. Wreghitt TG: Blood-borne virus infections in dialysis units—a review, *Rev Med Virol* 9(2):101-109, 1999.

230. U.S. Department of Labor, Occupational Safety and Health Administration: *Enforcement procedures for the occupational exposure to bloodborne pathogens,* OSHA Directives CPL 2-2.44D, Washington, DC, 1999, OSHA.

231. Cozanitis DA, Makela P, Grant J: Microorganisms in the hair of staff and patients in an intensive care unit, *Anaesthetist* 26:578-580, 1977.

232. U.S. Department of Health, Education and Welfare: *Minimum requirements of construction and equipment for hospital and medical facilities,* DHHS Pub No 81-14500, Washington, DC, 1981, U.S. Government Printing Office.

233. Ayliffe GS, Babb JR, Collins BJ, et al: *Pseudomonas aeruginosa* in hospital sinks, *Lancet* 1:578, 1974.

234. Lister J: An address on the effect of the antiseptic treatment upon the general salubrity of surgical hospitals, *Br Med J* 2:769, 1875.

WOUND HEALING

Mary Beth Flynn

15

The definition of trauma implies injury to tissues, including the possible involvement of supporting structures. The extent of wounding varies from minor abrasions, contusions, lacerations, and surgical wounds sustained during treatment to extensive avulsion in which tissue separates from underlying structures as a consequence of injury. After traumatic injury, tissue integrity is reestablished through integrated physiologic processes and careful therapeutic management. Traumatic wounds differ from wounds that occur as a consequence of surgery, and this has implications for both the healing process and treatment. In contrast to the controlled nature of surgical wounds, traumatic wounds are often multiple in nature, induce extensive stress with catecholamine release, are often concomitant with shock and hypoxemia, and lead to depletion of physiologic reserves as the body responds to the insult and attempts to normalize. These differences and the likelihood of bacterial contamination at the time of injury present the potential for impairment of wound healing. Therefore care is directed toward the avoidance of complications such as wound infection and delayed healing, in addition to maximizing postinjury function of the affected body part.

All wounds, regardless of their origin, heal through the interaction of a complex set of physiologic and biochemical responses. This chapter provides a basis for understanding treatment modalities by addressing the physical properties of the skin, the physiology of wound healing, and factors that affect healing. Selected aspects of wound assessment and management throughout the trauma cycle also are discussed.

ANATOMY OF SKIN

The skin has a surface area of 1.5 to 2 m^2 and accounts for one sixth of total body weight, making it the largest organ of the body. It is one of the fastest growing tissues of the body, evidenced by complete replacement every 4 to 6 weeks. Normal skin is critical to survival through its provision of thermal regulation, prevention of dehydration, and function as a barrier to external insults such as chemicals and microorganisms. The skin receives about one third of the circulating blood volume and plays an important role in homeostasis regulation.

The integumentary system is composed of the skin and its appendages: hair, nails, and sweat and sebaceous glands. The skin is divided anatomically into two major layers: the epidermis and the dermis. The epidermis is the external, protective layer, and the dermis, composed largely of collagen and elastic fibers, provides strength, elasticity, and protection against mechanical shearing forces. The epidermis is the outermost layer of the skin and is further divided into the *stratum corneum* (cornified layer), *stratum lucidum* (clear layer), *stratum granulosum* (granular layer), *stratum spinosum* (prickle cell layer), and *stratum basale* (basal layer). The stratum corneum makes up the most superficial skin layer and is composed of nonviable keratinized cells, desiccated cells that are shed continually. The stratum corneum is also referred to as the horny layer. The stratum lucidum, located below the stratum corneum, is the transitional layer. Cells in this layer release lipid granules into extracellular spaces before movement to the stratum corneum layer. This lipid-rich coating protects the epidermis against aqueous solutions. Stratum granulosum lies below the stratum lucidum and is known as the granular layer. The next layer is the stratum spinosum, in which cells have spinelike structures that create bridges between them.[1] Stratum basale, also called the stratum germinativum or basal layer, is the mitotically active layer. Keratinocytes divide and begin the process of differentiation in this layer. This single layer of cells runs along the dermis, creating epidermal rete ridges. These cells engage in mitotic division in response to multiple stimuli, such as growth factors, hormones, and vitamins. The columnar basal cells undergo continual mitosis and are the source of new cells that eventually reach the stratum corneum.

The epidermis provides the exit for hair follicles and glands. The thickness of the epidermis varies with body surface location and function, the eyelids having thinner layers and the soles of the feet and palms of the hands having thicker layers. The epidermis is avascular, receiving nutrients from the blood vessels in the dermis and subcutaneous tissues.[2,3]

Migrating cells—melanocytes, Merkel cells, and Langerhans' cells—are distributed uniformly throughout the basal and suprabasal layers of the epidermis.[1] Melanocytes are responsible for producing melanin and giving rise to skin color. Carotene, oxyhemoglobin, and circulating substances in the plasma (e.g., bilirubin) are also present in the epidermis and will influence skin color. Merkel cells make up a small part of the basal layer and are believed to participate in the sensation of touch. Langerhans' cells are macrophages that function primarily in delayed hypersensitivity reactions. They also produce interleukin-1, which aids T-cell activation,[2] and thus serve an important immune function.

The basement membrane zone lies below the basal keratinocytes and is a very thin layer separating the epidermis from the dermis. The basement membrane provides mechanical support for the epidermis and allows for the transport of material between the layers.

The dermis lies between the epidermis and the subcutaneous tissue. The dermis is a connective tissue composed of fibrous proteins (collagen and elastin) in a gel of ground substance (glycosaminoglycans).[1] The junction between epidermis and dermis is undulated with upward-projecting dermal papillae and downward-projecting epidermal rete ridges. The dermis nourishes the epidermis through its rich supply of vascular and lymphatic structures. There is a superficial layer, the papillary dermis, composed of interlacing fine collagen fibers, blood vessels, nerve endings, and thermoreceptors, and a deeper reticular layer of thicker bundles of collagen that provide the skin with structural support (Figure 15-1). Fibroblasts are the major differentiating cell type that becomes active during inflammatory conditions and wounding. Fibroblasts are responsible for the secretion of collagen and elastin. Sensory receptors within the papillary dermis respond to pain, cold, heat, touch, and pressure. Dermal appendages, hair follicles, and sweat glands reside within the reticular dermis and extend upward through the epidermis. These serve as an important source of epidermal regeneration during wound healing.

The subcutaneous tissue lies between the lower border of the dermis and the deeper fascia and muscle tissues. Although not generally considered a true part of the skin, it is closely associated with the dermis and is an important tissue to consider in terms of wound healing. The subcutaneous tissue functions to absorb shock, insulate, store nutrients, and shape the body contour. It is composed of many cells, including adipocytes, histiocytes, plasma cells, lymphocytes, and mast cells. Fat lobules of the subcutaneous tissue are surrounded by strands of collagen that contain nerves. Vascular and lymphatic networks travel from the fascia through the subcutaneous tissue and supply the dermis. There are few vascular connections between fat lobules and neighboring structures, which leaves the subcutaneous tissue vulnerable to decreases in vascular supply.[1-4] Altered vascular supply, or hypoperfusion of the subcutaneous tissue, has implications for wound healing. Complications of impaired healing such as infection often have their origin in subcutaneous tissue.

The integumentary system functions as a barrier and buffer zone against chemical, mechanical, and ultraviolet radiation insults. The skin maintains fluid and electrolytes within the body, provides thermal regulation, and provides

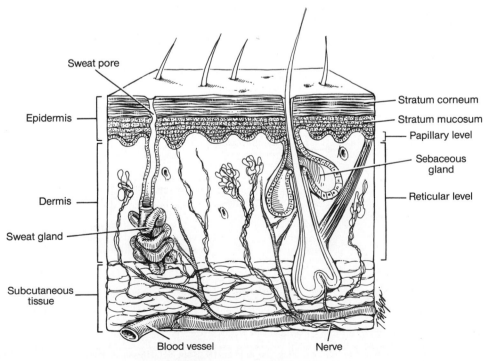

FIGURE 15-1 Anatomy of the skin.

Sweat pore
Epidermis
Dermis
Sweat gland
Subcutaneous tissue
Blood vessel
Nerve
Stratum corneum
Stratum mucosum
Papillary level
Sebaceous gland
Reticular level

an essential means of communication through sensation. Tactile stimulation is vital for normal growth and development and for normal psychophysiologic function.

Traumatic injury may result in damage to any or all layers of the integument. A superficial abrasion involves the epidermal layer of the skin. Partial thickness injuries, the most common wound, involve the epidermal layer and a portion of the dermal layer. Full thickness injuries involve all epidermal and dermal skin layers and may affect subcutaneous tissue, muscle, and bone.

PHYSIOLOGY OF WOUND HEALING

When the skin or internal organs are disrupted by trauma or surgery, a series of interdependent physiologic events occurs and results in tissue repair (Figure 15-2). They occur within the three major phases of healing—inflammation, proliferation, and remodeling. The tissue response has seven major components: (1) hemostasis, (2) inflammation, (3) fibroblast proliferation, (4) matrix deposition, (5) angiogenesis, (6) epithelialization, and (7) contraction.[5] Through these responses, the process of healing is initiated, directed, and finally completed.

Wound healing occurs through primary or secondary intention or, alternately, by delayed primary closure, also called tertiary intention. In primary intention healing there is limited tissue loss, the wound is clean, and the wound edges are easily approximated using suture material or staples. In secondary intention healing a large amount of

tissue has been lost or the wound may be heavily contaminated. The wound is left open, and healing occurs through formation of granulation tissue, contraction, and reepithelialization. In wounds with high bacteria counts, delayed primary closure is often used. The wound is cleaned and temporarily left open until the bacterial load decreases, at which point wound edges are approximated.

Tissue repair requires complex, overlapping, interdependent processes with multiple vascular, cellular, and biochemical responses. The actual time frame for healing varies depending on several factors, such as type of wound closure (e.g., primary or secondary intention) and host status (e.g., perfusion, nutritional status, edema, low oxygen tension, infection, and co-morbid metabolic diseases). Generally, in acute wounds, hemostasis and the inflammatory phase begin the first day after injury. Migration and the proliferation phase begin shortly after inflammation and peak at 7 to 21 days. Remodeling and wound contraction begin about 3 weeks after injury and may continue for 6 months to a year (Figure 15-3). The first days and weeks after injury are critical periods in the healing process because multiple cellular events occur.

HEMOSTASIS AND INFLAMMATION

When a wound extends through the epidermis, blood vessels are disrupted and a clot is formed, beginning the process of normal tissue repair. The initial response to injury activates the arachidonic acid-mediated cytokines of tissue complement that attract polymorphonuclear granulocytes (PMNs)

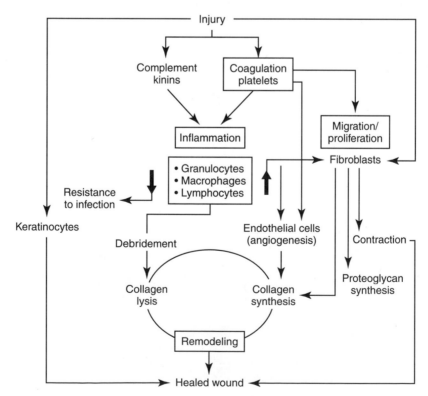

FIGURE 15-2 Schematic representation of wound healing. (From Hunt TK, Hopf HH, Hussain Z: Physiology of wound healing, *Adv Skin Wound Care* 13(2):6-11, 2000.)

to the injured site, serving as a defense against infection.[5,6] Exposed endothelial collagen activates Hageman factor, initiates platelet degranulation, and activates the coagulation cascade. Activated platelets release biochemical mediators, serotonin, and thromboxane A_2, which cause vasoconstriction and minimize blood loss. Platelets also interact with the injured tissue, causing the release of thrombin, which converts circulating fibrinogen to fibrin. Fibrin and platelets form the hemostatic "clot." Thrombin also stimulates the increased vascular permeability seen after injury, facilitating the extravascular migration of inflammatory cells.[7] The fibrin clot, in addition to hemostasis, provides a scaffold for the migration and proliferation of cells.[5-8] As platelets degranulate, their α-granules release cytokines and growth factors, which aid in the wound healing process. The cytokines include platelet-derived growth factor (PDGF), transforming growth factor β_1 and β_2 (TGF-β_1 and TGF-β_2), platelet activating factor (PAF), platelet-derived epidermal growth factor (PDEGF), insulin-like growth factor I (IGF-I), and fibronectin. These cytokines are chemoattractants for inflammatory cells (PMNs and monocytes) and mitogens for noninflammatory cells (fibroblasts and endothelial cells).[5-9]

Activation of the coagulation cascade also activates the plasma proteins of the complement system and the vasodilator peptides of the kinin cascade. Activation of the complement cascade produces biologically active molecules that opsonize and lyse bacteria, cause histamine release from mast cells, and act as chemotactic factors that attract inflammatory cells to the area of injury. Histamine, kinins, prostaglandins, and leukotrienes[7] act to relax vascular smooth muscle, producing vasodilation and increased blood flow to the area of injury. In addition, kinins attract inflammatory cells and increase capillary permeability. Once vasodilation and increased capillary permeability occur, intravascular elements (protein, enzymes, and cells) leak into the wound area and create edema, warmth, pain, and redness.

As the body establishes a clot, the inflammatory process also begins and lasts for a few days. The inflammatory process has implications for the entire healing process. PMNs phagocytize bacteria and digest the fibrin matrix in preparation for new tissue.[5,8-10] PMNs also secrete vasodilatory mediators and cytokines that activate fibroblasts and keratinocytes and attract macrophages.[5,7] PMNs are present during the first 48 hours of the inflammatory process.

Chemotactic factors, complement components, thrombin, and TGF-β_1 also recruit monocytes, which transform into macrophages. Tissue debris and PMNs are then phagocytized by macrophages. The destruction of the denuded tissue and bacteria creates an acidotic environment, decreased tissue oxygenation as a result of damaged blood supply, and pain at the wound site. Macrophages are the predominant cell in the wound bed at 72 hours; they remain in the wound for several days.[7,8] In addition to the immunologic response, macrophages also secrete cytokines and growth factors necessary for successful wound healing. Substances secreted include collagenase and elastase, which break down damaged matrix; fibroblast growth factors (FGF); epidermal growth factor (EGF); vascular endothelial growth factor (VEGF); tumor necrosis factor α (TNF-α); interleukin-1 (IL-1); and interferon-γ (IFN γ).[5,7-10] Macrophages also produce prostaglandins, oxygen metabolites, and arginine, which regulate healing processes.[5] These chemical messengers stimulate the infiltration, proliferation, and migration of fibroblasts and endo-

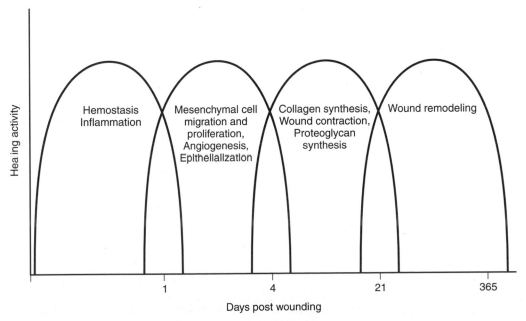

FIGURE 15-3 Phases of the healing wound. (From Lawrence WT: Physiology of the acute wound, *Clin Plastic Surg* 25(3): 321-340, 1998.

thelial cells. Molecular oxygen is converted to superoxide, which is important for wound resistance to infection. Because of their multiple functions, macrophages are essential to normal wound healing.[5-7,11-13]

Early physiologic responses to injury accomplish hemostasis through clot formation, increase blood flow to the wound, and initiate an inflammatory response that begins to clear the wound of cellular debris and provide substrates for tissue regeneration.

CELL MIGRATION AND PROLIFERATION

The processes of cell migration and proliferation predominate 2 to 4 days after wounding and are mediated by cytokines and growth factor (Table 15-1). This phase of healing is characterized by rapid cell mitosis, migration of cells, and synthesis of new tissue. The primary migratory cells are epithelial cells (keratinocytes), fibroblasts, and endothelial cells.

EPITHELIALIZATION. The migration of epithelial cells across a wound provides protection against entry of bacteria into the wound and wound fluid loss. Within 24 to 48 hours of wounding, epithelial marginal basal cells enlarge, flatten, undergo mitosis, and migrate over the defect. The epidermal covering, composed of primarily keratinocytes, begins to differentiate and reestablish the protective barrier. This process is referred to as epithelialization. Epithelialization promotes extracellular matrix production, cytokine and growth factor release, and angiogenesis. A predominant growth factor released during this process is keratinocyte growth factor (KGF)[5] (Figure 15-4). Cells migrate from one wound edge to an adjacent wound edge, as well as from appendages such as hair follicles. Cells move as a monolayer across the denuded area in a leapfrog fashion.[7,14] A moist wound environment enables the migrating cells to move across the wound surface more easily and quickly. Desiccation of wounds and eschar on the wound surface act as a deterrent to movement of epithelial cells. In wounds allowed to heal in a moist, protected environment, epithelial cells migrate on top of the wound. This is in contrast to wounds that epithelialize by cell migration under eschar that forms when a wound is allowed to become dry.

Keratinocytes stimulate angiogenesis by releasing FGF and VEGF.[5,7] TFG-α and PDGF are also present and assist in the matrix development. Once the monolayer of keratinocytes covers the wound surface, proliferation and migration slow and differentiation and stratification of epidermis with basal membrane are established.[5,7-10,13] This process is facilitated by contraction of the underlying connective tissues. Unfortunately, regenerated epithelium does not retain all the functional appendages and strength of normal epithelium.

FIBROPLASIA AND COLLAGEN SYNTHESIS. Concurrently, cytokines and growth factors attract fibroblasts to migrate to the wound site. Fibroblasts are the primary mesenchymal cells in dermis and are the most important cells involved in wound healing.[7] Fibroblasts are activated by PDGF, EGF,

TABLE 15-1	Cytokines and Growth Factors Involved in Wound Healing
Healing Function	**Cytokines and Growth Factors Involved**
Inflammatory cell migration	PDGF
	TNF-α
	TGF-β
	EGF
	VEGF
	IL-1
	IFN-γ
Fibroblast proliferation	PDGF
	TNF-α
	IL-1
	EGF
	IGF
	TGF-β
Angiogenesis	FGF-α
	FGF-β
	EGF
	VEGF
	IL-8
	PDEGF
	TNF-α
	TGF-β
Epithelialization	EGF
	TGF-α
	KGF
	FGF-β
	IGF
	HBEGF
	PDGF
	PDEGF
	VEGF
Fibroplasia and collagen synthesis	PDGF
	TGF-β
	FGF-β
	EGF
	CTGF
	AVTIVIN

EGF, Epidermal growth factor; *TGF-α,β,* transforming growth factor α and β; *TNF-α,* tumor necrosis factor α; *KGF,* keratinocytes growth factor; *FGF-β,* fibroblast growth factor β; *IGF,* insulin-like growth factor; *HBEGF,* heparin-binding epidermal growth factor; *PDGF,* platelet-derived growth factor; *PDEGF,* platelet-derived epidermal growth factor; *VEGF,* vascular endothelial growth factor; *CTGF,* connective tissue growth factor; *IL-1,* interleukin-1; *IL-8,* interleukin-8; *IFN-γ,* interferon-γ.

lactate, and oxidants to synthesize and deposit collagen and protoglycans (Figure 15-5). The migrating fibroblasts use strands of fibrin and fibronectin as a scaffold for migration across the wound. The major function of fibroblasts in wound healing is to synthesize the basic monomer of the collagen fiber (fibroplasias). Fibroblasts are sensitive to the partial pressure of oxygen (Po$_2$) and acidosis. Local acidosis and hypoxemia initially stimulate fibroblast activity and angiogenesis[7,11]; however, prolonged states of acidosis and hypoxemia will inhibit these same cells and their functions, slowing wound healing.

Collagen provides strength and support to new tissues

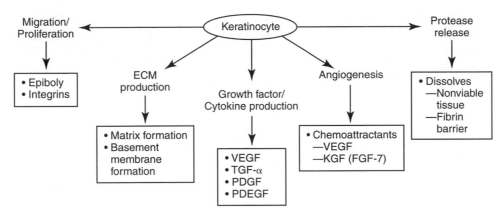

FIGURE 15-4 Role of keratinocytes in wound healing. (From Hunt TK, Hopf HH, Hussain Z: Physiology of wound healing, *Adv Skin Wound Care* 13(2):6-11, 2000.)

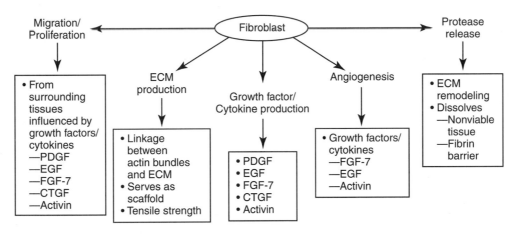

FIGURE 15-5 Role of fibroblasts in wound healing. (From Hunt TK, Hopf HH, Hussain Z: Physiology of wound healing, *Adv Skin Wound Care* 13(2):6-11, 2000.)

through its deposition and cross-linking in the injured area. There are several types of collagen with different tissue distributions. Type I is the predominant collagen in skin, tendon, and bone.[7] Fibroblasts synthesize the basic structural unit of collagen, procollagen. Collagen formation depends on the enzymes lysyl and prolyl hydroxylase and the presence of molecular oxygen. As collagen is formed on ribosomes, transfer RNA (tRNA) brings specific amino acids to the chain; there is no tRNA for the amino acids hydroxyproline or hydroxylysine.

Proline and lysine residues are incorporated into the growing collagen chains and are converted to hydroxyproline and hydroxylysine through enzymatic attachment of an oxygen atom by the hydroxylases.[7,15] Alpha-ketoglutarate, vitamin C, and ferrous iron[7,8,16] are other cofactors required for collagen synthesis. Deficiencies in vitamin C, or oxygen or suppression of enzymatic activity by corticosteroids may lead to underhydroxylated collagen, which is incapable of generating strong cross-links and is easily broken down.[7,17] The precursor chain of collagen is subsequently glycosylated and assembled into procollagen. Procollagen molecules are secreted into the extracellular wound space, where they become tropocollagen through enzymatic cleavage of peptidases. The tropocollagen then forms larger collagen fibers.

The fibers band together by cross-linking and overlapping.

Collagen is both synthesized and degraded in a continual process during wound repair. Scarring is greater when collagen synthesis is not balanced by lysing and contraction.[5,8,15] The strength of older collagen in the wound decreases with lysis as the strength of new collagen increases with synthesis. Over several weeks the collagen is remodeled, and the fibers that remain are those oriented parallel to lines of tension. By the third week after injury, the wound has its greatest mass and net collagen loss begins. The processes of collagen synthesis, lysis, and fiber cross-linking result in collagen with greater organization and a stronger, tighter matrix.

ANGIOGENESIS. Angiogenesis, the formation of new capillaries, follows the entry of fibroblasts into the wound. Angiogenesis is necessary for reestablishment of blood flow to the wound bed and successful healing. New capillaries result from endothelial budding of existing capillaries in tissues surrounding the wound and are supported by the collagen produced by fibroblasts. Tissue hypoxia, such as that occurring in the central space of a wound, stimulates angiogenesis along with cytokines and other growth factors released by fibroblasts, keratinocytes, and macrophages.[5-7,13,15] Hypoxic wound gradients stimulate macrophages to produce plasminogen activator, mitogenesis factors, and angiogenesis factors (FGF, VEGF, TGF-α, IGF, and PDGF), which in turn stimulate angiogenesis.[5-7,11] As endothelial cells grow toward the hypoxic wound edge, capillary buds join with other similar buds, forming new capillary loops and reestablishing blood flow. The new vasculature provides a continued supply of nutrients for wound healing and formation of the granulation bed consisting of fibroblasts, collagen, new vessels, and macrophages.

CONTRACTION. Wound contraction occurs in open wounds that are closing through the deposition of granulation tissue. It is the active process stimulated by PDGF, angiotensin, prostaglandins, bradykinins, and endothelins[10] by which the area of a wound is decreased by movement of the extracellular matrix and wound edges. In this process new tissue is not formed; inward movement of existing tissue at the wound edge closes the area of the wound. Myofibroblasts, the most abundant cells in granulation tissue, extend and retract pseudopods attached to collagen fibers, contracting the wound bed slowly (0.6-0.75 mm/day).[10] Wound contraction and remodeling occurs for 6 to 18 months after injury.

REMODELING

As healing progresses, edema decreases, and the numbers of fibroblasts and blood vessels recede. The local metabolic needs of the tissue decrease and no longer require the support of a dense cellular and vascular network. The tissue enters into the final repair process, remodeling. This begins approximately 3 weeks after injury and continues for 6 to 18 months. As described earlier, the scar tissue loses mass and gradually gains strength as collagen remodels into an organized and tighter matrix. As the scar tissue matures, it also generally changes color and form. The early red, edematous, firm scar softens, lightens to pink, and becomes smaller. The scar tissue is strengthened through remodeling; however, skin and fascia only achieve approximately 80% of their original strength.[5-8,10,13-15]

DETERMINANTS OF THE HEALING PROCESS

Physiologically, wound healing begins at the moment of injury and proceeds through cellular recruitment and interaction until tissue continuity is reestablished. Several local and systemic factors influence the healing process. These can be organized conceptually into a human response model that includes factors inherent in the person that increase vulnerability for impaired healing and environmental factors that present a risk for impairment of healing (Figure 15-6). Some factors may be modifiable, whereas others are not; all are worthy of consideration to provide appropriate therapy and an environment that supports healing.

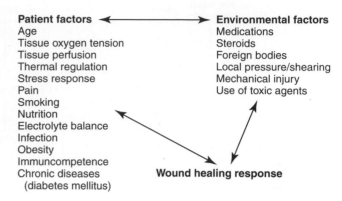

FIGURE 15-6 Human response model of factors that influence wound healing.

AGE

Advancing age influences healing. The elderly have slower cellular activity and multiple concurrent conditions, predisposing them to impaired healing.[14] In aging skin the epidermis thins gradually and is more easily stretched because of a decrease in elastin fibers.[16,18] The dermal layer experiences many changes with aging. There is a loss of approximately 20% in dermal thickness, which may account for the thinning appearance of elderly skin.[18] Decreases in dermal cells, blood vessels, nerve endings, and collagen alter thermoregulation, sensation, and protective functions (e.g., moisture retention) of the skin with aging. The subcutaneous layer atrophies, decreasing the mechanical protection and insulation provided to the dermis by the subcutaneous layer. Additional factors such as lowered immunologic resistance, circulatory changes, and poor nutritional status seen in the elderly also contribute to altered wound healing. Because of these changes, aging skin is more prone to traumatic injury and generally takes longer to heal.

TISSUE OXYGEN TENSION

Oxygen is essential to meet the energy needs of biologic activity. In wounds, oxygen and perfusion play critical roles in the healing process and are related to many host factors that influence healing. Ischemic and hypoxic tissues do not heal. An adequate supply of oxygen to the wounded area is needed for synthesis and accumulation of collagen, phagocytic activity of PMNs and macrophages, angiogenesis, and epithelialization.[5,13,14,17,19] Oxygen is necessary for the enzymatic hydroxylation of proline and lysine residue on the forming collagen chains.[13] Insufficient proline hydroxylation caused by low tissue oxygen levels (oxygen tension <25 mm Hg) will result in weaker collagen and decreased tensile strength in the repaired tissues. The rate of epithelialization is also dependent on tissue oxygen tension. Replication of keratinocytes and migration requires oxygen.

Initially the disruption of the blood vasculature creates a local hypoxemic state that stimulates cytokines and growth factors to begin angiogenesis. Once angiogenesis begins, the

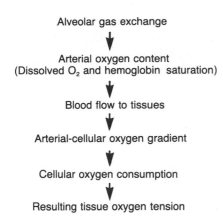

Alveolar gas exchange

↓

Arterial oxygen content
(Dissolved O_2 and hemoglobin saturation)

↓

Blood flow to tissues

↓

Arterial-cellular oxygen gradient

↓

Cellular oxygen consumption

↓

Resulting tissue oxygen tension

FIGURE 15-7 Determinants of tissue oxygen tension. (From Whitney JD: The influence of tissue oxygen and perfusion on wound healing. In Stotts NA, editor: *Wound healing: AACN clinical issues in critical care,* Philadelphia, 1990, JB Lippincott.)

success of new endothelial development is dependent on an adequate tissue oxygen tension.[5,13,17] Figure 15-7 depicts the physiologic system that determines tissue oxygen levels.

The relationship of adequate tissue oxygenation in the control of bacterial growth is important in the prevention of wound infection. Bactericidal activity by neutrophils is mediated by oxidative killing through the production of superoxide radicals from oxygen molecules.[8,13,17,19,20] The presence of oxygen molecules is directly dependent on the partial pressure of oxygen in the tissues. Research by Greif et al[20] suggests that improving arterial oxygen tensions beyond that required to saturate the blood will enhance tissue oxygenation and decrease the risk of infection. Greif[20] studied 500 patients undergoing colorectal surgery. Half the patients received standard oxygen supplementation (Fio$_2$ 30%) and the other half received 80% Fio$_2$ during the operation and for 2 hours after surgery. Results demonstrated that the incidence of postoperative wound infections decreased by half.

Tissue oxygenation is essential for normal wound healing. It has increased importance when subcutaneous tissue and fascia are involved in the wounding process. Wound healing is slower is these tissues because of limited vascular supply, which is further compromised in the presence of low oxygen tension.

PERFUSION

Oxygen delivery, along with the supply of neutrophils, monocytes, cytokines, growth factors, other cells, and nutrients, is closely linked to perfusion. Measurement of tissue oxygen tension has provided information about blood flow to peripheral tissues. Decreases in tissue oxygen reflect decreases in blood flow, provided pulmonary status is normal. This has become apparent through studies of human and animal systems, in which tissue oxygen was measured during blood volume changes. There was a clear response of decreased oxygen tension in the tissue, with a slow recovery to baseline once volume was replaced despite

the observation that both blood pressure and cardiac output returned to normal levels.[11] Subsequent studies support these findings, emphasizing the importance of adequate perfusion to ensure tissue oxygenation for optimal wound healing.[8,9,13,17,20]

Multiple factors influence perfusion in the trauma patient. Interventions to maximize perfusion to enhance wound healing should be addressed. Excessive catecholamine release with traumatic injury and hypothermia induce vasoconstriction, which will compromise tissue oxygen tension. Intraoperative and vasoactive agents used to support the cardiovascular system may compromise peripheral perfusion to tissues.[9,11,17] Sepsis and systemic inflammatory response syndrome (SIRS) may further alter tissue perfusion and oxygenation through maldistribution of blood flow and excessive cytokine release.[11] The management of trauma patients should include support of cardiovascular and pulmonary systems, sometimes above normal, to preserve wound perfusion and tissue oxygenation.[11]

In certain cases where tissue oxygen needs cannot be met through standard treatment modalities, hyperbaric treatment may be considered. Hyperbaric delivery of oxygen increases oxygen levels in soft tissues that are infected (e.g., necrotizing fasciitis) or slow to heal because of damage to the circulation. Although these tissues may be hypoperfused, at least some degree of blood supply must be present to effectively deliver oxygen to the wound site. The cellular use of oxygen is the same as in any wound; leukocytes, fibroblasts, endothelial cells, and other cells in their reparative roles of bacterial control, collagen synthesis, and angiogenesis also use oxygen.

INFECTION

Traumatic wounds are often contaminated with bacteria from the environment where the wound occurred. Wounds that contain more than 100,000 organisms per gram of tissue are at risk for subsequent infection. Fewer bacteria may result in wound infection in cases where local defense is compromised by necrotic tissue, dead space, or foreign bodies. Adequate and aggressive wound cleansing using controlled irrigation and nontoxic solutions will assist the healing process. Antiseptic agents such as povidone-iodine, sodium hypochlorite solution (Dakin's fluid), acetic acid, and hydrogen peroxide should not be used to cleanse the wound because they are toxic to fibroblasts and delay healing.[10,21,22] Normal saline is sufficient for wound cleansing; however, in the presence of suspected bacterial contamination, chlorhexidine gluconate (Hibiclens) is the agent of choice.[10,21,22]

Again, tissue oxygenation is essential to the prevention and treatment of wound infection. Oxygen is used in the aerobic pathway of leukocytes for the killing of bacteria that have been introduced or migrated to the wound site. Oxygen is converted into free radicals that form a system of bactericidal agents. As leukocytes phagocytose bacteria, a primary oxidase in the cell membrane is activated that catalyzes an oxidation reaction, with subsequent killing of the bacteria. Recent experimental evidence has shown that sufficient tissue oxygen levels are needed to resist infection.

Immuncompetence of the patient will also influence the ability to resist wound infection. States of chronic stress, sepsis, and disease or drugs that compromise immunologic cells will deter the healing process but not absolutely inhibit healing.[6] A patient with a compromised immune system may require more meticulous wound cleansing and vigilance in the assessment of wound infection and progression of healing. The ability of the patient to mount an inflammatory response is essential to normal healing. Equally important, the inflammatory process must cease. Wounds in which the inflammatory process is prolonged because of local or systemic factors heal more slowly and may be categorized as chronic.[6,7,14,16]

SEVERE ANEMIA, SMOKING, AND TEMPERATURE

Several factors can restrict tissue oxygen supply. Severe anemia and smoking are two patient elements that influence tissue oxygen and, potentially, healing. Because oxygen is transported primarily by hemoglobin, there is concern that oxygen supply will be limited in patients with severe anemia. However, a number of studies indicate that anemia is not as serious a threat to healing as once thought. Anemia in the presence of normal vascular volume and cardiac function does not impair wound healing until the hematocrit reaches a very low level (15%-18%).[5-7,16] At that point, transfusion is beneficial in terms of maintaining tissue oxygen supply.

Smoking has several detrimental effects, including decreasing the amount of functional hemoglobin, causing peripheral vasoconstriction, and lowering tissue oxygenation.[16] A study by Jensen et al showed that smoking lowers subcutaneous oxygen tension acutely, with oxygen levels remaining depressed for 30 to 50 minutes.[23] Fluid support and supplemental oxygen (nasal or hyperbaric) may support wound healing in patients who smoke.[16]

Hypothermia may indirectly influence healing through the thermoregulatory responses it elicits, with subsequent vasoconstriction and lowered tissue oxygen. During and after extensive surgery, body temperature may drop below 36° C, invoking cutaneous vasoconstriction and shivering mediated through the sympathetic nervous system. Energy and oxygen consumption rise above resting levels, further increasing the need for adequate oxygen supply to tissues. In addition, leukocyte activity is also adversely affected by decreases in body temperature.[19] It is well documented that prevention or correction of hypothermia decreases wound infection rates.[5,9,13,17,19]

PAIN

When patients are in pain, the sympathetic nervous system is activated and catecholamines are released, increasing vasomotor tone.[13,24] The resultant vasoconstriction depresses wound tissue oxygen tension, compromising the healing process. Local perfusion to the wound cannot be ensured until patients have normal volume, are warm, are receiving no vasoconstrictive drugs, and are pain free.[17] Cortisol is an adrenal glucocorticoid released in response to stimulation of the sympathetic nervous system. It is well documented that glucocorticoid impairs collagen synthesis[5,6,10,24,25]; however, it is not known whether physiologic levels of cortisol and adrenal glucocorticoids negatively affect the wound healing process.[13,25]

STRESS

Physical and psychologic stressors may impair healing. Physical stress to the edges of a wound can lead to partial or complete separation. The stress may be the result of strain, movement, or weight bearing on an injured extremity. Vomiting and abdominal distention also can disrupt chest or abdominal wounds. For this reason, adequate gastric decompression and drainage of bladder or wound cavities are important to avoid unnecessary stress on healing suture lines.

Psychologic stresses created by trauma evoke a neuroendocrine response. The sympathetic nervous system stimulation increases metabolic rate, catecholamine-induced vasoconstriction, oxygen consumption, and glucocorticoid levels. Collective responses decrease tissue oxygen tension and perfusion, negatively affecting wound healing.[13] Minimizing stressors may indirectly influence wound healing by reducing the stress response.

NUTRITIONAL STATUS

Nutritional assessment and maintenance of the trauma patient are discussed in detail in Chapter 16; however, several areas are notable for their effect on healing. Inadequate amounts of protein, fat, carbohydrates, calories, vitamins, and minerals contribute to impaired healing, impaired collagen formation, delayed development of wound tensile strength, and increased incidence of infection.[14,16]

Multiple trauma initiates a state of significant physiologic stress. The stress response is quite complex, encompassing inflammatory, endocrine, and central nervous system functions.[26] The collective result is a catabolic state, frequently leading to depleted protein status and lowered serum proteins. Fewer amino acids are available for neovascularization, fibroplasia, collagen synthesis, and the formation of antibodies and leukocytes. If a patient losses more than 10% of the usual body weight, administration of anabolic agents (human growth hormone, testosterone) should be considered to enhance protein synthesis and improve wound healing.[26-28] Glutamine and arginine are amino acids that assist the immune function and collagen deposition and may assist with normal wound healing.[26-29]

Hypoalbuminemia itself is not a direct cause of poor wound healing.[28] Hypoalbuminemia is associated with a decrease in plasma oncotic pressure, tissue edema, and slowed oxygen diffusion. Albumin also serves as a carrier for many substances, including cortisol and drugs. Hypoalbuminemia has been linked to increased morbidity and mortality.[28-30]

Carbohydrates are needed in wound healing to provide glucose as the main substrate for energy production. In the absence of glucose the body will continue the process of gluconeogenesis, further depleting protein stores and compromising wound healing. Glucose is also important as an energy source for leukocytes, cell proliferation, phagocytic activity, and fibroblast function.[28]

Vitamins and trace minerals are important for several biochemical processes. Collagen formation requires vitamin C, iron, and zinc as cofactors. Vitamin C is necessary for hydroxylation reactions involving proline and lysine during collagen synthesis. Collagen that is synthesized in conditions of vitamin C depletion is insufficiently hydroxylated and lacks strength because normal collagen fibers cannot be formed.[28,29] Iron and zinc are also involved in hydroxylation reactions. In addition, iron plays a critical role in oxygen transport. Zinc is present in all tissues and is necessary for metabolic pathways and enzyme functions.[28] Vitamin A is necessary for normal inflammatory response in wound healing. It stimulates cellular differentiation in fibroblasts and collagen, enhancing the healing process.[27,28] Vitamin A also enhances tensile strength of wounds and counteracts delayed healing caused by corticosteroids.[13,25,27,28] Vitamin E has been shown to interfere with collagen synthesis and wound repair and antagonizes the immune effects of vitamin A.[27] The trace elements copper and magnesium are important in the synthesis of polypeptide chains.

Water is a major constituent of the body and is required for oxidation of nutrients. Water intake needs to meet metabolic needs. It needs to be sufficient to replace insensible fluid losses, gastric and fistula fluid losses, and fluid lost with diarrhea. Estimated fluid needs are generally equivalent to 1 ml of water for each calorie provided.[28] Fluid intake should be sufficient to maintain good skin turgor and urine output.[26] Adequate nutrition is complex in the multiple trauma patient and has a profound impact on the success of wound healing.

ELECTROLYTE BALANCE

Normal serum electrolytes and acid-base balance are essential for cell function. Potassium is necessary for maintaining protein anabolism for wound repair and may be lowered through loss of body fluids and in response to adrenocortical hormone release in trauma. Release of aldosterone can result in potassium loss and sodium retention, which in turn alter cellular responses. Phagocytosis is inhibited by serum sodium levels in excess of 300 mmol/L and by elevated serum glucose levels. Serum pH has direct effects on cell motility. Acidosis decreases phagocytosis, thereby diminishing an essential component of the inflammatory response.

PREEXISTING HEALTH CONDITIONS

Primary vascular disease, diseases in which the immune system is compromised or depressed, states of malnutrition, and diabetes contribute to vulnerability to impaired healing.[31] Primary vascular disease interferes with the delivery of oxygen to the tissues. Immunocompetence is necessary for an appropriate inflammatory response and expression of macrophages for wound healing. Nutrition is essential for the anabolism required for tissue repair. Diabetes is associated with small vessel disease that can limit blood supply to the wound area, and hyperglycemia retards neutrophil function so that infection becomes a greater risk. Control of serum glucose levels to below 200 mg/dl is important in the prevention of wound healing complications.

PRINCIPLES OF WOUND ASSESSMENT THROUGHOUT THE TRAUMA CYCLE

Traumatic wounds result from the impact of an energy source applied against the skin and underlying structures. The initial assessment is focused on the treatment of life-threatening conditions and, of necessity, precedes the exterior wound assessment and subsequent treatment. Once the patient's condition is stabilized, wound assessment is done concurrently with the physical examination and the patient's history. Assessment information throughout all the phases of the trauma cycle provides the basis for development of the wound management plan. During this process, the patient is assessed thoroughly and is included as an active participant to the greatest extent possible. Patient involvement is generally limited only by physical condition. Many injuries that involve the skin are not life threatening, but they may have considerable psychologic impact, depending on a number of factors. For this reason, information about the patient's perception of the injury, its impact on daily living, and available support systems is included in the assessment.

WOUND HISTORY

The wound history includes the details of the incident, including the time and the mechanism of injury. The age of the wound and the environment in which it occurred must be identified. It is important to estimate the time at which inoculum was introduced into the wound. Efforts should focus on cleaning the contaminated wound before critical numbers of bacteria are reached and increase the likelihood of local and systemic infection.[32,33] The environment of the wound includes both the location on the body and the source of the injury. The distribution of microorganisms on the body varies; in general, moister body areas harbor greater numbers than drier areas.[34] Information about the physical environment in which the wound occurs helps to predict the existence of foreign bodies in the wound space, such as clothing fragments and types of soil and dirt, which vary depending on the source. Similarly, an injury caused by a clean knife from the kitchen has different implications than one caused by mechanical equipment on a farm or a motorcycle crash on a city street. The organic components of soil and inorganic clay fragments have been associated with the development of wound infections, presumably because of their inhibitory effect on host-defense systems. Organic fractions are heavily concentrated in swamps, bogs, and marshes; clay fractions are largely located in the subsoil.

Thus there is an increased risk of contamination and wound infection if injury occurs in swamps or excavation areas. Injuries that occur on farms have the potential for contamination with *Clostridium tetani;* the bacteria's natural habitat is the intestinal tract of domesticated animals, and it is consequently found in their excretions.[33,34]

The patient's history also includes an assessment of concomitant disease, which may influence the course of healing, as discussed earlier. History of medication use, allergies, previous healing impairment, and tetanus immunization status are also pertinent to the wound treatment regimen.

PHYSICAL EXAMINATION

The physical examination is intended to detect sensory, motor, and vascular complications that may have resulted from the injury in addition to the physical wound. It is followed by assessment of the wound status, location, and configuration and the viability of tissue, after which initial wound treatments are implemented.

NEUROVASCULAR ASSESSMENT. A comprehensive neurovascular assessment should be performed and documented before initiating wound treatment in order to document the existence of complications related to the injury itself as opposed to treatment-induced complications. The components of the assessment are movement, sensation, color, temperature, presence of pulses, and edema. Comparison of the affected wounded area with its contralateral anatomic site is useful to determine disruption in neurovascular function.

The patient is tested for both sensory and motor integrity in the affected area. Both gross and fine motor functions are tested, including the flexion and extension of each joint and full range of motion of each extremity. Sensation distal to the wound can be tested grossly by discrimination between sharp and dull sensations. Systematic evaluation is based on knowledge of the major nerves serving the extremities.

PERFUSION AND TISSUE OXYGENATION. The critical components of wound repair during the resuscitation phase, hemostasis, and initiation of the inflammatory process depend on perfusion and delivery of oxygen to the wounded tissues. Therefore clinical monitoring of circulation is essential. Distal and proximal pulses are assessed during the neurovascular examination to confirm the presence or absence of circulation to the affected area. Strong distal pulses provide a gross estimate of vascular supply to distal areas. Pulses are palpated bilaterally and documented using a 0 to 3+ scale, characterizing the pulse as absent (0), weak or thready (1+), normal (2+), or full or bounding (3+). Use of a Doppler ultrasound blood flow detector provides an auditory pulse when palpation is not possible. When wounds of the extremities cause tissue edema and diminished pulses, tissue pressure should be measured before the loss of pulses to detect complications associated with compartment syndrome.[34]

Arterial oxygenation should be assessed critically, both the saturation of hemoglobin with oxygen and the partial pressure of oxygen. As previously discussed, wound healing and prevention of infection rely on adequate tissue oxygenation.

Temperature of the wounded area is assessed by palpation using the dorsum of the hand. Wound area temperature is compared with the same region on the opposite side of the body. Temperature is significant to perfusion in the sense that cold elicits catecholamine release, which in turn decreases blood flow to connective tissues.

DEPTH OF WOUND INJURY. Assessment of the depth of tissue injury is necessary for the development of a plan of care. The location of the wound will also influence treatment choices (e.g., facial wounds versus lower extremity wounds). Assessment includes depth of wound bed: superficial, partial thickness, deep partial thickness, or full thickness. Assessment also includes evaluation of involvement of subcutaneous tissue, tendons, muscles, and bones. The extent of injury and tissue loss is considered, as well as the presence of nonviable tissue. There are many categories of soft tissue injuries. These categories are well described in Chapter 27 on soft tissue injuries.

WOUND ASSESSMENT IN THE RESUSCITATION PHASE. Initially wound location and configuration are assessed. The location is considered in terms of the distribution of microflora on the skin and also the proximity of the wound to sources of contamination, its vascular supply, weight bearing, and static and dynamic stress on the tissue. The natural static and dynamic skin tensions that occur after wound closure influence the final appearance of the scar. Noting the extent that the wound edges are retracted and the difficulty in which the edges are reapproximated can predict the final wound appearance. Wound edges that are retracted more than 5 mm are exposed to stronger static skin tensions and heal with wider scars than do wounds with edges separated less than 5 mm. Static tension is also influenced by wound configuration. It is sometimes not fully appreciated that jagged edged wounds, if carefully reapproximated, yield narrower scars than straight wounds because the magnitude of static tension is less per unit of wound length.[34]

WOUND ASSESSMENT IN THE CRITICAL CARE PHASE. Healing processes that coincide with the critical care phase include hemostasis, inflammation, fibroplasia and matrix deposition, angiogenesis, and epithelialization. Wounds that have been incised cleanly and closed will generally heal without problems; inflammation is minimal, and the distance required for new vessels to reestablish capillary networks is small. There is also relatively little need for matrix deposition and epithelial repair. These wounds present the patient with less of a metabolic burden than open wounds; however, in a compromised patient, healing may be problematic. Assessment of primary closure wounds includes observation initially for normal responses of inflammation, erythema, warmth, and induration along the suture line. Inflammation usually abates by the third to fifth day after injury, and by the seventh to ninth day a palpable healing ridge of collagen is present.[5] The wound edges should be approximated. Impaired healing is indicated by the absence of an inflammatory response, absence of a healing ridge by the ninth day, and continued drainage along the incision, which indicates the lack of an epithelial seal.

Assessment of open wounds is vital in order to evaluate the progress of healing and make decisions regarding therapy. The location, size, and depth of open wounds need to be documented. This can be accomplished with wound tracings or by measuring the wound width, length, and depth. When measuring the wound, the patient should be in the same position each time measurements are made to control for the influence of body position on wound shape and dimensions. The wound is also assessed for tracts and pockets, and the location and depth of these are noted. It is important to remember that when wounds are debrided, they will likely increase in size, and this need not be interpreted as a delay in healing but as a necessity for healing to proceed.

Critical aspects of the wound, including the character of tissue in the base and sides and new epithelium on the edges, as well as the presence of exudates, should be evaluated and assessment documented. The characteristics of tissue and exudate, including color, moisture, and distribution, are documented. Healthy granulation tissue is deep pink to bright red in color and moist, with minimal amounts of exudate. Exudate, when present, varies in consistency, color, and odor; these characteristics should be documented, as well as its distribution. Differences in exudate (purulent or serous) and amount of moisture may dictate different management regimens, such as dressings that are more absorbent, the need for irrigation, or dressings that simply protect the wound. Exudate or tissue that is very dark or black is necrotic and must be removed for healing to progress. True wound assessment cannot be completed in the presence of eschar.[22,35]

Growth of new epithelium is assessed on the wound edges. Its color and extent are important to note. Normally it is a light pink or pearl color. It should eventually be observable around the entire edge, extending across the wound as healing progresses. New epithelium also may be present, forming small pink islands around hair follicles.

A thorough wound assessment with documentation of the character of tissue, exudate, and epithelium is made daily or with each dressing change. Exceptions to daily assessment are made when the type of dressing dictates a less frequent changing schedule, which is the case with some of the biosynthetic dressings. In the acute care setting, wound size should be documented at least twice a week.

WOUND ASSESSMENT IN THE INTERMEDIATE AND REHABILITATION PHASES.   The extent to which a wound has healed after trauma is at best imprecise and depends on many factors. These include the balance between metabolic de-

mand and nutritional supply, cardiovascular and respiratory status, and the existence of pertinent patient and environmental factors (reviewed previously). As the patient enters the intermediate and rehabilitation phases, the process of wound healing should be well established. The biologic processes of collagen synthesis, angiogenesis, and epithelial regeneration will likely continue through the intermediate phase, whereas remodeling and contraction will be the predominant processes in the rehabilitation phase. Primarily closed wounds should at this point have an epithelial seal and be gaining strength. The tensile strength of wounds cannot be observed or measured. However, the wound can be assessed for complete closure and the absence of inflammation and infection. If the wound is healing by secondary intention, the assessment strategy used in the critical care phase remains appropriate. Generally the wound should decrease in both size and volume as granulation tissue accrues and contractile forces operate to close the wound.

WOUND MANAGEMENT THROUGHOUT THE TRAUMA CYCLE

SYSTEMIC SUPPORT

PERFUSION AND OXYGENATION.   In the resuscitation and critical care phases of recovery, adequate perfusion and supply of oxygen and nutrients to the wound area are crucial for optimal healing, in particular for the avoidance of infection. Systematic clinical assessment of perfusion, and in some cases oxygen tension and blood flow, as described in the section on assessment, remain appropriate evaluation strategies. Support of vascular volume is essential to ensure that needed nutrients reach the reparative cells. Clinical studies have documented that low tissue oxygen tensions are most common in the first 24 to 48 hours after surgery or injury, highlighting the necessity of maintaining tissue perfusion in the critical care period.[5,20] In the presence of adequate perfusion the use of supplemental oxygen is a rational therapeutic choice to sustain tissue oxygenation in patients who are at high risk for infection.[7,8,13,17,20] Treatment of hypothermia is important to consider, particularly if the patient has experienced surgery. Restoring normothermia will help prevent cutaneous vasoconstriction and may be important for resistance to infection by maintaining perfusion to injured tissues. An aggressive pulmonary hygiene plan, position changes, and ambulation if possible should also be considered in an effort to optimize tissue oxygenation.

As healing progresses in the intermediate and rehabilitation phases of recovery, perfusion and tissue oxygen supply remain important and should continue to be supported. The emphasis and extent of treatment depend on assessment of wound status. In primarily closed wounds that are healing without complications, interventions focused on optimal pulmonary status and adequate oral intake to support nutrition and avoid dehydration are likely to be sufficient. Wounds healing by secondary intention present greater metabolic demands. Regular clinical assessment of peripheral perfusion, with careful attention to volume status and in some cases supplemental oxygen, may be necessary to sustain healing.

NUTRITION.   Nutritional status should be assessed in the resuscitation phase and a plan for support developed. In the critical care phase it is important to provide energy for phagocytosis and the beginning reparative processes such as angiogenesis, collagen synthesis, and matrix deposition. Recall that vitamin C, iron, and zinc all contribute to the production of collagen. It is also critical to the support of wound healing that provision of nutrients be implemented quickly in the course of treatment and not be delayed. The reader is referred to Chapter 16 for detailed information on nutritional therapy during this phase.

Depending on the status of the wound, nutritional demands for healing will vary during subsequent trauma phases. Open wounds that continue to synthesize new tissue will naturally have greater energy requirements than wounds that are reapproximated. For wounds that are progressing, if the nutritional needs of the whole patient are met, it is likely that nutrition is adequate for the purposes of wound healing.

INFECTION CONTROL AND ANTIBIOTICS

The use of antibiotics can affect the outcome of healing, but successful therapy depends largely on when they are administered. Prophylactic antibiotics are considered when the risk of infection is high or when the results of an infection would be life threatening.[34] Wound infection must be treated regardless of when it occurs. However, heavy bacterial load is most commonly associated with the resuscitation phase, and infection is most likely to occur in the early trauma phases. Tissue in which repair is well established, with development of a healthy granulation bed or the presence of an epithelial seal, is usually resistant to infection. Ideally this situation exists by the time the patient enters the intermediate and rehabilitation phases of recovery. If the wound is healing by secondary intention, the presence of foul drainage, a pale wound bed, erythema surrounding the wound edges, leukocytosis, and pain are signs that should be evaluated to rule out infection. The presence of wound infection may be evaluated by clinical examination, swab culture, or tissue culture. Although swab cultures are the most frequently used method, they are easily contaminated and significantly underestimate bacterial counts in the wound bed.[36] Tissue cultures, although more invasive (requiring a sample of tissue), are more accurate in isolating wound bacteria.[36] Systemic antibiotics are most effective when they are given before injury (e.g., preoperatively) or, in the case of trauma, as soon after injury as possible and when they are matched to the sensitivities of the infecting organism.[8,10,33,34,37] Local antibiotics may be used to obtain high concentrations in the wound without systemic side effects. However, local antibiotics have several disadvantages: cutaneous sensitization, development of bacterial resistance, inhibition of wound healing, and inactivation of the antibiotic by the wound.[37]

PROGRESSIVE PHYSICAL ACTIVITY

The effects of activity on wound healing are not well documented. In the early phases of recovery from trauma some immobilization and physical support of the wound area to avoid stress on newly injured tissues are important. Wounds, when immobilized, should be in the position of maximal function. Splinting may be required to optimize wound positioning and function. At the same time, any activity that the patient can tolerate (e.g., turning) is likely to be beneficial through indirect cardiopulmonary effects. Physical activity improves oxygenation in peripheral tissues through improvement of the ventilation to perfusion, provided that cardiac output and peripheral flow are adequate.

In the intermediate and rehabilitation phases a progressive plan for physical activity may enhance healing. Motion and mild stress applied to wounds have been associated with increased wound strength, although the mechanism is not clear.

WOUND CLOSURE AND DEBRIDEMENT

WOUND CLOSURE.   Decisions about wound closure depend on the type of wound and amount of tissue loss. When tissue loss and contamination are minimal, primary closure is the likely method of choice. Factors that influence the decision regarding the type of closure material include wound location, configuration, tension that will be applied to the wound, and desired cosmetic result. Sutures are used most commonly for primary closure (Figure 15-8). Sutures that lose their tensile strength within 60 days are classified as *absorbable; nonabsorbable* sutures maintain their tensile strength beyond 60 days. Techniques of suture closure for skin include percutaneous (passing through epidermal and dermal layers) and dermal (epidermis is not penetrated). Small wounds that are not exposed to significant tension or stress can be closed using adhesive strips. Tape closure is useful for linear wounds in areas where tensions are low. If tissue loss is extensive, grafts or flaps will be required (see Chapter 27).

In some cases the wound heals by secondary intention through the processes of granulation tissue formation, contraction, and epithelial migration. However, the final scar is generally larger and the resulting deformity greater. The timing for wound closure is dependent to a large extent on the degree of contamination. Delayed primary closure, or tertiary closure, may be used with contaminated wounds. The benefits of delayed wound closure for contaminated wounds are well recognized; wound infection and dehiscence can often be avoided. The use of delayed primary closure enhances the development of a healthy granulation bed that resists infection and is prepared for subsequent grafting or closure, usually within a few days of the original injury.

DEBRIDEMENT.   Debridement is a traditional, accepted approach for the removal of necrotic tissue (eschar) and debris from the wound. Devitalized tissue promotes bacte-

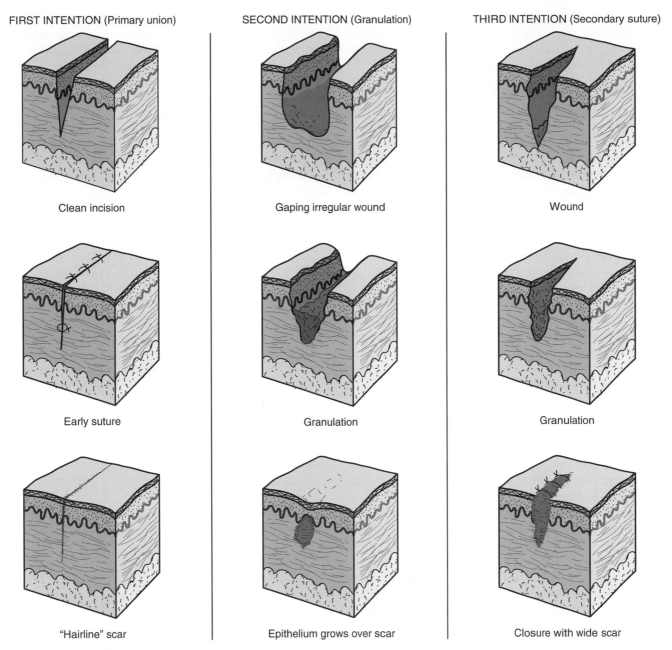

FIRST INTENTION (Primary union)

Clean incision

Early suture

"Hairline" scar

SECOND INTENTION (Granulation)

Gaping irregular wound

Granulation

Epithelium grows over scar

THIRD INTENTION (Secondary suture)

Wound

Granulation

Closure with wide scar

FIGURE 15-8 Wound healing by primary, secondary, and tertiary closure. (From: Lynn-McHale DJ, Carlson KK [eds]. *AACN Procedure Manual of Critical Care,* ed 4, Philadelphia, 2000, Saunders.)

rial growth and diminishes leukocyte function. Epithelialization cannot progress until the wound is free of eschar. Eschar may be removed via sharp, autolytic, mechanical, or chemical debridement.

The most rapid and efficient method of debridement is sharp surgical debridement.[38] Sharp debridement is the process of excising necrotic devitalized tissue from the wound bed. Healthy tissue is usually lost in the process, creating a larger wound. Sharp debridement gives the rapid result of a clean wound bed and is the method of choice in the face of potentially septic wounds. Disadvantages include pain and creation of a larger wound.

Autolytic debridement is a process initiated by covering the eschar with a synthetic dressing (gel, hydrocolloid, or film). The body's moisture, macrophages, and cytokines are trapped over the necrotic tissue and begin to rehydrate, soften, and, finally, liquefy the hard eschar.[39] Autolytic debridement is a selective process that destroys only the necrotic tissue. The process takes about 4 to 7 days, does not cause pain, and is the best option when a wound is not in need of immediate debridement.[39]

Mechanical debridement is a nonselective procedure in which wet dressings are placed in the wound bed, allowed to dry, and then removed. Upon removal of the dry dressing, healthy granulation tissue, as well as the necrotic tissue, is removed. The process is very painful and damaging to viable tissues. Mulder[40] compared the cost effectiveness of autolytic and mechanical (wet-to-dry gauze) debridement methods. Results from this study showed that, although mechanical debridement methods were less expensive in terms of the cost of gauze and saline, the costs of nursing time to perform the daily procedure, and pain medications and the length of time to achieve a debrided wound bed (average time to achieve a debrided wound bed was 11 days) caused this technique to ultimately be more expensive than autolytic methods.

Hydrotherapy is also considered a means of mechanical debridement. Irrigation uses mechanical force to remove debris and bacteria from the surface of wounds. Contaminants and particles are removed when irrigation pressure exceeds adhesive forces.[21] High-pressure irrigation, defined as 4 to 25 lb/in^2, will remove particulate matter and bacteria more effectively than low-pressure irrigation. Low-pressure syringe irrigation, such as with a bulb syringe, removes large particles but not smaller contaminants and bacteria. An effective high-pressure system can be created using a 19-gauge plastic needle, a 35-ml syringe, and sterile normal saline.[21,22] Concern has been raised about potential damage to tissues from high-pressure irrigation systems. The pressure needs to be sufficient to clean the wound effectively, but it should not traumatize the healing tissue. Pressure greater than 25 psi will traumatize the healing tissues and impair the wound's ability to resist infection.[21]

Chemical, or enzymatic, debridement is accomplished by applying topical debridement agents to remove devitalized tissues on the wound surface.[22,39] Enzymatic debridement may be used when the patient cannot tolerate sharp debridement and removal of necrotic tissue may be achieved more gradually. Debridement using enzymatic agents will be complete in 3 to 30 days, depending on the agent used.[22] Enzymatic agents are highly selective, causing debridement of only the devitalized tissue, thus promoting wound healing.

ANTISEPTIC AGENTS. Several solutions commonly used for wound cleansing (povidone-iodine, 1%; sodium hypochlorite [Dakin's]; hydrogen peroxide; acetic acid) are associated with toxic effects to leukocytes and fibroblasts and retard epithelial repair.[10,22] If an antiseptic is needed for cleaning, chlorhexidine (Hibiclens) has been shown to reduce bacterial counts and have less toxic effects on wound tissue.[10] The use of normal saline and high-pressure irrigation remains the best method for removing bacteria and particulate matter and cleansing a wound.[22]

DRESSINGS: PRINCIPLES AND TECHNIQUES

Once the wound has been cleansed, debrided if necessary, and assessed, appropriate dressing materials must be chosen. Before the early 1960s, wounds were thought to heal more quickly and better if kept open to the environment and allowed to form a dry crust. Classic work by Winter[41] and Hinman and Maibach[42] revealed that partial thickness wounds heal twice as fast under occlusion than wounds exposed to air. Numerous studies have since supported this early work, advocating the provision of a moist wound

environment to enhance and expedite the wound healing process.[10,39,42] In a dry environment epidermal cells are inhibited from migrating and resurfacing the wound because they must burrow between eschar and the underlying tissues. In a moist environment cells migrate more easily and enhance the resurfacing process. A moist environment enhances healing, but a wet environment may hinder healing by macerating healthy tissues that surround the wound. Excessive drainage and perspiration need to be considered when selecting a wound dressing to prevent excessive moisture in the wound bed. Infections are reduced in a moist wound environment. Wound occlusion actually reduces the risk of infection by maintaining the inflammatory cells that destroy bacteria and foreign materials in the wound bed.[43,44]

The dressing of choice during any phase of wound healing depends to a large extent on the characteristics of the wound, including whether it is closed primarily or left open. A myriad of wound-covering products are available, and it is probably best to make choices based on some simple but important moist wound healing principles. In general, wound treatments (dressings) should protect the wound from further injury, remove infection and necrotic tissue, support the body's tissue defenses, eliminate dead space, prevent excess exudates in the wound, and provide an optimal moist environment for healing.[43] Table 15-2 illustrates the basic characteristics and design of commonly available dressings. Dressings that come in contact with a wound bed are considered primary dressings. Secondary dressings are those dressings that cover a primary dressing or secure a dressing in place.[43] Dressings listed in Table 15-2 may be either primary or secondary dressings, depending on the application.

PRIMARY-CLOSURE WOUNDS. A primarily closed wound is most often covered with a protective dressing that may be layered if drainage is expected. A nonadherent dressing may be used as the first layer to avoid disruption of new epithelium when the dressing is removed. The next layer is absorbent to collect exudate, provide light pressure and support, and immobilize the local tissues. The top layer provides external support and protection. Coverings over primary-closure wounds are usually needed for 2 to 3 days until the wound surface is sealed with epithelial cells.

PARTIAL-THICKNESS WOUNDS. Wounds that are open will require different dressings depending on their characteristics. Partial-thickness wounds, such as dermabrasions, that mainly require epithelialization in order to heal and are not heavily exudative can be covered with a product designed to provide a moist environment that supports cell migration. Several types of semiocclusive/occlusive dressings may be used to heal a partial-thickness wound. Polyurethane film dressings trap fluid next to the wound, do not adhere to the wound surface, and do not absorb fluid. Hydrocolloid and hydrogel dressings absorb moderate amounts of fluid, do not adhere to the wound, provide

TABLE 15-2 Categories of Wound Dressings

Category of Wound Dressing	Characteristics/ Functions	Best Uses	Advantages	Disadvantages
Gauze	Coarse or fine mesh cotton dressing Size of pore in dressing will determine absorptive and debridement qualities of dressing	Primary dressing for wet-to-moist debridement May be used as a secondary absorptive layer	Economical Coarse gauze provides effective mechanical debridement	Nonspecific debridement Painful on removal May damage healthy granulation tissue with removal and cause minor bleeding
Nonadherent impregnated gauze (e.g., Vaseline gauze, Telfa)	Nonadherent fine-mesh gauze impregnated with emollient or hydrophic agent Does not adhere to wound May assist in creating moist wound environment that promotes autolytic debridement	Primary dressing over a wound closed by primary intention Requires secondary dressing to secure	Nonadherent Economical Provides moisture to wound surface	Nonabsorptive May require a secondary dressing
Transparent films	Semipermeable membrane dressings Waterproof yet permeable to oxygen and water vapor Prevent contamination of wound by exogenous bacteria Maintain moist wound environment, facilitate cellular migration, and promote autolysis of necrotic tissue by trapping moisture at wound surface	Superficial wounds Wounds with light exudates Wounds on elbows, heels, flat surfaces Covering blisters Retention of primary moist healing dressings Protects skin from exogenous moisture	Transparent, so wound progress can be evaluated without removal of dressing Waterproof and gas permeable Maintain moist environment Economical	Adhesive, so they can tear healthy tissue with removal Nonabsorptive Tend to roll off wounds in high friction areas (e.g., coccyx)
Hydrocolloid dressings	Occlusive and adhesive wafer dressings Combine absorbent colloidal materials with adhesive elastomers to manage light to moderate amounts of wound exudates Most react with wound exudates to form gel-like covering that protects wound bed and maintains moist wound environment Hydrocolloid powders and pastes also available for increased absorptive capacity; covered with wafer dressing	Cover granulating and epithelializing wounds draining low to moderate amounts of exudates Promote autolytic debridement	Waterproof Prevent bacterial and environmental contamination Comfortable for easy application to body sites with curves and creases (e.g., coccyx, heel) May reduce pain at wound site Avoid placing over wounds that are close to rectum	Moderate to heavy exudative wounds overwhelm hydrocolloid dressings and create leakage Impermeable to oxygen; not recommended for wounds with suspected or known anaerobic infections Odor on removal of dressing may be unpleasant (from mixture of wound fluid and dressing matrix materials)

Continued

Modified from Smith and Nephew, Inc.: *Physician's guide to moist wound healing*, Largo, Fla, 1998, Smith and Nephew.

TABLE 15-2   Categories of Wound Dressings—cont'd

Category of Wound Dressing	Characteristics/ Functions	Best Uses	Advantages	Disadvantages
Hydrogel sheet dressings	Most hydrogel sheets are cross-linked polymer gels in sheet form Generally waterproof and prevent bacterial and environmental contamination Some are available with adhesive borders and are covered with moisture vapor permeable films Most are manufactured with high water content, so they do not absorb much exudate Hydrophilic and will allow evaporation of exudate	Reepithelializing wounds with minimal exudate Aid in autolytic debridement by hydrating the eschar Abrasions, minor burns, and wounds	Comfortable dressings that help reduce pain Most are relatively transparent, allowing visualization of wound	Nonabsorptive May require secondary dressing to secure
Wound gels	Excellent for maintaining moist environment or creating one in a dry wound environment Some provide absorption, desloughing, and debriding Hydrate eschar and slough by increasing moisture at wound site	Providing and maintaining moist wound environment to reduce eschar formation and create environment for fast, safe, and painless healing Effective cleansing and debridement of necrotic and sloughy wounds by increasing moisture contents, aiding in autolytic debridement	Comfortable Cover sensitive nerve endings, decreasing pain Very effective in hydrating wound surfaces Assist autolysis of necrotic tissue Easy to use Nonadherent Can be removed from wound without discomfort or harming of fragile granulation tissue	Require secondary dressing Absorb only minimal exudate Difficult to keep in place on superficial wounds

	Description	Indications	Advantages	Disadvantages
Foam dressings	Highly absorbent dressings, generally made from hydrophilic polyurethane foam Some are waterproof and aid in prevention of bacterial contamination Some have adhesive backing; others require secondary dressing to secure to wound surface Foam dressings absorb large amounts of exudate, reducing maceration while promoting healing	Highly exudating wounds Deep cavity wounds as packing to prevent premature closure while absorbing exudate and maintaining moist environment	Comfortable and conformable Very absorbent Can be left on wound 3-4 days, depending on amount of drainage No dressing residue in wound bed on removal Some foams can absorb under compression bandages/stockings	Require secondary dressing Without waterproof covers, tend to soil and leak easily May dry wound if there is too little exudate
Alginates	Made of soft, nonwoven fibers derived from brown seaweed Available as wound pads and ropes for packing deep cavity wounds Absorb wound exudate and form moisture/vapor-permeable, gel-like covering over wound, maintaining moist environment Absorb many times their own weight Absorbancy directly related to weight of alginate applied to wound	Wounds with moderate to heavy wound exudate Granulating and epithelializing wounds in which some exudate is present	Very useful for packing wounds with exudate Easy to use Several have good wet strength and can be removed in one piece	Require secondary dressing Risk of drying wound bed with low volumes of exudate Will not debride hard eschar Wound will need to be well irrigated with some alginates to ensure full removal of product from wound cavity
Copolymer starches	Gel-like dressings that are packed, squeezed, or poured into wound Absorb moderate to heavy amounts of wound exudate while maintaining moist wound environment	Deep crater wounds Cavities where they can absorb while promoting granulation of wound bed without undermining	Conform easily to wound surface and obliterate dead space without need for gauze packing Irrigate relatively easily out of wounds Will not physically inhibit wound contraction	May require mixing and some type of secondary dressing Limited to deep cavity wounds Will not debride hard eschar

Modified from Smith and Nephew, Inc.: *Physician's guide to moist wound healing*, Largo, Fla, 1998, Smith and Nephew.

autolytic debridement, and can be used to cover partial-thickness wounds.

Although risk of infection is not increased with the use of occlusive dressing, caution should be used in the presence of gram-negative bacteria, which thrive in moist environments, and in patients who are immunosuppressed. More frequent assessment of the wound under occlusion may be necessary with contaminated wounds and immunosuppressed patients. Care also should be taken to avoid the entry of microorganisms from outside the wound, through the provision of a tight wound dressing seal.

An additional apparent benefit of semiocclusive/occlusive dressings is the relief of pain associated with the wound, particularly for dermabrasions and skin-graft donor sites. In addition to pain relief, there are advantages in terms of the final cosmetic result when semiocclusive dressings are used.[45] Although semiocclusive dressings may be more expensive, the cost for treatment is lowered by virtue of the decreased frequency of dressing changes.[45] The relevance of these benefits should not be minimized. Increasing patient comfort is a significant contribution to care, improved scar appearance and quality are particularly important for wounds in highly visible areas, and decreased cost is a ongoing health care concern.

HEALING OF DEEP PARTIAL-THICKNESS AND FULL-THICKNESS WOUNDS BY SECONDARY INTENTION OR DELAYED CLOSURE.

Deep partial-thickness and full-thickness wounds may require more extensive dressings that offer greater absorption in addition to maintaining wound moisture. In wounds that are not necrotic or heavily exudative but have some depth, a simple wet-to-damp saline, fine-mesh gauze dressing will provide a moist environment for the wound bed and margins. If removal of exudate is needed, coarse gauze is recommended, since fluids will move from the wound into the interstices of the gauze layers and then can be removed when the dressing is changed. Wet-to-damp or wet-to-wet dressings are removed before they dry, thus protecting fragile new capillaries from damage when dressings are allowed to dry and adhere to the wound bed.

Hydrocolloid, hydrogel, alginate, or foam dressings can be applied to deep partial-thickness and full-thickness wounds. In wounds with exudate, they are absorbent to the extent that there is gel available. These dressings, as discussed earlier, provide a moist healing environment, conform to the wound, occupy dead space, enhance healing, and increase comfort. Absorptive properties of these dressings vary, and the amount of wound exudate should determine which dressing is selected.

Open wounds that produce large amounts of exudate can be dressed traditionally with gauze packing and multiple superficial layers to absorb fluid. Frequent changes of these dressings will manage excess drainage and remove contaminants from highly exudative wounds. Absorbent dressings are also available. They are placed into the wound cavity and covered with a secondary dressing. Wound fluid and bacteria become trapped in the spaces of the absorbent materials and are removed from the surface of the wound, reducing mediators of inflammation and infection and improving the granulation bed.

GRAFTS AND BIOLOGIC/BIOSYNTHETIC TECHNIQUES FOR WOUND CLOSURE.

A deep partial-thickness or full-thickness wound may require 14 to 21 days to heal on its own.[46] Grafting of the wound may be necessary to decrease the risk of infection, speed healing, and provide better cosmetic results. Skin grafts may be full-thickness sheet grafts or meshed partial-thickness grafts. Location of the wound, donor sites available, and cosmesis are factors used to determine the type of autograft.[46]

A number of dressings categorized as biologic and biosynthetic dressings have been developed in recent years and may be used on deep partial-thickness and full-thickness wounds. Cultured epidermal autografts are created by collecting a tissue biopsy specimen from the patient and growing keratinocytes over a 3- to 4-week period in a cultured medium. The tissue is then grafted on to the patient's (host's) wound bed. Composite grafts are skin substitutes containing dermal and epidermal layers. Composite grafts are autografts grown from a dermal tissue culture and a biosynthetic biodegradable layer over 3 to 4 weeks and then grafted over the wound.[47] Composite grafts provide increased tensile strength. Cultured epidermal allografts use tissue such as neonatal foreskin as donor tissue for developing grafts.

Biosynthetic dressings consist of synthetic materials (nylon/silicone) that may be used to close a deep partial-thickness wound. Biosynthetic dressings have a prolonged shelf life and are intended for application on to a debrided wound bed until reepithelialization is complete. The dressing does not have adhesive materials but adheres to the wound surface by entrapment of fibrin.[10,48] Nonliving skin substitutes include chemically treated cadaver allografts and Integra artificial skin.[48] Chemically treated cadaver allografts are composed of acellular dermal matrix and intact basement membrane. Integra artificial skin is a synthetic composite graft that provides immediate wound coverage, promotes vascularization, and prepares the wound bed for grafting as it slowly biodegrades.[48]

Deep partial-thickness and full-thickness wounds should be closed as quickly as possible to decrease the chances of infection and optimize healing. Dressing choices will depend on patient factors (perfusion, oxygenation, nutritional status, immuncompetence) and available tissue donor sites.

ALTERATIONS IN HEALING

KELOIDS AND EXCESSIVE SCARRING.

Hypertrophic scarring and keloids are two alterations in healing that may become evident in the rehabilitation phase of trauma. They are significant because of their cosmetic and symptomatic consequences for the patient. Hypertrophic scars are an overgrowth of collagenous scar tissue within the wound margins; they may regress spontaneously. A keloid is distinguished as a fibrous growth resulting from abnormal connective tissue response, which extends beyond the wound margins and rarely regresses.[15] Management of hypertrophic scarring and keloids are discussed in Chapter 27, Soft Tissue Injuries.

SCAR CONTRACTURE. Scar contracture is the result of contractile processes in healed scars that result in a fixed, rigid scar that causes functional or cosmetic deformity. Wound contraction begins as a beneficial process that facilitates earlier wound closure by reducing the surface area of the wound bed. Continual contraction by myofibroblasts tends to pull points of flexion together, limiting movement and causing considerable disability.[15] The most common sites involve areas of flexion, such as fingers, arms, legs, and neck. Treatment modalities include physical therapy, splinting, and surgical release with grafting. Range-of-motion exercises affect the remodeling of collagen as it is deposited within the wound. Splinting procedures impede contraction mechanically. Split-thickness skin grafts are less effective than full-thickness grafts, which are less effective than flaps. Control of contraction appears closely related to elements of the dermis, so grafts containing dermis provide more effective therapeutic treatment.[15,46]

PRESSURE ULCERS. Although pressure ulcers are not the direct result of trauma, they are associated with acute illness and surgery. Immobility is the greatest risk factor for development of a pressure ulcer. Approximately 12% to 66% of patients with nosocomial pressure ulcers develop them during surgical procedures.[49,50] Trauma patients frequently undergo lengthy elective and emergent procedures that place them at risk of developing pressure ulcers.[51]

Pressure ulcers occur in areas where pressure, shearing force, friction, and moisture have damaged the epidermis, dermis, and underlying tissue layers. They occur over a bony prominence. The smaller the area over which the pressure is distributed, the greater the potential for the development of an ulcer. Shearing forces caused by sliding adjacent surfaces produce friction and tissue damage. Excess skin moisture from perspiration and incontinence increases the risk of skin breakdown and development of a pressure ulcer. Patients who remain immobile or have other factors that place them at risk of pressure ulcer development need to be assessed continually throughout all the phases of trauma care. Calianno[52] suggests vigilant assessment for the risk of pressure ulcers in the following groups of patients: those with spinal cord injuries, diabetes, multiple diseases, a history of pressure ulcer, low ejection fractions, malnutrition, and incontinence; patients undergoing orthopedic surgery; those in intensive care units; and elderly patients.

Guidelines for pressure ulcer prevention issued by the Agency for Health Care Policy and Research (AHCPR) stress the need for assessment of risk at admission. The AHCPR recommends the Braden and Norton scales, which incorporate the following categories for assessment of skin breakdown risk: level of consciousness (sensory perception), moisture, mobility (activity), nutrition, friction, and shear. If a patient is found to be at risk, risk reduction methods should be implemented. Lewicki et al[53] found the Braden scale to predict pressure ulcer risk in the acutely ill cardiac surgical population; however, a high index of suspicion and increased frequency of assessment were necessary. The trauma patient population would benefit from the bedside nurse completing a thorough assessment for risk of pressure ulcers on admission and at a set frequency throughout the hospital stay. Prevention of nosocomial pressure ulcers in trauma patients can be attributed to proactive nursing interventions.

Assessment is accompanied by preventive measures to relieve pressure through frequent turning,[22] avoiding friction and shearing forces, providing meticulous skin care, nutritional support, and patient education. The skin should be kept dry, warm, well moisturized, and protected with lubricants or protective coverings.[22] Regular use of a mild skin cleanser and the use of barrier sprays and creams to repel moisture when needed are suggested. Massage over bony prominences is contraindicated.[52] To relieve pressure, patients require repositioning every 2 hours at a minimum if on bed rest. Static support surfaces filled with foam, water, gel, or air can be used, as well as dynamic systems such as alternating-pressure mattresses, air-fluidized systems, low air loss support systems, viscoelastic, and elastic surfaces.[54] Smaller supports such as foam cushions, wedges, pillows, or blankets can keep knees, elbows, ankles, and heels from receiving too much pressure. To avoid shearing and friction during positioning, patients should be lifted with linens or a lifting device.

The principles of assessment for open wounds apply to pressure ulcers. Location, size, and tissue and exudate characteristics are evaluated on a regular basis. A plan of treatment is established, based on assessment of the wound and risk factors specific to the patient. In addition to choosing an appropriate dressing, a plan of care that incorporates positioning and pressure relief is essential.

SUMMARY

Development of knowledge in the area of wound healing has advanced rapidly in recent years. An increased understanding of this complex process and the effects of various therapies on its progression has altered some traditional beliefs about wound care and healing and has provided an empirical basis for treatment. There is still much to learn. Available data emphasize the need for early assessment of the patient's status and the wound and maintaining an optimal environment for wound healing. Steps taken to provide systemic support in the early trauma phases of care contribute significantly to the healing process and can prevent a number of complications, including infection. Many therapies for wound healing have yet to be studied to discern their mechanism of action and to define the limits of their use clinically to promote and improve healing. Continued research will extend the science of wound healing and provide a rational direction for optimal assessment and treatment strategies.

REFERENCES

1. Wysocki AB: A review of the skin and its appendages, *Adv Wound Care* 8(2):53-70, 1995.
2. Stotts NA: Integumentary clinical physiology. In Kinney MR, Dunbar SB, Brooks-Brunn JA et al, editors: *AACN's clinical reference for critical care nursing,* ed 4, St. Louis, 1998, Mosby, 1055.
3. Hess CT: Fundamental strategies for skin care, *Ostomy Wound Manage* 43(8):32-41, 1997.
4. Rijswijk LV: The fundamentals of wound assessment, *Ostomy Wound Manage* 42(7):40-52, 1996.
5. Hunt TK, Hopf HH, Hussain Z: Physiology of wound healing, *Adv Skin Wound Care* 13(2):6-11, 2000.
6. Kerstein MD: The scientific basis of healing, *Adv Wound Care* 10(3):30-36, 1997.
7. Lawrence WT: Physiology of the acute wound. *Clinics Plastic Surg* 25(3):321-340, 1998.
8. Witte MB, Barbul A: General principles of wound healing, *Surg Clin North Am* 77(3):509-523, 1997.
9. Hunt TK, Hopf HW: Wound healing and wound infection, *Surg Clin North Am* 77(3):587-606, 1997.
10. Cho CY, Lo JS: Dressing the part, *Dermatol Clin* 16(1):25-43, 1998.
11. Thorton FJ, Schaffer MR, Barbul A: Wound healing in sepsis and trauma, *Shock* 8(6):391-394, 1997.
12. Hess CT: Skin care basics, *Adv Skin Wound Care* 13(3):127-129, 2000.
13. Whitney JD, Heitkemper MM: Modifying perfusion, nutrition, and stress to promote wound healing in patients with acute wounds, *Heart Lung* 28(2):123-133, 1999.
14. Stotts NA: Promoting wound healing. In Kinney MR, Dunbar SB, Brooks-Brunn JA et al, editors: *AACN's clinical reference for critical care nursing,* ed 4, St. Louis, 1998, Mosby, 237.
15. Tredget EE, Nedelec B, Scott PG et al: Hypertrophic scars, keloids, and contractures, *Surg Clin North Am* 77(3):701-724, 1997.
16. Krasner D: Minimizing factors that impair wound healing: a nursing approach, *Ostomy Wound Manage* 41(1):22-30, 1995.
17. Hopf HW, Hunt TK, West JM et al: Wound tissue oxygen tension predicts the risk of wound infection in surgical patients, *Arch Surg* 132(9):997-1004, 1997.
18. Baranoski S: Skin tears: the enemy of frail skin, *Adv Skin Wound Care* 13(3):123-126, 2000.
19. Kurz A, Sessler DI, Lenhardt R: Perioperative normothermia to reduce the incidence of surgical wound infection and shorten hospitalization, *N Engl J Med* 334(19):1209-1215, 1996.
20. Greif R, Akca O, Horn EP et al: Supplemental perioperative oxygen to reduce the incidence of surgical wound infection, *N Engl J Med* 342(3):161-167, 2000.
21. Barr EJ: Principles of wound cleansing, *Ostomy Wound Manage* 41(7A):15S-21S, 1995.
22. Agency for Health Care Policy and Research: *Clinical practice guideline: treatment of pressure ulcers,* Washington, DC, 1994, U.S. Department of Health and Human Services.
23. Jensen JS, Goodson WH, Hopf HW et al: Cigarette smoking decreases tissue oxygen, *Arch Surg* 126(9):1131-1134, 1991.
24. Rook JL: Wound care pain management, *Adv Wound Care* 9(6):24-31, 1996.
25. Anstead GM: Steroids, retinoids, and wound healing, *Adv Wound Care* 11(6):277-285, 1998.
26. DeSanti L: Involuntary weight loss and the nonhealing wound, *Adv Skin Wound Care* 13(1):11-20, 2000.
27. Thomas DR: Specific nutritional factors in wound healing, *Adv Wound Care* 10(4):40-43, 1997.
28. Brylinsky CM: Nutrition and wound healing: an overview, *Ostomy Wound Manage* 41(10):14-24, 1995.
29. Flanigan KH: Nutritional aspects of wound healing, *Adv Wound Care* 10(3):48-51, 1997.
30. Clochesy JM, Davidson LJ, Caulkins EP et al: Use of serum albumin levels in studying clinical outcomes, *Outcomes Manag Nurs Pract* 3(2):61-66, 1999.
31. Chalk L: Wound prevention and healing: everyone's problem, *Surg Serv Manage* 5(11):35-38, 1999.
32. Robson MC: Wound infection: a failure of wound healing caused by an imbalance of bacteria, *Surg Clin North Am* 77(3):637-649, 1997.
33. File TM, Tan JS: Treatment of skin and soft tissue infection, *Am J Surg* 169(5A):27S-33S, 1995.
34. Stewart RM, Page CP: Wounds, bites, and stings. In Mattox KL, Feliciano DV, Moore EE, editors: *Trauma,* ed 4, New York, 2000, McGraw-Hill, 1115.
35. Kranser D: Wound care: how to use the red-yellow-black system, *Am J Nurs* 95:44-47, 1995.
36. Neil JA, Munro CL: A comparison of two culturing methods for chronic wounds, *Ostomy Wound Manage* 43(3):20-30, 1997.
37. Degreef HJ: How to heal a wound fast, *Dermatol Ther* 16(2):365-374, 1998.
38. Sieggreen MY, Maklebust JA: Debridement: choices and challenges, *Adv Wound Care* 10(2):32-37, 1997.
39. Smith and Nephew, Inc.: *Physician's guide to moist wound healing,* Largo, Fla, 1998, Smith and Nephew.
40. Mulder GD: Cost effective managed care: gel versus wet to dry for debridement, *Ostomy Wound Manage* 41(2):68-76, 1995.
41. Winter GD: Formation of the scab and the rate of epithelialization of superficial wounds in the skin of the young domestic pig, *Nature* 193:293-294, 1962.
42. Hinman CD, Maibach H: Effects of air exposure and occlusion on experimental human skin wounds, *Nature* 200:377-379, 1963.
43. Baranoski S: Wound assessment and dressing selection, *Ostomy Wound Manage* 41(7A):7S-14S, 1995.
44. Hutchinson JJ: Prevalence of wound infection under occlusive dressings: a collective survey of reported research, *J Hosp Infect* 17:83-94, 1991.
45. Bolton LL, Rijswijk LV, Shaffer FA: Quality wound care equals cost effective wound care: a clinical model, *Adv Wound Care* 10(4):33-38, 1997.
46. Ratner D: Skin grafting: from here to there, *Dermatol Clin* 16(1):75-89, 1998.
47. Choucair MM, Phillips TJ: What is new in clinical research in wound healing, *Dematol Clin* 15(1):45-55, 1997.

48. Johnson PC: The role of tissue engineering, *Adv Skin Wound Care* 13(2):12-14, 2000.

49. Norton E, Young MA: Perioperative patient positioning, *Surg Serv Manage* 4(11):14-20, 1999.

50. Stotts NA: Risk of pressure ulcer development in surgical patient: a review of the literature, *Adv Wound Care* 12(2): 127-136, 1999.

51. Rodeheaver GT: Pressure ulcers: a preventable tragedy, *Surg Serv Manage* 4(11):111-113, 1999.

52. Calianno C: Assessing and preventing pressure ulcers, *Adv Skin Wound Care* 13(5):244-246, 2000.

53. Lewicki LJ, Mion LC, Secic M: Sensitivity and specificity of the Braden scale in the cardiac surgical population, *J Wound Ostomy Continence Nurs* 27(1):36-41, 2000.

54. Brienza DM, Geyer MJ: Understanding support surface technologies, *Adv Skin Wound Care* 13(5):237-243, 2000.

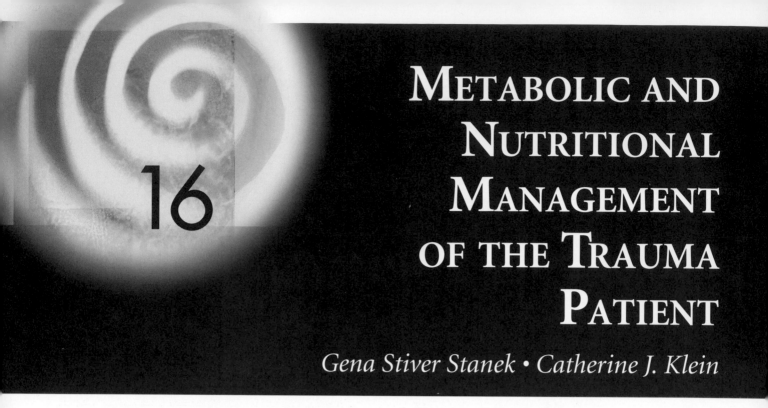

16

METABOLIC AND NUTRITIONAL MANAGEMENT OF THE TRAUMA PATIENT

Gena Stiver Stanek • Catherine J. Klein

OVERVIEW OF METABOLISM AND NUTRITION IN TRAUMA

In the healthy person a balance exists between anabolism and catabolism. Normal dietary intake replenishes the stores of carbohydrates and fat for oxidation and provides the proteins necessary for maintenance of enzyme function, muscle mass, and visceral proteins. Once a person is traumatically injured, the delicate balance between these processes is seriously disrupted. Trauma has a phenomenal impact on a patient's nutritional status. Critically ill trauma patients are characterized by metabolic alterations that favor catabolism (i.e., metabolic breakdown).

In trauma, glycogen stores are depleted rapidly, and the body must use endogenous substrates, protein, and fat to provide for the constant high energy needs that maintain physiologic functions. Increased demands coupled with the inability to ingest food set the stage for serious nutritional deficiencies. Despite the fact that a large number of patients admitted to trauma centers are young, previously healthy people who contain enough reserve to support the metabolic and healing processes for extended periods, severe trauma and sepsis can produce rapid weight loss and nutritional depletion. In fact, protein depletion may be accelerated in the athletic, muscular young trauma victim, and these patients eventually exhibit wasting from accelerated muscle catabolism. Protein depletion is common in the patient with a combination of severe catabolic stress and low nutrient intake. Protein malnutrition may result in decreased resistance to infection and poor wound healing. A well-planned, interdisciplinary nutritional assessment is needed for initial and ongoing evaluation of critically ill trauma patients.

Patients should be screened within 24 hours of admission to identify those who might benefit from a more in-depth evaluation of their nutritional needs. Nutritional assessments are conducted on high-risk patients to determine the appropriate nutritional interventions to prevent or correct malnutrition and promote healing. Nutritional assessment of the trauma patient is challenging. Traditional nutritional assessment strategies need to be validated for use in the trauma population. For example, mid-arm muscle circumference is not a valid indicator of nutritional status in a patient with edema. Similarly, serial weight measurements reveal little information regarding nutritional status in a critically ill trauma patient whose casts and Hoffman apparatus invalidate accurate interpretation.

When oral intake is prohibited, both enteral and parenteral nutrition support can provide substrates that may be lifesaving. The exact number of calories and the benefit of specific solutions (e.g., branched-chain amino acids, glutamine, and lipid composition) remain controversial and therefore need further research. Although total parenteral nutrition (TPN) has been vital in nutrient replacement, it is not a panacea. During TPN there is a marked reduction in the mass of the small and large intestines. Using the gut to some degree during TPN may be beneficial to retain intestinal mass and function. Specific nutrient formulations are being studied as they relate to improved gastrointestinal (GI) tract function and nitrogen retention. Numerous studies have described specific metabolic, mechanical, and infectious complications related to nutritional support.

Nutritional assessment and management are in a state of evolution. This chapter addresses state-of-the-art metabolic and technical management of the trauma patient. Familiarity with this information enhances the nurse's understanding of and ability to be actively involved in a truly interdisciplinary aspect of the trauma patient's care. Certain nutritional assessment techniques may be inappropriate in one phase of recovery yet be acceptable in another. Similarly, feeding modalities change as the patient begins to recover. Therefore this chapter addresses phase-specific patient alterations, nutritional assessments, nutritional goals, feeding modalities, and monitoring.

METABOLISM

NORMAL METABOLISM

Metabolism constitutes the cyclic physical and chemical changes that occur within cells during anabolism and catabolism. Normally there is a balance between the two processes. Anabolism is considered the process of food assimilation, or constructive metabolism. In contrast, catabolism involves a series of changes by which living matter is broken down into simple and less stable substances within a cell or organism. Energy metabolism is the transformation of fuel (food) into energy for work, such as breathing. Carbohydrates, protein, fat, trace elements, vitamins, and minerals all have integral roles in metabolism. These nutrients serve specific functions and have specific normal metabolic pathways.

ENERGY SUBSTRATE.   Carbohydrates, fats, and proteins are all used as energy fuel in the human body. These substrates are available from the digestion and absorption of food and from the breakdown of endogenous body tissue. In general, these substrates are allocated as follows: (1) protein compartments, (2) energy demand, and (3) excess calories to glycogen and adipose stores.

Glucose becomes the final compound for transport of almost all carbohydrates. The major purpose of carbohydrates is to supply direct and potential energy, sparing the use of protein and fat. Carbohydrates are the preferred energy source for the brain and formed blood elements. A lack of carbohydrates may lead to functional losses and ketosis and can cause potentially life-threatening problems. On the other hand, when intake of carbohydrates exceeds the amount needed, excess is stored in the form of glycogen in liver and muscle cells. This stored glucose is an important reservoir for maintaining constant blood glucose levels. The process of forming glycogen is called glycogenesis. Conversely, the breaking down of glycogen stores for energy is called glycogenolysis (Figure 16-1). The two principal hormones secreted by the pancreas, insulin and glucagon, control glucose metabolism.

Insulin affects the rate of glucose transport into the cells. When a person eats a meal, blood glucose levels rise and trigger increased insulin production from the beta cells of the pancreas. The presence of insulin facilitates transport of glucose into the cell, allowing more rapid transport. As glucose enters the cell, blood levels of glucose decrease to normal. In the opposite manner low levels of glucose

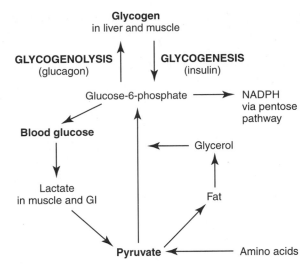

FIGURE 16-1 Glucogenesis and glycogenolysis.

stimulate production and secretion of the hormone glucagon from the alpha cells of the pancreas. Glucagon triggers glycogenolysis, stimulating the breakdown of glycogen stores into free glucose and increasing low blood glucose levels to normal.

A number of compounds in food are classified as lipids. These include (1) free fatty acids (FFA) and triglyceride, (2) phospholipids, and (3) cholesterol. After a meal, fatty acids are transported as triglyceride. Triglyceride is composed of three fatty acids bound to glycerol. Intravenous lipid contains triglyceride, phospholipid, glycerol, and some cholesterol. Some circulating lipid is taken up by reticuloendothelial cells, such as the hepatic Kupffer's cells. However, most fats are degraded by lipoprotein lipase (whose activity is stimulated by insulin) in the capillaries of adipose, cardiac, and skeletal muscle tissue. The resulting FFA can be further degraded for energy or reesterified into triglyceride and stored in adipose tissue. The triglyceride in fat cells is replaced every 2 to 3 weeks.

Excessive consumption of protein, carbohydrates, and fat promotes the synthesis and deposition of fat, whereas inadequate energy intake stimulates fat mobilization. The rate of turnover of FFA in the plasma is rapid (every 2 to 3 minutes). Any condition that increases energy demands also increases the concentration of FFA in the blood. When FFA leaves the fat cell for the purpose of providing energy, it combines with the plasma protein albumin to allow transport to other tissues. The exchange of fat from adipose tissue and blood is modulated by hormone-sensitive lipase. Fatty acids are used for fuel, particularly in the liver, heart, kidneys, and skeletal muscle. Once the FFA enters the cell, it is further broken down through the process of beta-oxidation to form molecules of acetyl coenzyme A (CoA), which can be oxidized for energy. The role of acetyl CoA as an energy intermediate is discussed in the following section on energy production.

Proteins can be broken down to amino acids, which are further broken down by deamination to form carbon chains that can generate energy. The amino groups (ammonia) removed during deamination are converted to urea for excretion.

The central nervous system (CNS) requires glucose as an energy substrate. When carbohydrate stores are low, a moderate quantity of glucose can be formed from certain amino acids and the glycerol portion of fat. This process of synthesizing glucose from amino acids and fat, gluconeogenesis, occurs in the liver and kidneys. The basic stimuli for gluconeogenesis are diminished amounts of carbohydrate in the cells and decreased blood glucose concentration. In addition, several hormones secreted by the endocrine glands, such as glucagon, are especially important in modulating this response.

In summary, carbohydrates, fats, and proteins are used as energy substrates. After meals, excess dietary carbohydrates are stored in the body as glycogen to provide a ready supply of glucose between meals. Fat serves as a vast reservoir of calories in times of stress. In contrast, only a small percentage of protein is used for energy. Multiple enzymes and hormones regulate the storage, use, and synthesis of these substrates.

ENERGY PRODUCTION.   Adenosine triphosphate (ATP) is the major chemical form of energy necessary for all aspects of cell life. Cellular and tissue functions dependent on the availability of ATP include muscle contraction, hormone secretion, membrane transport, and synthesis of new substances. The hydrolysis of high-energy phosphate bonds in ATP supply energy for biochemical reactions. When one phosphate bond is lost, ATP becomes adenosine diphosphate (ADP); similarly, the loss of a second high-energy phosphate bond yields adenosine monophosphate (AMP). Nutrients from food and body tissue are used to reform ATP from AMP and ADP.

The major function of glucose is to ensure adequate energy in the form of ATP. The breakdown of glucose or glycogen to pyruvic acid is called glycolysis. During glycolysis each mole of glucose yields two moles of ATP. After this, pyruvic acid is further broken down to acetyl CoA. If oxygen is available in the tissue, acetyl CoA enters the citric acid cycle, also known as the Krebs cycle or tricarboxylic acid cycle (TCA). Hydrogens (electrons) generated in the TCA cycle enter the electron transport (respiratory) chain, producing 34 ATP molecules. This occurs through a series of intricate oxidation-reduction reactions in which oxygen is the final electron acceptor. Energy production results in a net gain of 38 ATP molecules for each molecule of glucose degraded into carbon dioxide and water. The process of energy production results in oxygen consumption (Vo_2), heat, and carbon dioxide production (Vco_2). Carbon chains from the breakdown of fatty acids and amino acids are also used in the TCA cycle to produce ATP.

Under anaerobic conditions, energy production is extremely wasteful because only a small amount of the total energy in the glucose molecule is used. Glycolysis continues to produce two ATP molecules, since the conversion of glucose to pyruvic acid does not require oxygen. In the absence of oxygen, pyruvic acid and hydrogen ions (as $NADH + H^+$) build up and react with each other to form lactic acid, which diffuses out of the cells into extracellular fluids, creating a state of acidosis.

Proteins serve many essential functions: (1) enzymes catalyze chemical reactions; (2) transport proteins, such as albumin, provide a mode of transportation for nutrients and other substances; and (3) peptide hormones regulate metabolism and homeostasis. Because proteins serve specific metabolic functions, a low supply may have deleterious effects on health. General signs of protein deficiency include hair loss, loss of muscle mass, and edema. There are essentially two compartments of biologically available protein: somatic protein (skeletal muscle protein) and visceral protein (internal organ proteins and plasma protein). Proteins are constantly undergoing turnover; yet in a steady state the total body protein pool remains relatively constant. The synthesis of new protein from endogenous and exogenous amino acids is equal to degradation and loss of amino acids. Protein in the lining of the GI tract, liver, and kidneys turns over in approximately 3 days, whereas protein in skeletal muscle turns over in approximately 18 days. Some proteins are relatively inert, such as those that make up bone, cartilage, and tendons.

Most amino acids are conserved and reused to make new protein, yet a small amount is routinely catabolized and must be replaced. Of the 20 common amino acids, nine are considered essential because they cannot be synthesized in the body and must be supplied in the diet. The essential amino acids are histidine, lysine, phenylalanine, threonine, and tryptophan; the branched-chain amino acids (BCAA) isoleucine, leucine, and valine; and the sulfur-containing amino acid, methionine.[1] Dietary recommendations are expressed as protein because all food protein, except for gelatin, contains some of each essential amino acid.[1] The recommended dietary allowance (RDA) of protein for healthy adults is 0.8 g/kg of body weight, with an additional 10 g per day needed during pregnancy.[1] Protein intake in the United States far exceeds the minimum requirement and is usually not deficient in the diets of average persons, including vegetarians. Protein deficiency may be a problem for those who have limited access to food or severely restricted intake.

VITAMINS, MINERALS, AND ESSENTIAL FATTY ACIDS.   Energy production and protein synthesis depend on several vitamins and minerals, particularly the B vitamins, phosphorus, and magnesium (Figure 16-2). Vitamin coenzymes keep the process of energy production moving forward; phosphorus creates the bonds in ATP that store and release energy for metabolism; magnesium is required for glycolysis, fat oxidation, and protein synthesis. Table 16-1 outlines the role of macronutrients, vitamins, and minerals in wound healing.[1-3]

Two types of fatty acids are considered essential because they must be supplied in the diet: omega-6 linoleic acid and

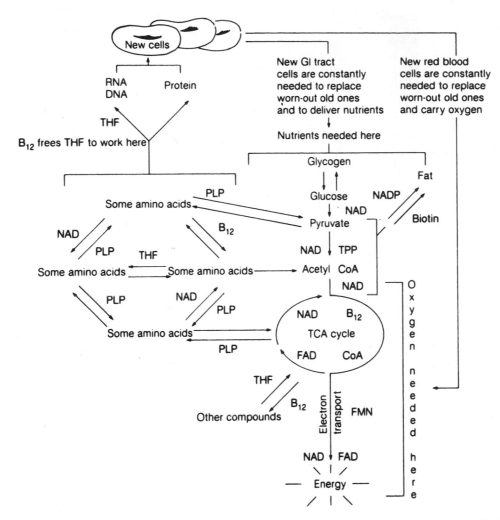

FIGURE 16-2 Role of vitamins in energy production and protein metabolism. (From Whitney EN, Hamilton EMN, Rolfes SR, editors: *Understanding nutrition*, ed 5, Pacific Grove, Calif, 1990, Wadsworth.)

omega-3 α-linolenic acid.[4] The body converts α-linolenic acid into docosahexaenoic acid (important for cell membrane structure in the brain and retina) and eicosapentaenoic acid (considered beneficial because of its antidysrhythmic, antithrombotic, and antiinflammatory effects).[4] Essential fatty acid deficiency (EFAD) can occur within days or weeks of administering fat-free TPN to trauma patients.[5] Signs of EFAD include hepatomegaly (from hepatic steatosis), elevated liver enzymes, hematuria, anemia, thrombocytopenia, scaly skin, and hair loss.[4,5] EFAD can interfere with wound healing and decrease resistance to infection. The Holman index is the ratio of 20:3n-9 to 20:4n-6 fatty acids. Amounts greater than 0.2 are indicative of EFAD.[4,5] Approximately 20 to 40 grams of linoleic acid and 2 to 10 grams of linolenic acid are needed each week. A minimum of 1 liter of a 10% soybean oil emulsion for intravenous use (2 × 500 ml bottles) can be administered during the course of a week to prevent EFAD in most adult patients who require TPN. Essential fatty acids are provided by most tube feeding formulas and parenteral lipid emulsions.

METABOLIC ALTERATIONS IN STARVATION

Tragic circumstances demonstrate that humans will not survive much past 60 days without intake of energy and protein. Death would ensue sooner if the body did not have the capacity to adapt to periods when food is scarce. A decrease or absence of nutrient intake alters how the body uses or conserves carbohydrates, fats, and proteins. Different mechanisms are at work, depending on the length of time the body is deprived of food. Starvation is the lack of food intake for several days to the time of death.

The effects of starvation lasting from several hours to several days are outlined in Table 16-2. Low nutrient intake causes blood glucose levels to decrease, with a concomitant fall in circulating insulin. Alpha cells in the pancreas respond to low levels of insulin by secreting glucagon, which stimulates glycogenolysis. Glycogen stores are used initially to increase blood glucose. Glycogen stores are depleted in approximately 24 to 72 hours. The body then relies on proteins and fat, which are oxidized for the purpose of supplying continued energy demands. Low levels of glucose

TABLE 16-1 Nutrition and Implications for Wound Healing and Recovery

Nutrient	Primary Functions	Indicators for Assessment	Outcomes of Nutrient Imbalance
Total energy	Sufficient ATP production to sustain metabolism, spare lean body mass, and promote wound healing	Indirect calorimetry; calorie counts; body weight; body mass index	Undernutrition: Local infection; slowed wound healing; weight loss; muscle wasting (amino acids used for energy); loss of fat pads increase risk of pressure ulcers at bony prominences; increased dependence on mechanical ventilation; slow progress in physical therapy Overnutrition: Increased body fat; health risk increases with increasing overweight
Amino acids (protein)	Protein synthesis, enzyme activity, growth of new tissue and maintenance of body cell mass, host defense, neural and muscular function, nutrient transport, and oncotic pressure	Albumin, transferrin, arm muscle area, nitrogen balance, blood urea nitrogen	Undernutrition: Delayed wound healing; muscle wasting; edema; dull, dry, sparse, depigmented hair; psychomotor changes; decreased resistance to local infection; weight loss Overnutrition: Dehydration, azotemia with possible alterations in acid-base balance
Glucose (carbohydrate)	Important energy source for tissues, particularly the central nervous system, red blood cells, leukocytes, and fibroblasts	Indirect calorimetry and RQ, blood glucose	Undernutrition: Muscle wasting (amino acids channeled to gluconeogenesis), loss of sodium and dehydration Overnutrition: Wound infection
Fiber (carbohydrate)	Gastrointestinal regularity and preservation of gut barrier as host defense	Diet analysis, stool consistency and regularity	Undernutrition: Constipation; strain of defecation may increase perianal wound dehiscence Overnutrition: Diarrhea with increased risk of stool contamination of perianal wounds
Fats	Constituent of cell membrane; needed for cell growth; source of energy for resting skeletal muscle; facilitates intestinal absorption of fat-soluble vitamins; substrate for synthesis of eicosanoids; role in visually cued learning	Triglyceride level, ratio of essential fatty acids in blood	Essential fatty acid deficiency: Impaired wound healing; decreased resistance to infection; disruption of epidermal water barrier; hair loss; possible decreased attention and cognitive processes Overnutrition: Congestion of reticuloendothelial system

Nutrient	Function	Assessment	Signs and Symptoms
Water	Nutrient transport, elimination of waste, matrix for chemical reactions, dissipation of metabolic heat, cellular growth and survival	Intake-output records: Abnormal fluid loss (seeping wounds, drains, diarrhea, sweating) or retention (renal failure); blood sodium; osmolality; urine volume	Water deficit: Decreased blood flow to skin, elevated body core temperature, headache and mental confusion, physical fatigue, renal failure. Overhydration: Cardiovascular stress, pulmonary edema and respiratory failure
Electrolytes (sodium, potassium, chloride)	Regulate blood volume; needed for normal blood pressure, acid-base balance, nerve transmission, muscle contraction, and hormone secretion	Blood electrolytes	Undernutrition: Physical weakness, anorexia, nausea, drowsiness, irrational behavior, gastric hypomotility, cardiac arrhythmia. Overnutrition: Edema, hypertension, cardiac arrest
Vitamin C	Collagen formation; needed for the function of leukocytes and macrophages; enhances iron absorption; protects DNA, proteins, and lipids from oxidation; preserves integrity of capillary structure; hormone biosynthesis; formation of norepinephrine from dopamine	Blood vitamin levels	Undernutrition: Collagen synthesis impaired; poor wound healing; infection; fatigue; ecchymoses and petechiae; hair follicles with a hemorrhagic halo; joint pain; swollen or bleeding gums; dry eyes and mouth. Overnutrition: False negative results for detection of occult blood; diarrhea; flushing; hyperuricosuria; hyperoxaluria; effects on red blood cell transfusions are still unknown; destruction of vitamin B_{12}
Vitamin B complex (thiamin, riboflavin, niacin, pyridoxine, folic acid, biotin, pantothenic acid, vitamin B_{12})	Integral component of ATP production and protein metabolism; drug metabolism; protects cell membranes and DNA from oxidation; nucleic acid synthesis and cell division for growth of new tissue; cell-mediated immune response; maintains integrity of hepatocytes, adrenal cortex, and nervous system; steroid synthesis and function; gluconeogenesis; neurotransmitter production	Blood vitamin levels; erythrocyte transketolase activity; urinary excretion of metabolites	Undernutrition: Slow growth of new tissue; fatigue, muscular weakness, and peripheral paralysis; tachycardia; respiratory distress; conjunctivitis; fissures at corners of mouth; swollen, beefy red tongue; papillary atrophy with smooth appearance; dermatitis; "burning feet" syndrome; neuropsychosis; nausea and abdominal distress; anemia. Overnutrition: Gastric upset; flushing; ataxia and sensory neuropathy; drug-nutrient interaction between folic acid and phenytoin

Continued

Modified from Food and Nutrition Board: *Recommended dietary allowances*, ed 10, Washington, DC, 1989, National Academy; Institute of Medicine, Food and Nutrition Board: *Dietary reference intakes for thiamin, Riboflavin, niacin, vitamin B6, folate, vitamin B12, pantothenic acid, biotin and choline*, Washington, DC, 1998, National Academy; and Ziegler EE, Filer LJ Jr, editors: *Present knowledge in nutrition*, ed 7, Washington, DC, 1996, ILSI.
RQ, Respiratory quotient.

TABLE 16-1   Nutrition and Implications for Wound Healing and Recovery—cont'd

Nutrient	Primary Functions	Indicators for Assessment	Outcomes of Nutrient Imbalance
Fat-soluble vitamins (A, D, E, K)	Cell differentiation and proliferation; integrity of the immune system, particularly the function of T lymphocytes; vision; calcium homeostasis and bone mineralization; protects cell membranes from oxidation; synthesis of prothrombin and clotting factors II, VII, IX, X; regulation of blood clotting	Blood vitamin levels	Undernutrition: Retardation of epithelialization, cross-linking of newly formed collagen, and impaired closure of wounds; dermatitis; peripheral edema; dry, rough inflamed skin; bruising; malaise; night blindness; higher incidence of severe infections; neuromuscular degeneration; anemia; impaired blood clotting. Overnutrition: Headache, emesis, alopecia, dryness of mucous membranes, blurred vision, muscular incoordination, calcification of soft tissue, altered platelet adhesion, nutrient-nutrient interaction between vitamin E and function of vitamin K
Calcium, phosphorus, and magnesium	Energy metabolism, protein synthesis, bone mineralization, nerve conduction, muscle contraction, blood clotting, beta oxidation of fatty acid	Blood and urine concentration	Undernutrition: Weakness; tetany, tremors, spasms; cardiomyopathy; anemia; nausea and gastrointestinal distress; hypokalemia, refractive to treatment; personality changes. Overnutrition: Nausea, hypotension, bradycardia
Zinc, iron, selenium, copper, manganese	Cross-linking of collagen and elastin, cell growth and repair, oxygen transport and energy production, defense against oxidative injury, formation and inactivation of hormones, biosynthesis of catecholamines, urea production	Blood minerals, ferritin, mean cell volume, hemoglobin, transferrin saturation, erythrocyte protoporphyrin	Undernutrition: Impaired thermoregulation, immune competence, wound healing, and growth of bone and cartilage; reduced life of erythrocytes; anemia; neutropenia; impaired taste; muscle weakness; cardiomyopathy. Overnutrition: Constipation, gastrointestinal discomfort, reduced immune function, nutrient-nutrient interaction of zinc and copper, psychiatric disorders, fatigue

Modified from Food and Nutrition Board: *Recommended dietary allowances*, ed 10, Washington, DC, 1989, National Academy ; Institute of Medicine, Food and Nutrition Board: *Dietary reference intakes for thiamin, Riboflavin, niacin, vitamin B6, folate, vitamin B12, pantothenic acid, biotin and choline*, Washington, DC, 1998, National Academy; and Ziegler EE, Filer LJ Jr, editors: *Present knowledge in nutrition*, ed 7, Washington, DC, 1996, ILSI.
RQ, Respiratory quotient.

	Starvation			
Characteristic	Early	Intermediate	Late	Injury
Metabolic rate		↓	↓	↑
Body temperature	No change	↓	↓	↑
Gluconeogenesis				
From protein	↓	↓	↑	↑
From fat	↓	↑	↓	↑
Blood glucose levels	↓	↓	↓	↑
Serum insulin	↓	↓	↓	↑ or no change
Glucagon levels	↑			↑
Catecholamines	Slight ↑			↑
Cortisol levels				↑
Blood lactate				↑
Free fatty acids	↑	↑		↑
Urine nitrogen excretion	↑	↓	↓	↑
Urine ammonia		↑		
Interleukin-1				↑
Body weight	↓	↓	↓	Varies
Muscle mass	↓	↓	↓	↓
Visceral protein		↓	↓	↓

TABLE 16-2   Characteristics of Starvation and Injury

and insulin continue to trigger the hormone-sensitive triglyceride lipase to mobilize fatty acids from lipid reserves in adipose tissue. A low concentration of insulin also stimulates muscle catabolism and release of amino acid from skeletal muscle. In addition, catecholamine (epinephrine, norepinephrine) excretion is increased during the first several days of starvation, further accelerating release of FFA and amino acids. Some amino acids are converted by the liver and kidneys into glucose, and other amino acids are used to replenish the four-carbon intermediate metabolites of the TCA cycle.[6] Amino acids are deaminated during this process, resulting in increased urinary nitrogen excretion, a byproduct of protein metabolism. To catabolize stored fat in the adipocyte, lipase cleaves the three fatty acids from the glycerol backbone of triglyceride. The released free fatty acids are carried in the bloodstream by albumin, and the freed glycerol travels to the liver for gluconeogenesis. The contribution of glycerol to gluconeogenesis equals that of all amino acids combined.[6]

The brain and central nervous system use about 80% of the glucose produced through gluconeogenesis in the liver. Other tissues that primarily use glucose are red cells, white cells, bone marrow, and cells of the renal medulla. Hepatic gluconeogenesis derives its energy from the oxidation of fat in the liver. Some fatty acids are only partially oxidized in the liver, forming ketone bodies. The remainder of the body, including skeletal muscle, will use both fatty acids and ketones as energy substrate. Therefore the need for glucose is minimized and protein is spared, resulting in decreased urea loss. Ammonia excretion increases and is highly correlated with ketonuria.[6]

The overriding goal of energy metabolism in starvation is to conserve energy while providing sufficient substrate to fuel processes that are vital for survival. As starvation continues, the brain and other glucose-dependent tissues begin to use even more ketone bodies to meet energy demands. Metabolic acidosis occurs, which is usually mild and of little consequence unless the patient is stressed; then buffer capacity is limited. Importantly, to conserve energy, overall body temperature and metabolic rate decrease gradually. Fat stores eventually become depleted, requiring even more endogenous proteins be destroyed to meet energy demands. Alanine and glutamine are the major glucogenic amino acids released from skeletal muscle. Alanine leaves the muscle by way of the blood, where it travels to the liver to form new glucose.

As prolonged starvation continues, protein compartments (both visceral and somatic) become severely depleted. Weight loss and muscle wasting are evident and excessive. Catabolism of body protein leads to decreased osmotic gradients, depressed enzymatic activity, and impaired immune competence. Thus the body is unable to respond efficiently to stressful situations such as infection or injury. At the very least, the body must have a continuous supply of amino acids or glucose to accompany fatty acid oxidation. Death ensues when one third of the endogenous protein supply is exhausted,[7] even if some fat stores remain available.[6] The optimal amount of dietary protein needed to treat severe starvation is not known, but the benefit of high-protein diets in the early phase of recovery has come into question.[8,9] Refeeding may need to start with 40% to 60% of the RDA for protein.[9]

In summary, fasting rapidly depletes glycogen stores, forcing the body to rely on gluconeogenesis from endogenous proteins and fat. With prolonged starvation, body tissues that depend on glucose to supply energy needs adapt and use ketone bodies (from fat catabolism) as energy substrate. The liver serves as the transformer, synthesizing glucose from protein and fat and using fatty acids as its main energy source. Protein depletion is minimized as much as possible. Continued starvation eventually leads to death after a critical amount of protein, vital for all body processes, is degraded and not replaced.

Unlike starvation, during which the body activates adaptive mechanisms that allow it to conserve energy for a prolonged period in the absence of food, the metabolic response to stress such as trauma, burns, or sepsis evokes a hypermetabolic response.

METABOLIC ALTERATIONS IN INJURY

Critically ill trauma patients are characterized by metabolic alterations that favor catabolism. Increased demands coupled with the inability to ingest food set the stage for serious nutritional deficiencies. Metabolic alterations occur immediately after injury because of increased neurohormonal activity. Unlike the starvation state, in which the body gradually adapts by lowering the metabolic rate and increasing utilization of fatty acids for energy while sparing protein, the physiologic milieu of critical illness results in rapid and accelerated proteolysis, gluconeogenesis, lipolysis, ketogenesis, and glycogenolysis. These catabolic processes occur in a population that needs energy to heal massive tissue injuries.

Various factors may elicit the metabolic response to injury. In the first 12 to 24 hours after traumatic injury, hypoxia, anoxia, decreased blood volume, pain, and anxiety trigger the "ebb phase." During the ebb phase, cardiac output, oxygen consumption, and temperature are decreased, whereas levels of catecholamines, glucagon, lactate, glucose, and FFA increase.[10] Once resuscitation occurs and these initial insults are managed effectively, the patient enters the "flow phase," a hypermetabolic period that may last for weeks. During this time cardiac output, oxygen consumption, and temperature may be elevated and lactate normalizes. Many factors contribute to the degree and duration of the hypermetabolic response. The mass of injured tissue, loss of normal barriers to infection, and starvation all play a role in the stress response to injury. In addition to the extent of primary injury and related complications, age, sex, and previous health influence the metabolic response to injury. Bloodborne chemical mediators, liberated directly from the site of injury by white blood cells as a result of the offending organisms, are of primary importance early in the stress response (Figure 16-3). In particular, endogenous pyrogens, such as interleukin-1 (IL-1) and tumor necrosis factor (TNF), produce fever, tachycardia, and leukocytosis and increase the hepatic uptake of amino acids, iron, and zinc.

After traumatic injury, the nervous system and these cytokines (IL-1, TNF) stimulate continued release of the stress hormones glucagon, catecholamines, and cortisol.[10] These hormones are responsible for the increased glucose turnover, oxidation, and metabolic rate. Sustained levels of cortisol and glucagon accelerate gluconeogenesis, leading to hyperglycemia. This hyperglycemia, known as the diabetes of stress, is resistant to control by insulin, probably because of the high hormone levels. Therefore the insulin level is normal or slightly elevated relative to the existing hyperglycemia. Lactate levels increase as a result of incomplete breakdown of glucose under anaerobic conditions. Cortisol and the catecholamines, epinephrine and norepinephrine, increase lipolysis, which increases circulating FFA.[10] Interestingly, cortisol's impact on metabolism is dependent on the CNS. If the spinal cord is transected above the level of tissue damage, the hypermetabolic response will be cancelled.[10]

Catecholamines increase the basal metabolic rate (hypermetabolism). Hypermetabolism means that the patient's energy expenditure at rest or under basal conditions is greater than if the person were healthy. A measured resting energy expenditure (REE) that is 110% greater than normal is indicative of hypermetabolism.[11] In most studies conducted up to 10 days after traumatic injury, REE is 120% to 155% above normal.[12-18] The body responds to traumatic injury with hypermetabolism in order to provide a steady supply of endogenous carbohydrates, proteins, and fats for use as substrate to support survival and recovery.

Fatty acids supply a considerable portion of energy in critical illness. Both basal concentrations of FFA and clearance of triglyceride are enhanced in septic patients compared with healthy persons.[19] The amount of fat mobilized from adipose tissue exceeds the amount that can be oxidized for energy. The leftover fatty acids increase the risk of hypertriglyceridemia.

All aspects of protein metabolism are accelerated in critical illness; however, protein catabolism is disproportionately increased relative to protein synthesis, resulting in a net loss of protein.[12,20,21] Protein synthesis is reprioritized; synthesis of acute-phase proteins (e.g., C-reactive protein, ceruloplasmin) that assist in immune function and wound healing increases. Other proteins (e.g., albumin, transferrin, and skeletal muscle) experience breakdown rates higher than synthesis rates. The catecholamines and the glucocorticoids act permissively, allowing an overwhelming release of alanine and glutamine from skeletal muscle.[22] These amino acids are shuttled to the liver for glucose production, resulting in increased production of urea (see Figure 16-3). In fact, nitrogen excretion parallels the severity of injury. The peak metabolic response and peak nitrogen excretion occur between 5 and 10 days after injury (Figure 16-4).[23,24] Previous nutritional status and age will influence the amount of protein catabolized. Young, healthy, muscular patients have a much greater degree of protein wasting. In contrast, an older, malnourished person

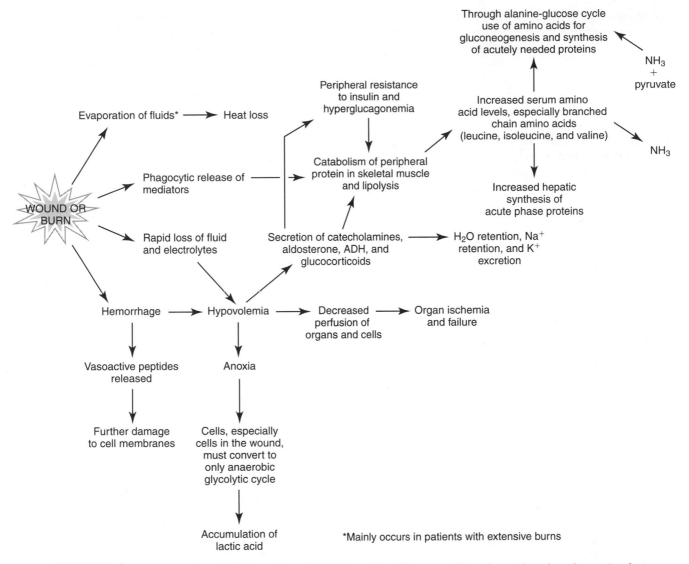

FIGURE 16-3. Physiologic and metabolic changes immediately after an injury. The extent of these changes depends on the severity of the trauma. (From Mahan LK, Escott-Stump S: *Krause's food, nutrition and diet therapy,* ed 9, Philadelphia, 1996, WB Saunders.)

has a lower rate of muscle catabolism. Although proteolysis can be modified slightly by feeding, this catabolic process cannot be altered significantly and lean body mass is sacrificed.[25]

If the hypermetabolic state is prolonged, greater amounts of lean body mass will be sacrificed, leading to cytokine-induced malnutrition. At this stage the immune system and wound healing could be impaired, and the sustained elevations in Vo_2, Vco_2, and energy expenditure may complicate recovery.[26] On the other hand, patients who are unable to maintain the manifestations of a hypermetabolic response and those who cannot mount a stress response in the first place, despite severe trauma, are likely to lose the battle and succumb to their injuries.[27,28] The metabolic responses to injury are summarized in Table 16-2.

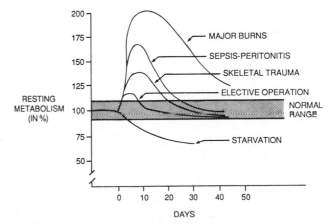

FIGURE 16-4 Stress-induced changes in resting metabolic expenditure. (Modified from Long CL, Schaffel N, Geiger JW et al: Metabolic response to injury and illness: estimation of energy and protein needs from indirect calorimetry and nitrogen balance, *J Parenter Enterol Nutr* 3:452-456, 1979. © American Society of Parenteral and Enteral Nutrition.)

THE NUTRITION CARE PROCESS

Nutritional care occurs as a process and is interdisciplinary in nature (Figure 16-5).[29,30] Initial baseline data are obtained from the patient and family. When this information is obtained early, it helps to predict whether the patient is at nutritional risk (phase I). Once the level of risk is established, appropriate referrals must be made.

Assessment strategies are determined individually, and nutritional goals and interventions are established. Nurses play a role in referral and planned intervention (phase II). More importantly, the nurse at the bedside provides constant surveillance and feedback, such as tolerance of tube feeding and complications of the implemented regimen. The evaluation process (phase III) involves subjective, objective, and biochemical data. If nutritional goals are not achieved, then a revised nutrition plan is developed. Once the goal is achieved, continued assessment by the health care team provides ongoing evaluation for maintaining goal and revisions as necessary. This process is dynamic because goals change throughout the trauma patient's recovery.

NUTRITION SCREENING

Current standards of the Joint Commission on Accreditation of Healthcare Organizations (JCAHO) specify that hospitalized patients must be screened for nutritional risk within 24 hours of admission by a qualified individual.[31] This screening will identify patients needing an in-depth nutritional assessment. Nurses are in a strategic position for identifying patients requiring further nutrition evaluation.

On admission a medical and dietary history should be taken. The nurse is frequently the person who obtains this information by way of a nursing database. In an intensive care unit (ICU) setting a family member is often the one who provides information; therefore the validity of this information may be questionable. Medical and dietary histories are focused on items that help to determine the patient's likelihood of nutritional deficiency before hospitalization. These include observations such as the following:

1. Recent weight loss or gain, with rationale
2. Diet history, special diets, food fadism, and types of foods eaten
3. Recent change in eating habits, with rationale
4. GI disorders
5. Chronic illness
6. Social factors, such as substance abuse or homelessness

These items help direct the assessor to dietary or medical imbalances that might result in nutrient deficiencies. Important clues include any other serious condition such as pressure ulcers or necrotizing fasciitis. Several nutritional deficiencies are associated with specific disease processes. Therefore knowledge of the disease (e.g., substance abuse) might lead one to suspect related nutritional deficiencies (e.g., protein, folate, niacin, thiamin, and riboflavin). These factors affect nutritional status and further complicate recovery. The susceptibility of malnourished patients to infection is well known. The combination of this scenario

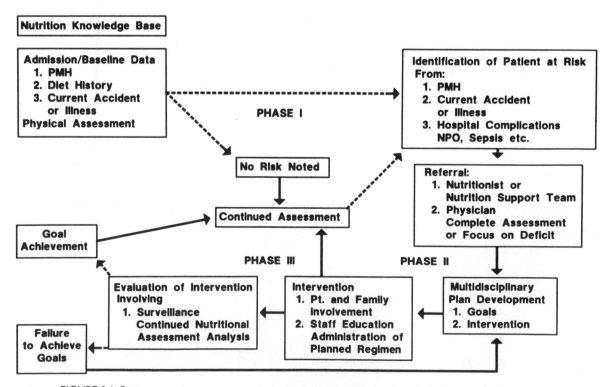

FIGURE 16-5 Nutritional care process. *Dotted lines* represent potential choices and *solid lines* are mandatory steps.

with a hypermetabolic trauma state increases the risk for complications.

Adults are considered nutritionally at risk if they have any of the following characteristics[30]:

1. Body weight change of 10% or more within the past 6 months, a change of 5% to 10% within the past month, being 20% above or below ideal body weight (IBW), or having an emaciated appearance
2. A restricted or required diet (e.g., diabetic diet, renal diet)
3. Inadequate intake for more than the past week

Identifying patients who are malnourished prior to admission is important because malnutrition is associated with poor long-term survival.[32] In addition, the traumatic event itself is critical to the risk assessment: The greater the magnitude of injury, the greater the risk for developing protein-calorie malnutrition. For example, patients who are not expected to consume food for more than 5 days because of severe traumatic brain injury, bowel resection, or other nutritionally disabling trauma should be categorized as at high risk for malnutrition. Patients in this group are provided with a full nutritional assessment to determine whether support is needed and, if so, what type. Most trauma centers have created their own admission screening forms to help nurses identify patients who are at high risk for malnutrition. The results of the nutrition screen need to be documented.[33] Patients considered not at risk must be rescreened for nutritional risk at regularly specified intervals or when nutritional or clinical status changes.[30]

Nutrition Assessment

Nutrition assessments are conducted to determine the patient's nutritional status and his or her nutritional needs. An evaluation of whether nutrition support is needed to correct nutritional imbalances (depletion or toxicity) and promote healing is included in the assessment. The assessment precedes the nutrition plan of care and intervention.[34]

All pertinent anthropometric, biochemical, clinical, dietary, energy, and psychosocial data are considered when assessing the patient's overall nutritional status. The patient's nutritional requirements are summarized, particularly the recommendations for protein and calories. An appropriate route of feeding and type of nutrition support formula, if needed, will be identified. The summary also includes fluid, electrolyte, and micronutrient requirements that will not be met by standard oral, enteral, or parenteral feedings. Psychosocial and socioeconomic factors that may influence prescription and administration of nutrition support are identified.[33] This evaluation is then translated into immediate and long-term nutrition goals. Special tests or procedures may be needed to follow up on nutrition-related concerns. The nutrition assessment is documented in the patient's chart and is used to develop the interdisciplinary plan for nutrition care.

Nutrition Plans

The nutrition care plan is developed by the patient's physician, nurse, and nutrition support service with input from other relevant health care personnel and family members. This effort produces a comprehensive interdisciplinary course of action.[31,33] Measurable and realistic patient-specific outcome goals are set. Interventions are planned to achieve these goals within an anticipated time frame. Nutrition therapy should be optimal, appropriate, and resource efficient. The care plan addresses patient and family education about nutrition therapy, discharge planning, and the need for home training. Reassessments are conducted to evaluate the efficacy of therapy, and goals and plans are changed as needed to enhance the patient's recovery.[31,33]

THE ABCs OF ASSESSMENT

Nutritionists may use a variety of techniques to assess a person's nutritional status. The most common measures for nutrition assessment will be discussed briefly. It is important to remember that nutritional indices may be influenced by nonnutritional factors, particularly in critically ill patients, and that standards derived from epidemiologic studies may not always be applicable to evaluation of a given person. Nutritional assessment should not depend on a single parameter but should involve multiple parameters, the interpretation of which must take into account the entire medical status of the patient. Typically the nutrition assessment is based on an evaluation of anthropometric measures (height and weight), biochemical data (composition of blood and urine), clinical data (from physical examination), dietary data (calorie counts), and measures of energy expenditure. These are collectively known as the ABCs of nutrition assessment.

ANTHROPOMETRICS AND BODY COMPOSITION TECHNIQUES

Anthropometric measures include all physical measures of the body, such as height, weight, weight history, triceps skin fold (TSF), and mid-arm circumference. In general, anthropometric data derived from a given individual are interpreted by comparison with normal values obtained from a healthy population of the same sex and age.

Prior height and weight estimates, when available, provide baseline information on current body weight. Weight relative to height is a measure of gross body composition and a valuable indicator of nutritional risk when compared with the patient's usual weight, desirable weight, or both. Weight is the most widely used measure of nutritional status because it is a general indicator of malnutrition. The main concern is evaluation of trends. Underweight is defined as having a body mass index (BMI) less than 18.5, whereas obesity is a BMI of 30 or greater[35] (Table 16-3).

Special attention must be paid to the obese patient, who commonly is mislabeled as overnourished for all nutrients. For example, an elderly obese woman was admitted to the trauma unit with severe protein malnutrition. Her calorie

TABLE 16-3   Equations Used in Nutrition Assessment

1. Body mass index (BMI) is used as an evaluation of weight status.[35]

   BMI = kg/(m)^2 where weight is in kilograms
   and height is in meters

2. Adjusted body weight is a combination of the ideal body weight (IBW) plus an estimate of the metabolically active weight of overweight.[33]

   Adjusted weight =
   [(Preadmission weight – IBW) × 0.25] + IBW

3. Hamwi equation for ideal body weight[38]

   IBW Men: 106 lb for the first 5 ft +
   6 lb for each additional inch

   IBW Women: 100 lb for the first 5 ft +
   5 lb for each additional inch

4. Percentage of usual body weight (UBW) is used as a reflection of weight change and the adequacy of energy intake.

   % UBW = (Actual body weight/usual body weight) × 100

5. Nitrogen (N) balance is a marker of severity of the acute phase response and a rough estimate of protein need in malnourished but otherwise healthy individuals.[55]

   N balance (g) = N intake – (N output in urine + 4)

   where 4 is an estimate of fecal and obligatory losses

6. The amount of nitrogen in protein is calculated using the following equation:

   $$\text{Nitrogen intake (g)} = \frac{\text{Protein (g)}}{6.25}$$

7. The Harris Benedict energy equation (HBEE) is an estimate of basal energy requirements.[53]

   HBEE Men: 66 + (13.8 × W) + (5 × H) – (6.8 × A)

   HBEE Women: 655 + (9.6 × W) + (1.8 × H) – (4.7 × A)

   where weight (W) is in kilograms, height (H) is in centimeters, and age (A) is in years

8. Total lymphocyte count (TLC) is calculated with the following equation.

   TLC = (% Lymphocytes × WBC)/100

intake was excessive; however, she had visceral protein depletion caused by a deficient protein intake. This patient's course was complicated by multiple infections, which are typical in people with visceral protein depletion. The energy needs of obese people are overestimated if body weights are not adjusted in calculations.[36] Traditionally body weight has been adjusted[37,38] for obese patients to minimize overfeeding (see Table 16-3).

Skin fold measures are a reflection of the body's energy storage (fat). Precise measurements for TSF are essential because the fat distribution in the upper arm is not uniform and limitations in accuracy depend primarily on location of the skin fold and intraobserver variability. Accuracy can be improved by marking the position of measurement directly on the skin, which also improves reliability. Mid-arm circumference and arm muscle area (derived from skin fold and circumference measures) are indicators of skeletal muscle protein mass. These measures cannot be used on edematous patients.

More technical methods to assess body composition are available in some hospital settings. These methods include duel-energy x-ray absorptiometry (DEXA) scanning to determine fat and muscle mass; gamma neutron activation analysis to measure total body protein; and in vivo tritiated water and sodium bromide dilution techniques to measure body water.[23]

BIOCHEMICAL TESTS AND NITROGEN BALANCE

The analysis of body fluids such as blood and urine yields a variety of biochemical data that are useful for nutrition assessments. Protein status, vitamin and mineral status, and essential fatty acid status may all be evaluated by numerous biochemical indices, although blood levels of minerals may not reflect tissue stores. Biochemical data, such as nitrogen balance, can be combined with dietary and anthropometric data for use in nutrition assessment.

An assessment of serum proteins helps to estimate visceral protein status. However, malnutrition should not be defined by visceral protein concentration alone; its assessment must include corroborating evidence from dietary and anthropometric data. Albumin, transferrin, prealbumin, and retinol-binding protein have varying sensitivities in estimating visceral protein depletion. Albumin levels in the serum do not decrease for some time during protein deprivation because albumin has a 14- to 20-day rate of turnover. Therefore serious protein deficits may exist before they are obvious. Various other factors, such as physical stress, infection, and hydration, are also associated with a decrease in serum albumin. Repeated studies have correlated hypoalbuminemia with increased morbidity and mortality.[32,39,40] Albumin has been used as a prognostic indicator because of this correlation.

Transferrin concentration varies widely in malnutrition and repletion. Interpretation of transferrin values is especially limited in the setting of iron deficiency anemia, when the production of transferrin is increased. Monitoring trends in prealbumin (transthyretin) can help answer questions about nutritional status and the adequacy of feeding. Prealbumin serves as a carrier protein for thyroxin (T$_4$) and retinol-binding protein. Because the half-life of prealbumin is only 2 to 3 days, prealbumin concentration decreases with even short periods of underfeeding and increases rapidly with diet therapy. Transferrin and prealbumin levels also decrease as part of the acute phase response after traumatic injury.

Nitrogen balance can be employed as an index of protein status because nitrogen is the primary component that differentiates protein from other basic nutrient moieties. Every 6.25 g of protein in a typical diet contains approximately 1 g of nitrogen. Nitrogen balance equals the nitrogen intake from protein, minus the nitrogen output as urine urea nitrogen plus obligatory nitrogen losses from skin, feces, drains, and menstruation (see Table 16-3). Typically, a factor of 4 is used to estimate obligatory losses from feces and skin. Total amount of nitrogen intake is calculated from the protein intake from enteral and parenteral routes in the 24-hour study period. Urine urea nitrogen is analyzed from a 24-hour urine collection to calculate nitrogen output.

Nitrogen balance is positive during anabolism when the body accumulates new tissue, such as during pregnancy or during growth in children. Nitrogen balance is negative when the body loses muscle mass, such as during weight loss. When body weight, body composition, and dietary intake are consistent during periods when intake is adequate, nitrogen balance is approximately zero. Numerous factors make nitrogen balance studies difficult to interpret:

- Nitrogen losses usually are lower in nutritionally depleted people.
- Accurate urine collection is required.
- The nurse must accurately maintain intake/output records.
- All nitrogen intake (oral, enteral, parenteral) must be calculated.
- All possible nitrogen losses (urinary, fecal, dermal) must be considered, and renal disease can confound the results.

CLINICAL EXAMINATION

Clinical data include the results of physical assessment and information about the patient's past and present medical status. A physical examination can contribute to identification of nutrient deficits, excesses, or fluid imbalance. During a physical assessment the clinician looks for abnormalities in skin, eyes, hair, nails, and oral and perioral body areas; these abnormalities are then evaluated with regard to nutritional status.[41] The clinical assessment also includes an evaluation of the impact of medical status on feeding and nutritional needs. Certain medical conditions might indicate a need to modify the route of feeding or the type of nutrients in the feeding solution/diet, such as restricting protein in the case of renal failure and restricting carbohydrates in the case of diabetes.[31]

FLUID AND DIET STATUS

Two main routes for water loss from the body are evaporation and urination. These losses need to be replaced. Evaporation from lungs and skin is known as insensible water loss. The amount of water lost in urine varies depending on the renal solute load.[42] The human body does not store water. Kidneys help to regulate water homeostasis by altering the concentration of urine to excrete more or less water as needed to maintain serum osmolarity around 300 mEq/L. Under average conditions, normal adults require

about 1 ml of water per kilocalorie of energy expenditure, or 35 to 40 ml/kg of body weight. Drinking in response to thirst sensation maintains water balance. Elderly persons whose thirst is blunted or whose kidneys have lost the ability to concentrate urine are at risk for dehydration.[1]

The dietary assessment evaluates the adequacy of current, previous, and required diets, including the number of days of restricted oral intake (NPO), the diet prescription, and eating disorders. Drug-nutrient interactions are considered. Food intolerance and allergies are taken into account, as are religious, cultural, ethnic, and personal food preferences.[31] Methods such as the 24-hour recall, food frequency questionnaire, and food records (calorie counts) help determine actual or usual intake. Standardized food composition tables are used to convert food into values of energy, protein, vitamins, and minerals. Dietary status is scored as part of calculating the Braden scale to categorize the patient's risk of developing pressure ulcers.[43,44]

ENERGY

ENERGY MEASURES.   Energy needs can be determined from actual measures of energy expenditure or from estimates based on published data. Classic investigations occurred during the first 25 years of this century, including those of Lusk, DuBois, and Benedict. Special populations of patients have stimulated research in the measurement of energy expenditure, such as patients with cancer, malnutrition-starvation syndromes, and critical illness. There is general acceptance that these acute conditions are associated with alterations in energy expenditure that favor weight loss, protein catabolism, and immunosuppression. Developments in TPN and new attempts at prophylactic nutritional regimens have prompted many new questions regarding energy expenditure and utilization by acutely ill or injured patients.

Basal metabolic rate (BMR), the thermogenic effect of food, and physical activity all contribute to the body's total energy expenditure. BMR is the amount of energy required to carry on the involuntary work of the body. This includes the functional activity of various organs, such as the brain, heart, liver, kidneys, and lungs; gland secretion; peristaltic movements of the GI tract; oxidation occurring in resting cells; and maintenance of muscle tone and body temperature. BMR is the measurement of caloric expenditure (heat production) in a person under specific controlled conditions, such as supine, at rest, with some muscle tone, and fasting a minimum of 12 hours in a thermally neutral environment. In normal people the BMR is depends on several factors, including body weight, body surface area, age, and sex. Body surface area best represents the metabolically active cellular component in the BMR. Studies show that females with the same body size as males have a lower BMR, primarily because women have a smaller proportion of lean muscle mass and therefore less active metabolic tissue. As people age, their metabolic rate decreases, which is also related to decreased lean body mass. The thermogenic effect of food represents the energy required for digestion and absorption of food and the stimulating effect of nutrients on metabolism. A major variable of energy expenditure in normal people is intensity and duration of activity.

Direct calorimetry measures the heat lost directly from energy expenditure. A kilocalorie is the amount of heat required to raise the temperature of 1 g of water 1° C at a pressure of 1 standard atmosphere (atm). Indirect calorimetry requires less equipment and is the method of choice in the clinical setting.

Indirect calorimetry determines energy expenditure using the quantification of gas exchange. It is based on the principle that a standard amount of oxygen is consumed for each mole of glucose oxidized; that is, Vo_2 and Vco_2 are quantified and related to heat production.[45] Typically subjects are measured at rest (resting energy expenditure [REE]) for 15 to 30 minutes; some patients are measured for a full 24-hour period (total energy expenditure [TEE]). REE is greater than BMR, but the difference is minimal. So, for practical purposes, REE is used to represent BMR. The equipment is calibrated before each use. In order for patients to be measured, they need to have an Fio_2 of less than 60% and there must not be any gas leaks in the collecting system, such as pleural leaks through chest tubes or leaks around endotracheal tubes. Tests begin once a steady state has been reached, meaning that average Vo_2, Vco_2, and respiratory quotient (RQ) vary less than 10% to 15% from minute to minute during 5 consecutive minutes.[46]

Indirect calorimetry has been widely accepted because of its close correlation to direct calorimetry.[3] Problems associated with the use of metabolic carts to perform indirect calorimetry are primarily related to the short duration of sampling periods, the expense of equipment for maintenance, and the need for trained personnel. Results from both direct and indirect calorimetry have been used to develop energy prediction equations.

The RQ is an additional gas exchange parameter obtained from a metabolic cart used in assessing nutritional status. The RQ is a ratio calculated by dividing the volume of CO_2 produced by the volume of O_2 consumed during the same period (Vco_2/Vo_2). If a mix of substrates (fat, carbohydrates, and amino acids) is used, the RQ will be approximately 0.85. This ratio will vary depending on the primary substrate being used. If glycogen is depleted and glucose is scarce, there is a gradual shift to oxidation of more fat and the RQ decreases to about 0.70. An RQ less than 0.70 has been associated with oxidation of ketones. Under other conditions where the intake of carbohydrates exceeds the requirements for glucose, glycogen stores are filled and cellular oxidation shifts to consume a greater percentage of carbohydrates. This produces proportionately more CO_2 than the amount of O_2 consumed, resulting in an RQ close to or slightly greater than 1. Extreme values for RQ may reflect methodologic error and should be regarded with skepticism.

A newer method to measure energy expenditure is the doubly labeled water technique. Water is labeled with ^2H and ^{18}O and given to the subject. After the labeled water equilibrates with body water, baseline samples of blood, saliva, or urine are collected to determine the ratio of ^{18}O to ^2H. After the study period, more samples are taken and compared with the baseline values to calculate daily energy expenditure. Although this method is accurate in healthy subjects, it is expensive, must be conducted over a period of many days, and requires specialized equipment for analysis.[3]

ENERGY ESTIMATES.   Over the years, numerous equations have been developed to predict energy expenditure, each with varying accuracy, such as the Fick equation and those by Fleisch,[47] the World Health Organization (WHO),[48] and others.[49-52] The Harris and Benedict energy equation (HBEE; see Table 16-3)[53] is the most widely used multiple linear regression formula to predict BMR because of its historical use and the ready availability of variables needed in the equation. The HBEE was developed by Harris and Benedict in 1919 from measures of indirect calorimetry. Weight, height, and age are included in the calculations. Because of gender differences, separate regression equations are used to determine metabolic rates for women and men. Several researchers have scrutinized the accuracy of the HBEE as a technique for determining energy needs. In fact, the HBEE has been validated as a method of predicting BMR in healthy older women[54]; predictions come within 114 calories of REE when analyzed by root squared prediction error. On the other hand, less than 74% of predictions from the HBEE come within 19% of REE for healthy, sedentary young adults, and predictions tend to overestimate REE.[55] Interestingly, predictions calculated using equations from the WHO came within 10% of the measured value for these young subjects.[55] Only five men older than 45 years of age were included in the HBEE study, so the validity of using the HBEE for older men is questionable.[53] There was also an insufficient number of subjects younger than 19 years of age to adequately represent BMR in teenagers. Furthermore, only 6 of 239 subjects were obese, so the original HBEE is not truly applicable to these groups. The HBEE can be modified by various factors to account for energy required for activity and the hypermetabolism of disease.

The Fick equation, used in combination with thermodilution techniques as an estimate of energy expenditure, requires hemoglobin concentration and simultaneous measurements of cardiac output and arterial and mixed venous oxygen saturations obtained from a pulmonary artery catheter.[46] Estimates derived from this method will most likely differ from indirect calorimetry by more than 20%, which means an unacceptable difference of 350 or more calories.[46,56] Substantial evidence exists to conclude that the Fick equation and thermodilution technique are unreliable and should not be used to determine nutritional support.

The REE for healthy, normal-weight adults is 23 to 24 kcal/kg of body weight. The recommended intake for older adults and sedentary adults is 30 kcal/kg, which is approximately the HBEE × 1.3. The average energy need for healthy, active younger adults is approximately 40 kcal/kg; it rises with increasing physical activity.[1] Of course, weight status will influence energy need: People who need to lose weight need to consume less than their energy expenditure, and those who need to gain weight need to eat more energy than they expend.

IMMUNOLOGIC TESTS

An intact immune system is of utmost importance in traumatically injured patients. Numerous clinical observations and epidemiologic data document a close association between protein-calorie malnutrition and increased susceptibility to infection. Immune functions are influenced by multiple factors, including nutritional status; therefore evaluation of such parameters is of nutritional importance. Protein-calorie malnutrition is recognized as the most common nutritional cause of immune dysfunction, although deficiencies of other nutrients, such as zinc and iron, can also change immunologic responses. Total lymphocyte count (TLC) is one way to assess immune function.

Multiple factors can alter TLC and must be considered before low counts are used to reflect the degree of protein depletion. For example, lymphocytopenia has been observed in well-nourished patients after anesthesia and operations; such depressed counts usually return to normal within 48 hours. In contrast, an elevation in white blood cells (leukocytosis) may be caused by a number of factors, including tissue necrosis or infection. Therefore the use of TLC as a nutritional parameter depends on excluding the influence of many possible nonnutritional factors. In general, this assessment parameter would be collected and used for noting trends in relation to the patient's clinical picture. Potential research also exists in this area.

The calculation for TLC is shown in Table 16-3. A level less than 1500 cells/mm³ indicates moderate nutritional depletion; a level less than 900 cells/mm³ indicates severe nutritional depletion. Considering the influence of nonnutritional factors such as sepsis, necrosis, and surgical interventions evident in most trauma patients, TLC is of limited use in the intensive care unit.

Loss of immune competence may also be evaluated by skin antigen testing. The inability to respond to an antigen challenge (anergy) is related to nutritional depletion. Delayed-type hypersensitivity reactions to common skin test antigens have been used to evaluate function of the cellular immune system. Subjects who are tested repeatedly may exhibit accelerated reactions, which start within several hours after injection, peak within 24 hours, and subside quite rapidly, indicating increased response without any nutritional treatment. However, after trauma, skin antigen testing is almost never sensitive because surgery and trauma blunt the normal response. Therefore this test should not be used as a method of nutrition assessment in the trauma setting.

Additional tests such as measurement of thymus-dependent lymphocytes (T cells) and lymphocyte mitogen assays are used in research settings as a means of assessing nutritional status. The T-cell count is decreased because of malnutrition but will increase after nutritional therapy. Results are expressed as the number of T cells per microliter of whole blood compared with normal control tests. Lymphocyte mitogen assays assess lymphocyte function in vitro. Lymphocytes are incubated with a mitogen such as concavalin A, phytohemaglutinin, or pokeweed mitogen and labeled with tritiated thymidine. The proliferation of lymphocytes is determined by counting the tritiated thymidine per culture. A low response, compared with normal control tests, indicates immune dysfunction.

PSYCHOSOCIAL ISSUES

Nurses collect the majority of psychosocial data during the initial medical history. Factors that may influence the patient's nutritional status include family dynamics, language barriers, psychiatric disorders, finances, and patient preferences and directives with regard to intensity and invasiveness of care.[33]

CRITICAL CARE MANAGEMENT

PATIENT CHARACTERISTICS

Catabolism is the most striking characteristic of the critical care phase of injury. Once the patient is hemodynamically stable, fat loss can be prevented and cell composition can be preserved with adequate feeding. However, the muscle protein compartment suffers considerable loss, exceeding what might be expected in relation to food intake.[23] This hypercatabolic response peaks approximately 10 days after injury, then gradually decreases (see Figure 16-4).[24] The degree of catabolism and hypermetabolism and the duration of negative nitrogen balance depend on the extent of injury, the nutritional status of the patient at the time of injury, and the medical course after injury. Patients recovering from blunt trauma lose an average of 6.4 kg of skeletal muscle over 21 days.[23] Prolonged protein catabolism could result in muscular weakness, contributing to inadequate pulmonary ventilation and cardiac insufficiency; reduced immune system potency; and, eventually, loss of wound strength and improper healing.

Most trauma patients have disruption of several physiologic systems and have undergone extensive surgical interventions. Massive blood loss results in coagulopathies and hemodynamic instability. Patients typically have subnormal blood albumin and prealbumin concentrations as a result of the stress response regardless of their nutritional status before injury. Depending on the degree of organ failure, patients may develop hyperglycemia and hypertriglyceridemia, which can limit their ability to tolerate certain types of feeding. The GI tract is rendered useless for the first 42 to 48 hours because of extensive surgeries and the resulting upper GI ileus. Abdominal trauma requiring bowel surgeries might eliminate the GI tract as a route for nutrient intake unless a jejunostomy tube for feeding can be used. Patients with severe head injury, altered levels of consciousness, and loss of the gag reflex may not be capable of oral intake for long periods. Similarly, paralytic ileus is common initially in the spinal cord-injured population because of autonomic disruption and ischemia at the time of injury.

The neurologically injured patient may exhibit increased energy expenditures greater than those of the general multiple-trauma patient, but they are extremely variable. Multiple nutritional assessment parameters need to be obtained and reviewed in relation to the total clinical picture to make an appropriate assessment and intervention.

The overall goal for nutritional intervention during this catabolic phase is provision of nutrients and energy requirements for maintenance. Halting the hypermetabolic response to injury is not yet possible. Fortunately the response is self-limiting, provided that wounds are debrided and closed, infections are prevented or treated, and supportive nutritional measures are maintained.

ASSESSMENT

ANTHROPOMETRICS. Weight, skin fold, and circumference measures may be impossible to obtain in the critical care phase because of orthopedic, neurologic, burn, and other injuries. Furthermore, traction, mental status, and edema make it difficult to measure patients who are unable to sit or stand upright. Even when measures are obtained, they are difficult to apply because standard tables for evaluating anthropometric data have not been developed for the trauma population. In contrast, preinjury weight and weight/height ratios, such as BMI, provide a baseline index and should be used for a general comparison of nutritional reserves in the patient with traumatic injuries.

If body weight is measured for nutritional purposes, the nurse will need to consider that body casts, braces, Hoffman apparatus, and other devices will falsely elevate body weight. Also, day-to-day variations in weight may occur because of edema. The early postadmission weight of the multiple-trauma patient is elevated above the preinjury weight as a consequence of fluid resuscitation. On average, nearly 5 L of resuscitation fluid will be retained by the time the patient is hemodynamically stable,[23] which adds approximately 10 kg in weight.[57] Body weight is then lost at a rate of approximately 0.8 kg/day until preinjury weight is restored around day 10.[57] Early weight changes may be more reflective of fluid status than muscle or fat status in the critically ill patient. Following long-term trends in changes in body weight may be more appropriate than using actual body weight.

Body weight should be adjusted after amputations. To estimate postamputation weight, 6% of preinjury weight is subtracted for a below-the-knee amputation and 12% of preinjury weight for an above-the-knee amputation.

In light of these findings, anthropometric measures should be used cautiously, if at all, during the critical phase of trauma. Their use is more appropriate during the intermediate and rehabilitation phases of recovery.

BIOCHEMICAL TESTS AND NITROGEN BALANCE. Blood minerals are checked repeatedly in critically ill patients and should be replaced if their levels are low, especially potassium, phosphorus, calcium, and magnesium. Iron itself is not directly regulated in the intensive care unit, but its related blood products (e.g., hemoglobin) are monitored. Albumin levels below 3 g/dl are common in critically ill trauma patients, who exhibit hypoalbuminemia for multiple reasons. Expansion of the extracellular fluid compartment will result in a reduction in serum albumin, as will excessive loss by way of kidneys, steroid administration, blood loss, and the stress response to injury. The concentrations of other serum proteins such as transferrin, retinol-binding protein, prealbumin, somatomedin-C, fibronectin, and C-reactive protein are altered in the acute phase of trauma. Their measure often reflects the stressed state, not nutritional status or adequacy of nutrition supplementation.[32] Blood products may contain prealbumin. Therefore, if the patient receives massive transfusions, the prealbumin test may reflect exogenous prealbumin rather than that synthesized in the patient's liver. Steroid medication such as methylprednisolone can also elevate prealbumin concentration. Therefore prealbumin measurements should be used cautiously and only for monitoring trends during this phase of recovery.

The physical stress of severe trauma and sepsis alters the balance between anabolism and catabolism, favoring protein catabolism. Nitrogen balance in this case would be negative because of the greater degree of protein degradation. Feeding will not prevent nitrogen depletion during this period. Nitrogen balance serves as an indicator of the magnitude of injury rather than as an indicator of the amount of protein needed.

CLINICAL EXAM. A review of systems for the purpose of assessing the patient's capacity to tolerate feeding and the likely start time for feeding should be made as soon as possible. Answers to the questions outlined in Table 16-4 will help to determine nutrient need and the route and composition of feeding.

DIETARY DATA AND NUTRIENT NEEDS. Past diet information, such as food allergies and preferences, collected during the initial medical history is reviewed. Length of time NPO or without adequate intake is determined. Diet orders, actual intake, intravenous fluids, repletion orders (particularly for phosphorus, potassium, and magnesium), and diet prescriptions are evaluated with regard to adequacy and appropriateness.

Obtaining 24-hour energy expenditure repeatedly through indirect calorimetry is the best method available to predict energy expenditure in critically ill patients. To prevent overfeeding, this measure is particularly useful in the elderly, in patients who are obese or unusually small, and in those who are severely malnourished or diabetic. Measures should also be obtained in patients who are having difficulty weaning from the ventilator. Patients who are difficult to wean include those with low cervical and upper thoracic spinal cord injuries, pulmonary contusions, rib

TABLE 16-4   Questions to Assist the Clinician in Planning the Appropriate Route and Composition of Feeding

1. Is the patient unconscious, mechanically ventilated, or otherwise unable to take in food safely or adequately?
2. Does the patient have high gastric residuals, a firm abdomen, a lack of bowel sounds, or other signs of ileus?
3. What access is currently available for feeding (e.g., gastric tube, triple lumen catheter)?
4. Is there a head-of-bed restriction, is the patient on a rotating bed, or are there other factors that would increase the risk of aspiration?
5. What organs and tissues are injured or impaired? Could this affect the patient's tolerance of certain substrates or limit the routes of feeding?
6. What other medical plans are being made, such as surgery, dialysis, or weaning from the ventilator? Could these plans impact nutrition?
7. How is the skin integrity? Does the patient have open or draining wounds? Are there pressure sores or necrotizing fasciitis?
8. What medications are being administered? How might they affect nutrition?
9. How does the patient look compared with all the information you have received in the chart and verbally from others? Does your visual assessment match the information? (Do the height and weight appear to be what was reported?)

TABLE 16-5   Clinical Factors Associated With Altered Energy Expenditure

Clinical Factor	Elevated Expenditure	Depressed Expenditure
Feeding	Glucose infusion Overfeeding	Underfeeding
Medication	Glucocorticoids	Neuromuscular blocking agents Sedation (nonspecific) Sodium pentobarbital
Activity	Dressing changes Agitation Motor activity (muscle rigidity, fine motor tremors) Shivering	Bed rest
Patient status	Traumatic injury Severe thermal injury Surgery Ventilator dependency Fever Sepsis (but no septic shock)	External cooling (no shivering) Protein-calorie malnutrition Spinal cord motor deficit

Modified from references 14, 16, 18, 28, 58-62.

fractures, or hemopneumothoraces and patients with premorbid pulmonary diseases.

Energy expenditure cannot be measured with a metabolic cart in all patients, only those in a relatively stable state (see Energy Measures). Indirect calorimetry is often conducted while the patient is being fed continuously. Therefore these measurements already include the thermogenic effect of food. Typically the subject is monitored for 15 to 30 minutes, and the values obtained are projected for a 24-hour period. Sample periods of short duration do not reflect changes that occur in the critical care environment. Anxiety-provoking and painful procedures are examples of the many variables that alter metabolic rate throughout the day. Chest physiotherapy may cause the most sustained increase in metabolic rate.[45] Readings taken over time help to minimize respiratory variation.

Hyperventilation can cause an inaccurate test. Initial REE measures taken during the ebb phase, soon after injury, are lower than later measures in the flow phase. REE can vary from day to day in any one patient and vary considerably between patients, particularly those with neurotrauma. Anthropometric factors such as body surface area, body weight, age, and sex contribute to intersubject variation[14,18]: Women and the elderly expend fewer calories than others.[14,17] Although patients with fever expend more energy,[14] body temperature fluctuates with medical intervention, and an elevation in it may not warrant modifying energy goals.

However, consistent temperature elevations increase energy needs. Factors that alter energy expenditure in hospitalized patients are listed in Table 16-5. In most studies that include patients with traumatic injuries, REE averages 2000 to 2600 kcal/day (approximately 28-30 kcal/kg).[12-14,16-18,63,64]

Trauma patients as a group are more hypermetabolic than other critically ill patients. Interestingly, injury severity is not even moderately correlated with energy expenditure when severity is scored by the Glasgow Coma Scale (GCS), Injury Severity Score (ISS), multiple diagnoses, or Acute Physiology and Chronic Health Evaluation II (APACHE II).[14,36,54,64] Energy expenditure does not always correlate with severity of illness because people who are severely and terminally ill may not be hypermetabolic. Oxygen consumption, and hence energy expenditure, is suppressed in patients who have a high risk of mortality,[27] resulting in REE approximately equal to normal (HBEE).[28] This does not support the practice of assigning ever increasing injury factors to amplify feeding as the injury severity and the number of failed organs increase. In fact, erring on the side of underfeeding would be best because macronutrient loads are less likely to be tolerated by the sickest patients.

Accurately assessing energy needs is important because complications from inappropriate feeding can be serious and prolong recovery. Regression equations, such as those developed by Ireton-Jones[65] and Frankenfield[18] to estimate

TABLE 16-6	Energy and Protein Recommendations	
Phase	Total Energy Needs	Protein Needs
Critical care	25-30 kcal/kg	1.2-1.5 g/kg
Intermediate	25-30 kcal/kg	1.0-1.5 g/kg
Rehabilitation	25-40 kcal/kg	0.8-1.5 g/kg
Normal	30-40 kcal/kg	0.8 g/kg

Modified from references 12-18, 63, 64.

REE in critically ill trauma patients, only approximate actual REE and offer little improvement in precision over other equations.[46,66] They do a good job of predicting mean REE for a group of patients, but their poor precision on estimates for any one patient (± 400 or more kcal) renders their clinical application inadequate and potentially harmful in those susceptible to complications from overfeeding.[46,66] Another method attempts to estimate hypermetabolism by multiplying the HBEE by an injury/stress factor. This method results in substantial overestimation or underestimation, particularly in patients with traumatic brain injury, and is not recommended.[67]

When actual measures are not possible, 25 kcal/kg can be used for adults over the age of 65 years and 30 kcal/kg for other adults of normal weight (Table 16-6) in place of the more traditional regression equations. For obese patients (BMI >30) and amputees, adjusted body weight is inserted into these equations (see Table 16-3).

The critical care phase may require more than 1 g of protein/kg of body weight[57]; amounts greater than 1.5 g/kg show no additional nutritional benefit[25,57] and may be detrimental. Protein requirements need to be monitored carefully in elderly patients and patients with acute renal failure (see Table 16-6).[68-70] Research by Braden supports an average daily protein intake of approximately 120% of the RDA (96 g/day) to protect patients from developing a pressure sore.[43] Supplementation of extra nutrients such as vitamin C and vitamin E remains controversial. Supplemental vitamin E, for example, can be detrimental to wound healing.[71,72]

Appropriate assessment, monitoring, and interventions by the interdisciplinary team in the critical care phase will minimize complications from both enteral and parenteral nutrition and allow early goal achievement. The patient's nutritional care plan should be reviewed by the interdisciplinary team regularly, and modifications should be made based on the patient's laboratory values and clinical status. Outcome goals should be an integral part of the plan, and specific target dates should be set for achievement of the goal.

RANGE OF MOTION

An important but often overlooked aspect of the patient's plan of care centers around range-of-motion activities. Feeding adequate diets will not necessarily increase muscle mass. To build muscle, one must exercise. Disuse not only causes muscles to weaken and atrophy, but causes bones to lose minerals, decreasing bone density. Promoting muscle activity, both initially as passive activity and later as more strenuous activity, may improve muscle function and growth. Frequent passive exercises should be incorporated into the patient's daily activities. The physical therapist should be consulted at the earliest possible date to assist in planning progressive activity.

SELECTING APPROPRIATE NUTRITION SUPPORT

Fluid and blood product resuscitation and control of major fluid, electrolyte, and acid-base disturbances should be achieved before nutrition support is initiated. Patients who are in shock and those requiring substantial amounts of fluids and inotropic agents are likely to have poor perfusion to the GI tract. Feeding increases the demand for oxygen, so feeding into a poorly perfused gut can exacerbate GI ischemia and even lead to bowel necrosis.[72] Patients with mild to moderate injuries who were previously well nourished can be provided with 5% dextrose in water (D_5W) if they are expected to resume oral intake within 5 to 7 days. This provides 120 to 180 g of glucose/day (400 to 600 kcal/day), an amount that should meet the glucose requirements of the brain and formed blood elements.

ROUTE OF FEEDING. The type of feeding modality used depends largely on the severity and type of injury and the expected recovery period. The physician usually has some idea how long patients will be NPO and whether a patient will tolerate a certain feeding modality. Most sources agree that a nutritional regimen should be initiated no later than 3 to 4 days after injury. The goal in feeding is to nourish the patients adequately and safely through the best route possible. The common rule of thumb for feeding is that oral is better than tube feeding, which is better than parenteral nutrition. Lipman[73] reviewed the evidence comparing tube feeding with TPN and concluded that with the exception of cost and possibly a reduced septic morbidity in abdominal trauma with tube feeding, appropriate TPN may be as safe and efficacious as enteral nutrition. According to Campbell,[74] there is no evidence to suggest that the route of feeding will improve outcome once multiple organ dysfunction syndrome (MODS) is established. Some theorize that atrophy of the gut related to delays in enteral feeds may be one of the precipitating factors for MODS. Bacterial translocation from the gut to the bloodstream can occur in rodents; however, not all studies conducted on these animals under conditions of stress found a favorable outcome with enteral feeding compared with intravenous nutrition.[75] The role, if any, of gut atrophy and translocation in the development of postinjury MODS in humans is not completely clear.[73,74]

In general the gut is not a dormant organ and therefore is considered vital to the patient's nutritional plan of care. Small bowel motility and absorption may remain intact despite surgery or injury, and feeding into the jejunum should be considered even if gastric or colon motility or peristalsis is impaired. Primary considerations in choosing

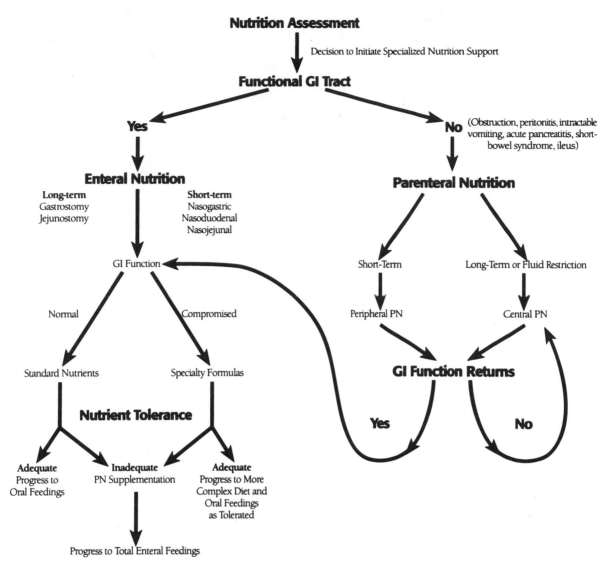

FIGURE 16-6 Routes to deliver nutrition support to adults: clinical decision algorithm. *GI,* Gastrointestinal; *PN,* parenteral nutrition. (From ASPEN Board of Directors: *Clinical pathways and algorithms for delivery of parenteral and enteral nutrition support in adults,* Silver Spring, Md, 1998, American Society for Parenteral and Enteral Nutrition.)

the feeding route and formula include degree of GI function, expected duration of nutrition therapy, aspiration risk, and degree of organ dysfunction.[30] A feeding algorithm was developed by the American Society for Parenteral and Enteral Nutrition (ASPEN) to assist clinicians in selecting the route and type of nutrition support (Figure 16-6).[30]

SPECIALIZED FORMULAS. Various formulas are available for feeding, and the dietitian recommends a specific formula based on the patient's condition. Several nutritional additives remain controversial. Administration of formulas enriched with branched-chain amino acids (BCAA) is promising but so far lacks conclusive evidence of benefit for trauma patients. Some studies fail to confirm any benefit to BCAA enrichment, whereas several others have demonstrated increased nitrogen retention,[76] improved protein synthesis,[77] greater visceral protein concentration, and decreased mortality.[78] Further research is

needed to replicate these findings, particularly the effect, if any, on outcome.

Some specialized enteral formulas have been called "immune enhancing" because they contain arginine and other supplements thought to promote healing.[79] However, more research is needed to determine whether any of these ingredients actually confers a beneficial effect. Arginine is an amino acid that enhances synthesis of nitric oxide in the endothelium. When produced in small amounts, nitric oxide plays a major role as a vasodilator.[79,80] However, when released in large amounts by macrophages, nitric oxide promotes autoimmune tissue damage. Another concern with arginine supplementation is that it can increase azotemia by 30% and raise the concentration of L-ornithine (a prosclerotic agent) in patients with renal failure.[80] Research about arginine is of interest because, under experimental conditions, arginine also increases insulin-like growth factor-1 plasma concentration, which increases the hydroxyproline content in wounds, promoting wound healing.[81] Yet in clinical studies, patients with traumatic injuries (ISS >13) who were given arginine along with extra trace elements and omega-3 fatty acids required considerably longer ventilator support and had longer lengths of stay compared with those fed a standard formula.[68] In another study[82] trauma patients (ISS >20) did not benefit from arginine-enriched diets. In fact, their infection rate, hospital stay, and mortality did not differ from those of patients in the control group.

Another supplement, glutamine, improved wound healing in rodents,[83] decreased infectious complications in patients after traumatic injury,[84] and improved long-term survival for patients with MODS.[85] Although these are impressive results, glutamine supplementation may not be beneficial for all patients. Glutamine supplementation might be contraindicated at least initially after focal contusions and ischemic events in the brain, particularly if there is a disruption of the blood-brain barrier.[86,87] Also, glutamine supplementation may not be appropriate for patients with hepatic insufficiency or those with glutamine-expansion disorders such as Huntington's disease.

ENTERAL SUPPORT AND MONITORING

Many patients require enteral nutrition support because they are mechanically ventilated or because diminished gag or cough reflex or altered consciousness puts them at risk for aspiration if they eat or drink. If the patient has a functional GI tract, enteral nutrition should be initiated. Feeding into the gut assists in maintaining a thicker gut barrier, which in turn protects the gut against the effects of stress and medications, such as inflammation, ulceration, and bleeding.[88] Enteral feedings benefit the GI absorptive structures by nourishing enterocytes at a local level. The gut resists invasion by pathogenic organisms by the physical barrier formed by its endothelium and by the submucosal collection of coordinated lymphatic tissue known as the gut-associated lymphatic tissue (GALT), which produces secretory IgA.[89]

SELECTING AN ENTERAL ROUTE.
Determining the length of time feeding is needed assists the clinician in deciding the most appropriate enteral route. However, the length of time that enteral nutrition support will be needed might not be evident initially. For example, a patient who has had traumatic brain injury and is comatose may wake up quickly or take weeks to months to be able to take in food voluntarily. Therefore the short-term approach of using an existing orogastric or nasogastric tube is often tried first, but this varies with the aggressiveness and expertise of the medical team.

Frequently the trauma patient has pulmonary injuries such as pulmonary contusions, aspiration at the scene, hemopneumothorax, or acute respiratory distress syndrome (ARDS). Injuries such as these make aspiration an even greater risk in a patient with an already compromised pulmonary system, particularly if the patient has a head-of-bed restriction, requires periodic alternating supine

and prone repositioning, or needs frequent chest physiotherapy. Therefore postpyloric feedings past the ligament of Treitz (in the fourth portion of the duodenum) are preferred to eliminate duodenogastric reflux of feeding.[88] The algorithm developed by ASPEN (see Figure 16-6) provides a template for nutrition teams to work from to select the appropriate route and tube.[30] Ideally an interdisciplinary nutrition support team uses an algorithm or a clinical pathway approach with clearly defined roles to guide the selection of feeding tubes and feeding route.

For patients needing long-term (>3-4 weeks) enteral nutrition support, gastrostomy or jejunostomy is preferred. In contrast, short-term (<3-4 weeks) enteral support can be administered via a nasogastric, nasodudodenal, or nasojejunal route. The nasal route is contraindicated for trauma patients who have coagulopathies and those with facial fractures, particularly nasal fractures, or CNS trauma. An orogastric/enteric route is usually chosen for patients with facial trauma or sinusitis. If risk of aspiration is not high, feeding into the stomach is ideal, since this is most natural.

TUBE SELECTION, PLACEMENT AND CARE.
The rigid, large-bore tubes that are initially placed for gastric decompression have several potential problems if they remain in use for long-term feeding. The trachea and esophagus are anatomically close, which can predispose the patient to a tracheoesophageal fistula. Thus the two rigid tubes create pressure, with eventual necrosis and fistula formation. Similarly, gastritis and esophagitis are not uncommon complications of rigid nasogastric tubes. The rigid tube may also prevent complete closure of the cardiac sphincter and therefore permit reflux of acidic gastric contents into the esophagus. Chronic esophagitis can lead to esophageal strictures. If enteral nutrition support is expected to be longer than 3 weeks, a jejunostomy or gastrostomy can be placed surgically. Tubes placed for postpyloric feeding may be inserted by blind passage or by operative, endoscopic, laporoscopic, or radiologic placement. A soft, small-bore tube should be used. Small tubes (8- to 10-gauge French) made of polyurethane or silicon are less irritating to mucous tissue, especially in the nasal passage. A tube at least 105 cm in length is required for postpyloric feedings past Treitz's ligament. Both weighted and nonweighted tubes are used, and neither has been proven superior to the other.[90] The method and route of insertion depends largely on the preference, training, and availability of staff. Feeding tube placement sites are portrayed in Figure 16-7.[91]

Several methods have been described in the general nutrition literature regarding cannulation of the duodenum. These methods include pH sensors, pharmacologic measures such as promotility agents, fluoroscopic and endoscopic insertion techniques, and bedside mechanical techniques. Initially some patients with small bowel feeding tubes also require a gastric tube for decompression and suction of fluids. Some newer tubes have two ports: a gastric port for suction, decompression, or medication delivery and

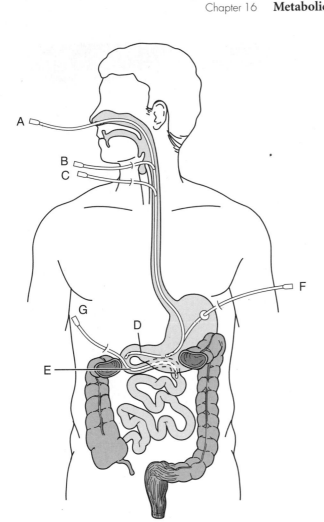

FIGURE 16-7 Tube feeding routes. **A,** Nasogastric; **B,** pharyngostomy; **C,** esophagostomy; **D,** nasoduodenal; **E,** nasojejunal; **F,** gastrostomy; **G,** jejunostomy. (From Veldee MS: Nutrition. In Tietz NW, Burtis CA, Ashwood ER, editors: *Tietz textbook of clinical chemistry,* ed 2, Philadelphia, 1994, WB Saunders, 1247.)

a separate, extended lumen for simultaneous small bowel feeding.

Before administering any tube feeding by way of a small-bore tube, a radiograph should be taken to confirm proper placement.[92] The radiograph remains the gold standard; however, interpretation can be difficult.[92] Auscultating the epigastrium for gurgling sounds to rule out respiratory tube placement should never be the sole method of determining feeding tube placement, because numerous authors have reported "pseudoconfirmatory" gurgling when tubes were placed improperly.[92] During and immediately after insertion, the following supportive methods should be considered to verify tube placement:

- Observing for respiratory distress
- Marking the point at which the tube exits the patient
- pH testing of aspirate
- Observing the color of the tube aspirate
- Auscultating sounds when injecting air into the tube
- Noting changes in residual volumes aspirated from the feeding tube[92]

The nurse should check daily for the external length of tube from the exit site and note any changes in the chart. The tubes should be stabilized and cleaned as needed with normal saline. Gastrostomy and jejunostomy tubes should be dressed daily with dry gauze and anchored. The exit site should be evaluated daily for redness, swelling, warmth, skin breakdown, and drainage. Verifying tube placement and patency is a routine but essential practice and should be performed at initial placement, before administering medications, after replacement, when proper placement is questioned, and routinely based on hospital protocols. Gastric leakage or tube displacement of more than 1 inch needs to be reported, and a radiograph should be taken if the tube has been misplaced or displaced.

Maintaining tube patency requires frequent tube irrigation. Water is the most effective irrigant. The ports should be flushed every 6 hours during continuous feeding, after any bolus feedings, and after residuals are assessed. If the enteral infusion is turned off for any length of time, the tube should be flushed before restarting the feeding. Medication should be given separately, and the tube should be flushed with 5 to 10 ml of water before and after medication administration.

ENTERAL FORMULAS. The registered dietitian is an integral part of the team and should be consulted on the type of formula each patient needs, rather than a decision being made arbitrarily based on availability. Various solutions are available for tube feeding, and their use is determined based on the nutritional assessment (Table 16-7).[93] Nurses should be aware of the osmolality of the formula. In general, tube feedings vary in osmolality from 300 mOsm (isotonic) for standard formulas to 850 mOsm (hypertonic) in elemental formulas. Isotonic formulas are better tolerated than more concentrated formulas, especially when tube feedings are initiated. Standard tube feeding solutions usually provide 1 kcal/ml, whereas concentrated formulas provide 1.5 to 2 kcal/ml. Most full-strength enteral formulas come with a standard mix of vitamins and minerals that meet the RDA when 1700 to 2400 ml of solution is provided.

INITIATION OF ENTERAL FEEDING. The pump-assisted method is strongly recommended for patients who are critically ill and is required for those who are continuously fed into the small bowel.[88] This method helps to minimize gastric complications such as nausea, cramping, and diarrhea.[88] In addition, this method allows for more accurate recording of intake and calculation of fluid balance and energy intake.

The head of the bed should remain at a 30- to 45-degree angle during enteral feeding for all patients to decrease the risk of aspiration. Dyes such as blue food coloring are frequently used to help detect aspiration. The reliability and validity of this method is not well tested.[88] If dye is added to the enteral formula, the smallest amount of dye possible should be used to avoid allergic reactions and changes in pH. The trauma patient who has pulmonary contusions,

TABLE 16-7   Classification of Enteral Tube Feeding Formulas

Product Category	Product Characteristics	Patient Indications	Examples of Product
Standard	• Intact macronutrients • Mimics typical American diet	• Fully functional GI tract	Isocal[*] Isosource[†] Nutren 1.0[‡] Osmolite[§]
High nitrogen	• Intact macronutrients • >14% total calories	• Malnourished • Catabolic • Elderly	Impact[†] Isocal HN[*] Nitro-PRO[**] Osmolite HN[§] Replete with fiber[‡] Entrition HN[‡]
Elemental/semi-elemental	• Hydrolyzed macronutrients • Hyperosmolar • Low in total fat; may contain 30% of calories as fat with <50% from long-chain triglyceride	• Severe maldigestion and malabsorption	Criticare HN[*] Glutasorb[**] Peptamen[‡] Pro-Peptide[**] Reabilan[‡] Vital HN[§] Vivonex Plus[†]
Concentrated	• Intact macronutrients • Mimics typical American diet	• Restricted fluid intake	Nutren 2.0[‡] ReSource Plus[†] TwoCal HN[§]
Fiber containing	• Fiber from natural food or added soy polysaccharide	• Bowel function regulation	Compleat[†] Ensure with fiber[§] Jevity[§] Probalance[‡] Ultracal with fiber[*]
Specialty products	• Varies depending on disease state	• Organ failure (renal or hepatic) or pulmonary compromise	Glytrol[‡] Pulmocare[§] Magnacal Renal[*] ReSource Diabetic[†] Travasorb MCT[‡]

Modified from Skipper A, editor: *Dietitian's handbook of enteral and parenteral nutrition*, Rockville, Md, 1989, Aspen.
[*]Mead Johnson Nutritionals
[†]Novartis
[‡]Nestle Nutrition
[§]Ross Products Division, Abbott Laboratories
[**]Gala Glen

atelectasis, and pneumonia may require chest physiotherapy and postural drainage. Tube feedings should be discontinued 1 hour before and during chest physiotherapy to decrease the risk of aspiration. In most cases the risk of aspiration is small relative to the benefit of feedings when appropriate nursing interventions are instituted.

When introducing feeding, small amounts should be used initially, especially in elderly, head-injured, and unconscious patients. If gastric motility is a problem, metoclopramide (Reglan) may be effective in increasing gastric motility. Feeding through a jejunal tube can begin as soon as the patient is hemodynamically stable, whereas gastric feeding must wait until the pylorus resumes normal function.

Gastric ileus is the major barrier to initiating enteral feeding into the stomach after traumatic injury. The nurse plays a key role in assessing bowel sounds and reporting these findings, along with the amount of gastric residuals, to the physician and dietitian. If for some reason there is a long delay before bowel sounds are present, an alternate route for feeding will need to be used, such as feeding into the jejunum or through the parenteral route. For many patients with neurotrauma, recovery from the initial posttraumatic paralytic ileus occurs within 72 hours of injury, and then gastric feeding is well tolerated. Enteral feeding can also be delayed because of surgery or radiologic procedures or because feeding tubes are dislodged.

Generally, full-strength enteral feeding is begun slowly (10-40 ml/hour). The rate is increased based on physician order or hospital protocol. Typically the rate is increased by 20 ml every 8 hours as tolerated until the target rate is achieved. Attempts should be made to assess residual GI contents every 2 to 4 hours and as needed. Tube feeding is generally withheld when residuals are two times the hourly rate, or 100 to 200 ml from orogastric or nasogastric tubes or 100 ml or more from gastrostomy tubes. Residual volumes greater than 100 to 200 ml consistently or gastric distention or vomiting may signify the need to change the feeding route.

It is the nurse's responsibility to ascertain whether the patient is tolerating the administration of formula and to communicate findings regarding vomiting, bowel sounds, residual volume, flatus, and amount and consistency of stools to the nutrition team. If the patient complains of any abdominal discomfort or if there is distention, diarrhea, nausea, or vomiting, the feeding should be discontinued for further evaluation. If the patient cannot communicate, abdominal girth can be measured every 4 hours.

CONSIDERATIONS FOR DRUG ADMINISTRATION. Drugs and nutrients can interact, altering nutrition status and the intended action of the drug. Tube feeding can interfere with the absorption of some medications, and some medications can clog the feeding tube.[88,89] The nurse, in consultation with the dietitian and pharmacist, is in a key position to ensure that medication has an optimal chance of absorption. Medications should not be mixed with formulas or other medications unless they have been shown to be compatible to avoid altering absorption or clogging the feeding tube.[88] Liquid forms of medicine are preferable for absorption; however, liquids with lower pH can cause clumping and clogging. Elixers and suspensions are a better choice for administering through a feeding tube than are syrups, because a number of syrups are incompatible with enteral formulas.[88,89] If only solid forms of medication are available, they should be crushed into a fine powder to ensure dissolution and to prevent clogs. Adequate drug dosage may be difficult to achieve with soft gelatin capsules, which must be poked open, squeezed of their contents, and diluted for administration down the enteral tube. Sustained release and enteric-coated pills are not appropriate for administration through feeding tubes. Tube feeding will need to be delayed 30 minutes to 2 hours before and after some medications are administered. For example, tube feedings are held for 2 hours before and after administering phenytoin (Dilantin). In this case therapeutic levels of the drug need to be monitored to maintain seizure prophylaxis. On the other hand, toxicity can occur when the patient is transitioned to oral feeding. The placement of the end tip of the tube is also important; some medications, such as sucralfate, must enter the stomach because they require a low pH to convert to an active form. The hospital pharmacist should be consulted when questions arise about drug-nutrient compatibility.

COMPLICATIONS. Common GI complications during tube feeding include inadequate gastric emptying, diarrhea, vomiting, nausea, and tube dislodgment or obstruction.

Obstruction of the feeding tube results from residual tube feedings and medications caking on the inner lumen; gastric acid coagulates the protein in enteral formulas. A clog may be loosened by flushing the tube with warm water, alternating attempts to irrigate and aspirate in a rhythmic motion, allowing for slight expansion of a flexible tube using a syringe of 20 ml or greater.[89,94] If this approach fails, a declogging device might be used to remove the clog mechanically. The nurse should never attempt to force a clog through the tube because the tube may rupture. Prevention remains the best solution to clogged tubes.

Diarrhea is a common complication in critically ill patients and is not usually related to the nutritional formula.[88,89,92,95,96] Common causes of diarrhea include infection, drug administration, toxins, and gastric surgery.[88] Diarrhea can be osmotic, secretory, or exudative. A concentrated hyperosmolar solution, such as an elemental feeding formula, introduced into the GI tract can cause water to remain in the intestinal lumen, resulting in osmotic diarrhea. Conditions of maldigestion and malabsorption, such as lactose intolerance or dumping syndrome after gastric surgery, can also cause accumulation of hyperosmolar substances in the intestinal lumen, leading to retention of fluid in the GI tract.

Continuous tube feeding rather than bolus tube feeding is preferred for postsurgical patients to promote adequate digestion and absorption. Osmotic diarrhea should resolve within 24 hours of stopping the concentrated feeding or medication. The pharmacist can assist with determining whether drugs may have induced diarrhea in tube-fed patients. Diluting hyperosmotic drugs with water decreases the risk of side effects.[88]

Secretory diarrhea is caused by bacterial or viral toxins, which trigger the enterocytes to secrete fluid and electrolytes into the intestinal lumen. Fasting will not resolve this type of diarrhea. Exudative diarrhea results from mucosal damage as a result of antibiotics, radiation enteritis, or ulcerative colitis. A thorough medical workup should be undertaken if the patient has prolonged diarrhea; dehydration should be prevented.

A large number of microorganisms can precipitate diarrhea.[96] *Clostridium difficile* toxin should be ruled out as the cause of diarrhea before administering antimotility agents, which can enhance bacterial overgrowth[88] and increase the risk of toxic megacolon. Changing the feeding bag every 24 hours and using clean techniques during administration help to minimize microbial contamination and growth. Similarly, feedings should be given in no more than a 4-hour supply, particularly if the formula was altered after the manufacturer's seal was opened. The maximal time a given lot of formula should hang is 8 to 10 hours.[89]

Once tube feedings are contaminated, rapid bacterial growth can occur with gram-negative bacilli.[96] Critically ill patients are particularly vulnerable to bacterial overgrowth in the GI tract if the gastric pH exceeds 4, which can occur with medicines that suppress gastric acid.[96] Bacterial overgrowth can damage the intestinal mucosa and lead to diarrhea.[96] Commercially prepared, ready-to-use formulas that do not require the addition of water or supplements are least likely to contribute to microbial growth. For this reason it is better to administer the tube feeding slowly and manage hydration with water boluses and intravenous fluid rather than by diluting the enteral formula. Proper handling and cleaning of the lid before pouring the formula into the feeding bag is important. Unused portions should be covered, labeled, and refrigerated.[95]

Many drugs, such as potassium chloride, are hyperosmolar and when given through the feeding tube can cause diarrhea. Control of peristalsis may be drug related. Tincture of opium or a more natural fiber bulk form (such as Metamucil) may be prescribed to slow down GI motility and diarrhea. A fiber-containing formula may solidify stools that are too loose.[88,89] Non-fiber-containing formulas typically produce a stool that is pasty in consistency.[88] Fiber gives form to and retains moisture in the stool. Also, neutral bacteria in the lower intestine consume the fiber and produce short-chain fatty acids, a source of energy for enterocytes. This improves the health of the intestinal lining, leading to better sodium and water absorption. In summary, when diarrhea occurs, drug administration and infection should be considered as possible causes in addition to feeding intolerances.

The need for fluid may be increased by mechanical ventilation, fever, wound drainage, neurosweats, diarrhea, and hyperventilation. Constipation may occur if the patient is not adequately hydrated.[96] Fluid, fiber, stool softeners, and bowel stimulants may help to regulate bowel movements. Tube feedings that are high in protein can cause urea diuresis with subsequent dehydration. Metabolic signs of dehydration include elevated blood urea nitrogen (BUN), increased BUN/creatinine ratio, and increased sodium. Clinical signs include poor skin turgor, dry mouth, and an elevated heart rate. Administer adequate amounts of water throughout the day.

Multiple mechanical, gastrointestinal, and metabolic complications of enteral feeding exist and should be resolved when possible. If the patient cannot be nourished adequately through the enteral route because of prolonged complications, parenteral nutritional support should be considered.

PARENTERAL SUPPORT AND MONITORING

A select group of patients may require parenteral nutrition. Parenteral nutrition should be considered if enteral feeding is expected to be delayed for 5 days or if the patient does not tolerate sufficient amounts of enteral feeding (see Figure 16-6).[30] Parenteral feeding modalities include peripheral (PPN) for short-term therapy and central (TPN) routes for patients who will require more than 7 days of parenteral support. A complete nutritional assessment should be made before initiating parenteral nutrition therapy.

PERIPHERAL PARENTERAL NUTRITION.

Patients who can tolerate approximately 3 liters of fluid each day, have peripheral access, have no history of hyperlipidemia, have adequate platelet counts, and will be able to transition to enteral nutrition in less than 1 week are potential candidates for PPN therapy. PPN was designed for short-term therapy (<10 days) and typically contains fat, carbohydrates, protein, electrolytes, vitamins, and trace minerals. It is less likely to cause metabolic complications of hyperglycemia, hypophosphatemia, and increased CO_2 production than TPN, since the calorie and carbohydrate load is relatively low (1000-1500 kcal).[97] On the other hand, there are several disadvantages to PPN therapy. A limited amount of protein

and calories can be infused into the small peripheral veins, and it requires more volume to deliver these calories and protein than does TPN.[97] Nursing responsibilities during PPN include careful observation of sites to prevent infusion into the subcutaneous space. In addition, using other peripheral sites to infuse medications such as antibiotics is better than having to stop PPN, flush the tubing, and infuse antibiotics and other medications in the PPN site. Veins can develop a thrombus, causing pain and fever. Rotating PPN sites every 72 hours decreases the risk of vein thrombosis.

CENTRAL LINE INSERTION AND INFECTION CONTROL.

Nurses should have full knowledge of infection control policies related to central line insertion, site preparation, care of site and dressing, tubing and fluid change protocols, and other practice-related issues. Hospitals should have established protocols for these line-care issues. Catheter-related infections remain one of the most important complications of TPN therapy.[98]

Risk factors for infections include the following:

- Method and site of catheter insertion
- Breaks in aseptic technique to maintain system
- Using a multiple lumen catheter
- Using the TPN line for fluids other than TPN
- Length of time the catheter remains in place

Proper preparation of the patient and good surgical technique reduce the risk of these complications. Standardizing insertion technique and care for all peripheral, central venous, and arterial catheters minimize catheter-related infections.[99] Dressings should be changed when the catheter is replaced; when the dressing becomes damp, loosened, or soiled; and when inspection of the site is necessary.[98] Careful observation of the site is recommended as frequently as every 8 hours and when fever develops.[99] The length of time the catheter remains in place is the most critical factor associated with the development of infections. Although the Centers for Disease Control and Prevention do not make specific recommendations regarding when the catheter site should be rotated, it is prudent to discontinue use of the site and TPN as soon as possible. TPN lines should be used only for TPN except in a life-threatening emergency. Maintaining a closed system minimizes the chance for contamination. Although TPN is more likely to support microbial growth than routine IV fluids, contamination from TPN fluids is rare. Even three-in-one admixtures do not appear to support microbial growth very well.[98] In contrast, undiluted lipid solutions have a greater chance of promoting bacterial growth, so they should be infused over a 12-hour period.[98] TPN tubing should be changed every 24 hours when lipids are administered through any portion of the line.[98] The lipid tubing should be discarded after the 12-hour infusion is complete.

COMPOSITION OF TPN.

Each liter of TPN usually contains 4% to 6% amino acids, 15% to 20% glucose, electrolytes, trace elements, vitamins, and sometimes insulin and H_2 blockers. Lipid emulsions (10% or 20%) are typically infused from a separate bottle. Lipids (fat) provide essential fatty acid (linoleic and linolenic acids) and are especially important for patients who receive long-term TPN. Fat calories typically constitute up about 25% to 30% of the total calorie intake in TPN administered to trauma patients. One 500-ml bottle of 10% lipid emulsion provides 50 g of fat and 550 kcal. A 500-ml bottle of a 20% lipid emulsion provides 100 g of fat and 1000 kcal. A minimum of 100 g of lipid (two bottles of 10% or one bottle of 20%) is given each week to prevent EFAD. Fluid-restricted patients may need the calorically dense lipid calories (9 kcal/g) to provide sufficient energy. There is little information available regarding safe administration of intravenous lipid emulsions to critically ill adult patients with hypertriglyceridemia.[100] Possible consequences of lipid administration concomitant with hypertriglyceridemia include pancreatitis, immune suppression, and altered pulmonary status.[100]

TPN is formulated with most nutrients in amounts that meet health needs. However, because of problems with compounding, some minerals, such as calcium, are provided in amounts less than may be needed for long-term health. Physicians can order varying amounts of electrolytes from day to day to tailor the prescription as much as possible to the patient's need. Omissions of vitamins and minerals in TPN have resulted in serious disorders and even death. Overdoses of nutrients can also be dangerous.

TPN ADMINISTRATION AND MONITORING. Serum samples for measurement of triglyceride, phosphorus, magnesium, and other standard electrolyte levels should be obtained before the start of TPN (Table 16-8). If the blood triglyceride concentration is mildly elevated, a trial dose of 10% lipids should be given and serial triglyceride levels should be followed daily. There have been some reports of patients developing cramping, tachypnea, and tachycardia and becoming diaphoretic during lipid infusions. This remains rare, and the cause is still under investigation. Infusing lipids over a 12-hour period appears to be well

tolerated by most patients, with minimal, if any, adverse effects. Lipid infusion protects the venous endothelium from injury related to hypertonic glucose solutions. TPN is hyperosmolar, so it must be infused into the superior vena cava, preferably via the subclavian route. Amino acids, glucose, and lipids can be infused concurrently.

The nurse will monitor the patient closely for signs and symptoms of infection that may be catheter related. If the patient suddenly develops an elevated temperature, blood cultures and a fever workup based on clinical signs and hospital policy should be done. If catheter-related sepsis is suspected, the line should be removed and a new catheter inserted.

Trauma patients are already stressed, and TPN can add to that stress if close monitoring is neglected. Intake and output, fluid and electrolyte status, results of kidney and liver function tests, and serum glucose and triglyceride levels should be recorded carefully and evaluated on a regular basis. Special attention to intake and output records is particularly important for patients with impaired renal function or impaired cardiac function because they are prone to fluid overload. Serum and urine osmolality are measured routinely to assess fluid status. Records of the volume of TPN administered are used with the TPN prescription to calculate the intake of energy, protein, and other nutrients.

Energy requirements and fluid and electrolyte status must be monitored closely in the acutely ill trauma patient. The frequency of specific laboratory tests varies depending on the patient's clinical status. Suggested guidelines for metabolic monitoring during stress and variables to be monitored during TPN are provided in Table 16-8.[88] Table 16-9[91] outlines possible electrolyte complications that may occur if close monitoring is neglected. In addition, acid-base balance studies assist the physician and dietitian in making necessary changes in TPN composition. The nurse is involved with assessing respiratory and metabolic acidosis as it relates to overfeeding. Trends in albumin and prealbumin are used to determine changes in metabolic response to

ₒTABLE 16-8 **Suggested Monitoring for Total Parenteral Nutrition**			
Parameter	Baseline	Critically Ill Patients	Stable Patients
Chemistry screen (Ca, Mg, LFTs, PO$_4$)	Yes	2-3 times/week	Weekly
Electrolyte, BUN, creatinine	Yes	Daily	1-2 times/week
Serum triglycerides	Yes	Weekly	Weekly
CBC with differential	Yes	Weekly	Weekly
PT, PTT	Yes	Weekly	Weekly
Capillary glucose	Yes	3 times/day until consistently <200 mg/dl	3 times/day until consistently <200 mg/dl
Weight	If possible	Daily if appropriate	2-3 times weekly
Intake and output	Daily	Daily	Daily until fluid status can be assessed by physical exam
Indirect calorimetry	As needed	As needed	As needed
Nitrogen balance	As needed	As needed	As needed

From Scouba WW Jr, Kohn-Keth C et al: *The ASPEN nutrition support practice manual*, Silver Spring, Md, 1998, American Society for Parenteral and Enteral Nutrition, Section 9-6.

TABLE 16-9   Possible Metabolic Complications of Parenteral Nutrition

Complication	Laboratory Indices	Cause
Fluid and Electrolytes		
Dehydration	↑ Serum Na, BUN, creatinine, osmolality, Hct	Inadequate fluid support; unaccounted fluid loss (e.g., diarrhea, fistulas, persistent high fever)
Overhydration	↓ Serum Na, osmolality, Hct	Excess fluid administration; compromised renal or cardiac function
Alkalosis	↓ Serum K	Inadequate K to compensate for cellular uptake during glucose transport; excessive GI or renal K losses
	↓ Serum Cl^-	Inadequate Cl^- in patients undergoing gastric decompression
Acidosis	↑ Serum K, ↓ HCO_3^-	Excessive K in TPN
	↑ Serum Cl^-, ↓ HCO_3^-	Excessive renal or GI losses of base; excessive Cl^- in TPN
Hypocalcemia	↓ Serum Ca	Excessive PO_4 salts, low serum albumin
	↓ Serum-ionized Ca	Inadequate Ca in TPN
Hypercalcemia	↑ Serum Ca, ionized Ca	Excessive Ca in TPN; can lead to pancreatitis
Hypomagnesemia	↓ Serum Mg	Inadequate Mg in TPN; excessive Mg losses; cellular uptake with induction of anabolism
Hypophosphatemia	↓ Serum PO_4	Excess losses (↑ urinary PO_4 in alkalosis, ↓ Mg, diabetes mellitus, steroid and diuretic therapy); cellular uptake with induction of anabolism
Carbohydrate Metabolism		
Hyperglycemic, hyperosmolar nonketotic coma	↑ Serum glucose, Na, osmolality	Sustained untreated glucose intolerance; easily prevented by frequent glucose monitoring; 40% mortality rate
Hyperglycemia	↑ Serum glucose	Stress response; occurs in approximately 25% of cases
Hypoglycemia	↓ Serum glucose	Sudden withdrawal of concentrated glucose; more common in children
Hypercarbia	↑ CO_2	Excessive caloric or carbohydrate load
Lipid Metabolism		
Essential fatty acid deficiency	↑ Triene:tetraene ratio	Inadequate provision of linoleic acid in TPN; release of linoleic acid from adipose stores prevented by continuous dextrose infusion and associated hyperinsulinemia
Hemolytic anemia	↓ Hct, ↑ triglycerides, ↑ cholesterol	Prolonged high serum level of triglycerides
Protein Metabolism		
Hyperammonemia	↑ Blood ammonia	Excessive protein load; arginine deficiency (urea cycle); hepatic dysfunction; preformed ammonia in amino acid solution; more common in children
Hepatic and Biliary Effects		
Tissue damage, fat infiltration	↑ Serum transaminases, alkaline phosphatase	Unclear etiology; may be related to excessive glucose or energy administration; L-carnitine deficiency
Cholestasis	↑ Conjugated bilirubin	Lack of GI stimulation; sludge present in 50% of patients on TPN for 4-6 wk; resolves with resumption of enteral feeding

From Veldee MS: Nutrition. In Burtis CA, Ashwood ER, editors: *Tietz textbook of clinical chemistry*, ed 2, Philadelphia, 1994, Saunders.

stress and to note when the anabolic building phase is beginning.

Important physical assessment strategies include assessing skin and sclera for jaundice, palpating the liver for tenderness or enlargement, and assessing urine color (liver dysfunction can produce urine with an orange tint). Patients who are malnourished before admission are more susceptible to abnormalities from nutritional support. TPN must be provided cautiously in this group.

TPN should be discontinued as soon as possible, and transition to enteral feeding should be considered. Patients may initially need parenteral nutrition as the primary source

of feeding, and most are able to progress partially or completely to enteral feedings. Patient and family teaching should be conducted. Many patients may think they are starving when they receive TPN; in fact, they are receiving maintenance nutrition until they can eat.

TRANSITIONING FROM PARENTERAL NUTRITION. Once the patient's condition stabilizes and the GI tract becomes a viable feeding route, either enteral or oral intake should be considered.[30] This transition should be planned in an organized fashion by the interdisciplinary team. Oral feedings may be initiated if the patient is awake, alert, and motivated. Before a patient returns to an oral diet, a speech therapist should conduct a swallowing evaluation. Disuse, general muscle weakness, endotracheal tube placement, and neurologic alterations can lead to swallowing problems, which increase the risk of aspiration. Calorie counts should be initiated to determine if intake is adequate. TPN can be reduced and then eliminated once tube feedings and oral feedings are meeting 60% of the goal for energy and protein.[88] Abrupt discontinuation of TPN without any oral or enteral intake may result in acute hypoglycemia and is not recommended. Administering $D_{10}W$ in these situations minimizes the potential for rebound hypoglycemia. Similarly, decreasing the rate of TPN by half for a few hours may reduce hypoglycemic events.

INADEQUATE NUTRITIONAL REPLACEMENT

Inadequate caloric replacement has been associated with complications and can alter the body's reparative process. Protein-calorie malnutrition (PCM) can develop rapidly in patients who have a combination of severe catabolic stress and prolonged low nutrient intake. PCM leads to depressed respiratory function and increased dependence on mechanical ventilation, impaired wound healing, decreased resistance to infection, decreased ability to tolerate surgery, and decreased sense of well-being. PCM significantly alters renal function, specifically decreasing glomerular filtration rate and renal plasma flow and lowering the capacity to concentrate urine, predisposing the patient to acidosis. Patients with protein malnutrition are more prone to metabolic acidosis because they have a reduced rate of urinary phosphate excretion, decreased proton secretion, and impaired sodium/hydrogen exchange.[101]

Morbidity and mortality are particularly severe in malnourished patients.[102-105] Protein malnutrition contributes to an impaired host-defense mechanism, depressed antibody production, impaired function of phagocytic cells, and altered levels of complement.[106] Viral and fungal infections are associated with depressed T-cell-mediated immunity, which is affected by malnutrition. Inadequate intake exacerbates weight loss and reduces subcutaneous tissue. A loss of fat padding between bones and skin allows bony prominences to compress and restrict circulation to the skin, increasing the likelihood of pressure sores.[107]

The hypermetabolic trauma patient who is dependent on others for feeding is at risk for development of PCM. PCM is evident as low visceral protein and emaciated fat and muscle stores. Trauma patients who are elderly or have preexisting nutritional deficits are at even greater risk of PCM, which can drastically alter recovery. Sullivan and Walls[108] categorized PCM in hospital patients, noting that an albumin concentration less than 3 g/dl or a BMI less than 19 signified high nutritional risk. They discovered that in older adults, PCM at discharge was a strong independent risk factor for subsequent mortality within 6 years.[108] The population with chronic illness is most susceptible to PCM. This portion of the trauma population needs early identification and intervention.

The idea that permissive underfeeding may be of some benefit has been discussed for many years. This idea is based on the notion that underfeeding some nutrients may confer a protective effect by depleting infecting organisms and impairing their ability to replicate. Further research is necessary to identify the specific nutrients (e.g., zinc, iron), the circumstances under which they would be restricted (e.g., fever), and the degree of restriction.

Periodic nutritional reassessment of energy and protein needs and delivery of necessary nutrients can positively influence the prognosis of the trauma patient. Inadequate intake is only one factor that can lead to PCM. Other factors include impaired digestion, malabsorption, and problems with utilization once the nutrient has been absorbed. Additionally, patients with increased needs, such as those with high-output fistulas, are at higher risk for malnutrition.

EXCESS NUTRITIONAL REPLACEMENT

Health professionals need to evaluate patients' energy/caloric needs carefully, since serious complications can occur with overfeeding. Chwals[109] defined overfeeding as the administration of energy and substrate in excess of the amount required for metabolic homeostasis. Multiple complications can occur if energy and nutrient needs are overestimated. If nurses have not been trained to recognize metabolic complications of overfeeding, a patient's symptoms may be attributed inaccurately to other causes, and this delays appropriate intervention. Klein, Stanek, and Wiles[110] summarized the detrimental effects of excess intake as it relates to major body systems. As depicted in Figure 16-8,[111] excessive carbohydrate administration (e.g., dextrose, glucose) can cause metabolic changes such as hyperglycemia, fatty liver (hepatic steatosis), hypercapnia (elevated CO_2), hypertriglyceridemia, and refeeding syndrome. Protein overfeeding increases the production of urea, which can lead to azotemia, hypertonic dehydration, and metabolic acidosis. Overfeeding fat can result in hypertriglyceridemia and congestion of the reticuloendothelial system, compromising immune function.

Patients at risk for overfeeding include very small, cachectic, or obese patients, and those whose weight was overestimated; elderly patients; patients receiving concentrated formulas (e.g., TPN dextrose >20%); and patients just beginning TPN or making the transition from TPN to tube feeding. Other patients at risk include those receiving propofol, steroids, or peritoneal dialysis with dextrose in the dialysate and patients at risk for MODS.

McClave et al[11] noted that "the signs of inappropriate feeding may not always be apparent to the clinician, because ventilator settings may be adjusted to correct blood gases, the duration and frequency of dialysis are increased to control azotemia, or insulin doses are increased to control hyperglycemia." Indeed, the job of monitoring the patient's response to feeding is particularly challenging in the critical care setting, especially when patients undergo numerous and unpredictable changes in medical status unrelated to nutrition support.

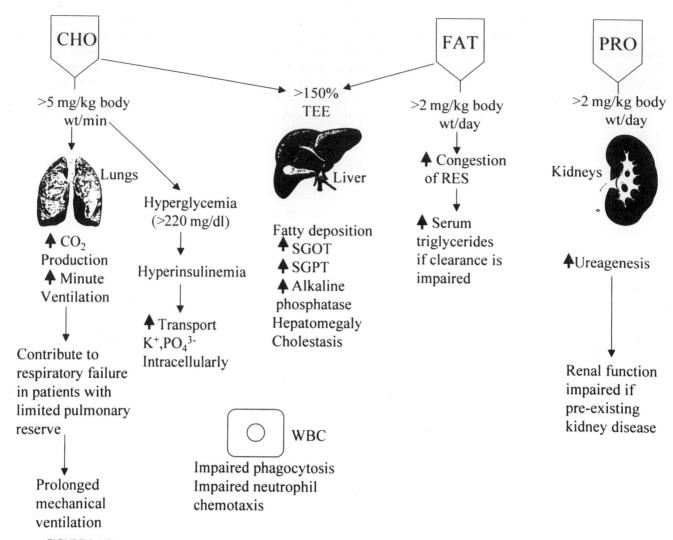

FIGURE 16-8 The potential consequences of overfeeding macronutrients to critically ill adults. (From Frankel WL, Evans NJ, Rombeau JL: Scientific rationale and clinical application of parenteral nutrition in critically ill patients. In Rombeau JL, Caldwell MD, editors: *Clinical nutrition: parenteral nutrition,* ed 2, Philadelphia, 1993, WB Saunders, 601.)

CARBOHYDRATE OVERFEEDING. Pathways leading to complications during carbohydrate overfeeding are summarized in Figure 16-8.[111] Hyperglycemia (e.g., >200 mg/dl) is an independent risk factor for morbidity and mortality,[39] particularly in patients with traumatic injuries. Nurses who provide good blood glucose control may decrease their patients' risk of infection,[112-114] even patients who do not have diabetes.[115] Good blood glucose control involves providing appropriate nutrition support, adequate blood tests, hypoglycemic agents when needed, and timely assessments by qualified staff.

The early stages of carbohydrate overfeeding are associated with sodium and water retention, which increases demands on the heart. Chronically malnourished patients, such as those who are anorexic or addicted to alcohol, have a nutritionally depleted cardiac mass and are not prepared to deal with the circulatory demand caused by aggressive nutrition support. Glucose feeding stimulates insulin production. Increased insulin triggers cells to rapidly take up circulating minerals, particularly phosphorus, magnesium,

and potassium. The decreased amount of available blood minerals combined with the expansion of blood volume increases the risk of respiratory distress and heart failure. This is known as refeeding syndrome, which is characterized by hypophosphatemia, arterial hypotension, tachycardia, and acute respiratory failure; it can be fatal. Blood minerals should be brought to normal levels before TPN is initiated in malnourished patients, and feeding should be advanced gradually as tolerated, with continued mineral repletion as needed.[116,117]

Excess carbohydrate feeding is a physiologic stress because it causes increases in minute ventilation, V_{O_2}, and V_{CO_2}. The increased levels of V_{CO_2} contribute to an increased workload, which may precipitate respiratory failure in the compromised host[118] or impair the patient's ability to wean from a ventilator. Patients with low cervical and upper thoracic spinal cord injuries are particularly vulnerable to being overfed because of their decreased energy needs combined with their inability to use intercostal, abdominal, and diaphragm muscles to compensate for increased V_{CO_2}.

Many patients have pulmonary contusions, rib fractures, and hemopneumothoraces, which can limit their ability to compensate for increased Vco_2. Avoiding excessive carbohydrate loads is therefore an important consideration for this population of patients. Furthermore, excessive carbohydrate loading may precipitate respiratory acidosis in patients who are unable to adequately improve alveolar ventilation when compensating for increasing Vco_2. Direct measurement of Vo_2 and Vco_2 by way of indirect calorimetry, when possible, is useful to assess the nutritional status of traumatically injured patients.

Aranda-Michel and Morgan[118] presented the case study of a patient who developed complications from carbohydrate overfeeding. The patient was a thin, 56-year-old woman who underwent cholecystectomy, bowel resection, and jejunocolostomy to treat mesenteric ischemia and gangrenous cholecystitis. She received TPN providing 2200 kcal/day (HBEE × 1.9). She developed tachycardia and hypercapnia, for which she had to be mechanically ventilated. Once ventilated, repeated measures of $Paco_2$ were normal at 35 mm Hg and pH remained greater than 7.4. One week later the physician decided the patient might need more calories and ordered TPN providing 2400 kcal/day (HBEE × 2.1). In addition to respiratory distress, the patient had a grade I sacral decubitus ulcer, two fistulae, sacral and pedal edema, and congestive heart failure. Her clinicians surmised that the respiratory distress and congestive heart failure developed in response to overfeeding. The plan was to consult a nutrition support team, who recommended feeding a mixed-fuel solution of carbohydrates, protein, and fat providing 1600 kcal/day (HBEE × 1.4). The outcome was dramatic; within a day of reducing the calories in TPN, the patient's heart rate improved and she was weaned from the ventilator.

What were the indications of carbohydrate overfeeding in this patient? First, although the actual amount of carbohydrates was not reported, we can assume by the amount of energy provided that the carbohydrate load was excessive for this woman, who weighed only 82% of ideal body weight. The nutrition support team would have calculated the actual rate of carbohydrate infusion in mg/kg/min for comparison with recommended rates. Second, she went into respiratory distress after TPN was initiated, and it resolved soon after the TPN was delivered at a more appropriate rate.

Carbohydrate overfeeding causes a shift in substrate oxidation over time, so that glucose oxidation increases and fat oxidation decreases. Despite the shift toward less fat oxidation, lipolysis persists in critical illness. This surplus of fatty acid increases the risk of hypertriglyceridemia and hepatic steatosis when the patient is overfed carbohydrates or lipids.

LIPID OVERFEEDING.   Complications can occur within days of lipid overfeeding or not appear until after weeks of apparent tolerance. Platelets can take up excess fat in the blood, which interferes with clotting function. Prothrombin time and partial thromboplastin time are prolonged. The patient may develop bloody diarrhea, bloody urine, bleeding gums, or other bleeding. As fat overfeeding continues, reticuloendothelial cells phagocytize blood lipids and giant platelets distended by fat, impairing immune function. Major organs can be severely affected by fat overload (see Figure 16-8).[111] Fat overload syndrome is the sudden onset of multiple complications associated with excessive lipid infusion; it leads to MODS and can be fatal. In addition to signs of coagulopathy, other early signs of fat overload syndrome include sudden and extreme hypertriglyceridemia, hypercapnia, tachycardia, hypertension, fever, elevated bilirubin, elevated liver enzymes, and decreased hemoglobin.

Some drugs, such as propofol (Diprivan), are administered in lipid solution. If lipid calories in medicines administered to the patient are substantial, they should be counted toward the nutrition prescription. The parenteral administration of lipids in excess of 2 g/kg/day is associated with hypertriglyceridemia.[119]

Roth et al[120] presented a case study of metabolic complications from fat overfeeding. The patient was a previously healthy 21-year-old woman who incurred epidural and subdural hematomas in a traffic crash. One 500-ml bottle of 20% lipid emulsion was administered daily, beginning on day 3, and provided 100 g of fat per day. Serum triglyceride was normal at that time. After 2 days of TPN the patient's systolic blood pressure increased above 170 mm Hg despite aggressive antihypertensive treatment. Temperature increased to 40° C and remained at 40° to 41° C. She developed minor bronchial bleeding and hematuria. After 3 days of TPN the patient's plasma became white, turbid, and viscous. Her triglyceride level rose to 753 mg/dl. Liver enzymes, bilirubin, and serum creatinine also became elevated. Hemoglobin level and platelet count decreased substantially. A bone marrow smear indicated substantial macrophage phagocytosis. All tests for bacteria were negative. The assessment was that overfeeding had led to fat overload syndrome, which contributed to the development of hematologic, hepatic, renal, and pulmonary failure. The plan was to discontinue the intravenously administered lipids and remove 2 L of blood for partial plasmapheresis. She was provided with transfusions of blood, fresh frozen plasma, and platelets. The patient responded well and survived, although weeks passed before her serum triglyceride returned to normal levels.

What were the indicators of fat overload in this patient? First, the actual amount of fat provided was excessive for a critically ill patient. This amount of fat probably provided 50% to 60% of the total energy required. The second indication was that she developed sudden and severe hypertriglyceridemia and her blood appeared lipemic. Next, she developed a fever, hypertension, and bleeding. In addition, her liver function tests were elevated and her hemoglobin level decreased. There was also evidence of increased hemophagocytosis. Finally, most symptoms responded fairly rapidly to the discontinuation of lipid administration.

PROTEIN OVERFEEDING. Urea is the end product of protein metabolism: The more protein catabolized, the more urea produced and the greater the risk of azotemia. Azotemia is an increased amount of nitrogen in the blood, particularly as urea (BUN). For each molecule of urea produced, one molecule of bicarbonate is consumed, contributing to pH imbalance. Therefore catabolic patients who are losing skeletal muscle proteins, which are degraded to urea, are at risk of developing metabolic acidosis if they are also fed excessive amounts of protein, which generates more urea and uses up greater amounts of base. Extreme acidosis with a pH less than 7.3 can produce symptoms similar to severe dehydration, including mental confusion, abnormal neuromuscular activity, and hypotension.[121] Increased urea production increases the renal solute load, necessitating increased urination. Because high-protein diets require increased urination, a patient could become dehydrated if fed a high-protein diet without sufficient water, particularly an elderly patient who has lost the ability to concentrate urine. For these reasons, protein overfeeding can lead to azotemia, hypertonic dehydration, and metabolic acidosis[11,121,122] (see Figure 16-8).

Gault et al[122] reported the case of a 65-year-old man who developed complications from protein overfeeding. The patient had undergone a total laryngectomy and tracheostomy. Four months later he developed dysphagia and underwent gastrostomy. After the operation the patient was provided with a high-protein enteral formula. He was fully conscious when the tube feeding was initiated. He began complaining bitterly of thirst. He was unable to swallow drinks given by mouth because of an obstruction in his esophagus. Additional water was not provided through his feeding tube. Later he ceased to complain of thirst. After 2 weeks he was less responsive; after 23 days he had become stuporous and cyanotic. He responded to painful stimuli but was unable to answer questions or respond to commands. Tube feeding provided 210 g of protein and 2 L of water per day. Urine output was 850 ml per day. His reflexes had become hyperactive and large muscle groups would jerk occasionally. His diastolic blood pressure was 70 mm Hg, his pulse was 96 beats/min, respirations were 26 breaths/min, and temperature was elevated at 38.3° C. Blood tests revealed severe hypernatremia, with a sodium concentration of 192 mEq/L. BUN was elevated at 92 mg/dl, yet serum creatinine was 1.7 mg/dl. An elevated BUN/creatinine ratio greater than 15 can indicate dehydration and protein overfeeding, since BUN rises disproportionately under these circumstances. An osmolality of 376 mOsm/kg suggested dehydration. The assessment was that the hypernatremia was primarily the result of a water deficit caused by protein overfeeding. Protein overload led to azotemia and osmotic diuresis. Sufficient fluid was not provided, and over time this led to severe dehydration. (This condition has been named *tube feeding syndrome.*) The plan was to decrease protein intake and gradually administer water as D_5W while monitoring vital signs and laboratory test results. In severe dehydration, water is administered slowly, over 1 to 2 days, to avoid too great a shift of water into brain cells, which could cause cerebral edema. The patient's outcome was dramatic. After 6 L of D_5W was administered over 48 hours, he became alert and cooperative.

What were the indicators of protein overfeeding in this case? First, the actual amount of protein fed was excessive. Second, the patient complained of thirst and there were other signs of dehydration. Third, the patient had azotemia with an elevated BUN/creatinine ratio. Last, symptoms resolved once protein was decreased and fluid was provided.

INTERMEDIATE CARE MANAGEMENT

PATIENT CHARACTERISTICS

The intermediate phase of the trauma patient's recovery is characterized by an overall gradual decrease in metabolic rate. Severe septic complications have resolved; however, bacteremia and wound infections are still potential problems that can increase metabolic rate. Skeletal muscle wasting may have occurred despite nutritional support, and it requires continued support and physical therapy. A generalized weakness is apparent as a result of multiple factors. Prolonged bed rest, anemia, muscle wasting, and psychosocial alterations contribute to general malaise. Most patients have been extubated and are capable of maintaining adequate oxygenation and ventilation. Similarly, patients have exhibited hemodynamic and fluid and electrolyte stability.

Chief nutritional concerns are (1) the transition to an intermediate phase of nutritional support, (2) the quantification of energy expenditure with new activity levels, (3) improvement of muscle and visceral protein compartments, and (4) maintenance of immune function. Frequently, patients are ready to begin learning more about nutritional requirements and interventions. Family members play an integral role in the patient's total recovery. Traumatic illness can cause psychologic stress, anger, dependence, and depression that can potentially alter the success of the prescribed nutritional regimen. Similarly, neurologic and physical deficits may prevent independent feeding. Interdisciplinary assessment, planning, and intervention are critical to successful achievement of goals.

NUTRITION ASSESSMENT

ANTHROPOMETRIC DATA. Accurate and consistent weight measurements need to be obtained. Anthropometric measurements of patients with traumatic injuries should be interpreted with caution. Height/weight ratios may be appropriate at this time if the patient is hemodynamically stable and without edema. Evaluating actual weight by comparing it with ideal body weight has been criticized because a patient may have a stable body weight that is below ideal and not be malnourished. On the other hand, an obese person may rapidly lose excessive amounts of weight from muscle tissue, still be overweight, and be malnourished. Calculating the percentage of usual body weight is helpful to assess the degree of depletion since admission (see Table 16-3). Serial weights can note trends, which are helpful when viewed in relation to other factors. When the patient is medically stable with adequate osmolarity, trends of small weight increases with specific nutritional support indicate adequate sustenance. Because of the time and equipment required, skin fold measures are of little clinical use during this phase. In comparison, mid-arm circumference is more easily measured and requires little time and training. Mid-arm circumference measures could be used as an adjunct in noting trends in nutritional status.

BIOCHEMICAL DATA AND NITROGEN BALANCE. Traumatic injury and surgery depress prealbumin and albumin concentrations, which may remain depressed as a result of the acute phase response despite adequate feeding. However, once prealbumin concentration begins to rise in response to a normalization of protein production by the liver, prealbumin becomes an excellent marker of nutritional status and adequacy of feeding, followed by a similar rise in albumin. The goal is for the patient to achieve and maintain prealbumin and albumin within normal limits.

Nitrogen balance might assume a greater priority in the intermediate phase of recovery. At this time, one would expect the patient to be moving toward a neutral or more positive nitrogen balance. Patients who have spinal cord injury will have additional losses in nitrogen, reflecting protein loss caused by denervation and disuse of paralyzed muscles. Persistent negative nitrogen balance studies or studies that are not showing progress toward a positive balance might reflect failure of the prescribed nutritional plan, necessitating reassessment of energy and protein requirements. Continuing efforts to clarify nitrogen balance in relation to protein flux with the use of isotope technology may provide even more promise for future interpretation of this parameter.

CLINICAL EXAMINATION. Although not quantitative, the physical examination may give clues to protein-calorie malnutrition and specific vitamin and mineral deficiencies (see Table 16-1). Astute observation of physical assessment findings may lead to changes in patient management. Patients whose Braden Scale score is less than 18 should have regular screening for nutritional risk.[123] A full nutritional assessment should be conducted on all patients with a Braden Scale score of 12 or less.[44] If muscle wasting continues after the nutritional goals are met, nitrogen balance studies or metabolic cart evaluations can helpful to assess the appropriate nutrient prescription.

Patients with severe head injuries are dependent on nutritional support and may not begin oral feeding until 1 to 2 weeks after they are extubated. The greater the neurologic injury, the greater the risk for swallowing impairment and aspiration, particularly if the patient was intubated for 2 or more weeks or had a trachcostomy.[124] A patient whose level of consciousness improves may be ready to convert from enteral to oral feedings. Maxillofacial trauma repair may limit the patient's ability to chew or to take nourishment in general.[125]

Monitoring hydration is especially important for elderly patients, who often have reduced thirst and a general tendency to become dehydrated. A decline in renal function with advancing age leads to excess water loss because the capacity to concentrate urine may be impaired.[125] On the other hand, if the patient develops signs of fluid overload, the amount of fluid provided must be adjusted and a more concentrated form of calories be considered, depending on the cause of the fluid imbalance.

DIETARY DATA. Intake and output records are an essential aspect of nutritional assessment. The dietitian reviews records when determining nitrogen balances and calculating actual substrate intake. The nurse has total control of this record and must make sure intake of all oral, enteral, and parenteral nutrition is documented. Similarly, ensuring that the patient has received prescribed feedings is a must. Feedings may be held for therapeutic interventions; attempting to minimize this loss of intake is an important responsibility. Information regarding excessive diarrhea, vomiting, or drainage from other sources assists in determining adequacy or complications that relate to prescribed nutritional regimens.

Calorie counts are another assessment tool used to determine protein, carbohydrate, fat, and caloric intake. Calorie counts provide information on patients' ability to take in adequate nutrients on their own. The nurse, patient, and, possibly, a family member may participate in accurately recording the type of food and quantity ingested. The dietitian or diet technician analyzes these records to determine whether intake is adequate and to make recommendations. For example, adequate calories may be consumed, but protein intake may be below ideal levels. In this case protein supplements are ordered to improve dietary intake. When several days of adequate oral intake are documented, enteral tube feeding may be decreased or discontinued.

ENERGY AND PROTEIN NEEDS. Determining energy (caloric) requirements is essential in this phase, as in any other phase of trauma recovery. The HBEE continues to provide an estimate for basal energy needs during this phase. Metabolic demands seem to decrease relative to denervation of muscle tissue and associated loss of lean body mass. It is possible for patients with significant spinal cord deficit to have caloric requirements lower than basal levels. Normal body weight in the spinal cord-injured population is less than normal weight in an uninjured population. It may be appropriate for the spinal cord-injured patient to be 10 to 20 pounds lighter than normal.

Patients' activity level varies much more during the intermediate phase than during the critical care phase. Although energy requirements associated with the metabolic effects of injury may gradually decrease, activity level probably increases. The HBEE is usually multiplied by a factor of 1.2 for a patient confined to bed, and the factor 1.3 is used for a patient who is out of bed. Caution must be applied when using these factors because they have not been rigorously tested. The nurse is responsible for relaying information that updates the dietitian's records on activity level.

Similarly, altered wound status and temperature are important factors that might alter the patient's energy expenditure. Infections frequently can occur, with associated temperature elevations. As previously mentioned, a 1° C temperature elevation is associated with a 13% to 14% increase in basal energy requirements. Feeding should not be adjusted based on day-to-day variations in body temperature unless the patient has a consistently elevated temperature. An open wound that is infected and in need of debridement may contribute to an elevated metabolic rate because of endogenous mediator release. Open communication regarding changes in activity, infection, and wound status assists in accurately assessing the patient's energy requirements. In addition, indirect calorimetry, if available, helps to quantify these changes in metabolic rate more accurately.

When utilizing nitrogen balance in the trauma patient, one must consider occult losses. Nitrogen excretion is underestimated in patients with burns, diarrhea, vomiting, fistula drainage, and other abnormal nitrogen losses unless all losses of body fluids are analyzed. C-reactive protein can be used to help interpret the results of nitrogen balance studies. For example, if C-reactive protein is elevated, indicating an active stress response, and nitrogen balance is negative, the goal is to provide calories relative to measured or calculated needs. If stress levels are high, it may be impossible to reach positive nitrogen balance. Conversely, if C-reactive protein is not elevated and negative nitrogen balance persists, energy expenditure may be exceeding energy intake and adjustments can be made to increase energy and protein intake.

Skeletal muscle protein can continue to breakdown at an accelerated rate during convalescence, even when stress hormones have returned to normal levels. The cause of the continuing protein catabolism remains unknown.[21] Protein requirements may vary significantly, depending on degree of stress and amount of tissue loss and healing. As with the acute phase, protein intake in the intermediate phase is between 1 and 1.5 g/kg/day. The calorie/nitrogen ratio is approximately 120 to 125 kcal to 1 g nitrogen. The dietitian frequently calculates actual caloric intake as part of the nutritional assessment.

NUTRITION SUPPORT

Feeding modalities during the intermediate phase may be similar to those in the critical care phase. For example, if a patient receiving parenteral nutrition is still undergoing multiple surgical interventions that require NPO status, parenteral nutrition should continue. In contrast, if a patient has been extubated and major wound problems resolved, enteral tube feeding or oral nutrition may be initiated. Ongoing nursing, dietary, and medical assessments are necessary to determine the earliest possible transition to the oral or enteral nutrition route.

Some reduction in the mass of the large intestine occurs during TPN; in fact, small bowel biopsies from long-term TPN patients have shown dramatic atrophy of the microvilli height mass and absorptive area. In addition, patients with preexisting malnutrition might have additional losses of absorptive GI surface and further depressed enzyme production, contributing to even greater malabsorptive problems and intolerance of some enteral feedings, particularly of milk products (lactose). Therefore patients who are being changed from parenteral to enteral tube feeding or oral feedings need special consideration. As use of the new route for feeding increases, feeding through the previous route is gradually decreased. It may take several days for the gut to readjust to enteral tube feeding or oral diets. This is why patients progress from ice chips to a clear liquid diet, then to a full liquid diet, and finally to a regular diet as tolerated. Patients started on tube feedings should be able to tolerate the goal rate within 72 hours of the start of tube feeding. Initially, high residuals caused by decreased peristalsis may occur when a patient is making a transition from TPN to enteral feeding. Medications that increase GI motility may decrease problems with high residuals.

The head-injured patient requires a creative approach to nutritional interventions for multiple reasons. Altered levels of consciousness, cranial nerve damage, and general weakness or paralysis may alter the patient's ability to take in food voluntarily or safely. Maintaining caloric needs is imperative to avoid underfeeding and associated complications; therefore feeding modalities must be tailored to each patient's specific needs. If cranial nerve damage exists, swallowing ability must be assessed. Speech therapists test the patient's swallowing ability with foods that vary in consistency, such as thin liquids, pudding, and mashed potatoes. Once safe swallowing ability has been confirmed, the patient can be switched to oral meals as tolerated. Some patients may be able to tolerate thickened liquids safely, but not thin liquids. Consistency restrictions may be recommended by the speech therapist, and these may be modified over time as the patient recovers function. Patients who have had their jaws wired shut will also require meals of special consistency (blenderized liquid). The dietitian needs to ensure that patients with consistency restrictions are provided with adequate and appropriate meals. Furthermore, the dietitian needs to educate patients and caregivers on how to select nutritious foods, plan meals, and prepare foods to achieve appropriate body weight after the patient is discharged.

Patients who complain of anorexia or poor chewing ability are at risk for inadequate intake and loss of muscle mass.[126] Patients with marginal intake should be provided with interventions to promote good nutrition, such as oral supplements. Shakes, puddings, and food bars, with or between meals, are examples of supplements that are high in calories and protein. Families can be encouraged to bring in special foods the patient may desire. Eating while family members visit may be helpful to the patient from a psychologic and physical standpoint. Family members may be included to help feed or encourage the patient during mealtimes. Their input may be valuable with regard to special likes, dislikes, and psychologic or cultural considerations.

Several methods have been used to help ensure an appetite when meals are delivered. Using enteral tube feedings at night, while the patient is sleeping, and discontinuing them during the day is one method to help the patient achieve an adequate intake. If appetite problems persist because of fullness from continued enteral tube feedings, a trial period in which tube feedings are discontinued may help. The nasogastric tube may stay in place for several days to ensure consistent feeding behaviors. Similarly, some institutions continue tube feeding throughout the day, turning it off 2 hours before meals and reinstituting it 1 to 2 hours after a meal. These methods are individualized to meet the patient's personal and metabolic demands. Negotiating feeding schedules when appropriate may help the patient gain control over feedings and increase motivation. Tube feeding is not stopped completely until calorie counts confirm that the patient is meeting 50% to 75% of the estimated nutrient and fluid needs by oral means.[30]

Gastrostomy tube feedings may be the choice for long-term feeding. Because these tubes exit from the stomach through a small external opening, there is increased risk of infection. Care should be given to the exit site. Checking for redness, edema, exudate, and leakage of acidic stomach contents that break down the skin barrier is important. Dry sterile dressings and antimicrobial ointments should be applied to protect the exit site. Patients who are nauseated or vomit during tube feeding are at risk for aspiration. Keep the head of the bed elevated during the infusion of tube feeding to reduce this risk.

EDUCATION AND RANGE-OF-MOTION EXERCISE

The health care team determines what nutrition education is appropriate for the patient based on the patient's needs, abilities, readiness, and length of stay. Education about proper diet and hydration should be included in the bowel management of patients with spinal cord injuries, particularly with those with neurogenic bowel dysfunction. Lesions of the lumbar and sacral spine may damage the defecation center, requiring the manual removal of stool (flaccid bowel dysfunction). Fractures of the T12 vertebra and above can eliminate the normal sensation to defecate (spastic bowel dysfunction).[127] Regularly scheduled, well-balanced meals with plenty of fiber and fluids are necessary for a good bowel program. The patient should be taught to avoid foods that cause gas (e.g., onions, cabbage) or include, as needed, foods that have a natural laxative effect (e.g., prune juice) or that stimulate defecation (e.g., tea, coffee).

Promoting muscle activity improves muscle function and growth. Patients who have been on long-term controlled

mechanical ventilation because of extensive trauma need encouragement to increase their respiratory muscle activity. Similarly, frequent, active range-of-motion exercises should be incorporated into daily assessment activities. Patients are often fearful of various tubes and drains and need to be encouraged to exercise as tolerated. The physical therapist should assist in maintaining appropriate progress in the patient's activity level. Physical therapists and nurses should provide ongoing range-of-motion activities to rebuild the muscle mass lost because of the catabolic processes associated with severe trauma. As activity increases and muscle is rebuilt, the patient's energy needs increase and protein status improves.

REHABILITATION PHASE

PATIENT CHARACTERISTICS

The rehabilitation phase of recovery is characterized by a more stable metabolic rate. The patient's basal needs are closer to normal. The type of rehabilitation necessary greatly affects the patient's overall metabolic needs. For example, a patient who has sustained major pelvic fractures requires weeks to months of rigorous physical therapy, necessitating high caloric intake. Anabolic processes such as muscle building are evident in this phase. Physical and occupational therapists are actively involved in assisting the patient to achieve levels of independent functioning. Teaching the patient to overcome disabilities and understand the rationale behind proper nutritional intake is essential. The patient may be transferred to a rehabilitation facility, which usually promotes greater freedom and independent functioning. Patients have usually begun to adjust psychologically to their situation, although depression may still be present; boredom may exist, and patients may be eager to return home. Most patients have advanced from parenteral or enteral nutritional support to a completely oral diet. Patients referred for home tube feeding are those whose diagnoses prohibit oral intake of normal food.

ASSESSMENT

During the rehabilitation phase of trauma recovery, assessment strategies focus on teaching and assessing patients' ability to be independent in their care. Weight measurements are much more valid in this stage of recovery and provide a gross assessment of body composition (fat and protein stores). Patients should be weighed and trends should be evaluated.

The spinal cord-injured population have a shift in weight associated with protein muscle loss from atrophy and disuse. Skin fold measures may be of clinical value during this phase if the patient is expected to have a long stay in rehabilitation. Over time, changes in body composition, fat distribution, and energy stores may be evident from the changes in fat folds. Also, measurements of mid-arm circumference and arm muscle area may be of benefit to assess anabolic growth of lean muscle mass. Many patients recovering from critical illness are able to regain body protein by 3 months.[74] However, patients with spinal cord injuries incur significant reductions in bone and muscle tissue during the year after injury.[128] Muscle paralysis and subsequent extreme inactivity contribute to changes in body composition.

Serum albumin is expected to be within the normal range. If a patient's protein and caloric needs do not appear adequate, nitrogen balance studies may be performed. At this stage, nitrogen balance studies may reflect protein status if intake has been steady, urine collection is complete, and occult losses are minimal. Serial nitrogen balances may prove useful for indicating the effectiveness of dietary intake or nutritional support. Patients whose treatment required partial or total gastrectomy should be followed with yearly serum vitamin B_{12} tests. Parietal cells of the stomach produce a factor that is required for vitamin B_{12} absorption. Irreversible neurologic disease from vitamin B_{12} deficiency has been documented, developing 10 years after gastric surgery.[129]

Typically the patient is on an oral diet during rehabilitation. Some patients still require dietary supplements. If patients are responsible for their own dietary requirements, they may need to be instructed on appropriate selection of food groups for a balanced diet. Before discharge the nurse or dietitian should provide patients needing diet instruction with appropriate education. The focus is on foods high in calories and protein if the patient's nutritional status is not adequate. Calorie counts (diet records) or 24-hour diet recalls can help determine the amount of energy and protein the patient is consuming. Patients who sustained neurotrauma, especially spinal cord-injured patients, need extensive health teaching because of their tendency to be malnourished, their increased risk for pulmonary infection and pressure ulcers, and their problems with constipation. Similarly, patients are reminded of the importance of dietary calcium to assist in bone healing and maintenance of bone structure.

ENERGY AND PROTEIN NEEDS.   Muscle paralysis, extreme inactivity, and wheelchair confinement reduce energy expenditure in patients with spinal cord injuries. Two or more years after a spinal cord injury, men who can perform all their own activities of daily living expend approximately 27 kcal/day.[128] Persons with high-level injuries, such as those with high quadriplegia, are expected to have lower energy expenditures.[128]

Nutritional deficits can support the development and impede the treatment of pressure ulcers. If the patient has problems chewing, swallowing, or self-feeding, corrective action can be taken by offering assistance with eating and supplements; nutritional support may be needed. Protein repletion is associated with less bone loss and shorter length of stay in rehabilitation for elderly persons recovering from osteoporotic hip fracture.[130] The nutrition plan should be updated periodically to meet the individual's needs and to remain consistent with the overall goals of therapy.[31,33]

NUTRITION EDUCATION AND PSYCHOSOCIAL CONCERNS

Problems related to the experience of traumatic injury, such as loss of friends, loss of employment, and depression, can diminish patients' self-esteem and their relationship with their caregiver. Family coping skills and financial status also affect rehabilitation. All these factors indirectly or directly affect the patient's capacity to achieve optimal nutritional status and should be addressed as appropriate to improve the patient's quality of life.[131] Insurance coverage should also be discussed to decrease financial concerns. Those who are going home with physician orders for special diets or nutrition support must be provided with teaching; home health care assistance may be required.

Preparing the patient and significant other for home nutrition support or special diets requires multidisciplinary coordination. Social workers, nursing staffs, dietitians, pharmacologists, and a home health agency may be required for an adequate transition to home.

Once the medical team has determined the patient to be an appropriate candidate for home nutrition support, the teaching process begins. First, an assessment of the patient's and support person's cognitive and motor skills must be completed. Similarly, psychologic concerns related to lifestyle changes must be discussed.

Most patients are anxious to go home but may be frustrated if all procedures are not mastered. Therefore adequate time for preparation is essential. The following should be done:

1. Identify patient's learning needs
2. Determine readiness to learn
3. Establish mutual goals and objectives
4. Choose appropriate method/plan for teaching

When preparing the patient for discharge, technical aspects of TPN or tube feeding must be taught. Topics to cover include material storage, line/tube care, site care, dressing changes, infusion pump functions, nutrient delivery systems, physical activities, catheter complications (infection), metabolic assessment (intake and output, urine testing), and preparation of solutions if premixed solutions are not used. Complications such as diarrhea, dehydration (as a result of inadequate free water), and feeding tube blockage should be discussed. Patients must be taught to report symptoms such as nausea, vomiting, and abdominal distention because these may indicate feeding intolerance. In addition, the patient should report weight loss or excessive weight gain because this could indicate inadequate feeding or overfeeding. Health personnel teach by demonstration, using a return demonstration by the patient to determine acquisition of skills. In addition, detailed written instruction is necessary. The nurse should document all aspects of the educational process. Keeping lines of communication open by reinforcing the need to communicate questions and concerns may prevent major problems. A coordinated approach to home nutrition support requires appropriate selection, training, and follow-up for effective and safe application.

INTERDISCIPLINARY STRATEGIES

Independent and collaborative research opportunities exist for improvement in the quality of nutrition-related care for the trauma population. Clinicians need to work together to provide quality nutrition care. The ultimate goal is to prevent malnutrition and nutrition-related complications by identifying patients at greatest risk and intervening before serious functional losses or conditions appear. Additionally, the demand to determine and select the most beneficial, risk-free nutrition interventions for the trauma population cannot be underestimated. To participate effectively in a team approach, nurses, physicians, pharmacists, and dietitians need a sound knowledge base in nutrition. Weaknesses in nutritional knowledge, such as in recognizing the symptoms of overfeeding, need to be addressed so that patients are provided with appropriate and timely interventions.

Interdisciplinary collaborative strategies are essential for a comprehensive, outcome-oriented nutritional program for the trauma population. Strategies should include clarifying interdisciplinary role responsibilities, identifying nutritional clinical pathways for various nutritional modalities, ensuring that assessment and monitoring strategies are outlined in the pathway, and establishing an interdisciplinary communication system. Once the nutrition team has defined its strategies, ongoing and appropriate education and training sessions are needed to educate interdisciplinary team members as they are hired. Finally, quality teams and clinical quality measures should be established to determine the effectiveness of the nutritional program and to make ongoing program improvements.

CLINICAL PATHWAYS

Clinical guidelines in the form of clinical pathways, algorithms, and protocols need to be developed by the interdisciplinary team. Ideally, if a pathway exists for a given population, the nutrition-related care should be integrated into the entire plan of care. This approach capitalizes on the collaborative expertise of the interdisciplinary team. Clinical pathways are an interdisciplinary strategy that articulate practice expectations along the continuum of care. The pathway document itself can serve as a mechanism for communication, an approach for documentation, and a method to evaluate processes and outcomes of care. A clinical pathway generally works best for select populations. If specific practice interventions or outcomes do not occur in the time frame specified, then a variance has occurred. Variances are outcomes, missed interventions, or complications that need to be reviewed and may represent opportunities for improvement. Complications such as hyperglycemia and diarrhea represent variances. All complications cannot be prevented. However, excessive rates for specific complications, such as hyperglycemia, represent an opportunity for nutritional care evaluation and improvement.

ASPEN has published *Clinical Pathways and Algorithms for Delivery of Parenteral and Enteral Nutrition Support in Adults.*[30] This document assists interdisciplinary teams in establishing a customized plan of care for the trauma population. Developing these approaches requires intense interdisciplinary work. During team meetings, roles and responsibilities (e.g., assessing, monitoring, and evaluating) will be clarified relative to the patient's nutritional plan of care. This type of process facilitates teamwork and keeps the team focused on patient care and clinical outcomes.

QUALITY MEASURES

Whatever method is used to articulate assessment, monitoring, and outcome measures of nutritional care, the team must work together in an organized approach. The assessment, monitoring, and outcome information should be reviewed to determine the most appropriate quality measures.[29,132,133] Quality indicators representing the three areas of structure, process, and outcome should be considered. The team should determine the quality measures that will be used to evaluate the overall nutrition program.

Structure indicators relate to the characteristics of the staff: Is there adequate dietitian support to cover the trauma service? Is the nutrition team following the JCAHO standards? Process indicators assist in verifying that the appropriate steps in the process or procedure have been performed: Were all procedures related to TPN central line care performed, such as site care, tubing changes, and correct hang times? Were enteral feedings administered appropriately? Were drug-nutrient interventions considered? Were patients at nutritional risk identified early?

Identifying outcome measures, such as complications relative to overfeeding, are essential measurements of quality clinical care. These quality indicators need to be determined by the interdisciplinary team and evaluated as needed based on the hospital's baseline quality data. Collected data should be compared with benchmark data available in the literature. If baseline data are not available, a brainstorming session with all the disciplines present should be held to set priorities for data to be collected and monitored (internal benchmark data).

ROLES, RESPONSIBILITIES, AND COMMUNICATION

Determining roles and responsibilities for the team members is a natural part of the pathway development process. If pathways are not used, the group can review the nutrition support activities (e.g., nutrition assessment, patient care rounds, daily assessment, and surveillance), clarify the specific associated tasks, and clearly assign responsibilities. This helps the team to have clear expectations. Many of the tasks can be reviewed from a quality perspective. The written document will serve as an educational and communication tool, reinforcing and clarifying role expectations. Further, patient care rounds should be scheduled and conducted in a mutually agreed upon format. Ideally, an interdisciplinary computerized medical record with a specific nutrition screen that is integrated with laboratory data and other nutrition-related information should be created. Computer support personnel can help the clinical staff create computer programs that automatically "dump" data within the system into an organized nutrition screen. During rounds this screen/printout can function as the interdisciplinary rounding structure.

Roles and responsibilities may vary from organization to organization. Major nursing responsibilities include identifying high-risk patients, ensuring that orders are executed correctly, being alert to drug-nutrient interactions, and providing patient and family education. Accurately documenting intake and output records, obtaining and reviewing laboratory data, and recording side effects and complications of nutrition support are essential aspects of the nurse's role.

The dietitian will be the overall coordinator of nutrition care, involved in screening high-risk patients; performing a detailed nutritional assessment; making recommendations related to the nutrition support plan; and calculating energy, protein, carbohydrate, and fat requirements. In addition, calculating actual intake, reviewing laboratory values, and assessing tolerance to the nutritional support are critical aspects of the dietitian's role.

The pharmacist is responsible for reviewing each parenteral nutrition prescription for dose, route of administration, and the potential for drug-nutrient interactions.[134] The pharmacist must evaluate the parenteral nutrition ordered. Any major deviations from the previous day's prescription, including omissions, should be questioned.[134] In addition, any enteral drug-nutrient interactions should be identified collaboratively with the nurse so that appropriate drug dosing can be altered.

It is important to have a trauma physician who has a special interest in nutritional care involved in the interdisciplinary team process. Physicians work collaboratively with the dietitian and pharmacist to finalize nutrition support orders; review laboratory values; and order additional lab work, indirect calorimetry, and vitamin, mineral, and electrolyte replacement or supplementation. Managing complications is an interdisciplinary function. The process of rounding, in which all disciplines pull together to discuss and evaluate each patient individually, is instrumental to fine-tune the nutritional plan of care so that optimal patient outcomes can be achieved.[135]

PERSONNEL EDUCATION AND TRAINING

An orientation to the nutritional care process should be provided to all new interdisciplinary staff members. Individual role responsibilities and collaborative activities (e.g., rounds) that are critical to successful patient outcomes should be specified and reinforced. For nursing staff, this education should include the following:

- A general overview of metabolic and endocrine response to injury
- The importance of nutritional status to wound healing and recovery

- Administration of nutrition support and assessing tolerance
- Metabolic complications of overfeeding and underfeeding
- Infection control principles related to nutrition
- Clinical guidelines, pathways, protocols, or algorithms with a description of the various interdisciplinary role expectations

Special considerations in the multitrauma, traumatic brain injury, and spinal cord-injured populations should also be addressed. Ongoing in-service education is needed to disseminate changes in the nutritional program, the latest nutrition research, and quality improvement issues or initiatives. Finally, physicians and nurses who are involved in inserting and caring for the vascular access devices should have hands-on experience and mentoring and supervision as part of their comprehensive nutrition support education.[90]

FUTURE RESEARCH

Energy prediction equations with various factors need to be further validated. Standard operational definitions need to be developed so that multiple institutional settings can consistently and accurately use a formula and factors based on objective criteria. Nurses' input regarding use of an assortment of activity factors and the objective criteria is essential because nurses are in the best position to validate these factors. Similarly, we need to validate the characteristics in trauma patients that have a high correlation with metabolic rate alterations.

Subgroups of trauma patients need further consideration. For example, elderly and obese people have more complications when traumatically injured. Are there specific metabolic or nutritional interventions that might improve prognosis? Are there differences in metabolic rate and injury response in specific subgroups (e.g., males versus females) that necessitate different nutritional interventions? The head-injured population has a variable metabolic rate. Can subgroups be identified that will help practitioners individualize nutrition support?

Can the nurse and physical therapist improve nitrogen retention and increase muscle mass by an active or passive range-of-motion program for patients who are not weight bearing and are receiving nutrition support?

What baseline complications occur in the trauma population related to enteral and parenteral nutrition support? Can we make quality improvements to decrease these complications?

An interdisciplinary team can evaluate the current literature, hospital blood stream infection (BSI) rates, and trends (specifically those associated with TPN) along with the hospital infection control office to customize policies and procedures that meet the needs of the trauma population. Any increased BSI rates related to TPN must be investigated thoroughly so that appropriate teams can be formed to identify the root cause and take appropriate actions. BSI infections are associated with a doubling of the intensive care unit stay and increase hospital length of stay by 24 days (for survivors). BSI can cost anywhere from $3,061 to $40,000.[136,137] BSI-associated mortality ranges from 23.8% to 50% (including pneumonia).

In conclusion, previous research emphasized the need to prevent underfeeding. Although this is an extremely important finding, recent studies suggest equally significant consequences related to overfeeding. It is possible that, because of the emphasis on hospital malnutrition in the past, distorted findings from unreliable energy measurements are being used without substantial validation. Future research will reveal ways to assess nutritional status accurately and to improve nutritional intake and energy prediction uniformly, thus improving overall outcome and reducing excessive costs caused by overfeeding critically ill trauma patients.

SUMMARY

This chapter has provided an overview of normal metabolism and metabolic alterations after injury. Various hormonal and humoral factors that favor catabolism are activated by injury. Combined with the inability to take in food, the trauma patient uses endogenous substrates to provide for high-magnitude energy needs during the hypermetabolic response. The protein compartment, the most functional compartment, is the most seriously depleted during recovery from injury. Complications related to depletion of this compartment have serious sequelae.

Traditional nutritional assessment parameters are of questionable validity in the critically ill trauma population. Various factors need to be assessed and viewed in relation to a patient's clinical picture to be meaningful. An interdisciplinary approach that involves close relationships among the nurse, dietitian, and physician is necessary to achieve nutrition goals. Prescribed nutritional regimens need accurate assessment and evaluation by an astute nursing staff.

Multiple nutritional modalities are used depending on specific patient criteria. Complications can occur related to excessive or deficient calories. The entire team must provide continuous monitoring of nutritional assessment parameters and fluid and electrolyte status. This continuous monitoring provides data necessary to institute different nutritional modalities as the patient progresses through the critical care, intermediate, and rehabilitation phases of recovery. Patients and families must be taught about nutritional modalities and the rationale and consequences associated with inadequate intake.

A number of research findings emphasize the need for individual and collaborative studies. Current practices must continue to be evaluated to provide the best possible comprehensive metabolic and nutritional care for seriously injured patients.

REFERENCES

1. Food and Nutrition Board: *Recommended dietary allowances,* ed 10, Washington, DC, 1989, National Academy.
2. Institute of Medicine, Food and Nutrition Board: *Dietary reference intakes for thiamin, Riboflavin, niacin, vitamin B6, folate, vitamin B12, pantothenic acid, biotin and choline,* Washington, DC, 1998, National Academic.
3. Ziegler EE, Filer LJ Jr, editors: *Present knowledge in nutrition,* ed 7, Washington, DC, 1996, ILSI.
4. Connor WE: Alpha-linolenic acid in health and disease, *Am J Clin Nutr* 69:827-828, 1999.
5. Adolph M, Hailer S, Eckart J: Serum phospholipid fatty acids in severely injured patients on total parenteral nutrition with medium chain/long chain triglyceride emulsions, *Ann Nutr Metabol* 39:251-260, 1995.
6. Owen OE, Smalley KJ, D'Alessio DA et al: Protein, fat, and carbohydrate requirements during starvation: anaplerosis and cataplerosis, *Am J Clin Nutr* 68:12-34, 1998.
7. Cahill GF Jr: Survival in starvation, *Am J Clin Nutr* 68:1-2, 1998.
8. Collins S, Myatt M, Golden B: Dietary treatment of severe malnutrition in adults, *Am J Clin Nutr* 68:193-199, 1998.
9. Caballero B: Optimal amount of dietary protein for treating adult malnutrition, *Am J Clin Nutr* 68:10-11, 1998.
10. Vitello JM: *Metabolic response to stress.* Presented at Nutrition Support in Stress and Sepsis, 23rd Clinical Congress of the American Society for Parenteral and Enteral Nutrition, San Diego, Calif, Jan 31-Feb 3, 1999.
11. McClave SA, Lowen CC, Kleber MJ et al: Are patients fed appropriately according to their calorie requirements? *J Parenter Enteral Nutr* 22:375-381, 1998.
12. Petersen SR, Holaday NJ, Jeevanandam M: Enhancement of protein synthesis efficiency in parenterally fed trauma victims by adjuvant recombinant human growth hormone, *J Trauma* 36:726-733, 1994.
13. Kiiski R, Takala J: Hypermetabolism and efficiency of CO_2 removal in acute respiratory failure, *Chest* 105:1198-1203, 1994.
14. Boulanger BR, Nayman R, McLean RF et al: What are the clinical determinants of early energy expenditure in critically injured adults? *J Trauma* 37:969-974, 1994.
15. Jeevanandam M, Petersen SR, Shamos RF: Protein and glucose kinetics and hormonal changes in elderly trauma patients, *Metabolism* 42:1255-1262, 1993.
16. Casati A, Colombo S, Leggieri C et al: Measured versus calculated energy expenditure in pressure support ventilated ICU patients, *Minerva Anestesiol* 62:165-170, 1996.
17. Hwang T, Huang S, Chen M: The use of indirect calorimetry in critically ill patients: the relationship of measured energy expenditure to injury severity score, septic severity score, and APACHEII score, *J Trauma* 34:247-251, 1993.
18. Frankenfield DC, Omert LA, Badellino MM et al: Correlation between measured energy expenditure and clinically obtained variables in trauma and sepsis patients, *J Parenter Enterol Nutr* 18:398-403, 1994.
19. Druml W, Fischer M, Ratheiser K: Use of intravenous lipids in critically ill patients with sepsis without and with hepatic failure, *J Parenter Enterol Nutr* 22:217-223, 1998.

20. Flakoll PJ, Wentzel LS, Hyman SA: Protein and glucose metabolism during isolated closed-head injury, *Am J Physiol* 269:E636-E641, 1995.

21. Wolfe RR: Herman Award Lecture, 1996: relation of metabolic studies to clinical nutrition—the example of burn injury, *Am J Clin Nutr* 64:800-808, 1996.

22. Lipp J: Glutamine and immune function: theory and clinical applications, *Support Line* 19(5):14-18, 1997.

23. Monk DN, Plank LD, Franch-Arcas G et al: Sequential changes in the metabolic response in critically injured patients during the first 25 days after blunt trauma, *Ann Surg* 223:395-405, 1996

24. Long CL, Schaffel N, Geiger JW et al: Metabolic response to injury and illness: Estimation of energy and protein needs from indirect calorimetry and nitrogen balance, *J Parenter Enteral Nutr* 3:452-456, 1979.

25. Bistrian BR, Babineau T: Optimal protein intake in critical illness? *Crit Care Med* 26:1476-1477, 1998.

26. Beisel WR: Herman Award Lecture, 1995: infection-induced malnutrition from cholera to cytokines, *Am J Clin Nutr* 62:813-819, 1995.

27. McClave SA, Snider HL: Understanding the metabolic response to critical illness: factors that cause patients to deviate from the expected pattern of hypermetabolism, *New Horiz* 2:139-146, 1994.

28. Kreymann G, Grosser S, Buggisch P et al: Oxygen consumption and resting metabolic rate in sepsis, sepsis syndrome and septic shock, *Crit Care Med* 21:1012-1019, 1993.

29. Kushner RF, Ayello EA, Beyer PL et al: National Coordinating Committee clinical indicators of nutrition care, *J Am Diet Assoc* 94:1168-1177, 1994.

30. ASPEN Board of Directors: *Clinical pathways and algorithms for delivery of parenteral and enteral nutrition support in adults,* Silver Spring, Md, 1998, American Society for Parenteral and Enteral Nutrition.

31. Joint Commission on Accreditation of Healthcare Organizations: *Accreditation manual for hospitals,* vol 1, Standards; vol 2, Scoring guidelines, Oakbrook Terrace, Ill, 1994, The Commission.

32. Hedund J: Community-acquired pneumonia requiring hospitalization. Factors of importance for the short and long term prognosis, *Scan J Infect Dis* 97(suppl):1-60, 1995.

33. American Society for Parenteral and Enteral Nutrition: Standards for nutrition support: hospitalized patients, *Nutr Clin Pract* 10:208-219, 1995

34. Posthauer ME, Dorse B, Foiles AA et al: Identifying patients at risk: ADA's definitions for nutrition screening and nutrition assessment, *J Am Diet Assoc* 94:838-839, 1994.

35. The National Heart, Lung and Blood Institute Expert Panel on the Identification, Evaluation and Treatment of Overweight and Obesity in Adults: Executive summary of the clinical guidelines on the identification, evaluation, and treatment of overweight and obesity in adults, *J Am Diet Assoc* 98:1178-1191, 1998.

36. Cutts ME, Dowdy RP, Ellersieck MR et al: Predicting energy needs in ventilator-dependent critically ill patients: effect of adjusting weight for edema or adiposity, *Am J Clin Nutr* 66:1250-1256, 1997.

37. American Dietetic Association: Adjustment in body weight for obese patients. In *Manual of clinical dietetics,* Chicago, 1988, The Association, 622-623.

38. Hamwi GJ: Therapy: changing dietary concepts. In Danowski TS, editor: *Diabetes mellitus: diagnosis and treatment,* New York, 1964, American Diabetes Association, 73-78.

39. Dunham CM, Damiano AM, Wiles CE et al: Post-traumatic multiple organ dysfunction syndrome: infection is an uncommon antecedent risk factor, *Injury* 26:373-378, 1995.

40. Koval KJ, Maurer SG, Su ET et al: The effects of nutritional status on outcome after hip fracture, *J Orthop Trauma* 13:164-169, 1999.

41. Kight MA, Kelly MP, Casillo S et al: Conducting physical examination rounds for manifestations of nutrient deficiency or excess: an essential component of JCAHO assessment performance, *Nutr Clin Pract* 14:93-98, 1999.

42. Cuffaro L, Levine AM, Harrison L et al: Fluid intakes and hydration status of institutionalized elderly nursing home residents, *J Am Diet Assoc* 97:A-79, 1997.

43. Braden BJ: Using the Braden scale for predicting pressure sore risk, *Support Line* 18:14-17, 1996.

44. Panel for the Predicting and Prevention of Pressure Ulcers in Adults: *Pressure ulcers in adults: prediction and prevention,* Clinical Practice Guidelines No. 3, AHCPR Publ No. 92-0047, Rockville, Md, 1992, Agency for Health Care Policy and Research, Public Health Office.

45. Porter C, Cohen NH: Indirect calorimetry in critically ill patients: role of the clinical dietitian in interpreting results, *J Am Diet Assoc* 96:49-54, 57, 1996.

46. Flancbaum L, Choban PS, Sambucco S et al: Comparison of indirect calorimetry, the Fick method, and prediction equations in estimating the energy requirements of critically ill patients, *Am J Clin Nutr* 69:461-466, 1999.

47. Fleisch A: Le metabolisme basal standard et sa determination au moyen du metabocalculator, *Helv Med Acta* 18:23-44, 1951.

48. World Health Organization: *Energy and protein requirements,* WHO Technical Report Series No. 724. Geneva, 1985, WHO.

49. Vinken AG, Bathalon GP, Saway AL et al: Equations for predicting the energy requirement of healthy adults aged 18-81 y, *A J Clin Nutr* 79:920-926, 1999.

50. Seale JL, Conway JM, Rumpler WV: Free-living and sleeping energy expenditure predicted from gender, weight, and fat mass, *FASEB J* 10:A212, 1996.

51. Yamasaki M, Irizawa M, Kanura T et al: Daily energy expenditure in active and inactive persons with spinal cord injury, *J Hum Ergol* (Tokyo) 21:125-133, 1992.

52. Gagliardi E, Brathwaite CEM, Ross SE: Predicting energy expenditure in trauma patients: validation of the Ireton Jones equation [abstract], *J Parenter Enterol Nutr* 19(Suppl):22S, 1995.

53. Harris JA, Benedict FG: *A biometric study of basal metabolism in man,* Publ No. 279, Washington, DC, 1919, Carnegie Institute of Washington.

54. Taaffe DR, Thompson J, Butterfield G et al: Accuracy of equations to predict basal metabolic rate in older women, *J Am Diet Assoc* 95:1387-1392, 1995.

55. Garrel DR, Jobin N, DeJonge LHM: Should we still use the Harris and Benedict equations? *Nutr Clin Prac* 11:99-103, 1996.

56. Ogawa AM, Shikora SA, Burke LM et al: The thermodilution technique for measuring resting energy expenditure does not agree with indirect calorimetry for the critically ill patient, *J Parenter Enterol Nutr* 22:347-351, 1998.

57. Ishibashi N, Plank LD, Sando K et al: Optimal protein requirements during the first two weeks after the onset of critical illness, *Crit Care Med* 26:1529-1535, 1998.

58. Muller T, Muller A, Bachem MG et al: Immediate metabolic effects of different nutritional regimens in critically ill medical patients, *Intensive Care Med* 21:561-566, 1995.

59. Harkin R, Brillon DJ, Matthews DE: The effects of glucocorticoids on energy expenditure [abstract], *Am J Clin Nutr* 61:913, 1995.

60. Bruder N, Lassegue D, Pelissier D et al: Energy expenditure and withdrawal of sedation in severe head-injured patients, *Crit Care Med* 22:1114-1119, 1994.

61. Poblete B, Romand JA, Pichard C et al: Metabolic effects of i.v. propacetamol, metamizol or external cooling in critically ill febrile patients, *Br J Anaesth* 78:123-127, 1997.

62. Royall D, Fairholm L, Peters WJ et al: Continuous measurement of energy expenditure in ventilated burn patients: an analysis, *Crit Care Med* 22:399-406, 1994.

63. Frankenfield DC, Smith JS, Cooney RN: Accelerated nitrogen loss after traumatic injury is not attenuated by achievement of energy balance, *J Parenter Enteral Nutr* 21:324-329, 1997.

64. Rodriguez DJ, Sandoval W, Clevenger FW: Is measured energy expenditure correlated to injury severity score in major trauma patients? *J Surg Res* 59:455-459, 1995.

65. Ireton-Jones CS, Jones JD: Why use predictive equations for energy expenditure assessment? *J Am Diet Assoc* 97(Suppl): A-44, 1997.

66. Amato P, Keating KP, Quercia RA et al: Formulaic methods of estimating calorie requirements in mechanically ventilated obese patients; a reappraisal, *Nutr Clin Pract* 10:229-232, 1995.

67. Sherman MS: A predictive equation for determination of resting energy expenditure in mechanically ventilated patients, *Chest* 105:544-549, 1994.

68. Mendez C, Jurkovich GJ, Garcia I et al: Effects of an immune-enhancing diet in critically injured patients, *J Trauma* 42:933-940, 1997.

69. Druml W: Protein metabolism in acute renal failure, *Miner Electrolyte Metab* 24:47-54, 1998.

70. DuBose TD Jr, Warnock DG, Mehta RL et al: ARF in the 21st century: recommendations for management and outcomes assessment, *Am J Kidney Dis* 29:793-799, 1997.

71. Breslow RA, Bergstrom N: Nutritional prediction of pressure ulcers, *J Am Diet Assoc* 94:1301-1304, 1994.

72. Weireter LJ Jr: Controversies in nutritional support of the surgical patient, *Surg Ann* 27:41-54, 1995.

73. Lipman TO: Grains or veins: is enteral nutrition really better than parenteral nutrition? A look at the evidence, *J Parenter Enteral Nutr* 22:167-182, 1998.

74. Campbell LT: Nutrition support in patients with multiple organ failure, *Curr Opin Clin Nutr Metab Care* 1:211-216, 1998.

75. Raina N, Cameron RG, Jeejeebhoy KN: Gastrointestinal, hepatic, and metabolic effects of enteral and parenteral nutrition in rats infused with tumor necrosis factor, *J Parenter Enteral Nutr* 21:7-13, 1997.

76. Cerra FB: Evidence-based analysis of nutrition support in sepsis. In Sibbald WJ, Vincent JL, editors: *Clinical trials for the treatment of sepsis*, New York, 1995, Springer-Verlag, 225-236.

77. Stein TP, Boden G: Attenuation of the protein wasting associated with bed rest by dietary branched chain amino acids, *Am J Clin Nutr* 61:904, 1995.

78. Garcia-de-Lorenzo A, Ortiz-Leyba C, Planas M et al: Parenteral administration of different amounts of branch-chain amino acids in septic patients: clinical and metabolic aspects, *Crit Care Med* 25:418-424, 1997.

79. Galban C, Celaya S, Marco P et al: *An immune-enhancing enteral diet reduces mortality and episodes of bacteremia in septic ICU patients.* Presented at American Society for Parenteral and Enteral Nutrition, 22nd Clinical Congress, Lake Buena Vista, Fla, Jan 18-21, 1998.

80. De Nicola L, Minutoto R, Bellizzi V et al: Enhancement of nitric oxide synthesis by L-arginine supplementation in renal disease: is it good or bad? *Miner Electrolyte Metab* 23:144-150, 1997.

81. Albina JE: Nutrition in wound healing, *J Parenter Enteral Nutr* 18:367-376, 1994.

82. Weimann A, Bastian L, Bischoff WE et al: Influence of arginine, omega-3 fatty acids and nucleotide-supplemented enteral support on systemic inflammatory response syndrome and multiple organ failure in patients after severe trauma, *Nutrition* 14:165-172, 1998.

83. Demetriades H, Botsios D, Kazantzidou D et al: Effect of early post-operative enteral feeding on the healing of colonic anastomoses in rats. Comparison of three different enteral diets, *Eur Surg Res* 31:57-63, 1999.

84. Houdijk APJ, Rijnsburger ER, Jansen J et al: Randomized trial of glutamine-enriched enteral nutrition on infectious morbidity in patients with multiple trauma, *Lancet* 352:772-776, 1998.

85. Griffiths RD: Outcome of critically ill patients after supplementation with glutamine, *Nutrition* 13:752-754, 1997.

86. Baldwin SA, Fugaccia I, Brown DR et al: Blood-brain barrier breach following cortical contusion in the rat, *J Neurosurg* 85:476-481, 1996.

87. Bullock R, Zauner A, Woodward JJ et al: Factors affecting excitatory amino acid release following severe human head injury, *J Neurosurg* 89:507-518, 1998.

88. Souba WW Jr, Kohn-Keeth C, Mueller C et al: *The A.S.P.E.N. nutrition support practice manual*, Silver Spring, Md, 1998, American Society for Parenteral and Enteral Nutrition.

89. Rombeau JL, Rolandelli RH: *Enteral and tube feeding*, ed 3, Philadelphia, 1997, WB Saunders.

90. Winkler MF, Watkins CK, Albina JE: Vascular access devices: one institutions teaching experience, *Nutr Clin Pract* 14: 205-207, 1999.

91. Veldee MS: Nutrition. In Burtis CA, Ashwood ER, editors: *Tietz textbook of clinical chemistry*, Philadelphia, 1994, WB Saunders, 1236-1274.

92. Kudsk KA: *Current issues in enteral nutrition support: report of the first Ross Conference on Enteral Devices*, Columbus, Ohio, 1996, Ross Laboratories.

93. Skipper A: *Dietitian's handbook of enteral and parenteral nutrition*, Rockville, Md, 1989, Aspen, 284.

94. Erickson A: Inquire here—what is the best method to prevent the development of clogs in feeding tubes? What are some techniques to unclog feeding tubes? *Support Line* 2:18-19, 1997.

95. Campbell SM: Guidelines for preventing contamination of enteral feedings. In *Preventing microbial contamination of enteral formulas and delivery systems,* Columbus, Ohio, 1995, Ross Products Division, Abbott Laboratories, 19-22.

96. Kirby DF, Dudrick SJ: *Practical handbook of nutrition in clinical practice,* Boca Raton, Fla, 1994, CRC.

97. Morrison G, Hark L: *Medical nutrition and disease,* Cambridge, Mass, 1996, Blackwell Science, 347-359.

98. Pearson ML: Guidelines for prevention of intravascular-device related infection, *Infect Control Hosp Epidemiol* 17: 438-473, 1996.

99. Tasota FJ, Fisher EM, Coulson CF et al: Protecting ICU patients from nosocomial infections: practical measures for favorable outcomes, *Crit Care Nurse* 18:54-64, 1998.

100. Sacks GS: Is IV lipid emulsion safe in patients with hypertriglyceridemia? *Nutr Clin Prac* 12:120-121, 1997.

101. Benabe JE, Martinez-Maldonado M: The impact of malnutrition on kidney function, *Miner Electrolyte Metab* 24:20-26, 1998.

102. Fiaccadori E, Lombardi M, Leonardi P et al: Outcome of malnutrition in acute renal failure, *J Am Soc Nephrol* 7:1372, 1996.

103. Jensen SA, Tygstrup N, Kondrup J: Effect of semistarvation and refeeding on plasma-macroglobulin and hepatic mRNA for APR in endotoxin-treated rats, *J Parenter Enteral Nutr* 22:S8, 1998.

104. Desai G, Sucher K, Chen MC: Impact of malnutrition in patients with pneumonia on length of stay, *J Am Diet Assoc* 97(suppl):A-50, 1997.

105. Naber THJ, Schermer T, de Bree A et al: Prevalence of malnutrition in nonsurgical hospitalized patients and its association with disease complications, *Am J Clin Nutr* 66:1232-1239, 1997.

106. Bower RH: Nutrition and immune function, *Nutr Clin Pract* 5:189-195, 1990.

107. Thomas B: *Manual of dietetic practice,* ed 2, London, 1994, Blackwell Scientific.

108. Sullivan DH, Walls RC: Protein-energy undernutrition and the risk of mortality within 6 years of hospital discharge, *J Am Coll Nutr* 17:571-578, 1998.

109. Chwals WJ: Overfeeding the critically ill child: fact or fantasy? *New Horiz* 2:147-155, 1994.

110. Klein CJ, Stanek GS, Wiles CE: Overfeeding macronutrients to critically ill adults: metabolic complications, *J Am Diet Assoc* 98:795-806, 1998.

111. Frankel WL, Evans NJ, Rombeau JL: Scientific rationale and clinical application of parenteral nutrition in critically ill patients. In Rombeau JL, Caldwell MD, editors: *Clinical nutrition: parenteral nutrition,* ed 2, Philadelphia, 1993, WB Saunders, 601.

112. Zerr KJ, Furnary AP, Grunkemeier GL et al: Glucose control lowers the risk of wound infection in diabetics after open-heart operations, *Ann Thorac Surg* 63:356-361, 1997.

113. Pomposelli JJ, Baxter JK III, Babineau TJ et al: Early postoperative glucose control predicts nosocomial infection rate in diabetic patients, *J Parenter Enteral Nutr* 22:77-81, 1998.

114. Verhofstad MHJ, Hendriks T: Complete prevention of impaired anastomotic healing in diabetic rats requires preoperative blood glucose control, *Brit J Surg* 83:1717-1721, 1996.

115. Wallace LK, Starr NJ, Leventhal MJ et al: Hyperglycemia on ICU admission after CABG is associated with increased risk of mediastinitis or wound infection, *Anesthesiology* 85:A286, 1996.

116. Perreault MM, Ostrop NJ, Tierney MG: Efficacy and safety of intravenous phosphate replacement in critically ill patients, *Ann Pharmacother* 31:683-688, 1997.

117. Olerich MA, Rude RK: Should we supplement magnesium in critically ill patients? *New Horiz* 2:186-192, 1994.

118. Aranda-Michel J, Morgan SL: Overfeeding in a patient with kwashiorkor syndrome, *Nutrition* 12:623-625, 1996.

119. Lowry TS, Dunlap AW, Brown RO et al: Pharmacologic influence on nutrition support therapy: use of propofol in a patient receiving combined enteral and parenteral nutrition support, *Nutr Clin Prac* 11:147-149, 1996.

120. Roth B, Nilsson-Ehle P, Eliasson I: Possible role of short-term nutrition with fat emulsions for development of haemophagocytosis with multiple organ failure in a patient with traumatic brain injury, *Intensive Care Med* 19:111-114, 1993.

121. Bauer B, Gardner L, Holdy K, Kalafer M: *Case report: metabolic acidosis associated with high protein enteral nutrition (EN).* Presented at American Society for Parenteral and Enteral Nutrition's 21st Clinical Congress: Nutrition and Metabolic Support: Challenges in the Age of Managed Care, San Francisco, Calif, Jan 26-29, 1997.

122. Gault MH, Dixon ME, Doyle M et al: Hypernatremia, azotemia, and dehydration due to high-protein tube feeding, *Ann Intern Med* 68:778-791, 1968.

123. Bergstrom N, Braden B, Kemp M et al: Prediction pressure ulcer risk, *Nurs Res* 47:261-269, 1998.

124. Mackay LE, Morgan AS, Bernstein BA: Swallowing disorders in severe brain injury: risk factors affecting return to oral intake, *Arch Phys Med Rehab* 80:365-371, 1999.

125. Marciani RD: Critical systemic and psychosocial considerations in management of trauma in the elderly, *Oral Surg Oral Med Oral Pathol Oral Radiol Endod* 87:272-280, 1999.

126. Incalzi RA, Gemma A, Capparella O et al: Energy intake and in-hospital starvation: a clinically relevant relationship, *Arch Intern Med* 156:425-429, 1996.

127. Hammond MC, Umlauf RL, Matteson B et al: *Yes, you can! A guide to self-care for persons with spinal cord injury,* ed 2, Washington, DC, 1994, Paralyzed Veterans of America.

128. Monroe MB, Tataranni PA, Pratley R et al: Lower daily energy expenditure as measured by a respiratory chamber in subjects with spinal cord injury compared with control subjects, *Am J Clin Nutr* 68:1223-1227, 1998.

129. Ukleja A, Scolapio JS, Tarrosa V et al: Irreversible neurologic disease following partial gastrectomy, *Nutr Clin Prac* 14:103, 1999.

130. Schurch MA, Rizzoli R, Slosman D et al: Protein supplements increase serum insulin-like GF-I levels and attenuate proximal femur bone loss in patients with recent hip fracture. A randomized double-blind, placebo-controlled trial, *Ann Intern Med* 128:801-809, 1998.

131. Smith CE: Quality of life in long-term parenteral nutrition patients and their family caregivers, *J Parenter Enteral Nutr* 17:501-506, 1993.

132. Winkler MF: Clinical indicators for nutrition support, *Top Clin Nutr* 10:17-24, 1995.

133. Klein CJ, Henry SM: Acute nutrition interventions help identify indicators of quality in a trauma service, *Nutr Clin Pract* 14:85-92, 1999.

134. National Advisory Group on Standards and Practice Guidelines for Parenteral Nutrition: Safe practices for parenteral nutrition formulations, *J Parenter Enterol Nutr* 22:49-66, 1998.

135. Klein CJ, Wiles CE: Evaluation of nutrition care provided to patients with traumatic injuries at risk for multiple organ dysfunction syndrome, *J Am Diet Assoc* 97:1422-1424, 1998.

136. Pittet D, Tarara D, Wenzel PP: Nosocomial blood stream infections in critically ill patients, *JAMA* 271:1598-1601, 1994.

137. Jarvis WR: Selected aspects of the socioeconomic impact of nosocomial infections: morbidity, mortality, cost and prevention, *Infect Control Hosp Epidemiol* 17:552-557, 1996.

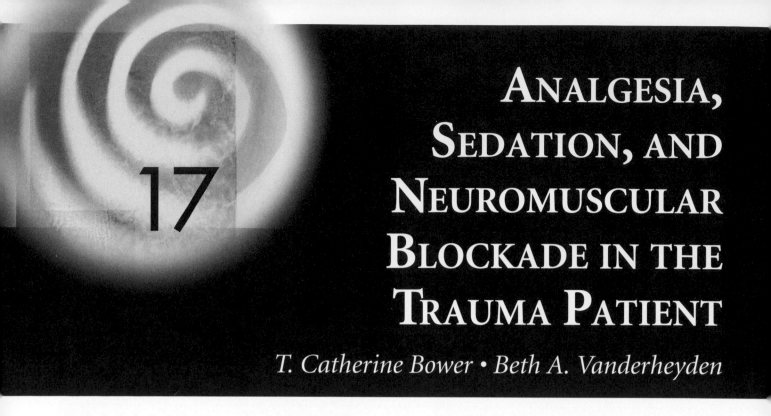

17

ANALGESIA, SEDATION, AND NEUROMUSCULAR BLOCKADE IN THE TRAUMA PATIENT

T. Catherine Bower • Beth A. Vanderheyden

Pain management, sedation, and neuromuscular blockade within the trauma population offer unique challenges to nursing care and require a multidisciplinary approach. Traumatic injuries are the consequence of external forces, and subsequent delayed sequelae are complex and painful. The purpose of this chapter is provide a comprehensive review and offer guidelines for managing trauma patients receiving analgesia, sedation, and neuromuscular blockade (NMB) through the phases of the trauma continuum. It should be stressed that although the topics are discussed separately, application of therapies described in each topic should be addressed holistically in defining a comprehensive plan, with individualization and ongoing reassessment. In the ever-changing climate of health care resource reduction, the practitioner caring for a trauma patient must apply a basic understanding of pain mechanisms and treatment strategies to provide patient-centered quality care throughout the acute and rehabilitative course.

INADEQUATE PAIN MANAGEMENT

Analgesics and sedatives are among the most frequently administered agents in the acute care setting, yet there is documentation that pain and agitation are inadequately controlled.[1-3] Obstacles to pain management in the critical care population include the inability to communicate pain rating, competing priorities of care, lack of documentation, and practitioners' lack of knowledge.[4] In the trauma setting some patients require immediate resuscitation, when priorities of oxygenation and circulation outweigh the administration of analgesic and sedative agents. Endotracheal intubation prohibits patient verbalization of pain intensity. Despite expressing high levels of pain when interviewed, patients in the critical care environment have reported satisfaction with their management of pain.[5-7]

DEFINITIONS

Pain has been described as "an unpleasant sensory and emotional experience associated with actual or potential tissue damage."[8] It is a sensation that is strictly subjective in nature. Caillet states that pain is the protective signal for the threat to survival.[9] Pain warns the individual that something is not right and that homeostasis is altered. The physiologic response to injury, with release of catecholamines, is not the only component influencing pain; emotion is strongly associated with painful stimuli.[10] Trauma patients experience unique behaviors after traumatic injury. Sudden, unplanned hospitalization and severe multisystem injuries causing alteration in body image create a stressful climate for both the trauma patient and family. Emotional behaviors, such as anger, fear, and anxiety, are displayed and can amplify the pain experience.[11]

Pain can be acute, chronic, or neuropathic in nature. Acute pain is brief, lasting less than 6 months. It subsides once the healing process is accomplished. Chronic pain involves complex processes and pathology. It is constant and prolonged, lasting longer than 6 months. Neuropathic pain involves alteration to the nervous system that produces unique features, such as constant burning sensations. Trauma patients can experience any of the mentioned types of pain, both singularly and in combination. The severity of injury, the presence of preexisting pain states, and subsequent complications all affect the overall pain experience. Trauma patients may experience chronic wound pain,[12] which can be cyclic or constant, especially after open tissue or degloving injury.

The nurse in the trauma setting must appreciate that pain is whatever the person says it is and that it occurs when that person says it does.[13] Pain assessment and treatment are challenging when the patient cannot communicate pain perceptions, particularly in the intubated and brain-injured populations. Maintaining pain management as a priority in overall care, whether the patient is conscious or unconscious, is the key to proactive management. Total quality management programs and customer satisfaction feedback place emphasis on pain management as a priority, incorporating pain into critical pathways and including pain assessment as the fifth vital sign.[14-16]

The undertreatment of pain is well documented.[17,18] The Agency for Health Care Policy and Research (AHCPR) recognized that inadequate pain management is widespread as a result of many factors, one being a lack of a comprehensive team approach.[19] The clinical practice guideline for acute pain management identified common barriers to postoperative pain management, such as lack of assessment, and offered health care providers principles and procedures to apply to daily practice. As we enter the new millennium, the challenge has shifted to the bedside caregiver to provide state-of-the-art, highly sophisticated assessment and analgesic delivery to complex trauma patients.

PAIN THEORY

Theories about the origin of pain have evolved from simplistic concepts to intricate systems involving the interplay of neurochemical and neurophysiologic mechanisms. The gate control theory, developed by Melzack and Wall in 1965, remains the most accepted theory of pain. It describes a complex neural mechanism in the dorsal horn at the site of the substantia gelatinosa. Modulation of pain from the periphery to the central nervous system occurs through A (large) and C (small) fiber balance. They hypothesized that the substantia gelatinosa acts like a gate. Activity in large afferent fibers blocks pain transmission (or closes the gate), and activity in small fibers enhances transmission (or opens the gate) (Figure 17-1). They further proposed that supraspinal descending systems and cognitive factors also influence the gate. Psychologic factors, such as attention span, anxiety, past pain experience, and personality, can modulate pain.[20] An explosion of pain research has occurred since the introduction of this theory.

In cases of chronic pain states after crush and traumatic tissue injuries, the concept of central neural plasticity may change the sensitivity of dorsal horn neurons to stimulation.[21] Mediators released after tissue injury sensitize the nociceptors, which include potassium, prostaglandins, bradykinins, and substance P. Neural discharge becomes more excited and frequent.[22] Hyperalgesia is the end result,

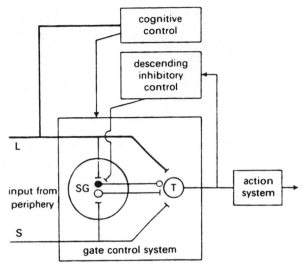

FIGURE 17-1 The gate control theory. Excitatory (*white circle*) and inhibitory (*black circle*) links from the substantia gelatinosa (*SG*) to the transmission (*T*) cells and descending inhibitory control from brainstem systems. L, large, nonpain fibers; S, small, pain fibers. (From Melzack P, Wall P: *The challenge of pain*, New York, 1983, Basic Books.)

occurring when the intensity of pain sensation induced by noxious stimulation is greatly increased.[23] Central sensitization to afferent impulses results from functional changes in spinal cord processing, termed *plasticity* or *neuroplasticity*.

Melzack describes the phantom limb phenomenon after amputation based on the concept of the *neuromatrix*.[24] This is a predetermined genetic network of neurons among the thalamus, limbic system, and cortex. A normal characteristic is a cyclic pattern, known as the neurosignature, in which repeated transmissions are imprinted in the neuromatrix to produce awareness of self. It is been hypothesized that after amputation reorganization of the primary somatosensory cortex occurs, which has been linked to the development of phantom limb pain.[25] In the absence of the amputated limb, the brain or "sentient neural hub" continues to process the message of the neurosignature and attempts to activate muscles to produce movement in the absent limb. Burning and cramping are perceived output messages as the attempt to produce movement persists.[24]

PAIN MECHANISMS

The peripheral nervous system contains nociceptors, or free nerve endings. These receptors transmit the sensation of painful stimuli from tissues that have been injured.[26] Nociceptors are located in skin, joints, and periosteum and surround blood vessel walls. Traumatic injuries usually occur in these areas. *Nociception* refers to the body's response to a noxious (or painful) stimulus. This stimulus activates nociceptors on tissue cells, causing them to depolarize. Pressure, thermal stimuli, and biochemical substances released from damaged cells can stimulate or sensitize nociceptors by acting like neurotransmitters or neuromodulators.[26] Neurotransmitters are chemicals that

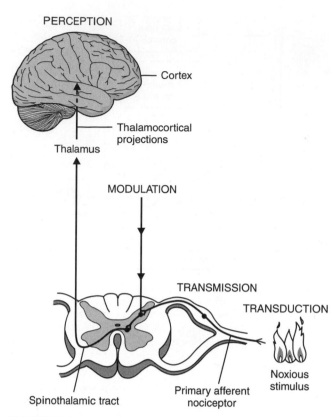

FIGURE 17-2 The four processes that make up nociception: transduction, transmission, modulation, and perception. (From Ferrante and VadeBoncouer, editors: *Postoperative pain management*, New York, 1993, Churchill-Livingstone.)

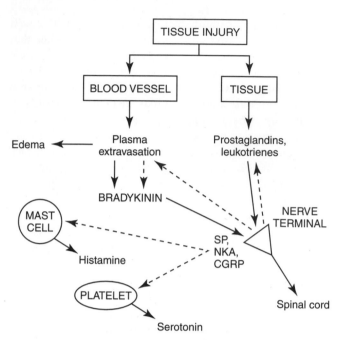

FIGURE 17-3 The peripheral activation of primary afferent fibers after tissue injury. *Solid lines,* initial responses; *dashed lines,* responses that occur after activation of the peripheral nociceptor. (From Sinatra R: *Acute pain: mechanisms & management,* Baltimore, 1992, Mosby Year Book.)

attach to cell receptors and cause change in the polarization of the cell membrane. Neuromodulator chemicals sensitize cells to make transmission of stimuli easier.

Nociception involves the processes of transduction, transmission, modulation, and perception[27] (Figure 17-2). Noxious stimuli are converted into electrical activity during the transduction process. Transmission uses the afferent (sensory) and efferent (motor) components of the peripheral nervous system. There are two types of peripheral nerve fibers: A delta and C fibers. They are classified according to their size and myelination (insulation). A delta fibers are large, myelinated, and transmit fast-moving impulses described as sharp and localized. C fibers are small, unmyelinated, and transmit delayed, dull pain. A alpha and A beta myelinated sensory fibers transmit nonnoxious (normal) sensory information, such as touch, pressure, and vibration.

Modulation involves the modification of nociceptive transmissions in the dorsal horn or spinal reflexes.[22] After peripheral injury, biochemical substances are released and interact to produce nociception. The initial insult results in the activation of the arachidonic acid cascade, which leads to the formation of prostaglandins and leukotrienes (Figure 17-3). These mediators are released from damaged tissue and act to sensitize primary afferent terminals.[28] Some

endogenous chemicals, which include bradykinin, histamine, serotonin, prostaglandins, arachidonic cascade byproducts, leukotrienes, and substance P, are released in the periphery. Many of these chemicals are also responsible for the inflammatory process after traumatic tissue injury, especially bradykinin and prostaglandins.[22] One modulating system, the spinal opioid receptors, are located in the dorsal horn of the spinal cord and include mu (μ), delta (δ), and kappa (κ) receptors. Perception is the interplay of mentioned processes, and it develops into a subjective, individualized experience. Perception involves supraspinal processing on descending inhibition.[22]

PHYSIOLOGIC EFFECTS OF PAIN

The triad of traumatic injury, surgical stress, and undertreated pain elicits a negative effect on many organ systems. A multitude of cardiovascular consequences are activated by the release of several substances. They include the catecholamines from sympathetic nerve endings and adrenal medulla, aldosterone and cortisol from the adrenal cortex, antidiuretic hormone from the hypothalamus, and activation of the renin-angiotensin system.[22] Direct effects on the myocardium by catecholamines include increased heart rate and contractility, causing an increase in oxygen delivery and myocardial oxygen consumption. Angiotensin II causes generalized vasoconstriction, resulting in hypertension, tachycardia, and arrhythmia. Salt and water retention caused by increased levels of aldosterone, antidiuretic hormones, and cortisol can precipitate congestive heart failure in patients with compromised cardiac reserve.[22] Respiratory sequelae include alterations in ventilation secondary to limited chest wall motion, splinting, and ineffective coughing; retention of secretions; and hypoventilation leading to pneumonia, atelectasis, and hypoxemia. Musculoskeletal effects of pain include contraction of skeletal muscles, muscle spasms, and rigidity.[26] The restriction of mobilization impedes activities such as deep breathing, coughing, and ambulation.

PATIENTS REQUIRING SEDATION

Anxiety, fear, and agitation are common in critically injured patients. The intensive care unit (ICU) environment and the various invasive procedures needed can be antagonistic and frightening. Patients in the ICU have multiple psychologic and physical stressors that are responsible for their anxiety and agitation.[29] Common indications for sedation in trauma patients include improving patient comfort,[30] facilitating mechanical ventilation,[30] inducing sleep,[31] decreasing oxygen consumption,[32] providing amnesia during neuromuscular blockade,[30] and controlling agitation. The use of sedatives for intracranial pressure control is discussed later in the chapter.

Sedation is almost always indicated to help patients tolerate the subjective and objective discomforts associated with mechanical ventilation. The discomforts experienced by patients during ventilatory therapy are anxiety and fear, inability to communicate, shortness of breath, persistent coughing, and difficulty with secretions.[33] Patients with severe respiratory failure may require ventilation modes that are especially uncomfortable, such as inverse ratio ventilation. As a result, these patients typically receive sedation and pharmacologic paralysis to facilitate optimal effect of the ventilatory mode. Advances in ventilatory technology such as airway pressure release ventilation (APRV), a positive pressure mode of ventilation that allows spontaneous breathing, may eliminate the need for heavy sedation in many patients requiring mechanical ventilation.

Physiologic sleep is an organized pattern involving distinct stages and successive cycles of slow-wave sleep and rapid eye movement (REM) sleep. Postoperative patients have disrupted or fragmented sleep patterns involving these stages and cycles of sleep.[31] Anxiety and pain further contribute to sleep deprivation by causing difficulties with initiation and maintenance of sleep. The ICU environment, which may lack clocks, calendars, windows, and a conducive environment for sleep, can disorient a patient's normal day-night cycle and produce poor-quality sleep. All these factors promote the development of sleep deprivation. Sleep deprivation can be exhibited as delirious behavior with auditory and visual hallucinations, paranoia, and disorientation.[34] Sedation is used to ensure a proper day-night cycle and prevent sleep deprivation. However, it is not known whether sedative agents like propofol and benzodiazepines produce physiologic sleep. In fact, benzodiazepines and opioids are known to disturb the normal balance between REM and slow-wave sleep.[35] Nevertheless, it seems appropriate to administer sedatives to prevent the disorientation attributed to undefined day-night cycles.

The use of sedatives to decrease oxygen consumption is controversial. Trauma patients often have increased oxygen consumption.[36-38] If oxygen delivery is insufficient to meet demand, tissue hypoxia can develop. Efforts are usually focused on achieving a balance between oxygen supply and demand. Sedation may decrease oxygen consumption.[39] This effect may be particularly useful in agitated patients with symptoms of tachycardia and hyperventilation, who may be exhausting their oxygen supply. However, studies are inconclusive with regard to whether sedatives bring the oxygen supply and demand into balance.[33] Sedative agents may depress cardiac output and decrease oxygen delivery, but these agents should not be withheld.

Sedation is always indicated in patients receiving neuromuscular blocking agents. Without sedatives, neuromuscular paralysis is a frightening experience. In the literature there are many patient accounts of the fear related to loss of muscle function and the nightmares that resulted after discharge.[40-42] Sedatives should be administered on a regular schedule to optimize their anxiolytic and amnestic effects.

Finally, agitation may be a symptom of physiologic conditions, such as hypoxemia, sepsis, brain injury, various electrolyte abnormalities, and drug use (e.g., opiates, digoxin). When the patient becomes agitated, the clinician must identify and treat the underlying cause. Medical conditions known to cause agitation are listed in Table 17-1. If the patient's agitation is not a result of a medical condition or its treatment, adequate pain control should be addressed. A conscious patient can respond appropriately to a pain assessment tool, and adequate analgesic relief can be provided. In an unresponsive patient a clinician must rely on nonspecific signs to indicate inadequate analgesia, such as restlessness, tachycardia, hyperventilation, and hypertension. Unfortunately, many times the specific cause of a patient's agitation is not established.

Delirium is a condition characterized by disorganized thinking, reduced attentiveness, and incoherent thought processes.[43] Delirious patients often exhibit random, purposeless movement and may harm themselves or others as a result of their agitation. It can be difficult to determine if patients are suffering from agitation or delirium, especially if they are intubated. One distinguishing feature is that delirious patients may have impaired short-term memory

TABLE 17-1 **Common Medical Causes of Agitation**	
Hypoxia	Sedative withdrawal
Hypercarbia	syndrome
Hypoglycemia	Narcotic withdrawal
Hyponatremia	syndrome
Hyperosmolar state	Drug intoxication
Hypercalcemia	Digitalis toxicity
Hypocalcemia	Paradoxic effect, sedative
Addisonian crisis	drugs
Cerebral event	Histamine blockers
Cerebral thrombosis,	Atropine, scopolamine
embolism	Others
Subarachnoid	Partial drug-induced
hemorrhage	paralysis
Intracranial bleed	Antibiotic induced
Cerebral vasospasm	Electrolyte disorders,
Cerebral edema	hypophosphatemia
Inadequately treated pain	Hypermagnesemia
Infection	Steroid psychosis
Meningitis	Thyrotoxicosis
Encephalitis	Organic brain syndrome
Brain abscess	Mental retardation
Sepsis syndrome	Fear
Delirium tremens	Anxiety disorders
Hepatic encephalopathy	ICU psychosis
Uremic encephalopathy	

From Durbin CG: Sedation of the agitated critically ill patient without an artificial airway, *Crit Care Clinics* 11:915, 1995.

and may hallucinate or misinterpret stimuli. These behavioral manifestations are often diagnosed as ICU psychosis; however, ICU delirium is a more appropriate term. Haloperidol is the preferred agent to reverse the behavioral manifestations of delirium because of its quick effect and lack of sedative qualities.[44]

SEDATION ASSESSMENT

Sedation assessment is more difficult and less reproducible than pain assessment for two reasons: (1) an optimal, well-defined state of sedation does not exist; and (2) sedation assessment tools have not been tested for reliability and validity.[45] The appropriate level of sedation is defined by the clinicians caring for the patient. Different practitioners caring for a patient may have different interpretations of sedation. A sedation goal should be defined daily and individualized for the patient's care needs. Patients with mild symptoms of anxiety require low doses for comfort, whereas others may need heavy sedation to facilitate mechanical ventilation. Additionally, levels of activity may vary throughout the day, necessitating customization of sedation to provide a cooperative patient for the more awake periods and a sleepy patient for the restful periods.

Sedative dose and frequency of administration need to be

TABLE 17-2 **Ramsay Scale**	
Level	Description
Awake Levels	
1.	Patient anxious and agitated, restless or both
2.	Patient cooperative, oriented, and tranquil
3.	Patient responds to commands only
Asleep Levels, Depends on Response to a Light Glabellar Tap or Loud Auditory Stimulus	
4.	Patient responds briskly
5.	Patient responds sluggishly
6.	Patient does not respond

Modified from Ramsay MAE, Savage TM, Simpson BRJ et al: Controlled sedation with alphaxalone/alphadolone, *Br Med J* 2:656, 1974.

evaluated daily. Daily assessment helps to prevent prolonged drug effects or increased length of stay. Patients receiving intermittent bolus dosing should be assessed before each dose to prevent a cumulative effect. A daily wake up or period without drug administration can be considered for those patients receiving continuous infusion therapy. If assessments are not routinely performed, patients may become oversedated, which causes disorientation, cardiovascular instability, and difficulty in weaning from the ventilator.

The most widely used sedation assessment tool is the Ramsay scale; however, many clinicians use scales developed by their own institutions.[46-48] The Ramsay scale (Table 17-2) was developed to quantitate an objective endpoint of therapy. For most patients a sedation level of 2 to 3 is considered desirable. Patients who are maintained at this level are at minimal risk for prolonged sedation after therapy is discontinued.[48] The Ramsay scale cannot be used to assess the adequacy of sedation in a patient receiving neuromuscular blocking agents (NMBAs) because it relies on verbal and motor responses to stimulation. Physiologic changes such as increases in heart rate, blood pressure, and diaphoresis may serve as the only measures of comfort. This is obviously suboptimal because other physiologic changes can affect vital signs.

The Ramsay scale is limited by its lack of description for degrees of agitation. A sedation-agitation scale[49] developed by Riker and colleagues may be more useful in settings that require both sedation and agitation assessment (Table 17-3). The acceptable goal of sedation on the sedation-agitation scale ranges from 4 to 2.

In the future, computer analysis of electroencephalogram (EEG) patterns may be used as an objective means of measuring sedation. Bispectral analysis of the EEG has been used to assess both midazolam-induced[50,51] and propofol-induced[52] sedation, and it has been successful in predicting a patient's ability to respond to commands. In the future, analysis of EEG patterns and response to various sedatives may be the most objective tool to assess the sedation needs of patients.

TABLE 17-3 Sedation-Agitation Scale

Score	Description	Example
7	Immediate threat to safety	Pulling at endotracheal tube or catheters, trying to climb over bed rail, striking at staff
6	Dangerously agitated	Requiring physical restraints and frequent verbal reminding of limits, biting endotracheal tube
5	Agitated	Anxious or mildly agitated, attempting to sit up, calms down to verbal instructions
4	Calm and cooperative	Calm, arousable, follows commands
3	Oversedated	Difficult to arouse, awakens to verbal stimuli or gentle shaking but drifts off again, follows simple commands
2	Very oversedated	Awakens to physical stimuli but unable to communicate or follow commands
1	Unarousable	Does not awaken to stimuli, unable to communicate or follow commands

From Riker RR, Picard JT, Fraser GL: Prospective evaluation of the sedation-agitation scale for adult critically ill patients, *Crit Care Med* 27:1325-29, 1999.

TABLE 17-4 Comparison of Opioid Adverse Effects

Drug	Analgesia	Constipation	Respiratory Depression	Sedation	Emesis
Morphine	++	++	++	++	++
Hydromorphone	++	+	++	+	+
Meperidine	++	+	++	+	nr
Fentanyl	++	nr	+	nr	+
Sufentanil	+++	nr	nr	nr	nr
Alfentanil	++	nr	nr	nr	nr
Codeine	+	+	+	+	+
Oxycodone	++	++	++	++	++

Modified from Kastrup E: *Facts and Comparisons*, St. Louis, 1999, Facts and Comparisons, 1376.
nr, not reported.

PHARMACOLOGIC AGENTS

OPIOIDS

Nurses routinely administer opioids for the effective management of pain. Knowledge of opiate receptors and their response to agonists is essential to monitor and treat adverse effects. Analgesia is thought to be the result of activation of the μ and κ receptors; the δ receptors may also be involved. The opioid receptors, located on presynaptic nerve terminals, are thought to exert an inhibitory modulation effect on the synaptic transmission of nociception by decreasing the release of neurotransmitters. Morphine stimulates two subtypes of μ receptors to produce its pharmacologic effects.[53] The μ_1 receptor mediates supraspinal analgesia and, to a lesser extent, euphoria. The μ_2 receptor is associated with respiratory depression, decreased gastric motility, and other adverse effects. The κ agonist and δ agonist drugs have not been developed for clinical use.

Currently available opioids produce their major effects on the central nervous and gastrointestinal systems. Some of these effects are analgesia, sedation, mood changes, respiratory depression, decreased intestinal motility, nausea, and vomiting[54] (Table 17-4). Opioids have no significant amnestic or anxiolytic properties. Co-administration of a benzodiazepine or propofol is necessary to achieve adequate levels of sedation and amnesia. Analgesia occurs without loss of consciousness. After administration of an opioid, patients describe the pain as less intense, less discomforting, or entirely gone; patients are more comfortable.

ADVERSE EFFECTS. Sedation, constipation, nausea, vomiting, and respiratory depression are the most common adverse effects of opioids. The major side effect of opioid administration is respiratory depression. Opioids depress ventilation, and the respiratory rate is unresponsive to increasing carbon dioxide tension. Within 5 to 10 minutes after intravenous (IV) administration of morphine, maximal respiratory depression occurs; this effect may extend beyond the duration of the analgesic effect.[54] After large doses of opioids, patients will breathe if told to do so. However, without instruction these patients may remain relatively apneic. Sedation precedes respiratory depression; therefore frequent nursing assessment for its presence is imperative. No patient has succumbed to respiratory depression while awake.[55] Sedation is best treated by reducing the dose and increasing the frequency of administration. Morphine and meperidine can also cause histamine-induced bronchospasm in susceptible patients, and all opioids depress cough reflex by affecting the cough center in the medulla.[54]

Opioids slow gastric emptying time by reducing peristalsis. Increased bile duct pressure may result from opioid-induced contraction of the sphincter of Oddi. The clinical significance of the increased bile duct pressure is unknown because biliary pain may not correlate with changes in pressure. All patients taking opioid analgesics are at risk for constipation and should be given stool softeners and laxatives so that enteral feeding administration is not complicated.

Fentanyl and its congeners, sufentanil, alfentanil, and remifentanil, can induce chest wall rigidity severe enough to compromise respiration. This centrally mediated muscle contraction is most frequent after large bolus doses and is effectively treated with muscle relaxants.[54]

Opioids do not seriously impair cardiovascular function. Meperidine, because of its anticholinergic effects, tends to increase heart rate, whereas high doses of morphine, fentanyl, and its congeners are associated with a vagus-mediated bradycardia. With the exception of meperidine, the opioids do not depress cardiac contractility. Nevertheless, arterial blood pressure often falls as a result of bradycardia, venous dilation, and decreased sympathetic reflexes. Furthermore, morphine, meperidine, and codeine evoke histamine release in some individuals that can lead to profound drops in arterial blood pressure and systemic vascular resistance. The effects of histamine release can be minimized in susceptible patients by slow opioid infusion and adequate intravascular volume. Fentanyl, sufentanil, alfentanil, and remifentanil do not release histamine and therefore do not induce this effect.

Regular use of opiates can produce tolerance to some effects, such as respiratory depression, sedation, and analgesia. *Tolerance* is defined as the requirement of increasing doses to produce the same effect; it is the result of decreased receptor density after prolonged exposure to a drug. *Innate tolerance* is a genetic insensitivity to a drug when administered.

Physical dependence, not to be confused with psychologic dependence, is revealed in patients taking chronic opioids when abrupt discontinuation of an opioid or the administration of an opioid antagonist produces abstinence syndrome. This syndrome is characterized by anxiety, irritability, chills alternating with hot flashes, salivation, lacrimation, rhinorrhea, diaphoresis, piloerection, nausea, vomiting, abdominal cramps, and insomnia. Abstinence syndrome can be avoided by slowly withdrawing chronically used opioids at a rate of approximately 50% every several days[55] (see Chapter 32).

Psychologic dependence or addiction is a pattern of compulsive drug use characterized by a continued craving for an opioid and the need to use the opioid for effects other than pain relief. The patient exhibits drug-seeking behavior and becomes overwhelmingly involved with using and procuring the drug. Although most patients who receive opioids several times daily for more than 1 month develop some degree of tolerance and physical dependence, data suggest that the risk of addiction is very small, and fear of opioid addiction should not be a primary concern in treating pain.[56] Nurses should make it clear to patients and other staff that tolerance and physical dependence are not the same as addiction.

SPECIFIC AGENTS
Table 17-5 lists the routinely used opiate agents and doses recommended in trauma patients.

TABLE 17-5   Opioid Agents and Doses*

Drug	Usual Dose Intermittent	Usual Dose Infusion	Advantages	Disadvantages
Morphine	1-5 mg IV every 1-2 hours	2-15 mg/hr	Inexpensive	Active metabolite Histamine release Vasodilation
Fentanyl	25-100 µg IV every 0.5-1 hours	50-200 µg/hr	Rapid onset No active metabolite Useful in morphine allergy Minimal CV effect	Single-dose short duration Lipid accumulation with continued use
Meperidine	Not recommended	Not recommended	Inexpensive	Active metabolite Drug interactions
Sufentanil	—	10-100 mg/hr	Short-acting	Expensive Chest wall rigidity with high dose
Alfentanil	—	250-2500 mg/hr	Short-acting	Expensive Chest wall rigidity with high dose
Remifentanil	—	Unknown	Continuation of intraoperative analgesia Very short-acting	Expensive Pain recurrence if stopped acutely Chest wall rigidity with high dose
Hydromorphone	0.15-1.5 mg IV every 1-2 hours	0.45-1.5 mg/hr	Potent Useful in morphine allergy	

CV, cardiovascular; *IV,* intravenous; *GI,* gastrointestinal.

*These are routinely used opiate agents and doses recommended in trauma patients. Patient needs may vary. Titrate to desired response.

MORPHINE. Morphine, a naturally occurring compound, is the most commonly used opiate analgesic agent and the standard with which all other analgesic agents are compared. It is considered the first agent recommended by the Society of Critical Care Medicine (SCCM).[57] Morphine may be administered by oral, subcutaneous, intramuscular, intravenous, epidural, and intrathecal routes. Peak effect after a single IV bolus of morphine occurs within 15 minutes, and the duration of clinical effects is 2 to 7 hours.[58] Morphine is poorly lipid soluble, a property that results in a slow onset and long duration when the drug is administered intravenously or epidurally. It is metabolized by the liver to form water-soluble glucuronides. Morphine-3-glucuronide (M3G) has no analgesic activity and is readily excreted by the kidney. Morphine-6-glucuronide (M6G) produces potent opioid effects, approximately four times more potent than morphine. In patients with normal renal function the elimination half-life is two to three times longer than morphine.[59] In patients with renal impairment, M6G accumulates and can result in persistent sedation and ventilatory depression after discontinuation of morphine.[59]

MEPERIDINE. Meperidine is less potent and has a shorter half-life than morphine. It has anticholinergic effects and can cause mydriasis rather than the usual miosis. Meperidine is not recommended for more than occasional use because of the active metabolite normeperidine. Normeperidine is a toxic metabolite capable of inciting central nervous system (CNS) excitement, tremor, myoclonus, and tonic-clonic seizures.[60,61] Normeperidine is excreted in the urine and accumulates in the elderly, in patients with renal insufficiency, and after high doses (400-600 mg/24 hours).[61] Seizures produced by normeperidine will not respond to naloxone and should be treated with anticonvulsants.[62] Another disadvantage of meperidine is its life-threatening interaction with antidepressants. An excitation syndrome of hypertension, hyperpyrexia, and convulsions can be observed after recent monoamine oxidase inhibitor use.[62] Meperidine can also cause excitation syndrome (serotonin syndrome) in combination with serotonin reuptake inhibitors such as fluoxetine, paroxetine, sertraline, and fluvoxamine through stimulation of central serotonin release and decreased reuptake.[63]

FENTANYL. Fentanyl is a synthetic opioid structurally similar to meperidine and is the second-line agent recommended by the SCCM, particularly in the event of hemodynamic instability.[57] Intermittent doses of fentanyl are used for procedures, but fentanyl is often administered as a continuous infusion for sustained effects. This opiate is 50 to 100 times as potent as morphine.[64] In comparison with morphine, fentanyl does not induce histamine release and produces minimal cardiovascular effects. However, hypotension can still occur in the volume-depleted patient. It has been suggested that fentanyl increases intracranial pressure in patients with head trauma, but clinically it is used in these patients with adequate monitoring.[65,66] Fentanyl is approximately 7000 times more lipophilic and significantly more protein bound than morphine.[67] These properties result in a very rapid onset (within 30 seconds) when single doses are administered parenterally or epidurally. However, these properties help to create a reservoir or depot effect with repeated administration and are responsible for the prolonged clinical effect observed after discontinuation of fentanyl.[68]

SUFENTANIL, ALFENTANIL, AND REMIFENTANIL. These fentanyl analogs have been used in trauma patients, but higher cost has limited their use. Sufentanil is 5 to 10 times more potent than fentanyl and approximately 1000 times more analgesic than morphine.[53,69] Similar to fentanyl, sufentanil has minimal cardiovascular effects. It is highly lipophilic and has a faster onset of action than fentanyl.[58]

Alfentanil is 30 times more potent than morphine; however, it is one eighth as potent as fentanyl.[70] This opioid's onset and duration of action are shorter than fentanyl. Alfentanil offers intense analgesia and is highly useful for potentially painful procedures like scheduled dressing changes.[71]

Remifentanil is a new, ultra-short–acting fentanyl congener that is slightly less potent than fentanyl. Unlike other opioids, the liver does not metabolize remifentanil. Instead, it is rapidly hydrolyzed by plasma and tissue esterases. It is indicated for operative use as part of balanced anesthesia; however, continuation of infusions into the ICU has been reported.[72] Routine use in the ICU will be limited by cost, risk of rapid loss of analgesia if the infusion is interrupted, and the potential development of tolerance. The ultra-short–acting agent (half-life of 3 minutes) is expected to produce tolerance more rapidly.

HYDROMORPHONE. Hydromorphone is a potent, synthetic derivative of morphine that produces more sedation with less euphoria than equivalent doses of morphine. It is five times more potent than morphine and can be given orally or parenterally. Hydromorphone offers no advantages over morphine in the ICU setting. It may cause cross-reaction in morphine-allergic patients. It is the third-line agent recommended by the SCCM and is ideal for use in patients with renal impairment because it causes no metabolite buildup.

METHADONE. Methadone is a long-acting equivalent to morphine. This agent is primarily used to suppress withdrawal symptoms in patients with physical chemical dependency. Because the half-life is 15 to 40 hours, respiratory depression can be observed for more than 24 hours after a single dose. Methadone is administered by slow IV push or orally. With repeated administration, cumulative effects are seen, so that lower doses or longer intervals between doses may be necessary. Side effects are similar to those seen with morphine. This agent can be given to patients in acute pain because of its analgesic benefits, particularly when opioid doses have increased over time. Administration of shorter-acting agents two or three times a day is used as "rescue" dosing to treat activity-related pain.

COMMONLY USED ORAL OPIOIDS.   Codeine, oxycodone, and hydrocodone are commonly administered as combination products with acetaminophen and aspirin. Because of differing mechanisms of action, these opiates in combination with aspirin or acetaminophen produce additive analgesic effects.

These opioids are mild analgesics used to relieve mild to moderate pain. Codeine is structurally related to morphine and exerts its analgesic effect through demethylation to morphine. In comparison with morphine these agents cause minimal sedation and rare respiratory depression as a result of their lower potency. These agents may cause a cross-reaction in morphine-allergic patients.

NALOXONE

Naloxone is a competitive antagonist at the μ, κ, and δ receptors. It is active against all available μ receptor agents. Naloxone has no significant agonist activity. Respiratory depression caused by overzealous opioid administration is rapidly antagonized (1-2 minutes). Low doses of intravenous naloxone reverse the side effects of epidurally administered opioids without necessarily reversing the analgesia.[73]

Abrupt reversal of opioid analgesia can result in sympathetic stimulation (e.g., tachycardia, ventricular irritability, hypertension, pulmonary edema) caused by pain perception, an acute withdrawal syndrome in narcotic-dependent patients, or vomiting. The extent of these side effects is proportional to the amount of opioid being reversed and the speed of the reversal. Careful titration of naloxone in small increments is advised. Intravenous naloxone (0.4 mg/ml) diluted to 0.04 mg/ml can be titrated in increments of 0.5 to 1 μg/kg every 3 to 5 minutes until adequate ventilation and alertness occur. Intravenous doses in excess of 0.2 mg are rarely indicated. Because naloxone has a brief duration of action (30-45 minutes), a more prolonged effect is almost always necessary to prevent the recurrence of respiratory depression from longer-acting opioids. Therefore a continuous infusion is recommended (4-5 μg/kg/hr).

CLINICAL USE OF OPIOIDS

Knowledge of the various methods used to administer opioids and of how opioids are absorbed is helpful in understanding why one technique of providing analgesia may be superior to another in certain phases of the trauma cycle. The methods discussed include oral, intramuscular, intravenous, neuraxial, transdermal, and rectal routes and patient-controlled analgesia.

ORAL ROUTE

The oral route usually is chosen because it is the easiest and most convenient route of administration. Absorption of orally effective opioids by the gastrointestinal (GI) tract usually is complete, but the rate of absorption varies. Peak drug effects occur after 1 to 2 hours for most analgesics, which may be a drawback for treating rapidly fluctuating pain. Most drugs undergo significant first-pass hepatic metabolism after absorption. First-pass hepatic metabolism is the effect seen after drugs are absorbed from the stomach and the intestine, thus passing through the liver before entering the systemic circulation. While in the liver, the drugs are metabolized, so that some of the active drug is inactivated before it is delivered to the tissue receptors. This effect explains the discrepancy between intravenous and oral doses.[55]

The oral route is not suitable for patients with severe pain because of the slower onset of action and the variability of absorption. In addition, it is not useful during the early phases of the trauma cycle if patients are to receive nothing by mouth, are unable to swallow, or are hemodynamically unstable. Oral analgesics are used in the intermediate and rehabilitation phases of the trauma cycle, when the pain is less severe and the patient is able to take oral medications.

INTRAMUSCULAR ROUTE

The traditional method of analgesia for postoperative patients has been intramuscular (IM) injection. This route enables the patient to receive a faster therapeutic drug effect and avoids the interference of the digestive system, which makes this route more predictable compared with the oral route. The rate of absorption after injection, however, is largely dependent on the blood flow to the muscle.[74] During states of hemodynamic instability, blood flow is shunted from the extremities to the central compartment; thus IM injections are not readily absorbed. Repeated administration can produce a depot effect. When circulation is improved, a large amount of the drug may be absorbed, resulting in toxic effects, including respiratory depression.

Many physician orders are written for as-needed (PRN) administration of IM injections. Peak opioid effects can take as long as 30 to 60 minutes to occur. The patient may be suffering so much pain and anxiety by the time the IM-PRN medication takes effect that there is little chance the medication will effectively relieve the pain.[75,76] Misinterpretation of the IM-PRN order, inadequate pain assessment, fear of addiction, administration of inadequate dose of opioids, and variable absorption rates are other factors cited for the ineffectiveness of the IM-PRN method of postoperative analgesia. This is the rationale for scheduled or regular IM injections. Regular IM injections given every 4 hours achieve serum levels that are equal to or exceed the minimum effective analgesic concentration for a short period in the 4-hour time frame.[76] Large doses given at longer intervals result in higher peak concentrations and lower trough levels. The high peak concentrations produce undesirable effects and the low troughs are associated with inadequate analgesia for a portion of the dosing interval. For these reasons, practitioners have increased the use of constant infusions and patient-controlled analgesia (PCA), because lower doses are given to provide a steady plasma concentration of opioid and avoid the adverse effects seen with large doses. Figure 17-4 compares the effects of opioids

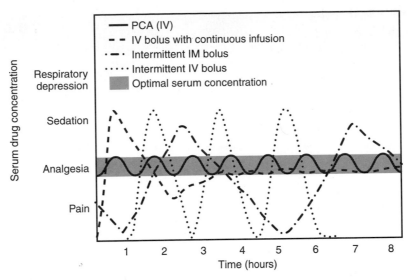

FIGURE 17-4 Administration methods and serum levels. Effects of opioids according to serum levels produced by different methods of administration. The appropriate dose and timing is important to produce effective serum levels and minimize unwanted effects. (From Lubenow TR, Ivankovich AD: Patient-controlled analgesia for postoperative pain, *Crit Care Clin North Am* 3:35, 1991.)

according to serum levels produced by different methods of administration.

INTRAVENOUS ROUTE

Although the most common method of providing analgesia after surgery remains the use of intramuscular injections of opiates, patients in critical care areas are often given analgesics by intravenous infusion or bolus. When morphine and other opioids are given intravenously, they quickly exert an effect. Time to peak effect varies with drug lipid solubility, ranging from 1 to 5 minutes for fentanyl to 15 to 30 minutes for morphine. The highly perfused, vessel-rich tissues absorb intravenous opioids first. As the plasma concentration of the opioid decreases below the level found in the vessel-rich tissues, the drug leaves these tissues and is consequently distributed in the less perfused sites, such as the skeletal muscles and fat. In addition to tissue perfusion, the physiochemical properties of the opioid govern its ability to be absorbed by certain tissues. For example, only small quantities of morphine, a relatively hydrophilic opioid, pass the blood-brain barrier compared with more lipid-soluble opioids, such as fentanyl, codeine, meperidine, and heroin.[53] Intravenous administration of opioids allows for more rapid access to the sites where they exert an effect, the central nervous system and the opioid receptors.

Intravenous infusions of opioids provide steady blood levels and the ability to rapidly titrate relief in patients with acute pain that is severe and continuous. When increased analgesia is necessary, an opioid bolus of about 1 hour's drug infusion should be administered in addition to increasing the infusion rate. Without the bolus dose, the full effect of an increased rate alone may not be felt for 12 hours or more. Activities, such as turning, chest physical therapy, or chest tube removal require additional analgesic coverage.[77]

Morphine and fentanyl are appropriate opioids to be used with continuous infusion because of their medium to high rate of systemic clearance. Morphine has traditionally been the drug of choice for continuous opioid infusions. It is slowly being replaced by fentanyl because less pruritus occurs with the latter agent. However, as a result of accumulation in muscle and fat, respiratory depression may occur when fentanyl is redistributed to the central circulation.[78] Advantages of fentanyl over other opioids include the abolished hyperglycemic response and decreased release of plasma cortisol and growth hormones in response to surgery. Histamine seldom is released with fentanyl use, which results in fewer complaints of pruritus.[79]

The intravenous route is used during the resuscitation and critical care phases and the early part of the intermediate phase of the trauma cycle. By the time the patient reaches the intermediate phase, the pain is manageable by other routes.

PATIENT-CONTROLLED ANALGESIA

Patient-controlled analgesia is a technique that allows the patient to self-administer small amounts of opioid in response to pain. Many patients experience superior pain relief with PCA than with intramuscular or intravenous administration because it maintains a more constant blood level of opioid. With PCA a computerized pump device is programmed to deliver a constant dose of drug to suit the needs of the individual patient. (Table 17-6 shows common PCA settings.) Most PCA pumps allow the administration of a bolus dose and delivery of the opioid at a constant basal rate. The patient presses a button on a cord attached to the pump to administer the bolus dose. The patient is instructed to self-administer the opioid when the constant basal rate is insufficient or when the patient anticipates the need for more opioid to ambulate or to perform pulmonary care

TABLE 17-6　Common PCA Settings

Analgesic (min)	Bolus Dose (mg)	Maintenance Dose	Lockout Interval
Fentanyl	0.02-0.1	15-60 µg/hr	3-10
Hydromorphone	0.1-0.5	0.1-0.3 mg/hr	5-15
Meperidine	5-30	5-20 mg/hr	5-15
Morphine	0.5-3.0	0.5-3.0 mg/hr	5-20
Sufentanil	0.003-0.015	2-8 µg/hr	3-10

Modified from Lubenow TR, Ivankovich AD: Pain and post anesthesia management, *Crit Care Nurs North Am* 3:35, 1991.

measures (e.g., cough, deep breathing, incentive spirometry). Some practitioners do not program the pump to deliver a basal rate, so that the only time the patient receives the opioid is when the button is pushed. An advantage to the use of a constant background infusion is that it allows the patient to sleep without waking in pain. Programmed into the pump are time and dose lockout features that do not allow the delivery of a bolus dose even if the patient requests it. In some pumps the computer records how often the patient requests a bolus dose and how often the request is honored. This feature helps to assess the effectiveness of PCA.

It is postulated that by allowing patients to control their own pain and suffering, they titrate the amount of opioids they want to receive with the degree of discomfort and adverse effects from the opioids they are willing to tolerate.[80] Egan[80] proposed that the belief in the controllability of pain, whether true or not, influences the patient's appraisal of the situation. Having control over one aspect, the level of pain, may have far-reaching influence on the patient's emotional and cognitive appraisal. The end result is that by allowing patients to control their level of pain, they suffer less and have less anxiety and distress. Patient participation in therapeutic regimens decreases the likelihood of developing postoperative complications that are a consequence of pain.

The effectiveness of PCA is only as good as the doses that are provided. The same problems inherent with other methods of analgesia occur with PCA if the doses or time frames used are inadequate. Figure 17-4 shows the importance of appropriate doses and timing in producing adequate serum levels without the unwanted effects.

NEURAXIAL OPIOIDS AND LOCAL ANESTHETICS

Epidural analgesic technique involves the administration of opioids and diluted local anesthetics into the epidural space. The resulting analgesia is superior and longer lasting. Studies have compared epidural with parenteral therapy and demonstrated that epidural analgesia improved pulmonary function after thoracic and abdominal surgery.[81] It has been attributed to reducing the neuroendocrine and metabolic responses to the stress of surgery and pain. Sympathetic stimulation and adrenal catecholamine release become attenuated. By altering the stress response, blood viscosity, clotting, and platelet aggregation are altered and the resultant tendency for thrombus formation decreases.

The epidural space lies within the spinal canal, which runs from the foramen magnum to the sacral hiatus. It is highly vascularized and contains fat, connective tissues, a lymphatic network, and dorsal and ventral roots of spinal nerves. Agents administered are proximal to the opioid receptors and diffuse across the dura. Peak drug concentrations are established in the cerebrospinal fluid within 10 to 20 minutes after administration. Morphine is a pure µ-agonist, and as a result of its hydrophilic properties, absorption is slow and prolonged. Respiratory depression, although rare, develops more often with hydrophilic agents and can occur within 30 minutes and up to 18 to 22 hours after injection into the epidural space.[82] Lipophilic opioids, such as fentanyl, have a shorter duration of action, and are commonly used for continuous infusions. Opioids combined with diluted local anesthetics reduce overall opioid requirements.[82]

Local anesthetics, such as lidocaine and bupivacaine, produce analgesia through blockade of impulse conduction along nerve fibers within the spinal nerves. There is an interference with the function of sodium channels during nerve conduction, when sodium ions enter and potassium ions exit the cell.[83] Blockade occurs first in the small C fibers to alter slow pain, then in the large A fibers for fast pain. High concentration anesthetics, such as 0.5% bupivacaine, block all types of fibers including sympathetic, pain, sensory and motor, and are used for surgical anesthesia neural blockade. Low concentrations, or dilute solutions, such as 0.1% bupivacaine, will selectively affect very fine sympathetic and pain fibers, with little effect on larger sensory fibers, responsible for touch and pressure. Large motor fibers are spared with low concentration local anesthetics, characterizing a differential nerve block, thus facilitating mobility and ambulation.

Factors that influence the onset of an epidural blockade include the site of injection and nerve root size, height and weight of the patient, positioning, and the volume, concentration, and dose of local anesthetic.[84] Dermatomes are cutaneous sensory bands that are 1 to 2 inches wide and correspond to a specific nerve root. Common landmarks include the nipple line at T4 level, the umbilicus at T10, and the groin at L1. After neuraxial injection the presence of an analgesic block is assessed through the loss of sensation and temperature discrimination along the dermatomal tracts. Temperature discrimination can be distinguished with the use of an alcohol wipe or ice bag.

TRANSDERMAL ROUTE

The transdermal route is appealing because it provides steady, therapeutic plasma levels without the peaks and troughs seen with intermittent dosing. The advantages of transdermal application include the avoidance of the first-pass effect, prolongation of effect, and its ability to be used when swallowing is a problem.

Fentanyl is the only opioid that possesses characteristics that make it suitable for transdermal use. The fentanyl patch come in 25-, 50-, 75-, and 100-μg doses. Steady-state concentrations are reached in 8 hours, and concentrations decrease slowly after removal.[85] Latasch and Luders[86] recommend application of the patch 5 hours before surgery. The long period necessary to reach analgesic concentrations and the apparent deposition of drug beneath the skin (which is responsible for the slow decline of fentanyl)[86] are two disadvantages of using this drug for acute pain.

The transdermal route may be effective in the latter part of the intermediate phase and in the rehabilitation phase of the trauma cycle. Transdermal opioids have been used successfully in patients who suffer chronic pain from cancer, but the use of transdermal opioids for critically ill trauma patients is not currently recommended.

RECTAL ROUTE

The effectiveness of drugs administered rectally depends on the rate of absorption, which can be variable. Drugs inserted into the proximal rectum are absorbed by the hemorrhoidal veins and then go to the portal circulation (first-pass effect). Drugs absorbed in the lower rectal area go directly to the general circulation without undergoing the first-pass effect. The unpredictable nature of drug absorption in the rectal area, along with possible local mucosal irritation, make this route less desirable.

Aspirin, acetaminophen, and some opioids (oxymorphone and hydromorphone) are available in suppository form. Aspirin and acetaminophen relieve mild pain, and the opioids are used for severe pain. Rectal suppositories occasionally are used in the intermediate phase of the trauma cycle.

NONSTEROIDAL ANTIINFLAMMATORY DRUGS

The nonsteroidal antiinflammatory drugs (NSAIDs) decrease levels of inflammatory mediators generated at the site of tissue injury. NSAIDs have central and peripheral actions that block the production of prostaglandins, which are proinflammatory mediators produced after tissue damage. These agents have been shown to be as effective as opioids for the relief of moderate to severe pain and lack the adverse effects of opioids. Even when insufficient alone to control pain, NSAIDs have a significant opioid dose–sparing effect on postoperative pain and can be useful in reducing opioid side effects.[87,88] The concurrent use of opioids and NSAIDs often provides more effective analgesia than either drug class alone.

Unfortunately, all NSAIDs have specific, predictable, and important side effects, of particular relevance after trauma, that may severely limit their usefulness. NSAIDs inhibit thromboxane A_2 production, creating an antiplatelet effect that prolongs bleeding time. Therefore these agents are contraindicated in the early phase of trauma management when hemorrhage is present and in the head-injured patient at risk for intracranial bleeding. Some evidence exists that two salicylates, salsalate and choline magnesium trisalicylate, do not profoundly affect platelet aggregation.[89,90]

NSAID-associated peptic ulceration and bleeding can be life-threatening. In addition, parenteral (as opposed to enteral) administration does not avoid the systemically mediated antiprostaglandin effect on gut mucosa. Recently, a selective coenzyme inhibitor (specifically cyclooxygenase-2 [COX-2]) NSAID was marketed. Agents with this property appear to be as efficacious as other NSAIDs; however, by not inhibiting the other coenzyme (COX-1) to any significant extent, it has been associated with a lower risk of severe GI complications and platelet effects.[91,92] The benefits of this selective NSAID may cause it to be the preferred agent for trauma patients in the future.

If renal function is likely to be compromised, as is often the case in trauma patients (with marked activation of the renin-angiotensin-aldosterone system), or in those with preexisting renal failure, NSAIDs are potentially dangerous and should not be given because they will often aggravate renal dysfunction.[93] NSAIDs block the protective effects that vasodilator prostaglandins (e.g., prostaglandin D_2 [PGD_2] and prostacyclin [PGI_2]) present to the renal circulation by opposing the vasoconstrictor effects of angiotensin during times of stress (e.g., hypovolemia, ischemia). Thus it is not recommended that NSAIDs be used in the resuscitation phase when hypovolemia, renal hypoperfusion, and major fluid shifts are present.

Ketorolac is most often used because of the availability of a parenteral form. It should be administered in doses appropriate for age, size, and renal function and continued for no more than 5 days. Use for more than 5 days increases the risk of renal failure and gastrointestinal bleeding. Lack of a response to a particular NSAID does not preclude response to another NSAID in the same or a different chemical class.

NONPHARMACOLOGIC PAIN INTERVENTIONS

Although there is much emphasis on the administration of pharmacologic agents to control pain, nurses can autonomously use nonpharmacologic techniques. The techniques discussed can be applied in the trauma setting, although no dedicated research has been reported specifically for the trauma patient. Individual innovation and refinement can be applied to the patient's unique pain experience. The patient must be willing to accept the application of these techniques. Eliciting family support can aid the nurse in the education and application of nonpharmacologic interventions and create a climate where education can take place. These techniques allow the patient to actively participate and control his or her pain experience.

Examples of nonpharmacologic interventions for postoperative and traumatic pain include two categories: cognitive-behavioral techniques and application of physical agents.[19] Some of the physical agents discussed may require a physician's order unless included in a clinical protocol. Examples of cognitive-behavioral techniques include relaxation, breathing techniques, imagery, music distraction, and biofeedback. Physical techniques include the application of moist heat or cold, massage, pressure, physical therapy, and transcutaneous electric nerve stimulation (TENS).

Relaxation is a form of distraction. Jaw relaxation, combined with slow breathing, requires only a few minutes of patient instruction and can be performed at regular intervals chosen by the patient.[94] Breathing exercises offer both relaxation and distraction. Slow, regular breathing, particularly during potentially painful interventions, helps reduce muscular tension. Music therapy is readily available and can be personalized to patient preference. Imagery is the use of the imagination to alter the present situation of emotional distress or pain. The patient must be in a state of relaxation in order to accept this form of distraction.[95] Thinking of a pleasant situation or a place associated with happy memories is a simple approach to imagery. Specialized training or consultant employment is required for complex imagery, hypnosis, and biofeedback techniques.

The application of cold through compresses or packs aids in the reduction of edema and pain. Cold application is usually recommended during the acute injury phase, particularly after muscle twisting and strain, except in patients with compromised vascular perfusion. Heat application increases blood flow and is usually reserved for postacute phases of injury, such as after physical therapy during the rehabilitation phase. Education in regard to application and the potential for damage to skin integrity and circulation must be provided before initiation of this therapy.

Massage can be accomplished by rubbing the affected area of discomfort. Mentholated ointments and lotion can also enhance the relaxing and sedative effects of massage and should be applied to intact skin. Pressure application to painful areas, especially with headache pain, is an instinctive mechanism to pain. It is a temporary measure that reduces blood flow, especially with the concurrent use of elevation. An individualized exercise and physical activity plan are best formulated with input from the patient and physical therapist.

TENS is a battery-operated device that transmits electrical impulses over a painful area. Individualized responses to TENS have been reported after postoperative incisional pain.[96-98]

Nonpharmacologic Therapeutic Approaches to Sedation

The stressful environment of the ICU can induce patient anxiety and fear because of a loss of independence, sensory overload, immobility, and loss of control.[99] Nonpharmacologic modalities can be used to decrease the anxiety associated with ICU care. Efforts to reduce night noise, lighting, and staff conversation promote regular sleep-wake cycles.[100,101] Physical contact, communication and education, clocks, and calendars can help prevent disorientation.[102] Reinstitution of patient control and family visitors can also help to relieve anxiety nonpharmacologically.[103,104] In addition, successful relaxation of ICU patients has been achieved with alternative therapies such as relaxation techniques, hypnosis, music therapy, breathing instruction, and massage.[105,106]

Pharmacologic Agents for Sedation

Sedative, anxiolytic, and amnestic effects can be achieved with a variety of medications. Sedatives do not provide analgesia; pain control must be addressed separately. The drug's onset, duration, side effects, and cost dictate the choice of sedative. Intermittent administration of sedatives is used to calm a patient and to induce amnesia before a procedure. Intermittent administration of long-acting sedatives like diazepam will provide a sustained state of sedation. However, with repetitive dosing there is a risk of drug accumulation that can prolong ventilatory support and length of stay.[107] The risk of accumulation can be minimized with short-acting agents (e.g., propofol), but these agents require either frequent administration requiring a great deal of nursing time or use of a continuous infusion. In addition, these agents can cause sudden awakening if the infusion is disconnected or interrupted.

Benzodiazepines

Benzodiazepines are the agents most commonly used to produce sedation in trauma patients. Benzodiazepines achieve their effects by binding to and activating a high-affinity benzodiazepine receptor within the γ-aminobutyric acid (GABA) receptor in the central nervous system. As the dose of a benzodiazepine is increased, anxiolysis progresses to sedation and sedation to hypnosis.[108] Three benzodiazepines are commonly used in the trauma setting: diazepam, midazolam, and lorazepam (Table 17-7).

Pharmacokinetics. The clinical differences observed with these benzodiazepines are primarily due to differences in potency, uptake, distribution, elimination, and the presence or absence of active metabolites. Benzodiazepines have a high degree of lipophilicity, and therefore distribute quickly into the central nervous system to induce sedation. Because of its lower lipid solubility, lorazepam has a slower onset and longer duration of action than midazolam and diazepam.[109-111] Termination of the effects of benzodiazepines is related to redistribution of the drug from the CNS to the peripheral compartments. As a result of redistribution, the clinical effects of benzodiazepines have a shorter duration than the plasma terminal elimination half-life. Benzodiazepines are metabolized in the liver with renal excretion of the metabolites. Diazepam and midazolam undergo hepatic microsomal oxidation, which is influenced

TABLE 17-7		Commonly Used Benzodiazepines in the ICU			
Drug	Onset (min)	Duration (hr)	Half-life (hr)	Advantages	Disadvantages
Midazolam	1-5	2	1-12.3	Rapid onset Easily titrated Soluble	Variable duration Expensive

Lorazepam	40	12-24	10-20	Preferred for
				  long-term sedation
				No active metabolites
					Limited solubility
					  for infusion
					Slow onset

Diazepam	1-5	0.25-1	20-50	Inexpensive Rapid onset	Long-acting metabolites Phlebitis

by age, liver disease, and some other drugs (e.g., cimetidine, phenytoin).[112] Because lorazepam is metabolized by glucuronide conjugation, it is less influenced by these factors.[110]

Midazolam is a short-acting agent with a duration of sedative effect that ranges from 30 to 120 minutes.[112,113] However, a continuous infusion for more than 24 hours in critically ill patients has led to prolonged effects.[114-122] The longer half-life (i.e., 39 hours) in critically ill patients is secondary to an increase in the volume of distribution and decreased elimination.[117-119] These parameters are difficult to predict in patients, and therefore nurses should be aware that patients receiving midazolam may have a prolonged recovery.[123]

Lorazepam has peak effects that are not observed for 30 minutes and a duration of 10 to 20 hours after a single bolus. This agent has the advantage of having no active metabolites.[124] Unlike midazolam and diazepam, elderly patients or patients with significant liver disease do not appear to have prolonged sedative effects after single bolus injection.[125]

Diazepam has slow elimination of both itself and its active metabolite, with half-lives of 20 to 50 hours for diazepam and 30 to 200 hours for the metabolite desmethyldiazepam.[126] Initially diazepam may promptly produce sedative effects, but sedation wanes rapidly as the drug moves to other tissues. Subsequently, as tissues are saturated, the sedative effects become dependent on metabolism and the duration of action is prolonged.

INDICATIONS AND ADMINISTRATION METHODS. Midazolam is the most widely used agent for short procedures, such as dressing changes and invasive procedures. A recent meta-analysis comparing the recovery from diazepam and midazolam when used for short duration found no clinically important differences in recovery time.[123] In the past the phlebitis and pain associated with administration of intravenous diazepam minimized its use. Recently the availability of a lipid formulation of diazepam has reduced these concerns. Therefore intermittent midazolam, 0.025 to 0.20 mg/kg, or diazepam, 0.1 to 0.2 mg/kg, administered 5 minutes before the procedure should provide safe and effective sedative and amnestic effects for short procedures.[127]

Sedation is provided to the ICU patient for the treatment of anxiety or agitation that is not produced by pain, hypoglycemia, hypoxemia, hypotension, or substance withdrawal. The SCCM practice parameters recommend pre-

ferred agents for treating anxiety in critically ill patients.[57] Continuous infusions of midazolam and propofol were selected as agents of choice for short-term therapy, defined as less than 24 hours. Propofol is an ultra-short–acting intravenous anesthetic agent. Sedation, anxiolysis, and some amnestic effects are produced at subanesthetic doses. Propofol is equally effective as a sedative agent when compared with midazolam.[128,129] SCCM's recommendation for the restricted use of propofol and midazolam was based on weighted consideration of the agents' rapid recovery after discontinuation (when used for short-term periods) and the greater expense occurred when using these agents. Midazolam may be initiated at 0.03 mg/kg/hr, with dosage titrated to effect.[57] Propofol is administered at an initial infusion rate of 0.5 mg/kg/hr and titrated rapidly in 0.5 mg/kg increments to a typical maintenance dose of 0.5 to 3.0 mg/kg/hr.[57]

Beyond the first 24 hours, the SCCM guidelines recommend lorazepam for prolonged treatment of anxiety. Because lorazepam is a longer-acting, slower-onset benzodiazepine, intermittent boluses are adequate to sedate most patients. An initial lorazepam dose of 0.044 mg/kg every 2 to 4 hours serves well as a starting point, with subsequent doses titrated to effect.[57] Some patients require a continuous infusion when their sedation needs become labor intensive. Midazolam and lorazepam, when administered by continuous infusion in critically ill patients, have been proven to be safe and effective.[130] However, two considerations should be taken into account when administering lorazepam infusions. First, lorazepam is not as soluble as midazolam. Precipitation is avoided when infusions are prepared with a final concentration of 0.2 to 1.0 mg/ml in glass containers.[131] Second, high doses (>10 mg/hr) of lorazepam have been associated with polyethylene glycol and propylene glycol toxicity.[132-134] The toxicity is characterized by lactic acidosis, nephrotoxicity, and hyperosmolarity with hypotension. Each milliliter of lorazepam contains 0.18 ml of polyethylene glycol 400 and 0.8 ml of propylene glycol. Patients receiving high doses of lorazepam should be monitored for these effects. Continuous infusion can be initiated at 0.01 mg/kg/hr.

Diazepam is a long-acting agent that can be useful in cases when a prolonged duration of sedation is anticipated, such as a patient with severe respiratory failure requiring intensive mechanical ventilatory support. Sedation levels must be monitored so that doses can be modified in anticipation of awakening the patient. If doses are not appropriately adjusted, the patient will have a prolonged recovery that may extend the need for mechanical ventilation and increase length of stay. Diazepam is rarely administered by continuous infusion because a large volume of diluent is needed to avoid precipitation. A dosage of 0.1 to 0.2 mg/kg every 2 to 4 hours is generally administered by slow intravenous injection.[135] SCCM's practice parameters did not recommend diazepam because of the concerns for phlebitis, its long half-life, and the need for large fluid volumes when given by continuous infusion.[57]

Enteral administration of lorazepam, midazolam, and diazepam is a cost-effective alternative and can be given intermittently or as a continuous dose mixed in feedings. However, dose and frequency should be evaluated daily to prevent the oversedation or undersedation that may occur when feedings are adjusted or interrupted.

TAPERING.   Long-term administration and high dosages of benzodiazepines are associated with tolerance and physical dependence. Unfortunately, data are limited on the development of tolerance and dependence with administration of continuous-infusion benzodiazepines in critically ill patients. The amount of time or dosage required to produce physical dependence that will predispose patients to withdrawal with abrupt discontinuation is unclear. Thus gradual tapering of the dosage is recommended when discontinuing therapy.[136] For patients who receive a continuous infusion for at least 2 weeks, a dosage taper of 10% per day over 10 days is advocated.[137]

There are currently no recommendations for tapering regimens for ICU patients who receive intermittent bolus doses of benzodiazepines for various lengths of time. Effective sedation monitoring is required to reduce the risk of withdrawal effects and the potential for prolonged drug effects as a result of long-term benzodiazepine therapy. Patients who are tolerant to the effects of alcohol are likely to be cross-tolerant to agents such as barbiturates and benzodiazepines that render the same physiologic response as alcohol. These patients will commonly require large doses of benzodiazepines before a pharmacologic effect is observed and anxiety is controlled. Withdrawal is characterized by anxiety, agitation, and symptoms of sympathetic stimulation (e.g., hypertension, tachycardia, or diaphoresis). Significant withdrawal reactions, including seizures, can occur with abrupt discontinuation of this regimen.[138] Slowing the benzodiazepine taper or reinstituting therapy may relieve these symptoms.

SIDE EFFECTS.   Benzodiazepines have a low incidence of side effects. The greatest concern is respiratory and cardiovascular depression. Benzodiazepines depress central respiratory drive; however, the effect is less profound than with opiates.[139] The somnolence associated with these agents can lead to a decrease in minute ventilation.[140]

Midazolam and diazepam have little hemodynamic effect. Sedative doses have produced a slight increase in heart rate and a mild decrease in blood pressure and systemic vascular resistance.[141-143] However, in a volume-depleted state the hemodynamic effects can be more pronounced as a result of venous pooling.

Flumazenil, the only benzodiazepine antagonist approved by the Food and Drug Administration (FDA), reverses the effects of benzodiazepines. Flumazenil competitively inhibits benzodiazepines from binding to its receptor site, facilitating reversal of the deleterious effects associated with benzodiazepine overdose. For prolonged benzodiazepine sedation in a patient who fails to awaken after an appropriate duration following discontinuation, low doses (0.1-0.2 mg IV over 1 minute) of flumazenil may be diagnostic. However, even if an improvement in level of consciousness is noted transiently, flumazenil should not be used for reversal of long-term benzodiazepine sedation because this may produce significant anxiety or more severe withdrawal effects. Withdrawal reactions, including seizures, can result from rapid reversal of benzodiazepines.[144] Flumazenil has been administered to critically ill patients via continuous infusion in doses of 0.5 to 1 μg/kg/min to provide ongoing reversal of a long-acting benzodiazepine.[145] However, this method should be avoided.

PROPOFOL

Propofol is an ultra–short-acting sedative hypnotic with anxiolytic and amnestic properties. Propofol does not provide analgesic effects, and patients require co-administration of an analgesic for pain relief. Propofol is highly lipophilic with a rapid onset and short duration of action. Sedation can be produced within 1 minute of injection, and recovery usually occurs within 10 to 15 minutes, allowing easy titration, control of sedation depth, and rapid awakening for frequent assessment of neurologic status. These characteristics differentiate propofol from other sedatives. It is ideal in trauma patients for the following indications: to facilitate rapid weaning from mechanical ventilation; short-term administrations for ICU-related anxiety; sedation and control of intracranial pressure in the head-injured patient; and deep sedation for surgical or diagnostic procedures.

Patients requiring short-term ventilatory support usually require sedation. The short-acting propofol may be preferred so that spontaneous ventilation can quickly resume, extubation is successful, and the patient is transferred from intensive care.

The SCCM practice parameters recommend propofol and midazolam as agents of choice for the short-term treatment of anxiety or agitation that is not produced by medical conditions such as pain or substance withdrawal.[57] The recommendation for restricted use was based on consideration of the agents' rapid recovery after discontinuation (when used for short-term periods) and the greater expense incurred when using these agents. Several trials have compared propofol and midazolam for the ability to achieve a desired level of sedation, and some have compared costs of therapy. Propofol and midazolam provide a comparable quality of sedation and are equally effective in achieving the desired sedation level.[128,129,146,147] A smoother and faster recovery was identified with propofol compared with midzolam.[146-148] In studies comparing the cost of therapy, propofol use for short-term sedation demonstrated a lower cost than midazolam because of more rapid weaning from mechanical ventilation and transfer out of intensive care.[146,147]

The neurologic examination is the gold standard for monitoring head-injured patients. Propofol, because of its rapid recovery, does not interfere with neurologic assessments.[149-151] Propofol also has been demonstrated to slightly decrease intracranial pressure and to slightly increase cerebral perfusion pressure.[152,153] Caution should be used in initiating or adjusting the dose of propofol to avoid significant hypotension and the resultant decrease in cerebral perfusion pressure.

Effective systemic sedation and analgesia have been achieved when propofol is used in conjunction with fentanyl for procedures including abscess incision and drainage, orthopedic reductions, and chest tube placement.[154] The rapid recovery did not interfere with ventilatory support weaning, and the agent provided adequate amnestic properties for the procedure.

The major disadvantage of propofol has been its expense. When used for short-term infusion, propofol ($151-$1187) has been slightly more expensive than midazolam ($90-$1183) but two to four times the cost of lorazepam ($10-$379).[30,155] The recent availability of a generic propofol product may minimize this concern and result in greater use of propofol.

AVAILABILITY AND DOSING. Propofol is a lipid-soluble agent and is commercially prepared in a 1% lipid emulsion, which provides 1.1 kcal/ml as lipid. The administration of the agent requires a dedicated IV line to prevent contamination and separation of the emulsion. Most indications in trauma patients do not require a loading dose. Infusions are initiated at a slow rate and titrated to therapeutic effect, with dosing adjustments every 5 to 10 minutes (Table 17-8). Critically ill, elderly, and obese patients have prolonged elimination half-life and an increase in volume of distribution, so they may require dosage adjustments.[156-158] Dosing

in obese patients should be based on lean body weight; elderly patients generally require a lower dosage.[158]

Aseptic technique must be observed during preparation and handling of propofol, including swabbing the stopper with alcohol before spiking. The manufacturer recommends discarding any unused portions of the vial and changing the tubing every 12 hours.[159] If syringes are prepared, any unused drug must be discarded and administration sets changed after 6 hours.[159] Lapses in aseptic technique resulting in contaminated propofol preparations have caused sepsis and death.[160] Recently the manufacturer added disodium edetate to the preparation to reduce bacterial growth in the event of accidental contamination; however, appropriate aseptic precautions and techniques for propofol still must be carefully followed.

ADVERSE EFFECTS. Adverse events with propofol include hypotension, bradycardia, hypertriglyceridemia, and greenish discoloration of urine. Hypotension is most common with the administration of large doses or rapid injection and co-administration of agents (i.e., opiates) capable of hypotension.[161-163] Patients who are elderly, hypovolemic, or suffer from severe cardiac disease are at increased risk for hypotension.[161,162] Hypotensive effects can be minimized by avoiding bolus dosing. Additional cardiovascular effects reported are bradycardia, heart block, and ventricular tachycardia.[162]

Although EEG studies demonstrate anticonvulsant activity, propofol has induced seizures in several cases during emergence from anesthesia.[164-166] Many of the seizures occurred in patients with a history of epilepsy, and the patients responded to phenytoin therapy.

Maximal dosing may be dictated by the ability to metabolize intravenous lipids. In some cases hypertriglyceridemia has necessitated discontinuation of the drug. The additional calories provided by propofol infusions should be considered when designing a nutritional regimen to minimize the risk of hypertriglyceridemia and overfeeding. Despite this, patients with disorders of triglyceride metabolism, such as diabetes mellitus, may still develop hypertriglyceridemia.

Long-term administration of propofol may produce tolerance and dependence. Tolerance to the sedative effects was reported in patients receiving the drug for longer than 7 days.[163] A delayed withdrawal pattern characterized by restlessness, confusion, hallucinations, and seizures occurred 5 to 6 days after discontinuation of infusion.[167-169]

HALOPERIDOL

Haloperidol is considered by many clinicians to be the drug of choice for reversing the behavioral manifestations of ICU delirium. The mechanism by which haloperidol reduces delirium is not clear. Actions other than blockade of central dopamine receptors are thought to be responsible for haloperidol's calming effect in patients with delirium.[170,171] Because of the need for rapid control of acute delirium, haloperidol should be given intravenously. Although the

TABLE 17-8	**Propofol Doses and Indications**	
	Sedation Dose	
Indication	µg/kg/hr	mg/kg/hr
Weaning from ventilator	6-53	0.4-3.2
ICU-related anxiety	9-131	0.5-7.9
Neurotrauma	13-37	0.8-2.2
Surgical or diagnostic procedures	100-150 for 3-5 min, then 25-75	6-9 for 3-5 min, then 1.5-4.5

intravenous route is not FDA approved, there is extensive literature demonstrating its safe and effective use.[44]

For the severely agitated patient, the recommended dosage regimen uses progressive dose doubling. Doses should be given at intervals of no less than 20 to 30 minutes.[44] If the desired calming effect is not produced after 30 minutes, the initial dose may be doubled and administered at 30-minute intervals until one of three endpoints is reached[172,173]: the patient is calm; the patient develops an adverse effect; or a total, arbitrary, cumulative dose has been administered.

After the delirious patient is calmed, haloperidol should be given on a scheduled basis every 4 to 6 hours. If agitation remains controlled, the dose is tapered over several days. Intravenous infusions have been reported for patients who require frequent IV administration for agitation control[49,174,175]; however, the agent is usually administered by intermittent IV push. A maximal dosage range has not been established for rapid haloperidol tranquilization. Individual doses up to 150 mg and daily doses as high as 945 mg are reported in the literature.[44]

Haloperidol should not be used as a single agent to control agitation in patients withdrawing from alcohol or benzodiazepines. Although haloperidol reduces some of the signs and symptoms associated with these withdrawal syndromes, it increases the risk of seizures by lowering the seizure threshold. Patients who cannot tolerate the hemodynamic effect of other sedatives or who are weaning from mechanical ventilation can be sedated with haloperidol alone.

Adverse effects associated with intravenous haloperidol include neurologic and cardiovascular toxicities. The neurologic toxicities are extrapyramidal effects such as akathisia and dystonia. Patients with akathisia often have the clinical symptoms of restlessness, irritability, and thought or speech disorders. Akathisia is often mistaken for continued or worsened delirium, and accurate differentiation is necessary for proper treatment. Both dystonia and akathisia respond to treatment with anticholinergic agents (e.g., diphenhydramine or benztropine).[176] However, in patients with akathisia who are unresponsive to anticholinergics, propranolol or amantadine may be useful.[177-181] The extrapyramidal effects are not dose related and are sudden in onset; however, the incidence of these symptoms after intravenous use is lower than it is after oral or intramuscular administration.[182]

Cardiovascular consequences consist of the rare occurrence of QT interval prolongation and the development of polymorphic ventricular tachycardia such as torsades de pointes.[183] The majority of these cases have occurred in patients receiving more than 50 mg per day.[49,183,184-187] Patients receiving intravenous haloperidol should have continuous electrocardiogram (ECG) monitoring. Haloperidol should be discontinued or the dose reduced if the QT interval is prolonged by 25% or more over baseline, the interval is longer than 440 ms, or polymorphic ventricular tachycardia is observed.[183] Hypotensive episodes after the administration of intravenous haloperidol are rare and almost always caused by hypovolemia.

The use of lorazepam in combination with haloperidol can be helpful for two reasons.[188,189] First, combination therapy may allow lower total doses of each to be used with increased efficacy and fewer adverse effects. Second, this combination may have a synergistic effect. Therefore the addition of a benzodiazepine can be considered to avoid the need for large haloperidol doses.

BARBITURATES

Barbiturates produce sedation by depressing excitable tissues throughout the CNS. They suppress transmission of excitatory neurotransmitters (e.g., acetylcholine) and enhance transmission of inhibitory neurotransmitters (e.g., GABA). Barbiturates are usually administered only when the usual agents have failed to produce the desired level of sedation. These agents are effective sedatives at low doses but have no amnestic or analgesic properties. In fact, they sometimes appear to have antianalgesic effects by lowering the pain threshold. These agents were once widely used in the ICU to control agitation and delirium through sedation. As agents with amnestic properties and a more favorable adverse effect profile have been developed, the routine use of barbiturates is no longer recommended.[57]

The highly lipophilic barbiturates have a rapid onset and short duration of action. For example, thiopental typically produces a loss of consciousness within 30 seconds, and recovery occurs within 20 minutes. Barbiturates are degraded by hepatic microsomal enzymes to inactive metabolites. Tolerance to the sedative effects quickly develops, and this tolerance is conferred to most CNS depressant drugs as well.

Thiopental and pentobarbital are used most often to treat seizure disorders. They have been used to manage intracranial hypertension in patients who do not respond to conventional therapy; however, a beneficial effect on outcomes has not been demonstrated.[190]

Complications associated with barbiturate administration include myocardial depression with hypotension and respiratory depression. Patients who are elderly or who are intravascularly volume depleted are especially prone to these adverse effects.

KETAMINE

Ketamine is an intravenous anesthetic agent that produces analgesia and sedation at low doses. It is occasionally used for repeated painful procedures such as dressing changes.[191] Ketamine causes a functional dissociation between the thalamus (which relays sensory impulses from the reticular activating system to the cerebral cortex) and the limbic cortex (which is involved with the awareness of sensation). The patient appears conscious (e.g., eyes opening, swallowing) but is unable to process or respond to sensory input. Because of its sympathomimetic properties, an increase in blood pressure and heart rate is typical. However, an unexpected hypotension can occur in critically ill patients as a result of a direct myocardial depressant property. Ketamine is used most often in children younger than 10 years of age. Use in adults is limited by an emergence phenomenon characterized by hallucinations and nightmares. Pretreatment with a benzodiazepine may minimize this reaction. Ketamine is a bronchodilator and has been used to treat severe asthma exacerbations.[192] Pretreatment with atropine may diminish upper airway secretions. The place of this agent in routine ICU sedation remains to be determined.

NEUROMUSCULAR BLOCKING AGENTS

Neuromuscular blocking agents (NMBAs) available for clinical use, including rapacuronium, a nondepolarizing relaxant that recently received FDA approval, are listed in Table 17-9. Rapacuronium has a very rapid onset and a recovery pattern close to that of succinylcholine.[193]

NMBAs are used to facilitate endotracheal intubation and help prevent laryngospasm. Once intubated, however, only a small fraction of ICU patients are treated with continuous infusion or scheduled NMBAs. Aggressive use of analgesia and sedation is preferred initially, and NMBAs are reserved for patients who fail to meet desired goals despite maximal sedative therapy. In the ICU setting, NMBA therapy is frequently used to paralyze mechanically ventilated patients in an attempt to improve chest wall compliance. NMBAs can assist ventilation therapy in at least three ways: (1) reducing or eliminating spontaneous breathing; (2) preventing motor activity that can dislodge catheters, surgical dressings, or chest tubes; and (3) reducing oxygen consumption by patients with severely diminished cardiopulmonary function.[30] However, patients who are maximally sedated may only experience minimal improvements in ventilatory mechanics and chest wall compliance with the addition of NMBAs.

NMBAs are often used during surgical procedures when complete muscle block is desirable, such as abdominal or cardiothoracic surgery, or in the setting of dislocations and fractures.[194] Postoperative neuromuscular blockade can be a useful adjunct to promote healing of specific surgical wounds (e.g., vascular anastomosis) by immobilizing the patient for a defined period.[194] Immobilization may prove of particular benefit when wound closure has been difficult or disruptive and loss of wound integrity would place the patient at great risk.

Apart from mechanical ventilation and postoperative indications, several situations in the ICU may justify the use of NMBAs. Neuromuscular blockade can prevent unacceptably high oxygen consumption as a result of the profound shivering that frequently accompanies rewarming from hypothermia.[195] Furthermore, therapeutic paralysis has been used in the treatment of tetanus,[196,197] status epilepticus,[198] and uncontrolled intracranial hypertension.[198,199]

PHYSIOLOGY

The neuromuscular junction consists of the motor nerve terminal, the synaptic cleft, and the muscle's end plate, which contains nicotinic receptors (Figure 17-5). The motor nerve terminal synthesizes and stores the neurotransmitter acetylcholine. Upon arrival of a nerve impulse at the nerve terminal, acetylcholine is released by the nerve terminal into the synaptic cleft and binds to the nicotinic receptor,

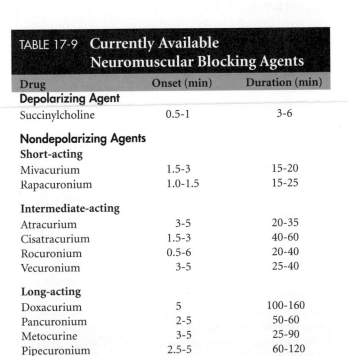

TABLE 17-9	Currently Available Neuromuscular Blocking Agents	
Drug	**Onset (min)**	**Duration (min)**
Depolarizing Agent		
Succinylcholine	0.5-1	3-6
Nondepolarizing Agents		
Short-acting		
Mivacurium	1.5-3	15-20
Rapacuronium	1.0-1.5	15-25
Intermediate-acting		
Atracurium	3-5	20-35
Cisatracurium	1.5-3	40-60
Rocuronium	0.5-6	20-40
Vecuronium	3-5	25-40
Long-acting		
Doxacurium	5	100-160
Pancuronium	2-5	50-60
Metocurine	3-5	25-90
Pipecuronium	2.5-5	60-120
Tubocurarine	3-5	35-45

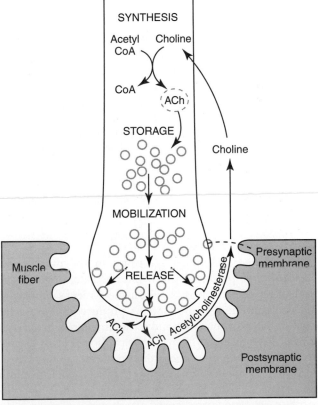

FIGURE 17-5 Neuromuscular junction. The neuromuscular junction consists of the nerve axon and the muscle fiber. The neurotransmitter acetylcholine is released from axonal vesicles in response to nerve action potentials. The combination of acetylcholine with the receptor results in a depolarization of the muscle cells and contraction of the muscle fiber.

initiating the opening of a potential channel. The opening of this channel allows the influx of sodium and calcium ions and the efflux of potassium ions, thereby triggering depolarization of the motor end plate. This depolarization leads to muscle contraction. Acetylcholine can attach to or detach from the receptor. Unbound acetylcholine is metabolized by the enzyme acetylcholinesterase, thus terminating the depolarization of the end plate and the resultant contraction.

NMBAs induce paralysis of the skeletal muscle by disrupting normal neuromuscular transmission. The currently available agents structurally resemble acetylcholine and occupy the nicotinic receptors on the muscle fiber, which prevents the binding of acetylcholine to the receptors. The NMBAs are classified as depolarizing or nondepolarizing relaxants according to their effect on the motor end plate. Succinylcholine, the only depolarizing agent currently used, attaches to the receptor and depolarizes the motor end plate. The depolarizing action of succinylcholine is more sustained than that of acetylcholine, and the end plate remains refractory to the effects of acetylcholine. Transient twitching of skeletal muscle (fasciculations) is briefly produced, followed by paralysis. Nondepolarizing relaxants bind to the same receptors as acetylcholine, establishing a competitive inhibition of the attachment of acetylcholine to the receptor. In contrast to succinylcholine, nondepolarizing agents do not depolarize the end plate and cause muscle contraction.

SEQUENCE OF ONSET

When an appropriate dose of an NMBA is injected intravenously, the onset of blockade is rapid. Motor weakness progresses to total flaccid paralysis. Small, rapidly moving muscles such as those of the eyes are involved before those of the limbs, neck, trunk, and abdomen. Ultimately, intercostal muscles and finally the diaphragm are paralyzed and respiration ceases. Recovery of skeletal muscles usually occurs in reverse order to that of paralysis, so that the diaphragm is the first to regain function. Intravenous injection of an NMBA to a person who is awake initially produces difficulty in focusing and weakness in the mandibular muscles, followed by ptosis, diplopia, and dysphagia. Consciousness and sensorium remain undisturbed even in the presence of complete neuromuscular blockade.

COMPARISON OF AGENTS

NMBAs can be classified according to the duration of blockade they produce—short, intermediate, or long (see Table 17-9). Selection is based on the patient's needs and medical condition. Some NMBAs produce cardiovascular effects such as hypotension and arrhythmia. In patients with cardiovascular impairments, the cardiovascularly stable NMBAs (vecuronium, pipecuronium, doxacurium, cisatracurium, and rocuronium) may be preferred. Pancuronium has vagolytic effects that produce tachycardia and an increase in blood pressure.[200] It should be avoided in patients who cannot tolerate a further increase in heart rate (coronary heart disease, valvular heart disease). However, in the absence of cardiovascular disease, the increase in heart rate is well tolerated by many young patients. Hepatic and renal failure should be considered when choosing a NMBA, but they are not contraindications to agents metabolized or eliminated by these routes as long as appropriate monitoring is performed. Atracurium and cisatracurium undergo Hoffman elimination, and because this elimination does not depend on organ function, these agents may be a good choice for patients with renal and hepatic failure. Asthmatic patients may be at increased risk when administered NMBAs that release histamine (tubocurarine, atracurium). Pancuronium, vecuronium, pipecuronium, rocuronium, cisatracurium, or doxacurium may be preferred for patients with asthma because they are not associated with significant histamine release.

The SCCM practice parameters recommend pancuronium as the preferred NMBA for most critically ill patients because the agent is inexpensive and the relative tachycardia and mild hypertension are seldom of clinical consequence and are presumed to be related to the dosage and rate of administration.[201] Vecuronium is the preferred NMBA for patients with cardiac disease or hemodynamic instability in whom tachycardia may be deleterious. The SCCM panel agrees that there are numerous theoretical advantages to the use of cisatracurium and atracurium in the ICU, but they feel the advantages are outweighed by the agents' expense. Therefore they are not recommended unless extenuating circumstances (e.g., multiple organ dysfunction) are present.

BOLUS DOSING VERSUS CONTINUOUS INFUSION

NMBAs are usually administered as a bolus-loading dose followed by repeat bolus or continuous infusion. With short-acting or intermediate-duration drugs such as mivacurium, rocuronium, atracurium, or vecuronium, continuous infusions may be preferred.

ENDOTRACHEAL INTUBATION

Succinylcholine is commonly administered as an IV bolus of 1.5 mg/kg in adults to facilitate endotracheal intubation because its onset of 60 seconds is faster than many of the nondepolarizing relaxants. Unfortunately, the side effects associated with succinylcholine may limit its usefulness for intubation in some patients (see adverse effects). Large doses of the nondepolarizing agents mivacurium and rocuronium approach the rapid onset of succinylcholine, with muscle relaxation occurring within 2 to 2.5 minutes and 1 to 1.5 minutes, respectively.[202,203] However, rocuronium is very expensive, and large doses of mivacurium may cause histamine release and hypotension in patients with preexisting cardiovascular instability.

The other nondepolarizing relaxants have an onset of about 3 to 4 minutes, limiting their use for rapid tracheal intubation. However, two techniques can speed the onset of neuromuscular blockade. The first technique involves the administration of a priming dose, one tenth of an intubating dose, several minutes before the bolus dose. Ideally, after the priming dose patients should be able to breathe spontaneously, maintain a patent airway, and avoid aspiration so that intubation can occur within 100 seconds. Some patients, however, experience weakness or respiratory distress and fear and anxiety from diplopia and dyspnea after the priming dose.

Another technique involves the administration of a dose two times the intubating dose of nondepolarizing relaxants. The large dose saturates the receptors and speeds up the onset of intubation. The risks of this method are related to the cardiovascular effects of the relaxant, which can be avoided by using a drug with a stable cardiovascular profile such as vecuronium, doxacurium, cisatracurium, or rocuronium.[204]

FACTORS AFFECTING PARALYSIS

Many factors affect the degree of paralysis induced by NMBAs.[205-234] These factors may inhibit or potentiate neuromuscular blockade depending on the degree of blockade induced, the agent used, and individual patient characteristics. Table 17-10 lists clinical conditions and medica-

tions capable of altering the effects of NMBAs. Because the trauma patient is at risk for these conditions and may require one or many of the interacting medications, close monitoring and assessment of the patient is recommended.

NURSING ASSESSMENT

Monitoring of NMBA therapy by train-of-four (TOF) stimulation is widely recommended.[235-242] Routine monitoring using this method helps avoid excessive or insufficient use of paralytics and may prevent prolonged effect of NMBAs. Changing organ function and addition of medications that potentiate NMBAs can foster accumulation of the NMBA or its active metabolites, which will be undetected without train-of-four monitoring. Investigators have documented that adjusting the dose of NMBAs by monitoring peripheral nerve stimulation versus standard clinical dosing in critically ill patients reduces drug requirements and allows a faster recovery of neuromuscular function and spontaneous breathing.[236] Nerve stimulators deliver an electrical current that is intended to activate a motor nerve while the mechanical response of a muscle enervated by that nerve is measured. Examples of peripheral nerve stimulators are shown in Figure 17-6. As the NMBA occupies an increasing number of postsynaptic acetylcholine receptors, the block becomes more profound and the muscle response to nerve stimulation diminishes.

Monitoring neuromuscular function can be uncomfortable for the patient. Therefore monitoring should begin after sedation and analgesia and, optimally, before any NMBA is given. This sequence shows that the nerve stimulator is functioning properly and that the electrodes are placed correctly and assesses baseline muscle contraction. The peripheral nerve stimulator delivers electrical current via

TABLE 17-10 **Factors Affecting Paralysis**	
Potentiate Blockade or Decrease Drug Requirement	**Antagonize Blockade or Increase Drug Requirement**
Drugs	**Drugs**
Halogenated anesthetics	Phenytoin
Local anesthetics	Carbamazepine
Antibiotics	Anticholinesterase agents
Aminoglycosides	Edrophonium
Clindamycin	Neostigmine
Vancomycin	Pyridostigmine
Antiarrhythmics	Theophylline
Procainamide	Azathioprine
Quinidine	Ranitidine
Bretylium	
Calcium channel blockers	
Beta-adrenergic blockers	
Cyclosporine	
Dantrolene	
Cyclophosphamide	
Lithium	
Mineralocorticoids	
Clinical	**Clinical**
Acidosis	Alkalosis
Electrolyte abnormalities	Hypercalcemia
Severe hyponatremia	Demyelinating lesions
Severe hypocalcemia	Peripheral neuropathies
Severe hypokalemia	Diabetes mellitus
Hypermagnesemia	
Neuromuscular diseases	
Myasthenia gravis	
Muscular dystrophy	
Amyotrophic lateral sclerosis (ALS)	
Poliomyelitis	
Multiple sclerosis	
Eaton-Lambert syndrome	
Hypothermia	
Acute intermittent porphyria	
Renal failure	
Hepatic failure	

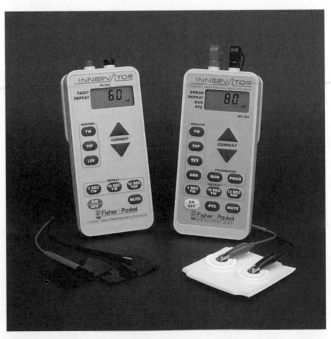

FIGURE 17-6 Peripheral nerve stimulators. (Courtesy Fisher & Paykel Healthcare.)

two electrodes placed over a peripheral nerve (ECG electrodes are most commonly used). Electrodes should be placed over skin that is clean, dry, and hairless and replaced every 24 hours. Substantial edema or obesity may result in insufficient current being delivered to the nerve by surface electrodes. Needle electrodes (23 gauge) are available if ECG electrodes are ineffective.

The ulnar nerve at the wrist is most frequently used to evaluate neuromuscular function (Figure 17-7). Stimulation of the ulnar nerve results in the adduction of the thumb. Peripheral nerve monitoring may be performed on the facial nerve, which results in movement of the orbicularis oculi muscle (Figure 17-8). Because it is blockade of the neuromuscular junction that needs to be monitored, direct stimulation of muscle should be avoided by placing electrodes over the course of the nerve and not over the muscle itself.

Train-of-four measurement is the most common method used to monitor NMBAs in the intensive care unit. Four stimuli are delivered along the path of the nerve at a frequency of 2 Hz for 2 seconds. Muscle response is measured to evaluate the number of stimuli blocked versus delivered. In the absence of NMBA, four equal muscle contractions should be observed in response to the four stimuli (4/4). In the presence of a nondepolarizing NMBA, a progressive loss of twitch height and number of twitches represent a progressive degree of neuromuscular blockade (Figure 17-9). When 90% of the receptors are blocked, the

muscle will only respond once (1/4). At greater than 90% blocked, no movement of the muscle may be seen (0/4). If two, three, or four twitches are observed, a block less than 90% has been quantified.

Although no prospective, controlled trials have determined the degree of neuromuscular blockade required to achieve optimal mechanical ventilation in patients, the recommended rate of infusion is that titrated to a minimal presence of one or two twitches (80%-90% blockade) at all times. TOF stimulation should be monitored and recorded every 8 hours or more frequently when patient status dictates. Ablation of all four twitches during continuous infusion is a sign of relative overdose of an NMBA. In this

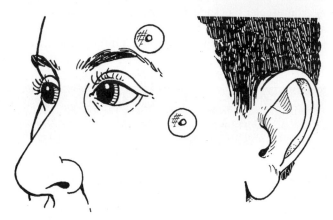

FIGURE 17-8 Facial nerve placement for train-of-four stimulation of the facial nerve. Electrodes are placed on either side of an imaginary line between the outer canthus of the eye and the tip of the ear. The muscles of the face will twitch when stimulated.

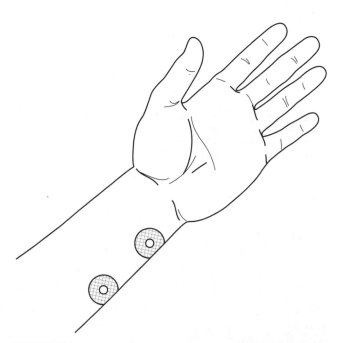

FIGURE 17-7 Ulnar nerve placement for train-of-four stimulation of the ulnar nerve. Electrodes are positioned in a direct line along the lateral side of the wrist. The thumb adducts to stimulation.

Strength of thumb adductions

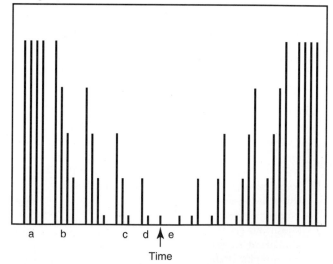

Time

FIGURE 17-9. **Train-of-Four Monitoring.** Quantifying the degree of neuromuscular blockade. **A,** Four strong twitches indicate an absence of blockade. **B, C, D,** As more receptors become occupied with an NMBA, fewer twitches occur in response to stimulation. A single twitch response indicates a 90% block to four stimuli (*arrow*). **E,** No observed twitches indicates 100% blockade and may represent an overdose situation. (From Davidson JE: Neuromuscular blockade: indications, peripheral nerve stimulation, and other concurrent interventions, *New Horiz* 2:77, 1994.)

situation the NMBA infusion should be discontinued until the one or two twitches return, then reinstated at a lower infusion rate.[243] If intermittent boluses are used, TOF should be repeated every 15 to 30 minutes and the next bolus not administered until at least a single twitch appears.

If TOF monitoring is not available, continuous infusion of the NMBA should be stopped once a day and the time for return of some neuromuscular function noted. If this time is longer than 1 hour, the rate of infusion is empirically decreased on reinstatement of the continuous infusion. The amount of the decrease is related to the duration of prolonged neuromuscular blockade. For example, if a 1-hour recovery was expected but if 4 hours were required before movement, the dose may be decreased by 25%, compared with 50% if 8 to 12 hours pass before movement. This prevents accumulation of the NMBA. Regardless of whether TOF is used, all patients who receive NMBA infusions should have their infusions stopped once daily to assess blockade and to provide an opportunity for clinical evaluation to assess the adequacy of concomitant sedation and analgesia.

PROBLEMS WITH TOF

Substantial edema or obesity are the most often identified factors affecting TOF monitoring. Electrode placement too far from the nerve and pressure applied to the electrodes can also affect response. Pressure decreases the electrode skin resistance and distance from the skin to the nerve, thus increasing the amount of current delivered and possibly leading to overstimulation. Use of surface electrodes and marking the location on the skin minimize variability between observers compared with the use of ball electrodes and conducting gel. Operator assessment of TOF is subjective and prone to misinterpretation. For example, two equal, strong thumb twitches with a faint third twitch may be interpreted as two twitches by one observer and as three twitches by another. Whether faint twitches should be included in the assessment is controversial and not addressed in the literature.

Equipment malfunction can produce a TOF error. Variability in current output has been documented at higher impedance with some peripheral nerve stimulators (PNS). Faulty connections of the stimulator to the electrodes, inadequate battery power, and improperly lubricated electrodes can contribute to erroneous TOF readings.

A major limitation to peripheral nerve stimulation is that the TOF of the ulnar nerve may not accurately reflect the depth of paralysis of the diaphragmatic and accessory respiratory muscle because of differences in sensitivities to neuromuscular blockade.[244,245] Some patients will have no response to TOF testing but may still demonstrate movement or response to stimulation, such as cough or gag when suctioned. Clinical assessment of patient response remains the standard when monitoring these patients, and TOF testing is performed to guide the maximal dose required. The maximal acceptable dose is determined by improvement in the parameter or condition being treated.

Because of the many chances to introduce errors into TOF monitoring, the SCCM guidelines recommend that even with the use of peripheral nerve stimulation, neuromuscular blockade should be stopped at least once daily for clinical evaluation to assess the adequacy of concomitant sedation and analgesia and determine if continued paralysis is needed.[201]

DISCONTINUATION AND REVERSAL OF BLOCKADE

Most patients receiving NMBAs are allowed to regain neuromuscular function spontaneously. Several clinical techniques can be used to assess the adequacy of recovery: ability to open the eyes wide, to sustain protrusion of the tongue, to maintain an effective handgrip, and to lift the head for 5 seconds.

In rare instances, waiting for the spontaneous recovery from nondepolarizing agents may be impractical and administration of reversing agents is necessary. Acetylcholinesterase inhibitors (ACIs) are administered to inhibit the destruction of acetylcholine by acetylcholinesterases. Acetylcholine concentration increases at the neuromuscular junction, and the binding of acetylcholine occurs more readily than the binding of the NMBA to the acetylcholine receptors. Neostigmine, edrophonium, and pyridostigmine are the ACIs frequently used. These antagonists are not specific for nicotinic receptors and, when administered, result in toxic effects from the stimulation of muscarinic receptors. These toxic effects include excessive oral secretions, bronchospasm, and potentially severe bradycardia, which can lead to heart block, nodal escape rhythm, and premature ventricular contractions. Anticholinergic agents, atropine, or glycopyrrolate are concurrently administered to minimize or prevent these effects. The half-life and duration of the anticholinergic should be matched to the ACI. Atropine should be administered with edrophonium, and glycopyrrolate is best administered with neostigmine or pyridostigmine. Table 17-11 summarizes the intravenous doses of anticholinergics and ACIs.

Because succinylcholine is not metabolized by acetylcholinesterase, it diffuses away from the neuromuscular junction and is hydrolyzed in the plasma and liver by another enzyme, pseudocholinesterase. Fortunately this is a rapid

TABLE 17-11	**Anticholinesterase Inhibitors and Anticholinergic Doses for Reversal of Neuromuscular Blockade**		
Neostigmine + glycopyrrolate 25-75 μg/kg + 5-15 μg/kg	Pyridostigmine + glycopyrrolate 100-300 μg/kg + 5-15 μg/kg	Edrophonium + atropine 500-1000 μg/kg + 10 μg/kg

process in most patients because there are no reversal agents available for depolarizing blockade. In rare instances patients may have a pseudocholinesterase deficiency that results in a prolonged duration of blockade after succinylcholine administration.[246] Supportive care is provided to these patients until muscle function returns.

ADVERSE EFFECTS

The undesired effects seen with NMBAs are generally of three different domains: (1) complications resulting from immobility, (2) adverse effects associated with individual NMBAs, and (3) residual paralysis extending after discontinuation of the NMBA. The immobility produced by extended use of muscle relaxants increases the risk of pressure injury to nerves, pressure necrosis and ulceration, cough failure and retention of secretions, impaired ability to perform abdominal and neurologic examinations, and disuse atrophy.

Succinylcholine is associated with many adverse effects.[247-254] Most serious of these is malignant hyperthermia syndrome. Massive muscle depolarization occurs, causing hypermetabolism and hyperkalemia. Although pretreatment or early treatment with dantrolene is effective, malignant hyperthermia syndrome can be fatal.

Depending on the patient's autonomic nervous system, succinylcholine may increase or decrease heart rate and blood pressure. Additionally, succinylcholine commonly increases the serum potassium level 0.5 to 1 mEq/L. In rare cases serum potassium levels exceeding 5.0 mEq/L can occur. Medical conditions associated with this include upper motor neuron lesions or spinal cord injury, large burns, and massive trauma, including closed head injury. Patients become vulnerable within days of the injury and remain at risk for months. The subsequent cardiac arrest can be refractory to resuscitative efforts. Table 17-12 lists absolute contraindications to succinylcholine.

Succinylcholine-induced fasciculations cause increases in intraocular and intragastric pressure. The cause of increased intracranial pressure is less understood. Increased intraocular pressure might extrude vitreous from a ruptured globe. Increased intragastric pressure may cause a patient with residual gastric contents to regurgitate and possibly aspirate. Cricoid pressure is applied when securing the airway to avoid aspiration. Whether succinylcholine should be avoided because of these increases is controversial. Uncoordinated muscle fasciculations are also thought to be responsible for the myalgias experienced by some patients.

The adverse effects associated with nondepolarizing relaxants involve the cardiovascular and respiratory system. Tubocurarine, atracurium, rapacuronium, and mivacurium cause the release of histamine, which can cause hypotension and tachycardia in hypovolemic patients and wheezing in some patients.[255,256] Pancuronium has vagolytic activity that in some patients results in hypertension and tachycardia.[206,257] Vecuronium, doxacurium, pipecuronium, cisatracurium, rocuronium, and rapacuronium have minimal cardiovascular effects.

The literature contains many reports of prolonged weakness in the ICU. Several distinct clinical syndromes of prolonged weakness have been identified. Critical illness polyneuropathy is both a sensory and motor polyneuropathy commonly observed in seriously ill, septic, and elderly patients.[258] Presently the development of this syndrome is not thought to be directly related to NMBAs.

In contrast, critical illness myopathy is most likely a direct myotoxic effect from combining steroids and NMBAs.[258] The syndrome is characterized as a persistent moderate or severe flaccid, generalized weakness that becomes apparent after the NMBA is discontinued. Sensory function is preserved.

Prolonged neuromuscular blockade occurs when neuromuscular transmission remains impaired and weakness persists after NMBAs are discontinued. The mechanism of prolonged weakness is thought to be caused by residual NMBA or active metabolites.[194,258-260] Routine TOF monitoring of the degree of neuromuscular blockade produced by the muscle relaxant and discontinuing the relaxant once daily to assess the patient can prevent overdose of the NMBA and prolonged paralysis.[201,236,261]

The greatest problem associated with prolonged neuromuscular blockade is the delay in weaning patients from mechanical ventilation as a result of diaphragmatic or intercostal muscle weakness. No specific therapy is available, so the goal is prevention. Although TOF monitoring may prevent prolonged paralysis from NMBA, there is no evidence that it prevents critical illness myopathy or polyneuropathy. NMBA use and duration should be minimized. Most trauma patients requiring mechanical ventilation should be managed with maximal use of sedatives and analgesics.

TABLE 17-12	Contraindications to Succinylcholine Commonly Encountered in the ICU	
Burns	Disuse atrophy
Spinal cord injury	Massive trauma
Hyperkalemia	Septic or hemorrhagic shock
Peripheral nerve injury	

NURSING CARE THROUGH THE PHASES OF TRAUMA

PAIN ASSESSMENT IN THE ADULT TRAUMA PATIENT

Adequate assessment of pain in the trauma setting is difficult based on the complexity of injury and need for immediate resuscitation. Pain assessment must be individualized, and basic principles of a comprehensive analgesic plan can be applied using the ABC method as described by the AHCPR[262] (Table 17-13).

A comprehensive approach to postoperative pain assessment requires the careful evaluation of key elements. They include patient perception and physiologic, behavioral, and cognitive responses.[19] In addition to identifying obvious injuries, such as open wounds, fractures, and soft tissue disruptions that cause pain, the nurse must also explore past pain experiences and trauma, especially with patients who have surgical scars. The mechanism of injury and potential for delayed complications, especially in patients with orthopedic trauma at risk for development of compartment syndrome, are important considerations. Identifying individual coping responses and cultural interpretations are important; input from family members is beneficial. Patient personality and expectations concerning pain and its management must be considered. History of polysubstance abuse requires further investigation in regard to pattern of use and duration of intake (Table 17-14).

The PQRST mnemonic is a quick and lenient method for the trauma nurse to apply the key elements of the comprehensive pain assessment. Obtaining information from a patient who can speak regarding what **p**rovokes/**p**alliates pain, the **q**ualities of the pain, the **r**egion of **r**adiation of pain, the **s**everity and **s**trength of the pain, and length of **t**ime the pain has persisted ensures a thorough assessment.[263]

The provoking aspects and causes of pain must be investigated thoroughly. Inquiries should include what triggers the pain (such as movement or deep breathing), specific treatments (such as wound dressing changes), and its duration: Is the pain constant or episodic? Does tactile stimulation, such as pressure from orthopedic appliances or bed linens, cause discomfort? Elevation, realignment, and support of the injured body part are a few nursing interventions to apply while investigating provoking aspects of pain.

The quality aspect of assessment uses the patient's own descriptors. Request of the patient, for example, "Tell me how your discomfort feels." Verbal rating scales or the McGill Pain Questionnaire (see Figure 17-10 for examples) aid the practitioner to further evaluate traumatic pain complaints. Certain clusters of words alert the assessor to unique pain states. Pain that is excruciating with passive motion may indicate early development of compartment syndrome.

Encourage the patient to point to the region of pain or use a body diagram to locate pain. Obvious injuries may not be the source of pain; for example, nasal drainage tubes can cause more distress than surgical incisions. Further explore reports of phantom limb sensation and pain by the amputee population. Investigate any report of pain radiating to other areas besides that of obvious injury.

Severity of pain can be quantified by asking the patient to rate his or her pain between 0 and 10, where 0 is no pain and 10 is the worst pain imaginable. Consistently using the same rating tool is imperative throughout the trauma continuum. Many pain intensity rating tools are available, and some use horizontal or vertical linear orientation or variations of color. The Wong-Baker FACES pain rating scale can be used in patients older than 3 years of age and those with cognitive impairment (see Figure 17-10 for examples).

Timing refers to when pain occurs and how long it lasts. Does it vary with activity or intensify during certain time frames? Episodic or procedure-related pain can be corre-

---

TABLE 17-14   Pain Assessment Factors in the Critical, Intermediate, and Rehabilitative Phases of Trauma

1. Patient report of pain
   a. Rating on 0-to-10 scale
   b. Description (in own words: continuous, intermittent, percentage of time in pain, sharp, dull, burning, aching)
2. Blood pressure, pulse, respiratory rate
3. Mobility (sit, stand, lift, bend)
4. Food and fluid intake
5. Elimination
6. Sleep and rest
7. Location of injury/injuries
8. Type of injury (fractures, ruptured viscera, head, nerve, burn, infection, loss of body part)
9. Affect (anxious, worried, oblivious, happy, sad, fearful, angry)
10. Behavior (crying, lethargic, restless, motionless)
11. Energy level (patient report)
12. Past experience with pain
13. Meaning of pain (to patient and family)
14. Cultural beliefs with pain
15. Orientation to person, place, date, and situation
16. Memory functioning
17. Ability to follow instructions
18. Knowledge of injuries
19. Health history
    a. Chronic pain history
    b. Physical illnesses
    c. Emotional illnesses
    d. Medications (name, dose, frequency, last taken)
20. Social functioning
    a. Education, occupation
    b. Family history (parent and sibling functioning)
    c. Behavioral problems
    d. Substance abuse (name, amount, length of time used, last used, treatment, withdrawal reactions)

TABLE 17-13   Pain Assessment and Management Mnemonic

A   Ask about and Assess pain regularly and systematically.
B   Believe the report of pain.
C   Choose the best pain control options.
D   Deliver pain interventions consistently and timely.
E   Empower the patient and family to control the course.

Modified from Jacox A, Carr DB, Payne R et al: *Management of cancer pain*, Clinical Practice Guideline No. 9, AHCPR Pub No 94-0592, Rockville, Md, 1994, Agency for Health Care Policy and Research, U.S. Department of Health and Human Services, Public Health Service, 24.

10-cm Visual Analogue Scale

No Pain ██ Worst Pain

Directions: Explain to the patient that one end of the line equals no pain and the other end is the worst pain. Have the patient mark or point to the place that shows how much pain he or she is experiencing.

Graphic Rating Scale

No Pain   0 1 2 3 4 5 6 7 8 9 10   Worst Pain

Directions: Have patient circle or point to the number that best represents how much pain is experienced.

Verbal Rating Scale   0 (No Pain) through 10 (Worst Pain)

Directions: Ask the patient to verbalize a number between 0 and 10 that represents how much pain is experienced.

Faces Pain Rating Scale

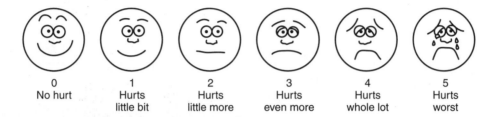

0	1	2	3	4	5
No hurt	Hurts little bit	Hurts little more	Hurts even more	Hurts whole lot	Hurts worst

Directions: Explain to the patient that each face is for someone who feels happy because he has no pain or sad because he has some pain. Ask the patient to choose the face that best describes how he is feeling.

Children's Hospital of Eastern Ontario Pain Scale (CHEOPS)

Item	Behavior	Score	Definition
Cry	No cry	1	Child is not crying.
	Moaning	2	Child is moaning or quietly vocalizing silent cry.
	Crying	2	Child is crying, but the cry is gentle or whimpering.
	Scream	3	Child is in a full-lunged cry; sobbing; may be scored with complaint or without complaint.
Facial	Composed	1	Neutral facial expression
	Grimace	2	Score only if definite negative facial expression.
	Smiling	0	Score only if definite positive facial expression.
Child	None	1	Child not talking.
Verbal	Other complaints	1	Child complains, but not about pain, e.g., "I want to see Mommy" or "I am thirsty."
	Pain complaints	2	Child complains about pain.
	Both complaints	2	Child complains about pain and about other things, e.g., "It hurts; I want Mommy."
	Positive	0	Child makes any positive statement or talks about other things without complaint.
Torso	Neutral	1	Body (not limbs) is at rest; torso is inactive.
	Shifting	2	Body is in motion in a shifting or serpentine fashion.
	Tense	2	Body is arched or rigid.
	Shivering	2	Body is shuddering or shaking involuntarily.
	Upright	2	Child is in a vertical or upright position.
	Restrained	2	Body is restrained.
Touch	Not touching	1	Child is not touching or grabbing at wound.
	Reach	2	Child is reaching for but not touching wound.
	Touch	2	Child is gently touching wound or wound area.
	Grab	2	Child is grabbing vigorously at wound.
	Restrained	2	Child's arms are restrained.
Legs	Neutral	1	Legs may be in a position but are relaxed; includes gentle swimming or serpentine-like movements.
	Squirming/kicking	2	Definitive uneasy or restless movements in the legs or striking out with foot or feet.
	Drawn up/tensed	2	Legs tensed or pulled up tightly to body and kept there.
	Standing	2	Standing, crouching, or kneeling.
	Restrained	2	Child's legs are being held down.

Directions: This tool is specifically for children. Look at each item and assign the score that corresponds to the observed behavior. The scores denote: behavior that is the antithesis of pain (0); behavior not indicative of pain and is not the antithesis of pain (1); behavior indicating mild or moderate pain (2); and behavior indicating severe pain (3).

FIGURE 17-10 **Pain Rating Scales.** (Wong-Baker Faces pain rating scale from Wong DL: *Wong's essentials of pediatric nursing,* St. Louis, 2001, Mosby; Children's Hospital of Eastern Ontario Pain Scale [CHEOPS] from McGrath P, Johnson G, Goodman JT et al: CHEOPS: a behavioral scale for rating post operative pain in children. In: *Advances in pain research and therapy,* vol 9, New York, 1985, Raven, 398.)

lated with therapeutic activities, such as turning, endotracheal suctioning, and removal of drains from wound beds.

In the critical care environment nurses must rely on behaviors and physiologic indicators to diagnose pain.[26] Behavioral responses and some physiologic parameters to pain are absent in the chemically paralyzed patient. The nurse must assume that pain is present and provide prophylactic analgesic therapies. Use of a sedation assessment tool, such as the Ramsay Sedation Rating Scale, is appropriate. A behavioral rating scale was applied in a postanesthesia care unit (PACU) study of patients unable to quantify their pain intensity during emergence from general anesthesia. A positive correlation resulted between cues measured by PACU nurses and a retrospective patient self-report of pain.[264] Pain behaviors included restlessness, muscle tension, facial grimacing, and patient sounds. In the trauma environment where there is a high incidence of altered level of consciousness, behavioral manifestations such as restlessness, moaning, crying, or protecting an injured body part can cue the nurse to the presence of pain or discomfort.

Nursing assessment of pain must be adopted as a standing routine, incorporating it within the vital sign routine. Frequency of assessment is directly related to its presence and severity.[265] If the intensity rating is high, pain assessment should be performed more frequently, as often as every 2 hours. As pain is controlled and becomes less acute, frequency of assessment can decrease. It is imperative to explore new reports of pain and the effectiveness of analgesic therapeutics. Reevaluation of analgesic effectiveness is recommended within 30 minutes of parental administration and within 1 hour of oral administration.

Documentation is facilitated by inclusion of pain assessment on a vital sign sheet, where trends can be identified. Institution of specific pain flow sheets or pain rating with medication recording are other options. Consistency with recording pain rating is important. If the numerical scoring system is used, the patient rating over the range is suggested. For example, if a patient rate's pain as 5 on the 0 to 10 scale, nursing documentation would be "5/10."

Pain assessment and history should be included with the initial survey. Clarification of a pain rating system requires patient instruction and understanding. Foreign language tools are available or can easily be devised with input from an interpreter. Validation of pain rating scale education will ensure consistent use of the same rating tool throughout the trauma continuum. Behavioral presentations indicating pain may be the only aspect to rely on if the patient is unable to communicate pain because of neurologic insult.

A pain history should include information regarding pain medication allergies or sensitivities. A true allergy to an analgesic agent involves the IgE immune response of raised red rash, urticaria, wheezing, airway swelling, or edema. Prophylactic medications can be administered for reports of nausea and vomiting in response to previous administration of analgesics. Current use of analgesics, whether over-the-counter products or prescription analgesics and

sedatives, should be investigated. Preexisting pain conditions, chronic pain, and enrollment in detoxification programs for substance abuse are important aspects to explore during the history-taking phase. In regard to previous hospitalizations, previous surgical interventions and analgesia methods that were favorable should be noted. Coping behaviors and patient response to stressful situations can be obtained from the patient, with significant others' validation.

RESUSCITATIVE PHASE

Nursing competency for administration of agents and patient monitoring is institution specific. Practice guidelines and standards of care for sedation and analgesic administration have been established by specialty organizations such as the American Society of Anesthesiologists (ASA). Nursing responsibilities include validation of appropriate preparation of the patient, effectively monitoring the patient during the procedure, and demonstration of appropriate actions in the event of complications. Access to and readiness of reversal agents and resuscitative equipment are imperative. Documentation of patient response, return to baseline level of consciousness, and vital signs determines the reduction in intensive nursing monitoring.

During the intake process, priorities of care regarding airway, ventilation, and circulation are paramount. The nurse can apply the mechanism of injury to patient presentation with associated injuries and anticipate potential areas of pain or discomfort. After the neurologic examination, short-acting analgesics and sedatives can be titrated in small doses to effect. Careful monitoring of patient response to agents is important. Verbal reassurances also play a significant role. Continuous pulse oximetry, respiratory monitoring, and sedation level are priorities during this phase of care.

Administration of analgesic agents and sedatives will greatly depend on the acuity of the patient and the need to perform pain-producing interventions. The goal of procedural analgesia is to minimize adverse psychologic responses. The intravenous route is the preferred method during this phase of care because a more predictable response can be attained. Analgesic and sedative agents should be titrated to a desired endpoint. The desired endpoint for analgesics is reduction in pain rating to an acceptable level, defined by the patient, without compromised ventilation.[266] A decrease in pain behaviors, such as resolution of thrashing movements, would be an example in the patient unable to verbalize pain location. The root cause of agitation must be explored before administration of sedative agents. Hypoxemia must always be ruled out. The frequency of analgesic and sedative administration will be individualized; protection from self-harm during combativeness warrants prompt action.

Before the administration of analgesic and sedative agents in the nonemergent situation, a thorough history and physical are indicated in order to establish any preexisting medical conditions, with focus on airway condition. With the presentation of complex medical conditions, an evaluation by an anesthesiologist may be indicated for ASA rating. Fasting from solid food for 6 hours and liquids for 2 hours is recommended before elective procedural analgesia and sedation.[266]

Preemptive administration of short-acting analgesics and sedation should be practiced before the start of pain-producing procedures, such as joint relocation or orthopedic realignments. Verbal reassurance and explanation of procedures, along with nonpharmacologic interventions, can be used with some patients. Nursing interventions after administration of agents include intensive monitoring to ensure safe recovery from the effects of the procedure and agents used. Institution-specific standards regarding monitoring the level of consciousness, blood pressure, pulse, respiratory rate, and oxygen saturation should be established. Minimal frequency should be every 15 minutes for 1 hour, and then every 30 minutes until preprocedure baseline is attained.

PREEMPTIVE ANALGESIA IN THE OPERATIVE PHASE

Preemptive analgesia is defined as delivering pain medications before the start of surgery, which significantly reduces pain after surgical interventions.[267] The rationale involves the central blockage of pain before the stimulation of pain. Principles of preemptive analgesia can be applied after trauma, especially during the intraoperative phase of care. Preemptive analgesia provided during perioperative epidural blockade has been linked to the prevention of chronic stump and phantom limb pain.[268]

CRITICAL CARE PHASE

Assessment and management of pain and sedation within the critically injured population must be individualized and ongoing. An optimal analgesic plan considers several factors, including the presence of preexisting medical conditions, the potential for complications, and the hemodynamic stability of the patient.[269] Previous medical conditions, such as diabetes, peripheral and cardiovascular disease, and chronic alcohol consumption, must be identified during pain assessment. Differentiation among pain and states of peripheral neuropathy, ischemic extremity pain, and angina is essential. Anatomic distribution of injuries, along with location of surgical incisions, must be considered if neuraxial techniques are to be applied to analgesic management.

The patient's hemodynamic, coagulation, and neurologic conditions influence the choice of treatment options during the critical care phase. Concurrent administration of a variety agents is the basis for multimodal analgesia, in which the synergistic effects of the agents used interfere with painful transmission in multisystem injury.[268] Pharmacologic agents that affect the hemodynamic system, such as morphine, are contraindicated in shock states and persistent hypotension. The use of fentanyl in the presence of hemodynamic instability (and the absence of increased intracranial

pressure) is endorsed. Contraindications to epidural catheter insertion in trauma patients are clotting abnormalities, septicemia, and altered mental status changes.[270]

An analgesic plan for the multi-injured patient includes consideration of the anatomic distribution of injury, the stability of the patient, and the presence of complications.[269] Analgesic techniques used in the critically ill include administration of opioids through continuous infusions, intravenous bolus dosing, and PCA or patient-controlled epidural analgesia therapies. The therapeutic window for attainment of effective analgesic effects is between a minimal effective concentration (MEC) and maximal effective concentration (MaxEC) (see Figure 17-4). Insufficient analgesia or the perception of pain occurs below the MEC. Side effects of agents, or toxicity, such as respiratory depression occur above the MaxEC. The attainment of pain relief within the therapeutic window involves repeatedly titrating or front-loading small doses of analgesic agents until the desired effect is achieved. The amount of the loading dose and the pain score during the initiation of PCA are useful in assessing overall response to postoperative pain management.[271] An example would be reaching a pain rating acceptable to the patient or a pain rating score below 5/10. Maintaining the therapeutic analgesic level can be accomplished via a basal infusion, with availability to achieve the therapeutic level through "rescue" dosing if analgesic effect decreases below MEC.

In the awake and cooperative patient, PCA therapy can be used during the critical care phase. The patient must be able to understand how to use the technology and be able to trigger the PCA button. PCA devices have features to deliver continuous infusion, PCA demand only, or a combination of both. This therapy gives the patient the ability to titrate his or her opioid dose to achieve an acceptable pain rating.

Studies comparing epidural therapy with parenteral therapy have demonstrated that epidural analgesia improved pulmonary function after thoracic and abdominal surgery.[81,272] The strategic placement of the catheter is planned to deliver analgesia to selected areas of painful injury. Thoracic-level epidural catheters can be used for chest and higher abdominal incision discomfort, and lumbar catheters cover lower abdominal, upper thigh, and hip pain.

Nursing assessment during use of analgesic infusion devices is paramount. Assessment parameters include pain score rating, respiratory rate, sedation score, and the presence of side effects from analgesic agent. After the initiation of PCA therapy, assessment of these parameters every 30 minutes for 1 hour, then every 2 hours for 8 to 16 hours, and then every 4 hours is appropriate. A standard for treatment of respiratory depression must be part of the standing orders. Discontinuance of the agent and reversal with titrated doses of naloxone for respirations below 8 breaths/min are immediate actions to be taken by the nurse. Institutional policy and procedures based on position statements from national nursing organizations and local nurse practice acts guide care of the patient receiving analgesics by way of epidural catheter technique. Elements for nursing competency include patient assessment, prevention of side effects, and management of potential complications related to epidural catheter technique therapy. Assessment of respiratory rate and sedation every 1 to 2 hours during epidural therapy is appropriate. Pain score assessment, side effect monitoring, and inspection of the catheter dressing site are ongoing nursing actions during neuraxial therapy. Side effects, such as nausea and vomiting, urinary retention, itching, and constipation, are narcotic related and can be treated during therapy. Offering prophylactic medications to combat uncomfortable side effects should be included in the standing orders.

An algorithm or institution-specific protocol can be used to differentiate the need for analgesia, sedation, or anxiolytic therapy in the critically injured patient. Figure 17-11 is an example of a systematic approach to diagnosis and treatment of anxiety and agitation.[273] An algorithm allows the nurse to choose interventions based on the current patient presentation and to provide consistency.

Sedative and analgesic medications should be maximized before the institution of neuromuscular blockade. Adjunct agents providing sedation, analgesia, and anxiolysis reduce awareness and relieve anxiety and pain. Johnson et al reported patient recall after therapeutic paralysis as being vague and dreamlike, with little recall of pain or painful procedures.[274] Sedatives cause retrograde amnesia, so frequent reorientation to place and time is important. Professional staff must monitor bedside conversation, and verbal reassurances and explanations of care should occur frequently and consistently. A visual reminder for staff and family that the patient is chemically immobilized should be placed near the patient's bedside.

Other nursing care measures for the patient receiving neuromuscular blockade include frequent position changes and turning at least every 2 hours to prevent atelectasis and pressure injuries to skin and nerves. Specialty beds that rotate and soft or air mattresses can be instituted. Maintaining good body alignment to promote comfort and obtaining consultation from physical and occupational therapists for positioning splints and joint support are important interventions during neuromuscular blockade. Disuse muscle atrophy occurs, and scheduled range-of-motion exercises for extremities are indicated on a regular basis. Deep vein thrombosis (DVT) prophylaxis through extremity compression devices and anticoagulant therapy will minimize the risk of DVT and pulmonary embolus. The blink reflex is absent during neuromuscular blockade, necessitating administration of artificial tears or ophthalmologic lubricant and securing of the eyelid with tape across the lid to prevent formation of corneal abrasions. Train-of-four assessments are recommended every 4 hours.

Environmental control of temperature, lighting, and excessive noise are nursing measures to decrease unnecessary stimulation during this phase of care. Time for rest and promotion of sleep should be provided at scheduled intervals. Liberal visiting policies offer friends and family the opportunity to provide verbal reassurances and support.

INTERMEDIATE PHASE

Pain in the intermediate phase remains acute, with varying degrees of intensity, and may become episodic in nature as a result of operative or therapeutic procedures. When planned surgical interventions occur, patient preparation and inclusion of an analgesic plan is recommended. This allows the patient to establish acceptable levels of pain and expectations of analgesia postoperatively. Preoperative teaching offers preparation for patients to effectively communicate their pain rating and to operate PCA devices that may be used postoperatively. Repetitive procedures are causes of episodic pain, and pretreatment with short-acting opioids and nonpharmacologic strategies may be warranted. Pain may linger after the procedure, and reassessment of analgesic requirements is indicated.

Patients who have required opioid analgesia may develop tolerance. Trauma patients who have been receiving therapeutic doses of morphine for 7 to 14 days may develop physical dependence.[275] Abrupt discontinuance of the opioid can elicit withdrawal syndrome. Tapering or weaning the dose of the agent over time helps to alleviate withdrawal symptoms. If tolerance is present after the critical care phase and the route of administration changes, for example from intravenous to neuraxial opioid delivery, the patient will still require intravenous coverage with opioids to prevent possible withdrawal symptoms. Addiction is a complex syndrome, involving psychologic craving and dependence on an opioid. Opioid use is compulsive and uncontrollable, and use of the substance continues despite its negative effects (see Chapter 32).

Pain management strategies for a known substance abuser offers unique challenges for the health care team. A multidisciplinary approach to management is required, with dedicated members involved in prescribing and managing analgesic prescriptions. Opioid doses often need to be increased because of preexisting physical tolerance and should be individualized. PCA therapy is a recommended option for individualized titration. Addiction specialists and pain management teams can offer support to the health care team through scheduled team meetings and daily interaction with the patient. Consistent caregivers and mutual goal formulation in regard to analgesic plans will decrease potential problematic behaviors. Use of pain relief therapies as a bargaining tool and the use of placebos are strongly discouraged in this patient population.

As the control of pain stabilizes and if the patient has effective gastrointestinal mobility, analgesic coverage can be converted to an equivalent oral route. This is especially important when invasive intravenous access becomes limited or is no longer indicated. Pharmacologic principles of equianalgesia can be applied to facilitate the transition from one route or agent to another. *Equianalgesia* refers to the dose of one agent producing the same analgesic effect as

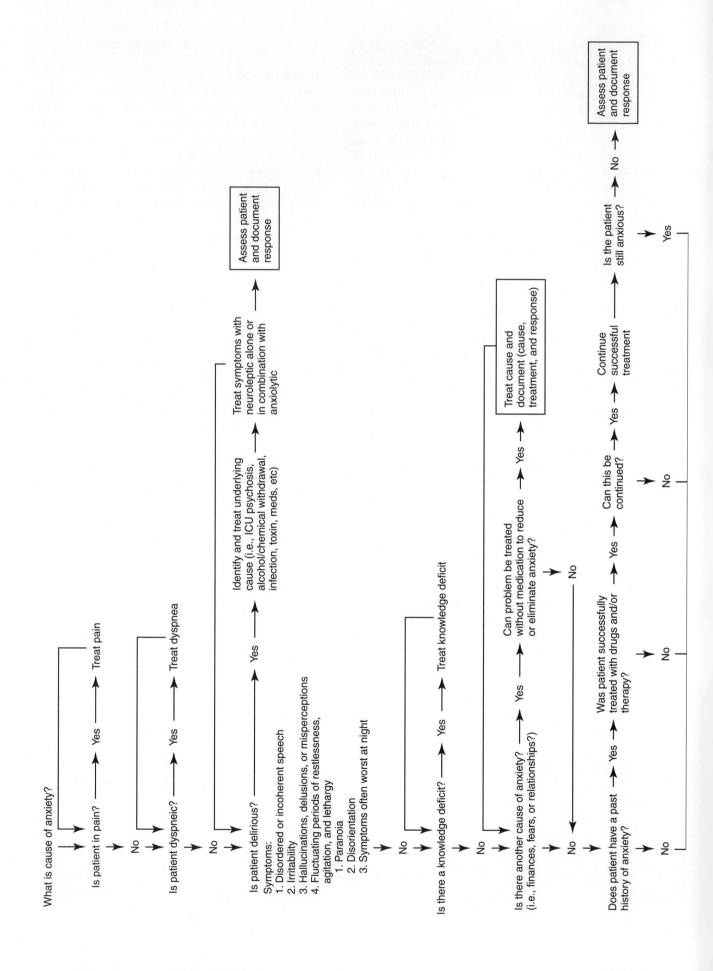

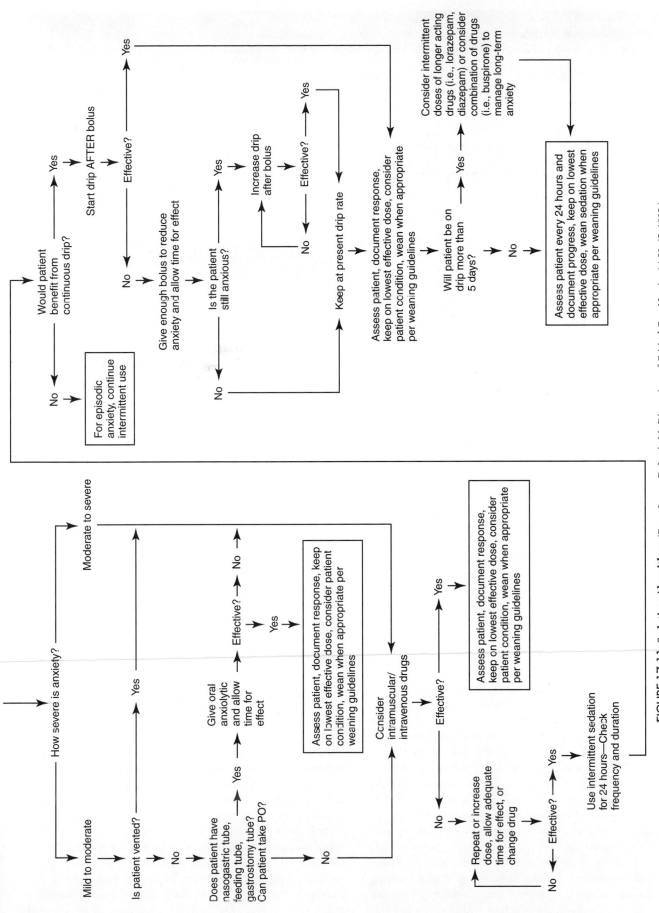

FIGURE 17-11 **Sedation Algorithm.** (From Jensen D, Justic M: *Dimensions of Critical Care Nursing* 14:58-65, 1995.)

TABLE 17-15   Equianalgesic Doses of Commonly Used Analgesics*

Drug	Route	Equianalgesic Dose	Comments
Fentanyl (Sublimaze)	IV	100 μg	Highly potent; monitor for chest wall rigidly
Hydromorphone (Dilaudid)	IV/IM	1.5 mg	
	PO	7.5 mg	
Methadone (Dolphine)	IV/IM	10 mg	Duration of action 4-8 hr
Meperidine	IV/IM	100 mg	Toxic metabolite normeperidine
Morphine	IV/IM	10 mg	
	PO	30 mg	
Oxycodone	PO	30 mg	Usually in combination with acetaminophen or aspirin

*All doses are equal to 10 mg IV/IM morphine.

another agent or route. An equianalgesia chart or opioid conversion chart (Table 17-15) is a guide to establish doses of another agent based on morphine equivalent. The practices of preemptive dosing before painful events and automatic around-the-clock dosing occur during the intermediate phase of care. Patient reluctance to switch from one effective route to another may be encountered. Patient education regarding the method and agent delivery schedule may decrease anxiety related to change.

Nonpharmacologic measures are alternatives to enhance comfort and can be used alone or concurrently with the administration of analgesic agents. Patient participation and interest in using alternative modalities require exploration, and family members can be involved in the process of teaching and application of techniques. Relaxation and music therapy can be used if the patient is receptive. Progressive relaxation involves contracting and relaxing muscle groups, allowing tension release, starting from the head and progressing downward to the toes. A quiet environment is required, and nursing instruction is recommended. Music therapy, used as a distraction modality, has been reported to reduce analgesic requirements during painful procedures and decrease anxiety and stress.[276-278] Massage of painful joints, along with the application of heat and cold, can also be used to promote comfort and relaxation.

REHABILITATION PHASE

Pain during the rehabilitative phase of care is usually still acute in nature, particularly from injuries requiring lengthy healing and repetitive reconstructive surgery. Patients with complex orthopedic injuries continue to experience significant pain, and oral narcotic opioid administration is indicated. The choice of agent should be individualized, and pharmacologic safety is important. For the patient requiring increasing doses of products containing acetaminophen or aspirin, a sustained-release opioid preparation may be indicated. Long-acting opioid preparations include morphine formulations (MS Contin), oxycodone hydrochloride controlled release (Oxycontin), and methadone. Equianalgesic dose conversion, careful monitoring, and a tapering plan can be coordinated with a pain management team. Reassessment of pain in conjunction with healing is para-

TABLE 17-16   Common Skeletal Muscle Relaxants

Single Agents

Baclofen (Clofen)
Carisoprodol (Soma)
Chlorzoxazone (Paraflex)
Cyclobenzaprine hydrochloride (Flexeril)
Diazepam (Valium)
Methocarbamol (Robaxin)

Combination Skeletal Muscle Relaxants

Carisoprodol with aspirin (Soma Compound)
Chlorzoxazone with acetaminophen (Parafon Forte)
Methocarbamol with aspirin (Robaxisal)

mount, especially when the patient is seen in an outpatient environment. Nursing pain assessment should be detailed, and formalized pain questionnaires are useful in obtaining a comprehensive pain history after traumatic injury.

Physical therapy is an important aspect of this phase of care. Complaints of dull pain with muscle ache and spasm may occur as a result of muscle stretching and activity. Rest, elevation, massage, and the application of moist compresses are nonpharmacologic interventions that can decrease the stress and strain of exercise and activity. Adjunct medications can be offered if pain is not relieved by nonpharmacologic interventions and nonopioid analgesics. Muscle relaxants (Table 17-16) decrease muscle spasm and tension that could be the cause of pain. Major side effects from these agents include drowsiness, sedation, and gastrointestinal upset.

After complex traumatic injuries, some patients may develop chronic pain, which requires specialized assessment and care. By definition, chronic pain is pain lasting longer than 6 months.[94] Many injuries have healed within 6 weeks, so pain complaints require investigation. The incidence of chronic pain syndromes after traumatic injuries is high. Specific injuries, such as amputation and spinal cord injury, are reported to yield chronic pain complaints.[28] The International Association for the Study of Pain (IASP) has classified, defined, and described chronic pain syndromes and terms. Table 17-17 offers a synopsis of terms and

TABLE 17-17	Descriptions of Chronic Pain Syndromes and Definitions of Pain Terms

Allodynia: pain from a source that normally does not provoke pain.

Causalgia: a cluster of symptoms resulting from a traumatic nerve lesion (e.g., burning, allodynia, hyperpathia).

Central pain: pain resulting from a lesion or malfunction in the CNS.

Dysesthesia: an unpleasant sensation.

Hyperalgesia: an increased sensation after a painful stimulus.

Hyperesthesia: increased sensitivity.

Neuralgia: pain following the path of a nerve.

Neuropathic pain: pain caused by a CNS lesion or malfunction.

Paresthesia: abnormal sensation.

Modified from Merskey H, Bogduk N: *Classification of chronic pain: descriptions of chronic pain syndromes and definitions of pain terms,* ed 2, Seattle, 1994, ISAP.

syndromes. In-depth discussion is beyond the scope of this chapter.

After an amputation, nociceptive activity becomes overactive and abnormal impulses are discharged from the region of injury and the dorsal root ganglion in the dorsal horn. Central sensitization occurs at the site of the spinal cord and is projected to the brain, where pain perception is processed. Approximately 70% of amputees experience burning, cramping, and shooting pain in the first weeks after amputation.[279] Many mechanisms are involved in phantom limb pain, particularly the peripheral and central nervous systems and psychologic aspects. The nurse caring for the amputee must fully investigate all complaints of pain from the absent limb. It is not unusual for a lower leg amputee to complain of toes that are curling in an awkward position and ask for the nurse to straighten them out. The grieving experience will most likely be a part of the patient's adaptation to a new self, and support appropriate to the stage of grief is indicated.

The distinction among phantom sensation, stump pain, and phantom pain is important. Phantom sensation is a continued perception of the missing limb. The phenomenon of telescoping is described as the shortening of the sensation over time and has been reported more frequently with nonpainful upper extremity amputations.[280] Stump pain is the experience of localized pain near the end of the stump after amputation. Phantom pain is the distressing pain felt in a missing body part. Patients who have experienced a traumatic amputation will probably develop phantom limb pain.[270] During the acute phase of injury, epidural blockade has been reported to minimize the severity and decrease the incidence of phantom limb pain.[270]

Phantom pain has been classified into four categories, Group 1 through Group 4.[280] In the first group, patients experience mild paresthesia that does not interfere with daily routine. In Group 2, paresthesia becomes uncomfortable but does not interfere with normal daily activity. In Group 3, pain is bearable but interferes with daily routines. Conservative treatment measures are usually introduced at this point, and patients report effective relief with treatment measures. In Group 4, patients experience severe pain that interferes with daily activity and sleep, and they require aggressive therapy.

Treatment options for phantom pain are multifocal. Physical therapy promotes strength and conditions the stump in preparation for prosthesis application. Nonopioid analgesics and the application of TENS are some therapies for stump pain. Relaxation therapy and psychologic support are also useful in the patient who is able to accept these interventions. Adjuvant medications, particularly certain antidepressant and anticonvulsant agents, have been used. Amitriptyline and carbamazepine have been instituted when phantom pain starts to interfere with daily activity and sleep. Amitriptyline dosing starts at the lower end and can be titrated upward, with the added benefit of sleep enhancement. Carbamazepine blood level monitoring is required, and several weeks may be required to establish analgesic benefit.

Gabapentin is a fairly new anticonvulsant agent that has been used, according to case reports, to effectively treat chronic neuropathic pain syndromes. It is related structurally to γ-aminobutyric acid (GABA), a neurotransmitter that plays a role in pain transmission and modulation, and has been effective in animal models of chronic neuropathic pain.[281] More definitive studies are required to establish its effectiveness in the trauma patient population.

Outpatient specialized therapies for persistent phantom pain are available and require specialized practitioners and experts. Nerve blocks at trigger points and surgical interventions for neuroma removal can be employed. Alternative methods such as acupuncture have also been used with some anecdotal success. Neurosurgical interventions involving the insertion of dorsal column and posterior column stimulators have given some patients relief from pain that is refractory to the therapies mentioned.

Pain experienced with spinal cord injury is complex and is categorized as nociceptive or neurogenic.[282] Nociceptive pain occurs from normal noxious stimuli occurring above or at the level of the cord lesion. Neurogenic pain is directly related to nerve injury at the cord level. An example of pain above the level of the cord injury is pain related to excessive use of the upper extremities during self-care and wheelchair powering.[283]

After spinal cord injury, 10% to 20% of patients develop central neuropathic pain.[284] Burning and cramping sensations are common complaints.[285,286] Central pain usually occurs with complete or partial lesions of the spinothalamic tract, which carries pain and temperature discrimination.[287] It has been theorized that the origin of central pain evolves from abnormal activity of the sensory neurons that have lost sensory input, hyperactivity of the sensory neurons, or oversensitivity of the spinothalamic neurons.[288] Nociceptive pain can be perceived above or at the cord lesion, whereas neuropathic pain is felt below the cord injury. Neuropathic pain can be classified as radicular or segmental central pain.[289] Radicular pain is caused by damage to the nerve roots at the level of the cord injury and distributes along the respective dermatome. Segmental pain is related to damage to the gray matter, resulting in hyperactivity. Tingling, burning, and aching are sensations that have been reported.[289] Neuropathic pain associated with allodynia tends to be more common with incomplete cervical lesions and central cord syndrome.[290]

Treatment remains quite difficult for this patient population. The focus of pain management is to decrease discomfort and offer psychologic support. The role of opioids in treatment of neuropathic pain requires further randomized controlled clinical trials.[291] Pain management, particularly with intensive psychologic therapy, aids in the prevention of unnecessary emotional stress that can occur with neuropathic pain. Amitriptyline or anticonvulsant agents such as phenytoin, carbamazepine, gabapentin, or divalproex sodium are commonly prescribed to effectively reduce neuropathic pain.

SPECIAL POPULATIONS

ELDERLY

Patients in the category of "advanced age"[292]—older than 65 years of age—present unique factors in the management of their pain. Pain management is affected by the misconceptions that pain perception decreases with age, that pain is an inevitable result of aging, and that pain is expected with surgery.[77] The reluctance to use analgesics in the elderly is twofold: the fear of addiction and the fear of overdose. With the use of more technology for analgesic delivery, the older individual may underuse devices such as PCA machines because of unfamiliarity and fear of overuse.

Some common ailments affecting pain assessment in older patients include memory disruption, depression, decreased vision and hearing, and cognitive impairment. All affect effective pain assessment. Alternative assessment tools may need to be applied for the elderly patient who cannot articulate pain using the common method of numerical rating. Simplification of a word descriptor scale can be used, employing patients' own words to quantify their pain. The Face Scale is also an alternative tool to sample. Exploring a patient's perception of pain, especially with family input, offers the health care team another perspective on the patient's discomfort or soreness.

As the aging process occurs, the metabolism and elimination of drugs are altered. By age 70 there is a decrease in lean body mass, a 15% to 30% increase in body fat, a decrease in muscle and soft tissue mass, and a reduction of body water.[77] The use of NSAIDs needs careful monitoring. NSAIDs, based on their effect on reduction of prostaglandin formulation in the stomach, the incidence of gastric irritability, and the development of peptic ulcers, warrant judicious administration. Hydrophilic opioids such as morphine have a lower volume of distribution, resulting in higher peak plasma concentrations that decline more slowly.

Lipophilic agents such as fentanyl are more widely distributed, resulting in a slightly delayed onset of action and an increased risk of drug accumulation with repeated doses. Meperidine should be avoided because of the decline of glomerular filtration and delayed elimination of its active metabolite, normeperidine.

A rule of thumb in the advanced age population is to lower the dose and administer agents slowly. Opioid dosages should be 25% to 50% lower than those recommended for the young, healthy patient.[77] Dosing intervals should be longer, and diligent nursing assessment for sedation and confusion is imperative. Agents with short half-lives are recommended in this patient population. Around-the-clock dosing with widened intervals, such as every 6 to 8 hours, is an example of an acceptable starting dose regimen.

Nursing strategies for this patient population include articulating pain assessment with concise, slow vocalizations that can be heard by the patient. Offering clear explanations regarding how to communicate pain to the nursing staff, ensuring that hearing and sight aides are within reach, and enlarging pain intensity rating tools greatly enhance pain communication. Addressing issues of addiction and overdose with patient and family, along with encouraging analgesic use, will decrease fears and improve overall comfort.

PEDIATRIC PAIN AND SEDATION MANAGEMENT

The nurse plays an important role in the relief of pain in children. One barrier to effective pain management in the hospitalized child is the assumption that children do not perceive or will not remember the perception of pain.[293] Analgesic use monitored in an emergency setting identified that 53% of children (and 75% of adults) with long bone fractures received no analgesics.[293] Another barrier to early pain management is the fear of masking symptoms of progressive injury. Proactive pharmacologic and nonpharmacologic management in the pediatric population after traumatic injury is imperative and considered a priority of care.

Expectations, parental response, and the cognitive-developmental level influence children's perceptions of pain.[294] Expectations of pain are imprinted from previous painful experiences. Parental input and support when indicated during the intake phase elicit past experiences and reactions to painful procedures. Sharing information with a parent alleviates anxieties and focuses support on the injured child. Appreciating the child's age and stage of development aids the nurse in assessing and planning analgesic strategies after traumatic injury.

The toddler's stage of development evolves, encompassing the concepts of self-awareness, autonomy, and control. Pain at this stage of development may be perceived as a form of punishment. By the age of 3, children are able to report pain, probably in their own words, such as "owie" or "booboo." The Face Scale is an example of an age-appropriate tool for this stage.[294] Nonverbal children can be assessed with a behavioral tool such as the Children's Hospital of Eastern Ontario Pain Scale (CHEOPS) (see

Figure 17-10). Specific behaviors measured include crying, facial expressions, body positions, and activity.

The preschool child's awareness of self continues to expand. The body and its function are a major focus of learning. Linguistic skills have developed, and dramatic play is used to process life experiences. Pain is perceived as the child's fault, as a consequence of real or fantasy play. When a preschooler requires painful procedures, diffusing fear and anxiety can be accomplished through the use of a stuffed animal or toy. Demonstrating the procedure on a neutral toy gives the child some control over expected events and an outlet for emotions. The stuffed animal can also be used as a support tool by offering comfort during a painful episode. The Oucher scale is an age-appropriate assessment tool for this age group. It consists of a group of six photographs with different facial expressions indicating varying degrees of distress.

School-age children have a broader sense of understanding about life and painful events. At this stage there is a firm belief in following rules, and pain can be perceived as punishment for transgression of set rules in their daily routine. The pondering of life's mysteries, such as mortality and death, has began.[294] From about age 5 and beyond, the concept of numbers is understood, and a number intensity scale can be used for pain assessment.

Adolescence is a time of sexual maturity and conflict. Body image, peer relationships, and personal control are major themes. Respecting the adolescent's privacy and having candid conversations about alcohol and illicit drug consumption and experimentation enhances communication between the nurse and the adolescent. Devastating injuries and prolonged hospitalization separate the adolescent from peer socialization. Sadness and anxiety influence pain perception. Support from family and friends promotes the adjustment to traumatic injury. The numerical pain rating tool can be used during the assessment of pain.

Nursing strategies with the pediatric population include offering positive support to enhance self-esteem. Saying "You were brave" or "You did a fantastic job" during a painful event reinforces positive pain coping. Colorful stickers are excellent tangible rewards. Offering procedural information before and during the event in terms that the child understands, with a loved one's support if indicated, will greatly enhance the outcome. Distraction methods such as counting, singing, or storytelling can be used to ease pain for procedural events. The use of restraints represents loss of control and confinement and should be avoided if possible.

The use of topical EMLA cream is recommended before the elective insertion of invasive lines or intramuscular injections in children. This preparation consists of prilocaine and lidocaine in an emulsion and should be applied with a clear occlusive dressing 60 to 90 minutes before a painful invasive technique. Oral transmucosal fentanyl citrate (OTFC) has been reported to improve pain ratings before wound care and enhance anxiolysis during wound procedures in children.[295] The recommended dosage is 10 to 15 µg/kg,[295] with onset of action between 5 and 15 minutes and the duration of analgesia lasting 1 to 2 hours. Parenteral morphine and fentanyl are other analgesic agents of choice. The recommended dose of morphine is 0.05 to 0.15 mg/kg, and the dose of fentanyl is 2 µg/kg. PCA therapy can be used in children as young as 4 years of age.[296]

The American Academy of Pediatrics (AAP), the American Society of Anesthesiologists, and the American College of Emergency Physicians (ACEP) have established sedation guidelines for monitoring and treating children. Sedative agents should be administered with extreme caution to patients with preexisting medical conditions, such as asthma. The incidence of respiratory depression, airway obstruction, and apnea increase in children under the age of 5 after sedative administration.[266] Preparation of children before the administration of procedural sedatives mirrors the adult standards of care. In reference to monitoring guidelines it is recommended that a pediatric advanced life support (PALS) certified clinician be in attendance.

PAIN AND SEDATION MANAGEMENT IN THE HEAD-INJURED PATIENT

After traumatic brain injury the goal of care is to preserve neurologic function. Sedative techniques are widely used to prevent secondary neurologic insult by stabilizing cerebral blood flow and metabolism.[269] Patients receiving analgesia and sedation require frequent neurologic and hemodynamic assessment. Assessment of pain in the head-injured patient is limited by the inability to self-report. Behavioral and physiologic manifestations cannot be relied upon because of concurrent presentations with cerebral pathology. The proactive treatment of pain may decrease the physiologic sequelae of the stress response after multisystem injury.[297]

Pharmacologic pain management in the head-injured patient has a direct effect on the central nervous system, blood flow, metabolism, and intracranial pressure, and signs of neurologic deterioration must be appraised immediately. For example, restless behaviors, hypoxia, hypercarbia, or acidosis may indicate that cerebral metabolism is compromised and immediate correction is indicated.

Fentanyl and sufentanil have been linked to a significant but transient increase in intracranial pressure in patients with head trauma.[298-301] Use of short-acting agents should be individualized and titrated in small increments. Patient response to sedatives should be assessed and documented after each administration, including level of consciousness, respiratory rate, blood pressure, and pulse rate. Use of a sedation algorithm or the Ramsey Sedation Scale is recommended to provide consistency among different practitioners. Hypotension must be avoided after head injury to prevent secondary brain injury; thus close monitoring of hemodynamic and volume status is indicated with analgesic or sedative use. Narcotic effects are reversed by the antagonist naloxone, which may be needed for a neurologic exam. Careful titration of naloxone, between 40 to 80 µg, is recommended.[297]

Nonpharmacologic interventions can be used when systemic agents are restricted to preserve the possibility of neurologic examination. Positioning injured extremities in correct alignment and massage of uninjured areas to promote relaxation are effective strategies, especially during the critical care stage. Analgesics such as acetaminophen can also be used when centrally acting agents are restricted.

Summary

Cost-effective protocol- and pathway-driven pain and sedation management must become standard in the current climate of health care cost containment. Consistent monitoring for appropriate response and side effects related to therapies requires specialized skill and knowledge. Trauma patients often require aggressive analgesia and sedation management. Maintaining a current knowledge base of new agents, particularly the COX-2 inhibitors and NMBAs, will enable the nurse to offer patients safe, quality care.

References

1. Webb MR, Kennedy MG: Behavioral responses and self reported pain in postoperative patients, *J Post Anesth Nurse* 9:91-95, 1994.
2. Puntillo KA, Miaskowski C, Kehrle K et al: Relationship between behavioral and physiological indicators of pain: critical care patient's self-report of pain, and opioid administration, *Crit Care Med* 25:1159-1166, 1997.
3. Carroll KC, Atkins P, Herold GR et al: Pain assessment and management in critically ill postoperative and trauma patients: a multisite study, *Am J Crit Care* 8(2):105-117, 1999.
4. Stannard D, Puntillo K, Miaskowski C et al: Clinical judgment and management of postoperative pain in critical care patients, *Am J Crit Care* 5:433-441, 1996.
5. Desbiens NA, Wu AW, Brosste SK et al: Pain and satisfaction with pain control in seriously ill hospitalized adults: findings from the SUPPORT research investigations, *Crit Care Med* 24:1953-1961, 1996.
6. Kuperberg KG, Grubbs L: Coronary artery bypass patient's perceptions of acute postoperative pain, *Clin Nurse Spec* 11:116-122, 1997.
7. Afilalo M, Tselios C: Pain relief versus satisfaction, *Ann Emerg Med* 27:436-438, 1996.
8. Mersy H: Classification of chronic pain: description of chronic pain syndromes and definitions of pain terms, *Pain Suppl* 3:S1-S226, 1986.
9. Caillet R: *Pain: mechanisms and management,* Philadelphia, 1993, FA Davis.
10. Puntillo K: Physiology of pain and its consequences in critically ill patients. In Puntillo K, editor: *Pain in the critically ill: assessment and management,* Gaithersburg, Md, 1991, Aspen, pp 9-64.
11. Grossman S, Labedzki D, Butcher R et al: Definition and management of anxiety, agitation, and confusion in ICUs, *Nursing Connect* 9:49-55, 1996.
12. Krasner DL: The chronic wound pain experience: a conceptual model, *Ostomy Wound Manage* 41:20-25, 1995.
13. McCaffery M: *Nursing management of the patient in pain,* ed 2, Philadelphia, 1979, JB Lippincott.
14. Joel LA: The fifth vital sign, *Am J Nurs* 99:9, 1999.
15. Gordon DB: Critical pathways: a road to institutionalizing pain management, *J Pain Symptom Manag* 11:252-259, 1996.
16. Caswell DR, Williams JP, Vallejo M: Improving pain management in critical care, *Jt Comm J Qual Improv* 22:702-712, 1996.
17. Bostrom BM, Ramberg T, Davis BD et al: Survey of postoperative patient's pain management, *J Nurs Manag* 5:341-349, 1997.
18. Barnason S, Merboth M, Pozehl B et al: Utilizing outcome approach to improve pain management by nurses: a pilot study, *Clin Nurs Spec* 12:28-36, 1988.
19. Public Health Service Agency for Health Care Policy and Research: *Acute pain management: operative or medical procedures and trauma,* Clinical Practice Guideline No. 1, Publ No. 92:0032, Rockville, Md, 1992, U.S. Department of Health and Human Services.
20. Horn S, Munafo M: *Pain: theory, research, and intervention,* Philadelphia, 1997, Open University.
21. Coderre TJ, Katz J, Vaccarino AL et al: Contribution of central neuroplasticity to pathological pain, *Pain* 52(3):259-285, 1993.
22. Lubenow TR, Ivankovich AD, McCarthy C: Management of acute postoperative pain. In Barash PG, Cullen BF, Stoelting RK, editors: *Clinical anesthesia,* ed 3, Philadelphia, 1997, Lippincott-Raven.
23. Dubner R, Ruda MA: Activity-dependent neuronal plasticity following tissue injury and inflammation, *Trends Neurosci* 15:96-103, 1992.
24. Melzack R: Pain: past, present, and future, *Can J Exp Psych* 47:615-629, 1993.
25. Birbaumer N, Lutzenberger W, Montoya P: Effects of regional anesthesia on phantom limb pain are mirrored in changes in cortical reorganization, *J Neurosci* 17:5503-5508, 1997.
26. Puntillo KA: Pain. In Kinney MR, Packa DT, Dunbar SB (editors) et al: *AACN's clinical reference for critical care nursing,* ed 3, St. Louis, 1993, Mosby-Yearbook, 329-439.
27. Fine PG, Ashburn MA: Functional neuroanatomy and nociception. In Rice L, Ashburn MA: *The management of pain,* New York, 1998, Churchill Livingstone, 1-28.
28. Sinatra RS, Herd AH, Ginsberg B et al: *Acute pain: mechanisms and management,* St. Louis, 1992, Mosby.
29. Dantzer R: Peptides and anxiety, *Encephale* 9:1778-1782, 1983.
30. Hansen-Flaschen JH, Brazinsky S, Basile C et al: Use of sedating drugs and neuromuscular blocking agents in patients requiring mechanical ventilation for respiratory failure: a national survey, *JAMA* 226:2870-2875, 1991.
31. Aurell J, Elmquist D: Sleep in the surgical intensive care unit: continuous polygraphic recording of sleep in nine patients receiving postoperative care, *Br Med J* 290:1029-1032, 1985.
32. Moritz F, Petit J, Kaeffer N et al: Metabolic effects of propofol and flunitrazepam given for sedation after aortic surgery, *Br J Anaesth* 70:451-453, 1993.
33. Tung A, Rosenthal M: Patients requiring sedation, *Crit Care Clin* 11:791-802, 1985.
34. Simons C, Parks H: Understanding human behavior in health and illness, Baltimore, 1977, Williams & Wilkins, 633-635, 637-652.
35. Kay DC, Blackburn AB, Buckingham JA et al: Human pharmacology of sleep. In Williams RL, Karacan I, editors: *Pharmacology of sleep,* New York, 1976, John Wiley & Sons, 83-188.

36. Shoemaker WC, Appel PL, Kram HB et al: Prospective trial of supranormal values of survivors as therapeutic goals in high-risk surgical patients, *Chest* 94:1176-1186, 1988.

37. Shoemaker WC, Appel PL, Kram H: Role of oxygen debt in the development of organ failure, sepsis, and death in high-risk surgical patients, *Chest* 102:208-215, 1992.

38. Abramson D, Scalea TM, Hitchcock R et al: Lactate clearance and survival following injury, *J Trauma* 35:585-589, 1993.

39. Bruder N, Lassegue D, Pelissier D et al: Energy expenditure and withdrawal of sedation in head-injured patients, *Crit Care Med* 22:1114-1119, 1994.

40. Parker MM, Schubert W, Shelhamer JH et al: Perception of a critically ill patient experiencing therapeutic paralysis in an ICU, *Crit Care Med* 12:69-71, 1984.

41. Perry SW: Psychological reactions to pancuronium bromide, *Am J Psych* 142:1390-1391, 1985.

42. Blacker RS: On awakening paralyzed during surgery: a syndrome of traumatic neurosis, *JAMA* 234:67-68, 1975.

43. Wagner BKJ, Zavotsky KE, Sweeney JB et al: Patient recall of therapeutic paralysis in a surgical critical care unit, *Pharmacotherapy* 18:358-363, 1998.

44. Cassem EH, Lake CR, Boyer WF: Psychopharmacology in the ICU. In Chernow B, editor: *The pharmacologic approach to the critically ill patient,* ed 3, Baltimore, 1994, Williams & Wilkins, 651-665.

45. Hansen-Flascher J, Cowen J, Polomano RC: Beyond the Ramsay scale: need for a validated measure of sedating drug efficacy in the intensive care unit, *Crit Care Med* 22:732-733, 1994.

46. Ramsay M, Savege T, Simpson B et al: Controlled sedation with alphaxolone-alphadolone, *Br J Med* 2:656-659, 1974.

47. Wang DY, Med M: Assessment of sedation in the ICU, *Intensive Care World* 10:193-196, 1993.

48. Avramov MN, White PF: Methods for monitoring the level of sedation, *Crit Care Clin* 11:803-826, 1995.

49. Riker RR, Fraser GI, Cox, PM: Continuous infusion of haloperidol controls agitation in critically ill patients, *Crit Care Med* 22(3):433-440, 1994.

50. Buhrer M, Maitre PO, Crevoisier C et al: Pharmacodynamics of benzodiazepines. II. Pharmacodynamic modeling of the electroencephalographic effects of midazolam and diazepam, *Clin Pharmacol Ther* 48(5):555-567, 1990.

51. Buhrer M, Maitre PO, Hung O et al: Pharmacodynamics of benzodiazepines. I. Choosing an EEG parameter to measure the CNS effect of midazolam, *Clin Pharmacol Ther* 48(5): 544-554, 1990.

52. Schwilden H, Stoeckel H, Schuttler J: Closed-loop feedback control of propofol anaesthesia by quantitative EEG analysis in humans, *Br J Anaesth* 62(3):290-296, 1989.

53. Reisine T, Pasternak G: Opioid analgesics and antagonists. In Hardman JG, Goodman Gilman A, Limbird LE et al, editors: *Goodman and Gilman's the pharmacologic basis of therapeutics,* ed 9, New York, 1996, McGraw-Hill, 521-555.

54. Stoelting RK: *Pharmacology and physiology in anesthetic practice,* ed 2, Philadelphia, 1991, JB Lippincott, 1-32.

55. American Pain Society: Principles of analgesic use in the treatment of acute and chronic pain, ed 2, *Clin Pharm* 9:601-612, 1990.

56. Kanner RM, Foley KM: Patterns of narcotic use in a cancer pain clinic, *Ann N Y Acad Sci* 362:161-172, 1981.

57. Shapiro BA, Warren J, Egol AB et al: Practice parameters for intravenous analgesia and sedation for adult patients in the intensive care unit: an executive summary, *Crit Care Med* 23:1596-1600, 1995.

58. Balestrieri FJ, Fisher S: Analgesics. In Chernow B, editor: *The pharmacologic approach to the critically ill patient,* ed 3, Baltimore, 1994, Williams & Wilkins, 643-650.

59. Milne RW, Nation RL, Somogyi AA et al: The influence of renal function on the renal clearance of morphine and its glucuronide metabolism in intensive care patients, *Br J Clin Pharmacol* 34:53-59, 1992.

60. Goetting MG, Thirman MJ: Neurotoxicity of meperidine, *Ann Emerg Med* 14:1007-1009, 1985.

61. Buck ML, Blumer JL: Opioids and other analgesics. Adverse effects in the intensive care unit, *Crit Care Clin* 7:615, 1991.

62. Wood MM, Cousins MJ: Iatrogenic neurotoxicity in cancer patients, *Pain* 39:1-3, 1989.

63. Martin TG: Serotonin syndrome, *Ann Emerg Med* 28:520-526, 1996.

64. Barr J, Donner A: Optimal intravenous dosing strategies for sedatives and analgesics in the intensive care unit, *Crit Care Clin* 11:827-847, 1995.

65. Jones R, Gage A: Use of fentanyl in head-injured patients, *Ann Emerg Med* 23:385-386, 1994.

66. Sperry RJ, Bailey PH, Reichman MV et al: Fentanyl and sufentanil increase intracranial pressure in head-trauma patients, *Anesthesiology* 77:416-420, 1992.

67. Herz A, Teschenmacher HJ: Activities and site of antinociceptive action of morphine-like analgesics and kinetics of distribution following intravenous, intracerebral and intraventricular application, *Adv Drug Res* 6:79-119, 1971.

68. Murphy MR, Olson WA, Hug CC Jr: Pharmacokinetics of 3H-fentanyl in the dog anesthetized with enflurane, *Anesthesiology* 50:13, 1979.

69. Dubois-Primo J, Dewatcher B, Massaut J: Analgesic anesthesia with fentanyl and sufentanil in coronary surgery, *Acta Anaesthesiol Belg* 2:113-126, 1979.

70. Clotz MA, Nahata MC: Clinical uses of fentanyl, sufentanil, and alfentanil, *Clin Pharm* 10:581-593, 1991.

71. Tarantino DP, Baker CR, Bower TC: Patient-administered alfentanil for wound dressing changes in a non-intensive care unit setting, *Anesth Analg* 80:191-193, 1995.

72. Patel SS, Spencer CM: Remifentanil, *Drugs* 52:417-427, 1996.

73. Rawal N, Schott U, Dahlstrom B et al: Influence of naloxone infusion on analgesia and respiratory depression following epidural morphine, *Anesthesiology* 64:194-201, 1986.

74. Austin KL, Stapleton JV, Mather LE: Multiple intramuscular injections: a major source of variability in analgesic response to meperidine, *Pain* 8:47-62, 1980.

75. Belatti RG: Patient-controlled analgesia, *Nebr Med J* 74(3): 49-54, March 1989.

76. Lubenow TR, Ivanovich AD: Patient-controlled analgesia for postoperative pain, *Crit Care Clin N Am* 3:35-41, 1991.

77. Pasero CL, Reed B, McCaffey M: How aging affects pain management, *Ann Neurol* 98:12-13, 1998.

78. Bailey PL, Pace NL, Ashburn M et al: Frequent hypoxemia and apnea after sedation with midazolam and fentanyl, *Anesthesiology* 73:826-830, 1990.

79. Wood M: Opioid agonists and antagonists. In Wood M, Wood AJJ, editors: *Drugs and anesthesia-pharmacology for anesthesiologists,* ed 2, Baltimore, 1990, Williams & Wilkins, 152-153, 156.

80. Egan KJ: What does it mean to be "in control"? In Ferrante FM, Ostheimer GW, Covino CG, editors: *Patient-controlled analgesia,* Boston, 1990, Blackwell Scientific, 17-26.

81. Furrer M, Rechsteiner R, Eigenmann V et al: Thoracotomy and thoracoscopy: postoperative pulmonary function, pain, and chest wall compliance, *Eur J Cardiothorac Surg* 12(1): 82-87, 1997.

82. Boysen PG, Blau WS: Pain management and sedation in the intensive care unit. In Gallagher TJ, editor: *Postoperative care of the critically ill patient,* Baltimore, 1995, Williams & Wilkins, 76.

83. Strichartz GR: Neural physiology and local anesthetic action. In Cousins MJ, Bridenbaugh PO, editors: *Neural blockade in clinical anesthesia and management of pain,* ed 3, Philadelphia, 1998, Lippincott-Raven.

84. Cousins MJ, Veering BT: Epidural neural blockade. In Cousins MJ, Bridenbaugh PO, editors: *Neural blockade in clinical anesthesia and management of pain,* ed 3, Philadelphia, 1998, Lippincott-Raven.

85. Nimmo WS: The promise of transdermal drug delivery, *Br J Anaesth* 64:7-10, 1990.

86. Latasch L, Luders S: Transdermal fentanyl against postoperative pain, *Acta Anaesthesiol Belg* 40:113-119, 1989.

87. Hodsman NB, Burns J, Blyth A et al: The morphine sparing effects of diclofenac sodium following abdominal surgery, *Anaesthesia* 42:1005-1008, 1987.

88. Martens M: A significant decrease of narcotic drug dosage after orthopaedic surgery. A double-blind study with naproxen, *Acta Orthop Belg* 48:900-906, 1982.

89. Estes D, Kaplan K: Lack of platelet effect with the aspirin analog, salsalate, *Arthritis Rheum* 23:1301-1307, 1980.

90. Danesh BJ, Sania badi AR, Russell RI et al: Therapeutic potential of choline magnesium trisalicylate as an alternative to aspirin for patients with bleeding tendencies, *Scot Med J* 32:167-168, 1987.

91. Mengle-Gaw L, Hubbard RD, Karim A et al: A study of the platelet effects of SC-58635, a novel COX-2-selective inhibitor [abstract 374], *Arthritis Rheum* 40(suppl):S93, 1997.

92. Simon LS, Lanza FI, Pipsky PE et al: Preliminary study of the safety and efficacy of SC-58635, a novel cyclooxygenase 2 inhibitor: efficacy and safety in two placebo-controlled trials in osteoarthritis and rheumatoid arthritis, and studies of gastrointestinal and platelet effects, *Arthritis Rheum* 41: 1591-1602, 1998.

93. Murray MD, Brater DC: Adverse effects of nonsteroidal anti-inflammatory drugs on renal function, *Ann Intern Med* 112:559-560, 1990.

94. McCaffery M, Beebe A: *Pain: clinical manual for nursing practice,* St. Louis, 1989, Mosby.

95. Atsberger DB: Relaxation therapy: its potential as an intervention for acute postoperative pain, *J Post Anesth Nursing* 1:2-8, 1995.

96. Chen L, Tang J, White PF et al: The effect of location of transcutaneous electrical nerve stimulation on postoperative opioid analgesic requirement: acupoint versus nonacupoint stimulation, *Anesth Analg* 87:1129-1134, 1998.

97. Jain S, Datta S: Postoperative pain management, *Chest Surg Clin N Am* 7:773-799, 1997.

98. Carroll D, Tramer M, McQuay H et al: Randomization is important in studies with pain outcomes: systemic review of transcutaneous nerve stimulation in acute postoperative pain, *Br J Anaesth* 77:798-803, 1996.

99. Bryan-Brown CS, Dracup K: Alternative therapies, *Am J Crit Care* 4:416-418, 1995.

100. Meyer TJ, Eveloff SE, Bauer MS et al: Adverse environmental conditions in the respiratory and medical ICU settings, *Chest* 105:1211-1216, 1994.

101. Edwards GB, Schuring LM: Sleep protocol: a research-based practice change, *Crit Care Nurse* 13:84-88, 1993.

102. Estabrooks C: Touch: a nursing strategy in the intensive care unit, *Heart Lung* 18:392-401, 1989.

103. Krapohl GL: Visiting hours in the adult intensive care unit: using research to develop a system that works, *Dimensions Crit Care Nursing* 14:245-258, 1995.

104. Harvey MA, Ninos NP, Adler DC et al: Results of the consensus conference on fostering more humane critical care: creating a healing environment, *Clin Issues Crit Care Nurs* 4:484-507, 1993.

105. Richards K: Sleep promotion in the critical care unit, *Clin Issues Crit Care Nurs* 5:152-158, 1994.

106. Guzetta CE: Effects of music therapy on patients in a coronary care unit with presumptive acute myocardial infarction, *Heart Lung* 18:609-616, 1989.

107. Mazzeo AJ: Sedation for the mechanically ventilated patient, *Crit Care Clin* 11:937-955, 1995.

108. Amrein R, Hetzel W, Hartmann D et al: Clinical pharmacology of flumazenil, *Eur J Anaesthesiol* 5(suppl 2):65-68, 1988.

109. Greenblatt DJ, Shader RI, Franke K et al: Pharmacokinetics and bioavailability of intravenous, intramuscular, and oral lorazepam in humans, *J Pharm Sci* 68:57-63, 1979.

110. Greenblatt DJ: Clinical pharmacokinetics of oxazepam and lorazepam, *Clin Pharmacokinet* 6:89-105, 1981.

111. Arendt RM, Greenblatt DJ, DeJong RH et al: In vitro correlates of benzodiazepine cerebrospinal fluid uptake; pharmacodynamic action and peripheral distribution, *J Pharm Exp Ther* 227:98-106, 1983.

112. Reves JG, Fragen RJ, Vinil HR et al: Midazolam: pharmacology and uses, *Anesthesiology* 62:310-324, 1985.

113. Ziegler WH, Schalch E, Leishman B et al: Comparison of the effects of intravenously administered midazolam, triazolam, and their hydroxymetabolites, *Br J Clin Pharmacol* 16: 63S-69S, 1983.

114. Byatt C, Lewis L, Dawling S et al: Accumulation of midazolam after repeated dosage in patients receiving mechanical ventilation in an intensive care unit, *Br Med J* 289:799-800, 1984.

115. Dundee JW, Collier PS, Carlisle RJ et al: Prolonged midazolam elimination half-life, *Br J Clin Pharm* 21:425-429, 1986.

116. Mathews HM, Carson IW, Collier PS et al: Midazolam sedation following open heart surgery, *Br J Anaesth* 59: 557-560, 1987.

117. Maitre PIO, Funk B, Cervoisier C et al: Pharmacokinetics of midazolam in patients recovering from cardiac surgery, *Eur J Clin Pharmacol* 37:161-166, 1989.

118. Malacrida R, Fritz ME, Suter P et al: Pharmacokinetics of midazolam administered by continuous infusion to intensive care patients, *Crit Care Med* 20:1123, 1992.

119. Oldenhof H, de Jong M, Steenhoek A et al: Clinical pharmacokinetics of midazolam in intensive care patients: a wide interpatient variability? *Clin Pharmacol Ther* 43: 263-269, 1988.

120. Patel IH, Soni PP, Fukuda EK et al: The pharmacokinetics of midazolam in patients with congestive heart failure, *Br J Clin Pharmacol* 29:565-569, 1990.

121. Shafer A, Dose VA, White PF: Pharmacokinetic variability of midazolam infusions in critically ill patients, *Crit Care Med* 18:1039-1041, 1990.

122. Wills RJ, Khoo KC, Soni PP et al: Increased volume of distribution prolongs midazolam half-life, *Br J Clin Pharmacol* 29:269-272, 1990.

123. Ariano RE, Kassum DA, Aronson KJ: Comparison of sedative recovery time after midazolam vs diazepam administration, *Crit Care Med* 22:1492-1496, 1994.

124. Greenblatt DJ, Ehrenberg BL, Gunderman J et al: Kinetic and dynamic study of intravenous lorazepam: comparison to midazolam and diazepam, *J Pharmacol Exp Ther* 250:134-140, 1989.

125. Kraus JW, Desmond PV, Masrshall JP et al: Effects of aging and liver disease on disposition of lorazepam, *Clin Pharmacol Ther* 24:411-419, 1978.

126. Klotz U, Avant GR, Hoyumpa A et al: The effects of age and liver disease on the disposition of diazepam in adult man, *J Clin Invest* 55:347-359, 1975.

127. Van Houten JC, Crane SA, Janarden SK et al: A randomized, prospective, double-blind comparison of midazolam (Versed) and emulsified diazepam (Dizac) for opioid-based, conscious sedation in endoscopic procedures, *Am J Gastroenterol* 93:170-174, 1998.

128. Aitkenhead AR, Pepperman ML, Willatts SM et al: Comparison of propofol and midazolam for sedation in critically ill patients, *Lancet* 2:704-709, 1989.

129. Wolfs C, Kimbimbi P, Colin L et al: A comparison of propofol/fentanyl and midazolam/fentanyl for ICU sedation after abdominal surgery, *J Drug Dev* 4(suppl 3):69-71, 1991.

130. Pohlman AS, Simpson KP, Hall JB et al: Continuous intravenous infusions of lorazepam versus midazolam for sedation during mechanical ventilatory support: A prospective, randomized study, *Crit Care Med* 22:1241-1247, 1994.

131. Trissel LA: Lorazepam. In Trissel LA, editor: *Handbook on injectable drugs,* ed 10, Bethesda, Md, 1998, American Society of Health System Pharmacists, 728-734.

132. Seay RE, Graves PJ, Wilkin MK: Comment: possible toxicity from propylene glycol in lorazepam infusion (letter), *Ann Pharmacother* 31:647-648, 1997.

133. Laine GA, Hossain SMH, Solis RT et al: Polyethylene glycol nephrotoxicity secondary to prolonged high-dose intravenous lorazepam, *Ann Pharmacother* 29:1110-1114, 1995.

134. D'Ambrosio JA, Borchardt-Phelps P, Nolen JG et al: Propylene glycol-induced lactic acidosis secondary to a continuous infusion of lorazepm, *Pharmacotherapy* 13:274, 1993.

135. Amstrong DK, Crisp CB: Pharmacoeconomic issues in sedation, analgesia, and neuromuscular blockade in critical care, *New Horiz* 2:85-93, 1994.

136. Anonymous: Recognition, assessment, and treatment of anxiety in the critical care patient, *Dis Mon* 5:299-359, 1995.

137. Schweizer E, Rickels K, Case GW et al: Long term therapeutic use of benzodiazepines. II. Effects of gradual taper, *Arch Gen Psychiatry* 47:908-915, 1990.

138. Teboul E, Chouinard G: A guide to benzodiazepine selection. II. Clinical aspects, *Can J Psychiatry* 36:62-73, 1991.

139. Forster A, Gardaz JP, Suter PM et al: Respiratory depression by midazolam and diazepam, *Anesthesiology* 53:494-497, 1980.

140. Paulson BA, Becker LD, Way WL: The effects of intravenous lorazepam alone and with meperidine on ventilation in man, *Acta Anaesthesiol Scand* 27:400-402, 1983.

141. Marty J, Gauzit R, Lefevre P et al: Effects of diazepam and midazolam on baroreflex control of heart rate and on sympathetic activity in humans, *Anesth Analg* 65:113-119, 1986.

142. Samuelson PN, Reves JG, Kouchokos NT et al: Hemodynamic responses to anesthetic induction with midazolam or diazepam in patients with ischemic heart disease, *Anesth Anlg* 60:802-809, 1981.

143. Samuelson PN, Lell WA, Kouchokos NT et al: Hemodynamics during diazepam induction of anesthesia for coronary artery bypass grafting, *South Med J* 73:332-334, 1980.

144. Spivey WH: Flumazenil and seizures: analysis of 43 cases, *Clin Ther* 14:292-305, 1992.

145. Murray MJ, DeRuyter ML, Harrison BA: Opioids and benzodiazepines, *Crit Care Clin* 11:849-873, 1995.

146. Barrientos-Vega R, Sanchez-Soria MM, Morales-Garcia C et al: Prolonged sedation of critically ill patients with midazolam or propofol: impact on weaning and costs, *Crit Care Med* 25:33-40, 1997.

147. Carraso G, Molina R, Costa J et al: Propofol versus midazolam in short-, medium, and long-term sedation of critically ill patients: a cost benefit analysis, *Chest* 103:557-564, 1993.

148. Ronan KP, Gallagher TJ, George B et al: Comparison of propofol and midazolam for sedation in intensive care patients, *Crit Care Med* 23:286-293, 1995.

149. Roekaerts PMHJ, Huygen FJPM, de Longe S: Infusion of propofol versus midazolam for sedation in the intensive care unit following coronary artery surgery, *J Cardiothoracic Vasc Anesth* 7(2):142-147, 1993.

150. Beller JP, Pottecher T, Lugnier A et al: Prolonged sedation with propofol in ICU patients: recovery and blood concentration changes during periodic interruptions in infusions, *Br J Anaesth* 61:583-588, 1988.

151. Ireland P, Monsour D, Lund N et al: A new agent for controlled sedation in closed head injury. In *Proceedings, Annual Meeting of the American Association of Neurological Surgeons,* San Francisco, 1992.

152. Farling PA, Johnstone JR, Coppel DL: Propofol infusion for sedation of patients with head injury in intensive care, *Anaesthesia* 44:222-226, 1989.

153. Herregods L, Verbeke J, Rolly G et al: Effect of propofol on elevated intracranial pressure: preliminary results, *Anesthesia* 43:107-109, 1988.

154. Swanson ER, Seaberg DC, Mathias S: The use of propofol for sedation in the emergency department, *Acad Emerg Med* 3:234-238, 1996.

155. Hadbavny AM, Hoyt JW: Promotion of cost-effective benzodiazepine sedation, *Am J Hosp Pharm* 50:660-661, 1993.

156. Bailie GR, Cockshott ID, Douglas EJ et al: Pharmacokinetics of propofol during and after long term continuous infusion for maintenance of sedation in ICU patients, *Br J Anaesth* 68:486-491, 1992.

157. Kirkpatrick T, Cockshott ID, Douglas EJ et al: Pharmacokinetics of propofol in elderly patients, *Br J Anaesth* 60:146-150, 1988.

158. White PF: Propofol: pharmacokinetics and pharmacodynamics, *Semin Anaesth* 7:4-20, 1988.

159. *Product information: Diprivan,* Propofol, Wilmington, Del, 1998, Stuart Pharmaceuticals.

160. Bennett SN, McNeil MM, Bland LA et al: Postoperative infections traced to contamination of an IV anesthetic, propofol, *N Engl J Med* 333:147-154, 1995.

161. Dixon J, Roberts FL, Tachley RM et al: Study of the possible interaction between fentanyl and propofol using a computer controlled infusion of propofol, *Br J Anaesth* 64:142-147, 1990.

162. Foex P, Diedericks J, Sear JW: Cardiovascular effects of propofol, *J Drug Dev* 4(suppl 3):3-9, 1991.

163. Fulton B, Sorkin EM: Propofol: an overview of its pharmacology and a review of its clinical efficacy in intensive care sedation, *Drugs* 50:636-657, 1995.

164. Herrema IH: A 10-second convulsion during propofol injection? *Anaesthesia* 44:700, 1989.

165. Collier C, Kelly K: Propofol and convulsion—the evidence mounts, *Anaesth Intensive Care* 19:573-574, 1991.

166. Makela JP, Iivanainen M, Pieninkeroinen IP et al: Seizures associated with propofol anesthesia, *Epilepsia* 34:832-835, 1993.

167. Thomas JS, Boheimer NO: An isolated grand mal seizure 5 days after propofol anesthesia, *Anesthesia* 46:508-511, 1991.

168. Valente JF, Anderson GL, Branson RD et al: Disadvantages of prolonged propofol sedation in the critical care unit, *Crit Care Med* 22:710-712, 1994.

169. Au J, Walker WS, Scott DHT: Withdrawal syndrome after propofol infusion, *Anaesthesia* 45:741-742, 1990.

170. Tesar GE, Stern TA: Rapid tranquilization of the agitated intensive care unit patient, *J Intensive Care Med* 3:195-201, 1988.

171. Baldessarini RJ: Drugs and the treatment of psychiatric disorders. In Hardman JG, Goodman Gilman A, Limbird LE et al, editors: *Goodman and Gilman's the pharmacologic basis of therapeutics*, ed 9, New York, 1996, McGraw-Hill, 399-459.

172. Lund N, Papadakos PJ: Barbiturates, neuroleptics, and propofol for sedation, *Crit Care Clin* 11:875-886, 1995.

173. Fish DN: Treatment of delirium in the critically ill patient, *Clin Pharm* 10:456-466, 1991.

174. Stern TA: The management of anxiety and depression following myocardial infarction, *Mt Sinai J Med* 52:623-633, 1985.

175. Fernandez F, Holmes VF, Adams F et al: Treatment of severe, refractory agitation with a haloperidol drip, *J Clin Psychiatry* 49:239-241, 1988.

176. Dubin WR, Feld JA: Rapid tranquilization of the violent patient, *Am J Emerg Med* 7:313-320, 1989.

177. Van Putten T, Marder SR: Behavioral toxicity of antipsychotic drugs, *J Clin Psychiatry* 48:13-19, 1987.

178. Marsden CD, Jenner P: The pathophysiology of extrapyramidal side-effects of neuroleptic drugs, *Psychol Med* 10:55-72, 1980.

179. Fann WE, Lake CR: Amantadine versus trihexyphenidyl in the treatment of neuroleptic-induced parkinsonism, *Am J Psychiatry* 133:940-943, 1976.

180. Allen RM, Lane JD, Brauchi JT: Amantadine reduces haloperidol-induced dopamine receptor hypersensitivity in the striatum, *Eur J Pharmacol* 65:313-315, 1980.

181. Adler L, Angrist B, Peselow E et al: A controlled assessment of propranolol in the treatment of neuroleptic induced akathesia, *Br J Psychiatry* 149:42-45, 1986.

182. Menza MA, Murray GB, Holmes VF et al: Decrease extrapyramidal symptoms with intravenous haloperidol, *J Clin Psychiatry* 48:278-280, 1987.

183. Lawrence KR, Nasraway SA: Conduction disturbances associated with the administration of butyrophenone antipsychotics in the critically ill: a review of the literature, *Pharmacotherapy* 17:531-537, 1997.

184. Zee-Cheng CS, Mueller CE, Seifert CF et al: Haloperidol and torsades de pointes, *Ann Intern Med* 102:18-19, 1985.

185. Fayer SA: Torsades de pointes ventricular arrhythmia associated with haloperidol, *J Clin Psychopharmacol* 6:375-376, 1986.

186. Kriwisky M, Perry GY, Tarchitsky D et al: Haloperidol induced torsades de pointes, *Chest* 98:482-484, 1990.

187. Zeifman CWE, Friedman B: Torsades de pointes: potential consequence of intravenous haloperidol in the intensive care unit, *Intensive Care World* 11:109-112, 1994.

188. Garza-Trevino ES, Hollister LE, Overall JE et al: Efficacy of combination of intramuscular antipsychotics and sedative hypnotics for control of psychotic agitation, *Am J Psychiatry* 146:1598-1601, 1989.

189. Adams F, Fernandez F, Andersson BS: Emergency pharmacotherapy of delirium in the critically ill cancer patient, *Psychosomatics* 27(suppl 1):33-37, 1986.

190. Rockoff MA Marshall LF, Shapiro HM: High dose barbiturate therapy in humans: a clinical review of 60 patients, *Ann Neurol* 6:194-199, 1979.

191. Aitkenhead AR: Analgesia and sedation in intensive care, *Br J Anaesth* 63:196-206, 1989.

192. Park GR, Manara AR, Mendel L et al: Ketamine infusion, *Anaesthesia* 42:980-983, 1987.

193. Bartkowski RR: Recent advances in neuromuscular blocking agents, *Am J Health Syst Pharm* 56(S1):S14-17, 1999.

194. Fleming NW: Neuromuscular blocking drugs in the intensive care unit: indications, protocols, and complications, *Sem Anesthesia* 13:255-264, 1994.

195. Rodriguez J, Weissman C, Damask M et al: Physiologic requirements during rewarming: Suppression of the shivering response, *Crit Care Med* 11:490-497, 1983.

196. Powles AB, Ganta R: Use of vecuronium in the management of tetanus, *Anaesthesia* 40:879-881, 1985.

197. Trujillo MJ, Castillo A, Espana JV et al: Tetanus in the adult, *Crit Care Med* 80:419-423, 1980.

198. Durbin CG: Neuromuscular blocking agents and sedative drugs, *Crit Care Clin* 7:489-506, 1991.

199. Werba A, Weinstable C, Plainer B et al: Vecuronium prevents increases in intracranial response during routine tracheobronchial suctioning in neurosurgical patients, *Anaesthetist* 40:328-331, 1991.

200. Larijani GE, Gratz I, Silverberg M et al: Clinical pharmacology of the neuromuscular blocking agents. DICP, *Ann Pharmacother* 25:54-64, 1991.

201. Shapiro BA, Warren J, Egol AB et al: Practice parameters for sustained neuromuscular blockade in the adult critically ill patient: an executive summary, *Crit Care Med* 23:1601-1605, 1995.

202. Bartkowski RR, Witkowski TA, Azad S et al: Rocuronium onset of action: a comparison with atracurium and vecuronium, *Anesth Analg* 77:574-578, 1993.

203. Goldberg MF, Larijani GE, Azad SS et al: Comparison of tracheal intubating conditions and neuromuscular blocking profiles after intubating doses of mivacurium or succinylcholine in surgical outpatients, *Anesth Analg* 69:93-99, 1989.

204. Lennon RL, Olson RA, Gronert GA: Atracurium or vecuronium for rapid sequence endotracheal intubation, *Anesthesiology* 64:510-513, 1986.

205. Cabel LA, Siassi B, Artal R et al: Cardiovascular and catecholamine changes after administration of pancuronium in distressed neonates, *Pediatrics* 75:284-287, 1985.

206. Kelman GR, Kennedy BR: Cardiovascular effects of pancuronium in man, *Br J Anaesth* 43:335-338, 1971.

207. Barnes PK, Thomas VJE, Boyd I et al: Comparison of the effects of atracurium and tubocurarine on heart rate and blood pressure in anesthetized man, *Br J Anaesth* 55:91S-94S, 1983.

208. Zaidan JR, Kaplan JA: Cardiovascular effects of metocurine in patients with aortic stenosis, *Anesthesiology* 56:395-397, 1982.

209. Lee Son S, Waud BE, Waud DR: A comparison of the neuromuscular blocking and vagolytic effects of ORG NC45 and pancuronium, *Anesthesiology* 55:12-18, 1981.

210. Savarese JJ, Basta SJ, Ali HH et al: Neuromuscular and cardiovascular effects of BW 33A (atracurium) in patients under halothane anesthesia [abstract], *Anesthesiology* 57: A262, 1982.

211. Funk DI, Crul JF, Pol FM: Effects of changes in acid-base balance on neuromuscular blockade produced by ORG NC45, *Acta Anaesthesiol Scand* 24:119-124, 1980.

212. Gencarelli PJ, Swen J, Koot HWJ et al: The effects of hypercarbia and hypocarbia on pancuronium and vecuronium neuromuscular blockades in anaesthetized humans, *Anesthesiology* 59:376-380, 1983.

213. Waud BE, Waud DR: Interaction of calcium and potassium with neuromuscular blocking agents, *Br J Anaesth* 52: 863-866, 1980.

214. Baraka A, Yazigi A: Neuromuscular interaction of magnesium with succinylcholine-vecuronium sequence in the eclamptic parturient, *Anesthesiology* 67:806-809, 1987.

215. Buzello W, Noeldge G, Krieg N et al: Vecuronium for muscle relaxation in patients with myasthenia gravis, *Anesthesiology* 64:507-509, 1986.

216. Nilsson E, Meretoja OA: Vecuronium dose-response and maintenance requirements in patients with myasthenia gravis, *Anesthesiology* 73:28-32, 1990.

217. Flusche G, Unger-Sargon J, Lambert DH: Prolonged neuromuscular paralysis with vecuronium in a patient with polymyositis, *Anesth Analg* 66:188-190, 1987.

218. Thomas D, Windsor JRW: Prolonged sedation and paralysis in a pregnant patient: delivery of an infant with a normal Apgar score, *Anaesthesia* 40:465-467, 1985.

219. Sokollo MD, Gergis SD: Antibiotics and neuromuscular function, *Anesthesiology* 55:148-159, 1981.

220. Singh YN, Marshall IG, Harvey AL: Pre- and postjunctional blocking effects of aminoglycosides, polymyxin, tetracycline and lincosamide antibiotics, *Br J Anaesth* 54:1295-1306, 1982.

221. Huang KC, Heise A, Schrader AK et al: Vancomycin enhances the neuromuscular blockade of vecuronium, *Anesth Analg* 71:194-196, 1990.

222. Azar I, Cottrell J, Gupta B et al: Furosemide facilitates recovery of evoked twitch response after pancuronium, *Anesth Analg* 59:55-57, 1980.

223. Miller RD, Sohn YJ, Matteo RS: Enhancement of d-tubocurarine neuromuscular blockade by diuretics in man, *Anesthesiology* 45:442-445, 1976.

224. Argov Z, Mastaglia FL: Disorders of neuromuscular transmission caused by drugs, *N Engl J Med* 301:409-413, 1979.

225. Chang CC, Chiou LC, Hwang LL et al: Mechanisms of the synergistic interactions between organic calcium channel antagonists and various neuromuscular blocking agents, *Jpn J Pharmacol* 53:285-292, 1990.

226. Jelen-Esselborn S, Blobner M: Potentiation of nondepolarizing muscle relaxants by nifedipine during isoflurane anesthesia, *Anaesthesist* 39:173-178, 1990.

227. Azar I, Kumar D, Betcher AM: Resistance to pancuronium in an asthmatic patient treated with aminophylline and steroids, *Can Anaesth Soc J* 29:280-282, 1982.

228. Doll DC, Rosenberg H: Antagonism of neuromuscular blockage by theophylline, *Anesth Analg* 58:139-140, 1979.

229. Ornstein E, Matteo RS, Schwartz AE et al: The effect of phenytoin on the magnitude and duration of neuromuscular block following atracurium or vecuronium, *Anesthesiology* 67:191-196, 1987.

230. Roth S, Ebrahim ZY: Resistance to pancuronium in patients receiving carbamazepine, *Anesthesiology* 66:691-693, 1987.

231. Borden H, Clarke MT, Katz H: The use of pancuronium bromide in patients receiving lithium carbonate, *Can Anaesth Soc J* 21:79-82, 1974.

232. Gramstad L: Atracurium, vecuronium and pancuronium in end-stage renal failure: dose-response properties and interactions with azathioprine, *Br J Anaesth* 59:995-1003, 1987.

233. Crosby E, Robblee JA: Cyclosporine-pancuronium interaction in a patient with a renal allograft, *Can J Anaesth* 35:300-302, 1988.

234. Meyers EF: Partial recovery from pancuronium neuromuscular blockade following hydrocortisone administration, *Anesthesiology* 46:148-150, 1977.

235. Earl G, McMahon MB, Bartley M et al: Development of a policy for patients receiving neuromuscular blocking agents, *J Trauma Nursing* 4:76-81, 1997.

236. Rudis MI, Sikora CA, Angus E et al: A prospective, randomized, controlled evaluation of peripheral nerve stimulation versus standard clinical dosing of neuromuscular blocking agents in critically ill patients, *Crit Care Med* 25:575-583, 1997.

237. Coursin DB: Neuromuscular blockade: should patients be relaxed in the ICU? *Chest* 102:988-989, 1992.

238. Coursin DB, Prielipp RC, Meyer D: Doxacurium infusion in critically ill patients tachyphylactic to atracurium, *Am J Health Syst Pharm* 52:635-639, 1995.

239. Gooch JL, Suchyta MR, Balbierz JM et al: Prolonged paralysis after therapy with neuromuscular junction blocking agents, *Crit Care Med* 19:1125-1130, 1991.

240. Hansen-Flaschen JH, Cowan J, Raps EP: Neuromuscular blockade in the ICU: more than we bargained for, *Am Rev Respir Dis* 147:234-237, 1993.

241. Prielipp RC, Wood KE, Coursin DB et al: Complications associated with sedation and neuromuscular blockade in the critically ill, *Crit Care Clin* 1:983-1003, 1995.

242. Segredo V, Matthay MA, Sharma ML et al: Prolonged neuromuscular blockade after long-term administration of vecuronium in two critically ill patients, *Anesthesiology* 72:566-570, 1990.

243. Rudis MI, Guslits BG, Zarowitz BJ: Technical and interpretive problems of peripheral nerve stimulation in monitoring neuromuscular blockade in the ICU, *Ann Pharmacother* 30:165-172, 1996.

244. Harper NJN: Neuromuscular blocking drugs: practical aspects of research in the intensive care unit, *Intensive Care Med* 19(suppl 2):S80-S85, 1993.

245. Erickson LI: Ventilation and neuromuscular blocking drugs, *Acta Anaesthesiol Scand Suppl* 102:11-15, 1994.

246. Prielipp RC, Coursin DB: Applied pharmacology of common neuromuscular blocking agents in critical care, *New Horiz* 2:34-47, 1994.

247. Bali IM, Dundee JW, Doggart JR: The source of increased plasma potassium following succinylcholine, *Anesth Analg* 54:680-686, 1975.

248. Bourke DL, Rosenberg M: Changes in total serum Ca^{++}, Na$^+$, and K$^+$ with administration of succinylcholine, *Anesthesiology* 49:361-363, 1978.

249. Tolmie JD, Joyce TH, Mitchell GD: Succinylcholine danger in the burned patient, *Anesthesiology* 28:467-470, 1967.

250. Gronert GA, Theye RA: Pathophysiology of hypercalcemia induced by succinylcholine, *Anesthesiology* 43:89-99, 1975.

251. Feingold A, Velazquez JL: Suxmethonium infusion rate and observed fasciculations. A dose-response study, *Br J Anaesth* 51:241-245, 1979.

252. Horrow JC, Lambert DH: The search for an optimal interval between pretreatment dose of d-tubocurarine and succinylcholine, *Can Anaesth Soc J* 31:528-533, 1984.

253. Pandey K, Badola RP, Kumar S: Time course of intraocular hypertension produced by suxamethonium, *Br J Anaesth* 44:191-196, 1972.

254. Minton MD, Grosslight K, Stirt JA et al: Increases in intracranial pressure from succinylcholine: prevention by prior nondepolarizing blockade, *Anesthesiology* 65:165-169, 1986.

255. Abel M, Book WJ, Eisenkraft JB: Adverse effects of nondepolarinzing neuromuscular blocking agents, *Drug Saf* 10:420-438, 1994.

256. Coursin DB, Prielipp RC: Use of neuromuscular blocking drugs in the critically ill patient, *Crit Care Clin* 11:957-981, 1995.

257. Montgomery CJ, Steward DJ: A comparative evaluation of intubating doses of atracurium, d-tubocurarine, pancuronium and vecuronium in children, *Can J Anaesth* 35:36-40, 1988.

258. Gorson KC, Ropper AH: Generalized paralysis in the intensive care unit: emphasis on the complications of neuromuscular blocking agents and corticosteroids, *J Intensive Care Med* 11:219-231, 1996.

259. Op de Coul AAW, Lambregts PCLA, Koeman J et al: Neuromuscular complications in patients in Pavulon (pancuronium bromide) during artificial ventilation, *Clin Neurol Neurosurg* 87:17-22, 1985.

260. Henning RH, Houwertjes MC, Scaf AHJ et al: Prolonged paralysis after long-term high dose infusion of pancuronium in anesthetized cats, *Br J Anaesth* 71:393-397, 1993.

261. Hoyt JW: Persistent paralysis in critically ill patients after the use of neuromuscular blocking agents, *New Horiz* 2:48-55, 1994.

262. Agency for Health Care Policy and Research: *Management of cancer pain*, Clinical Practice Guideline No. 9, Publ No. 94-0592, Rockville, Md, 1994, U.S. Department of Health and Human Services.

263. Laskowski-Jones LA: First-line emergency care: what every nurse should know, *Nursing* 25:34-43, 1995.

264. Mateo O, Krenzichek D: A pilot study to assess the relationship between behavioral manifestations and self-report of pain in postanesthesia care unit patients, *J Post Anesth Nurs*, 7:15-21, 1992.

265. Thorpe D: Pain management in the critically ill patient. In Ruppert SD, Kernicki JG, Dolan JT, editors: *Dolan's critical care nursing: clinical management through the nursing process*, ed 2, Philadelphia, 1996, FA Davis, 109.

266. Innes G, Murphy M, Nijssen-Jordon C et al: Procedural sedation and analgesia in the emergency department: Canadian consensus guidelines, *J Emerg Med* 17(1):145-156, 1999.

267. Pasero C, McCaffery M: Postoperative pain management in the elderly. In Ferrell BR, Ferell BA, editors: *Pain in the elderly*, Seattle, 1996, ISAP, 47.

268. Sinatra RS: Acute pain management and acute pain services. In Cousins MJ, Bridenbaugh PO, editors: *Neural blockade in clinical anaesthesia and management of pain*, Philadelphia, 1998, Lippencott-Raven, 823.

269. Young Y, Fletcher SJ: Sedation and analgesia for the trauma patient. In Park GR, Slade RN, editors: *Sedation and analgesia in the critically ill*, Philadelphia, 1995, Blackwell Scientific, 203.

270. Rauck RL: Acute pain syndromes: trauma. In Raj PP, editor: *Pain medicine: a comprehensive review*, St. Louis, 1996, Mosby, 353.

271. Stamer UM, Grond S, Maier C: Responders and non-responders to post-operative pain treatment: the loading dose predicts analgesic needs, *Eur J Anaesthesiol* 16:103-110, 1999.

272. Ferguson M, Luchette FA: Management of blunt chest injury, *Respir Care Clin N Am* 2(3):449-466, 1996.

273. Jensen D, Justic M: An algorithm to distinguish the need for sedative, anxiolytic and analgesic agents, *Dimens Crit Care Nurs* 14(2):58-65, 1995.

274. Johnson KL, Cheung RB, Johnson SB et al: Therapeutic paralysis of critically ill trauma patients: perceptions of patients and their family members, *Am J Crit Care* 8:490-498, 1999.

275. Collett BJ: Opioid tolerance: the clinical perspective, *Br J Anaesth* 81:58-68, 1998.

276. Cunningham MF, Monson B, Bookbinder M: Introducing a music program in the perioperative area, *AORN J* 66:674-82, 1997.

277. Evans MM, Rubio PA: Music: a diversionary therapy, *Today's OR Nurse* 16(4):17-22, 1994.

278. Miller EB, Redmond P: Music therapy and chiropractic: an integrative model of tonal and rhythmic spinal adjustment, *Alter Ther Health Med* 2:102-104, 1999.

279. Melzack R: Psychological aspects of pain: implications for neural blockade. In Cousins MJ, Bridenbaugh PO, editors: *Neural blockade in clinical anesthesia and management of pain*, ed 3, Philadelphia, 1998, Lippincott-Raven, 785-786.

280. Hord AH: Phantom pain. In Raj PP, editor: *Pain medicine: a comprehensive review*, St. Louis, 1996, Mosby, 483-484.

281. Backonja M, Beydoun A, Edwards K et al: Gabapentin for the symptomatic treatment of painful neuropathy in patients with diabetes mellitus: a randomized controlled trial, *JAMA* 280:1831-1836, 1998.

282. Ragnarsson KT, Stein AB, Kirshblum S: Rehabilitation and comprehensive care of the person with spinal cord injury. In Capen DA, Haye W, editors: *Comprehensive management of spine trauma,* St. Louis, 1998, Mosby.

283. Apple DF, Cody R, Allen A: Overuse syndrome of the upper limb in people with spinal cord injury. In Apple DF: *Physical fitness: a guide for individuals with spinal cord injury,* Baltimore, 1996, Department of Veterans Affairs.

284. Eide PK: Pathophysiological mechanisms of central neuropathic pain after spinal cord injury, *Spinal Cord* 36:601-612, 1998.

285. Ness T, Saredoro E, Richards JS et al: A case of spinal cord injury-related pain with baseline rCBF brain SPECT imaging and beneficial response to gabapentin, *Pain* 78:139-143, 1998.

286. New PW, Lim TC, Hill ST et al: A survey of pain during rehabilitation after acute spinal cord injury, *Spinal Cord* 35:658-663, 1997.

287. Demirel G, Yllmaz H, Gencosmanoghu R et al: Pain following spinal cord injury, *Spinal Cord* 36:25-28, 1998.

288. Loar CM: Central nervous system pain. In Raj PP, editor: *Pain medicine: a comprehensive review,* St. Louis, 1996, Mosby, 449-451.

289. Ragnarsson KT: Management of pain with spinal cord injury, *J Spinal Cord Med* 20:186-199, 1997.

290. Siddell PJ, Taylor DA, McClelland JM et al: Pain report and relationship of pain to physical factors in the first 6 months following spinal cord injury, *Pain* 81:187-197, 1999.

291. Dellemijn P: Are opioids effective in relieving neuropathic pain? *Pain* 80:453-462, 1999.

292. Ferrell BR, Ferrell BA: *Pain in the elderly,* Seattle, 1996, IASP.

293. Petrach EM, Christopher NC, Krinwinsky J: Pain management in the emergency department: patterns of analgesic utilization, *Pediatrics* 99:711-714, 1997.

294. Joseph MH: Pediatric pain relief in trauma, *Pediatric Rev* 20(3):75-83, 1999.

295. Sharar SR, Bratton SL, Carrougher GJ et al: A comparison or oral transmucosalfentanyl citrate and oral hydromorphone for inpatient pediatric burn wound care analgesia, *J Burn Care Rehabil* 19:516-521, 1998.

296. Kerschbaum G, Altmeppen J, Funk W et al: Patient controlled analgesia: PCA in a three year old after traumatic amputation, *Anaesthesist* 47:238-242, 1998.

297. Mirski MA, Muffelman B, Utatowsk JA et al: Sedation for the critically ill neurologic patient, *Crit Care Med* 23:2038-2053, 1995.

298. Sperry RJ, Baily PL, Reichman MV et al: Fentanyl and sufentanil increase intracranial pressure in head trauma patients, *Anesthesiology* 77:416-420, 1992.

299. Albanese J, Durbec O, Viviand X et al: Sufentanil increases intracranial pressure in patients with head trauma, *Anesthesiology* 79:493-497, 1993.

300. Weinstabl C, Spiss CK: Fentanyl and sufentanil increase intracranial pressure in head trauma patients, *Anesthesiology* 78(3):622-623, 1993.

301. Albanese J, Viviand X, Potie F et al: Sufentanil, fentanyl, and alfentanil in head trauma patients: a study on cerebral hemodynamics, *Crit Care Med* 27:407-411, 1999.

PSYCHOSOCIAL IMPACT OF TRAUMA

18

Jocelyn A. Farrar

A traumatic injury is a potentially devastating event that can produce physical or cognitive disability. There is tremendous potential for the creation of severe crisis for the patient, family, or caregiver. Trauma is often an event that occurs rapidly and is unanticipated. Both patients and families are often left vulnerable, feeling ill prepared to deal with the ramifications of the injury. Those involved suddenly experience an overwhelming amount of stress. Critical decisions must be made and resources mobilized, tasks that often overwhelm the patient and family. Psychologic consequences of traumatic injury often lead to long-term complications such as social isolation, job loss, economic problems, and decreased pleasure in leisure activities. In addition, depression, posttraumatic stress disorder (PTSD), and other psychologic morbidity contribute to postinjury functional limitations. Long-term ramifications of trauma are significant, leaving many patients and families with long-lasting physiologic scars.[1-5]

This chapter focuses on the psychologic impact of a traumatic event on the patient and family and the potential role of the trauma nurse in both crisis and long-term intervention with these individuals. Crisis intervention theory will be used as a framework for patient management. The Bowen family systems theory is used as a basis for the exploration of families experiencing crisis proneness and dysfunctional coping. Research is used to identify recommended intervention strategies.

TRAUMA AS A CRISIS

Crisis is defined as a situation that produces emotional strain for the individual. As a result, stress is experienced and adaptive mechanisms are put into play in an attempt to master the new situation. Failure of this adaptation results in impairment of function, and a crisis ensues.[6] A traumatic injury may produce crisis at any point in the continuum. Initially, during the phases of resuscitation and critical illness, the crisis may focus on whether the individual will survive the injury. Later, during the intermediate phase, the

patient and the family may experience a crisis as they attempt to adjust to physical or emotional disabilities. During the rehabilitation phase, crisis may ensue as the patient and family face the difficulties of reintegrating the injured individual into the family and the community.[7]

Infante[8] proposes a model of crisis that provides an understanding of crisis production and the potential for growth after the event (Figure 18-1). Before being injured the individual is experiencing an ongoing level of function, which allows management of his or her daily needs and provides a sense of equilibrium. The individual suddenly experiences a hazardous event, perhaps a traumatic injury, and will attempt to deal with the event using familiar coping mechanisms, which have been effective in the past. In the current situation, however, these coping mechanisms prove to be inadequate, resulting in crisis. There is always potential for the development of crisis if appropriate interventions are not initiated in a timely fashion. This crisis may result in the individual functioning at a lower level than before the crisis. He or she may experience disruption of the family, divorce, depression, or failure to return as a productive member of society. Intervention by the trauma nurse, however, can produce more positive outcomes. Although the minimal goal of crisis intervention is resolution and restoration to at least the precrisis level of functioning, the nurse should strive for the maximal goals of improvement of functioning above the precrisis level. This is possible through the acquisition of new skills and the adoption of enhanced coping mechanisms. A crisis, effectively managed, can strengthen adaptive capacity, promote growth and learning, and enhance problem-solving abilities. This potential growth depends on the timing and appropriateness of the intervention. In terms of the angle of recovery, the wider the angle, the longer the time the individual remains in crisis. Prolonged crisis without appropriate intervention can be devastating to the individual. Therefore timely intervention provided by the nurse and other members of the health care team ensures the potential for rapid and effective crisis intervention.

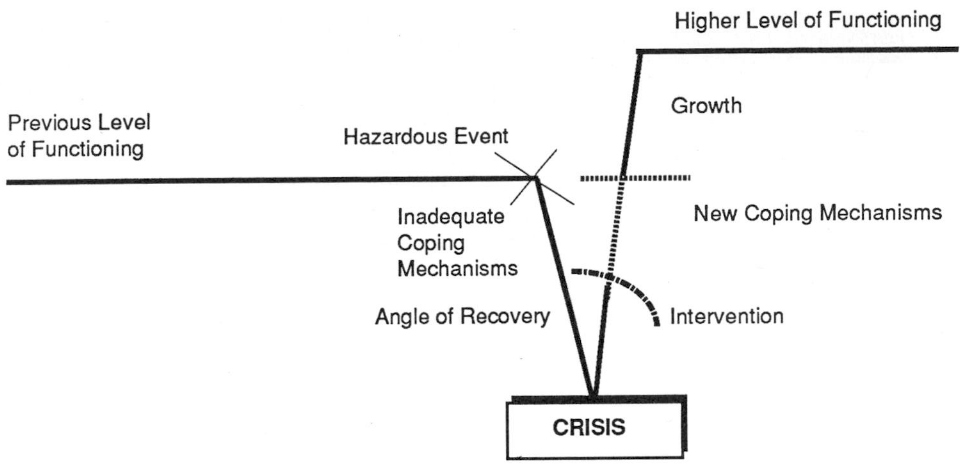

FIGURE 18-1 Potential growth curve of crisis. Modified from Infante MS: *Crisis theory: a framework for nursing practice,* Englewood Cliffs, NJ, 1982, Prentice Hall, 119.

CRISIS INTERVENTION

Traumatic injury can be defined as a situational crisis for both the patient and the family.[9] Individuals will respond to this event in their own unique manner. What one person perceives as stressful and overwhelming is perceived as a challenge to another. Therefore it is critical that the nurse obtain a thorough understanding of the meaning of the event to the individuals involved. Similarly, it is essential that the nurse accept the event as a stressor for the individual, being cautious not to interpret the event from his or her own viewpoint. For example, a patient experiencing an isolated femur fracture may view this injury as a crisis-producing event. The nurse, who in the past has cared for patients experiencing more severe injuries, may interpret the isolated injury as a minor event. The failure to interpret the seriousness of the situation from the patient's perspective may result in the failure to provide adequate psychologic intervention for the patient. Consequently the patient experiences additional stress, anxiety, and depression.[3]

Aquilera[9] presents a model of crisis intervention that incorporates three critical factors of crisis: (1) perception of the event, (2) adequacy of situational supports, and (3) effectiveness of coping mechanisms. These critical balancing factors determine whether an event will produce a crisis for the individuals involved (Figure 18-2). When caring for an individual experiencing a crisis, assessment of the three balancing factors will provide direction for intervention. A deficit in one or more balancing factors places the individual at risk for crisis. For example, after a traumatic spinal cord injury, Patient A may perceive the event as being completely overwhelming and one with which he can never cope. He may have functioned in isolation in the past and may feel that there is no one upon whom he can call for support. In addition, he may have a history of heavy alcohol use and poor coping abilities, providing him with few effective coping mechanisms to deal

with the current crisis. Patient A demonstrates deficits of all three balancing factors and is at risk for crisis development. Appropriate interventions would assist him to establish a more realistic perception of the event, use appropriate situational supports, and identify effective coping strategies. By providing support in each area of deficit, the nurse strengthens Patient A's balancing factors, reduces tension, and effectively intervenes to prevent a crisis. In contrast, Patient B has experienced a similar spinal cord injury. This patient, however, views her injury as a challenge, one she can overcome with support from the environment. In the past Patient B has established a solid support system of friends and family upon whom she can call on for help with the current event. In addition, her strong faith has assisted her to cope with past stressors and is also effective with the current stressor. Because Patient B has strengths in all three balancing factors, she is not currently crisis prone. Appropriate interventions would include support of her current resources and identification of future events that might generate a crisis.[9]

PERCEPTION

The first balancing factor is perception. Perception is defined as the subjective, individualized meaning of the stressful event and is determined by the individual's unique way of taking in, processing, and using information from the environment.[9] When confronted with an event, the individual will first perform a primary appraisal. This process allows the individual to judge whether the outcome of the event will be a threat to significant future values or goals. A secondary appraisal is then performed to determine the range of coping behaviors needed to either overcome the threat or achieve a positive outcome. If, during the appraisal stage, the stressor is perceived to be to overwhelming and not able to be handled successfully with available coping mechanisms, the individual may feel forced to deny, distort, or repress the reality of the situation to cope. If, however, the appraisal process indicates that the available coping mecha-

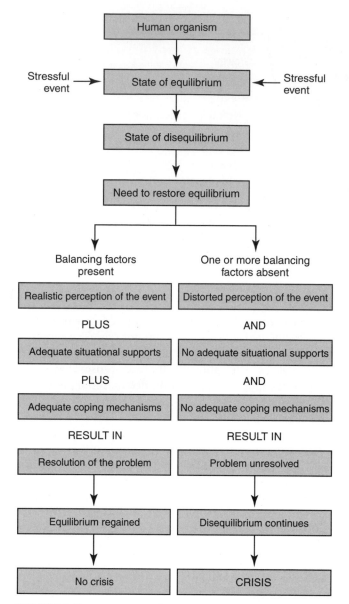

FIGURE 18-2 Paradigm: The effect of balancing factors in a stressful event. From Aguilera D: *Crisis intervention: theory and methodology,* St. Louis, 1998, Mosby, 33.

nisms are adequate to meet the threat, more efficient coping mechanisms may be used. If the individual chooses to distort or deny the reality of the event, attempts to deal with the stressor will be unsuccessful, tensions will escalate, and the stress will not be reduced.[9]

The goal of intervention is to clarify the individual's perception and to focus the individual on the immediate situation. Useful questions to ask include the following:

- What does this mean to you?
- Do you understand what was just explained?
- How does it affect you right now?
- What does it mean for the future?

Intervention is directed toward determining whether the individual's perceptions are realistic or distorted. If perception is found to be realistic, support of the perception is indicated. However, if perception is distorted, it is important

to use education and support to assist the individual to redefine the perception.

SITUATIONAL SUPPORTS

The second balancing factor, availability of situational supports, focuses on the evaluation of the availability of individuals in the environment who can be counted on to assist in the management of the problem. The individuals may include family members, friends, health care workers, support groups, and church or community resources. Adequate situational supports provide the individual with a source of advice, advocacy and strength. Inadequate situational support, however, leads to feelings of isolation, loss, and vulnerability. The individual then experiences increased stress and a sense of overwhelming isolation.[9]

The goals of intervention focus on assisting the individual to identify sources of emotional, physical, social, and spiritual support that may be tapped during the crisis. When assessing this balancing factor, useful questions to ask include the following:

- Are there people in your family or in your community on whom you can depend or call on for help right now?
- Who are they?
- Can/should they be contacted?
- Who can you most trust?
- Who is your most comfortable source of support?
- With whom do you have the closest ties?

Interventions focus on connecting the individual with the most accessible and most effective sources of support and encouraging their consistent use.

COPING

The third balancing factor, availability of effective coping mechanisms, focuses on the usefulness of current coping mechanisms to deal with the stressful event. Typically individuals use a spectrum of coping mechanisms on a daily basis to handle perceived stressors. These coping mechanisms may include prayer, exercise, discussion, or crying. Others include smoking, alcohol or drug use, verbal battles, anger, swearing, or violence. When confronted with a stressor, the individual attempts to deal with it by using familiar coping mechanisms that have been effective in the past. A crisis is initiated when the individual realizes that these coping mechanisms no longer reduce the stress or provide resolution of the event. This perception of inadequate coping leads the individual to feel overwhelmed. Tension and anxiety increase, and a crisis ensues. The goal of intervention is to assist the individual to delineate methods of new or previously used coping methods to decrease anxiety and enhance coping.[9] When assessing an individual for adequacy of coping mechanisms, it is useful to ask the following questions:

- Have you ever experienced anything like this before?
- How is this situation similar or different?

- Have you ever coped with high-anxiety situations in the past?
- What did you try? What worked? What didn't?
- What do you usually do when you feel like this?

Intervention focuses on assisting the individual to identify and use effective coping strategies.

PREVENTION PHASE

CRISIS PRONENESS IN TRAUMA VICTIMS

For some individuals, traumatic injury is a recurrent event, making one wonder if some individuals are more crisis or injury prone than others. The high rate of recidivism in trauma care has prompted researchers to attempt to identify social and psychologic factors that increase the risk for traumatic injury.

Poole and colleagues[10] attempted to identify the relationship between specific psychosocial factors and the likelihood of traumatic injury. It was discovered that individuals experiencing a traumatic injury are most likely young men who have not graduated from high school. Patients experiencing intentional injury have a higher rate of illicit drug and alcohol use than do those experiencing a nonintentional injury. In addition, patients experiencing intentional injury have a higher unemployment rate than those experiencing nonintentional injury. The average intelligence score for victims of intentional injury is lower than both the national median and the scores of nonintentional trauma victims. Psychopathology is evident in the intentional trauma group, with 63% of the sample meeting diagnostic criteria for psychiatric diagnoses, including antisocial personality, depression, illicit drug abuse, and mental retardation. Results from this study indicate that, for some individuals, traumatic injury may not be a random accident, but rather a result of the victim's high-risk behaviors and level of psychopathology. Social forces, such as unemployment and low education levels, may also influence the potential for traumatic injury.[10]

Jelalian and associates[11] examined the relationship among traumatic injury, risk taking, and personal perception of injury risk in adolescents ages 14 to 18 years. They found than younger adolescents' perception of the risk for traumatic injury in the future was higher than that of older adolescents. Differences in actual rates of risk-taking behaviors or injuries was not significant, demonstrating that older adolescents may perceive less risk for traumatic injury related to their high-risk behaviors than younger adolescents. Increased reports of risk-taking behavior correlated positively with increased rates of injury. The knowledge that risk-taking behaviors may be a predictor of traumatic injury reinforces the importance of targeting at-risk younger adolescents for trauma prevention programs to decrease the incidence of future traumatic injury. Males were more likely to experience both risk-taking behavior and injury than were females, and there was a stronger positive correlation between risk-taking and injury for the male group. It was hypothesized that these findings related to the fact that males, in general, linked positive self-esteem with risk-taking and reckless behavior. Individual adolescents often mimic their peers by participating in similar risk-taking behaviors, increasing the likelihood that the adolescent will experience a similar injury. Of concern is the possibility that peer injury somehow serves as a model of behavior for other adolescents, giving the trauma victim a higher level of importance or status within the peer group. It was also discovered that previous injury and increase in the number of reports of risk-taking behavior were the most significant predictors of higher expectation for traumatic injury in the future. The finding that adolescents who experienced a particular injury in the past had an increased expectation for experiencing the same injury in the future reinforced the potential for recidivism.[11]

It is well known that alcohol use is a contributing factor in traumatic injuries. Ankney and colleagues[12] analyzed the relationship among selected medical, social, and psychologic factors and alcohol-related trauma in a rural population. Their findings suggest that there are significant differences in the psychologic and social factors and medical histories of trauma victims with positive blood alcohol content (BAC) versus those with negative BAC. Patients with positive BAC were significantly more likely to be males age 21 to 50 who were unemployed or who had recently changed job status. In addition, this population was known to the criminal justice system in that they reported a history of more arrests and criminal charges than did the BAC-negative group. The BAC-positive group also had an increased rate of inpatient mental counseling and positive drug screens. The finding that an increased number of BAC-positive patients reported having incurred a traumatic injury in the past reinforced the concept of recidivism. Several other factors approached statistical significance for the BAC-positive group: recent conflicts, interpersonal problems, or criminal sentencing; changes in financial status; and significant personal changes. The researchers conclude that trauma patients experiencing premorbid alcohol abuse should be targeted for treatment in an effort to reduce the risk of recidivism. Trauma centers and emergency department health care professionals can play a key role by referring these patients for evaluation and treatment.[12]

Interestingly, a study by Gentilello, Donovan, and Dunn[13] of 346 victims of traumatic injury found that none was referred for alcohol counseling. It is recommended, at the least, that brief interventions for alcoholism be instituted as an attempt at low-cost intervention for BAC-positive trauma victims.[13] A more effective strategy would be the use of in-house alcohol counselors who could counsel the trauma victim and refer him or her for extensive outpatient or inpatient interventions as appropriate.[14]

CRISIS PRONENESS IN FAMILIES

Some families exhibit certain characteristics, functional levels, and abilities that constitute a predictable crisis proneness in family members.[15] These same characteristics may herald a family's dysfunctional coping with the stress of traumatic injury or critical illness once it occurs. Four general functional areas are discussed in light of crisis proneness and assessment of potential dysfunctional coping: (1) levels of chronic anxiety in the family, (2) family emotional relationship structure, (3) communication process, and (4) multigenerational heritage and patterns (Table 18-1).

LEVELS OF CHRONIC ANXIETY. Families prone to crisis and dysfunctional coping usually have very intense relationship systems: highly positive, highly negative, conflicting, or a combination. They are frequently characterized by a lesser ability to distinguish feeling process from intellectual process and are caught in a cycle of automatic emotional responses to each other, over which they perceive they have no control.[16] Their behaviors are reactive and impulsive, with the goal of "feeling better" being paramount. Their emotional responses are frequently chaotic and repetitive, reflecting a controlled, rigid, and limited repertoire of skills with which to deal with one another. In these families chronic anxiety tends to be absorbed by one family member, and that individual comes to be focused on in excess of either positive attention (i.e., "golden girl") or negative attitudes (i.e., "black sheep"). In this way the level of chronic anxiety between two family members, such as spouses, is somewhat lessened by the focus and diversion of energy on to a third person in the system. The member who is focused on in this way is the one who comes to be the most at risk for development of physical, emotional, and social problems throughout life.[17]

EMOTIONAL RELATIONSHIP STRUCTURE. Crisis-prone families and those likely to cope dysfunctionally tend to have a predominantly fixed and inflexible relationship structure dominated by dependence and adaptiveness to one another. There is a strong sense of "we" and a loyalty to the family as a blended unit, with autonomy of individuals often sacrificed to preserve harmony.[18] "Differentness" is not tolerated well, and members need approval from one another. Relationships tend to get fixed around one person underfunctioning in most of life's tasks and another reciprocally overfunctioning; there comes to be very little, if any, reciprocity within this pattern (i.e., one person always underfunctions and one always overfunctions). Members of this type of enmeshed, emotionally based family feel responsible for what another feels, whereas they do not feel much responsibility for themselves. Rather than being sensitive to another, these individuals find that they allow their behaviors to often be determined by another's desires. There is a problem distinguishing "needs" from "wants," and even though family loyalty is rewarded, there may be an overall low caring index on the part of individuals for one another.

COMMUNICATION PROCESS. Crisis-prone families have few hierarchical boundaries and rules between the generations in communication and tend to be sensitive to praise or criticism for one another.[18] Communication sequences are predictable, rigid, and reactive, with low levels of conflict resolution. Confrontation of issues tends to be avoided, and

many conflicting issues either are never discussed or are fought about but never resolved. Communication is closed, with little taking in of new information, and is impoverished in affect. Generalizations are frequent, and blaming is heavily used to hold someone in the family, the school, the law, the society, or the institution at fault. Others are often told what to do rather than being encouraged to find their own solutions.

MULTIGENERATIONAL HERITAGE AND PATTERNS. Often crisis-prone families are cut off from previous generations, being either geographically distant or, more frequently, emotionally disconnected. Boundaries around the family are closed, with little relationship network or few social supports available to help diffuse the family's chronic anxiety. There is a strong passing down of family "myths" and expectations for behavior and feelings on the part of individuals. Most often there are multigenerational patterns of various physical, emotional, and social dysfunctions such as chronic physical illnesses, depression, violence, substance abuse, and repeated accidents.

Although an assessment of these four functional areas may not prevent a future crisis or totally forestall dysfunctional family coping in light of a crisis, it can provide the nurse with a reasonably accurate predictor of what can be expected and what major areas for intervention will need to be targeted. In recent years public education has played a crucial role regarding developmental family issues, parenting, adolescence, and appropriate need for counseling. More and more families are aware, as a result, of their own strengths and weaknesses and their need for appropriate direction in seeking to improve function.

On the other hand, certain family characteristics are indications of potential ability to cope adaptively to the crisis of trauma or critical illness. They include low to moderate levels of anxiety, which allow the family to hear, understand, and repeat information; decreased reactivity to issues, which allows action rather than reaction and the adoption of a solution-oriented approach; high motivation and sense of personal identity distinct from collective identity with the patient; ultimate belief in one's ability to gain eventual control over one's life again; and evidence of role flexibility and high levels of family caring and cohesion. These characteristics can be assessed by evaluating the family members' responses to the sample questions provided in Table 18-1 for the assessment of crisis proneness and dysfunctional coping. Additional useful questions may include the following:

- What will it take for you to be able to do what you have to do?
- What do you think is the most important next step for you?
- How do you see yourself as distinct from _____ ?
- How does _____'s condition influence you the most?

TABLE 18-1 Assessment of Family Crisis Proneness and Dysfunctional Coping

Level of Chronic Anxiety	Sample Questions*/Observations
How many intense relationship systems are there (either highly positive or highly negative)?	How do people in your family relate to one another generally? Are they very supportive? Are there a lot of conflicts? Who is most concerned over whom? Is your family loyal to one another? Who is most likely to be critical when they don't agree?
Who absorbs most of the anxiety?	Who in your family seems to be the most special? Who is the most protected? Who seems to have the most problems? Who seems the most stressed?
How able is the family to distinguish *feelings* from *thinking*? Are they likely to do what feels better and impulsively react rather than measuring responsiveness for the future? Are they on the *defense* instead of the offense? Are they "out of control" instead of "in control?"	When there is a crisis in the family, what do you generally do first? How do you routinely react? How much do your "insides" rule what your behavior is in response to the problem? Is it important for you that problems/issues are settled immediately? What goes into that? Can you see problems coming before they hit, or are you often surprised and caught off guard?
How often do they tend to pull in others to blame or to help solve problems (i.e., police, school, alcohol, etc.)?	Who do you seek out when there is a crisis in your family? Who can you most depend on? Who would you try to keep the problem from? Where else might you go for help?
How many alternatives can they see to a problem, or do they see few choices and have fixed ways of responding?	What do you see as the possibilities here? What other kinds of approaches might help in resolving this problem? If that doesn't work, which might you think about trying next?

Emotional Relationship Structures	Sample Questions†/Observations
How much of a sense of "we" versus a sense of "I" exists in the family? Does the "I" tend to get lost in the "we-ness?"	Do you sense that people in your family are respected for their own unique characteristics? How important is it in your family that people get along? How different can someone in your family be from everyone else without causing conflict?
What is the basic "caring index" of the family (emotional climate connoting affectional caring for one another)?	Describe how you feel about _____ ? How would you describe _____ ? (Note use of adjectives, tone of voice, vividness versus ambiguity of description.) How do you show each other concern? caring?
How much *need* versus *want* exists within significant relationship structures?	What is it that you know you really need from this relationship? What would it be "nice to have/get?" What can't you do without?
Is being different accepted or rejected?	How would your family react if you decided not to adopt their ideas about _____ ? How much leeway for disagreement would be given?
Are individuals' behaviors determined by other family members' desires?	What would it take for _____ to influence _____ to change his mind on that? to act differently? Who would be most likely to hold his ground no matter what the pressure from others?
Is sameness required to prove loyalty?	What are your family expectations for members' behavior? How does _____ know you care for them? What is required of you by _____ ?
Who functions for whom? How often? In what capacities?	If things are going haywire, who can you always depend on? Who can you never depend on? If _____ is in trouble, who fills in? For how long? Who is most likely to pick up extra responsibilities in the family?
How sensitive are family members to one another?	How do you know when someone in your family doesn't agree with you? approve of your behavior? How influential is that in changing how you think or act? Can you criticize each other openly and honestly? How do people respond?

Communication Process	Sample Question/Observations
Is process flexible or rigid?	How are problems handled in your family? Is the process always the same or can it vary? What always happens? What never happens? What alternatives are tried? What if that doesn't work?
Is conflict resolution high or low? Can issues be confronted without threat to self or others?	How are issues resolved in your family? How do individuals respond to that? Who tends to feel the most threatened? the most in control? the most stressed? the most misunderstood?
How many issues are avoided or never discussed?	What do you discuss comfortably? Frequently? What is never discussed in your family?
Are there hierarchical boundaries between the generations? Are the appropriate generations "in charge?"	Who establishes the rules in your family? How are they enforced? By whom? For whom?

*These are suggested questions that may be useful in eliciting the information under each of the four areas. They are not meant to be all-inclusive or exhaustive, and alternate phraseology may be appropriate depending on the individual case.

†Blanks are included where specific family members' names or relationships would be inserted by the nurse (i.e., Blanche, your mother, etc.).

Continued

TABLE 18-1 **Assessment of Family Crisis Proneness and Dysfunctional Coping—cont'd**	
Communication Process—cont'd	**Sample Question/Observations—cont'd**
Is family affect impoverished? hysterical?	How would _____ react to a crisis with _____? How would they behave? How would you know something was wrong?
How much are members told what to do versus deciding for self?	Who tells who what to do? How much of what you ultimately do is left up to you? How do members of your family give you advice and direction?
How much generalization is made to include all family members?	How are you like _____? How is _____ like _____? How are you different?
How much criticism exists (i.e., what is the "critical index")?	How much disagreement do you usually have with _____? How do you know there is disagreement?
Are there deceptions within the communication process?	(Observe for incongruities between family members' information.) _____ indicated that this often occurs; do you see it that way or do you see it differently?
Multigenerational Heritage and Patterns	**Sample Questions‡/Observations**
How much a part of the current generation is the previous generation?	How often do you see _____? How do you keep in touch with _____? How many times a week? a month? a year? What kinds of things do you let them know about you?
How available is the relationship network?	Do you sense that you can seek _____ out when you need to? How comfortable would that be? How much do you do it?
Are there open or closed boundaries between the generations?	With whom do you have the most open relationship? the most closed? With whom do you not communicate?
What myths, expectations have been handed down? Are there "secrets?"	What are the things in your family past that no one is supposed to know? How did you find out? What is expected of you by your grandparents? Are there certain beliefs/attitudes that have been handed down to you through the generations?
Are there patterns or repeated chronic physical, emotional, or social problems within the family?	From the genogram information, the nurse can observe multigenerational patterns of suicide, alcoholism, depression, heart trouble, and delinquency.

‡Questions here would refer to those family members who had preceded the present family generation—aunts, uncles, grandparents, great-grandparents, second cousins, and others.

- How much control in what happens do you think you have?
- How can you go about assuming some of the responsibilities usually handled by _____ ?

If the nurse can accurately assess the presence or absence of these characteristics and plan interventions accordingly, many of the subsequent difficulties inherent within the prolonged course of treatment may well be avoided or sufficiently reduced in duration and scope.

RESUSCITATION PHASE

THE PATIENT

During the resuscitation phase the trauma victim experiences an instantaneous, overwhelming threat to life. A study by Morse and O'Brien[19] describes a four-stage process of self-preservation experienced by trauma victims (Table 18-2). The first stage of the process begins at the time of injury, and the remaining stages continue to the point of recovery.[19]

STAGE I: VIGILANCE: BECOMING ENGULFED.   Stage I is termed *vigilance: becoming engulfed.* During this stage the

trauma victim initially experiences a significant increase in cognitive abilities. There is a heightening of senses, and survivors are able to provide extremely detailed descriptions of the incident. Time seems to slow, and the individual has difficulty with the sense of time. The patient may relate that the extrication from the vehicle took hours, when in fact it took only minutes. The trauma victim often recalls the exact moment of impact of the traumatic event and immediately becomes aware of the seriousness of the injuries and that his or her life is in danger. During the prehospital phase the conscious individual becomes an active participant in his or her own care, instructing bystanders who are attempting to assist in the initial rescue. He or she will, however, relinquish control to the paramedic team if they appear to be competent.[19]

In the emergency department or resuscitation area the patient may surrender the vigilant role and assume the role of detached observer. At this point, patients in Morse and O'Brien's study reported feeling calm, detached, or in a dreamlike state. Despite the fact that externally the individual may be demonstrating intense anxiety and panic, the internal state is described as one of detached calmness. Some revealed that they experienced an internal dialog between their objective and subjective selves.

TABLE 18-2 The Stages of Preserving Self

Stage I Vigilance: Becoming Engulfed	Stage II Disruption: Taking Time Out	Stage III Enduring the Self: Confronting and Regrouping	Stage IV Striving to Regain Self: Merging the Old and the New Reality
Being vigilant	Being in a shattered reality	Learning to endure	Making sense
Experiencing clarity of thought	Experiencing memory gaps, "fog"	Living through pain and treatments	Seeking information about the incident
Experiencing the expansion of time	Dreaming vividly, frequently bizarre, confused with reality	Grasping the implications of the injury	Recognizing it could be worse
Being directive, protecting the living, breathing self	Vacillating sleep/wake cycles	Trying to "bear it," learning to "take it"	
	Perceiving the world as changing and hostile	Learning to accept dependence	
Distancing subjective from objective body	Anchoring onto the significant other	Latching onto the significant other	Getting to know and trust the altered body
Observing dispassionately	Trying to "keep myself together"	Not tolerating being left alone	Learning limitations
Becoming two-personned		Seeking distraction	Viewing life beyond self
		Seeking encouragement	Revising/modifying life goals
		Seeking entertainment	
		Learning physical limitations	
Relinquishing to caregivers	Recognizing reality	Doing the work of healing	Accepting the consequences of the experience
			Realizing they can "hack it"
Surrendering	Beginning the struggle	Living with setbacks and discouragement	
Becoming calm		Keeping a score card	Evaluating meaning
		Refusing to accept the damage	Redefining self

Morse JM, O'Brien B: Preserving self: from victim, to patient, to disabled person, *J Adv Nurs* 21:888, 1995.

One participant in the study described her experience as follows:

I remember lots of nurses and doctors or whatever around me. I don't remember feeling pain. I remember hearing a woman screaming for _____ , who was my son who died 9 years ago. I remember wondering, "Who is that woman screaming for my son? Doesn't she know he's dead? Doesn't she know he died 9 years ago? Why is she screaming?" I could feel that it was actually me screaming and I remember thinking, it's not _____ you want. Why aren't you screaming for _____ and _____ ?[19]

Visual input generates fear for patients. They may have only their own damaged body to explore; the sight of tubes and machinery to which they are attached contributes to increased anxiety. If they are able to see other patients, their visual sense will be bombarded by the overwhelming mutilation of others around them. Privacy is minimal and control nonexistent. As the stage of intense vigilance ends, the individual may experience gaps in conscious awareness. These gaps may be a result of administered analgesic or deterioration in the patient's physical state.[19]

The intensity and degree to which the injury and resuscitation process affects the patient depend largely on the person's perception and appraisal of the situation and the level of intactness of the person's biopsychologic state. Hence, response to traumatic injury is not directly related to the severity of the injury but to the unique perception and interpretation of events and stressors and the coping strategies trauma patients are able to call forth. In effect, then, it is feasible that a minimally injured trauma patient may in fact experience and respond more intensely to stressors than a severely physiologically impaired person. The inverse also is possible: The more severely injured the patient is, the less able he or she may be to mediate the stress. It becomes clear that the nurse's assessment and understanding of the patient's perception of stressors are what guide interventions, not simply the severity of the injury.

The nursing goals during this cycle are aimed at supporting patients in diminishing their anxiety level by providing them with information concerning their environment and making the environment understandable and as safe as possible for them. By speaking calmly, empathetically, and slowly; by gently touching the patient; and by helping the patient focus their attention, the nurse begins a relationship with the patient that allows them to trust someone in a foreign and chaotic situation. Eye contact is crucial when this mode is accessible. The nurse, in fact, may have to physically hold the patient's head with her hands, look him or her in the eyes, and give short, succinct bits of information. "I'm Ann, I'm a nurse. You're in the hospital. You've been in a car accident. You've been hurt and the doctors and I are going to take care of you." Telling the patient what is going to be done before doing it allows the patient to anticipate and process what is happening. Because many people often are performing procedures on the patient simultaneously, the painful stimuli can be overwhelming.

THE FAMILY

During the resuscitation phase the family also experiences a state of crisis after the injury of a loved one. Fear and uncertainty regarding the severity of the patient's condition and lack of communication from the trauma team produce increased stress.[20] The crisis of trauma is unique in that it often does not follow the time-limited range of a few minutes to 6 weeks' duration that is identified in the crisis literature. Hospitalization of trauma patients may extend for months, with alternate periods of stabilization and physical emergency, often followed by extended rehabilitation. Recovery is often unpredictable and unstable and requires that families adapt to long-term chronic levels of anxiety, uncertainty, unpredictability, and lack of overall resolution. For these reasons, a unique type of crisis assessment and intervention is indicated with these families.[20,21]

This assessment not only involves taking into consideration the immediate needs for assistance and direction with acute crisis, but also requires an intervention framework that assists the family toward enhanced self-reliance and functional coping above that of the precrisis level. The skills needed by the nurse during this acute phase incorporate a mixture of crisis intervention and beginning family system assessment as family members are struggling with the uncertainty of whether their loved one will survive.

This phase involves particularly high anxiety levels for family members, which may be exhibited in a number of ways and which are capable of being maintained for prolonged periods. Individuals may be unable to sit still; they may pace, have trouble processing verbal messages, shake, sigh deeply, or clench their fists, have difficulty breathing, not be able to complete a sentence, have flight of ideas, seem labile in mood swings, and exhibit a host of other anxious behaviors. They feel overwhelmed, powerless, out of control, and frightened and have a sense of immobilization. Even the most stable individual in the face of sufficient anxiety may behave in a bizarre fashion. One very reserved middle-aged male executive, known for his usual calm demeanor in the face of business problems, was so anxious during the first 48 hours of his son's admission to the trauma center with multiple injuries from a hit-and-run incident that he would periodically erupt from his chair in the waiting room and shout that he could not stand to hear one more announcement over the loudspeaker. His behavior frightened his family and himself because it was so out of character, yet everyone could be more calm about it and accepting when the nurse cast it within a normal range for the initial anxiety attendant to what he was experiencing.

Along with this high level of anxiety there may be accompanying shock, fright, disbelief, numbness, feeling of responsibility or blame, guilt, and distrust. It is important for the nurse to remember that a family's reaction to the present situation may be accentuated or blunted by previous experience with similar circumstances, and an initial question regarding whether the family has ever experienced anything of this nature or magnitude before may provide valuable initial direction. It is very important that families be afforded the opportunity to share all these initial responses because they must be dealt with in order for the family to move on with the crisis resolution.

In a classic study of families of trauma victims, Epperson identified a six-phase recovery process that families under severe and sudden stress undergo.[22] How individuals within the same family respond remains unique and diverse, although there does seem to be an identifiable course that is common (Figure 18-3).

HIGH ANXIETY. During periods of high anxiety, family members often need repeated clarifications and restatements of information. This information should be brief, explicit, and straightforward, and it may be more useful if it is actually written. To accurately ascertain that the family has heard what was being said, they should be asked to repeat what they understand at various points, what they have been told, and what that means to them. Even the most functional families may become dysfunctional for a time in light of enough stress, and an initial period of confusion and the need for precise reinforcement and repetition of information are normal. Often the identification of one key family member with whom the health care team communicates regarding the patient's status is useful in limiting the confusion and defusing some of the anxiety.[22]

DENIAL. Denial within the resuscitation phase serves a somewhat useful purpose for family members in that it may provide the time necessary to adapt and adjust to the actual reality of what has happened. Denial, as such, buys the family "psychologic time." The nurse needs to recognize the purpose and function of denial while at the same time recognizing the family's need to deal with the reality of the present situation and still maintain hope. Statements such as, "Mrs. _____ , your daughter has never been ill before and I know it must be very difficult for you to believe that she is in a coma from the car crash" are often useful. In this way the message is transmitted that the nurse is aware of the struggle between what is hoped for and what is the current reality.

If denial is prolonged and hampers the carrying out of necessary actions on the part of family members, additional interventions may have to be incorporated that are more directly unsupportive of the denial and much more directive and confrontational. In the case of one 36-year-old mother of an 11-year-old daughter who was a drowning victim and had been in a coma with no physiologic indication of functional improvement, the mother waited by the bedside every day for the child to wake up. She would say, "I just know that today Claudia's going to open her eyes and be OK." Her denial stemmed from the fact that the daughter's friend, who was with her and also had drowned and been initially unresponsive, had begun to respond and improve 3 weeks after the initial accident. Also, on the news that month was the story of a woman who had awoken after 11 years in a coma. Hence the mother's natural inclination toward denial and hope was buttressed by two cases evidencing improvement. However, given all medical indications, this was not predicted for Claudia, and her mother would make no perceptible move to investigate the possible institutional placements made available to her by the nurse and the rest of the team. A decision had to be made, and the mother had to be gently but firmly told that her daughter's case was different from the other little girl's. Clear distinctions were made in easily understandable terms as to the differences in initial signs and symptoms and the sequencing of return of function. She was shown visual pictures of the extent of brain damage and told that all indications of what was known at this time indicated that this was the state in which Claudia would remain. Hope is an important ingredient and should not be totally removed, but to break through prolonged denial that may become pathologic, a factual representation is essential, along with the notion that miracles are always possible; in this case that is what was necessary.[22]

ANGER. Families need to be able to verbalize their anger without the health care professional's personalizing it; they may be angry at the patient, at themselves, at the institutions giving care, at the physicians, at the nurses, at God, at society, and at life in general. Diffuse anger is often present and helps forestall the pain inherent in the grief that follows. Anger needs to be given expression and accepted by the nurse, while at the same time direction is given in the form

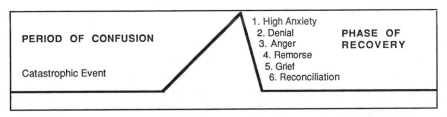

**Six-Phase Recovery Process for Families
Under Sudden, Severe Stress**

PERIOD OF CONFUSION

Catastrophic Event

1. High Anxiety
2. Denial
3. Anger
4. Remorse
5. Grief
6. Reconciliation

**PHASE OF
RECOVERY**

FIGURE 18-3 Six-phase recovery process for families under sudden, severe stress. From Epperson MM: Families in sudden crisis: process and intervention in a critical care center, *Soc Work Health Care* 2:205-273, 1977.

of questions that help families identify the actual legitimacy of the focus of their anger. When the "real thoughts behind the anger" can be pulled out by the family, they often realize that fear, guilt, and loss of control are driving the anger. They can then put that to rest and move on with the necessary grief work before reconciliation.[22]

REMORSE.   Epperson[22] refers to the remorse stage as the "if only" stage. Families struggle with sorrow and guilt over the part they played in the accident or injury or in not preventing the possibility of it. It is important not to rationalize this phase as problem-solving questions are asked to help families reason out the thoughts, fears, and misperceptions they have. A mother's remorse and guilt over allowing her 19-year-old son to buy and ride the motorcycle on which he was struck by a truck should be listened to without judgment and without rationalization. Statements and questions such as, "19-year-olds make their own choices," "No family is without conflict," "Have your efforts to control his use of his motorcycle worked before?" and "Is it possible for even a mom to control a 19-year-old's behavior?" may be helpful in this phase. The more verbalization the better because this will defocus the issue and work toward problem solving. However, bear in mind that wide fluctuations in mood are normal within these early phases, and they may change rapidly. Many family members share the fear that they are "going crazy" because of the lability of their emotional responses during the critical care phase, and it is crucial for the nurse to share the "norm" in ranges of feelings experienced by most families in similar situations.[22]

GRIEF.   Watching a family experience the necessary pain of the grief phase is especially difficult. Too often nurses intervene too rapidly to support, take care of, fix, or make better. Pain is a necessary component of grief work, and it must be allowed to run its course. To the extent that the nurse can be comfortable with staying connected to others' discomfort, the essential work for families within this phase will be augmented. This, in turn, allows the mobilization of resources and the realistic putting together of family life required for reconciliation. Table 18-3 summarizes the basic interventions for each of these initial family responses within the phases of recovery after a crisis.[23]

Throughout these phases, the art of nonjudgmental listening is essential. It is easy to allow oneself to get pulled in by emotions to giving too much support, assuming too much responsibility for others' feelings, and siding and blaming. Nontherapeutic responses, questions, and statements made by the nurse such as, "You shouldn't blame yourself," "How can you think you caused that to happen?" "Things will work out," "All things happen for a reason," and "I would agree that _____ was wrong to do that!" do nothing to assist in long-term coping and may do much to alienate the nurse from the family she or he is endeavoring to support. It is not important to know the answers to many of the unanswerable questions that families pose but rather to ask the right questions so that families

may begin to generate their own solutions, coping mechanisms, and resources. Questions such as "I hear what you say about _____ ; how do you see that as changeable?" "What goes into your thinking about that in that fashion?" "What would it take for you to feel less guilty? less hostile? less _____ ?" are examples of the types of thought-producing stimuli that facilitate the family's own problem solving and ensure the transmission of a nonjudgmental attitude on the part of the nurse.

CRITICAL CARE PHASE

THE PATIENT

The critical care phase is one of great challenges to the trauma patient. Described as a time of great fear and confusion, this phase demands both physical and emotional strength. The trauma patient must deal with the pain and uncertainty of injury, separation from significant others, alteration in body image as a result of injury and treatment, inability to communicate with family and staff, impaired thinking processes, sleep deprivation, and loss of control.

STAGE II: DISRUPTION: TAKING TIME OUT.   During the critical care phase, the trauma victim enters stage II of the process of self-preservation as described by Morse and O'Brien.[19] Stage II, defined as *disruption: taking time out,* is described by trauma survivors as an overwhelming phase with which they had difficulty coping. The stage is often described as consisting of episodes of vivid, terrifying dreams interspersed with periods of excruciating pain. Burn patients in particular were found to experience the most terrifying and confusing of dreams. One patient describes his experience as follows: "I had a nightmare of this little kid. I was in Vietnam and I was half blown away and this kid dragged me to his mother and his mother dissected a cow and used the cow's parts and put me back together."[19]

Patients experiencing spinal cord injuries with deficit often dream of the "old me," a dream in which the patient is intact and fully functional. Upon awakening, the patient is suddenly again confronted with the reality of the injury. Patients in this stage also describe intense difficulty defining reality, uncertainty as to which event is real and which is a dream. Both sleep and wakefulness are described as being intolerable. Patients describe this period as a vicious cycle wherein they attempt to escape from the terrifying sleep state by awakening and, in contrast, escape from the pain by sleeping. The result is a state of confusion or fog in which the patient cannot determine wakefulness from sleep or sometimes life from death. During this stage, patients are most often in critical condition, receiving pain medication and sedation, both of which contribute to the confusion. The period is often recalled as one of vague, dreamlike memories or flashbacks. Patients experience altered perceptions of the environment, believing that the furnishings of their rooms are changed frequently or that they have been moved from room to room. Health providers are often viewed as hurtful, hostile, and not to be trusted. Patients

TABLE 18-3   Interventions for Initial Family Responses to Crisis

Family Responses	Interventions
Anxiety, shock, fright	Give information that is brief, concise, explicit, and concrete.
	Repeat and frequently reinforce information—encourage families to record important facts in writing.
	Ascertain comprehension by asking family to repeat back to you what information they have been given.
	Provide for and encourage or allow ventilation of feelings, even if they are extreme.
	Maintain constant, nonanxious presence in the face of a highly anxious family.
	Inform family as to the potential range of behaviors and feelings that are within the "norm" for crisis.
	Maximize control within hospital environment, as possible.
Denial	Identify what purpose denial is serving for family (e.g., Is it buying them "psychological time" for future coping and mobilization of resources?).
	Evaluate appropriateness of use of denial in terms of time; denial becomes inappropriate when it inhibits the family from taking necessary actions or when it is impinging on the course of treatment.
	Do not actively support denial but neither dash hopes for the future (e.g., "It must be very difficult for you to believe your son is nonresponsive and in a trauma unit.").
	If denial is prolonged and dysfunctional, more direct and specific factual representation may be essential.
Anger, hostility, distrust	Allow for ventilation of angry feelings, clarifying what thoughts, fears, and beliefs are behind the anger; let them know it's OK to be angry.
	Don't personalize family's expression of these strong emotions.
	Institute family control within the hospital environment when possible (e.g., arrange for set time(s) and set person(s) to give them information in reference to the patient and answer their questions).
	Remain available to families during their venting of these emotions.
	Ask families how they can take the energy in their anger and put it to positive use for themselves, for the patient, and for the situation.
Remorse and guilt	Do not try to "rationalize away" guilt for families.
	Listen, support their expression of feeling and verbalizations (e.g., "I can understand how or why you might feel that way; however, . . . ").
	Follow the "howevers" with careful, reality-oriented statements or questions (e.g., "None of us can truly control another's behavior."; "Kids make their own choices despite what parents think and want."; "How successful were you when you tried to control _____'s behavior with that before?"; "So many things have happened for which there are no absolute answers.").
Grief and depression	Acknowledge family's grief and depression.
	Encourage them to be precise about what it is they are grieving and depressed about; give grief and depression a context.
	Allow the family appropriate time for grief.
	Recognize that this is an essential step for future adaptation—do not try to rush the grief process.
	Remain sensitive to your own unfinished business and, hence, comfort/discomfort with family's grieving and depression.
Hope	Clarify with families what their hopes are, individually and with one another.
	Clarify with families what their worst fears are in reference to the situation. Are the hopes/fears congruent? realistic? unrealistic?
	Support realistic hope.
	Offer gentle factual information to reframe unrealistic hope (e.g., "With the information you have or the observations you have made, do you think that is still possible?").
	Assist families in reframing unrealistic hope in some other fashion (e.g., "What do you think others will have learned from _____ if he doesn't make it?" "How do you think _____ would like for you to remember him/her?").

Modified from Kleeman KM: Families in crisis due to multiple trauma, *Crit Care Nurs Clin North Am* 1:25, 1989.

report that they expected their family members to protect them from these caregivers and are hurt and confused when the family leaves at the end of the visiting session.[19]

During stage II a critical need expressed by trauma survivors is to have family members readily accessible. Patients view their family members and significant others to be essential sources of support and a safe haven in their world of pain and confusion. Often the patient is afraid to be alone and the significant other represents a sense of security, reality, and safety. The family member helps anchor the patient to reality, assists the patient to regain a sense of self and "humanness," and contributes to the healing process. Patients describe the presence of a family member as being the most important intervention during stage II.[19]

ALTERATION OF BODY IMAGE.   As the critical care phase progresses, the patient shifts from a major fear of death to increasing concerns about alterations of body function and significant losses. When it is established that life itself will not be suddenly lost, patients gradually come to terms with their altered body and with the pain that seems unceasing. At the same time, other struggles emerge; the patient must develop new ways of expressing self in relating to family, significant others, and, increasingly, the nurse.

Mutilation of the body through both trauma and subsequent treatment is stressful for the patient and the nurse. Patients recognize that their once intact body now may have holes in it, tubes that emerge from their skin, and wires and pins that hold together their flesh and bone. They must address this change by coming to terms with the reality that these apparitions are now part of self.

In a society in which youthful physical attractiveness is valued, disability, disfigurement, and scarring are likely to produce anxiety and problems with self-esteem. Sudden changes in body image, such as those brought about by unexpected traumatic injury, place the patient at risk for loss, depression, sexual problems, guilt, and grief.[24]

It is important to assist the patient with integration of this changed body image into his or her concept of self. Interventions such as facilitating open communication; conveying an empathetic, caring approach; and providing acceptance are useful. It is important to remember that patient has a personal perception of his or her wounds. A massive abdominal wound that to the nurse is healing well may be of great worry to the patient. He or she may become anxious that the wound will not heal without great scarring or that abdominal organs will be exposed. It is important that the nurse carefully assess patient's perceptions of his or her wounds. The patient should be asked if they have any questions about his or her wound. His or her knowledge of his or her wound, its care, and the potential for healing should be assessed. The nurse should allow the patient to achieve control by answering only those questions they raise. This allows him or her to control the amount of potentially anxiety-producing information he or she receives at any one time. Answers to their questions should be conveyed in an accurate, factual, truthful, and reassuring manner. The provision of concrete information helps the patient become focused on reality and reduces uncertainty. The information should be communicated in easy-to-understand language.[24]

The manner in which friends, family, and staff react to the wound also greatly influences the patient's sense of self-esteem. Nonverbal body language is a powerful tool, and the health care team must be aware of its unconscious use. If the patient interprets this communication as negative, he or she will experience increased anxiety and self-doubt. In contrast, the patient will be able to begin to positively integrate the wound into his or her body image if he or she senses that the staff conveys a positive and accepting manner when caring for the wound.[24]

As a response to the mounting anxiety related to the wound and the altered body image, the patient may attempt to cope by putting into play defense mechanisms such as withdrawal, avoidance, and suppression in an attempt to maintain psychologic balance. Dressing changes and wound care are constant reminders of both the changes in the appearance of the body and the traumatic event that produced those changes. It is not unusual for the patient to respond by refusing to cooperate with dressing changes or being noncompliant with wound care. The health care team needs to be sensitive to these issues when caring for the wound. Relief from pain is a priority for the patient during dressing changes. Pharmacologic and nonpharmacologic strategies should be instituted to manage pain. Adequate relief from anxiety must be provided. Referral to a psychiatric liaison, use of relaxation techniques, and pharmacologic methods should be explored.[24]

IMPAIRED VERBAL COMMUNICATION.   In the critical care phase many patients are unable to verbalize their needs because they are intubated, have experienced facial trauma, or have tracheostomies. This compounds the problems of communication regarding the patient's psychologic needs. It is important that the nurse support patients in finding ways that they can make their needs, concerns, and feelings known. An environment that gives patients permission, creative options, and time to communicate at their own pace and in their own manner is crucial.

A major component of the nursing assessment is determining the ability of patients to comprehend what is said to them. Because the patient's sensorium fluctuates in response to physiologic shifts, pain, sedation, and environmental stimuli, a reliable assessment is best achieved when these factors are taken into account. Asking patients to respond to simple commands that they are physically capable of performing, such as "Raise your left arm" or "Blink your eyes twice if you understand what I'm saying," aids in determining patients' ability to comprehend information. Once the nurse assesses that the patient comprehends what is being said, creative modes for communicating must be devised.

It is frustrating for patients as well as the nurse when patients have to repeat their communications because the nurse is not able to read their lips. It is important to acknowledge that frustration and to keep trying. Questions that require short answers should be asked, so as not to tire the patient. Health professionals have a tendency to speak loudly to patients who are unable to talk, forgetting that the patient's comprehension and hearing are not altered. Speaking in a normal tone, facing the patient, modifying environmental stimuli, and being patient all facilitate communication. If a patient can write or use word and picture boards, these vehicles need to be incorporated into his or her care and made known to all those interacting with the patient. Mechanisms for contacting the nurse, such as call bells or buzzers, must also be identified because the patient's sense of helplessness and level of anxiety are compounded when he or she cannot call for help. In addition, the use of therapeutic listening skills such as maintaining eye contact, sitting at eye level with the patient, and leaning forward can communicate a supportive, caring attitude to the patient.[7]

IMPAIRED THINKING PROCESSES.   The trauma patient's thinking processes may be radically impaired secondary to physiologic, psychosocial, and environmental factors. Hypoxia, kidney failure, electrolyte imbalances, and medications in concert with anxiety, sensory overload and deprivation, social isolation, sleep deprivation, and immobility all affect the patient's cognitive functions, resulting in disorganized thinking and behavioral patterns.

Assessment of orientation may reveal that the patient frequently is not oriented to place, time, and situation. Testing of memory functioning reveals that the patient's short-term memory and immediate recall abilities are impaired. The patient's thinking processes, as assessed through spoken or written word, reflect unclear and loose association of ideas, indicative of scattered thinking processes. The flow of speech may be slow and hesitant, slurred, or mumbled. Response time to questioning often is retarded. The content of thought may indicate that the patient is misperceiving environmental stimuli, thus experiencing delusions. Repetitive themes often are present in verbalizations. Illusions or hallucinations in any of the sensory modalities may be present. The patient's affect may also be inappropriate to thought content. The patient's mood is labile: one minute the patient is crying, the next he or she is angry and hostile.

In assessing the patient whose thought processes are impaired, the nurse recognizes that the patient's attention span is minimal and that the patient is easily distracted by environmental stimuli. The patient's behavior is not goal-oriented. Because he or she misperceives stimuli, the patient may attempt to pull out tubes and tear off dressings. Eye contact is also poor, and the patient may not be responsive to touch.

When patients demonstrate that their thinking processes are impaired, the nursing goals are aimed at helping differentiate what is real from what is not. Frequently providing patients with information that supports orientation to place, time, and situation is paramount. Consistently modifying and interpreting the environment for patients using their intact sensory modalities supports patients in differentiating real from unreal. Respecting patients' inappropriate thinking and asking for clarification in a calm, interested manner often allows the nurse to understand patients' confusion. Because patients are at risk for paranoid ideation, the nurse needs to explain all that she is doing.[25] Being cognizant of body posture and facial expressions is key. Patients' concerns are real, as is their fear, and must be taken seriously. Interpreting events realistically may not diminish patients' concerns, but they rely on the nurse to support them in gaining clarity and control of their situation.

SLEEP DEPRIVATION. Physiologic systems function on a cyclical basis, with activity cycles being followed by seemingly quiescent periods. The evidence of this rhythmic pattern is seen throughout nature: all life exhibits phases of activity counterbalanced by periods of inactivity. In humans, inactivity is exemplified most clearly in sleep cycles. During this period of rest, all physiologic functions are maintained with a minimum expenditure of energy. The

process of sleep occurs in stages, with gradual withdrawal from the environment and its stimuli. People usually get 5 to 8 hours of uninterrupted sleep. During this period a person passes through the stages of sleep several times, with each cycle decreasing in length until the person awakens. Trauma patients experience abnormalities in sleep patterns and duration. Procedures and excessive stimulation frequently prevent extended periods of sleep, with the result that sleep deprivation occurs in a matter of days. The importance of providing meaningful sleep time rests in the awareness of nursing staff in scheduling care. Sleep-inducing medication, primarily barbiturates, blocks the REM stage of sleep and only contributes to sleep deprivation.[26]

In addition to excessive stimulation, medications, anxiety, fear, pain, and immobility all contribute to disruption of sleep patterns. Trauma patients who are experiencing sleep deprivation frequently are irritable and disoriented and display memory and thinking impairments. Many trauma patients doze for brief periods and claim that they are unable to fall asleep.[26]

Assessment data that are critical to determining sleep disturbances must be collected from family and nursing staff. A reliable sleep history from before the trauma establishes the patient's baseline sleeping patterns and requirements. Information elicited from family or significant others should include usual bed and arising times, use of naps, use of adjuncts to sleep, bedtime rituals, problems in the past with falling asleep, and fears. A running database of the actual time the patient sleeps in a 24-hour span can be collected and recorded by nursing staff. The nursing staff is also able to identify and address factors that contribute to sleep disturbances.[26]

The goal of the trauma nurse is to provide an environment that not only is conducive to sleeping but also allows maximal quantity and quality of sleep. Interventions focus on minimizing interruptions when the patient is attempting to rest. This requires the nurse to structure care and treatments so that the patient has blocks of uninterrupted sleep time. Decreasing environmental noise and lighting also facilitates sleep. Relaxation techniques such as back rubs, guided imagery, and music facilitate onset of sleep. Reassuring the frightened patient that the presence of the nurse remains while the patient is sleeping diminishes anxiety and the need for constant vigilance. Many trauma patients calmly drift off to sleep in the presence of someone they trust. Taking the time to sit and do charting quietly at the bedside provides the patient with a sense of security. Because patients need between 70 and 100 minutes of uninterrupted sleep to complete one full cycle of quality sleep, an ongoing chart that documents how well this is achieved is valuable. Quality sleep renews the patient both physically and psychologically and does much to enhance the healing process.[7,26]

LOSS OF EMOTIONAL CONTROL. Because traumatic injuries are accompanied by situations and procedures that cause pain and loss of normal emotional control of behavior, the patient, in an attempt to allay anxiety, may react with loud crying, dependent behavior, use of obscenities, and questioning of the staff's ability. This may not be the person's normal repertoire of responses. The person feels extremely vulnerable to this lack of personal control because it may lead to further isolation by staff and loss of self-esteem. If the response of the staff is one of ridicule of the behavior rather than insight into the emotional needs being expressed by the behavior, anxiety and fear are increased.

As the patient moves through the critical care phase, the magnitude of the number and variety of losses experienced is startling. Throughout this cycle patients have seen losses regarding their usual communication modalities, physical functioning, interpersonal relationships, environmental issues, alterations in roles, and invasion of boundaries of the self. The threat of powerlessness is profound. Patients respond with a variety of behaviors ranging from hostility and dependence to withdrawal and lack of motivation and interest in their environment. The inability to make simple decisions or take an interest in what is happening to them reflects the deep sense of helplessness and hopelessness they are experiencing.[27]

Throughout the patient's stay in the intensive care unit, the nurse constantly assesses and balances when and to what extent the patient can actively or passively make decisions and participate in his or her own care. A sense of personal autonomy is enhanced every time the nurse solicits the patient's views, preferences, and opinions. As the nurse selects opportunities that allow and support the patient's decision making and control over his or her environment, personal control is enhanced. Small achievements are consistently pointed out and hope is renewed. The nurse's ability to diagnose, assess, and intervene in this phase of trauma sets the groundwork for psychologic restoration.

THE FAMILY

The family also faces overwhelming stresses during the critical care phase. These include the realization that their loved one is critically ill with a potentially life-threatening injury; the stresses of the critical care environment; and the disruption of family roles, routines, and plans for the future.[5] The fear of death is foremost in the minds of family members and should be acknowledged and addressed by the nursing staff.

The foreign environment, frightening noises, lack of privacy, and presence of strangers further contributes to the high stress levels. Family members often judge the seriousness of the patient's condition based on the number of tubes, drains, intravenous pumps, and other equipment at the bedside. Conversely, the family may interpret the removal of these items as improvement in the patient's condition.[5]

Family routines become disrupted, and key roles may have to be delegated to other members. Dreams for the future may be destroyed, producing a sense of profound loss. The need to balance household and daily routines with the demands of the hospitalization often increase anxiety for family members.[5]

Treatment goals include the establishment of a trusting relationship with the staff. This relationship should begin as soon as possible after the patient's admission. The family should be assessed for feelings of helplessness or loss of hope, and interventions should be put in place to strengthen coping and increase hope.

Information regarding the patient's status should be provided on an ongoing basis. This information must be understandable and concise, using simple terminology. It is also critical to assess the family for informational overload and provide a balance of information.

Time should be set aside when possible to allow the family to participate in storytelling. This experience allows the family to discuss the impact of the injury on the patient and family system. The discussion promotes ventilation of feelings of loss, allows the family to begin the mourning process, and legitimizes the unique emotions they are experiencing.[5]

Spiritual needs must also be addressed. Referral to a chaplain or other spiritual leader may provide a sense of support to family members. Grieving members may find a spiritual leader essential to the grief process. Assisting the family to locate the hospital chapel may provide them with a quiet spot to meditate or pray.[28]

Cultural issues surrounding treatment and death must also be addressed. Culturally based grief reactions must be identified and supported. Death must be addressed based on the cultural traditions of the patient and family.[28,29]

Unfortunately, the ability and willingness to effectively incorporate the family into the plan of care is not uniformly found in the critical care unit environment. A study by Chesla[30] revealed that some staff have difficulty balancing the need for family care with the demands of technologic care. It was found that intensive care unit (ICU) staff and policies often impede the involvement of the family. The architectural design of the ICU makes it a closed environment, shutting out families. Frequently, entrance is allowed only after a phone call to the unit. Visiting hours are often restrictive and inflexible. Families are often asked to leave when the patient's condition deteriorates or when painful procedures are to be performed. Chesla[30] studied families and nursing responses in the intensive care unit setting. Interestingly, it was found that the practice of family care is most evident during birth and death, events to which the nurses are sensitive to the need for family presence. During the acute stage of illness, family care was generally less evident. Not surprisingly, some nurses described families as intrusive, meddlesome, pathologic, or a burden. The ideal family was described as compliant, passive, and uninvolved.[30]

It is vitally important, however, that family care be a priority in the critical unit. Appropriate interventions include adequately preparing the family for entrance to the care environment, for the patient's appearance, and for the surrounding equipment. This preparation will facilitate family responses to strange and frighteningly unfamiliar sights and sounds. It is often the nurse's role modeling that is most instrumental in helping families cope with seeing a loved one. The nurse should indicate that it is okay to touch the patient ("It's okay to touch _____ and talk to her") and should model how to do that, taking family members through the experience one by one. The nurse can tell family that it is okay to show emotion in front of the patient, to be demonstrative with affection toward him or her, and in other ways "give permission" for them to be as natural as possible while helping them to feel as unafraid as possible. No matter what the appearance of the patient, it is often the actual "seeing" that is instrumental in family coping, breakdown of denial, and commencement of necessary grief work.

Families need to feel that they are being helpful to the patient. This may be accomplished by actually providing some aspect of care; by performing tasks for the patient outside the hospital setting; or even by providing valuable information to the nurse regarding the patient's previous, usual functioning. This is an area where the nurse can use creativity in getting family members involved in ways most meaningful for them.

Families also need to be with or see the patient frequently. Although this is often difficult within the rigorous care schedules of a trauma unit or an ICU, family visiting is viewed as critical to the overall adaptation of family members to the crisis. As the patient's condition worsens or the family perceives that there is an increase in severity, the family's need to see the patient usually increases.[30] Visiting within a trauma unit or critical care area poses procedural difficulties for staff, but it is widely recognized and established that family members need routine and frequent access to the patient. Contact does not have to be lengthy but should be scheduled, predictable, and allowed. Within the uncertainties of this particular phase, one of the few things that families may count on is a visual verification of the status of their loved one. There is strong clinical evidence and substantial research to show that there are probably numerous beneficial psychophysiologic responses on the part of the patient to the presence of family.[7]

Special care should be taken to alert family members to any changes, positive or negative, in the patient's status or appearance before visits. Family members should be encouraged to communicate freely with patients even though they cannot respond; many patients, on recovery, report that communication by the bedside was critical to their sense of orientation and well-being, even though they could not respond.

If family members live a great distance away, or if there are too many teenage friends of an adolescent patient to allow all to visit, innovative ways of communication and contact can be instituted. Tapes can be made by friends or family members to be played at the bedside; telephone communication can be arranged with the aid of the nurse for logistics; pictures, cards, and letters or written corre-

spondence can all be used as effective means of communicating support and encouragement to a loved one when visiting is not possible or advisable.

Families also identify that they need support and allowance for ventilation of feelings. Families consistently identify their own personal needs as having low importance. Although this is important for the nurse to be aware of, families also should be apprised that they are just as much a part of the plan of care as the patient and that attention to their own personal needs can ultimately benefit the patient. Family members need to maintain adequate rest and nutrition in order to mobilize the energy required during the hospitalization course, and pointing this out in terms of their overall, long-term contribution to the patient is frequently beneficial.

Information regarding the patient's condition is also critical to the family. An overworked nursing staff, however, may perceive interruptions from family members requesting information as a burden. One strategy to meet these information needs is the distribution of pagers to family members. In this manner the family can leave the bedside, secure in the knowledge that the ICU staff can communicate with them when necessary.[31] An additional strategy is the use of structured communication programs. These programs offer focused discussion with the ICU staff within 24 hours of the patient's admission, provision of an information pamphlet describing the ICU staff and environment, and daily scheduled phone calls from the nurse caring for the patient. These strategies have been found to increase communication between the family and the ICU staff and increase family satisfaction.[32]

Intense bonding usually occurs between family members and the nurse/health care team on the first nursing unit to which a patient is sent. This is due to the high emotional intensity and extreme interdependence that exist in the first days of the critical care phase. As patients progress, they are often transferred to a different nursing unit with strange faces, different surroundings, and divergent rules for visiting. This is an extremely difficult time for both the patient and the family, who have grown secure in the familiarity and predictability of the previous unit. It is not uncommon for families to have greatly increased levels of anxiety and even anger over the transfer, largely as a result of a lack of control and fear of the unknown once again. Special care should be taken by the primary nurse of the first nursing unit to formally introduce the patient and family to the nurse taking over on the next unit. Families should be told that an extensive report will be provided to the new team on the patient's course and that they are still available to the patient and family even though in a different capacity. Every effort should be made to inform families ahead of time of the transfer, allowing them to verbalize their feelings about the move and providing a viable explanation as to why the transfer is necessary. Adequate preparation ahead of a transfer can alleviate a multitude of adjustment problems on the part of patients and families and is well worth planned time and effort.

Many times the only other people who share in the particular horror of a traumatic injury or sudden catastrophic illness are the other families experiencing similar situations within the institution. Other families who have made it through the labile course of the first 72 hours, lived through a transfer, survived two or three emergency surgeries for their loved one, and are also struggling to hold life and limb together can prove to be invaluable resources to one another. There is little so powerful as the support gained from others who have actually lived through a similar experience. It behooves the trauma nurse to link families whom she identifies as having had experiences that could be shared to benefit others. This often provides one family with the support they need and another with a sense of usefulness in providing aid and something tangibly positive and productive as an outcome of their pain.

The establishment of a trauma support group may provide the family with an opportunity to share their experiences. Led by a trained health care member, the support group brings together families at various stages of the critical care process. Information is shared among family members regarding the trauma experience. Experiences and feelings are explored. Misconceptions are clarified and reality is supported. In addition, it is a forum for the trauma family to network with other families who are currently living a similar stressful experience.[33]

INTERMEDIATE CARE PHASE

THE PATIENT

As the patient's condition stabilizes and becomes less critical, he or she is confronted with reality. Wounds and injuries become more real and patients must make a decision about whether or not to continue to strive for survival. Patients may begin to view themselves as victims. They are now challenged by the intense work required to heal and rehabilitate. They again mourn their losses as they begin to view life as it will be after injury. Physical and psychologic challenges arise as the patient and family become fully aware of the real impact and meaning of the injuries. Morse and O'Brien call this stage *enduring the self: confronting and regrouping.*[19] Important themes during the intermediate care cycle include learning to endure the injury, learning physical limitations, latching on to significant others, doing the work of healing, and mourning losses.

STAGE III: ENDURING THE SELF: CONFRONTING AND REGROUPING.   During stage III patients continue to experience periods of anxiety, especially when they perceive that the nurse is not available to them. Often patients are afraid of being left alone. Patients requiring increased dependence on the nurse find themselves watching the clock and fearing they have been abandoned.[19]

In the Morse study, patients emphasized that they counted to bring order to their days. This task allowed them to maintain a sense of control in an environment where they perceived no control. One participant states, "I would count

the days. I would ask them how long I would stay in the hospital, every time they would change my bandages. . . .I must have driven them crazy. . . . I'd keep bugging the [the nurses]. How long do you figure? How long do you figure?"[19]

Participants in this study reported that they counted surgeries, dressing changes, days, hours, treatments, physical therapy sessions, and baths. Treatments that produced pain were also counted as one less to endure or a step closer to discharge. Sometimes counting was used as a mechanism to defend against having to focus on the future. The intense concentration needed to count ceiling tiles or bricks in the wall prevented them from focusing on the trauma or the difficulties that were in the future.[19]

During stage III patients continue to use family support as an anchor to maintain identity and begin to look to therapists and others as a source of encouragement and support. Acceptance and encouragement from the health care team takes on particular significance as patients struggle to regain independence. Patients also begin to identify with and depend on other patients.[19]

The intense therapy required during the intermediate care phase requires an enormous amount of energy expenditure by patients. Patients may view the movement toward recovery as a slow, tedious, frustrating, and exhausting process. They may find themselves on an emotional roller coaster. On one day they may be elated at a small step in the healing process. The next may find them in a deep depression, as they perceive their condition to be worse, with little progress being made on the road to independence. To deal with the stresses of rehabilitation, the patients in the Morse study described the use of mental scorecards. Each foot walked with the prosthesis was a step closer to recovery. Each dressing change was a step closer to complete healing. These imaginary scorecards assisted the patients to begin to envision life after trauma.

As patients face the challenges of the intermediate care phase, it is important for the nurse to assist them to identify small, incremental milestones of success and to celebrate these. Encouragement of independence is essential. Independence in activities of daily living such as brushing teeth or self-feeding often help patients feel a sense of accomplishment.

During the intermediate care stage, patients may cling to the hope that a miracle will return them to their preinjury level of function. Morse and O'Brien[19] found that spinal cord-injured patients were especially prone to this type of magical thinking. One patient stated, "But I'm not going to sit down and accept the fact that I have to stay in [the wheelchair] all my life, because I might not. And I think people who accept being paralyzed defeat themselves. . . . cause if you accept it, you shut your mind down. . . . to working towards getting better, or getting things back. So I was coming here with, uh, expectations of getting back. . . . getting as much as I could do, try to get back on my feet."[19] Maintenance of hope is critical during this stage of the healing process. Research has shown that this type of coping behavior may prompt patients to work intensely to achieve a maximal level of recovery.[19]

LOSS AND GRIEF. A major task during this phase is the task of grieving for losses incurred by self and others involved in the traumatic event. Patients who have lost family members during the traumatic event begin the task of mourning.

Patients face loss of body integrity with all its attendant meanings: loss of control over their body, loss of control of the environment, and loss of control of their affective responses. Loss of function leads to loss of roles as well. Patients perceive themselves as powerless. One means of coping with these numerous losses is to become dependent on the power of others and to regress to early phases of development when the psyche could tolerate such dependency.

Patients' responses to actual or perceived losses are to mourn or grieve for them. Grieving begins the moment patients are cognitively aware that a change has occurred. The work of grief is displayed effectively by patients throughout each of the phases of trauma. The most frequently verbalized or displayed affects are denial, anger, guilt, bargaining, depression, and hope. Because the expression of grief is unique for each person, it is important that the trauma nurse be cognizant of the process and recognize each of the themes that patients are expressing. Grief work is not a systematic process consisting of stages that occur sequentially. Rather, it is a complex array of affects and cognition that patients are sorting out and attempting to make sense of to integrate the changes in their life. Patients are struggling to hope and find meaning in their life. Mourning reflects the profound conflict that arises from patients' attempts to consolidate what was valuable in their past and preserve it from loss while simultaneously reconstructing a present and a future in which the loss is integrated.[34]

The patient who is grieving reflects this process in both verbalization and behavior. It is important for the nurse to obtain from either the patient or some significant other information regarding the patient's previous coping patterns when he or she experienced a significant loss. Did the patient deny the loss initially? How did the patient reflect this denial? Did his or her motor and psyche activity diminish? Was the patient verbal or nonverbal? Did he or she cry frequently? Was the patient hostile or agitated? Did he or she stop functioning in other roles, such as work? Did the patient withdraw from the people and activities in his or her environment? Did the patient's sleeping and eating patterns change? If so, how? Did the patient become dependent on others to direct his or her activities? Did the patient verbalize feelings of hopelessness? Did he or she become quiet, withdrawn, or apathetic? Was the patient preoccupied with the loss? What or who was significant in supporting the patient? What did they do or say that was helpful?[24] As the patient's history of responding to previous losses is obtained, the nurse integrates this information into workable interventions with the patient.

For patients who use denial, the nurse recognizes that their behavior serves a purpose: They are indeed buying time and preparing themselves intrapsychically to address the magnitude of the traumatic event. It is important that the nurse not strip away this defense. Reflecting verbalized content back to patients confronts their thought processes in a nonthreatening manner. For example, if a patient in traction is inappropriately attempting to get out of bed to go to the bathroom, sincerely asking him a question such as, "Do you think you would be able to walk with all that traction attached to your broken left leg?" helps the patient to focus on pieces of reality and allows the nurse to intervene with specific factual information. Simple explanations regarding the environment and procedures bring reality to the patient without forcing it on him.

Trauma patients often are hostile to and critical of staff. Anger exists because patients have lost control and are dependent on others and because what has happened to them is perceived as unfair. Because patients are virtually unable to change what has happened, by externalizing the anger to the environment they at least maintain some sense of control by finding what is at fault externally. Frequently this anger is reflected outwardly by complaining about unresponsiveness of staff to patients' needs, by questioning of staff's ability to care for patients adequately, and by constant demanding of attention from the staff. There are few, if any, answers to the question, "Why did this happen to me? It's so unfair." Blaming others initially relieves some of the patients' frustration. The astute nurse looks behind the angry verbalizations and recognizes the need they serve. The nurse must be nondefensive toward patients, recognize and acknowledge with them that they are feeling angry, and help them focus on the reasons for the anger. It is also important that nurses not be punitive in their actions or verbalizations.

Part of grief work is retreating from the environment by withdrawing invested energy from it. This internal retreat from external stimulation provides time for patients to put the pieces together. Recognizing affects of sadness and depression and verbalizing them for patients support them in acceptance of those feelings. The nurse supports this necessary introspection by minimizing environmental input and by spending quiet time with patients. When patients are depressed, small goals and choices that are achievable need to be set.

As the loss begins to take on perspective for the patient, he or she comes to recognize abilities that he or she does retain. Hope becomes a bigger piece of the picture at this point, and the nurse now actively presents positive aspects of his or her life situation and acknowledges independent functioning and strengths. As the patient's self-image is beginning to integrate the changes that have occurred, renewed energy is applied to the task of healing. Often at this point, the patient shifts to more independent functioning; however, the patient moves back and forth in his or her use of coping behaviors throughout the phases of trauma as he or she mourns for his or her loss.

Affective coping behaviors such as denial, regression, anger, and depression do not alter the stressors, but they alter the perception of the patient experiencing them. At this juncture in the journey to recovery is the seed of a major conflict between nurse and patient. Patients may appear less anxious because they have often transformed the stressor, such as loss of control, by becoming markedly more dependent, and they tolerate this position by regressing to a level of development when it was appropriate; the nurse, on the other hand, perceives the situation without the aid of dependent and regressive eyes. The nurse often cannot tolerate a patient's level of dependency once there are physical signs that the patient's functioning can allow more autonomous behavior. In effect, nurse and patient may no longer be moving in the same direction. To cope with anxiety the patient has transformed the anxiety so that it is no longer experienced. The nurse becomes more anxious as a result of a need for the patient to continue progressing in their previously mutual direction and goals. This apparent dilemma can cause an alteration in the nurse-patient relationship, as evidenced by increased conflict in their interactions. Acknowledgment of the tension by the nurse allows examination of causative factors, which in turn allows dialog and resolution. Although there are probably alterations in the patient's other relationships, the interactions that the creative, skilled nurse has with the patient can pave the way for further healing and rehabilitation.

During this stage the nurse is the dominating force that shapes the patient's experience. The nurse can tolerate the patient's dependency and regressive behavior and respond to it in such a way that hopelessness, helplessness, and powerlessness are not the patient's predominant experiences. Rather, the resourceful nurse continues to provide choices for the patient to act on. The patient's decisions in these matters of choice counteract the everpresent threat of powerlessness and helplessness. The nurse combats the patient's regressive tendencies by constantly presenting reality in terms of necessary treatments but leaves room for the patient to determine when and, as much as possible, how. The enterprising nurse constantly assesses the patient's functional level of responsibility, stepping in when the patient falters; when the patient is more active, the nurse withdraws, giving the patient freedom and legitimating these efforts to become more autonomous.

Nurses need to be extremely flexible to respond to patients' psychosocial needs. Because of pain and monotony and the constant danger of coping by regression, patients tend to be in flux. The nurse who intervenes as though patients were constantly in the same position does either too much or too little for these persons. Evaluation of patients' status is easily accomplished by assessing their capacity to problem solve. This occurs when the nurse frames the day's schedule and seeks patients' input about these events. A patient who is more regressed might simply wash her hands of the whole thing or say, "I don't care. Do what you want," or "You're going to do it anyway. Go away!" Each of these responses is a reasonably accurate reflection of the patient's willingness to act on her own behalf that day.

The reality of the impact of the injuries is evident as patients begin to realize how much time and work will be involved to achieve independence. Patients often experience a sense of loss of control because they are forced to depend on health care providers for everyday activities. As strength is regained, patients will begin to attempt to function as they did before their injury. Grief and loss are again experienced as patients discover the limitations of their level of function. During this stage patients realizes that their disability is permanent. On another level, however, they reject the reality of the disability and the fact that it is permanent. This notion of temporary disability is often reinforced for spinal cord-injured patients as they experience sudden spasticity and muscle contractions.

THE FAMILY

ADAPTING TO THE INJURY.   During the intermediate care phase the family is also confronted with the enormous physical and emotional impact of the patient's injuries. During the critical care phase the focus of the family is on the survival of the patient. The focus now shifts to the realization that the patient will indeed survive, but with associated, often devastating disabilities and disfigurement. One relative of a severely head-injured patient stated, "For weeks we prayed he'd live. Now we know he'll live and, my God, now what do we do?"

As the crisis of the critical care phase subsides, the family may discover that their own emotional and physical resources have been depleted. Fatigue and irritability may be noted, as energy runs low. It is important for the nurse to encourage the family to focus on its own restoration. The family may have to be "given permission" by the health care team to reduce visiting time to allow for refueling. Education regarding the long-term effects of chronic stress, stress management techniques, nutrition, rest, and health promotion is essential at this stage.

The intermediate care stage is the setting in which the family must become involved in the plan of care. Visiting hours should be flexible to allow the family to be present during dressing changes and therapies. Patient and family discharge education should be initiated early in this phase, not delayed until the day of discharge.

During this phase it may be apparent and become a source of conflict that the patient and family are at different points in their grief work. In most cases family members are ahead of the patient because all the patient's energy has gone into fighting for life while so acutely ill. Although families may have moved through denial and resolved anger, patients may just be starting with those responses. The nurse can educate the family about the stages of grief and the fact that it is not uncommon for patients to fall behind the family in their progression through grief work. The nurse can encourage family members to be patient and tolerant, giving the patient the time necessary to progress. It is important that the nurse take an active role in supporting both the patient and the family with information regarding what the differences in responses reflect and how to understand the divergence and work with it. This is an active time in terms of education and teaching of the family by the nurse. In contrast to the empathic support and direct guidance given in the critical care cycle, the intermediate cycle necessitates a higher level intervention skill, with restructuring of family patterns, renegotiation of tasks, and more advanced application of family systems theory. Families tend to be calmer during this period but less eager for intervention and more emotionally distant from the health care team and from the patient. Once again, this is a natural progression and should not be misinterpreted. There is nothing "magic" about the time that a family has had to cope with a situation. The course of coping for families on a trauma trajectory is often erratic rather than linear, and allowances for shifts in family function should be made and accounted for on the basis of what the nurse understands regarding the need for some emotional distance and temporary emotional disengagement.

FUNCTIONAL VERSUS DYSFUNCTIONAL COPING. Ambiguity and lack of resolution still remain for family members in this phase as coping demands continue to vary from day to day; however, in this phase most families who are functionally progressing have established a general system for the prolonged incorporation of the unexpected. Depending on the nurse's assessment of whether the family is functional or dysfunctional in coping at this point, consultants may be called in to deal with particular family issues of a more complex nature. Most trauma and critical care centers have highly skilled family service departments, psychiatric social workers, liaison psychiatric nurses, alcoholic counselors, and others to assist the nurse once a more complex need is identified. Also families can be directed to professional and nonprofessional support groups for additional assistance.

Table 18-4 presents 12 characteristics useful in identifying a family system as basically functional. In contrast, dysfunctional progression may be heralded by the following behaviors:

- Prolonged denial
- Blaming—increased conflict
- Forgetting critical facts or necessary information
- Not hearing—decreased crisis or nonresolution of crisis
- Scapegoating—projecting all the problems onto one family member to relieve the overall anxiety in the system
- Unhealthy communication patterns:

Secrets—keeping facts from the nurse or from other family members

Deception—usually to protect a family member or an image; hiding information that is necessary to plan intervention course (e.g., social stigmas like drug abuse, alcohol addiction)

Double messages—saying one thing and meaning another

Evasiveness—vague answers or no answer; yes or no answers with no elaboration

---

TABLE 18-4 Fogerty's Model of the Functional Family

The family has the kind of balance that adapts to and welcomes change.

Emotional problems are seen as existing in the family unit, with components in each person.

Connectedness is maintained across generations with all members of family.

Minimum of fusion; distance is not used to solve problems.

Each twosome can deal with problems occurring between them; triangling is discouraged.

Differences between people are not only tolerated but encouraged.

Each can operate selectively using thinking and emotional systems with other members of family.

Each knows what is gotten from self and from others.

Awareness of emptiness in each family member, and there is no attempt to fill it up.

The preservation of a positive emotional climate takes precedence over what "should" be done and what is "right."

Each member can say it is a pretty good family to live in over time; if one or more members say there is a problem, there is a problem.

Members of the family use each other for feedback and learning, *not* as the enemy.

Modified from Fogarty T: System concepts and the dimensions of self. In Guerin P, editor: *Family therapy: theory and practice,* New York, 1976, Gardner, 149.

The theory best suited for working with families, especially during the course of a prolonged traumatic or critical illness with the various cycles, is Bowen's Family Systems Theory.[16] This is a theory of human functioning based on relationship systems and patterns present in all families to some degree. How intense these patterns are is related to the level of anxiety within the system and to what degree individuals within the system can distinguish between feeling process and intellectual process. A very brief overview of the major concepts of this theory is presented, including only those aspects with the most relevance for trauma nurses in working with families in their settings.

NUCLEAR FAMILY EMOTIONAL SYSTEM. Emotional forces within a family bind it together; that is, the emotional influence occurs between any two people who are important to each other. A high emotional meshing between two people is called *fusion*. When two people are fused, they have difficulty seeing themselves as distinct from the other, and what is experienced by one family member is perceived as experience for all. There is an "emotional oneness," with no clear boundary definition. This, in turn, causes anxiety as a result of potential loss of self, and family members may seek distance to reestablish self boundaries. So the counterbalancing forces of the need for togetherness (fusion) and for individuality (differentiation) are found in varying degrees within different families. These patterns are often the result of learning with one's original family (family of origin). If fusion is very high, four major mechanisms may be used to handle the attendant anxiety:

1. Conflict: There is open fighting and high level of disagreement.
2. Emotional distance: Family members seek space by involvement in other things (e.g., sports, work, excessive TV watching, extramarital affairs).
3. Physical, emotional, or social dysfunctions: One family member serves as the symptom bearer and is adaptive and somewhat submissive to another family member who is more dominant. The adaptive person is less decisive and more dysfunctional. This may be exhibited by chronic physical problems, depression, or alcohol or drug abuse.
4. Projection to other family member: This usually involves a child who is the targeted focus for the transmission of system anxiety. It may involve more than one child or other person in the system; typically, this person becomes symptomatic, thus expressing the anxiety for the family. Families often describe projected children as "different," "special," "the problem one," or "the perfect one." Projection may be highly positive or highly negative.

Most families use a combination of these four mechanisms at various times. The problem of a rigid, inflexible family system exists when only one mechanism is used exclusively.

TRIANGLES. These are the basic emotional building blocks of the family in the face of tension. A triangle involves a three-person system that has definite patterns in relationships that are predictable and repetitive. Two members of the triangle are usually close and one member is somewhat distant or closed out. The normal movement is toward closeness, except when anxiety runs high, at which point people seek the outside position. Families are composed of a series of interlocking triangles and may even call in other persons from the outside to duplicate the same patterns (e.g., therapist, nurse, school authority, police). There is a constant emotional movement with triangles, and often families come to have fixed roles in how they relate within various triangles. It is essential for the nurse to identify how these triangles operate and what the automatic and repetitive emotional responses are for various family members. Families can be helped to identify those automatic responses ("triggers") and thus gain more control over relationship patterns and dynamics.

DIFFERENTIATION. *Differentiation* refers to how family members distinguish between feeling and thinking and how one person sees himself or herself as distinct and autonomous from another. How well one person in a family can self-define in the face of the emotional climate depends on the degree of fusion present. Those individuals who are more feeling dominated (i.e., make decisions based on what "feels" right) tend to be less adaptable, less flexible, and more dependent on those around them. They are easily stressed and become dysfunctional more quickly than those who are more intellectual in function (i.e., more purposeful, principle oriented, and goal directed). Persons who are more highly differentiated are more adaptable, more flexible, and less ruled by emotions. They hold solid convictions and beliefs and do not give way on these in light of relationship conflict. Less differentiated family members, on the other hand, acquire their beliefs from others and are influenced greatly by external pressures or relationship conflict.

SIBLING POSITION. Toman[35] has identified roles based on ranks of sex (male or female) and age (eldest, middle, youngest, only) that a person learns in his or her own family and tends to assume in future situations outside the original family.[35] Sibling position implies certain behavioral tendencies, personality traits, social inclinations, and attitudes. Although it is outside the purview of this chapter to highlight the various characteristics of the sibling positions identified by Toman, knowledge of one's sibling position can be useful in understanding function and in gaining an overall picture of the entire family system.

MULTIGENERATIONAL TRANSMISSION PROCESS (MGTP). Successive generations are dynamically linked to the preceding ones and to subsequent generations through family relationships. Issues, problems, patterns, and beliefs are passed on from one generation to another, with relationship patterns remaining amazingly stable over generations. As relationship systems are traced across generations, current issues become clearer in the light of historical developments, and projections for the future of the family are feasible. Alcoholism, violence, depression, and many similar patterns may become quite graphic when one explores the tradition of a family. The MGTP is the mechanism by which a family transmits relationship system patterns, tendencies, functioning, and habits from generation to generation. Families often find the tracking of these patterns exciting and freeing, in that it provides a context for understanding current problems and issues in light of the past. In many cases the result is less blaming, less guilt, and enhanced awareness and understanding of behaviors.

EMOTIONAL CUTOFF. Family members within intense relationship systems may exhibit high or extreme amounts of emotional disengagement. There is little, if any, person-to-person relating, and interactions may cease totally through separation, withdrawal, cessation of all contact, or denial of attachment to or importance of that relationship. Emotional cutoffs always indicate unresolved emotional attachments, and the more intense this is within primary relationships, the more likely a person is to be symptomatic in present relationships. Viable emotional contact with previous generations is important to how one comes to define oneself and how roles and patterns within future relationships are established.

When the nurse is aware of some of these basic patterns and tendencies, there is much more likelihood of instituting the type of intervention that a given family would most likely require. Without an accurate and adequate knowledge of the context of family relationships, both past and present, long-term intervention and change for families within this phase may turn out to be superficial and transitory. Discharge planning is often instituted during this phase and should be done based on adequate assessment of the family's coping (whether functional or dysfunctional). Appropriate referrals can be made to providers of specialized services, community groups, and other resources. Plans for follow-up with the patient and family should also be established.

REHABILITATION PHASE

The rehabilitation phase is a time of active growth for the trauma patient and family. During this phase the patient makes the transition from trauma victim to rehabilitated individual. Interventions to address ongoing physical and psychologic problems become critical to a positive outcome. Chronicity becomes an issue as the family faces the great challenge of integrating the patient back into the home setting and into society.

THE PATIENT

STAGE IV: STRIVING TO REGAIN SELF: MERGING THE OLD AND THE NEW REALITY.   Morse and O'Brien[19] identified the rehabilitation stage as the fourth and final stage in the trauma victim's journey to self-preservation. Stage IV is identified as *striving to regain self: merging the old and the new*. During this stage patients strive to regain the self as they perceived it to be before the traumatic injury. Goals include becoming acquainted with the new, altered body image; making sense of the trauma experience; and accepting the consequences of the traumatic event.[19]

During the rehabilitation stage, patients will attempt to piece together the details of the event leading to the injury. They will attempt to clarify the details and piece together the parts they cannot remember.[19]

For some patients the rehabilitation phase allows the first opportunity to compare injuries. Morse and O'Brien found that participants in their study identified this as the time when they became thankful their injuries were not more severe.[19]

During this phase patients become acutely aware of their disabilities and must begin to face the fact that life as they knew it before the injury has changed and that many dreams must be abandoned. With the support of staff and family, patients begin to make new plans for the future as they integrate a new self-image. The rehabilitation cycle is a critical phase for trauma patients because it is the setting in which the patient is reintegrated into the family and society. Major issues are addressed during this phase, including the internalization of a new, altered body image; resumption of prior roles and functions with modifications as appropriate; a shift from dependence to independent functioning; and a refocusing on the future.

During the rehabilitation phase it is important to continue to address both the physical and the psychologic nature of the injury. In a study by Ponzer and colleauges,[36] patients who did not feel recovered 1 year after the trauma reported higher levels of pain and anxiety than did patients who perceived themselves recovered. In addition, depression after traumatic injury has been found to be a negative predictor of functional outcome.[37]

Van der Sluis et al[38] found that some trauma patients report continued persistent physical problems even 6 years after injury. These problems were predominantly related to head, spine, and extremity injuries. These ongoing problems have been identified as risk factors for failure to return to work after trauma. The primary psychologic deficits reported were poor memory, mental slowness, fatigue, and loss of initiative. The researchers conclude that rehabilitation treatment should focus extensively on the psychologic aspects of the traumatic injury in addition to physical needs.[38]

For the spinal cord-injured patient in particular, depression is a common outcome and can impede the rehabilitation process. Spinal cord-injured patients are faced with monumental challenges such as mourning the loss of body function and independence, developing new roles, and establishing an altered self-concept. Many also battle chronic pain. The rate of depression after spinal cord injury is five times higher than that of the general population and the rate of suicide is five to seven times greater than the general population. Substance abuse is also a problem.[39] Patients who experience depression after spinal cord injury are more likely to feel hopeless, neglect themselves, and be less motivated to participation in rehabilitation activities.[39]

The incidence of depression after spinal cord injury may be moderated by the degree of social support the patient perceives, the presence of conflict within the family, the presence of sustained hopelessness and despair, and the patient's coping resources and personality.

Nursing interventions include identification of patients whose personality style, coping skills, interpersonal relations, or other factors place them at increased risk for depression. A multidisciplinary team approach should be used, incorporating the expertise of the nurse, physician, psychiatric team, and rehabilitation team members. Medications that could produce side effects mimicking depressive symptoms should be discontinued. Trained psychiatric clinicians should manage the diagnosis of depression. Social support should be assessed and supportive social interactions fostered. Therapy may assist families in improving communication skills, readjusting roles, and promoting maximal independence for the patient.[39]

Patients experiencing traumatic wounds are also at risk for depression and the development of posttraumatic stress disorder. Nursing interventions include empathetic communication, support, and referral to a psychiatric clinician.[24]

THE FAMILY

Leske[5] identified eight essential family outcomes following the critical care experience:

- Seeking manageable reactions to the injury
- Reframing the injury experience as a challenge

- Redefining what constitutes maximal recovery
- Maximizing family resources
- Using adaptive coping resources
- Promoting strong bonds within the family
- Maintaining family involvement in the patient's care
- Mobilizing family strengths

Achievement of these outcomes continues to be essential during the rehabilitation phase. An additional outcome during the rehabilitation phase is managing the chronicity of the injury. During this phase the family begins to better comprehend the enormous task that must be addressed in order to reintegrate the patient into the family. For the family of the spinal cord-injured patient, the focus becomes the development of a long-term caregiver role. A study by Weitzenkamp et al[40] demonstrated that significantly more caregiver spouses of spinal cord-injured patients experienced physical stress, emotional stress, burnout, anger, and resentment than did non-caregiving spouses. Interestingly, the caregiver, who was not disabled, reported more significant depression than did the disabled patient.[40]

Families of head-injured patients also struggle with the issue of chronicity. A study by Knight et al[41] demonstrated that caregiver burden is determined, in part, not by the severity of the head injury but by the caregiver's subjective perception of his or her ability to meet the challenges of the caregiver role. Caregivers who perceived their role as overwhelming and negative reported increased physical and emotional distress than did those who viewed the role in a more positive light. In addition, families reported that the most distressing problems when caring for the head-injured family member was dealing with mood disturbances such as anxiety, lability of emotion, anger, depression, and aggression.[41] It was found that the caregivers of head-injured patients reported significant changes in family routines, financial states, social roles, and leisure activities. Perception was again an important variable. Caregivers who perceived the patient to be highly disabled reported more negative life changes than did caregivers who had a more positive appraisal of the patient's outcome. In addition, it was found that the perceived degree of social support combined with the perception of the functional deficits was a better predictor of caregiver life change than was the actual degree of head injury itself.[42]

Nursing interventions include the recognition that family involvement or lack thereof can have a powerful impact on the rehabilitation process. Assessment of family dynamics is critical, especially when family problems or conflict take precedence over the rehabilitation process. Positive communication can be achieved by inviting the family to team rounds or to the therapy sessions. Emotional support and guidance should be offered to both the patient and the family. The family should be actively involved in the development of the discharge plan.[43]

In addition, nursing care of families during the rehabilitation period must focus on providing information and networking to the family. These resources will enable the family to establish a more realistic perception of the patient's injury and rehabilitation outcomes. Preparation for discharge to home must begin early in the rehabilitation process. Too often patients are sent home to families who are ill prepared to deal with their extensive needs, or intensive family education is provided on the day of discharge. Because of the stresses inherent in the discharge process, little learning is retained at that time. Families must be invited to rehabilitation therapy sessions where they are encouraged to be actively involved. Instruction regarding wound care or other procedures should be initiated early enough to allow the caregiver several practice sessions with nursing supervision available.[43]

Families of head-injured patients must establish new communication styles and relationships. Communication skills training and counseling sessions will reduce the resentment, frustration, and isolation often experienced by these caregivers.[41] Networking with other families, attending support group sessions, and contacting specialty agencies will provide a source of support to families of trauma patients.

SPECIAL SITUATIONS

POSTTRAUMATIC STRESS DISORDER

Posttraumatic stress disorder (PTSD) has been recognized as a major health problem after physical or emotional trauma during the past 20 years. Research indicates that this phenomenon places the victim at risk for long-term mental health problems. Also known as battle fatigue, shell shock, and accident neurosis, PTSD is often misdiagnosed after the traumatic event. Patients and families exposed to the event may initially complain of symptoms that seem to be part of the normal response to overwhelming trauma. Symptoms can begin anytime after the event and persist for months. Individuals experiencing PTSD may have experienced or witnessed an event that produced actual or threatened injury or death. Spinal cord injuries and facial injuries are two types of trauma that place patients at particular risk for PTSD.[9,44,45]

Individual experiencing PTSD will describe their response to the traumatic event as one of intense fear, helplessness, or horror. Victims will describe episodes of intrusion during which they experience sudden intense, vivid memories, or flashbacks of the event. These memories are so real that the persons may feel as if they are reliving the trauma. Stressful emotions such as fear, grief, and anger are felt. Intense emotional energy is needed to attempt to deal with these flashbacks.

In addition, individuals may demonstrate avoidance phenomena. Relationships with family and friends often disintegrate because individuals experiencing PTSD avoid close emotional ties. They may describe themselves as numb and emotionless. As this behavior continues, significant others may feel rebuffed and view victims as cold, indifferent, or preoccupied.[9]

Victims of PTSD experience a state of chronic hyperarousal and a biologic alarm reaction. A gunshot victim may experience extreme distress when hearing a car backfire.

Panic attacks and extreme fear may be experienced when individuals are in situations that remind them of the traumatic event.

Other symptoms described by victims of PTSD include somatic complaints such as gastric upset and headaches, irritability, difficulty concentrating, and insomnia. Relationships with family and friends may deteriorate, and family and work relationships may suffer.[9]

All trauma patients experiencing a traumatic event that they perceive to be stressful should be screened for PTSD. Time is of the essence because the sooner the patient receives intervention, the better the chance for recovery. Goals of intervention include restoring a sense of control to the individual; diminishing the power of the traumatic event; reducing chronic hyperarousal; reducing feelings of guilt, anger, and self-blame; and restoring a sense of equilibrium for the victim.[9]

Interventions may include pharmacologic measures such as the use of benzodiazepines and serotonin reuptake inhibitors. Many patients also benefit from nonpharmacologic measures. These include counseling sessions by trained psychiatric professionals and involvement of the family to ensure additional support.[9]

DEATH

The death of a patient creates tremendous stress for the significant others and for the health care team. Initially some family members may experience numbness and shock after the death announcement. Others may demonstrate no response whatsoever. Later, as the reality of the situation becomes apparent, family members may respond with crying, anger, guilt, and anxiety. Denial of the event may be forcibly expressed, and the family may ask for proof of death. Some individuals may become restless and move about aimlessly. Family members may experience profound physical distress, including nausea, chest pain, palpitations, lightheadedness, and syncope. Waves of physical distress may be experienced that last 20 to 60 minutes. Other members will begin raising questions regarding the details of the death. Some will find the need to express an obsessional review of the patient's life.

Immediate interventions include placing the family in a private area from which the body of the loved one is accessible. The pronouncement of death should be made in an empathetic manner. The term *death* should be used, rather than abstract words such as *passed away*. The spirituality of the family must be assessed and clergy consulted if appropriate. Emotional support must be provided. Consultation with a social worker or psychiatric nurse liaison may be appropriate. Information should be provided in an open, honest manner. Because of the family's stress level, information may have to be repeated and reinforced.[46,47]

The family should be given the option to view the body. This offer should be made in a nonjudgmental manner, allowing the family to feel supported in their decision. The viewing should take place after the body has been washed and as much invasive monitoring equipment as possible removed. All attempts should be made to present the body in as normal a condition as possible. Disfiguring wounds should be covered with a clean dressing when possible. This viewing should take place in a clean, well-lit, quiet environment. Initially the family may decline the opportunity to spend time with the deceased loved one because they need more time to adjust to the profound stresses inflicted on them. It is important to give the family time to reconsider their decision. Once the family has been allowed to mobilize resources and absorb the initial shock of the situation, they may desire a viewing. Research has shown that families who initially refuse to view the body often regret the decision at a later time. It is recommended that multiple offers be made to the family to allow them to change their mind. If, however, a family ultimately refuses a viewing, the health care team should support the decision.

The amount of time spent with the loved one should be determined by the family. Some family members may wish to remain at the bedside, whereas others come and go. Chairs should be placed at the bedside for the comfort of the family. Identified clergy should be summoned as the family desires, and cultural rituals should be observed when possible.

When the decision to leave is made, the family should be escorted gently from the unit. In a quiet area all necessary paperwork and funeral home arrangements should be completed. The unit phone number and the name of a contact person should be provided to the family in the event that they have questions in the future. An additional supportive family intervention includes sending a sympathy card to the family 2 months after the death of the patient. This intervention provides the family with a sense of comfort and caring and provides closure for the health care team.[47]

TRAUMATIC GRIEF

The unexpected death of a loved one as a result of a motor vehicle collision, homicide, drunk driving event, or community disaster produces a profound grief event for the family. The course of bereavement is complicated by the traumatic and often violent manner of the death. Traumatic grief is defined as a complicated bereavement in which the death takes place unexpectedly, in an unfamiliar environment, often violently, allowing the family no opportunity for anticipatory grief. The surviving members experience a vicarious traumatization as a result of the death. Traumatic grief is often viewed as a combination of complicated bereavement and PTSD.[48]

The individual experiencing traumatic grief often describes an overwhelming rage, terror, and depression in response to the death of the loved one. There is an affective flooding of emotion whenever the death is remembered, often incapacitating the individual with anger, fear, and profound depression. If the individual was present during the death, as a bystander or a passenger in the vehicle, he or she may experience flashbacks of the event. Cognitively the surviving individual is preoccupied with the loss. He or she may spend inordinate amounts of time reliving the experience. Often the individual may experience a morbid obsession with the loved one's thoughts and feelings at the time of the death. Whether accurate or not, these images of the loved one's physical suffering and terror and thoughts of the violent nature of the death produce significant stress for the survivor. Thoughts of real or imagined blame may be directed toward the alleged perpetrator or toward the health care team members who were not successful in saving the individual. Plans of revenge may be formed. The survivor may also experience cognitive dysfunction such as memory impairment. Physiologically the surviving individual may experience a chronic state of hyperarousal in which feelings of rage and anger are intensified. The individual experiences an exaggerated startle response to specific cues. For example, a passenger in a motor vehicle in which the driver was killed may experience feelings of acute anxiety, tachycardia, tachypnea, and hypertension when attempting future rides in motor vehicles. Behaviorally the surviving individual may experience a phobic avoidance of the stimuli related to the death. Fear exists that the traumatic event will be repeated. Family members may avoid driving on a road where a loved one was killed, taking an out-of-the way detour instead. The death event is examined to determine what could have been done to change the outcome. Often survivors experience extreme guilt over the fact that they survived the event and the loved one did not. There is real or imagined guilt over not preventing the death. Resentment toward the dead loved one is often identified as a theme after a traumatic event. The surviving individuals experience anger toward the dead loved one for not trying harder to survive and for leaving the survivors behind. Surviving individuals also report appetite disturbances, altered sleep patterns, episodes of depression, and relationship conflicts.[1,48]

In an attempt to control the intensity of the overwhelming grief, surviving individuals may experience prolonged denial after the death of the loved one. Repression of the events of the death and psychic numbing may follow, preventing survivors from effectively working through the normal grief process. Survivors may experience social isolation, overwhelming fears about the safety of self and others, and magical thinking related to keeping others safe. As a form of self-protection, survivors may use avoidance behaviors such as emotional distancing from others or the use of drugs or alcohol. On a more positive note, some survivors attempt to make sense out of the tragedy. Support groups such as Mothers Against Drunk Drivers may be joined or formed. Family members may become involved in attempting to change laws or public policies to prevent further deaths. Memorials or scholarships may be established to honor the dead individual.

Traumatic grief is further complicated by involvement with the criminal justice system. Survivors often report that they feel victimized twice: once by the actual event and again during the course of the trial. During the court process, survivors often come face to face with the alleged perpetrator. The loved ones experience a sense of loss of control and intense rage. The resolution of the grief process is interrupted as the survivors must again relive the events surrounding the death. During the course of the trial, the defendant and his or her attorney may present the deceased in a negative light. Blame for the event may be directed toward the dead loved one, producing additional pain for the survivors. Philosophic conflicts may arise if the surviving members do not believe that justice has prevailed.[49]

Individuals experiencing traumatic grief must receive intervention as early as possible after the death. Immediate intervention includes guiding the survivors through the grief process. Immediate referral to a social worker or clergy is appropriate. Additionally, individuals experiencing traumatic grief may require the services of professional psychologists or grief counselors. The names and phone numbers of competent individuals in the area should be provided to survivors before they leave the hospital setting. Education regarding the issues of traumatic grief should be provided to all survivors who have experienced the unexpected, violent death of a loved one. Professional counseling focuses on crisis intervention, stabilization, and psychosocial adaptation. Assessment is made for the presence of PTSD. Substance abuse is addressed. Systematic desensitization, stress management techniques, and biofeedback are incorporated into the plan of care. Treatment goals include allowing the survivor to ventilate, helping to identify symptoms of emotional distress, educating the individual about the normal grief process, validating the survivor's experiences, restoring control, reducing self-blame, providing support, and helping the survivor say goodbye.[50]

RESEARCH INDICATIONS

Although significant theories exist describing the experience of traumatic injury, little solid research is available to clearly define the psychosocial impact of the event. It is imperative that future research describe the psychologic experiences of trauma patients and families and identify the needs of these populations. Interventional studies are needed to identify the most effective interventions to assist the patient and family to overcome the crisis experience. Studies are needed to assist in clearly identifying crisis proneness in patients and families. In addition, research targeting preventative measures will assist at-risk individuals.

SUMMARY

A traumatic injury is a devastating event that produces both physical and psychologic injury. Both the patient and the family are affected by the injury, and significant crisis often ensues. The nurse, along with other members of the health care team, plays a significant role in assisting the patient and family survive the crisis experience. It is clear that the psychologic impact of injury must be addressed throughout the trauma cycle. Timely application of crisis interventions assist the patient and the family as they deal with the stresses of the injury. Use of family system theory helps the health care team better meet the needs of challenging or dysfunctional families. Finally, appropriate referrals to psychiatric clinicians, clergy, spiritual advisors, social workers, and outside resources promote positive outcomes for patients and families.

REFERENCES

1. Michaels AJ, Michaels CE, Moon CH et al: Psychosocial factors limit outcomes after trauma, *J Trauma* 44:644-648, 1998.
2. Holbrook TL, Anderson JR, Sieber WJ et al: Outcome after major trauma: discharge and six month follow up results from the trauma recovery project, *J Trauma* 45:315-324, 1998.
3. Anderson A, Bunketorp O, Allebeck P: High rates of psychosocial complications after road traffic injuries, *Injury* 28:539-543, 1997.
4. Winje D: Long-term outcome of trauma in adults: the psychological impact of a fatal bus accident, *J Consult Clin Psychol* 64:1037-1043, 1996.
5. Leske J: Treatment for family members in crisis after critical injury, *AACN Clin Issues Crit Care Nurs* 9:129-139, 1998.
6. Lindemann E: The meaning of crisis in individual and family, *Teaching Coll Rec* 57:310, 1956.
7. Jastremski C, Harvey M: Making changes to improve the intensive care unit experiences for patients and their families, *New Horiz* 6:99-109, 1998.
8. Infante MS: *Crisis theory: a framework for nursing practice*, Englewood Cliffs, NJ, 1982, Prentice Hall, 117-127.
9. Aguilera D: *Crisis intervention: theory and methodology*, ed 8, St. Louis, 1998, Mosby, 26-42.
10. Poole G, Lewis J, Devidas M et al: Psychopathologic risk factors for intentional and nonintentional injury, *J Trauma* 42:711-715, 1997.
11. Jelalian E, Spirito A, Rasile D et al: Risk-taking, reported injury, and perception of future injury among adolescents, *J Pediatr Psychol* 22:513-531, 1997.
12. Ankney RN, Vizza J, Coil JA et al: Cofactors of alcohol-related trauma at a rural trauma center, *Am J Emerg Med* 15:228-231, 1997.
13. Gentilello CM, Donovan DM, Dunn CW et al: Alcohol interventions in trauma centers, *JAMA* 274:1943-1948, 1995.
14. Bein TH, Miller, WR, Tonigan JS: Brief interventions for alcohol problems: a review, *Addiction* 88:315-336, 1994.
15. Hoff, LA: Families in crisis. In Getty C, Humphreys W, editors: *Understanding the family: stress and change in American family life*, New York, 1981, Appleton-Century-Crofts, 418-434.
16. Kerr ME, Bowen M: *Family evaluation: an approach based on Bowen theory*, New York, 1988, WW Norton.
17. Kerr ME: Chronic anxiety and defining a self, *Atlantic Monthly*, 35-38, Sept 1988.
18. Minuchin S: Structural family therapy, Cambridge, Mass, 1976, Harvard University.
19. Morse JM, O'Brien B: Preserving self: from victim to patient, to disabled person, *J Adv Nurs* 21:886-896, 1995.
20. Cross ML, Wright SW, Wrenn KD et al: Interaction between the trauma team and families: lack of timely communications, *Am J Emerg Med* 14:548-550, 1996.
21. Leske JS, Heidrich SM: Interventions for aged family members, *Crit Care Nurs Clin North Am* 8:91-102, 1996.
22. Epperson MM: Families in sudden crisis: process and intervention in a critical care center, *Soc Work Health Care* 2:265-273, 1977.
23. Kleeman KM: Families in crisis due to multiple trauma, *Crit Care Nurs Clin North Am* 1:23-31, 1989.
24. Magnan MA: Psychological considerations for patients with acute wounds, *Crit Care Nurs Clin North Am* 8:183-193, 1996.
25. Schnapper N: The psychological implications of severe trauma: emotional sequelae to unconsciousness: a preliminary study, *J Trauma* 15:94-98, 1975.
26. Fontaine DK: Sleep. In Kinney MR, Dunbar SB, Brooks-Brunn J et al, editors: *AACN's clinical reference for critical care nursing*, ed 4, St. Louis, 1998, Mosby.
27. Schrader KA: *Stress and immunity after traumatic injury: the mind-body link*, *AACN Clin Issues Crit Care Nurs* 7:351-358, 1996.
28. Hart C, Matorin S: Collaboration between hospital social work and pastoral care to help families cope with serious illness and grief, *Psychiatr Services* 48:1549-1552, 1997.
29. Arsenault S: Assessing the family: the importance of culture, *Crit Care Nurs* 17:96, 1997.
30. Chesla C: Reconciling technologic and family care in critical care nursing, *Image J Nurse Sch* 28:199-203, 1996.
31. Olson D: Paging the family: using technology to enhance communication, *Crit Care Nurs* 17:37-41, 1997.
32. Medland J, Ferran SC: Effectiveness of a structured communication program for family members of patients in an ICU, *Am J Crit Care* 7:24-29, 1998.
33. Hsu S: Trauma support groups, *Imprint* 43:45-48, 1996.
34. Marris P: *Loss and change*, New York, 1974, Pantheon, 31-32.
35. Toman W: *Family constellations*, ed 2, New York, 1982, Springer.
36. Ponzer S, Bergman B, Brisman B et al: A study of patient-related characteristics and outcome after moderate injury, *Injury* 27:549-555, 1996.
37. Holbrook TJ, Hout DB, Anderson JP et al: Functional limitation after major trauma: A more sensitive assessment using the quality of well-being scale—the trauma recovery pilot project, *J Trauma* 36:74, 1994.
38. van der Sluis CK, Eisma WH, Groothoff JW et al: Long-term physical, psychological and social consequences of severe injuries, *Injury* 29:281-285, 1998.
39. Boekamp JR, Overholser JC, Schubert DS: Depression following a spinal cord injury, *Int J Psychiatry Med* 26:329-349, 1996.
40. Weitzenkamp DA, Gerhart MS, Charlifue SW et al: Spouses of spinal cord injury survivors: the added impact of caregiving, *Arch Phys Med Rehabil* 78:822-827, 1997.
41. Knight RG, Devereaux R, Godfrey HP: Caring for a family member with a traumatic brain injury, *Brain Inj* 12:467-481, 1998.
42. Wallace CA, Bogner J, Corrigan JD et al: Primary caregivers of persons with brain injury: life changes one year after injury, *Brain Inj* 12:483-493, 1998.
43. Rintala DH, Young ME, Spencer JC et al: Family relationships and adaptation to spinal cord injury: a qualitative study, *Rehabil Nurs* 21:67-74, 90, 1996.
44. Binks TM, Radnitz CL, Moran AI et al: Relationship between level of spinal cord injury and posttraumatic stress disorder symptoms, *Ann N Y Acad Sci* 821:430-432, 1997.
45. Bisson JI, Shepherd JP, Manish D: Psychological sequelae of facial trauma, *J Trauma* 43:496-500, 1997.

46. Harrahil M: Giving bad news compassionately: a 2-hour medical school educational program, *J Emerg Nurs* 23:496-498, 1997.

47. Furukawa MM: Meeting the needs of the dying patient's family, *Crit Care Nurs* 16:51-57, 1996.

48. Spray G, McNeel J: A theoretical overview of traumatic grief. In Spray G, McNeel J, editors: *The many faces of bereavement: the nature and treatment of natural, traumatic, and stigmatized grief,* New York, 1995, Brenner/Mazel, 55-64.

49. Spray G, McNeel J: The process of grief following a murder. In Spray G, McNeel J, editors: *The many faces of bereavement: the nature and treatment of natural, traumatic, and stigmatized grief,* New York, 1995, Brenner/Mazel, 65-85.

50. Spray G, McNeel J: The treatment of traumatic grief. In Spray G, McNeel J, editors: *The many faces of bereavement: the nature and treatment of natural, traumatic, and stigmatized grief,* New York, 1995, Brenner/Mazel, 118-135.

SINGLE SYSTEM INJURIES

19

TRAUMATIC BRAIN INJURIES

Karen A. McQuillan •
Pamela H. Mitchell

Brain injury is the leading cause of all trauma-related deaths. It constitutes the primary cause of death and long-term disability among young Americans.[1,2] Survivors of the initial brain insult remain at risk for various multisystem complications that can exacerbate the initial brain injury and increase mortality and morbidity. The prevention, recognition, and immediate treatment of these complications in the prehospital, resuscitation, critical care, intermediate care, and rehabilitation phases of care are of utmost importance. Recovery is often a lifelong process beset with physical, mental, emotional, and social obstacles. Brain injury and the potential long-term disabilities it creates also have a tremendous impact on the family and cost society billions of dollars each year. Because of its high incidence, mortality and morbidity, economic cost, and demand for medical resources, brain injury is a major public health problem in the United States.

This chapter provides the trauma nurse with a comprehensive review of traumatic brain injury (TBI) and its sequelae. An overview of brain injury epidemiology, mechanism of injury, and related neuroanatomy increases the nurse's knowledge about the magnitude of this disease, as well as its etiology and neurologic impact. Explanation of the various types of brain injuries and pathophysiology provide the scientific basis for interventions used to treat traumatic brain injury (TBI). Strategies to monitor and assess the injured brain are reviewed so the nurse can collaborate with the other members of the health care team to properly guide and evaluate the effectiveness of treatment. Therapeutic interventions used by the multidisciplinary health care team to manage brain injury are described for each phase of trauma care. With knowledge about related anatomy and brain injury pathophysiology, assessment, and treatment, the trauma nurse can best promote optimal outcomes for patients with craniocerebral trauma.

EPIDEMIOLOGY

Historically it has been difficult to accurately determine the exact incidence of TBI, because of inconsistencies in the definitions of head injury, lack of a central head injury database, failure of some patients to seek medical treatment after head trauma, and varied methods for collecting data.[3] Public Law 104-166, the Traumatic Brain Injury Act of 1996, mandates the Centers for Disease Control and Prevention (CDC) to develop a uniform reporting system to tract the incidence, severity, causes, and outcomes of TBI.[2] Guidelines for surveillance of central nervous system injury are now established, and at least 15 states receive funding and participate in the CDC's TBI Surveillance Program.[4] Consistency in the documentation of the occurrence and causes of TBI assist in tracking trends and determining which prevention and treatment strategies are most effective.

The CDC estimate that 1.5 million persons sustain TBI each year in the United States.[5] The average annual incidence of TBI mortality and hospitalization is 95 per 100,000 population, based on analysis of preliminary data collected from 12 states.[6] The National Hospital Ambulatory Medical Care Services Survey revealed that approximately 1 million persons (392 persons per 100,000 population) visited an emergency department but were not hospitalized for TBI from 1995 to 1996.[7] Approximately 80% of persons evaluated for TBI in emergency departments are not admitted to the hospital.[8] The highest incidence of TBI-related emergency department visits occurs among children under 15 years; the two leading causes of injury are falls and motor vehicle-related incidences.[7] An estimated 230,000 U.S. residents are hospitalized because of TBI and survive.[1] The estimated incidence of annual TBI-related hospitalizations decreased 51% from 1980 to 1995. This reduction in hospitalizations occurred primarily among persons sustaining a mild TBI rather than those with moderate or severe injury.[8] This trend suggests that changes in hospital admission practices has led to fewer patients with mild TBI being admitted to the hospital. Motor vehicle-related crashes constitute the leading cause of traumatic brain injuries that result in hospitalization.[1,3]

The CDC estimate that 35% of all persons who survive hospitalization for TBI experience long-term disabilities. This means that approximately 80,000 to 90,000 persons each year are disabled by TBI. An estimated 53 million Americans (2% of the population) live with disabilities resulting from TBI. This estimate does not consider patients who were not admitted to the hospital and may still suffer long-term sequelae from TBI, so this estimate may be low.[1]

Approximately 50,000 Americans die each year from TBI, which accounts for about one third of all trauma-related deaths. This estimate may be low, because it does not account for persons who die of massive, multiple trauma and also have significant brain injury involvement.[6,9] TBI-related deaths declined 20% between 1980 and 1994, from 24.7 per 100,000 to 19.8 per 100,000.[1] This decline can be attributed to a 38% decrease in motor vehicle-related deaths and a decline in deaths related to falls and other incidents during this period. However, during this time the number of TBI deaths caused by firearms increased 11%.[1] As a result, since 1990 firearm use has surpassed transportation-related incidents as the leading cause of death from TBI.[1,9] Close to 17% of the deaths caused by TBI occurred in the prehospital setting, and 5.6% of deaths occurred while the person was receiving acute care. Approximately 22.6% of all reported TBIs result in death.[1]

Economic costs of TBI are staggering. Direct costs include initial and follow-up diagnosis, treatment, and rehabilitation. Indirect costs include societal losses secondary to restricted or lost productivity. The Brain Injury Association estimates the annual cost of TBI in the United States to exceed $48 billion.[10] The physical and psychosocial suffering from lifelong disabilities endured by brain-injured persons and their significant others is tremendous and the costs incalculable.[1]

CORRELATIVE NEUROANATOMY AND PHYSIOLOGY

The brain, which is part of the central nervous system, provides most of the control functions for the entire body. Like a computer, the brain receives thousands of bits of information from the sensory organs and then integrates them to determine the response to be made by the body. In general the brain maintains the quality and uniqueness of human life and behavior. The major divisions of the brain are the cerebrum, brainstem, and cerebellum (Figure 19-1), which are housed within multiple protective coverings.

COVERINGS OF THE BRAIN

Numerous protective coverings surround the brain. Outermost on top of the skull is the scalp, composed of five layers: skin, subcutaneous fascia, galea aponeurotica, loose connective tissue, and periosteum. The rigid, nondistendible cranium that encases the brain is made up of the sphenoid, ethmoid, frontal, and occipital bones, two parietal bones, and two temporal bones (Figure 19-2). Beneath the skull are three layers of connective tissue (the meninges), which surround the brain and the spinal cord. The meningeal layers include the outermost thick, fibrous dura mater; the fine, elastic arachnoid mater; and the innermost vascular membrane, the pia mater, which adheres to the brain's surface (Figure 19-3).

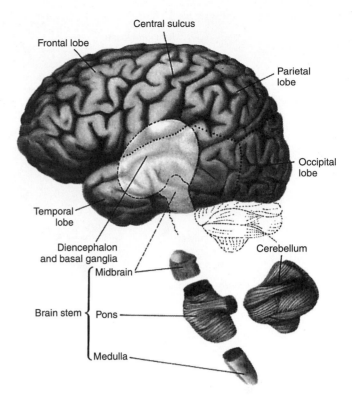

FIGURE 19-1 **Major Parts of the Central Nervous System.** (From Kandel E, Schwartz J: *Principles of neural science,* ed 3, New York, 1991, Elsevier/North-Holland.)

CEREBRUM

The cerebrum includes the cerebral hemispheres and the diencephalon. It is capped by gray cortex (neuronal cell bodies), under which lies extensive white matter (axons). The two large cerebral hemispheres are partially separated by the great longitudinal fissure and a vertical dural fold within the fissure that creates the falx cerebri. A thick tract of white interhemispheric nerve fibers at the base of the longitudinal fissure, the corpus callosum, is the primary connective pathway between the two hemispheres.

CEREBRAL HEMISPHERES. The two cerebral hemispheres are divided into four pairs of lobes: the frontal, temporal, parietal, and occipital (Figure 19-4). Knowledge of the primary functions of the lobes (Table 19-1) and lesion location can alert the nurse to the most likely assessment findings. For example, it can be anticipated that a lesion in the prefrontal region may result in altered behavior, whereas a lesion in the posterior frontal region of the dominant hemisphere may result in language dysfunction. Nursing assessment and the patient plan of care should anticipate and focus on the actual or potential problems associated with lesions in specific anatomic locations.

The cerebral hemispheres are responsible for sensory and motor processes of the contralateral side of the body. Sensory information entering the spinal cord from the right side of the body crosses over to the left before reaching the cortex. Similarly, motor impulses originating from the right cerebral cortex cross over to the left before synapsing in the

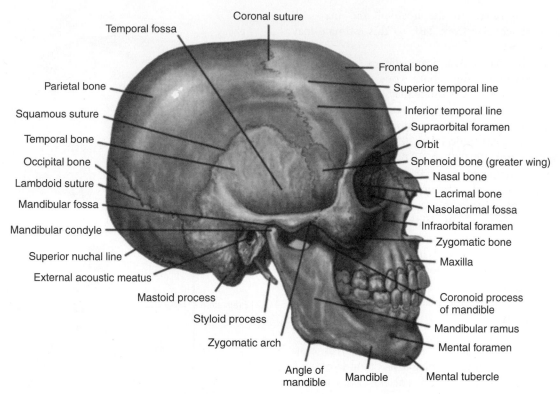

FIGURE 19-2 **Right Side View of the Skull.** (From Lindsay DT: *Functional human anatomy,* St. Louis, 1996, Mosby, 147.)

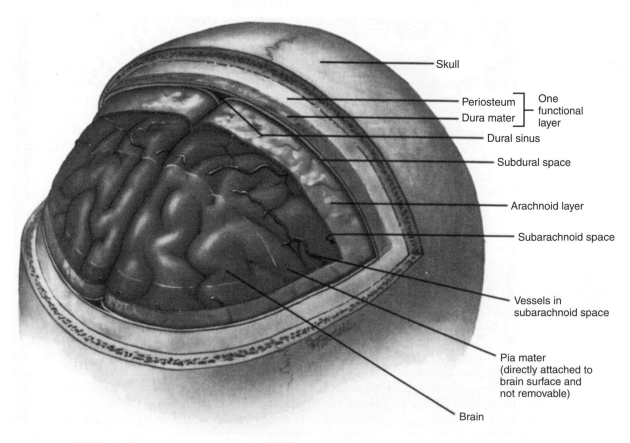

FIGURE 19-3 **Cranial Meninges.** (From Lindsay DT: *Functional human anatomy,* St. Louis, 1996, Mosby, 585.)

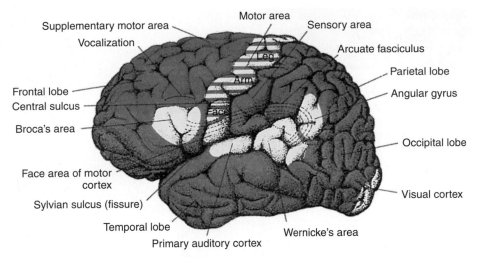

FIGURE 19-4 Lobes of the Brain. (From Kandel E, Schwartz J: *Principles in neural science,* ed 3, New York, 1991, Elsevier/North-Holland.)

cord. This explains one of the fundamental principles of motor assessment; that is, structural lesions causing compression of descending motor tract fibers will almost always result in contralateral motor signs.

DIENCEPHALON. The diencephalon is a complex of structures consisting of the hypothalamus, thalamus, epithalamus, and subthalamus. The hypothalamus, situated deep within the brain and just above the brainstem, is one of the most notable of the diencephalic structures. It is the primary regulator of autonomic function and controls numerous visceral and metabolic activities, including regulation of body temperature, blood pressure, heart rate, pupil size, shivering, sweating, gastrointestinal peristalsis, appetite, sleep-wake cycle, and water balance. Through its connection with the pituitary gland via the hypophyseal stalk, the hypothalamus directly influences pituitary hormonal activities and, in conjunction with the pituitary, mediates the body's stress/adaptation response.

BRAINSTEM

The brainstem is a midline structure situated beneath the diencephalon. The brainstem has three sections: the midbrain is the uppermost structure, the pons lies in the middle and the medulla is the lowest segment (see Figure 19-1). The descending medulla is contiguous with the spinal cord, which begins at the level of the foramen magnum.

The brainstem performs a variety of vital functions. It is the center of the brain that controls basic and reflexive activities such as visual and auditory motor reflexes, sleep and wakefulness, sneezing, coughing, breathing, vasomotor activity, and heart rate regulation. It is the pathway used by sensory fibers as they ascend from the cord to the cortex. Motor tract fibers on their descent from their cerebral or brainstem origin also traverse the brainstem, and many cross over (decussate) in the medulla before exiting down the spinal cord. Many cerebellar tracts also pass through the

brainstem, which allows formation of extensive connections between the cerebrum and cerebellum in this region. The reticular activating system responsible for consciousness originates in the brainstem as a dense bundle of fibers and ascends, coursing out over the cerebral cortices (Figure 19-5). The brainstem also controls many of the special senses, motor functions, and reflexes that are mediated by the cranial nerves, which arise and exit from this structure.

CEREBELLUM

The cerebellum lies within the posterior fossa behind the brainstem and beneath the cerebral hemispheres. It is separated from the cerebral hemispheres by a dural fold called the tentorium cerebelli and is attached to the three brainstem sections by three pairs of cerebellar peduncles. Cerebellar functions include control of muscle tone and fine motor movement, coordination of muscle activity, regulation of postural reflexes, and use of feedback loops to make appropriate corrections in motor activities and to maintain equilibrium.[11]

CEREBROVASCULATURE

The carotid and vertebral arteries deliver blood to an extensive capillary system that supplies the brain. The capillaries of the brain have a unique membranous structure that has tight junctions between the vessel wall network of endothelial cells and is surrounded by astrocyte end-feet projections. These unique capillary features, known as the blood-brain barrier, help maintain homeostasis for the neurons by limiting the transfer of substances from the intravascular space into the extracellular fluid and cerebrospinal fluid (CSF). From the capillaries, blood drains into the venous system, which differs from other veins of the body in that it lacks valves. Cerebral blood is carried by an internal and external venous system into large dural sinuses located between the dural layers, which empty into the jugular veins exiting the brain.

TABLE 19-1	**Primary Functions of the Cortex by Lobes**
Lobe	Function
Frontal	Prefrontal
	Short-term memory
	Emotional responsiveness
	Abstract thinking
	Foresight/judgment
	Behavior/tactfulness
	Primary motor cortex
	Broca's speech area (dominant hemisphere)*
	Expressive speech/vocalization
	Intellect
	Personality
Temporal	Primary auditory cortex
	Visual task learning
	Dominant hemisphere*
	Wernicke's speech area
	Receptive speech/comprehension
	Interpretive area
	Intellect
	Emotion
	Long-term memory
	Dominant hemisphere: verbal
	Nondominant hemisphere: sensory
Parietal	Primary sensory cortex
	Sensory interpretation
	Tactile and kinesthetic sense
	Body awareness
	Body image
	Spatial orientation/relations
	Dominant hemisphere
	Language
	Object perception/recognition
	Nondominant hemisphere
	Neglect syndrome
Occipital	Primary visual cortex
	Visual association

*Dominance: The majority (80%) of both right- and left-handed people have left hemispheric dominance for speech. A small percentage of left-handed people have both right and left hemispheric speech control. The preponderance of left cerebral dominance is felt to be due to anatomic asymmetry of the human brain. Sixty-five percent of people have a larger speech area (Wernicke's) surface on the left hemisphere; in 11% the right is larger, and in 24% the right and left sides are equal in size. Hemispheric lateralization or dominance is also found in functions related to mood and affect, as well as verbal, auditory, and visuospatial tasks.

CEREBROSPINAL FLUID

CSF supports and cushions the central nervous system. It is theorized that CSF also has nutritive qualities and aids in the removal of metabolic waste products. CSF plays an important role in intracranial dynamics and management of intracranial pressure (ICP) after severe TBI.

Cerebrospinal fluid is a clear, colorless liquid produced primarily within the choroid plexuses of the ventricles at a rate of approximately 20 ml/hr (480 ml/day).

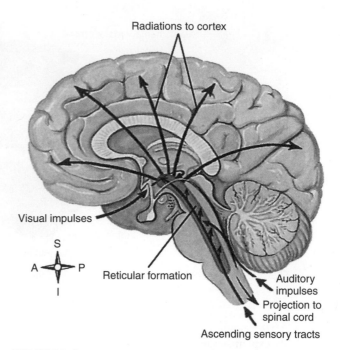

FIGURE 19-5 Reticular Activating System. Consists of centers in the brainstem reticular formation plus fibers that conduct to the centers from below and fibers that conduct from the centers to widespread areas of the cerebral cortex. Functioning of the reticular activating system is essential for consciousness. (From Thibodeau GA, Patton KT: *Anatomy & physiology*, ed 3, St. Louis, 1996, Mosby, 442.)

CSF contains small amounts of protein, glucose, oxygen, carbon dioxide, and potassium and relatively large amounts of sodium chloride. In adults the volume of CSF circulating through the ventricular system and subarachnoid space of the brain and spinal cord at any one time is 125 to 150 ml.

The CSF pathway (Figure 19-6) is a free-flowing system whereby CSF passes from the lateral ventricles (hollow cavities within each cerebral hemisphere) through the foramina of Monro (intraventricular foramina) into the third ventricle. From there it flows into the fourth ventricle via a small, narrow opening known as the aqueduct of Sylvius. CSF exits the fourth ventricle through the foramina of Magendie and Luschka to enter the cisterna magnum and the subarachnoid space (SAS). CSF within the subarachnoid space flows upward over the convexity of the brain and downward around the spinal cord.

Because there is continuous synthesis of CSF, it is essential that both a functional outlet system and a patent pathway be maintained to facilitate absorption and prevent fluid buildup. Arachnoid granulations or villi, outpouchings of the arachnoid membrane that herniate through the dura into the large venous sinuses, absorb most of the CSF into the venous system. These structures are pressure-dependent, one-way valves that open when CSF pressure exceeds venous pressure, allowing unidirectional flow of CSF from the subarachnoid space into venous blood.

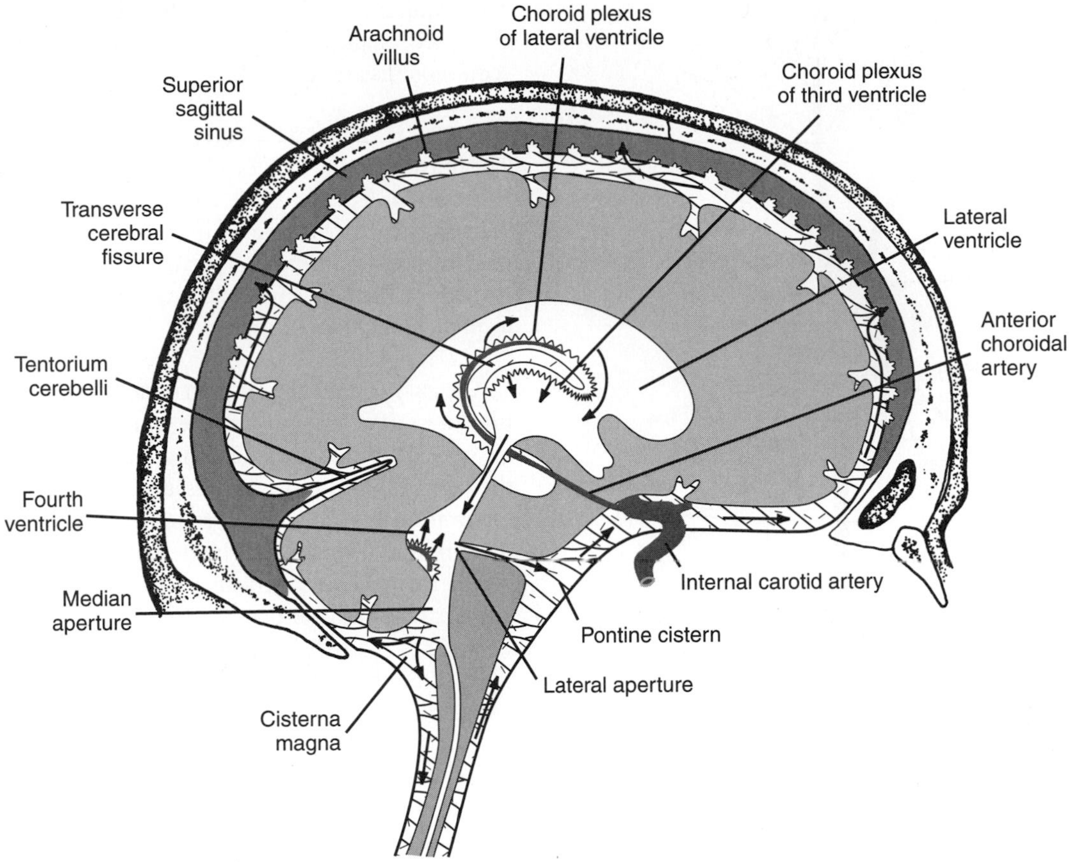

FIGURE 19-6 **Path of CSF Circulation.** (From Nolte J: *The human brain: an introduction to its functional anatomy,* ed 4, St. Louis, 1999, Mosby, 107.)

CELLS OF THE BRAIN

The central nervous system contains two types of cells: the neuroglial, or glial cell, and the nerve cell, or neuron. Glial cells outnumber neurons by approximately 9 to 1 and are generally classified as astrocytes, oligodendroglia, microglia, or ependymal cells. Glial cells lack axons and function primarily to nourish, support, and protect the nerve cells.

The neuron is the functional unit of the nervous system that transmits nerve impulses. This type of cell consists of a cell body, axon, presynaptic terminals of the axon, and dendrites (Figure 19-7). Each of these cell components has a distinctive function. The cell body synthesizes and packages the products of neuronal metabolism and transports them to other regions of the cell. It exchanges nutrients, ions, and other metabolically active substances with the extracellular environment through the cell membrane. This lipoprotein membrane is crucial for depolarization of the neuron through such mechanisms as the energy-dependent sodium-potassium pump, ion-selective channels, and voltage-sensitive channels. The myelin-covered axon, a tubular extension of the cell body, is responsible for rapid nerve conduction away from the cell body. The presynaptic terminals are specialized endings at the distal portion of the axon that transmit information by chemical or electrical means to other neurons or effector cells. The specialized contact zone between the transmitting (presynaptic cell) and the receiving (postsynaptic cell) neuron is the synapse. The dendrites, unmyelinated fibers that branch extensively as they extend from the cell body, receive incoming impulses and transmit them to the cell body. The physiologic and anatomic properties of the nerve cell account for its unique ability to communicate with other cells. In general the neuron is responsible for processing, analyzing, and acting on all incoming and outgoing information, which culminates in all our behavioral responses. Neurons differ from other cells not only in their communicative ability but also in their lack of mitotic ability. Without mitosis, neurons cannot multiply. With CNS maturity, the number of neurons is fixed and no new neurons are added. Injury to neurons is significant because it results in cell loss with no new cell replacement.

CEREBRAL METABOLISM

The average brain weighs 3 pounds and accounts for 2% of the adult body weight. Despite its relatively small size, the brain uses about 20% of the total-body resting oxygen consumption.[12] The primary energy source for the brain is glucose, which is converted by aerobic or oxidative metabolism into a high-energy phosphate form, adenosine triphosphate (ATP). Most of the energy is used for neuronal

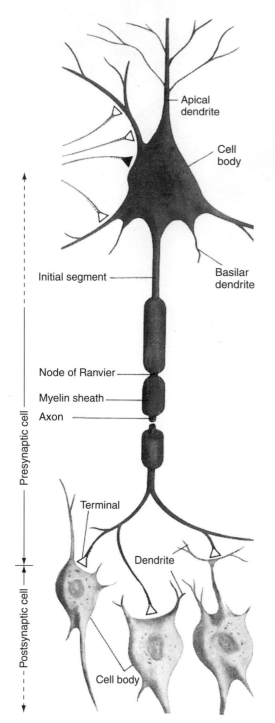

FIGURE 19-7 The Neuron. (From Kandel E, Schwartz J: *Principles in neural science,* ed 3, New York, 1991, Elsevier/North-Holland.)

metabolic and conductive activities. Oxygen and glucose are in continuous demand, since the brain has minimal storage capacity for either substrate. The brain's dependency on energy is so great that, without its nutrient supply, neuronal function fails within seconds of energy deprivation.

The need for oxygen and its rate of delivery depend on the degree of metabolic activity coupled with the rate of oxygen consumption. If metabolism is increased, as occurs with seizures, hyperthermia, or decerebrate posturing, oxy-

gen requirements increase. When cerebral metabolism is decreased, such as with coma or hypothermia, oxidative requirements are reduced.

CEREBRAL BLOOD FLOW

The normal brain receives 750 ml of blood, or 50 ml/100 g of brain tissue, per minute. The disproportionate flow is necessitated by the brain's incessant need for oxygen and glucose delivery. Cerebral perfusion pressure and intrinsic regulatory mechanisms influence and help maintain sufficient cerebral blood flow.

CEREBRAL PERFUSION PRESSURE. Cerebral perfusion pressure (CPP) is the pressure gradient in the brain—the difference between the incoming intra-arterial pressure and the outgoing intravenous pressure—that drives blood into the brain tissue.[13] Because pressure in the cerebral veins is the same as ICP, CPP can be determined by calculating the difference between the mean arterial blood pressure (MAP = 1/3 [systolic – diastolic] + diastolic) and ICP. The formula is CPP = MAP – ICP. For example, if the MAP is 90 and the ICP is 15, the CPP is 75. The normal range of cerebral perfusion in healthy adults is 50 to 150 mm Hg.

AUTOREGULATORY MECHANISMS. Pressure, or myogenic autoregulation, is the brain's ability to maintain a constant rate of blood flow over a wide range of perfusion pressures despite changes in arterial blood pressure and ICP. The cerebral arterioles or resistance vessels have an inherent self-regulatory (autoregulatory) mechanism contained within their muscular walls that allows them to change vessel diameter in response to changes in transmural pressure (Figure 19-8). As a result, an increase in arterial pressure causes vasoconstriction of the vessels and a decrease in arterial pressure causes vasodilation. This mechanism keeps cerebral blood flow essentially constant for a range of MAP from approximately 50 to 150 mm Hg. Intact autoregulation safeguards the brain from fluctuations in arterial pressure and ICP.

Several metabolic factors have a marked effect on cerebral blood flow, including partial pressure of arterial oxygen (Pao_2), pH, and partial pressure of arterial carbon dioxide ($Paco_2$). A decrease in Pao_2 below 50 mm Hg causes vasodilation, which increases cerebral flow and volume.[11] Extracellular reduction in pH (cerebral acidosis) caused by hypercarbia or acid byproducts of anaerobic cellular metabolism induces vascular dilation and increases cerebral flow and volume. Carbon dioxide (CO_2) is the most potent vasoactive agent known to cerebral vessels. An increase in CO_2 causes vasodilation, increasing cerebral flow and volume. Inversely, a decrease in CO_2 constricts the cerebral vessels, decreasing cerebral flow volume. Normocapnic individuals have about a 3% alteration in cerebral blood flow for every 1 mm Hg change in CO_2.[14]

Metabolic autoregulation causes the rate of cerebral blood flow to vary depending on neuronal metabolic activity. Gray matter, which contains the metabolically active

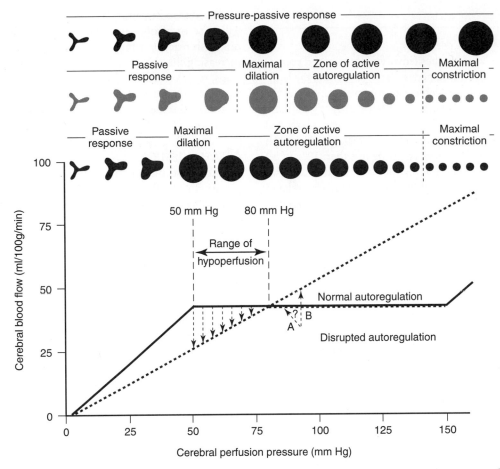

FIGURE 19-8 Normal pressure autoregulation and two possible degrees of disruption after severe traumatic brain injury. The relationship between CPP and cerebral blood flow (CBF) for these three states is represented by the graph. The status of the vascular system during the various stages of normal and disrupted autoregulation is represented by the *row of solid circles at the top* of the figure. The *bottom row of solid circles* represents intact autoregulation, the *middle row* corresponds to partially disrupted autoregulation (elevated lower breakpoint of active autoregulation), and the *top row* represents complete disruption of autoregulation (pressure-passive system). Cerebral blood volume (CBV) is represented by the *area of the circles.*

The solid line represents normal pressure autoregulation, with lower and upper breakpoints of active autoregulation at 50 and 150 mm Hg, respectively. Within this range, CBF is maintained at a stable value by varying the degree of vasoconstriction (zone of active autoregulation, *bottom row of circles*). A concomitant of this vasoconstriction is a progressive decrease in CBV as CPP is raised within the active range.

Disrupted pressure autoregulation is represented by the *dashed line*. The pressure-passive nature of complete disruption is illustrated by the straight curve *(line B)* where CBF is directly proportional to CPP. In a pressure-passive system, raising the CPP results in vasodilation, increased CBV, and elevated ICP throughout the range of CPP.

In the situation of partial disruption, the system is pressure-passive up to the reset breakpoint (80 mm Hg in this figure), after which pressure autoregulation occurs between 80 to 150 mm Hg *(line A)*. The situation of cerebrovascular response and CBV changes resembles the normal situation with the exception that the transformation from pressure-passive to active occurs at a higher breakpoint.

Note that in either pathologic case there is a range of hypoperfusion between 50 and 80 mm Hg, wherein ischemia may occur despite CPP values that appear to be "within normal limits." (Courtesy Randall M. Chesnut, MD.)

cell bodies, normally receives three to six times more flow than white matter. Cerebral blood flow (CBF) decreases globally in coma and increases regionally with activation or specific activities (e.g., hand movement, mental processing). In coma, both cerebral metabolism and blood flow are normally depressed. Even with a blood flow reduction of as much as 40%, neuronal integrity can still be maintained as long as metabolism is equally reduced.

Neurogenic factors and mediators released from the endothelium can also affect the cerebral vasculature. Neurogenic factors work in synergy with the pressure, chem-ical, and metabolic factors but seem to have a less significant impact on cerebral blood flow. Multiple neurogenic systems, such as the sympathetic and parasympathetic systems, innervate cerebral arteries and may exert a vasoactive effect on these vessels.[11,13] Stimuli such as shear stress and certain neurotransmitters can trigger the release of vasoactive mediators from the endothelium. Endothelin and thromboxane A_2 are examples of endothelium-derived mediators that cause vasoconstriction, whereas nitric oxide and prostacyclin dilate the cerebral vessels.[13]

ETIOLOGY

CAUSES AND RISK FACTORS

Transportation-related crashes (involving motor and recreational vehicles, bicycles, and pedestrians) constitute the leading cause of TBI. Motor vehicle occupants constitute the group that sustains brain injury most frequently.[1,3,8] Falls are the second leading cause of TBI, followed by firearm-related injuries and assaults not involving firearms. Although firearm-related brain injuries constitute less than 10% of all TBI, they are usually fatal, making them the leading cause of TBI deaths.[1,9,15] An estimated 90.4% of all firearm-related brain injuries result in death. Most of the firearm-related brain injuries are self-inflicted and slightly more than 25% result from intentional assaults by others.[1] Sports and recreational activities are another significant cause of TBI.[3]

Gender, age, ethnicity, and socioeconomic status can influence the risk of TBI. Males are twice as likely to sustain a TBI as females, and the death rate from TBI is 3.3 times higher in males than in females.[1] The highest incidence of TBI occurs among persons between 15 to 24 years and older than 75 years of age.[1] Falls are the most common cause of TBI in persons under 5 years and those older than 75 years, whereas motor vehicle crashes are the leading cause of TBI among adolescents and young adults.[1,16] African-Americans reportedly have the highest death rate from TBI, which is primarily due to the high rate of firearm-related deaths in this racial group.[1] Lower socioeconomic status may increase the risk of injury because of greater dependence on less safe housing and vehicles, higher likelihood of having a more physically demanding occupation, and increased exposure to personal violence.[3,17]

Certain medical conditions and behavior patterns may also increase risk of TBI. Persons with medical conditions that alter level of consciousness, impair neuromuscular function, decrease visual capacity, or result in seizures are more prone to injury and therefore are more likely to sustain TBI. Use of alcohol or other drugs can impair judgment, diminish reaction time, and reduce neuromuscular control, increasing the risk of TBI. Failure to employ safety precautions, such as not using occupant restraint systems, refusing to wear helmets when cycling or riding a motorcycle, or exceeding the speed limit, may also increase the likelihood of sustaining TBI.[3,18,19]

MECHANISM OF INJURY

SKULL DEFORMATION. Direct impact to the head can distort the skull's contour and injure the underlying brain tissue (Figure 19-9A). High-velocity blows to the head are most often associated with deformation injuries. Cranium indentation, fracture, or outward bowing can precipitate contusions or lacerations of the underlying brain tissue and intracranial hemorrhage.

ACCELERATION-DECELERATION INJURY. Acceleration-deceleration injuries occur when the head is thrown rapidly forward or backward, resulting in sudden alterations in movement of the skull and brain in a straight linear path (see Figure 19-9B).[11] Acceleration injuries occur when a moving object strikes the head (e.g., a baseball bat, fist, or hammer) and the skull and the brain are set in motion. Deceleration injuries occur when a head that is in motion hits a stationary object such as a wall or windshield, causing the skull to decelerate rapidly. The semisolid brain moves slower than the solid skull; therefore, the brain collides with the cranial surface and the rough bony prominences within the skull, causing brain tissue injury. Injury caused when the brain makes contact at the site of head impact is referred to as coup injury. Brain injury may also occur as the brain is thrown in the direction opposite the impact, causing collision with the contralateral skull surface; this is known as contrecoup injury.[20]

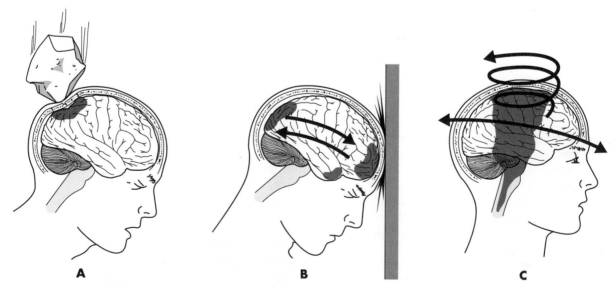

FIGURE 19-9 **Mechanisms of Injury. A,** Deformation; **B,** Acceleration-deceleration; **C,** Rotation.

ROTATION. Brain injury may also occur when acceleration or deceleration of the brain follows a nonlinear path, resulting in twisting or rotation of the brain within the skull (see Figure 19-9C). Rotation forces produce compressive, tensile, and shearing strains that cause distortion and injury of involved brain tissues and possible vascular disruption. Maximal stress from rotational forces is directed toward areas where tissues with different densities interface (e.g., between cerebral and fibrous tissue, between gray and white matter). The degree of injury from these rotational forces depends on the extent, rate, and direction of angular acceleration.[21] Motor vehicle crashes are a common cause of this type of injury.

PENETRATION. Penetrating brain injuries occur when a missile is projected, typically by a firearm, or an object is forced through the scalp and skull into the brain tissue. The penetrating object may cause brain laceration, contusion, hemorrhage, and subsequent cerebral edema and tissue necrosis. The severity of a penetrating injury depends on the size, shape, velocity, direction, and action of the foreign object that enters the brain, as well as the area of the brain involved.

A gunshot may create a single injury tract or, when a low-velocity missile is involved, it may ricochet within the cranial cavity and create multiple destructive missile tracts within the brain. A bullet projected through the skull and brain creates shock waves and a cavity that may expand to many times the bullet's diameter and then collapse, causing extensive local and remote tissue damage. High-velocity bullets that strike with much energy tend to cause greater tissue destruction from the temporary cavitation and shock waves than do low-velocity missiles, which wound primarily by direct tissue destruction.[12,22,23] Death associated with firearm-related TBI is the result of extensive structural damage and uncontrolled intracranial hypertension associated with intracranial hemorrhage and extensive cerebral edema. Patients may remain conscious immediately after gunshot wounds to the head, only to deteriorate rapidly with the onset of edema around the missile tract.

PATHOPHYSIOLOGY OF TRAUMATIC BRAIN INJURY
ASSOCIATED SCALP AND SKULL INJURIES

SCALP INJURIES. Injuries to the scalp may occur in isolation or may be associated with an underlying skull fracture or brain lesion. The scalp is very prone to profuse hemorrhage as a result of its rich vascular supply and the poor ability of the scalp vessels to vasoconstrict.[12] Blood may collect within the layers of the scalp (i.e., within the subcutaneous or subgaleal layers), or the scalp may be lacerated or avulsed, causing external hemorrhage. Subcutaneous and subgaleal hematomas generally resolve on their own without specific treatment.[11] Direct pressure over a scalp laceration is usually sufficient to decrease bleeding until a more thorough investigation of the site can be performed to ligate any major bleeding vessels and repair the wound. Before closure, scalp wounds should be cleansed well to prevent onset of infection. If the scalp is totally avulsed, vascular reanastomosis is required to restore circulation to the segment being replaced. Skin grafts or musculocutaneous flaps may be necessary to repair areas where the scalp is missing.

SKULL FRACTURES. Skull fractures are present in approximately half of all individuals with trauma-related intracranial anomalies.[24] Generally the more severe the brain injury, the greater likelihood that skull fracture is present.[25] Fractures of the cranial vault are three times more common than fractures of the base of the skull.[26] The degree of skull injury depends on the mass, characteristics (e.g., shape), velocity, momentum, and direction of the object that impacts the head and the thickness of the skull at the point of contact.[11]

A linear fracture is a simple break or crack in the continuity of the skull that dissects both the outer and inner table. Linear fractures are essentially benign and require no treatment. Even though direct treatment is not required, this type of injury warrants a computed tomography (CT) scan to rule out an underlying brain lesion. This is particularly true of linear fractures in the temporal and occipital regions, since arteries lying particularly close to the bones in these regions are susceptible to injury.

Depressed fractures are the result of the cranial bone being forced below the line of the normal skull contour. These fractures typically result from high-velocity contact sustained over a small surface area. The fragmented bone particles may be embedded into the brain tissue, resulting in cortical laceration and hemorrhage. A depressed skull fracture associated with a scalp laceration is called a compound or open fracture. These injuries are associated with an increased incidence of posttraumatic seizures and a high risk for intracranial infection.[25] Treatment of these fractures consists of debridement, evacuation of clots and bone fragments, elevation of the depressed bone, and repair of the lacerated dura.

Basilar skull fractures are located at the base of the cranium. The five bones that form the skull base are the occipital bone, the cribriform plate of the ethmoid bone, the orbital plate of the frontal bone, the sphenoid bone, and the petrous and squamous portions of the temporal bone (Figure 19-10). Basilar skull fractures are most common in the anterior and middle fossae. Fractures of the cranium base may be linear, compound, or depressed; most commonly they are linear fractures that extend downward into the base of the skull.[11] Basilar skull fractures can be difficult to detect with routine radiographic studies. Clinical examination findings typically identify their presence. Common symptoms of an anterior fossa fracture include periorbital ecchymosis (raccoon's eyes), rhinorrhea (CSF or blood draining from the nose), and conjunctival hemorrhage without evidence of direct ocular trauma. Physical findings common in the presence of a middle fossa fracture include

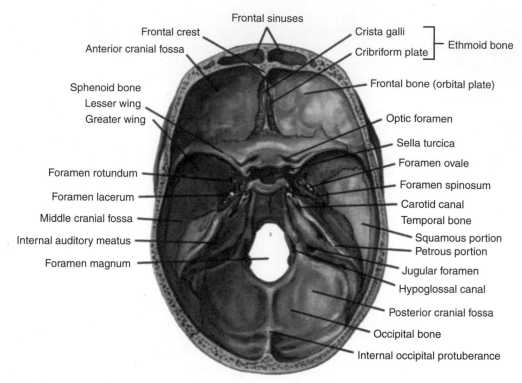

FIGURE 19-10 **Floor of Cranial Cavity with Anterior, Middle, and Posterior Cranial Fossae.** (From Lindsay DT: *Functional human anatomy*, St. Louis, 1996, Mosby, 151.)

mastoid ecchymosis (Battle's sign), otorrhea (CSF or blood from the ears), hemotympanum, facial nerve paralysis, and hearing loss.[11,27]

The presence of CSF otorrhea or rhinorrhea indicates not only that a basilar skull fracture exists but also that the dura is lacerated, which substantially increases the risk for intracranial infection. The CSF should be permitted to drain freely by only applying a loose sterile dressing over the drainage site. Medical management typically includes bed-rest and occasionally placement of a lumbar drain for a few days to relieve CSF and encourage closure of the dural laceration. Although 80% of CSF fluid leaks stop spontaneously, those that persist after 7 to 14 days may require dural repair. Use of prophylactic antibiotics in patients with basilar skull fractures to prevent intracranial infection remains controversial.

In addition to the possibility of intracranial infection, other potential complications associated with basilar skull fractures include cranial nerve injuries and cerebrovascular injuries. Because of their location at the base of the cranium, the cranial nerves are in jeopardy of direct injury when the basilar skull is fractured. The olfactory nerve is particularly vulnerable to fractures of the frontal bone, and the facial and auditory nerves are often injured in conjunction with temporal bone fractures.[11] Cerebral vessels that pass through or near the base of the skull, such as the internal carotid artery, may also be injured when the cranial base is fractured, causing hemorrhage, obstruction of vessel flow, or formation of aneurysms or fistulae.

TYPES OF BRAIN INJURIES

Brain injuries can be classified as focal or diffuse. Focal brain injuries occur in a localized region, and diffuse brain injuries involve a large generalized area. Many patients with TBI, especially severe injury, have a combination of focal and diffuse injuries.

FOCAL BRAIN INJURIES. Focal lesions cause local brain damage at the site of injury and eventually may expand to elevate intracranial pressure and compress, shift, and damage more remote areas of the brain. Focal brain injuries are associated with lateralizing or localized signs such as unilateral pupil dilation, hemiparesis, cranial nerve dysfunction, and speech deficit. These signs may help in localizing the site of injury. Focal injuries include cerebral contusion, subarachnoid hemorrhage, and epidural, subdural, and intracerebral hematomas.

Cerebral Contusions. Contusions are bruises of the brain tissue with associated hemorrhage and edema formation that may lead to subsequent tissue necrosis and infarction. These lesions constitute the most common type of brain injury. Contusions may occur beneath an area of skull deformation or secondary to acceleration-deceleration, rotation, or penetrating mechanisms of injury. Although contusions may occur anywhere in the brain, the most common sites are the frontal and temporal lobes.[26,28] Movement restrictions created by the cranial walls, dural folds, and irregular bony projections on the basilar skull

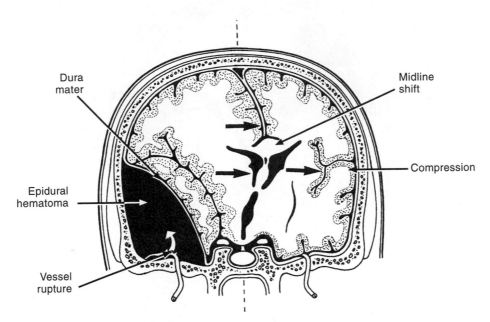

FIGURE 19-11 **Epidural Hematoma.**

surface in the frontotemporal regions explain the prevalence of brain injury in these areas. Contusions are most often multiple and frequently occur in association with other lesions.

Signs, symptoms, and severity of the injury depend on the site and extent of the contused brain. Isolated contusions generally do not produce immediate loss of consciousness. When coma is present, it is usually the result of an associated diffuse injury. Because the majority of contusions occur in the frontal and temporal lobes, patients usually present with localizing personality, behavior, motor, and speech deficits. Progressive edema formation can cause an abrupt mass effect, resulting in ICP elevation, brain compression, and eventually herniation.

Patients with brain contusions warrant close monitoring of their neurologic status to detect evidence of expanding mass effect and increased ICP. Special attention should be paid to patients with temporal lobe contusions, which may expand, causing brainstem compression without the warning of ICP elevation. The nurse must remain vigilant for subtle neurologic changes rather than focus solely on ICP values. Extensive contusions with mass effect require surgical evaluation as early as possible.

Epidural Hematoma. An epidural hematoma (EDH), also known as an extradural hematoma, is an accumulation of blood between the skull and dura mater (Figure 19-11). Epidural hematomas are most commonly located in the temporal region. These hematomas usually are associated with a linear fracture of the thin temporal bone that lacerates the underlying middle meningeal artery, causing an accumulation of blood in the extradural space. Less frequently, the source of hemorrhage is venous. As the hematoma accumulates, it strips the dura from the inner table of the skull and compresses the underlying brain. This local mass effect eventually causes brain herniation and can lead to death.

Signs and symptoms of EDH depend on the source and rate of blood accumulation. Clinical manifestations are usually seen within 6 hours of injury. The classic clinical presentation of a patient with an EDH is described as a period of unconsciousness, believed to occur because of a concussion, followed by a lucid period of variable length, after which the level of consciousness deteriorates as the hematoma expands. The lucid interval is not pathognomonic of EDH, since it reportedly occurs in as few as one third of patients with epidural hematomas.[29] Other common manifestations of an expanding hematoma are pupil abnormalities (e.g., unilateral and eventual bilateral pupil dilation and decreased reactivity to light), hemiparesis or hemiplegia, and flexion or extension posturing.

Any EDH creating a significant mass effect requires immediate surgical evacuation and ligation of bleeding vessels. If this is not possible and a neurologic emergency is in progress, a burr hole may be placed ipsilateral to the dilated pupil or contralateral to the motor deficits to evacuate the hematoma. Although significant brain injury may result from brain compression by the hematoma, there typically is little or no underlying primary brain damage.[25]

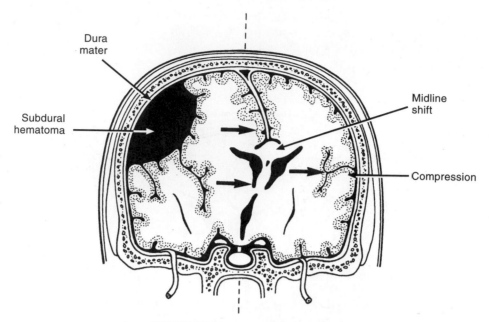

FIGURE 19-12 **Subdural Hematoma.**

Therefore, early diagnosis and treatment may yield a good prognosis.

Subdural Hematoma. Subdural hematoma (SDH) is a collection of blood beneath the dura mater and above the arachnoid layer of the meninges (Figure 19-12). These lesions are usually caused by rapid acceleration-deceleration mechanisms that tear veins bridging the subdural space, where they connect the brain's cortical surface to the dural sinuses.[25,27] Rupture of small cortical arteries may also be the source of subdural hemorrhage, which may extend over the entire hemisphere.

SDHs may be classified as acute, subacute, or chronic depending on the timing of symptom onset. Signs of acute SDHs become apparent within 48 hours after injury. These include indications of an expanding mass lesion, including pupil abnormalities, motor deficits, cranial nerve dysfunction, and altered level of consciousness. Patients who sustain a severe acute SDH are usually comatose on admission, with a Glasgow Coma Scale score below 8. Other patients with acute SDH of lesser severity may be conscious or experience a lucid period during their unconscious state.

Patients with acute SDHs have one of the highest reported mortality rates of all types of TBI, averaging around 50% to 60%.[30,31] High mortality associated with acute SDH is believed to be associated with the large amount of primary brain damage (i.e., contusion, laceration, and vascular disruption) underlying the clot, as well as the brain compression that occurs as the lesion expands. Mortality can be reduced substantially if timely surgical intervention takes place.[32]

Acute SDH creating a mass effect requires rapid clot evacuation, hemorrhage control, and resection of underlying nonviable brain. The operative procedure generally involves initial trephines or burr holes to locate the clot, followed by conversion to a craniotomy flap for optimal evacuation. A soft drain such as a Jackson-Pratt may be left in the subdural space for 24 to 48 hours. Postoperative complications include brain swelling with subsequent increased intracranial pressure, clot reaccumulation, delayed intracerebral hemorrhage, and seizures. Small acute SDHs producing no significant mass effect may not require surgical intervention and are absorbed spontaneously.

Subacute SDHs have similar but slower developing symptomatology than that seen with acute SDHs. Symptoms of a subacute SDH become apparent 2 days to 2 weeks after head injury. These symptoms tend to be more benign and the prognosis is generally better than with acute subdural hematoma. The improved prognosis is associated with less severe underlying brain contusion and the decreased likelihood that the patient will deteriorate to the point of brainstem compression. Like acute SDH, subacute SDH typically requires surgical evacuation.

Chronic SDHs do not demonstrate symptoms for at least 2 weeks after relatively low impact trauma. After the traumatic event, blood slowly fills the subdural space. Over the next 2 to 4 days, that blood congeals and becomes thick and jellylike. After about 2 weeks, the subdural clot begins to breakdown and becomes the consistency of thick oil. The clot then becomes more organized and encasing membranes surround the now xanthochromic fluid. Eventually the hematoma may calcify, ossify, or be absorbed. The hematoma increases in size slowly, most likely as a result of repeated small hemorrhages, causing more brain compression and eventual onset of symptoms. Signs and symptoms may include increasing headache, progressive decrease in level of consciousness, ataxia, seizures, incontinence, and eventually pupil and motor function alterations. Chronic SDHs are common among patients with brain atrophy, such as the elderly and chronic alcoholics.[11,25] Cerebral atrophy allows a significant volume of subdural blood to accumulate, possibly resulting in considerable brain distortion, before clinical evidence of neurologic decompensation becomes apparent. Surgical evacuation of the chronic subdural hematoma usually requires craniotomy to dissect the gelatinous or calcified clot and its encasing membranes. A subdural drain may be necessary for a short time after hematoma evacuation to prevent reaccumulation of fluid.

Intracerebral Hematoma. An intracerebral hematoma (ICH) is a well-defined clot located within the brain parenchyma (Figure 19-13). Most likely the bleeding originates from cerebral vessels that rupture at the time of injury.[25] Similar to contusions, most intracerebral hematomas occur in the frontal and temporal lobes and, less frequently, deep within the cerebral hemispheres or in the cerebellum.[11,33] Intracerebral hematomas may be multiple and associated with other lesions, particularly contusions. When an ICH is in continuity with a SDH, it is known as a burst lobe. Evidence of a single ICH after head trauma should cause health care providers to consider if a hypertensive bleed or an aneurysm rupture may be the source of the hemorrhage.[25]

Symptoms of intracerebral hematomas are similar to those of contusions, with the course and outcome dependent on the size and location of the hematoma. Signs and symptoms may include progressive deterioration in level of consciousness, headache, contralateral hemiplegia, and pupil abnormalities. Dominant hemispheric lesions are frequently associated with speech deficits.

ICHs are complicated by aggressive focal edema and increasing mass effect, which leads to elevations in intracranial pressure and further neurologic deterioration. Deterioration can occur as late as 7 to 10 days after injury, although the majority of neurologic deterioration typically occurs in the first 48 to 72 hours. Surgical evacuation of the ICH is not always beneficial or possible, and prognosis for these patients is poor.

Subarachnoid Hemorrhage. Subarachnoid hemorrhage (SAH) is bleeding between the arachnoid and pia mater layers of the meninges. This type of hemorrhage is seen commonly in patients with severe TBI. A preexisting vascular anomaly (i.e., cerebral aneurysm) needs to be ruled out as the source of SAH. Blood from the subarachnoid space or from a coexisting ICH may extend into the ventricular system of the brain.

Signs and symptoms of SAH include decreased level of consciousness, motor deficits (e.g., hemiparesis), pupil abnormalities, and evidence of meningeal irritation such as headache and nuchal rigidity. Potential complications of SAH include ICP elevation, posttraumatic hydrocephalus, and cerebral vasospasms. Patients demonstrating SAH on CT scan tend to have a significantly worse outcome than patients without evidence of SAH.[34-36] Treatment for SAH includes placement of an intraventricular catheter to drain

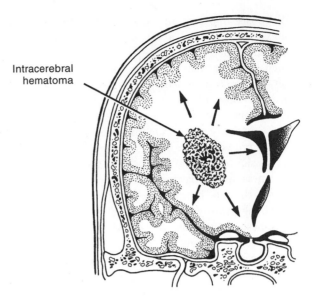

FIGURE 19-13 **Intracerebral Hematoma.**

bloody CSF, management of intracranial pressure if necessary, and possible vasospasm prophylaxis.

DIFFUSE BRAIN INJURY. Diffuse brain injuries include concussion and diffuse axonal injury (DAI). Unlike focal injury, which is well demarcated and usually can be seen on CT scan, diffuse injury involves microscopic damage to cells deep in the white matter and may be impossible to visualize with routine imaging modalities. Acceleration-deceleration and rotational forces, usually associated with motor vehicle crashes, are the most common mechanisms that cause diffuse injuries to the brain.[11,21] These forces create tension and compression on, and shearing of, nerve fibers, resulting in variable amounts of axonal damage. Although a portion of axons may be disrupted physically (axonotomy) at the time of injury, others may remain structurally intact but be functionally impaired. Axons that retain structural integrity but sustain internal damage and functional disruption may recover; experimental models suggest they may suffer delayed or secondary axonotomy hours after the injury.[25,37,38] The amount, severity, and location of axonal damage will determine the clinical severity and outcome of diffuse brain injury.[25,33,39] Diffuse brain injuries lie on a continuum of severity ranging from a concussion, with little or no sustained brain dysfunction, to diffuse axonal injury that may produce disabling deficits.[39]

Concussion. Concussion is a transient disturbance of neurologic function caused by rapid acceleration-deceleration or a sudden sharp blow to the head. Axonal shear, tension, or strain occur, resulting in conduction impedance and transient loss of function. No anatomic evidence of brain injury is evident on CT scan, although magnetic resonance spectroscopy, positron emission transaxial tomography (PET), and single-photon emission computed tomography (SPECT) scans are occasionally able to identify abnormalities after this type of axonal injury.[40-43]

The diagnosis is based on the patient's history, clinical neurologic findings, and a CT scan that rules out other intracranial lesions.

Concussions are categorized as mild or classic based on whether or not consciousness was lost. Mild concussion produces no loss of consciousness but causes a brief period of confusion and disorientation. Patients may or may not experience retrograde amnesia (inability to recall events just preceding the injury) or posttraumatic amnesia. A classic concussion involves a temporary loss of consciousness, usually lasting fewer than 5 minutes but for no longer than 6 hours. Retrograde or posttraumatic amnesia is always present, and the duration of posttraumatic amnesia is considered a good measure of the injury severity.[26] Signs and symptoms associated with both mild and classic concussions include headaches, dizziness, vertigo, nausea, visual disturbances, subtle personality changes, difficulty in concentration, poor memory, behavioral disorders, irritability, fatigue, increased anxiety, and insomnia. These manifestations, which can vary considerably among patients and may persist for days, weeks, or even months after the concussion, are collectively known as postconcussive syndrome (PCS). Persistence of these problems may be related to the degree of neuronal damage, emotional distress (e.g., anxiety or depression), motivational issues, cognitive factors, or a combination of these factors.[44-46]

Concussions are very common but, because of their apparently benign nature, medical attention is often not sought or there is a delay in seeking treatment for persistent symptoms. Patients who do seek medical care for an isolated concussion usually are not admitted to the hospital and receive no follow-up treatment at outpatient facilities. Patients and their families should receive information and supportive counseling on PCS, especially about the potential difficulties that may become evident after return to home, work, or school. Patients with persistent or disabling postconcussive symptoms may benefit from referral to a specialist (e.g., a neuropsychologist) for more extensive assessment and treatment. Early follow-up by skilled specialists (e.g., a nurse or clinical psychologist) to provide information, support, and advice related to PCS has been shown to reduce the severity of postconcussive symptoms and social disability 6 months after injury.[47] Patients should be advised to avoid activities (e.g., contact sports) that present a high risk for repeat concussion during their recovery period, since another concussion before resolution of the initial injury may cause cerebral autoregulatory dysfunction, progressive cerebral edema, neurologic deterioration, and possibly death.[48,49]

Diffuse Axonal Injury.   DAI is the more severe form of diffuse brain injury, which differs from concussion in degree rather than in type of brain injury. Tension, shearing, and compression strains created by rotational acceleration forces cause widespread axonal cytoskeletal and functional disruption in the cerebral hemispheres, the corpus callosum, the brainstem, and, less commonly, the cerebellum. Areas of the brain that are particularly susceptible to these shearing strains include the deep subcortical white matter throughout the hemispheres, the corpus callosum, and the dorsolateral aspect of the upper brainstem (Figure 19-14).[11,21,28] Severity and outcome depend on the extent and degree of structural damage.

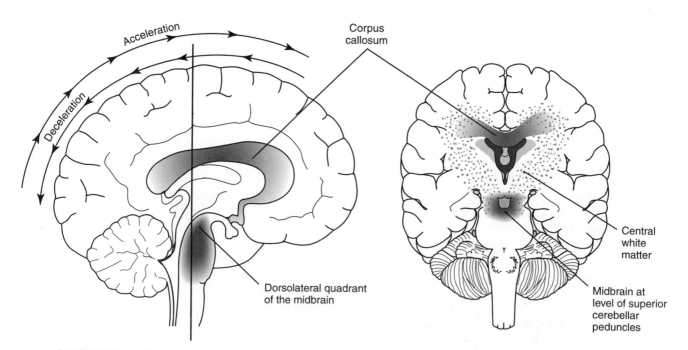

FIGURE 19-14 **Diffuse Axonal Injury.** Areas of the brain most often affected include the corpus callosum, the dorsolateral area of the upper brainstem adjacent to the superior cerebellar peduncles, and the parasagittal white matter.

The hallmark of DAI is immediate and prolonged coma lasting longer than 6 hours. The prolonged coma results from severe widespread damage to conducting white matter (axons), which disrupts the brain's reticular activating system. Because diffuse axonal injury is microscopic, the severity of injury is not determined radiographically but by the patient's clinical characteristics and duration of coma. Diffuse axonal injury can be classified as mild, moderate, or severe.

Mild diffuse axonal injury is associated with coma lasting 6 to 24 hours. Emergence from coma may be followed by prolonged periods of restlessness or stupor and mild to moderate memory impairment. Decerebrate or decorticate posturing is present transiently in approximately 30% of patients, but all patients with mild DAI generally follow commands within 24 hours.[38] Most patients with mild DAI recover and have relatively mild to moderate disabilities.[11,38]

Moderate diffuse axonal injury is more common and is distinguished by a coma lasting more than 24 hours. Confusion and long-lasting amnesia typically follow coma emergence. Most patients with moderate DAI move purposefully or withdraw from pain, but some may exhibit transient decorticate or decerebrate posturing. Mild to severe memory, behavioral, cognitive, and intellectual deficits usually persist.[38] The percentage of patients experiencing good outcomes after moderate DAI is lower and mortality is higher than seen with mild DAI.

Severe diffuse axonal injury results in extensive anatomic and functional disruption of axonal white matter fibers. Small tissue and vessel tears may appear on CT scan as small focal lesions typically located centrally in the corpus callosum and dorsolateral areas of the upper brainstem adjacent to the superior cerebellar peduncles.[25,28] Hemorrhagic lesions of the basal ganglia may also be visible on CT scan.[21] Because these lesions are small, they may be missed or difficult to realize on initial CT scan, and early resolution makes detection difficult in subsequent scans. Magnetic resonance imaging (MRI) is more effective than CT in visualizing small lesions associated with DAI, including lesions deep in the white matter of the cerebral hemispheres.[28,50] Diffuse cerebral edema may also be seen with severe diffuse axonal injury. Extensive neuronal loss eventually results in brain shrinkage. Follow-up CT scans typically show cerebral atrophy, as evidenced by enlarged sulci and ventricular dilation.

Clinically, severe DAI is manifested by deep prolonged coma lasting days to months. Signs of severe cerebral and brainstem dysfunction, including decorticate and decerebrate posturing, are often present on admission or develop with 24 hours of injury. Diencephalic involvement usually results in onset of tachycardia, systemic hypertension, hyperpyrexia (as high as 104° F to 105° F [40° C to 40.5° C]), and profuse diaphoresis (hyperhidrosis) covering the face and, less frequently, the neck and upper thorax. Manifestations of diencephalic involvement are often called neurosweats, diencephalic fits, or dysautonomia. Dien-cephalic signs and abnormal posturing usually resolve a few weeks after injury.[38]

Because of the extensive structural damage to neurons, severe DAI has a high mortality. The majority of severe DAI survivors typically have major residual disabilities. Major sequelae of severe DAI include deficits in cognition, memory, speech, sensorimotor function, and personality. Severe DAI is the most common cause of major disability and persistent vegetative state after TBI.[28,51]

PRIMARY VERSUS SECONDARY BRAIN INJURY

Injury to neurons can be classified as primary or secondary. Primary injury to the brain tissue or brain vasculature occurs immediately on impact of mechanical force. Once primary injury occurs, the damage is done and cannot be reversed. Because there is currently no direct treatment for primary brain injury, prevention remains the only effective intervention. Not all brain injury occurs immediately at the time of initial impact. Within seconds, hours, or days after primary brain injury a cascade of pathologic biochemical events is initiated within the injured or ischemic cells, leading to further cell death and secondary brain injury. Numerous neurologic and systemic complications after primary brain injury can also cause or exacerbate secondary brain injury.

CELLULAR RESPONSE TO INJURY. Injury, hypoxia, and ischemia are the fundamental initiators of the biochemical cascade that results in further cell death and secondary brain injury. Primary brain injury causes depolarization and halts aerobic metabolism and ATP production, quickly depleting the affected cells' energy stores, causing energy failure.[11,37] When the supply of oxygen or other nutrients is inadequate to meet cellular metabolic demands, ischemia results.

Cellular ischemia or hypoxia resulting from injury causes breakdown of the energy-dependent sodium-potassium and calcium pumps, with subsequent flux of sodium, water, and calcium into the cell and potassium out of the cell.[11,52] Influx of sodium and water causes cellular swelling. Acidosis is produced by conversion to anaerobic metabolism, as well as ionic fluxes. Disruption of intracellular calcium homeostasis is believed to be associated with many of the pathologic mechanisms that lead to further cell death, although the exact mechanisms by which calcium causes neurodegeneration remain poorly defined.[52] Calcium imbalance activates proteases (i.e., calpains) and lipases, which break down cytoskeletal proteins and lipids, respectively.[53] Phospholipases, which hydrolyze membrane phospholipids and result in accumulation of free fatty acids (e.g., arachidonic acid), are also activated by disruption of calcium homeostasis. Cellular energy failure and calcium imbalance may also trigger production of toxic eicosanoids (i.e., prostaglandins, leukotrienes and thromboxanes) and free radicals, which cause further cell damage.[11,52]

Free oxygen radicals (extremely reactive atoms or molecules that have an unpaired electron in their outermost orbit[52]) are generated in excess after injury, ischemia, or

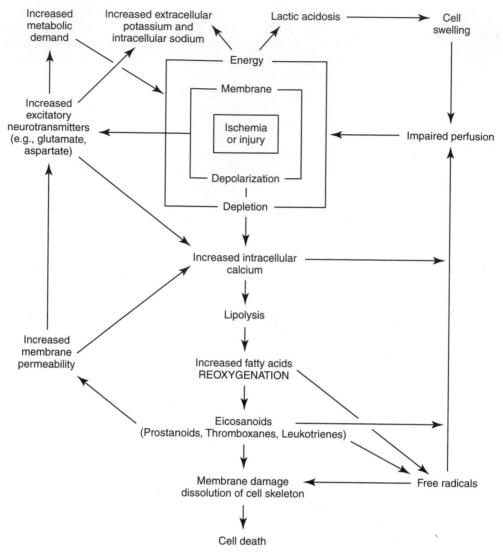

FIGURE 19-15 Some of the pathologic responses to brain injury or ischemia that lead to secondary cell death. (Modified from Teasdale G. The treatment of head trauma: implications for the future, *J Neurotrauma* 8(Suppl 1):S53, 1991.)

hypoxia and can overwhelm the cell's disposal mechanisms. Superoxide and hydroxyls are two potentially important free-radical species involved in the pathologic cascade initiated by brain injury or ischemia.[52] Oxygen-derived free radicals oxidize and eventually destroy the cell membrane by lipid peroxidation.[11,53]

Numerous neurotransmitter system alterations, such as increased excitatory neurotransmitter release, also accompany brain cell injury and energy failure. Excitatory neurotransmitters called excitatory amino acids (EAA), including glutamate and aspartate, are found in high amounts around injured and ischemic brain cells. Extracellular levels of glutamate, the major excitatory neurotransmitter, are particularly high surrounding focal brain contusions, when CPP falls below 70 mm Hg, and after ischemic events.[54-56] Excessive activation of glutamate receptors, namely, N-methyl-d-aspartate (NMDA) receptors, as well as non-NMDA receptors, triggers processes (e.g., opening of ion channels) that move sodium and calcium into the cell, increasing subsequent destructive processes.[11,52]

All these events disrupt cell structures and function. A vicious cycle is created as pathologic processes foster cellular changes that encourage further influx of extracellular ions, increased production of toxins, and eventually increased ischemia and cell death. One hypothesized scheme of how these pathophysiologic events interact to result in loss of cell integrity and neuronal death is shown in Figure 19-15. Refer to numerous reviews for a detailed description of the various processes involved in the secondary injury pathologic cascade.[37,52,53]

Definition of the intracellular pathologic cascade initiated by injury or ischemia has prompted numerous studies investigating pharmacologic agents that may target and halt these biochemical mechanisms and reduce secondary brain damage. Examples of agents that have been investigated extensively include oxygen-derived free-radical scavengers, antioxidants, excitatory amino acid antagonists, and ion-channel blockers.[57-61] Despite positive findings in numerous preliminary investigations, Phase III clinical trials have failed to identify an agent that demonstrates efficacy in the treatment of TBI. More research is needed to determine which therapy or combination of therapies is useful in improving outcomes and which targeted populations benefit from their use.

Other pathologic mechanisms that may contribute to delayed brain injury are currently being investigated. Apoptosis is a genetically regulated, active form of cell self-destruction that normally takes place during development and natural cell turnover but has also been identified as a likely contributor to cell death after TBI.[62,63] Apoptosis has distinct morphologic, biochemical, and pharmacologic features that differentiate it from the previously described necrotic cell death.[63] Although inflammatory responses initiated by TBI are believed to have some reparative functions, evidence suggests that these processes may also mediate delayed neuronal injury.[64-66] Speculation that TBI may be a neurodegenerative process has been fueled by evidence that links TBI to Alzheimer's disease (AD).[37,67] TBI has been identified as a risk factor for AD, and β-amyloid deposits, characteristic of AD, have been identified in the brain after injury.[53,68] Patients with the genotype predictive of AD onset, apolipoprotein E4, appear to have poorer outcomes after TBI.[69,70] As research provides greater clarity about the various mechanisms involved in brain injury and their interactions, new opportunities to better monitor and treat TBI can be developed.

OUTCOME OF THE INJURED NEURON: DEATH OR REPAIR AND REGENERATION.   Once a neuron has been injured, distinct morphologic changes occur throughout the cell in reaction to the injury. Proximal to the site of injury, the cell body undergoes chromatolysis. Chromatolytic changes result in cessation or impairment of cellular metabolism. Degenerative changes (Wallerian degeneration) occur distal to the zone of trauma and involve the axon and terminals, resulting in lost or impaired nerve conduction. Depending on the severity of injury, the neuron may progress in one of two directions:

1. When injury is extensive and the damage is irreversible, progressive degeneration of the nerve cell occurs, followed by glial cell phagocytosis. The loss of relatively few neurons may be insignificant, but substantial loss results in marked cortical atrophy as brain cells literally disappear. The degree of functional disability correlates with the extent of neuronal loss.

2. When neuronal injury is less extensive, the nerve cell has the potential to restore its functional capabilities. Neurons that are functionally disrupted but have not suffered irreversible mechanical damage are particularly vulnerable to secondary insults and must be provided an environment free of these complications for recovery to occur. Restoration of function is believed to occur through neuronal rearrangement of the injured neurons themselves or of neighboring uninjured neurons.

After neuronal injury, glial cells mobilize and proliferate at the injury site. They act as scavenger cells and aid in the healing process by phagocytizing cellular debris and toxic products left by injured degenerating neurons. This proliferation of glia at the zone of trauma also results in obstructive scar tissue formation, which can block the course of regenerating axons and prevent the formation of new synaptic connections.[71,72]

Neuronal Repair and Regeneration.   Injury to the neuron results in loss of synaptic contact or denervation. Generation of a new synapse (synaptogenesis) is essential for function to return. When synaptogenesis is accomplished, the injured nerve cell has regained the potential for receiving and transmitting messages. Structural and functional repair of the injured axons requires axonal regrowth or sprouting that extends in the appropriate direction through the lesion to reinnervate the specific target neurons. Regenerating axons must also reestablish functional electrophysiologic properties.[72] This process is thought to play a major role in promoting recovery of function after CNS injury.

Two types of axonal regeneration may occur after neuronal injury: spontaneous sprouting from the lesioned axon terminal and collateral sprouting. Spontaneous axonal regeneration occurs in response to neuronal injury or axotomy and consists of neurite outgrowths, or axonal sprouts, that extend from the proximal segment of the injured axon. The neurites eventually form axons and nerve terminals if an appropriate target cell membrane is contacted. Growth of neurites appears to be directed by protein substances called tropic, or nourishing, factors. Collateral sprouting involves the outgrowth of neurites from adjacent uninjured neurons in response to loss of neighboring injured neurons.[72] These new branches, or axon collaterals, establish new sites of innervation in close proximity to the denervated site. Whether collateral sprouting is always functional is still questionable, since sprouting fibers may arise from a different location and react in a different manner from the original nerve cell. Sprouting has been observed within a few days after injury and continues over several months. Sprouting appears to occur more readily in the immature nervous system, an observation that is reinforced by the fact that children make better recoveries than adults do after CNS injury. Mechanical barriers such as scar tissue formation, hematomas, and infection are thought to hamper sprouting by inhibiting or blocking effective regrowth or causing misdirected growth away from the target area.

Neuronal repair and axonal sprouting offer significant potential for CNS recovery and have become major foci of TBI research. Current research includes investigation of (1) neurotropic agents, such as nerve growth factor (NGF), to enhance sprouting by stimulating and guiding outgrowing neurites; (2) therapies to reduce scarring at the lesion site; (3) gene therapy to enhance neuronal growth; (4) hormones to promote neuronal regeneration; (5) reduction or neutralization of neurite growth inhibitors; (6) grafting of neural tissue or other growth supportive material at the lesion site; and (7) a combination of these approaches.[71-73]

FACTORS THAT CAUSE OR EXACERBATE SECONDARY BRAIN INJURY.

Any systemic or neurologic complication that compromises adequate oxygen and nutrient delivery to the brain's cells, causing hypoxia or ischemia, can cause or exacerbate the pathologic cascade of events that leads to secondary brain injury. Systemic complications that cause secondary brain insult include hypotension, hypoxia, hypercapnia, hypocapnia, hyperthermia, anemia, fluid and electrolyte imbalance, acid-base alterations, systemic inflammatory disorders, hypoglycemia, and hyperglycemia. Neurologic complications that may serve as causative factors for secondary brain injury include intracranial hypertension (any complications that may increase ICP, such as hydrocephalus, intracranial hemorrhage, cerebral edema), vasospasm, seizures, and intracranial infection.[12,74] Complications such as hyperthermia and seizures do not directly impair nutrient delivery, but they can elevate ICP and increase the brain's oxygen and nutrient requirements, making ischemia more likely. Although the healthy brain may sustain no permanent consequences with such complications, the injured brain is extremely vulnerable and can suffer irreversible damage with onset of such events.[75,76]

Complications that cause secondary brain injury are not uncommon after TBI and can contribute significantly to increased mortality and morbidity. Systemic hypotension and hypoxia are two of the most predominant causes of secondary brain injury.[77-82] When hypotension (systolic blood pressure <90 mm Hg [<95 mm Hg in study by Miller and Becker[82]]) or hypoxia (Pao_2 <60 mm Hg) is present upon patient admission to the hospital after TBI, mortality doubles.[80,82] Analysis of 717 patients with severe TBI from the Trauma Coma Data Bank found that systemic hypotension (systolic blood pressure <90 mm Hg), present in approximately 35% of patients, doubled mortality and significantly increased morbidity. Hypoxia (Pao_2 <60 mm Hg, apnea or cyanosis in the field) was present in almost 46% of hospital admissions with severe TBI but had a less detrimental effect on mortality and morbidity, especially if this complication was remedied in the prehospital setting.[81]

Factors that cause secondary brain injury continue to be problematic for the vast majority of patients with moderate or severe TBI during the critical care phase. The duration of hypotension, hypoxia, and pyrexia during this phase are significant predictors of mortality.[79] In one study, systemic hypotension, present in about one third of patients with severe TBI after 8 hours in an intensive care unit, tripled the rate of death or vegetative outcome.[80] Intracranial hypertension is another factor often associated with severe TBI that can lead to secondary brain damage and poorer patient outcomes.[77,82,83] One study indicated that an initial ICP reading of more than 20 mm Hg triples the risk of neurologic deterioration, resulting in higher mortality and morbidity.[83] Ischemia may be the single most important secondary event affecting outcome after severe TBI. Early ischemia correlates with poor outcome and early mortal-

ity.[75] Fortunately, complications that cause secondary brain injury are usually amenable to treatment.

INTRACRANIAL PRESSURE RESPONSE

ICP, the pressure within the cranial vault, has a normal range of 0 to 15 mm Hg. Sustained pressures greater than 15 mm Hg constitute increased intracranial pressure or intracranial hypertension.

The intracranial cavity is filled with three components: brain tissue, which makes up 80% of intracranial volume; blood, 10%; and CSF, 10%. The rigid skull restricts expansion of the intracranial contents. An increase in volume of any one of the components must be offset by a reciprocal decrease in one or both of the remaining components to maintain a constant total volume. If the volume begins to exceed the normal content within the skull, the pressure starts to rise within the enclosed compartment. This is the basis of the modified Monro-Kellie hypothesis, or box theory.

Intracranial volume can be increased after TBI for a number of reasons that add intracranial mass, blood, or CSF. Most mass or bulk is in the form of a blood clot or hematoma or, in the case of an associated infection, a superlative process. Brain volume is also increased when there is an excess of cerebral water (cerebral edema). Cerebral edema is a sequela that often accompanies tissue damage and can occur locally around an injured site, such as a contusion, or can be diffuse throughout the brain (DAI). Cerebral edema generally maximizes approximately 3 to 5 days after the primary TBI, but it may persist much longer or worsen if secondary brain insults occur.[11,25]

The two types of cerebral edema most commonly associated with TBI are vasogenic edema and cytotoxic edema. Vasogenic edema occurs when a breakdown in the blood-brain barrier allows osmotically active proteins and electrolytes (e.g., sodium) to move out of the intravascular space into the interstitial space, which in turn attracts fluid into the extracellular space. Cytotoxic edema occurs when cerebral tissues are deprived of adequate oxygen and glucose, resulting in cellular energy depletion and failure of the ATP-dependent sodium-potassium pump. Sodium-potassium pump failure permits accumulation of sodium and water inside the cell, eventually causing cell destruction.

An elevation in cerebral blood flow (hyperemia) may contribute to increased cerebral blood volume after TBI. Kelley et al found that hyperemic responses associated with intracranial hypertension were most prevalent in younger patients (under age 35) with more severe brain injuries, who may have had significant metabolic vasoreactivity and pressure autoregulation impairment.[84] Hypercarbia and hypoxemia can cause cerebral vasodilation, resulting in increased intracranial blood volume. Any obstruction of venous outflow, including simple neck flexion or rotation, also can also transiently contribute to increases in cerebral blood volume.

Cerebral spinal fluid volume can be increased after TBI as a result of obstruction of CSF flow or insufficient reabsorption. Blood in the subarachnoid space after brain injury can obstruct the arachnoid villi, impairing reabsorption of CSF. This is known as communicating hydrocephalus. Accumulation of CSF may also occur from noncommunicating hydrocephalus, in which CSF flow is obstructed by cerebral edema or hematoma, for example, preventing the CSF from reaching the villi to be reabsorbed.

Mechanisms to compensate for increased intracranial volume include cerebrovascular vasoconstriction, compression of the venous system, reduced CSF production, and movement of CSF to the more dispensable spinal subarachnoid space.[11] When these compensatory mechanisms are exhausted and volume continues to increase, a critical point is eventually reached, when the pressure within the skull starts to rise. When this occurs, even small increases in additional volume cause dramatic increases in ICP and brain tissue is displaced.

The relationship between pressure and volume within the skull is best illustrated with an ICP/volume curve, which depicts the exponential growth of ICP in response to volume increases (Figure 19-16). The flat portion of the curve represents the compensatory phase, when vascular and CSF volume displacement buffers increased intracranial volume. During this period, intracranial homeostasis is maintained. The inflection point indicates that the displaceable volume has been exhausted, and a sharp rise in ICP is precipitated by a minimal increase in volume. The brain's ability to yield under pressure is exceeded as volume and pressure rise. This decreased ability to yield is called decreased compliance, and the brain is said to be "tight" within the skull.

In the clinical setting, there are two established methods for estimating compliance—the pressure volume index (PVI) and the volume-pressure response. The PVI is determined by adding small volumes of saline or removing small volumes of CSF from the intracranial space and using a mathematical model to calculate the volume that would be needed to raise or decrease the ICP tenfold.[85] A large PVI indicates a soft, compliant brain, whereas a small PVI indicates a tight system with decreased compliance. The normal adult PVI is approximately 25 ml.[86] The volume-pressure response is determined by observing the ICP response after rapid addition of volume (usually 1 ml saline in 1 second) into the CSF space. A pressure increase of 5 mm Hg or greater indicates intracranial decompensation.[85] These invasive methods of estimating compliance are not routinely used in most institutions. Less invasive methods to serially measure intracranial compliance have been investigated.[85]

Patient observation may provide a rough approximation of brain compliance. Brain-injured patients who show substantial or sustained ICP elevations in response to changes in head position, turning, suctioning, or noxious stimulation should be suspected of having decreased compliance and should be treated accordingly. The patient's ICP waveform can also demonstrate specific morphologic changes that indicate poor intracranial compliance.[87] These alterations are described later in this chapter.

CEREBRAL HERNIATION. Cerebral herniation, the distortion and displacement of the brain from one intracranial compartment to another, eventually occurs if volume expansion continues within the intracranial cavity. Expanding mass lesions or hematomas are the primary causes of brain shift and herniation. The location of the lesion often determines the direction in which the brain is forcibly moved and consequently the type and pattern of herniation that occurs.

The majority of trauma-related mass lesions are hemispheric or supratentorial (located within the cerebral hemispheres above the tentorium). Three types of herniation are associated with supratentorial lesions: cingulate (or subfalcine), central, and uncal. All three herniation patterns can occur simultaneously as pressure gradients shift the brain laterally and eventually downward through the tentorium (Figure 19-17).

Cingulate herniation occurs when the cingulate gyrus (a convolution of brain tissue at the medial aspect of the hemispheres) is distorted beneath the falx cerebri (the dural fold that longitudinally separates the cerebral hemispheres). This type of herniation is fairly common and is caused by an expanding mass lesion in one cerebral hemisphere.[11] Intracranial volume displaced across the midline compresses the opposite side of the brain, eventually causing more edema and ischemia. Midline shift greater than 5 mm correlates with poorer patient outcome.[88]

Central transtentorial herniation consists of downward displacement of portions of the cerebral hemispheres, diencephalon, and midbrain through the tentorium into the posterior fossa (infratentorial compartment).[11] Clinical signs of central herniation are a reflection of compression and dysfunction of the displaced structures. These include impaired consciousness; initial contralateral hemiparesis

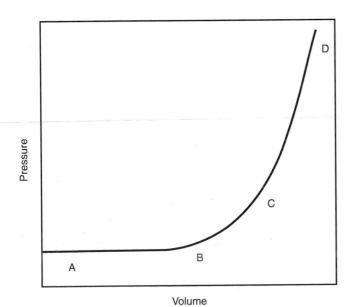

FIGURE 19-16 Pressure-Volume Curve. From *point A* to *point B*, ICP remains constant with addition of volume and brain compliance is high. At *point B* the brain compliance begins to change and ICP rises slightly. From *point B* to *point C*, compliance is low and ICP rises with increases in intracranial volume. From *point C* to *point D*, small increases in volume cause significant ICP elevations.

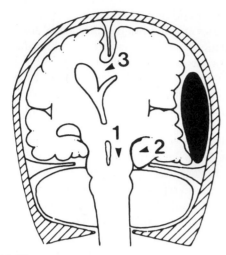

FIGURE 19-17 Brain Displacement From Supratentorial Hematoma. *1,* Central: downward displacement of brainstem. *2,* Transtentorial: herniation of the uncus of the temporal lobe into the tentorial notch. *3,* Cingulate: herniation of cingulate gyrus below the falx. (From Jennett B, Teasdale G: *Management of head injuries,* Philadelphia, 1982, FA Davis.)

evolving into bilateral motor dysfunction; small, equal, and reactive pupils progressing to be nonreactive and dilated; cranial nerve deficits; and vital sign alterations. Diffuse cerebral swelling, bilateral hemispheric lesions, and lesions in the midline have the greatest probability of causing central herniation.

Uncal or lateral transtentorial herniation occurs when the medial aspect of the temporal lobe (the uncus) is shifted toward the midline and then over the edge of the tentorium cerebelli. Like central herniation, uncal herniation causes life-threatening brainstem compression. Uncal herniation is most commonly associated with a unilateral hemispheric lesion, particularly epidural and subdural hematomas. Classic signs of uncal herniation include little early effect on consciousness followed by rapid deterioration, unilateral (usually ipsilateral) fixed and dilated pupils, contralateral (occasionally ipsilateral) hemiparesis or abnormal posturing, progressive dysfunction of cranial nerves III through XII, and vital sign alterations. Infratentorial or posterior fossa mass lesions are less common with TBI. When infratentorial lesions do occur, symptoms of brainstem compression typically are evident and death is imminent. Clinical signs of infratentorial herniation include coma, motor dysfunction, abnormal eye and pupil signs, vomiting, cranial nerve dysfunction, and vital sign alterations.

CEREBROVASCULAR RESPONSE

CEREBRAL PERFUSION PRESSURE AND AUTOREGULATION.
Increased ICP or decreased systemic blood pressure reduces cerebral perfusion pressure. With cerebrovascular autoregulation intact, the healthy brain can maintain a constant adequate cerebral blood flow despite these pressure changes unless the normal limits of CPP are exceeded. Once outside the normal CPP range, autoregulation is impaired, CBF becomes passively dependent on the CPP, and delivery of

metabolites is impaired (see Figure 19-8). Surpassing the upper CPP limit of 150 mm Hg causes passive vasodilation, which increases cerebral blood flow and fosters edema formation. When CPP falls below 50 mm Hg, cerebral blood flow is reduced. For example, if MAP is 60 mm Hg and ICP is 30 mm Hg, then CPP is only 30 mm Hg and the brain is being deprived of adequate blood flow. When MAP is 80 mm Hg and ICP is 80 mm Hg, there is no blood flow and brain death is imminent.

Cerebral autoregulation is typically lost or impaired regionally or globally after TBI. This occurs in patients with mild TBI, as well as those with more severe brain injury.[89,90] Failure of the pressure autoregulatory mechanism signifies that reactivity and responsivity of the resistance vessels are lost, so changes in blood pressure and cerebral perfusion pressure cause passive changes in cerebral blood flow (see Figure 19-8).[74] The nurse may recognize this loss of autoregulation when ICP fluctuations correlate with alterations in systemic blood pressure. When autoregulation is impaired, it is believed that the lower limit of CPP may reset itself so that the brain requires a minimal CPP of 70 or even 80 mm Hg to prevent cerebral blood flow compromise (see Figure 19-8).[13,74,89] Alterations in cerebral vascular autoregulation and cerebral blood flow after TBI are believed to contribute to the vulnerability of the injured brain to secondary insults.[13,75]

CEREBRAL BLOOD FLOW. TBI and subsequent alterations in CPP and autoregulation have a profound effect on cerebral blood flow, which greatly influences patient outcome. A number of researchers have attempted to define a pattern of blood flow changes that occur after TBI. Cerebral blood flow studies indicate that 45% of patients with severe TBI have subnormal CBF, possibly related to reductions in cerebral metabolic rate, and 55% demonstrate a hyperemic response at some time after injury.[91] Global or localized reductions in CBF to ischemic levels (less than 18 ml/100 g brain tissue/minute) were noted in approximately one third of patients within the first 6 hours after severe brain injury. Evidence of low cerebral blood flow had a strong correlation with poor outcome.[92] A number of studies suggest a triphasic pattern of cerebral blood flow change after TBI.[93] Within hours of injury, blood flow is lowest (reduced as much as 50%), then increases to reach or exceed normal levels for 4 to 5 days, and subsequently decreases again for up to 2 weeks after injury.[92-95] Phasic cerebral blood flow elevation within the first 5 days after moderate to severe brain injury has a strong correlation with functional recovery.[93] Optimal outcomes from TBI depend on prevention, early identification, and treatment of any factors that may compromise adequate CBF.

NEUROLOGIC ASSESSMENT

Once airway patency, effective ventilation, and adequate circulation have been ensured, the trauma patient's neurologic status can be assessed. Neurologic assessment after brain injury includes a comprehensive baseline evaluation followed by ongoing serial reassessment to detect changes in the patient's condition. As in all types of trauma, the assessment should include an initial injury database that provides information about the traumatic event and the probable mechanism of injury. A previous health history should be obtained from a family member or significant other as soon as possible. Neurologic assessment of the brain-injured patient also includes a clinical examination and analyses of data provided by monitoring devices and diagnostic studies.

CLINICAL NEUROLOGIC ASSESSMENT

The clinical neurologic examination is a basic yet incredibly important strategy used to assess and monitor the function of the injured brain. The nurse plays an essential role in performing a thorough baseline and serial follow-up neurologic examinations. The four components of the examination are of level of consciousness, motor and sensory function, eye and pupil signs, and vital signs.

LEVEL OF CONSCIOUSNESS.   Level of consciousness is the most sensitive indicator of brain injury. There are two components of consciousness: arousal and cognition or awareness. Arousal is mediated by the ascending reticular activating system, which carries sensory stimuli from the environment to the cortex, activating consciousness. This system is so diffuse that injury in just about any part of the brain can disrupt or compress the reticular activating system, resulting in alteration of consciousness (see Figure 19-5). Comatose states occur when there is pressure on the dense bundle of reticular fibers that course through the brainstem or when bilateral cortical injuries affect the reticular activating system.

Arousal is assessed by determining the type of stimulus necessary to arouse the patient. The patient may be alert and responsive as soon as he or she is approached. If the patient is not alert, the assessor should begin with the least noxious stimulus (i.e., voice) to attempt to elicit a response from the patient. If that is unsuccessful, slight shaking can be attempted, then peripheral pain or nail bed pressure, and finally central pain. Central pain can be applied by sternal rub or exerting pressure to the superior aspect of the periorbital region of the eye. Injuries to these specific areas obviously contraindicate application of pressure. The assessor should document what type of stimulus was necessary to elicit a response and what the patient's response was to the stimulus (e.g., moving away from or toward the stimulus, flexing, extending, giving no response). Words such as *lethargic, semicomatose,* and *obtunded* are vague and should not be used to document the patient's arousal. If the patient is arousable, awareness can also be assessed. This entails evaluation of the various cerebral cortical functions, such as memory; affect; ability to perform intellectual functions (e.g., calculations); and orientation to person, place, time, and situation.

Duration and depth of coma have been identified as markers of brain injury severity.[96] The longer the patient remains comatose, the greater likelihood of extensive severe neurologic dysfunction. Duration of coma tends to be longest in patients with severe diffuse axonal injury.

Other causes of altered level of consciousness need to be ruled out. Drug intoxication, shock, epilepsy, metabolic imbalances, infection, cerebral hypoxia, preexisting brain disease, and psychiatric disorders may alter the patient's level of consciousness. Even if underlying causes of altered mentation are identified, the examiner should still determine if the patient has sustained a brain injury.

MOTOR AND SENSORY FUNCTION.   Motor abnormalities in brain-injured patients are primarily related to upper motor neuron dysfunction (e.g., compression of the descending pyramidal or corticospinal pathways). Corticospinal fibers normally originate in the motor strip located in the posterior aspect of the frontal lobes and descend from the cortex through the cerebral hemispheres. They are arranged in bundles as they pass through the cerebral peduncle and into the brainstem. At the level of the medulla, the fibers decussate or cross over and terminate in the opposite side of the spinal cord. This crossing over at the medullar level results in contralateral motor dysfunction when TBI affects these tracts. Occasionally motor deficit is on the same side as the lesion. This occurs when the medial temporal lobe herniates, shifting the brainstem and compressing the contralateral cerebral peduncle against the tentorium. This ipsilateral motor deficit phenomenon is known as the Kernohan-Woltman notch phenomenon.[97]

The first aspect of motor function to be evaluated is the patient's response to stimuli applied to assess arousal. The best possible response is that the patient consistently follows motor commands (e.g., the patient is able to hold up two fingers or protrude the tongue). It is inappropriate to evaluate ability to follow commands by asking the patient to grasp your hand, because the primitive grasp reflex, typically absent after early childhood, may return in the adult with cortical damage. Patients may be unable to follow commands but are able to localize (i.e., find offending stimuli and attempt to remove it). Localization is indicative of cortical damage. Patients in a deeper state of unconsciousness are unable to reach for stimuli and instead withdraw or pull the limb away with a normal flexor movement (Figure 19-18). This type of flexion withdraw indicates extensive cortical damage. Considerably worse motor signs are abnormal flexion (decortication), abnormal extension (decerebration), and flaccid motor responses, which are typically associated with deep coma and significant brain dysfunction. Decortication or abnormal flexion (see Figure 19-18) indicates damage to the corticospinal tracts just above the brainstem within or near the cerebral hemispheres. Extension or decerebration (see Figure 19-18) typically indicates damage to the midbrain and upper pons regions of the brainstem. These abnormal decorticate and decerebrate postures may be elicited by noxious stimuli or

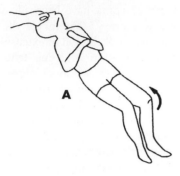

Bilateral Withdrawal
__(Flexion)__

Arms flexed
Legs flexed
Knees come up

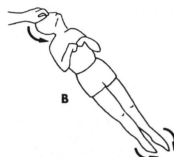

Bilateral Decortication
__(Abnormal Flexion)__

Arms flexed
Wrists flexed
Legs extended

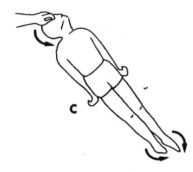

Bilateral Decerebration
__(Extension)__

Arms extended
External rotation of wrists
Legs extended
Internal rotation of feet

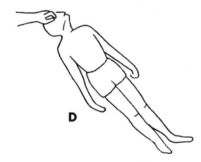

__Bilateral Flaccidity__

No response in any extremity to
noxious stimuli
Note: Spinal cord injury must be
ruled out as cause of flaccidity

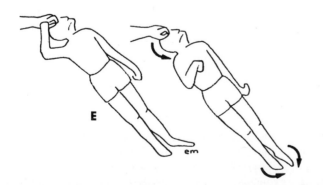

__Lateralization*__

Left Figure: Purposeful right side
          Decorticate left side
Right Figure: Decorticate right side
           Decerebrate left side

*These figures show how responses can
vary from limb to limb and stress the
importance of checking all
extremities for motor response.

FIGURE 19-18 **Abnormal Motor Responses. A,** Bilateral withdrawal (flexion). **B,** Bilateral decorticate posturing (abnormal flexion). **C,** Bilateral decerebrate posturing (extension). **D,** Bilateral flaccidity. **E,** Lateralization. (From Marshall SB et al: *Neuroscience critical care,* Philadelphia, 1990, WB Saunders, 102.)

may occur spontaneously. Posturing may be transient or prolonged. Flaccidity with lack of a motor response after resuscitative measures is associated with lower brainstem dysfunction (death is usually imminent) or high spinal cord injury. These motor responses may be observed on one or both sides of the body. Changes in motor responsiveness may occur as the patient's condition improves or deteriorates. In general, decortication is better than decerebration and decerebration is better than flaccidity. Deterioration in motor responsiveness indicates worsening neurologic status and warrants physician notification.

Corticospinal tract function in the awake patient is best evaluated by assessing motor tone and strength. Muscle tone is increased in patients with upper motor neuron lesions, such as brain injuries. Increased tone and spasticity can precipitate additional complications such as flexor extensor deformities and contractures in involved limbs.

Muscle strength is best evaluated by asking the awake patient to pull his or her limb in opposition to the examiner (resistance measures) or by testing hand grasp. It is important to compare both sides of the patient's body to determine equality of the strength. The best way to evaluate for early motor weakness is to ask the patient to extend his or her arms outward with palms up and eyes closed and observe for "pronator drift." This response is evident when the weak or hemiparetic limb begins to pronate and drift downward, indicating the presence of motor tract compression.

If the patient is unable to follow commands, the assessor should observe the strength and equality of spontaneous movement. If no spontaneous movement is present, a noxious stimulus is presented and motor response strength and equality of movement are evaluated. Awake and unconscious patients should also be evaluated for the presence of abnormal movements such as seizures, tics, and tremors. Location and description of any abnormal movements should be well documented and reported to the physician.

Cerebellar functions (namely, coordination and balance) can be assessed in the awake patient. Bedridden patients can have coordination and balance evaluated by having them close their eyes and touch their finger to their nose and move the heel of one foot down the opposite shin bilaterally.

The extensor plantar reflex (Babinski's reflex) is a pathologic response that is assessed by stroking the lateral sole of the foot from the heel upward and then medially across the ball. Great toe dorsiflexion and fanning of the other toes in response to this stimulus indicates dysfunction of the corticospinal tract anywhere between the cortex and the anterior horn cell of the spinal cord. Its presence does not localize dysfunction along this tract.

The range and complexity of the sensory examination are directed by the overall clinical status of the patient. If the patient is alert and stable, complete testing of sensory function is carried out. This includes evaluation of the patient's cortical discriminatory sensation (e.g., recognition of common objects and textures by touch, discrimination

between two points touched), which evaluates parietal lobe functions. The sensory examination is much more cursory if the patient is comatose or unable to communicate sensations. The practitioner makes note of the patient's response to painful or noxious stimuli applied to different areas of the body while performing different interventions (e.g., placing an intravenous catheter in an extremity).

CRANIAL NERVE DYSFUNCTION. Another aspect of the clinical neurologic examination involves evaluation of the cranial nerve functions. Table 19-2 lists the 12 pairs of cranial nerves, their site of origination, their function, and anticipated deficit in the presence of altered function. A helpful mnemonic for naming the nerves is "On Old Olympus Towering Tops, A Finn And German Vied At Hops," in which the first letter of each word represents the ordered sequence of nerves. With the exception of cranial nerves I and II, all other cranial nerves originate in and exit from the brainstem. Cranial nerve assessment not only gives the evaluator information regarding the function of a specific nerve or nerves being tested but also, and more importantly, provides vital information about general functioning of the brainstem itself. Cranial nerve dysfunction often provides substantive evidence of impending or actual brain herniation.

Cranial nerve injuries are not uncommon in patients with brain injury. Cranial nerve injuries can result from direct mechanical trauma; increased ICP; brain herniation; ischemia; and fractures of the face, temporal bone, or basilar skull. Documentation of cranial nerve dysfunction is an essential part of the nursing record so that deficits requiring specific nursing intervention (e.g., loss of the gag reflex, visual field deficits, or impaired hearing) receive appropriate attention and follow-up.

EYE AND PUPIL SIGNS. Pathologic eye and pupil findings can be ominous signs of neurologic deterioration, especially in the presence of concomitant motor and sensorial changes. Frequent eye and pupil checks are extremely important in nursing assessment of the brain-injured patient so that early and subtle signs of dysfunction can be recognized and reported immediately to the physician. A brief review of pupillary innervation and ocular motor function provides a better understanding of pathologic eye signs.

The oculomotor nerve (cranial nerve III) originates from the midbrain and performs the following functions: (1) moves the eyes medially (toward the nose), upward and inward, downward and outward, and upward and outward; (2) elevates the upper eye lid; and (3) enables ipsilateral parasympathetic pupil constriction. Compression of the nerve causes partial or complete loss of related functions. A patient with a complete third cranial nerve deficit has an eye that does not move in at least four of the six fields of gaze, an eyelid that droops, and a pupil that is dilated and does not react to light or accommodate.

Both parasympathetic and sympathetic fibers innervate

TABLE 19-2 Cranial Nerves: Origin, Function, and Anticipated Deficits

Cranial Nerve	Origin	Function	Anticipated Deficits
I Olfactory	Olfactory receptor cells in the nasal mucosa	Smell	Anosmia/hyposmia
II Optic	Retina	Vision	Visual loss • Blindness • Field cuts

III Oculomotor	Midbrain	Moves eyes (medially, upward and outward, upward and inward, downward and outward)
		Elevation of upper eyelid
		Pupil constriction (parasympathetic innervation)
			Loss of eye movements controlled by this nerve
			Eye "down and out"
			Diplopia (double vision)
			Ptosis
			Pupil:
			  Dilated
			  Unreactive to light

IV Trochlear	Midbrain	Moves eyes (downward and inward)	Impaired downward gaze Diplopia
V Trigeminal	Pons (with branches in the midbrain and medulla)	Sensation to face, scalp, nasal and oral cavities Corneal reflex Chewing muscles (masseter/temporalis)	Loss of sensation Absent blink/corneal reflex Muscle atrophy
VI Abducens	Pons	Moves eyes (laterally outward)	Eye fails to abduct Diplopia
VII Facial	Pons (with connections in the medulla)	Facial muscle movement Taste, anterior two thirds of tongue Lacrimation/salivation	Lower motor neuron • Ipsilateral weakness of the entire side of face • Loss of corneal reflex Upper motor neuron • Contralateral weakness of lower half of face Lost, delayed, or metallic taste Impaired/excessive salivation and lacrimation
VIII Acoustic (also known as vestibulocochlear)	Pons (with connections in the medulla)	Vestibular: balance Cochlear: hearing	Dizziness Hearing loss
IX Glossopharyngeal	Medulla	Taste, posterior third of tongue Sensation for posterior tongue, soft palate, and pharynx Pharyngeal reflex Sensation to carotid body and carotid sinus	Loss of taste in posterior third of tongue Loss of sensation in posterior tongue, soft palate, pharynx Loss of gag reflex Impaired blood pressure regulation
X Vagus	Medulla	Motor innervation to soft palate, pharynx, larynx Parasympathetic innervation of thoracic and abdominal viscera Conveys sensory impulses from pharynx, larynx, external auditory meatus, digestive tract, heart, and lungs	Unilateral lesion: Ipsilateral paralysis of soft palate, pharynx, and larynx • Impaired gag • Impaired palatal reflex • Dysphagia • Vocal cord impairment • Hoarseness Bilateral lesion: • Complete paralysis of pharynx and larynx • Death as a result of asphyxia • Vocal cord paralysis • Atonia of stomach and esophagus—vomiting • Dysphagia
XI Accessory (also known as spinal accessory)	Medulla	Sternocleidomastoid and trapezius muscle movement	Inability to shrug shoulders or rotate head

XII Hypoglossal	Medulla	Motor innervation of tongue musculature	Ipsilateral tongue paralysis and atrophy
			• Tongue deviation to side of lesion
			   • Dysphagia
			   • Dysarthria

the eye to control pupillary size. Parasympathetic influence provided by the oculomotor nerve normally causes pupillary constriction, but with midbrain or third cranial nerve compression the parasympathetic innervation is blocked and the sympathetic fibers act unopposed, causing pupillary dilation (mydriasis). Inversely, if sympathetic innervation is interrupted, the parasympathetic fibers act unopposed and the result is small (miotic) pupils. There are three nuclei or points of origin for sympathetic innervation—the hypothalamus, the pons, and the cervical ganglion. A lesion at any one of these sites can result in pupillary constriction. Because the cervical ganglion is an extracranial site, miosis of intracranial origin is due to pontine or diencephalic dysfunction. Pupil constriction secondary to hypothalamic or metabolic dysfunction retains reactivity to light, whereas pontine pupils are unreactive and fixed to light.

Pupils are assessed for shape, size, equality, and reactivity to light. Pupils are normally round and regularly shaped. An early warning sign that a pupil will progress to become fixed or dilated is a change in the shape from round to oval. An oval or irregularly shaped pupil is a significant sign of impending transtentorial herniation and third cranial nerve compression.[11] Irregularly shaped pupils may be seen when a patient has a history of an iridectomy or has sustained ocular trauma.

Depending on the amount of light that is entering the eye, pupils can vary in diameter from 1.5 to 8 mm but generally average about 3 mm. Variation in light should be taken into consideration when assessing pupil size. Consistency in room lighting is important when performing pupil assessments that are being compared. Variation in size is generally not significant as long as both pupils are the same diameter. Pupil inequality, asymmetry, or anisocoria can have pathologic importance. A small percentage of people (11%-16%) normally have anisocoria (inequality of the pupils), usually with a pupil size difference of less than 1 mm. Pupillary asymmetry of 1 mm or more is significant and often forewarns of subsequent progressive dilation. Unilateral pupil dilation is most commonly caused by third cranial nerve or midbrain compression but may also be due to seizures, direct orbital trauma, or optic nerve injury. Bilateral pupil dilation is seen after systemic or bilateral ophthalmic administration of mydriatics (e.g., scopolamine hydrobromide or atropine sulfate), instillation of cycloplegic agents, cerebral anoxia or ischemia, or amphetamine use.

Causes of pupillary miosis are pontine or hypothalamic dysfunction, cervical ganglion lesions, instillation of ophthalmic miotic agents, and use of opiates.

Pupillary reactivity to light is mediated by the parasympathetic fibers of the oculomotor nerve, which constrict the pupil when light stimulates the optic nerve (cranial nerve II). When the light is shined in one eye, both pupils should constrict. Constriction of the pupil with a direct light stimulus is the direct response to light, and the constriction of the contralateral pupil is the indirect response. Both the direct and the indirect response to light should be evaluated in both eyes. Absence of the direct response indicates either compression of the third cranial nerve or an optic nerve lesion resulting in blindness. An oculomotor nerve lesion causes loss of the direct and consensual light responses. A blind eye has no direct reaction to light, but the consensual response remains intact. Normal pupillary light response is brisk constriction of the pupils to light stimulus. Pupil size and reactivity normally decrease with age, especially in those older than age 60. The smaller the pupil, the smaller the amplitude of light reaction, so miotic pupils should be assessed carefully in a dim or darkened room to determine optimal reactivity. An early foreboding sign that a pupil will become unreactive to light is a delayed or sluggish response to light.

Abnormal pupils are important because of their localizing value. Table 19-3 describes the areas of brain dysfunction related to specific pupil abnormalities. Pupil reactivity also has prognostic importance and has been identified as an independent predictor of survival.[98] At least one nonreactive pupil noted just after resuscitation or at the time of the worst Glasgow Coma Scale score is prognostic of poorer neuropsychologic outcome at 1 year after severe TBI.[99]

Each eye is also evaluated to determine if the corneal reflex is intact. Testing this reflex entails lightly touching the cornea with a fine piece of cotton or a drop of saline and observing for a blink response. This reflex is mediated by two cranial nerves that both originate from the pons region of the brainstem: the trigeminal nerve (cranial nerve V), which provides sensation to the cornea, and the facial nerve (cranial nerve VII), which enables the eye to blink in response to the corneal stimulation. If the corneal reflex is absent, care must be taken to protect the eye from corneal abrasion or ulceration by instillation of ophthalmic lubricants, use of eye shields, or taping the eyelid closed.

TABLE 19-3   **Pupil Abnormalities Related to Specific Areas of Brain Dysfunction**

Pupil Findings	Related Brain Dysfunction
Fixed and dilated pupil	Ipsilateral oculomotor nerve (cranial nerve III) compression or injury
Bilateral fixed and dilated pupils	Severe brain anoxia and ischemia; bilateral cranial nerve III compression
Pinpoint, nonreactive pupils	Pons damage
Small, equal, reactive pupils	Bilateral diencephalic damage affecting sympathetic innervation originating from the hypothalmus; metabolic dysfunction
Nonreactive, midpositioned pupils	Midbrain damage

Prolonged contact lens use can weaken or obliterate the corneal reflex.

Other eye signs assessed as part of the clinical neurologic examination of the unconscious patient may include the oculovestibular and oculocephalic reflexes. Both these reflexes assess three cranial nerves: the oculomotor nerve (cranial nerve III), the abducens nerve (cranial nerve VI), and the acoustic nerve (cranial nerve VIII). Each of these nerves originates from a different portion of the brainstem. By evaluating these reflexes, the integrity of the three cranial nerves, as well as the brainstem, is assessed. However, the oculovestibular reflex is considered more sensitive than the oculocephalic reflex in assessing brainstem function.[11]

After ensuring that the tympanic membrane is intact, a physician can assess the oculovestibular or caloric reflex by injecting at least 20 ml of ice water into the patient's ear while holding the patient's eyes open. During the irrigation, if the reflex is intact, the eyes should deviate first slowly toward the irrigated ear and then rapidly away from the irrigated ear. The initial deviation toward the irrigated ear is controlled by the brainstem, and the rapid movement away from the irrigated ear is controlled by the cerebral cortex. Absence of eye movement toward the irrigated ear correlates strongly with brain death or a vegetative state. Preexisting disorders of the vestibular branch of the acoustic nerve (cranial nerve VIII), such as acoustic neuroma or Meniere's disease, cause an abnormal response to this test.[11]

The oculocephalic (doll's eye) reflex is examined by turning an unconscious patient's head rapidly from side to side while the eyes are held open and noting if the eyes move from side to side in the opposite direction of the head movement. If the eyes move asymmetrically or if there is no eye movement, the integrity of cranial nerves III, VI, or VIII or the brainstem (from which they originate) is disrupted. *Assessment of the doll's eye reflex is contraindicated if the cervical spine has not been cleared of possible injury.*

In addition to the oculomotor nerve, which controls four of the six fields of gaze, the abducens nerve (cranial nerve VI) controls the ability to look outward and the trochlear nerve (cranial nerve IV) enables the eye to look inward and downward. Eye movements are observed to determine if the eyes move together or conjugately. Gaze deviations, which are often associated with lesions in specific areas of the brain, should be noted. In awake and cooperative patients, more detailed assessment of extraocular movements, including gaze-holding and gaze-shifting capabilities, can be assessed when time permits.[100]

VITAL SIGNS.   Vital signs are monitored routinely in all critically ill neurotrauma patients to rapidly detect abnormalities that may cause unacceptable brain tissue hypoperfusion, hypoxemia, or hypercapnia. Abnormal respiratory patterns may have localizing value and serve as indicators of neurologic deterioration. Abnormal respiratory patterns and locations of associated anatomic lesions are described in Table 19-4. Progressively less effective patterns of respiration, characterized by slower rates and longer periods of apnea, are seen as the respiratory centers in the pons and medulla become dysfunctional. Abnormal respiratory patterns associated with brain injury may not be recognized in the patient on mechanical ventilation, and alterations in respirations may not be evident until death is imminent.[11] Many nonneurologic factors, such as anxiety, medications, acid-base imbalance, myocardial dysfunction, shock, pulmonary injuries, hypoxia, or hypercapnia, can also influence respiration.

Brain injury can cause variations in heart rate and rhythm, as well as blood pressure. Bradycardia, tachycardia, and various cardiac arrhythmias may be noted after brain injury. Onset of bradycardia and increased systolic blood pressure with a widening of the pulse pressure (Cushing's response) occurs as a late sign of intracranial hypertension and brain herniation, resulting in medullary compression and imminent death.[101] Other nonneurologic causes of heart rate and blood pressure change must also be considered. Change in blood pressure and heart rate without accompanying changes in level of consciousness indicates a nonneurologic etiology (e.g., shock).

TABLE 19-4	Respiratory Patterns Associated with Specific Areas of Brain Dysfunction	
Name	**Description**	**Neuroanatomic Brain Lesions**
Cheyne-Stokes respirations	Regular cycles of respirations that gradually increase in depth to hyperpnea and then decrease in depth to periods of apnea	Usually bilateral lesions deep within the cerebral hemispheres, diencephelon, or basal ganglia
Central neurogenic hyperventilation	Deep, rapid respirations	Midbrain, upper pons
Apneustic respirations	Prolonged inspiration followed by a 2- to 3-second pause, occasionally may alternate with an expiratory pause	Pons
Cluster respirations	Clusters of irregular breaths followed by an apneic period lasting a variable amount of time	Lower pons or upper medulla
Ataxic or Biots respirations	Irregular, unpredictable pattern of shallow and deep respirations and pauses	Medulla

Alterations in body temperature may indicate dysfunction of the hypothalamic temperature-regulating center caused by a lesion or intracranial hypertension. Patients can have rapid alterations in body temperature, with fluctuations between hyperthermic and hypothermic states. An infectious process should be ruled out as the cause of hyperthermia.

STANDARDIZED ASSESSMENT TOOLS

Standardized assessment tools are an important adjunct to the clinical neurologic examination. Many of these tools were created during clinical research to consistently document one or more aspects of the patient's initial condition, overall neurologic status, and response to therapy. Comparisons among groups of patients can be made using these tools. Two such tools widely used in the care of brain-injured patients are the Glasgow Coma Scale (GCS) and the Rancho Levels of Cognitive Functioning: a Clinical Case Management Tool.

GLASGOW COMA SCALE.   Brain injury severity and degree of consciousness are most commonly assessed with the internationally recognized Glasgow Coma Scale (Table 19-5).[102] The possible scores on this scale range from 3 to 15. The score is calculated by adding the values determined on three subscales: eye opening, motor response, and verbal response. The total GCS is used to classify the severity of brain injury. A score of 13 to 15 is defined as mild injury, a score of 9 to 12 is classified as moderate injury, and a score of 8 or less indicates severe head injury and coma. The lower the GCS score, the deeper the coma and the higher the associated mortality and morbidity. This tool enables clinicians and researchers to make meaningful comparisons among series of patients and more accurately predict brain injury outcome.

Eye Opening Assessment.   Assessment of eye opening, a measure of spontaneous arousal, is most accurate within the first 5 to 7 days after brain injury. Thereafter, many patients have return of the normal sleep-wake cycle, with associated spontaneous eye opening. Crediting such a patient with reflexive eye opening erroneously increases the GCS score by 3 points despite lack of true neurologic improvement. When the patient has facial trauma and periorbital edema that inhibit voluntary eye opening, the examiner should make note of the inability to evaluate eye opening by recording a "C" next to the total GCS score.[11]

Verbal Response Assessment.   Patients with brain injuries may require endotracheal intubation, preventing the practitioner from assessing the patient's verbal response. When scoring an intubated patient, a "T" should be placed next to the total GCS score, indicating that verbal response could not be evaluated because of endotracheal intubation.[11,26] It is controversial whether points should be awarded to the intubated patient who nods his or her head or displays other behaviors indicating that he or she would speak appropriately if able.

Motor Response Assessment.   The best motor response correlates most closely with outcome and provides greater interrater reliability. A patient who exhibits two different motor responses is always given credit for the best response, although it may be evident in only one extremity. Motor responses can be ambiguous, particularly when the initial flexor response becomes an extension response. Examiners need to be consistent in both the type of painful stimulus and limb position used to avoid influencing the patient's response.

Considerations and Limitations of the GCS.   Drug intoxication; aphasia; endotracheal intubation; periorbital swelling; and therapeutic use of sedatives, analgesics, and paralytic agents can all interfere with accurate interpretation of GCS responses. It is important therefore that the presence of these variables be noted when reporting the score. For infants and young children who are unable to produce normal adult verbal and motor responses, age-appropriate versions of the GCS must be used to accurately assess degree of coma and severity of brain injury (see Table 29-7).

Although the GCS has been the dominant scale used internationally and has demonstrated usefulness in predicting outcome from brain injury, there have been many criticisms of its relative insensitivity to significant clinical change in the early period and to the subtleties of neurologic function in recovering patients.[103,104] The developers of the GCS emphasize that it cannot stand alone in evaluating overall neurologic function in the acute period but must be

TABLE 19-5	**Glasgow Coma Scale**			
Eyes	Open	Spontaneously	4
		To verbal command	3
		To pain	2
		No response	1
Best motor response	To verbal command	Obeys	6
	To painful stimulus	Localizes pain	5
		Flexion—withdrawal	4
		Flexion—abnormal (decorticate rigidity)	3
		Extension (decerebrate rigidity)	2
		No response	1
Best verbal response		Oriented and converses	5
		Disoriented and converses	4
		Inappropriate words	3
		Incomprehensible sounds	2
		No response	1
Total			3-15

From Teasdale G, Jennett B: Assessment of coma and impaired consciousness: A practical scale. *Lancet* 2:81, 1974.

supplemented with neurologic evaluation of pupillary and eye movement and brainstem and cerebral function.[105] Critics have expressed concern over solely using the total GCS score versus considering patient performance on each subscale.[103,104] The reliability and validity of the GCS scale in comparison with other coma scales has also been questioned.[103]

OTHER COMA SCALES.   Many other scales have been proposed to replace or be used in conjunction with the GCS. Several scales incorporate indicators of brainstem function together with evaluation of consciousness and, in some cases, other aspects of neurologic function. Examples of such tools include the Glasgow-Pittsburgh Coma Scoring Method,[106] Glasgow-Liege Scale,[107] Innsbruck Coma Scale,[108,109] Comprehensive Level of Consciousness Scale,[110] Coma Recovery Scale,[111] Clinical Neurological Assessment Tool,[112] Edinburgh-2 Coma Scale,[113] and Reaction Level Scale (RLS85).[114,115]

RANCHO LOS AMIGOS LEVELS OF COGNITIVE FUNCTIONING SCALE.   The Rancho Levels of Cognitive Functioning: a Clinical Case Management Tool (Rancho Tool) is a multidisciplinary tool that places the patient in one of eight categories based on observed behavioral responses to stimuli and cognitive capabilities.[116] The scale has standardized evaluation criteria for each of the eight levels, which range from nonresponsive to independent functioning (Table 19-6). Patient cooperation is not necessary during scoring. Several disciplines frequently use the Rancho Tool, so implications for care based on the patient's level on the scale can be coordinated among speech, occupational, and physical therapy, as well as the nursing and physician staff. This scale is also useful when educating family members about the stages of recovery typically seen after TBI.[117] It can be used in all phases of brain injury management but is most widely used in the intermediate care and rehabilitative phases. It offers adequate reliability, but mixed findings regarding its validity have been documented.[117]

NEURODIAGNOSTICS AND MONITORING STRATEGIES

Alterations in results of the clinical neurologic examination typically trigger use of other neurodiagnostic and monitoring strategies. Information from these various diagnostic and monitoring strategies is used to guide therapeutic decision making and to evaluate the patient's response to treatment. Neurodiagnostics and monitoring employ tools that can evaluate the brain's anatomy, pressure, function, oxygenation, biochemical environment, blood supply, metabolism, and electrical activity.

RADIOGRAPHIC EVALUATION AND NEUROIMAGING.   Skull x-ray films have limited value in evaluating a patient with craniocerebral trauma. These films allow visualization of bony abnormalities (e.g., fractures), pneumocephalus, and metallic objects. Brain tissue and any uncalcified lesions cannot be seen on skull films.

Computed tomography (CT) scanning is the initial imaging modality of choice for the patient with craniocerebral trauma. It is recommended that a CT scanner be readily available at all times in trauma facilities that treat patients with moderate or severe TBI.[118] CT scanning provides anatomic localization for the majority of traumatic brain lesions. This diagnostic technique is very sensitive to the presence of intracranial hemorrhage and is superior to MRI in the diagnosis of acute hemorrhage, especially subarachnoid hemorrhage.[27,119,120] Space-occupying lesions, contusions, cerebral edema, and brain herniation are also identifiable. Most intracranial pathologic conditions, particularly injuries requiring surgical or medical intervention, can be diagnosed within several minutes of scanning, which has been a significant factor in reducing mortality from mass lesions. Follow-up CT scans are often indicated in patients with severe or moderate brain injuries to evaluate them for the evolution of pathologic brain conditions,[121] to diagnose possible causes of any neurologic deterioration, or to determine treatment effectiveness. CT scanning is safe, relatively inexpensive, and easy to perform, even on patients who require life support and stabilization devices. Trauma patients, who may require contrast for an abdominal CT scan, should have a head CT scan done first without contrast to avoid obscuring any intracranial pathologic conditions (e.g., an underlying contusion).[122] The base of the brain, brainstem, posterior fossa, and nonhemorrhagic lesions seen with diffuse axonal injury are usually difficult to visualize with CT scan.[27,28,50,122]

MRI uses the interaction of atomic nuclei in a static magnetic field that is moved about by radio waves to produce an excellent anatomic composite of the brain. The base of the brain, brainstem, posterior fossa, and gray and white matter differentiation are viewed better on MRI than CT scan. Compared with CT scanning, MRI is better able to detect the presence and extent of nonhemorrhagic lesions associated with diffuse axonal injury; extraaxial hematomas (i.e., subdural hematomas); and subacute or chronic intracranial hemorrhage.[27,28,50,120,122] Ischemic strokes tend to be evident sooner on MRI than on CT scan. MRI scanning may be indicated when CT findings do not explain the patient's neurologic deficits and the patient has no contraindications for the test to be performed.[120]

Several technical disadvantages to MRI hinder its use in the unstable brain-injured patient. The magnetic field is disrupted by ferrous containing compounds, which restricts the use of most ventilators and infusion pumps in the imaging suite. Radio frequency waves can interfere with unshielded monitoring devices. Patients with known or suspected metallic or electronic implants are prohibited from having an MRI. MRI is also more costly and takes longer to complete than CT.

Angiography may be indicated as an adjunct to CT when a vascular injury or disease is suspected. Angiography is

TABLE 19-6 The Rancho Levels of Cognitive Functioning: A Clinical Case Management Tool

Level of Function	Behavioral Characteristics
Level 1 No Response Total Assistance	• Complete absence of observable change in behavior when presented visual, auditory, tactile, proprioceptive, vestibular, or painful stimuli.
Level 2 Generalized Response Total Assistance	• Demonstrates generalized reflex response to painful stimuli. • Responds to repeated auditory stimuli with increased or decreased activity. • Responds to external stimuli with physiological changes, generalized gross body movement, and/or not purposeful vocalization. • Responses noted above may be same regardless of type and location of stimulation. • Responses may be significantly delayed.
Level 3 Localized Response Total Assistance	• Demonstrates withdrawal or vocalization to painful stimili. • Turns toward or away from auditory stimuli. • Blinks when strong light crosses visual field. • Follows moving object passed within visual field. • Responds to discomfort by pulling tubes or restraints. • Responds inconsistently to simple commands. • Responses directly related to type of stimulus. • May respond to some persons (especially family and friends) but not to others.
Level 4 Confused—Agitated Maximal Assistance	• Alert and in heightened state of activity. • Purposeful attempts to remove restraints or tubes or crawl out of bed. • May perform motor activities such as sitting, reaching and walking but without any apparent purpose or upon another's request. • Very brief and usually nonpurposeful moments of sustained alternatives and divided attention. • Absent short-term memory. • Absent goal directed, problem solving, self-monitoring behavior. • May cry out or scream out of proportion to stimulus even after its removal. • May exhibit aggressive or flight behavior. • Mood may swing from euphoric to hostile with no apparent relationship to enviromnental events. • Unable to cooperate with treatment efforts. • Verbalizations are frequently incoherent and/or inappropriate to activity or environment.

Level 5
Confused—
    Inappropriate—
    Non-Agitated
 	
Maximal Assistance
	• Alert, not agitated but may wander randomly or with a vague intention of going home.
	• May become agitated in response to external stimulation and/or lack of environmental structure.
	• Not oriented to person, place, or time.
	• Frequent brief periods, nonpurpseful sustained attention.
	• Severely impaired recent memory, with confusion of past and present in reaction to ongoing activity.
	• Absent goal directed, problem solving, self-monitoring behavior.
	• Often demonstrates inappropriate use of objects without external direction.
	• May be able to perform previously learned tasks when structure and cues provided.
	• Unable to learn new information.
	• Able to respond appropriately to simple commands fairly consistently with external structures and cues.
	• Responses to simple commands without external structure are random and nonpurposeful in relation to the command.
	• Able to converse on a social, automatic level for brief periods of time when provided external structure and cues.
	• Verbalizations about present events become inappropriate and confabulatory when external structure and cues are not provided.

From Hagen C, Malkmus D, Stenderup-Bowman K: Los Amigos Research and Education, Ranchos Los Amigos Hospital, Downey, Calif, 1973. Revised by Hagen CC, 1998.

Continued

TABLE 19-6   The Rancho Levels of Cognitive Functioning: A Clinical Case Management Tool—cont'd

Level of Function	Behavioral Characteristics
Level 6	
Confused— Appropriate	• Inconsistently oriented to person and place. • Able to attend to highly familiar tasks in non-distracting environment for 30 minutes with moderate redirection. • Remote memory has more depth and detail than recent memory. • Vague recognition of some staff.
Moderate Assistance	• Able to use assistive memory aide with Max assist. • Emerging awareness of appropriate response to self, family and basic needs. • Emerging goal directed behavior related to meeting personal needs. • Moderate assistance to problem solve barriers for task completion. • Supervised for old learning (e.g. self-care). • Shows carry over for relearned familiar tasks (e.g., self-care). • Maximum assistance for new learning with little or no carry over. • Unaware of impairments, disabilities, and safety risks. • Consistently follows simple directions. • Verbal expressions are appropriate in highly familiar and structured situations.
Level 7	
Automatic— Appropriate	• Consistently oriented to person and place, within highly familiar environments. Mod. assistance for orientation to time. • Able to attend to highly familiar tasks in a nondistraction environment for at least 30 minutes with minimal assistance to complete tasks.
Minimal Assistance For Routine	• Able to use assistive memory devices with minimal assistance. • Minimal supervision for new learning.
Daily Living Skills	• Demonstrates carry over of new learning. • Initiates and carries out steps to complete familiar personal and household routine but has shallow recall of what he/she has been doing. • Able to monitor accuracy and completeness of each step in routine personal and household ADLs and modify plan with minimum assistance. • Superficial awareness of his/her condition, but unaware of specific impairments and disabilities and the limits they place on his/her ability to safely, accurately and completely carry out his/her household, community, work, and leisure ADLs. • Minimal supervision for safety in routine home and community activities. • Unrealistic planning for the future. • Unable to think about consequences of a decision or action. • Overestimates abilities. • Unaware of others needs and feelings. • Oppositional/uncooperative. • Unable to recognize inappropriate social interaction behavior.
Level 8	
Purposeful and Appropriate	• Consistently oriented to person, place, and time. • Independently attends to and completes familiar tasks for 1 hour in a distracting environment. • Able to recall and integrate past and recent events.
Stand-by Assistance	• Uses assistive memory devices to recall daily schedule, "to do" lists and record critical information for later use with stand-by assistance. • Initiates and carries out steps to complete familiar personal, household, community, work, and leisure routines with stand-by assistance and can modify the plan when needed with minimal assistance. • Requires no assistance once new tasks/activities are learned. • Aware of and acknowledges impairments and disabilities when they interfere with task completion but requires stand-by assistance to take appropriate corrective action. • Thinks about consequences of a decision or action with minimal assistance. • Overestimates or underestimates abilities. • Acknowledges others needs and feelings and responds appropriately with minimal assistance. • Depressed. • Irritable. • Low frustration tolerance/easily angered. • Argumentative.

ADLs: Activities of daily living.

From Hagen C, Malkmus D, Stenderup-Bowman K: Los Amigos Research and Education, Ranchos Los Amigos Hospital, Downey, Calif, 1973. Revised by Hagen CC, 1998.

essential in identifying trauma-related vascular injuries, such as vessel laceration or occlusion and aneurysms. Posttraumatic vasospasms may also be detected. Interventions to treat or repair the injured or spasmodic vessels may be performed during angiography.

INTRACRANIAL PRESSURE MONITORING. Placement of an ICP monitor provides a direct measure of pressure within the intracranial vault. Presumptive evidence of increased pressure can be obtained from clinical examination and diagnostic study, but these findings may not be apparent until after a neurologic disaster has occurred and the brain has herniated. Compressed ventricles, absent or compressed cisterns, brain shift, and vessel displacement, as demonstrated on CT, MRI, or angiography, indirectly support the diagnosis of increased ICP but do not measure the actual level of pressure.

ICP monitoring is useful in the early detection of intracranial lesions that raise intracranial pressure and may cause brain herniation. ICP serves as a guide for therapy and enables the practitioner to determine the effectiveness or response to treatment provided. Monitoring ICP is particularly helpful in patients whose clinical neurologic examination is obviated by use of excessive analgesia, paralytic agents, or anesthesia.

ICP monitoring is indicated for patients with a GCS score less than 8 after resuscitation and an abnormal admission CT scan. Placement may also be indicated when patients have a GCS less than 8 with a normal CT scan if two or more of the following are noted on admission: (1) the patient is more than 40 years of age, (2) the patient has unilateral or bilateral abnormal posturing, or (3) the patient's systolic blood pressure is less than 90 mm Hg.[118] Physician discretion may also determine the use of ICP monitoring. For example, a patient with a GCS score greater than 8 and at risk for brain swelling or hematoma expansion may require prolonged surgery, during which neurologic status cannot be monitored by clinical examination.

Methods of Transducing Intracranial Pressure. Three systems are currently available for transducing the pressure from the intracranial vault to the bedside monitor: the hydraulic or fluid-filled system, the fiberoptic system, and the microstrain gauge system.

Fluid-Filled or Hydraulic System. A fluid-filled or hydraulic system employs a static fluid column to transmit pressure from within the intracranial vault to an external strain-gauge transducer, which then transmits the pressure reading to a bedside monitor. This system has been used extensively for monitoring hemodynamic, pulmonary, and intracranial parameters in critically ill patients. A fluid-filled system is inexpensive and can be recalibrated after insertion. Inherent problems of the fluid-filled system include possible entry of air bubbles, blood clots, brain tissue, or other debris within the tubing or transducer; kinked tubing; and loose connections. These problems can dampen or distort the ICP

waveform and give inaccurate measurements of ICP. Other components of the system—external transducers, stop cocks, flushing devices, and pressure tubing—are prone to technical malfunction. Even when the system is functioning well, inaccurate readings can result from changes in the patient's position that cause the transducer to come out of alignment with the external anatomic reference point corresponding to the intracranial location of the fluid-filled system's distal tip.

It is essential that the fluid-filled system be maintained optimally to reduce risk of complications and to ensure the accuracy of the ICP values. The system should be zeroed, balanced, and calibrated routinely, and the level of the transducer should be reassessed frequently to ensure that is in alignment with a predetermined and consistently used external landmark. When the waveform becomes dampened, the system should be inspected carefully for kinks; leaks; and the presence of air, tissue, blood clots, or other debris. If there is no improvement in the waveform after the transducer is zeroed and rebalanced, the physician should be notified. The system may need to be changed or irrigated according to institution protocol. Unlike hemodynamic pressure measuring systems, a bag of flush solution should not be hung, to prevent inadvertent infusion of a large volume of fluid into the cranial vault. Interruptions to the system should be minimized, and all connections should be kept snug to avoid risk of infection.[123,124]

Fiberoptic Transducer-Tipped Monitoring System. Fiberoptic ICP monitoring systems employ fiberoptics to transmit pressure from a transducer at the distal tip of the ICP monitoring catheter to a bedside monitor. This eliminates the need for a fluid-filled system and thus eliminates the problems inherent in a hydraulic system. Measurements are accurate and reliable compared with simultaneous standard intraventricular hydraulic system values, and the waveforms are excellent.[125] One problem in this system stems from the inability to recalibrate the transducer after implantation and the possibility of drift in measured pressures over time.[118] The fiberoptics within the system are relatively fragile, but breakage can be avoided by carefully securing the cables and avoiding kinks in the catheter. Securing the cables to the patient and not the bed is important to prevent dislodging the transducer.

Miniature Strain-Gauge Transducer-Tipped System. Miniature strain-gauge transducer-tipped systems use a miniature strain-gauge pressure sensor mounted in a titanium case at the tip of the flexible nylon tube to sense ICP. ICP is transmitted electronically from within the cranial vault to a bedside monitor. ICP values obtained with this system have been shown to be accurate and stable compared with measures obtained with fluid-filled external strain-gauge transducer systems.[126,127] Like the fiberoptic system, this system cannot be recalibrated after insertion. It also needs to be well secured, and kinking should be avoided to prevent catheter breakage or transducer dislodgment.

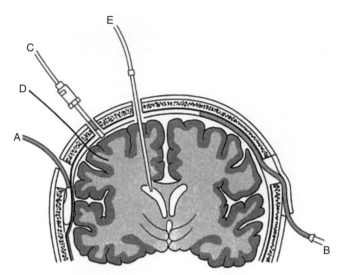

FIGURE 19-19 Coronal Section of Brain Showing Potential Sites for Placement of ICP Monitoring Devices. *A,* Epidural. *B,* Subdural. *C,* Subarachnoid. *D,* Intraparenchymal. *E,* Intraventricular. (From McNair ND: Intracranial pressure monitoring. In Clochesy JM, Breu C, Cardin S et al, editors: *Critical care nursing,* ed 2, Philadelphia, 1996, WB Saunders, 296.)

Location of ICP Monitoring Device. ICP can be monitored with a device placed in the epidural space, subdural/subarachnoid space, brain parenchyma, or intraventricular space (Figure 19-19). The advantages and disadvantages of each monitoring location are discussed next.

Epidural Monitoring. Epidural sensors are placed easily between the skull and the dura mater (Figure 19-19). Because the dura is not penetrated, this method is considered relatively noninvasive, reducing the risk of infection and inadvertent injury to the cerebral vasculature or brain tissue. CSF cannot be drained using this system. Because the sensor may not achieve perfect placement within the plane of the dura and it must detect pressure transmitted across the inelastic dura, the measurements obtained may be inaccurate and the waveform poor.[11,128] Epidural placement for ICP monitoring is the least desirable means of monitoring ICP when considering accuracy, stability, and ability to drain CSF.[118]

Subdural/Subarachnoid Monitoring. Fiberoptic, fluid-filled strain-gauge, or miniature strain-gauge systems can be used to monitor ICP in the subarachnoid or subdural space (see Figure 19-19). The fluid-filled system requires a hollow bolt or screw to be inserted via a twist drill through a hole in the skull and dura into the subarachnoid or subdural space. Fiberoptic and miniature strain-gauge systems can be placed with or without a bolt. Advantages of a subdural/subarachnoid monitoring system include the relative ease of insertion, even in the presence of small compressed ventricles; the lack of brain penetration; the reduced risk of infection compared with intraventricular monitoring; and the relative accuracy of the measurements. Disadvantages include possible hemorrhage or hematoma at the insertion site, risk of intracranial infection, and inability to withdraw

CSF. CSF leakage from the insertion site is a possible complication with subarachnoid placement. The skull must be intact for insertion and stabilization of a bolt. Protruding bolts may be inadvertently dislodged.

Intraparenchymal Monitoring. Fiberoptic or miniature strain-gauge systems can be inserted into the brain tissue to monitor intracranial pressure (see Figure 19-19). Intraparenchymal insertion is quick and easy even when the ventricles are small and compressed. There is little brain penetration, and the readings in this location tend to be accurate and yield a good waveform. Parenchymal transducer-tipped monitoring devices are considered second only to intraventricular monitoring techniques based on their accuracy, stability, and CSF drainage capability.[118] Intracranial infection and the possibility of hemorrhage or hematoma on insertion are potential complications associated with placement of ICP monitors into the brain tissue. CSF cannot be withdrawn with systems placed into the brain parenchyma.

Intraventricular Monitoring. Monitoring intraventricular pressure involves inserting a catheter through the scalp, skull, meninges, and brain tissue into the anterior horn of a lateral ventricle (see Figure 19-19). The ventricular method is used for both diagnostic and therapeutic purposes. It is considered the most accurate and reliable of all ICP monitoring techniques and serves as the reference standard.[118] Intraventricular catheter (IVC) placement also permits CSF removal for analysis, to evaluate brain compliance, or to reduce intracranial volume and decrease ICP.

A fluid-filled, fiberoptic, or miniature strain-gauge transducer system can be used to transmit the ICP from the intraventricular location. When a fluid-filled system is used, the transducer is leveled at a designated external anatomic landmark corresponding to the location of the foramen of Monro, where the IVC tip is situated. Suggested landmarks include the tragus of the ear, the outer canthus of the eye, the external auditory canal, and halfway between the outer canthus and tragus. Consistent use of the same landmark for leveling the transducer is most important.

CSF may be drained continuously or intermittently through the IVC. A continuous drainage system is open at all times to facilitate the automatic egress of CSF when ICP exceeds a predetermined level. The air-fluid interface of the CSF drip chamber is leveled a prescribed number of centimeters above the designated external landmark for the foramen of Monro. It is recommended that CSF drainage be briefly stopped to obtain an ICP measure, because pressure shunted through the outflow portal may cause artificially low readings.[129] The intermittent method of drainage is essentially a closed system that is opened periodically for drainage when the ICP rises to a specific level. The physician determines the ICP value that prompts drainage, as well as how much CSF should be drained or for how long the drainage should be continued. The nurse should monitor the amount and character of CSF drainage and notify the physician if there is a change in character of the drainage, a sudden increase in drainage, or a lack of CSF drainage.

Several disadvantages are associated with monitoring ICP in the intraventricular space. Insertion can be difficult, particularly when there is ventricular compression or shift. Each repeated attempt to pass the IVC through brain tissue increases the risk of brain or cerebrovascular injury. Excess drainage of CSF may cause ventricular collapse. This complication can be avoided by properly securing and positioning the CSF bag and draining the CSF only as prescribed. Intraventricular ICP monitoring has the highest risk of intracranial infection.[130,131] Timely removal of these invasive devices is important to reduce infection risk.[131] Nurses should ensure that the intraventricular drainage system remains closed, with all portals of entry covered, and that only strict aseptic technique is used if any interruption to the system is necessary.

Extracranial Monitoring.   Research is underway to develop a system capable of determining ICP or measuring ICP waveforms with a transducer applied to the outside of the head.[132,133] This type of monitoring system would virtually eliminate any substantial risks associated with the more invasive techniques used to monitor ICP and associated waveforms. The success of such a device could expand the use of ICP monitoring to the prehospital setting and outside the critical care environment.

Interpretation of ICP Data.   ICP monitoring provides a digital ICP measure. Various interventions and activities (e.g., suctioning, repositioning) may cause transient elevations in ICP. A sustained ICP elevation that reaches or exceeds 20 to 25 mm Hg typically indicates the need for therapeutic intervention. Although 20 to 25 mm Hg is the recommended upper threshold for ICP treatment,[118] thresholds may vary among institutions and between patients.

Several limitations should be considered when interpreting ICP. Pressure gradients may exist within different intracranial compartments, which may cause higher ICP in unmonitored compartments to go unnoticed. For example, ICP gradients between the supratentorial and infratentorial compartments and transient interhemispheric pressure gradients have been found in some patients after TBI.[134,135] Neurologic deterioration and CPP insufficiency can occur in the presence of normal ICP.[118] It is essential that nurses not focus solely on the ICP but also consider the neurologic examination, neuroimaging findings, and other monitored parameters when evaluating the patient's condition.

Waveforms displayed during ICP monitoring also require close evaluation. ICP waves originate from cerebrovascular pulsations and correlate with each cardiac systole and diastole. The upward sweep of the wave reflects cardiac systole followed by the diastolic slope and dicrotic notch (Figure 19-20). Natural fluctuations in the ICP pulse wave are caused by small amounts of blood added to the intracranial volume with each systolic ejection. This natural volume stress causes the ICP to increase by 2 mm Hg with each cardiac cycle. Slow oscillation of the entire waveform by a few millimeters of mercury may also be noted, and

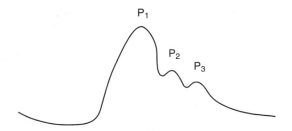

FIGURE 19-20 Components of the Intracranial Pressure Wave.

these fluctuations correlate with the changes in intrathoracic pressure that occur during respiration.

Each individual ICP wave usually has three peaks. First is P_1, the percussion wave, which has fairly consistent amplitude and is believed to originate from pulsations of the choroid plexus and intracranial arteries. P_2, the tidal wave, usually has a lower but more variable amplitude. P_3, the dicrotic wave, follows the dicrotic notch. The dicrotic wave has the lowest amplitude and usually tapers back to baseline.[11,87,136] Smaller peaks caused by retrograde venous pulsations may be noted after the initial three peaks.

As the ICP rises, so do the amplitudes of the various waveform components. P_2 wave elevations typically exceed the P_1 and P_3 wave elevations, causing a more rounded appearance of the pressure waveform as the brain's blood volume increases and compliance decreases (Figure 19-21). P_2 waves are thought to be a reflection of the brain's compensatory capacity or compliance. When the P_2 wave amplitude is equal to or greater than P_1, the brain's compliance is believed to be poor, indicating that the brain's ability to compensate for added volume is exhausted.[87,136]

Nurses should remain cognizant of ICP waveform configurations because evidence of poor brain compliance indicates that the patient is at significant risk for ICP elevations. This should be taken into consideration when preparing to perform interventions known to elevate ICP (e.g., suctioning, repositioning the patient). Advanced ICP waveform analysis (i.e., spectral analysis) techniques require further investigation as a means of dynamically assessing brain compliance.[87]

A dampened ICP waveform configuration usually indicates problems with the monitoring system, and every attempt should be made to troubleshoot the system and alleviate any problem if possible. If the problem cannot be resolved and an acceptable waveform regained, the physician should be notified. Never assume that the readings are accurate when the waveform is dampened.

In addition to the shape of each waveform, there are three patterns of collected waves or ICP trends: C waves, B waves, and A (plateau) waves. C waves are rapid (4-8 minute), rhythmic, and small in amplitude and correspond to changes in blood pressure (Figure 19-22). No clinical significance has been ascribed to C waves.

B waves are characterized by sharp, rhythmic elevations of variable amplitude. These elevations occur at 30-second to 2-minute intervals and may reach levels as high as 50 mm Hg (Figure 19-23). Elevations occur from a normal baseline

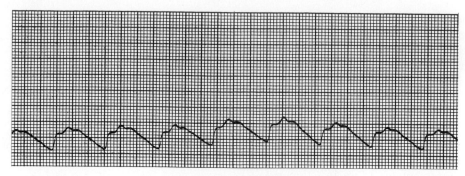

FIGURE 19-21 Intracranial pressure waveforms demonstrate elevation of the P_2 wave component.

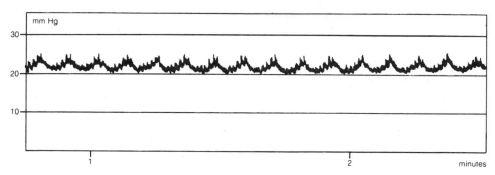

FIGURE 19-22 C Waves.

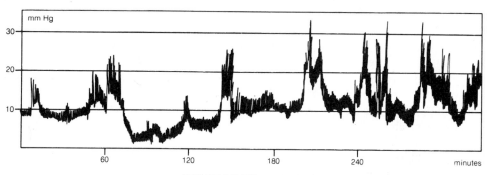

FIGURE 19-23 B Waves.

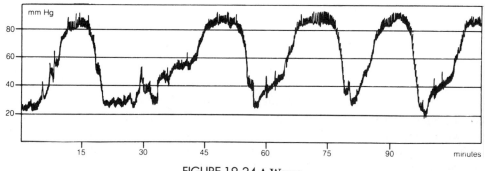

FIGURE 19-24 A Waves.

(<15 mm Hg) and are only a few seconds in duration. B waves have been associated with changes in respiration and may precede the more pathologic plateau or A waves, indicating decreasing intracranial compensation.

A, or plateau, waves are characterized by sustained elevations in ICP as high as 50 to 100 mm Hg, gener-ally lasting 5 to 20 minutes. These elevations, which typically arise from an elevated baseline, can happen at varying intervals and are precipitated by physiologic alterations or occur spontaneously (Figure 19-24). Dur-ing these elevations, CPP is compromised, possibly caus-ing cerebral ischemia and neurologic deterioration. The presence of A waves demands immediate intervention to control ICP.

CEREBRAL BLOOD FLOW.   Cerebral blood flow disturbances leading to cerebral ischemia may be the most significant pathophysiologic cause of disability or death following brain injury.[13,37,75,80,93] Unfortunately, there is no clinical symptom associated with reduced CBF until it decreases to a level that is unacceptably close to the threshold of permanent neuronal damage. Multiple techniques exist that enable practitioners to evaluate CBF directly or indirectly, although no one technique is perfect and without limitations or disadvantages.

Cerebral Perfusion Pressure.   Currently the most frequently used indirect index of global cerebral perfusion is cerebral perfusion pressure. CPP is easily monitored and calculated at the bedside by subtracting the ICP from the mean arterial blood pressure. Although normal CPP is considered to be 50 to 150 mm Hg, after TBI it is desirable to maintain the CPP above 70.[74,118]

CPP is not a specific or sensitive measure of CBF. CPP values may be within normal limits even though blood flow to the brain is inadequate. This measure also does not consider regional distribution of brain perfusion.

Clinicians have questioned if therapy for the patient with severe TBI should be targeted toward minimizing ICP or maximizing CPP and CBF. Rosner et al[137] advocated use of a management protocol that employed volume expansion, vasopressors, CSF drainage, and mannitol to maintain the CPP above 70 mm Hg, citing favorable patient outcomes using this treatment strategy. More recently, Robertson et al[138] compared a CBF-targeted protocol for TBI management, in which CPP was maintained higher than 70 mm Hg and $Paco_2$ was kept at approximately 35 torr, with an ICP-targeted protocol, in which CPP was maintained at more than 50 mm Hg and the $Paco_2$ was kept between 25 and 30 torr. Treatment was provided for ICP greater than 20 mm Hg or jugular venous oxygen saturation (Sjo_2) less than 50% for patients randomized to either treatment group. Results showed that the risk of brain ischemia more than doubled with the use of the ICP-targeted protocol and secondary ischemic insults could be prevented with the CBF-managed protocol. However, there was no difference in neurologic outcome. A fivefold increase in the frequency of acute respiratory distress syndrome (ARDS) was found in patients treated with the CBF-targeted protocol. Therefore, although ischemic insults were reduced substantially with the CBF-targeted protocol, the adverse effects of ARDS may offset these beneficial effects.[138] Juul et al,[83] in an analysis of prospectively collected data from 407 patients with severe brain injury, determined that ICP greater than 20 mm Hg was the most powerful predictor of neurologic deterioration. CPP, as long as it was maintained at more than 60 mm Hg, had no correlation with neurologic decompensation and little influence on outcome. As a result, it was recommended that treatment protocols for management of severe TBI focus on

maintaining the ICP at less than 20 mm Hg and maintaining the CPP at more than 60 mm Hg.[83] Desirable therapeutic endpoints for the patient with severe TBI should include minimizing ICP while ensuring adequate CPP. Other parameters, such as measures of CBF and oxygenation, may also serve as useful therapeutic guides.

Intermittent Measures of Cerebral Blood Flow: Clearance Techniques.   CBF can be quantified directly by measuring the brain's uptake and clearance of an inert, diffusible gas. These techniques are based on the principle that the rate of gas uptake and clearance is proportional to blood flow.[139] The first technique for accurately quantifying global CBF in humans used inspired nitric oxide as the measured gas tracer and analyzed arterial and jugular venous blood samples for nitric oxide concentrations.[140] Although this method of measuring CBF is relatively inexpensive and can be done repeatedly at the bedside, it largely has been replaced by the use of less invasive xenon clearance methods that provide information about regional CBF.

Xenon, a highly lipid-soluble gas that diffuses freely across the blood-brain barrier, can be used as a tracer to measure CBF using external detectors or a CT scan method. The noninvasive xenon technique employs radioactive xenon administered to the patient by inhalation or intravenous injection. Multiple detectors positioned outside the skull measure the washout of xenon to allow determination of global and regional CBF.[14] This technique is relatively low risk and can be performed at the bedside, making repeated follow-up measures fairly easy to obtain.[14,139] However, noninvasive xenon studies have poor resolution and therefore can be insensitive in detecting focal areas of low blood flow.[14,141] Flow to deep structures in the brain cannot be measured with this technique, and measures may be contaminated by extracerebral flow.[14,139,142]

Stable xenon CT is performed by having the patient inhale a mixture of oxygen and nonradioactive xenon while sequential CT scans are obtained for measurement of the uptake and clearance of the gas. From these measures, estimates of regional CBF are derived and correlated with the anatomic CT image.[14] This technique has better spatial resolution than the technique that uses external detectors, allowing identification of relatively small areas of brain ischemia.[139] Blood flow in and around lesions, on the cortical surface, and in deeper brain structures (e.g., brainstem, basal ganglia) can be evaluated with this method.[14,139] This technique requires transport of the patient to the CT suite, which may already be indicated for routine intracranial evaluation after brain injury. CBF results obtained using this technique may be affected significantly by artifact associated with patient movement during the test.[14,142] Xenon administered in a 30% concentration can cause cerebral vasodilation and augmentation of CBF, which may also affect study results.[143] Administration of relatively high-dose xenon for this test may produce sedation and possibly elevate ICP.[139,142]

Continuous Bedside Monitoring of Cortical Blood Flow.   Regional cerebral cortical blood flow can be monitored continuously using thermal diffusion flowmetry or laser Doppler flowmetry techniques. Thermal diffusion flowmetry uses a thermal diffusion sensor placed directly on the brain cortex, away from large blood vessels. Temperature differences between two plates on the sensor can be detected, providing an inverse measure proportional to CBF.[144] Laser Doppler flowmetry uses a low-power laser light positioned on the cortical surface or in the brain parenchyma to provide a nonquantitative measure of regional CBF.[142] Continuous measure of CBF can be used to detect regional ischemia, monitor autoregulation, provide prognostic insights, and serve as an additional guide for treatment of TBI.[145,146]

Continuous regional cerebral cortical blood flow monitoring devices evaluate blood flow in a small focal area and do not provide information about perfusion in other areas of the brain. Both devices are invasive and therefore carry the risk of intracranial infection and CSF leakage. Loss of probe contact with the cerebral cortex or contact with large surface vessels causes data to be unreliable. Artifacts caused by probe movement, strong external light, and change in hematocrit can also alter laser Doppler flowmetry measurements.[142,146]

Functional Neuroimaging.   Functional neuroimaging studies, including positron emission tomography and single-photon emission computed tomography, provide measures of regional cerebral blood flow and metabolic activity and thus furnish information about the functional status of brain tissue.[43,147] These measures can be useful in detecting cerebral blood flow and biochemical and physiologic abnormalities resulting from TBI.[147,148] PET or SPECT scans may detect areas of brain ischemia, metabolic abnormality, and cerebral dysfunction not identified on CT scan or MRI.[40,41,43,149,150] PET and SPECT findings may have some significance in determining prognosis after TBI.[150-152] A number of studies have used PET or SPECT studies to evaluate the effect of therapeutic interventions and to determine changes in cerebral blood flow and metabolism during recovery from TBI.[153-155]

Positron emission tomography employs positron-emitting radionuclide tracers, which are injected into the patient and then interact with electrons in the tissues to emit photons. Detectors positioned outside the head record the presence of photons, and a computer analyzes the data, calculating global and regional cerebral blood flow and providing quantitative measures of other physiologic functions such as regional variations in cerebral oxygen utilization and glucose metabolism.[11,141,144,147] PET scanning provides quantitative cross-sectional or three-dimensional images depicting cerebral blood flow and metabolism.[147] Production of the positron-emitting tracers for PET is complex and requires specialized instrumentation, which is expensive and available only at a limited number of centers in the United States. Therefore, PET lacks routine clinical utility, and it is currently employed primarily for research in patients with TBI.[11,43,148]

Single-photon emission computed tomography employs commercially available radionuclide tracers and a rotating gamma camera (available in many nuclear medicine departments) to measure and provide cross-sectional and three-dimensional images of regional cerebral blood flow distribution.[11,156] Because metabolism is directly linked to regional blood flow, this method provides an indirect measure of brain metabolism.[43,148]

Functional neuroimaging studies provide only a snapshot of cerebral blood flow and metabolic activity. Patients require transport to the scanner used for the imaging study, and the patient's head must remain immobilized during the test. Despite these limitations and disadvantages, the ability of functional neuroimaging studies to provide helpful information about the physiologic status of the injured brain is likely to expand their use in the future.

Transcranial Doppler Ultrasonography.   Transcranial Doppler (TCD) ultrasonography uses a low-frequency pulsed ultrasonic signal that penetrates thin areas of the cranium to measure the velocity and direction of blood flow in major intracranial arteries.[157,158] A TCD study cannot quantify blood flow to the brain, but its measures are affected by CBF. Flow velocity is proportional to CBF as long as the vessel diameter remains constant. If CBF remains constant, the flow velocity is inversely proportional to the cross-sectional area of the vessel being examined.[158,159] The pulsatility index, describing variability in maximal systolic and diastolic flow velocities, can be calculated to provide an indirect measure of the resistance in distal vessels.[157,158]

This noninvasive, portable technique can be performed repeatedly or continuously (with a Doppler probe secured to the patient's temporal scalp) to detect posttraumatic cerebral hemodynamic changes and complications (e.g., vasospasms, hyperemia, intracranial hypertension, cerebral blood flow reduction, and circulatory arrest).[157,158,160] TCD studies can also be used to evaluate the status of cerebral metabolic and vasomotor autoregulation and to confirm clinically diagnosed brain death.[158,160] This assessment strategy may also be valuable in detecting emboli or identifying vascular anomalies that may be premorbid or occurred as a result of cerebrovascular injury.[159] Despite its benefits, the measures are technician sensitive and the study is difficult to perform on uncooperative patients who do not remain still. Factors that influence CBF (e.g., $Paco_2$, hematocrit) must be considered when interpreting TCD findings.[157,158]

CEREBRAL OXYGENATION MEASURES

Jugular Venous Oxygen Saturation and Arteriojugular Oxygen Content Difference.   Jugular venous oxygen saturation (Sjo_2) is a measure of the hemoglobin's oxygen saturation level as the venous blood exits the brain.[160] Sjo_2 reflects the relative balance between cerebral oxygen consumption and cerebral oxygen delivery as long as hemoglobin levels, oxygen saturation of hemoglobin in the arterial blood (Sao$_2$), and the oxyhemoglobin dissociation curve remain constant.[161,162] Monitoring Sjo$_2$ allows detection of the coupling or uncoupling of oxygen delivery (flow) and oxygen use (metabolism) in the brain.[160]

Sjo$_2$ is monitored via a catheter placed into an internal jugular vein, with the catheter tip threaded retrograde to the jugular bulb, where the jugular vein curves before descending from the cranial vault. A lateral skull film typically is performed after insertion to confirm placement of the catheter tip in the jugular bulb.[141] Intermittent jugular venous blood samples can be obtained from the catheter and sent to the lab for Sjo$_2$ determination, or a fiberoptic oximetric catheter may be inserted into the jugular bulb to measure Sjo$_2$ continuously.

Sjo$_2$ values may be affected by factors that alter cerebral oxygen delivery or the cerebral metabolic rate of oxygen. When cerebral oxygen delivery is insufficient to meet the brain's metabolic need for oxygen, cerebral hypoxia and ischemia occur and Sjo$_2$ declines. Factors that reduce the oxygen supply to the brain include systemic hypoxemia, anemia, and reduced cerebral perfusion caused by intracranial hypertension, hypotension, hypovolemia, or cerebrovascular constriction.[160,163,164] Factors that increase the cerebral metabolic rate of oxygen include seizures, pain, agitation, and hyperthermia. Multiple studies have shown that Sjo$_2$ desaturations (<50% for longer than 10 minutes) are most common within the first 24 hours after TBI and are most prevalent in patients with low CBF.[161,165,166] Sjo$_2$ desaturations, particularly if the episodes are multiple or prolonged, are associated with poorer neurologic outcome after TBI.[165,166] If cerebral oxygen delivery exceeds the metabolic demand for oxygen in the brain, the Sjo$_2$ rises. Sjo$_2$ becomes elevated when there is an increased supply of oxygen to the brain, as seen with hyperemic or hyperoxia states, or when there is a decreased demand for oxygen

utilization in the brain, as seen with sedation, hypothermia, anesthesia, or large areas of cerebral infarction.[160] Elevations in Sjo$_2$ caused by reduction in the cerebral oxygen metabolism rate have been associated with poor outcomes.[161]

With knowledge of the Sao$_2$ and Sjo$_2$, the cerebral extraction of oxygen (CEo$_2$) can be calculated easily (Table 19-7).[140,160] A low CEo$_2$ indicates that the brain's supply of oxygen is greater than its demand for oxygen. A high CEo$_2$ indicates that the supply of oxygen is less than the demand.[160]

Arteriojugular venous oxygen content difference (Avjdo$_2$) is calculated by subtracting the content of jugular venous oxygen from the content of arterial oxygen (see Table 19-7). Although partial pressure of oxygen and oxygen saturation of the arterial and jugular venous blood are necessary to calculate this value, hemoglobin is a major determinant of content values. Avjdo$_2$ provides an indication of the overall balance between oxygen consumption and cerebral blood flow. Cerebral blood flow is normally coupled with cerebral metabolism, but this coupling is often lost after TBI.[162] Elevations in Avjdo$_2$ occur when the cerebral blood flow and oxygen delivery are inadequate for the brain's demand for oxygen.[160,167] When the Avjdo$_2$ is reduced, cerebral blood flow and oxygen delivery are excessive for the brain's demand for oxygen.[160,167] If the cerebral metabolic rate is constant, which is generally true in a stable patient with neurologic injury, then relative changes in cerebral blood flow can be reflected and are inversely proportional to changes in Avjdo$_2$.[167,168]

Direct and derived measures obtained by Sjo$_2$ monitoring can be extremely helpful in the clinical setting, where practitioners are striving to ensure adequate supply of oxygen to meet the brain's metabolic demand in an effort to reduce brain ischemia and secondary injury. When measures indicate that oxygen supply is excessive for the demand, as

TABLE 19-7 Sjo$_2$, CEo$_2$, and Avjdo$_2$ Normal Values and Calculations for Derived Parameters

Parameter	Source	Normal Values
Jugular venous oxygen saturation (Sjvo$_2$)	Directly measured	55% to 75% <50% for 10 min considered absolute desaturation
Cerebral extraction of oxygen (CEo$_2$)	Calculated Sao$_2$ − Sjo$_2$	24% to 40% <24% oxygen supply greater than demand >40% oxygen supply insufficient for demand
Arteriojugular venous difference of oxygen (Avjdo$_2$) = CMRo$_2$/CBF	Calculated Cao$_2$ − Cjvo$_2$ Cao$_2$ = (Sao$_2$ × 1.34 × Hb) + (Pao$_2$ × .0031) Cjvo$_2$ = (Sjo$_2$ × 1.34 × Hb) + (Pjvo$_2$ × .0031) OR (Sao$_2$ − Sjo$_2$) × 1.34 × Hb + (Pao$_2$ − Pjvo$_2$) × 0.0031 (Sometimes the relatively small contribution of dissolved oxygen in *italics* is ignored to simplify calculation and value is expressed in vol %)	4.5 to 8.5 ml/dl <4.5 ml/dl oxygen supply greater than demand >8.5 ml/dl oxygen supply insufficient for demand

Sao$_2$, oxygen saturation of hemoglobin in the arterial blood; Pao$_2$, Partial pressure of oxygen in arterial blood; Hb, hemoglobin; CMRo$_2$, Cerebral metabolic rate of oxygen; CBF, Cerebral blood flow; Sjo$_2$, jugular venous oxygen saturation; Pjvo$_2$, partial pressure of oxygen in jugular venous blood; Cao$_2$, arterial oxygen content; Cjvo$_2$, jugular venous oxygen content.

NOTE: Normal values and calculations reported in the literature vary.

noted by an elevation in Sjo_2 or a reduction in CEo_2 or $Avjdo_2$, consideration must be given to why the cerebral oxygen demand is low or why the cerebral supply of oxygen is excessive. Treatment of excessive systemic blood pressure may be warranted in this situation if hyperemia is present. Increasing ventilation to further reduce CO_2 would likely be best to treat intracranial hypertension if the patient is hyperemic.[160,162] When the oxygen supply is insufficient for the demand, as evidenced by a reduction in Sjo_2 or an elevation in the CEo_2 or $Avjdo_2$, consider why the demand for oxygen is excessive or why the supply is inadequate. It is important to ensure an adequate systemic blood pressure. Administering mannitol and possibly increasing the CO_2 may best manage intracranial hypertension.[160,162] In addition to serving as a guide for selecting the most appropriate ICP management and for optimal titration of therapeutic hyperventilation,[169] Sjo_2 monitoring parameters may assist the clinician in defining the patient's most desirable CPP and in detecting possible vasospasm or cerebral arteriovenous fistulas.[162] Cruz compared the outcomes of TBI patients with intracranial hypertension whose therapy was guided by CPP only with the outcomes of similar patients whose therapy was guided by CPP and CEo_2. The use of both CPP and CEo_2 as therapeutic guides yielded better outcomes, as measured by the Glasgow Outcome Scale.[170]

Potential complications of this monitoring technique include infection, vascular injury, and vascular thrombosis.[162,171] Nurses need to be proficient at maintaining, calibrating, and troubleshooting the oximetric monitoring system. Artifacts are common with oximetric Sjo_2 monitoring, which necessitates that any desaturation be verified by laboratory analysis of Sjo_2 from a jugular venous blood sample before therapeutic action.[172] Catheter malposition or breakage or formation of a fibrin clot on the tip of the catheter may make the readings inaccurate. Extracranial blood contamination can artificially elevate Sjo_2.[162]

This monitoring strategy provides a global view of cerebral oxygenation in the hemisphere where the catheter is placed. Therefore, relatively small focal areas of ischemia may go undetected, and Sjo_2 may not decline until significant cerebral ischemia has occurred.[160,162] The Sjo_2 reading may not reflect oxygenation changes in the hemisphere opposite where the catheter is placed.[162,173]

Near-Infrared Cerebral Spectroscopy. Another less invasive means of evaluating the regional cerebral oxygen saturation is near-infrared cerebral spectroscopy (NIRS). This technique requires application to the scalp of a probe emitting near-infrared light that penetrates the scalp and skull to measure the oxygen saturation of hemoglobin in the underlying cerebral tissue.[160,174,175] This noninvasive, portable device provides a continuous real-time measure of regional intracerebral oxygen saturation values.[141] Normal values have not been well defined for NIRS-monitored cerebral oxygen saturation, but changes in measured trends may indicate alterations in arterial oxygen saturation and cerebral perfusion.[160,174] NIRS measures are prone to distor-

tion by stray light interference, drift, temperature changes, probe disruption, contamination from extracranial tissue circulation, and movement artifacts.[141,174]

Partial Pressure of Brain Tissue Oxygen. Continuous partial pressure of brain tissue oxygen ($Pbro_2$) can be measured after introduction of an electrode into the brain parenchyma. This monitoring technique has been touted as a safe and reliable method for continuous measure of regional brain oxygen tension.[176-178] Brain Po_2 is a predictor of outcome, with the duration and depth of brain tissue hypoxia related to unfavorable patient outcome and death.[176,179-182] Although some researchers cite the $Pbro_2$ threshold for cerebral ischemia as less than 20 mm Hg, most report the critical value to be less than 10 mm Hg.[179,182-186] This technique shows much promise as a therapeutic guide for patients with severe TBI.[182]

BIOCHEMICAL MONITORING OF THE INJURED BRAIN. Brain injury and ischemia produce numerous biochemical byproducts, which can be measured in the brain tissue, cerebral spinal fluid, or blood. Examples of substrates that are elevated in response to brain tissue damage include creatinine kinase–BB,[187,188] neuron-specific enolase,[187,189-191] and protein S-100.[189-192] Measurement of these proteins in the serum or CSF may provide information about the extent or severity of primary TBI, detect ongoing secondary brain injury, and help predict the patient's outcome.[187] When a retrograde jugular venous catheter is in place, the arteriovenous difference in the levels of certain metabolites, such as glucose and lactate, can be measured to detect cerebral ischemia or metabolic dysfunction.[160] A multiparameter sensor is available that can be placed into the brain parenchyma to provide continuous measures of tissue pH and partial pressure of CO_2, in addition to $Pbro_2$ and brain temperature.[181]

The biochemical milieu of the brain tissue can be monitored directly at frequent intervals by use of cerebral microdialysis. Substances from local extracellular fluid diffuse across a semipermeable membrane into perfusate that flows continuously through a microdialysis probe inserted into brain tissue. Dialysate coming from the probe is sampled at regular intervals and analyzed to determine its chemical composition, which reflects that of the extracellular fluid.[193-195] The TBI-precipitated neurobiochemical events that are most commonly studied with microdialysis are energy metabolic disturbances (measuring pH, lactate, pyruvate, glucose, potassium, purines [e.g., adenosine, hypoxanthine]), transmitter release (measuring amino acids, catecholamines), excitotoxicity (measuring glutamate, aspartate), and oxidative stress (measuring ascorbate, glutathione, purines, uric acid oxidation products).[195,196] Monitoring the neurochemical composition of the brain may provide insight into the pathophysiologic mechanisms of TBI, the nature and magnitude of cerebral damage, the response to therapy, and the prognosis of the patient.[193] Currently, cerebral microdialysis is expensive and labor intense, limiting its use to research endeavors, but developments in this monitoring technique may expand its future clinical application.[141,193,194]

Proton magnetic resonance spectroscopy (^{1}H-MRS) allows noninvasive measurement of brain metabolites (e.g., *N*-acetylaspartate, choline, creatine, lactate) using standard MRI technology. This technology has the potential to detect neurochemical alterations associated with TBI.[42,197,198] ^{1}H-MRS may be particularly useful in revealing metabolite alterations associated with diffuse axonal injury that are not apparent on CT scan or routine MRI scanning.[197] ^{1}H-MRS findings may be valuable in evaluating the severity of brain injury and predicting patient outcomes.[42,197-199] MRS does have technical limitations that prohibit its use with certain patients, including those with metallic implants and those who cannot remain still during the test.

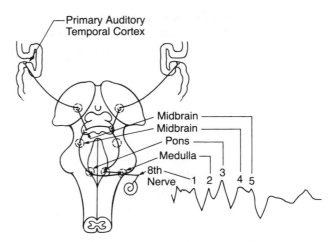

FIGURE 19-25 Neural Generator Sites of the Auditory Brainstem Response and Its Corresponding Waveform.

ELECTROPHYSIOLOGIC MONITORING

Electroencephalogram. Using scalp electrodes, an electroencephalogram (EEG) measures the spontaneous electrical activity of the superficial layers of the cerebral cortex.[141] Electroencephalographic findings are influenced by cerebral metabolism and brain ischemia or hypoxia but can also be affected by electrical, biologic, environmental, and movement artifacts, as well as drug therapy administered to the patient.[200] After TBI an EEG may be used to detect electrical abnormalities associated with insufficient cerebral perfusion, cortical dysfunction, or seizure activity.[200,201] The degree of cerebral suppression achieved with induction of a drug-induced (e.g., barbiturate) coma for the management of intracranial hypertension or status epilepticus may also be determined using electroencephalographic monitoring.[200] An EEG may be used as an adjunct study in the determination of brain death.[11]

A quantitative processed or computerized EEG, often used for continuous bedside electroencephalographic monitoring, employs a computer that manipulates and compresses data so that it can be displayed in a fashion that is easier to interpret by the bedside practitioner.[200,201] This technique allows evaluation of trend data and may enhance abnormalities difficult to visualize on a raw EEG, but it may miss short-lived events. In addition, results can be affected by numerous physiologic and technical variables.[200,202] Nurses caring for a patient on a continuous electroencephalographic monitor should be knowledgeable about the normal and abnormal EEG patterns and understand what action should be taken if abnormalities become apparent.

Sensory Evoked Potentials. Sensory evoked potentials (SEP) are small electrical responses generated along a sensory pathway in response to direct stimulation. Functional integrity of the visual, somatosensory, and auditory brainstem pathways can be assessed by evaluating the evoked potentials generated as each of these pathways is stimulated. SEPs are quantified by measuring the amplitude, latency from stimulation to response, and conduction time of the waveform generated by computer analysis of numerous evoked potentials (Figure 19-25).[11,202] Auditory brainstem evoked potentials, activated by tones and clicking sounds, and somatosensory evoked potentials, activated by peripheral nerve (e.g., median nerve) stimulation, are most commonly evaluated after severe TBI.[201,202] These studies can be performed at the bedside by a skilled technician, and results are relatively immune to the effects of sedatives (e.g., barbiturates).[201] SEPs, particularly somatosensory evoked potentials, correlate well with patient outcome after severe TBI.[201-204]

MANAGEMENT

PRIMARY PREVENTION

Because there is no treatment currently available to effectively treat primary brain injury, prevention of TBI is of utmost importance. The reduction in TBI deaths and hospitalizations is thought to be due in part to some success in primary prevention efforts.[1] Improvements in roadway safety measures, such as lowering speed limits and installing better lighting, roadside barriers, and traffic signage, contribute to reductions in motor vehicle crashes.[1,3] Improvements in motor vehicle safety (e.g., better ability to absorb impact, occupant restraint systems, and air bags) and helmet protection standards assist in decreasing the number and severity of injuries.[3,18] These safety initiatives, as well as legislative and educational efforts to increase the use of seat belts, child safety seats and helmets and to decrease the incidence of driving while intoxicated, have likely combined to reduce motor vehicle-related TBI deaths by an estimated 40% since 1980.[1,3] Despite this impressive decline in deaths caused by transportation-related TBI, the increase in violence-related TBI deaths indicates a need to focus strategies on curbing this problem.[1,9] Improved data about circumstances surrounding falls of the elderly will assist in establishing successful strategies to prevent falls among this high-risk population.[1] Development of new, more effective, targeted strategies to prevent TBI and continuation of initiatives with proven success require ongoing, standardized surveillance of TBI incidence, risk factors, causes, and outcomes.[1,6] Refer to Chapter 7 on injury prevention for more information on this topic.

GOALS OF CARE

There are three goals that nurses, together with the rest of the multidisciplinary health care team, strive to achieve when caring for a patient who has sustained TBI. First is to restore or maintain brain function, which focuses interventions on preventing secondary brain injury. The second goal is to prevent, recognize, and treat potential neurologic and systemic complications, which may increase mortality and morbidity and can exacerbate secondary brain injury. Third is to maintain and enhance the brain-injured patient's cognitive, psychosocial, and emotional processes. Achievement of these goals fosters optimal patient outcomes.

ESTABLISHED GUIDELINES AND RECOMMENDATIONS FOR CARE

Historically there has been much inconsistency among hospitals regarding which interventions should or should not be used to treat patients with TBI. In 1995 Ghajar et al published the results of a survey of 261 randomly selected hospitals that cared for patients with TBI about the care routinely provided. Considerable variations in treatment existed among the institutions. Based on these findings, it was suggested that research-based guidelines for treatment of TBI be established.[205] In response to this recommendation, the Brain Trauma Foundation, the American Association of Neurological Surgeons, and the Joint Section on Neurotrauma and Critical Care formed a panel of experts to compile research-based guidelines for management of severe TBI. "Guidelines for the Management of Severe Traumatic Brain Injury" was first published in 1995 and updated in 2000.[118] More recently, North American Neurosurgeons certified by the American Board of Neurosurgeons were asked about their views on the care of patients with severe TBI. The study revealed significant changes in the management of these patients, bringing clinical practice closer to the research-based guidelines.[206]

The Cochrane Collaboration performs similar research reviews on specific topics related to management of acute TBI. Conclusions based on these reviews are published on the Internet.[207]

RESUSCITATION PHASE

Priorities during resuscitation of the patient with severe TBI are the same as those used with any trauma patient—that is, ensuring adequate airway, breathing, and circulation. Accomplishing these priorities is essential so that adequate oxygen is delivered to the brain and secondary brain insult is avoided. The "Guidelines for Management of Severe Traumatic Brain Injury" reaffirm that the first priority of care should be a complete and rapid physiologic resuscitation focused on establishing airway, breathing, and circulation. It is recommended that no specific treatment for brain injury

be initiated unless symptoms of transtentorial herniation or progressive neurologic deterioration not attributed to an extracranial source are present.[118] If symptoms of neurologic deterioration become evident, intracranial hypertension is likely and aggressive treatment with therapeutic hyperventilation and mannitol should be considered.[118] Once these initial priorities are accomplished, efforts can be directed toward neurologic assessment and continued treatment of the TBI.

INJURY DATABASE. As with any trauma, an injury database is obtained from the prehospital care providers. The database includes all possible information about the onset and cause of injury, as well as significant events surrounding the traumatic event. It is important to document the patient's baseline neurologic status while in the field and changes that occur during transport to the hospital. Intervention provided by prehospital care providers and the patient's responses to these efforts should be noted.

AIRWAY PATENCY. Airway obstruction causing inadequate ventilation can transform a potentially mild brain injury into a severe brain injury as a result of hypoxia and hypercapnia. TBI sequelae put the patient at risk for airway obstruction. When level of consciousness decreases, the patient's upper airway relaxes and the tongue can prolapse back, obstructing the airway. Cough, swallow, and gag reflexes may be diminished or absent after TBI, which leaves the airway unprotected and puts the patient at increased risk for aspiration and secretion retention. Vomiting at or near the time of injury is common and increases the likelihood of aspiration. Associated maxillofacial injuries also heighten predisposition for airway obstruction.

When airway patency is impaired, interventions to alleviate the problem take precedence and are instituted immediately. Because 5% to 10% of patients with TBI also have spinal cord injury, great care must be taken to maintain cervical alignment during any attempt to reestablish airway patency.[208] The chin-lift or jaw-thrust maneuver may be all that is needed to open the airway. The oropharynx should be suctioned to clear secretions and foreign debris.

Care must be taken when using devices that assist in maintaining airway patency. Oral airways are used to prevent the tongue from falling back and occluding the airway, but they may stimulate coughing and gagging, thereby exacerbating intracranial hypertension. Nasopharyngeal airways are contraindicated in patients with suspected basilar skull fractures, because intracranial intubation may result. If protective airway reflexes are depressed or the patient's decreased level of consciousness impairs airway control, tracheal intubation is required. Patients with an initial GCS score of 8 or less generally require immediate endotracheal intubation. Intubation is usually performed in the resuscitation phase using an endotracheal tube, preferably via the orotracheal route, while maintaining inline manual cervical immobilization.[74] Cricothyroidotomy or tracheostomy may be necessary to establish an airway if an endotracheal tube cannot be placed. Sedative or paralytic agents are frequently required to facilitate intubation. Short-acting or easily reversible agents are preferable. If possible, a rapid neurologic assessment should be performed before administration of these pharmacologic agents.

Once a patent airway is established, measures to maintain a clear airway must be initiated. Endotracheal suctioning is provided as needed. Bronchoscopy may be used to clear secretions, vomitus, blood, teeth, and other debris from the airway. Gastric decompression using an orogastric tube in addition to early intubation greatly reduces the risk of aspiration.

SUPPLEMENTAL OXYGEN. Supplemental oxygen should be administered to ensure adequate cerebral oxygen supply. The initial fraction of inspired oxygen (Fio_2) delivered to patients with severe TBI is usually 100%.[74] Once an arterial blood gas reading can be obtained, the Fio_2 can be adjusted to maintain the Pao_2 above 70 mm Hg, optimally around 100 mm Hg.[11,26] Unnecessary excessive oxygen administration should be avoided. Pulse oximetry can be used to titrate oxygen administration to maintain a desired oxygen saturation of 100% throughout the resuscitation phase.[74] A Pao_2 less than 60 mm Hg must be avoided because outcome from severe TBI is likely to be compromised.[81,82,118] Administration of 100% oxygen before and after intermittent tracheal suctioning or intubation is important to prevent hypoxemia during these interventions.

ADEQUATE VENTILATION. Central nervous system injuries frequently result in abnormal and ineffective breathing patterns. Not only CNS dysfunction but also drugs with respiratory depressant effects and chest injuries can impair ventilation. Impaired ventilation leads to hypoxia and hypercapnia. Because hypoxia and hypercarbia potentiate intracranial hypertension and exacerbate secondary brain injury, prevention or immediate resolution of insufficient ventilation is a priority in brain injury management.

Nurses should assess the patient's respiratory status, paying particular attention to the respiratory rate and rhythm, chest excursion, breath sounds, and gas exchange effectiveness. Use of bedside devices such as pulse oximetry or end-tidal CO_2 monitoring to continuously evaluate oxygenation and carbon dioxide levels or monitoring with serial blood gases is essential in guiding oxygen and ventilatory therapy in the resuscitation phase. Once an airway is established, if ventilation is still deemed inadequate, the patient should be given assistance. Initially an Ambu bag can be used for manual ventilation. Mechanical ventilation may be required until the patient is able to breathe sufficiently without assistance. Carbon dioxide levels should be normalized, but hyperventilation of the patient is not indicated unless the patient shows evidence of neurologic deterioration or presents with refractory intracranial hypertension.[74,118]

ADEQUATE SYSTEMIC AND CEREBRAL PERFUSION. Once airway patency and adequate ventilation have been established, the priority becomes circulatory stabilization. Circulatory instability resulting in hypotension rarely occurs secondary to brain injury itself unless there has been prolonged medullary compression and brain death is imminent. Hemorrhagic shock as a result of blood loss from extracranial injury is the primary cause of systemic hypotension and consequent cerebral hypoperfusion during brain injury resuscitation. Hypotension (systolic blood pressure <90 mm Hg), present in approximately 35% of brain-injured patients from the time of injury through resuscitation, is predictive of a poorer outcome and should be corrected immediately.[74,80,81,118]

Intravascular volume must be restored and cardiac pump function must be optimized to restore circulatory stability. External and internal hemorrhage must be identified and controlled. Isotonic crystalloids, colloids, and, when appropriate, blood products should be infused to achieve a euvolemic state. Hypotonic solutions such as D_5W should be avoided because they reduce the osmolarity of the intravascular volume, which encourages fluid leakage out of the intravascular space, thereby exacerbating cerebral edema. Multiple animal and human studies have demonstrated positive effects when hypertonic saline and dextran-containing solutions are used during resuscitation of patients with TBI.[209-212] The use of hypertonic solutions to achieve cardiovascular stability is associated with a need for smaller fluid volumes and with fewer complications (e.g., cerebral edema and intracranial hypertension).

The patient's hemodynamic status (e.g., heart rate, blood pressure, central venous pressure) and clinical findings indicating sufficiency of tissue perfusion (e.g., capillary refill time, urine output, acid-base balance, lactate levels) should guide the volume of fluid resuscitation provided. Care should be taken to avoid fluid overload, which may exacerbate cerebral edema. If the patient's hypotension is unresponsive to fluid therapy, other causes, such as spinal shock, must be ruled out. Once adequate intravascular volume replacement has been ensured, consideration should be given to administration of inotropic and vasoactive agents in order to support blood pressure. Refer to Chapter 13 for additional information on the management of traumatic shock.

BASELINE AND ONGOING CLINICAL EXAMINATION. It is imperative that a baseline neurologic assessment is obtained as soon as possible and that the patient is monitored closely to determine if brain function deteriorates or improves over time. If cerebral hypoperfusion and hypoxia are contributing to the patient's altered mentation, sensorium should improve as oxygenation and perfusion deficits are corrected. Responses to various therapeutic interventions should be noted. Alterations in mental status caused by drug use generally resolve as the drugs are metabolized. If there is a high suspicion that the patient took an excessive amount of narcotic before injury, naloxone (Narcan) may be administered during resuscitation to reverse the narcotic effects. Metabolic disorders, such as hypoglycemia and electrolyte imbalances, should be corrected promptly. However, glucose should not be administered routinely or indiscriminately to unconscious patients, because hyperglycemia may worsen outcome after cerebral ischemia and TBI.[213]

A CT scan is obtained as soon as possible for patients who present with an altered level of consciousness. If an operable lesion is confirmed, the patient should be prepared immediately for surgery. Delay in surgical intervention to remove an acute subdural hematoma can escalate patient mortality and morbidity.[32]

ANALGESIA, SEDATION, AND CONTROL OF AGITATION. Pain and agitation must be controlled in order to decrease cerebral metabolic requirements, reduce ICP, facilitate effective ventilation, provide patient comfort and safety, and allow diagnostic and therapeutic procedures. Severe pain is most likely caused by extracranial sources, because the brain tissue itself lacks pain receptors. Agitation frequently accompanies TBI; however, other causes for agitation such as hypoxia or electrolyte imbalance must be ruled out before attributing the altered mental status solely to craniocerebral trauma.

Sedatives and analgesics should be administered judiciously to brain-injured patients, because their use can blunt clinical indications of neurologic deterioration. Management of pain and or agitation is based on individual patient assessment. Before administration of sedatives or analgesia, a complete baseline neurologic examination should be completed and precise anatomic areas of pain or tenderness identified when possible.

If the patient is awake and complaining of mild discomfort, the first drug of choice for pain relief should be a non-CNS depressant (i.e., a mild analgesic such as acetaminophen [Tylenol]). Codeine, a short-acting analgesic with minimal CNS effect, is used occasionally in stable, awake patients with mild or moderate pain of extracranial origin. When other agents are necessary to control pain, the smallest possible dosages of short-acting or easily reversible analgesic agents are preferred.[214] Morphine is one preferred agent for pain management because it is easily reversed with naloxone, has a minimal effect on cardiac output, and does not interfere with pupillary dilation if oculomotor nerve compression occurs. Fentanyl (Sublimaze), a rapid-acting synthetic opioid with a short half-life, is also reversible with naloxone, making it another option in the armamentarium of analgesic agents that may be used after brain injury. Short-acting agents such as thiopental, midazolam (Versed), or propofol (Diprivan) may be used to control agitation in the mechanically ventilated patient. No one analgesic or sedative agent has been proven most effective for all patients with TBI.

Extreme caution should be exercised when administering sedation or analgesia to patients with mild or moderate head injury who lack ventilatory support or ICP monitoring capabilities. The threat of respiratory depression inherent in the use of these agents contradicts rapid or high-dose intravenous administration in the spontaneously breathing patient. Large doses or rapid administration of analgesia or sedation may also lower blood pressure to unacceptable levels. Blood pressure response to administration of these medications should be noted, and care should be taken not to use excessive doses that may threaten hypotension.

Nursing interventions to reduce pain and agitation should complement pharmacologic agents used for these purposes. The nurse should attempt to calm, reassure, and comfort the patient. Physical restraint may become necessary to protect the patient from harm and should be applied according to institution protocol if needed.

PATIENT AND FAMILY PSYCHOLOGIC SUPPORT. During resuscitation, emphasis is placed on treating and maintaining the patient's physical being, but the psychologic, emotional, and spiritual welfare of the patient and family must not be overlooked. Even the patient who is confused or partially responsive may be aware of the environment and treatment events. The nurse, as well as other trauma team members, should take the time to explain procedures in simple terms, offer emotion support, and reorient the patient frequently.

The patient's family is typically in crisis and requires support and information. Repeated simple and clear explanations of the patient's condition and progress must be provided at timely intervals. Family coping mechanisms and support systems should be evaluated and mobilized whenever possible.[215]

CRITICAL CARE PHASE

Nursing care in the critical care phase continues to focus on preventing or minimizing secondary brain injury in order to optimize functional recovery. Avoidance of factors known to exacerbate secondary brain injury (e.g., hypoxemia, hypercapnia, systemic hypotension, and intracranial hypertension) continues to be the key physiologic priority. The critical care nurse is responsible for collaborating with the other trauma team members to prevent, recognize, and treat both intracerebral and systemic complications of TBI. Complications may arise in response to brain injury, nonneurologic injury, or treatment. Early aggressive intervention directed toward prevention and treatment of secondary complications reduces mortality and morbidity.*

Meticulous monitoring is essential to detect clinical changes and guide treatment. Ongoing comprehensive physical examination remains an essential aspect of assessment. Findings should be documented on a time-oriented flow sheet to facilitate rapid recognition of changes in the patient's status. In addition to physical examination findings, data from neuroimaging tests, ICP monitoring, cerebral blood flow measures, cerebral oxygenation assessment, CSF analysis, and electrophysiologic evaluation may be used in the critical care environment to guide therapy.

---

*References 74, 77, 80, 81, 83, 138.

Analyses of clinical findings permit the development of a multidisciplinary plan of care appropriate for the brain-injured patient.

ADEQUATE GAS EXCHANGE. It remains essential that hypoxia and hypercapnia be prevented and treated aggressively during the critical care phase to avoid secondary brain injury. Maintenance of adequate respiratory gas exchange during this phase can be challenging because of the onset of respiratory complications, which are common after TBI. Maintaining airway patency, adequate ventilation, and sufficient oxygenation are all important to ensure adequate respiratory gas exchange.

Airway patency is maintained by providing appropriate care for any artificial airway device in place (e.g., endotracheal tube or tracheostomy), employing aspiration precautions, and performing vigorous pulmonary toilet. The spontaneously breathing patient with a natural airway needs to be monitored carefully for any evidence of airway insufficiency. All necessary equipment for emergency intubation should be kept in close proximity. The patient who is beginning to localize to stimuli but is not yet ready for removal of the artificial airway may require soft protective restraints or hand mittens to prevent self-extubation.

Aspiration Precautions. During the critical care phase the patient with brain injury remains at high risk for aspiration, so precautions against this complication must be employed. The endotracheal or tracheostomy tube cuff should remain inflated with a minimal air leak, and secretions above the cuff should be cleared before cuff deflation.[216] Gastric decompression through a gastric tube should be continued until the patient has adequate gut function to achieve stomach emptying. Patients who receive enteral alimentation require assessment of gastric content residuals at regular intervals (usually every 4 hours) and before intermittent gastric feedings. If residuals exceed a predetermined amount, enteral feedings should be withheld. When possible the head of the bed should be elevated during enteral feedings, and the feeding should be discontinued at least 30 minutes before and during head-down positioning.

Respiratory Care. Aggressive respiratory care, including positioning, suctioning, and, when possible, chest physiotherapy (CPT), is important for removal of pulmonary secretions and prevention of atelectasis, which can compromise respiratory gas exchange. These respiratory care interventions are all known to have a potentially detrimental effect on the patient's cerebrovascular status, specifically by elevating ICP elevation and possibly compromising CPP.[217-220] Therefore, neurologic status, including ICP, CPP, and, when possible, cerebral blood flow or oxygenation parameters, should be monitored closely while performing these activities. If monitored neurologic parameters exceed acceptable limits, pulmonary care measures should be discontinued and then reinstituted when cerebro-vascular variables are brought under control. Maintaining good head and neck alignment and premedicating the patient with a prescribed sedative before performing these interventions may enhance his or her tolerance of these activities.[217,220,221]

Chest physiotherapy, including chest percussion, vibration, and postural drainage, is performed as tolerated by the patient's cerebrovascular status. Because most pathologic lung conditions in patients with severe TBI occur in the lower lobes, Trendelenburg's position (30-degree head-down position) is often indicated for postural drainage during CPT. The nurse should always confirm with the neurosurgeon that there is no contraindication for use of Trendelenburg's position. Research exploring the cerebrovascular effects of CPT (i.e., chest percussion and vibration, head-down postural drainage, and suctioning) on severely brain-injured patients with normal ICP and CPP at rest demonstrated that, although ICP increases during the treatment, CPP may remain adequate.[220] Studies evaluating the effects of CPT on cerebral blood flow and oxygenation are needed. Continuous monitoring of ICP, CPP, and, if available, oxygenation and CBF variables during chest physiotherapy allows rapid recognition of clinically significant changes that warrant aborting the intervention, thereby avoiding detrimental intracerebral effects.

Suctioning is performed through the established airway as necessary. Nasopharyngeal suctioning should be avoided until the possibility of a basilar skull fracture has been ruled out. Nursing research findings provide the basis for establishing research-based endotracheal suctioning protocols that minimize cerebrovascular compromise during this procedure (Table 19-8).[218,219,222-225] Studies have demonstrated that although suctioning increases ICP, CPP values can remain sufficient.[218,222-225] Using measures of SjO_2, MAP, and middle cerebral artery velocity, Kerr et al[218] demonstrated that cerebral oxygen delivery was maintained and cerebral oxygenation was preserved during endotracheal suctioning. The suctioning protocol employed by Kerr et al delivered four ventilator breaths at 135% of the patient's tidal volume, with 100% FiO_2 at a rate of four breaths in 20 seconds before and after two suction catheter passes.[218]

TABLE 19-8   Research-Based Recommendations for Suctioning Patients With Traumatic Brain Injury

- Pass the suction catheter for no longer than 10 seconds.
- Limit the number of suction catheter passes, preferably to no more than 2 passes per suctioning episode.
- Hyperoxygenate the patient before and after each passage of the suction catheter (e.g., deliver 4 ventilator breaths at 135% of patient's tidal volume on 100% FiO_2 at a rate of 4 breaths in 20 seconds).
- Minimize airway stimulation (i.e., stabilize endotracheal tube, avoid passing the suction catheter all the way to the carina).

Ventilator Management. Most patients with significant brain injury require mechanical ventilation to promote adequate respiratory gas exchange. Associated lung injury and onset of pulmonary complications may necessitate use of ventilator support that generates high intrathoracic pressures (e.g., high levels of positive end-expiratory pressure [PEEP]). Although mechanical ventilation techniques that increase intrathoracic pressure may be necessary for adequate oxygenation and to prevent hypercapnia, they can eventually impede cerebral venous return, causing ICP elevations. Patients with reduced intracranial compliance are at especially high risk for onset of intracranial hypertension from raised intrathoracic pressure.

Monitoring Respiratory Gas Exchange. Effectiveness of respiratory gas exchange should be evaluated frequently by monitoring oxygen and carbon dioxide levels. Use of pulse oximetry, a jugular bulb fiberoptic oximetric catheter (Sjo_2 monitoring), NIRS, and $Pbro_2$ monitoring facilitate continuous evaluation of oxygenation. End-tidal CO_2 can be monitored continuously with a capnometer that fits in line with the ventilator system. Serial blood gas analysis may also be used to evaluate respiratory gas exchange. When monitored parameters are verified to be outside acceptable limits, they should be reported immediately so that appropriate interventions to promote adequate gas exchange can be promptly instituted.

ADDITIONAL MEASURES TO CONTROL INTRACRANIAL PRESSURE

Therapeutic Hyperventilation. Therapeutic hyperventilation decreases $Paco_2$, which causes cerebral vasoconstriction and a decline in CBF, subsequently reducing ICP.[226,227] When cerebral reactivity to CO_2 is intact, the effectiveness of therapeutic hyperventilation is typically apparent within 2 to 3 minutes. Eventually the cerebral vasculature adapts to prolonged periods of hyperventilation as the CSF bicarbonate level and pH return to baseline.[228] CBF returns to prehyperventilation levels despite continued CO_2 reduction, typically within 24 hours of initiating this therapy.[228,229] An abrupt end to therapeutic hyperventilation, especially when used for prolonged periods, can cause vasodilation of the cerebral vessels beyond the baseline diameter, thereby elevating cerebral blood flow and increasing intracranial pressure.[228]

There is concern that the vasoconstriction and marked reduction in CBF induced by therapeutic hyperventilation may actually worsen cerebral ischemia in the injured brain. A prospective, controlled, randomized clinical trial conducted by Muizelaar et al[230] demonstrated that patients with a GCS motor score of 4 or 5 receiving prophylactic hyperventilation ($Paco_2$ of 24-28 mm Hg) had a worse outcome at 3 and 6 months than patients who had their $Paco_2$ maintained between 30 and 35 mm Hg.[230] Numerous studies have demonstrated that aggressive therapeutic hyperventilation can reduce CBF or cerebral oxygenation parameters (i.e., Sjo_2, $Avjdo_2$, $Pbro_2$) to levels at or below ischemic thresholds.[146,164-166,182,186,231]

Based on a review of current research findings, the "Guidelines for Management of Severe Traumatic Brain Injury" recommend that chronic prophylactic hyperventilation ($Paco_2$ ≤25 mm Hg) be avoided in the absence of ICP elevations during the first 5 days after severe TBI.[118] Lowering the $Paco_2$ to 35 mm Hg or less should be avoided during the first 24 hours after severe TBI because it can compromise brain perfusion at the time when cerebral blood flow is particularly low. Brief periods of therapeutic hyperventilation may be necessary when the patient has deterioration of neurologic status, and longer periods may be needed to treat refractory intracranial hypertension.[118] It is also recommended that, when $Paco_2$ is normalized, it be done gradually to avoid a rebound increase of cerebral blood flow and ICP. Measures of cerebral oxygenation (i.e., Sjo_2, $Avjdo_2$, $Pbro_2$) and cerebral blood flow may be helpful in guiding the appropriate use of therapeutic hyperventilation.[118]

Diuretic and Fluid Management

Osmotic diuretics are commonly used to control intracranial hypertension. Mannitol is widely accepted as the osmotic diuretic of choice. Mannitol's exact mechanism of beneficial action remains controversial. It creates an osmotic gradient between the blood and brain and draws fluid out of the brain, across the semipermeable blood-brain barrier, and into the intravascular space, subsequently reducing overall brain volume. Mannitol is also believed to cause hemodynamic changes that may reduce intracranial pressure while increasing CBF and oxygen delivery.[232-234] Hemodilution, reduced blood viscosity, and decreased red blood cell adhesiveness caused by mannitol improve CBF and oxygen delivery.[232,233] A transient elevation in intravascular blood volume and systolic blood pressure, together with ICP reduction, can improve CPP.[232-234] The plasma-expanding effects of mannitol probably best explain why mannitol is able to reduce ICP within minutes after administration. Mannitol may also exert a beneficial effect by scavenging oxygen free radicals, which are known to be cytotoxic and exacerbate secondary brain injury.[232,235]

Mannitol is typically administered to control intracranial hypertension, but it also may be indicated for a volume-resuscitated patient whose ICP is not being monitored but who has clinical evidence of transtentorial herniation or progressive neurologic decline that lacks an extracranial cause.[118] Bolus dose administration (rather than continuous infusion) is preferable for optimal effectiveness.[118,236] The smallest effective dosage of mannitol is recommended, with the effective dosage ranging from 0.25 to 1 g/kg body weight.[118] It is preferable to administer mannitol through a central line, because extravasation of the drug can cause skin sloughing.

There is concern that mannitol may get on the wrong side of the blood-brain barrier when administered to a patient with brain injury. If this occurs, fluid could be pulled into instead of out of the brain, causing a rebound ICP elevation.[232,237] Prolonged circulation of mannitol (which occurs with repeated doses or continuous infusion of the drug) may exacerbate this problem, further supporting use of intermittent bolus doses as the preferred method of administration.[118,237] Despite these concerns, mannitol continues to be a mainstay in the care of patients with severe TBI because of its effectiveness in reducing intracranial pressure.

Furosemide (Lasix) is the primary nonosmotic diuretic used for ICP reduction. Furosemide is a loop diuretic that reduces ICP by several possible mechanisms: it decreases sodium and water transport into the brain, reduces total body fluid volume by renal tubular diuresis, and inhibits CSF production.[238,239] Despite the beneficial effects of furosemide, it is slower acting and reduces ICP to a lesser extent than mannitol; therefore, mannitol remains the first-line diuretic of choice for lowering ICP, particularly in emergent situations.[240]

Some researchers have suggested that a combination of mannitol and furosemide may enhance the degree of diuresis, produce more pronounced brain shrinkage, and enhance the degree and duration of ICP reduction.[236,238,239] Currently there is limited data to support use of this combination therapy.[118]

Diuretic use has multiple implications for nursing practice. The nurse should ensure that the patient is not hypovolemic before administration of diuretics and must frequently monitor the patient's fluid, electrolyte, and hemodynamic status while diuretics are in use. A Foley catheter should be in place to better monitor urine output. Although a hyperosmolar state may be desirable to discourage intravascular fluid extravasation and reduce risk of cerebral edema, serum osmolality should be maintained below 320 mOsm to avoid onset of renal failure.[118] Even more importantly, administration of diuretics and subsequent fluid loss must be monitored to avoid an undesirable reduction in systemic blood pressure. Fluids must be administered to replace fluids lost by diuresis so that the patient's overall volume status is not compromised.[241]

Fluid Therapy.   Fluids should be administered with the goal of achieving and maintaining normovolemia. The practice of keeping the patient dehydrated in an effort to reduce brain swelling has largely been abandoned because severe dehydration compromises blood pressure, cardiac output, and renal function and increases the risk for cerebral vasospasms. Maintaining adequate intravascular volume is important to enhance perfusion to the injured brain. The patient's clinical assessment and hemodynamic parameters should continue to guide the volume of fluid administered. Patients with TBI may have multiple avenues of fluid loss that need to be accounted for, such as hemorrhage and fluid loss from associated injuries and surgical interventions, third-spaced fluid, and diuresis from diabetes insipidus or aggressive diuretics use. Generally, isotonic crystalloids (e.g., normal saline, plasmalyte-A) are administered to patients with TBI and hypotonic solutions (e.g., D_5W) are avoided unless severe hypernatremia dictates judicious use. Colloids may also be used for fluid replacement. If the patient is anemic or coagulopathic, blood products serve as excellent replacement fluids.

Numerous researchers have explored the efficacy of bolus doses or continuous infusion of hypertonic saline (3% to 23.4%) for the treatment of intracranial hypertension after TBI.[209,210,242-246] Hypertonic saline solutions have an osmotic effect, pulling fluid from the brain's interstitial spaces into the intravascular space, reducing brain water volume and effectively reducing ICP elevations refractory to other therapy.[210,242,247] These solutions may also provide benefits through a number of other mechanisms, such as exerting a hemodynamic effect that improves CBF and oxygen delivery and modifying the inflammatory response associated with injury.[209,210] Administration of hypertonic saline solutions may be particularly useful for patients in whom intravascular volume depletion (caused by osmotic diuretics) is undesirable. Rare complications associated with hypertonic saline solutions include electrolyte imbalance, phlebitis, coagulopathies, congestive heart failure, hyperosmolarity, acid-base imbalance, central pontine myelinolysis, renal insufficiency, and subdural hematoma formation.[209,210,244] Despite preliminary evidence that support use of hypertonic saline solutions to reduce ICP, additional controlled clinical trials are needed.[210]

Steroids.   Glucocorticoids (e.g., dexamethasone or methylprednisolone) were introduced into head injury treatment with the hope that they would reduce cerebral edema and thus ICP. However, randomized controlled trials have failed to substantiate the benefit of steroids in the management of TBI. Therefore, administration of steroids is not recommended for reducing ICP or improving outcomes in patients with severe TBI.[118] An extensive review of randomized controlled trials exploring corticosteroid use in acute TBI patients found that there is continued uncertainty about the effects of corticosteroids and that no beneficial effects on outcomes were evident.[248] A large randomized, prospective, controlled trial evaluating the effectiveness of a synthetic aminosteroid, tirilazad mesylate, also failed to detect any overall benefit on the outcome of patients with TBI.[60]

Measures to Reduce Cerebral Stimulation and Metabolic Demand.   A host of interventions can be performed in an effort to reduce cerebral stimulation and metabolic demand of the patient with severe TBI. When cerebral stimulation and metabolic demand are reduced, cerebral metabolic rate and cerebral oxygen consumption are decreased. As a result, CBF is diminished and ICP reduced. Minimizing unnecessary noxious stimuli; reducing body temperature; and using sedation, analgesia, and paralytic agents appropriately are examples of these interventions.

Noxious Stimuli Minimization. ICP can become elevated by the painful stimuli used in the neurologic examination and clinical procedures that cause discomfort (e.g., venipuncture, tube insertion, suctioning, manipulation of an injured area). Less obvious stimuli may also increase ICP, such as conversations at the bedside or the lighting in the room. It is the nurse's responsibility to evaluate what stimuli cause ICP elevations and to eliminate or reduce them whenever possible.

Body Temperature Normalization. Hyperthermia, with body temperature as high as 104° F to 105° F (40° C-40.5° C), may be caused by dysfunction of the hypothalamic temperature-regulating mechanism. Hyperthermia can be present on admission or appear within the first few days after injury and then subside, only to sporadically reappear throughout the recovery process or until hypothalamic control is reestablished. Never assume that fever in a patient with severe brain injury is of cerebral origin until other potential treatable sources of fever (e.g., infection, atelectasis, thromboembolism, seizures, drug reaction) are ruled out. Hyperthermia can be problematic because it increases the cerebral metabolic rate. For every 1° C rise in body temperature there is approximately a 10% elevation in cerebral oxygen consumption and a 6% increase in CBF.[11]

Nurses should monitor the patient's body temperature closely, recognizing that brain temperature is often 1° C to 2° C higher than rectal or bladder temperatures.[249,250] Differences between brain and body temperature are greatest when patients are hypothermic or hyperthermic.[249] Once hyperthermia is recognized, measures to reduce body temperature, such as administration of acetaminophen (Tylenol), cool baths, ice packs, and cooling blankets, should be implemented. Rapid cooling of the patient or prolonged use of hypothermia blankets may precipitate shivering, which also elevates ICP. Shivering can be avoided by slowly reducing body temperature, discontinuing hypothermia use when the body temperature reaches approximately 100° F, and, in severe cases, administering sedatives such as chlorpromazine (Thorazine).

Moderate Hypothermia. Multiple clinical studies have demonstrated that cooling the brain to 32° C to 34° C soon after injury for 24 to 48 hours can effectively lower the cerebral metabolic rate for oxygen, decrease ICP, and reduce mechanisms causing secondary brain injury.[251-255] Some of these studies suggest a trend toward improved outcomes when patients with severe TBI were treated with mild to moderate hypothermia.[253-255] Despite these findings, a large, multicenter, randomized, controlled, clinical trial failed to demonstrate any improvement in the outcomes of patients with severe TBI who were treated for 48 hours with induced hypothermia to 33° C within 8 hours of injury.[256]

Sedation, Analgesia, and Control of Agitation. As in the resuscitation cycle, pain and agitation must be adequately controlled in the brain-injured patient by the appropriate use of sedation and analgesia. Sound judgment is required in managing sedation and analgesia. The patient's neurologic and cerebral vascular status should be monitored closely to recognize the need for sedation when acute intracranial hypertension arises. Recognition of the need to withhold sedation when the patient must be evaluated clinically is equally important. Care must be taken to prevent systemic hypotension associated with sedation or analgesia administration. Nurses should continually evaluate the effectiveness of prescribed sedatives and analgesics and work in collaboration with the physician to find a drug and dosages that best meet the patient's needs. Small, frequent dosages of short-acting or easily reversible agents are typically preferred.

High-Dose Barbiturate Therapy. High-dose barbiturates have been used in the management of severe TBI to reduce elevated ICP and protect the brain against hypoxia and ischemia. High-dose barbiturate therapy is believed to decrease ICP by suppressing neuronal activity and reducing the cerebral metabolic rate, which subsequently decreases CBF and volume.[118,257,258] Barbiturates may also have a direct cerebral hemodynamic effect that is beneficial in decreasing ICP.[258] This therapy is also thought to inhibit certain intracellular pathologic events that play a role in secondary brain injury (e.g., scavenges free radicals, stabilizes plasma and lysosomal membranes, reduces release of excitotoxic amino acids).[258]

Barbiturates can reduce intracranial hypertension that is otherwise refractory to other interventions.[258-260] A case series by Rea et al[260] and a randomized controlled trial by Eisenberg et al[259] demonstrated that mortality is substantially less among patients with refractory intracranial hypertension that can be controlled with barbiturate therapy than among those whose elevated ICP is unresponsive to barbiturates. Clinical research does not support the prophylactic use of barbiturates in management of severe TBI.[261]

High-dose barbiturate therapy may be considered in the hemodynamically stable patient who has a survivable brain injury and refractory intracranial hypertension.[118] Pentobarbital, a short-acting barbiturate, is usually the drug of choice. An initial loading dose of the barbiturate (e.g., 10 mg/kg over 30 minutes and then 5 mg/kg every hour for 3 hours) is typically prescribed, followed by a maintenance dose (e.g., 1-2 mg/kg/hr).[258,259] The maintenance dose and additional loading doses are titrated to reach a desired therapeutic endpoint, which is ICP control while maintaining a blood pressure that preserves sufficient CPP. A reliable method of monitoring barbiturate effectiveness is continuous EEG.[118,262] Burst suppression on EEG indicates neuronal suppression with near maximal cerebral metabolism and CBF reductions.[118] Serum barbiturate levels may be measured routinely, but there is a poor correlation between serum drug levels, drug effectiveness, and onset of complications.[118,262]

High-dose barbiturate therapy is plagued with potential adverse effects. Most undesirable, barbiturates may cause myocardial depression and hypotension, which can precipitate detrimental reductions in cerebral perfusion pressure and eventually CBF ultimately worsening patient outcome. Continual assessment of hemodynamic parameters with an arterial blood pressure line and a pulmonary artery catheter permits early recognition and prompt treatment of hypotension or myocardial depression. Vasoactive and inotropic agents (e.g., dopamine, phenylephrine hydrochloride) are frequently necessary to support the hemodynamic state of the patient receiving barbiturates. High-dose barbiturates also obscure the results of the neurologic examination. Motor function, eye opening, and verbal response cannot be assessed reliably, and most brainstem and motor reflexes are suppressed. The pupillary dilation response to brainstem compression typically remains intact; therefore, pupil size should continue to be assessed. Suppression of most motor and sensory reflexes, including the corneal and protective airway reflexes, means that the patient is completely dependent on nursing care to protect his or her eyes, skin, and airway. High-dose barbiturates also induce respiratory depression, making the patient ventilator dependent. Meticulous pulmonary care must be provided. Gastrointestinal tract motility is also typically depressed by barbiturate use, which may limit use of enteral alimentation. High-dose barbiturate administration may also cause immunosuppression and increase risk of infection,[263] necessitating close surveillance.[241] Hypothermia, reversible leukopenia, and cardiovascular complications induced by high-dose barbiturates may mask early recognizable signs of infection, including fever, leukocytosis, and a hyperdynamic state.[241,263]

Paralytic Agents. Paralytic agents may be used to eliminate posturing and other movement that can elevate ICP or interfere with therapeutic interventions. Paralytics also prevent reflexive motor responses to tracheal stimulation (i.e., coughing) that can elevate ICP. Neuromuscular blockade can also facilitate patient control on mechanical ventilation. Early routine use of neuromuscular blocking agents is generally not indicated and has not been shown to improve overall patient outcomes.[264] Hsiang et al found that early routine long-term use of neuromuscular blocking agents increased rates of pneumonia and sepsis and ICU length of stay.[264] Therefore, neuromuscular blockade is generally reserved for patients requiring escalation in treatment intensity for intracranial hypertension.

Paralytic agents obliterate most of the neurologic examination, making the clinician dependent on pupillary activity, results of neuroimaging studies, and intracranial monitoring devices to evaluate the patient's neurologic status.[74] Paralytic agents can also mask the motor movement associated with seizures. An unexplained elevation in ICP, heart

rate, or blood pressure in the paralyzed patient may indicate an underlying seizure.[241] The patient requires mechanical ventilation while receiving paralytic agents, and there is always a concern about prolonged weakness after discontinuation of neuromuscular blocking agents. Nurses should ensure that adequate sedation is provided, because paralytics do not block the patient's perception of painful stimuli.

Lidocaine. Lidocaine reduces cerebral oxygen consumption and increases cerebral vascular resistance, thereby reducing CBF and subsequently decreasing ICP.[265] This drug can serve as an effective cough suppressant and has been used to attenuate ICP elevations associated with respiratory maneuvers (e.g., endotracheal intubation, endotracheal suctioning).[265-267] Typically lidocaine is administered intravenously or endotracheally in a dose of 1.5 mg/kg.[265] The practitioner should wait approximately 5 minutes after intravenous administration before performing a respiratory maneuver; however, respiratory maneuvers can be performed immediately after endotracheal administration.[265] Caution needs to be taken when administering lidocaine, because it can depress the myocardium and decrease the seizure threshold.[241] Frequent administration can lead to toxicity. Further controlled clinical trials evaluating lidocaine's effectiveness in the management of TBI are necessary, including studies of its effect on cerebral oxygenation parameters and definitions of its the most desirable dosage, frequency, and route of administration.

Removal of Intracranial Volume
Surgical Intervention. Surgical intervention may be necessary to reduce intracranial hypertension by removing mass lesions or necrotic brain tissue from within the cranial vault. The evacuation of mass lesions is often a life-saving measure, with speed of treatment being crucial. A study of comatose patients with acute SDH demonstrated that those undergoing surgical evacuation within 4 hours of injury had a mortality of 30% compared with a 90% mortality in those with surgical intervention after 4 hours.[32] When intracranial hypertension has been refractory to all other therapies and there is no focal or localized lesion that can be removed, consideration may be given to performing a unilateral or bilateral decompressive craniectomy. This entails removing the cranium from the frontal to temporal parietal region to decompress the edematous brain and reduce ICP.[268-270]

Cerebral Spinal Fluid Drainage. Reduction of CSF volume effectively but temporarily reduces ICP. Use of an intraventricular catheter allows measurement of ICP and continuous or intermittent CSF drainage. In patients with posttraumatic hydrocephalus, long-term CSF drainage via the intraventricular catheter may be necessary until a ventricular shunt can be placed.

Positioning. Adhering to research-based recommendations for positioning of patients with TBI may reduce ICP or prevent intracranial hypertension. Patient position can affect ICP, CPP, and other cerebrovascular parameters. Changing the patient's position may elevate the ICP and possibly compromise CPP.[217,271] To minimize adverse effects associated with repositioning, rapid unexpected turning, head and neck malalignment, neck compression, and sharp hip flexion should be avoided.[217,271,272] The patient should be turned slowly (after being informed of the pending change) while cardiovascular, respiratory, and cerebrovascular parameters are monitored. It is important to maintain head and neck alignment. Head rotation and neck flexion, extension, or compression can inhibit cerebral venous outflow, increasing cerebral vascular volume and elevating ICP.[217,221,273] Head and neck alignment can be maintained with bilateral rolled towels, small sandbags, or other immobilization devices.

As the head of the bed is elevated, ICP typically decreases, and as the head of the bed is lowered, ICP tends to rise.[271,274-278] This ICP response is believed to occur because the head-up position facilitates cerebral venous outflow. The opposite effect is usually seen with systemic blood pressure, which decreases as the head of the bed is raised and increases as the head of the bed is lowered. Although ICP may be lower with the head of the bed elevated, CPP and CBF may be reduced.[278] The nurse should keep in mind that elevating the head of the bed raises the cerebral circulation higher than the heart; therefore, arterial pressure at the head may be as much as 20 mm Hg lower than arterial pressure referenced at the heart level. In studies comparing a 0-degree versus 30-degree head-of-bed elevation on various cerebral, hemodynamic, and oxygenation parameters, CBF remained unchanged in some people and was reduced in others as the head was raised to 30 degrees; brain tissue oxygenation parameters demonstrated no significant change.[276,277,279] Studies comparing the cerebral vascular responses with various head-of-bed positions have suggested that a 30-degree head-of-bed elevation tends to be optimal for a majority of patients with TBI, although there are many individualized responses to head-of-bed position.[217,274,277,279] Optimal head-of-bed position should be selected based on the patient's individualized response, considering which position best minimizes ICP and optimizes CPP, CBF, and cerebral oxygenation.

Specific Nursing Interventions.   Nursing plays a pivotal role in preventing, recognizing, and treating intracranial hypertension. Nurses must remain extremely cognizant of which interventions, activities, or stimuli reduce ICP and which cause ICP elevations. There is wide variation in patient response to interpersonal, auditory, and tactile stimuli, and such responses should be considered when planning and implementing care aimed at minimizing ICP and optimizing neurologic outcome. Studies evaluating the effects of various stimuli and specific nursing interventions on cerebral oxygenation and CBF parameters are needed.

Evidence of decreased intracranial compliance (e.g., baseline ICP elevations or P_2 ICP wave amplitude that exceeds the P_1 wave) is also important to recognize.[87] In patients with decreased intracranial compliance, activities such as coughing, straining, and sneezing and variations in head and body position that normally cause transient ICP elevations may provoke prolonged increases that may compromise cerebral perfusion. Respiratory care procedures, positioning, and noxious stimuli are often responsible for abrupt elevations in ICP in patients with decreased brain compliance. Effects of such activities should be anticipated, and nursing interventions to attenuate the ICP elevation should be initiated. It may be useful to medicate the patient with a prescribed sedative or analgesic before implementing interventions. Proper body positioning, rest periods, and removal of any unnecessary noxious stimuli are other important nursing interventions that may foster the patient's ability to tolerate a procedure.

Other Measures to Reduce Intracranial Pressure. Other measures to reduce ICP include minimizing intra-abdominal pressure and preventing Valsalva's maneuver. Elevations in intra-abdominal pressure can be translated to the intrathoracic cavity, whereby cerebral venous outflow is inhibited and ICP increases. Gastric and bladder decompression should be performed when these hollow organs do not empty spontaneously to keep intra-abdominal pressure minimized. Valsalva's maneuver can be avoided by using stool softeners to prevent straining during bowel movements and to avoid having the patient push against the side rails while in bed.

Adequate Systemic Blood Pressure.   It is essential that the patient's systemic blood pressure be sufficient to ensure an adequate CPP. Care should be taken to avoid a systolic blood pressure below 90 mm Hg, which can double mortality in patients with severe TBI.[81] Optimally the mean arterial blood pressure should be maintained higher than 90 mm Hg.[118] Adequate intravascular volume should be maintained. Once adequate intravascular volume is ensured, vasoactive and inotropic medications may be needed to maintain blood pressure. The nurse should remain cautious when administering drugs that may cause systemic hypotension, such as diuretics and sedatives. Blood pressure should be monitored frequently during administration of such agents in order to rapidly detect and treat any subsequent hypotensive episode.

Management of excessive hypertension is controversial. Systemic blood pressure should be maintained to ensure adequate cerebral perfusion, but excessive hypertension may cause cerebral venous engorgement, subsequent ICP elevations, and exacerbation of cerebral edema.[280,281] Such patients may benefit from normalization of the systemic blood pressure. Patients with cerebral ischemia (i.e., vasospasm or cerebral infarct) may benefit from a higher than normal blood pressure to enhance cerebral perfusion. The health care team must be extremely cautious when deciding to treat systemic hypertension, remembering that elevations in blood pressure occur as a compensatory response to brainstem compression. When the brain-injured patient presents with hypertension, particularly if other symptoms of brainstem compression are evident, ICP must be controlled first and CPP evaluated before considering antihypertensive therapy.[281]

Extreme caution should be used when administering antihypertensives to prevent systemic hypotension at all costs. The patient's cerebrovascular and cardiovascular response to the antihypertensive agent should be monitored closely. Short-acting antihypertensives are often preferred when initiating treatment.[280] Nurses should also be cognizant that certain antihypertensives (e.g., nitroprusside) cause cerebral vasodilation and may increase ICP. α-Adrenergic and β-adrenergic receptor antagonists (e.g., labetalol) may be preferred because they reduce blood pressure with little to no effect on ICP within the range of autoregulation.[281]

RECOGNIZING, PREVENTING, AND TREATING POTENTIAL COMPLICATIONS

Neurologic Complications. Cerebral edema, delayed intracerebral hemorrhage, reaccumulation of an evacuated hematoma, and posttraumatic hydrocephalus are possible sequelae of TBI that directly increase intracranial volume, eventually increasing ICP and possibly causing secondary brain injury. Symptoms of these complications become evident as ICP rises and brain compression occurs. Other potential complications originating in the brain that can lead to secondary brain injury are cerebral vasospasms, seizures, and intracranial infections.

Posttraumatic Vasospasm. Cerebral vasospasms can occur after TBI, reducing blood flow and potentially causing ischemia to the region of the brain perfused by the artery in spasm. Vasospasm-induced ischemic injury may adversely affect patient outcome.[282-284] The reported incidence of posttraumatic vasospasms diagnosed by angiography or detected by transcranial Doppler varies but has been documented to be as high as 42%.[34,282-287] Occurrence of posttraumatic vasospasms is related to the presence of SAH, although vasospasms have been noted in brain-injured patients without evidence of blood in the subarachnoid space.[282,284,286,288] Patients with all levels of TBI severity may suffer vasospasms.[282,285,288,289] Posttraumatic vasospasms may become evident as soon as 2 days after brain injury, typically peaking between days 5 and 11 and normalizing within 2 to 3 weeks after the trauma.[282,285,286,288]

Nimodipine, a calcium channel blocker, has been used in an attempt to prevent and treat posttraumatic vasospasms. Multiple European brain-injury trials done in the early 1990s suggest a more favorable outcome when patients with subarachnoid hemorrhage were treated prophylactically with nimodipine, although the exact mechanism by which nimodipine favorably influences outcome is unclear.[35,36] Nurses administering nimodipine should be aware of the drug's potential adverse effects, such as hypotension. Considerable uncertainty about the effects of calcium channel

blockers on patients with acute TBI still exists.[289] Angioplasty or administration of "triple H" therapy (hypervolemia, hemodilution, and hypertension) may be considered for treatment of severe refractory vasospasms, keeping in mind the potential complications related to these therapies.[282,284] Further clinical research is needed to determine the efficacy of these treatments for posttraumatic vasospasm.

Seizures. Traumatic brain injury can trigger the onset of seizures, which may occur immediately (i.e., within hours of injury), early (i.e., within 7 days of trauma), or late (i.e., more than 7 days after injury). Severity of brain injury is a powerful risk factor for onset of early and late seizures.[290,291] Other risk factors identified for onset of late seizures include penetrating brain injury, intracranial hematoma, cortical contusion, depressed skull fracture, prolonged loss of consciousness, and presence of early seizures.[290,292] Seizures increase the cerebral metabolic rate, which may cause ischemia and intracranial hypertension, especially in the acute phase after TBI, when the brain is vulnerable to secondary insult and may have poor compliance. Hemodynamic instability, changes in oxygen delivery, and excessive neurotransmitter release associated with seizures may also have adverse effects on the patient with TBI.[118] Seizure activity may also result in patient injury or adverse psychosocial, emotional, or cognitive sequelae.[118,291]

Although it is desirable to prevent posttraumatic seizures, the anticonvulsants used to prevent or treat seizures may have numerous adverse side effects. Reviews of the research evaluating the benefits and efficacy of anticonvulsants administered to prevent posttraumatic seizures do not recommend the prophylactic use of phenytoin, carbamazepine, sodium valproate, or phenobarbital for prevention of late posttraumatic seizures.[118,293,294] There is evidence that phenytoin and carbamazepine are effective in preventing early seizures.[295,296] Therefore, it is recommended as a treatment option that phenytoin or carbamazepine be administered for the first week after TBI to patients at high risk for seizures.[118,293] Haltiner et al[297] demonstrated that administration of phenytoin for the first week after TBI to prevent posttraumatic early seizures can be done without significant increase in drug-related side effects. Routine use of valproate to prevent early posttraumatic seizures is not recommended, because it has no benefit over short-term phenytoin administration and may be associated with a higher mortality rate.[298] Currently there is no evidence that preventing early seizures improves outcome by reducing death or neurologic disability after TBI.[118,293,297]

Patients with a preinjury history of seizures should have their anticonvulsant therapy continued during and after hospitalization for brain injury. Seizure precautions should be instituted in all brain-injured patients. These precautions generally include keeping an airway, suction, and anticonvulsants readily available, siderails padded and upright, and the environment free of sharp or hazardous items. In the event of a seizure the nurse should observe and document its onset, characteristics, and duration. Maintenance of a patent airway remains the first treatment priority. Any objects in the patient's physical proximity should be removed to prevent injury, but no attempt should be made to restrain the patient. Prescribed anticonvulsants should be administered to halt the seizure activity, followed by a loading and maintenance dose of the antiepileptic agent desired for long-term seizure treatment. The nurse caring for the patient receiving anticonvulsants should monitor for adverse drug effects and ensure therapeutic drug levels are maintained.

Intracranial Infection. Meningitis and brain abscesses are examples of intracranial infections that may occur after TBI. Severe TBI is associated with depressed immune function, which can increase risk of infectious complications.[299-301] Administration of high-dose barbiturates to treat intracranial hypertension can also cause immunosuppression.[263] Patients with open head injuries are at greater risk for intracranial infection than are patients with closed injuries. Intracranial surgical procedures and placement of invasive intracranial monitoring devices also predispose the patient to CNS infection.

Every effort should be made to prevent, recognize, and appropriately treat intracranial infections to minimize adverse effects on patient outcome. Strict aseptic technique is imperative when manipulating intracranial monitoring devices. The nurse should monitor the patient closely for evidence of infection, including continued assessment of body temperature and white blood cell count trends. ICP elevations, focal neurologic deficits, and development of brain shift, which is usually visible on CT scan or MRI, are signs of a brain abscess. Meningitis is a more diffuse intracranial process characterized by signs and symptoms of systemic infection, meningeal irritation (e.g., nuchal rigidity, photophobia), deteriorating neurologic status, and a pathogen cultured from the CSF.

When an intracranial infection is confirmed or suspected, prescribed antibiotics should be administered. Antibiotics are selected based on the sensitivity pattern of the cultured organism and the ability of the agent to penetrate the blood-brain barrier. If drainage of an abscess is required, the patient and family should be prepared for upcoming surgery. Penetrating brain injuries (e.g., missile injuries) generally require immediate debridement of the wound, closure of CSF leaks, and administration of prophylactic antibiotics to reduce the risk of intracranial infection.[302] Prophylactic antibiotic therapy for open brain injuries associated with pneumocephalus or basilar skull fractures and dural tears that result in CSF leakage is much more controversial. Some practitioners feel that the adverse effects of the intracranial infection warrant prophylactic use of antibiotics; however, many others concerned about the onset of antibiotic-resistant infection, and drug side effects suggest that no antibiotics should be given until infection is evident.

Pulmonary Complications. Respiratory complications are prevalent after moderate and severe brain injury. Brain-injured patients with a decreased level of consciousness frequently have suppressed protective airway reflexes, with consequent increased susceptibility to secretion retention and aspiration. A decreased level of consciousness in concert with immobility and potentially abnormal respiratory patterns can lead to atelectasis and secretion retention. Endotracheal intubation is often necessary in the patient with severe TBI, causing bypass of the protective upper respiratory tract. Prolonged immobility and venous stasis pose a threat of pulmonary emboli. Severe head injury, often associated with intracranial hypertension, may trigger the onset of neurogenic pulmonary edema. Although the exact etiology of neurogenic pulmonary edema remains poorly defined, it is hypothesized that neurologic injury, possibly associated with disturbance of the hypothalamus and medulla, triggers a massive sympathetic discharge, causing severe pulmonary and systemic vasoconstriction.[216,303,304] The result is left ventricular failure, which, together with increased pulmonary capillary permeability, leads to pulmonary edema.[216,303] Direct or indirect pulmonary injury can trigger onset of acute respiratory distress syndrome, a cascade of pathologic inflammatory/immune reactions that leads to acute lung injury and respiratory failure.[216,305] Associated thoracic trauma may also impair pulmonary function.

Pulmonary complications can increase mortality and morbidity.[304] All respiratory complications increase the likelihood of detrimental hypoxia and hypercarbia and risk subsequent secondary brain injury. Aggressive pulmonary toilet, aspiration precautions, and appropriate ventilator management help to reduce the incidence of these complications. Close monitoring of respiratory status and respiratory gas exchange is imperative in order to detect the onset of these complications. Once recognized, appropriate therapy should be instituted to resolve the complications immediately.

Fluid and Electrolyte Imbalance. A number of conditions leading to fluid and electrolyte imbalance may exist after TBI. Diuretics used in the treatment of increased ICP may create fluid and electrolyte imbalance. The metabolic response to stress and injury can result in the release of the adrenocorticotropic hormone (ACTH) and aldosterone, resulting in sodium and water retention and hypothalamic release of antidiuretic hormone (ADH), which also causes water retention. Brain injury can cause fluid and electrolyte imbalance directly by increasing or decreasing ADH output by the hypothalamus-neurohypophyseal system or by triggering excessive sodium and water loss.

Nurses must closely monitor the brain-injured patient's urine and serum electrolytes and osmolarity, fluid intake and output, and hemodynamic parameters (e.g., central venous pressure, pulmonary artery pressures) to readily detect fluid and electrolyte imbalance. Once an imbalance is recognized, the physician should be alerted and appropriate interventions (e.g., administration of diuretics, electrolytes, or fluids) can be instituted to reestablish equilibrium quickly. The goal is to achieve a euvolemic state with a balance of fluid and electrolyte levels.

Neurogenic Diabetes Insipidus (DI). Brain injury that affects the hypothalamic/posterior pituitary system may cause partial or complete cessation of ADH production or secretion, resulting in neurogenic DI. ADH is normally released in response to hyperosmolarity, hypovolemia, stress, or any stimulus that signals the body to conserve water. This hormone acts on the kidneys to stimulate water reabsorption. Insufficient ADH decreases water reabsorption by the renal tubules, causing an increased loss of free water and hypotonic urine output. This loss of free water leaves behind a concentrated intravascular volume with increased serum osmolarity and sodium levels. Diabetes insipidus is typically recognized in the clinical setting when large volumes (≥200 ml/hr for 2 consecutive hours) of diluted urine output is noted (Table 19-9).[306]

Treatment varies according to the patient's mental status and degree of DI. Patients who are alert with mild DI can preferably regulate themselves by drinking in response to thirst. In patients with an altered level of consciousness, who are unable to self-regulate fluid intake, and with more severe degrees of DI, this disorder is treated with fluid and ADH replacement (see Table 19-9). Aqueous vasopressin (Pitressin) is typically the drug of choice to replace ADH in the critical care phase.

Syndrome of Inappropriate ADH. Syndrome of inappropriate ADH (SIADH) is a complication of CNS trauma that disrupts the hypothalamic-neurohypophyseal system, resulting in abnormal excretion of ADH. Abnormally elevated levels of ADH occur despite lack of a hypovolemic or hyperosmolar state that would normally trigger ADH release. This inappropriate increase in ADH secretion causes continuous reabsorption of water from the renal tubules, resulting in serum hypotonicity and hyponatremia without evidence of dehydration or peripheral edema.[307,308] High urine sodium levels and urine osmolality greater than the serum osmolarity are also noted.[308] As hyponatremia worsens, others symptoms become evident, such as neurologic deterioration, nausea, vomiting, and muscle weakness (see Table 19-9).[306] The ultimate consequence of SIADH is water intoxication with cerebral edema.

TABLE 19-9 Clinical Manifestations and Treatment of Neurogenic DI, Syndrome of Inappropriate ADH, and Cerebral Salt Wasting

Parameter	Diabetes Insipidus	Syndrome of Inappropriate ADH	Cerebral Salt Wasting
Urine specific gravity	Low	Elevated	Elevated
Urine osmolality	Low	Increased	Increased
Urine sodium	Low in relation to serum	Elevated	Elevated
Serum osmolality	Elevated	Decreased	Decreased
Serum sodium	Elevated	Decreased	Decreased
Clinical manifestations	Hypovolemia, dehydration, Intensive thirst (if mechanism is not impaired) Large volumes of poorly concentrated urine Aqueous Pitressin administration causes urine osmolality increase of 9% or more	Euvolemic or hypervolemic Usually low urine output, low BUN Muscle cramps, weight gain without edema, lethargy, confusion, personality change, irritability, sluggish deep tendon reflexes, anorexia, nausea/vomiting, diarrhea, abdominal cramps, fatigue, headache, restlessness Severe signs—coma, seizures, death	Hypovolemia, dehydration Increased BUN, High urine output, Net sodium loss
Treatment	Replete fluid volume • Hypotonic fluids usually indicated • Administer fluid to replace urine output and insensible losses • Administer exogenous ADH: • Aqueous Pitressin—commonly used in critical phase • Pitressin tannate in oil • 1-Deamino, 8-D-arginine vasopressin (dDAVP, desmopressin) • Nasal lysine vasopressin	Fluid restriction For severe symptoms: Give hypertonic saline solution Diurese with furosemide (Lasix) Give demeclocycline (Declomycin) to produce renal resistance to ADH	Replete salt and fluid volume

BUN, Blood urea nitrogen.

Treatment depends on the severity of SIADH and typically starts with strict fluid restriction (as little as 800 ml/day). Furosemide may be used to diurese the patient and, in severe cases, hypertonic saline solutions (usually 3% sodium chloride) may be administered judiciously. Demeclocycline hydrochloride (Declomycin) may be used to produce renal resistance to ADH.[306]

Cerebral Salt Wasting.   Brain injury may also trigger cerebral salt wasting (CSW), which causes primary sodium loss and subsequent reduction in extracellular fluid and intravascular volume. The exact etiology for this abnormal sodium loss is unknown. Like SIADH, cerebral salt wasting results in hyponatremia and serum hyposmolarity, but, unlike SIADH, there is a decrease in extracellular fluid volume and a negative salt balance (see Table 19-9).[306,308,309] High blood urea nitrogen levels, excessive loss of sodium in the urine, and evidence of fluid volume deficit are noted with CSW. Treatment of CSW entails replacing fluid, as well as sodium.[306-308]

Coagulopathy.   Severe TBI with massive brain tissue damage can activate coagulation systems, causing an increase in clotting and consumption of clotting factors, which results in coagulopathy and excessive bleeding. The degree of abnormality in coagulation parameters has been correlated with the severity of and morbidity from TBI.[310,311] Coagulopathy can increase the risk of delayed intracranial hemorrhage.[311,312] It can also be cause for delay in necessary neurosurgical procedures.[311] Nurses should monitor coagulation values to detect coagulopathy. Once recognized, treatment with appropriate blood products, such as fresh frozen plasma, platelets, and other sources of clotting factors, should be instituted as appropriate.

Gastrointestinal Mucosal Erosion.   Erosion of the gastrointestinal mucosa is common after severe brain injury.[313] The pathogenesis of this gastrointestinal process as it relates to intracranial injury is still unclear. Posttraumatic stress and autonomic nervous system disruption associated with brain injury are thought to be two potential causes of mucosal erosion. Venkatesh et al[314] demonstrated that significant gastric intramucosal acidosis occurred in 9 of the 10 patients studied who had isolated severe TBI. Proton pump inhibitors, mucosal protective agents (sucralfate), H2 antagonists, and antacids are usually routinely administered to prevent gastrointestinal erosion and possible bleeding. The character of gastric drainage and stool should be monitored for overt or chemical presence in blood.

Cardiac Rhythm Abnormalities.   Repolarization abnormalities and cardiac arrhythmias may occur after TBI. Repolarization abnormalities may include ST- and T-wave changes, prolonged QT waves, short PR intervals, Q or U waves, and myocardial infarction-like changes. Arrhythmias may include sinus bradycardia, caused by ICP elevations and resulting brainstem compression. Tachycardia and supraventricular tachycardia are often noted in the terminal phase during brainstem compression. Atrial fibrillation, atrial flutter, premature ventricular contractions, ventricular tachycardia, and atrioventricular blocks are other arrhythmias that may be seen after TBI.[315] These repolarization abnormalities and arrhythmias associated with brain injury may be linked to catecholamine release or autonomic nervous system disruption.

Patients with acute brain injury should be monitored with continuous electrocardiogram. Effort should be made to rule out other physiologic causes for the cardiac rhythm abnormalities, such as fluid and electrolyte imbalance, hypoxemia, heart disease, myocardial trauma, or hypovolemia. Treatment should be initiated for cardiac rhythm abnormalities as necessary.

Protein-Calorie Malnutrition.   Severe TBI triggers a metabolic response characterized by hypermetabolism, hypercatabolism, increased nitrogen excretion, and hyperglycemia.[118,316,317] The energy expenditure of patients with brain injury is increased an average of 40% above expected.[317] Nitrogen excretion is two to three times higher in brain-injured patients than uninjured persons.[118] Elevated catabolic hormone and cytokine levels and increased muscle tone associated with brain injury are believed to contribute to this hypermetabolic response.[317] This metabolic response to TBI can quickly lead to protein-calorie malnutrition, which increases the likelihood of multisystem organ dysfunction and impairs wound healing and immune function.[316]

Nutritional assessment and management are multidisciplinary, involving the nutritionist, physician, and nurse. Consultation with a registered dietitian is helpful for determining the patient's individualized nutritional requirements. The "Guidelines for Management of Severe Traumatic Brain Injury" recommend replacing 140% of the resting metabolism expenditure in brain-injured patients who are not paralyzed and replacing 100% of the resting metabolism expenditure in patients receiving paralytics or high-dose barbiturates within 7 days after injury.[118] Enteral or parenteral formulas containing at least 15% of their calories as proteins should be started within 72 hours of injury to achieve full caloric replacement by the seventh day after brain injury.[118] Although there are multiple advantages in using enteral nutrition, delayed gastric emptying may necessitate use of parenteral nutrition.[316] A jejunal route for enteral feedings is preferred, because risk of aspiration is reduced, gastric intolerance is avoided, and risks of parenteral nutrition are absent.[118] Nurses should remain cognizant of how well the patient is tolerating feedings. Hyperglycemia should be minimized to avoid a potential adverse effect on the patient's outcome.[317] See Chapter 16 for a complete review of the metabolic and nutritional management of the trauma patient.

Complications Related to Immobility.   Motor deficits caused by brain injury, as well as therapy employed to manage this disease (e.g., sedatives and paralytic agents), render the patients immobile, making them prone to a plethora of complications. Meticulous skin care and regular turning aid in the prevention of skin breakdown. Minimizing time on unpadded bed surfaces, adequately padding and relieving pressure on bony prominences, and avoiding placement of hypothermia blankets beneath the patient are other nursing measures that aid in preserving skin integrity. The incidence of deep vein thrombosis may be reduced by (1) use of lower extremity pneumatic compression devices to decrease venous stasis and (2) initiation of prophylactic heparin or low-molecular-weight heparin therapy, as directed by the neurosurgeon. Frequent passive range-of-motion exercises are needed to reduce venous stasis and prevent contractures. Once a patient is stable and approval has been obtained from the neurosurgeon, consideration should be given to getting the patient out of bed and properly supported in a bedside chair for a limited time to help prevent complications related to immobility. Serial lower extremity casting and upper extremity splints may be used in the critical care setting to prevent or treat spasticity-induced contractures. Early initiation of physical therapy and occupational therapy in the critical care phase can be vitally important for prevention of many complications associated with immobility.

COGNITIVE REHABILITATION.   Once the patient has been stabilized and ICP is well controlled, cognitive retraining can begin during the critical care phase. The nurse should work collaboratively with speech, physical, and occupational therapists to evaluate the patient's level of functioning and then plan appropriate therapies. In the critical care phase a patient with severe TBI is often unresponsive to stimuli, nonpurposeful, and demonstrates an inconsistent generalized response or an inconsistent localized purposeful response to stimuli. These behaviors are synonymous with the descriptors in the first three levels of the Rancho Tool. The goal for a patient with this low level of function is to elicit behavioral responses to external stimuli and to evoke higher level motor responses (i.e., arm or leg movement). Cognitive retraining proceeds by providing meaningful stimuli to the five senses. Sensory stimulation and all components of brain rehabilitation are based on the theory that repetition and consistency of stimuli strengthen recessive or alternative pathways through which function may be regained. Sensory stimulation therapy is designed to arouse only one sense at a time for a brief period to minimize confusion and sensory overload.[318,319] Most stimulation occurs naturally during routine nursing interventions. For example, tactile stimulation can be provided when performing hygiene measures. Soft, smooth speech patterns during reorientation or explanation of needed procedures, as well as intermittent music or television, provide auditory stimuli. Taste can be stimulated during mouth care with the use of flavored mouth swabs or by touching the tongue with a popsicle. Placing substances with pleasant odors near the patient provides olfactory stimulus. Family photos and familiar items can be shown to the patient to provide visual input. The nurse should identify particular and preferably familiar stimuli that best elicit a response. Each period of stimulation should be followed by a rest period.

The family should be included in the cognitive retraining program. Their ability to provide familiarity for the patient is invaluable. If family members are unable to visit, they can be encouraged to make audio tapes and supply personal items that have pleasant associations for the patient.

CARE OF THE FAMILY.   Crisis intervention that began in the resuscitation phase should continue in the critical care phase of care. Family members must be taught how to interact with a patient who is unresponsive or may respond inappropriately. The nurse should demonstrate how to speak and provide tactile stimulation to the patient. The patient's physiologic response to family interaction should be noted.

INTERMEDIATE CARE AND REHABILITATION PHASES

Numerous complications can continue to plague the brain-injured patient throughout the intermediate care and rehabilitation phases of care. Interventions aimed at prevention, recognition, and treatment of potential complications remain important. Therapy aimed at optimizing cognitive function and resolving psychologic and emotional disturbances associated with brain injury is also important during these phases.

MAINTAINING AIRWAY PATENCY.   Maintaining a patent airway remains a priority during the intermediate care and rehabilitation phases. The patient's airway can be partially or completely obstructed by improper positioning, collection of secretions in the respiratory tract, or aspiration. The patient should be positioned so that the upper airway is completely open. A side-lying or upright position with good head and neck alignment is advisable. Aggressive pulmonary toilet, including postural drainage and chest physiotherapy, should be continued as necessary to prevent atelectasis and possible retention of secretions. Aspiration precautions initiated during the critical care phase, when enteral tube feedings were likely started, should be continued in the intermediate care and rehabilitation phases. Before beginning feedings by mouth, a swallowing evaluation should be preformed to determine if swallowing dysfunction exists, which would increase the risk of aspiration.[320]

PREVENTING AND TREATING COMPLICATIONS RELATED TO IMMOBILITY.   Prevention and treatment of complications related to immobility, including pulmonary complications, venous thrombosis, skin breakdown, loss of joint mobility, and bowel and bladder complications, continue to be a high priority during the intermediate and rehabilitation phases of care. Occupational and physical therapists continue to play a pivotal role in prevention of immobility-related complications during these phases of hospitalization. Realistic goals to increase patient mobility should be set by the multidisciplinary health care team, taking into account the patient's tolerance of increased movement and any limitations cited by the neurosurgeon. Getting a patient out of bed at least twice a day as tolerated is helpful in preventing complications of immobility. Active and passive range-of-motion exercises remain important, and strengthening exercises can be started once the patient is actively involved in his or her therapy.

Spasticity.   Spasticity is the sustained increase in involuntary muscle tone that occurs in response to muscle stretch. Tone is increased as the rate of muscle stretch increases.[321] Spasticity occurs as a complication of an upper motor neuron injury. Spasticity may be beneficial because it can reduce the development of deep vein thrombosis or osteoporosis, maintain muscle mass, and assist the patient with minimal motor function in performing transfers.[322] Spasticity can also increase patient disability by reducing range of motion, decreasing the patient's functional capabilities, increasing energy requirements for movement, and causing contractures and severe pain.[322,323]

If spasticity becomes problematic for the brain-injured patient, treatment is indicated. Clear goals should be established when considering treatment options. Decisions about treatment should consider the distribution, severity, and chronicity of the spasticity; the support systems available to the patient; and the presence of co-morbidities (e.g., cognitive deficits, contractures).[323] Range-of-motion exercises are important for all patients because they help prevent contractures, desensitize nerve receptors, and may reduce motor unit activity by resetting the interneuronal pool.[323] Other physical modalities used to treat spasticity include cold and heat application, muscle stretching, vibration, splinting, casting or bracing, proper positioning, functional electrical stimulation, relaxation techniques, and biofeedback.[322] If oral antispasmodics are indicated, dantrolene sodium (Dantrium) is typically the initial drug of choice, because it has a peripheral site of action and has less sedative and cognitive effect.[322,324] Baclofen and diazepam are two other drugs that may be used to reduce cerebral spasticity, although sedative and adverse cognitive effects make them less attractive options.[324] Continuously infused intrathecal baclofen therapy has good long-term effect in reducing spastic dystonic hypertonia.[325,326] Chemical denervation using phenol or botulinum toxin has also been used to control spasticity.[323]

Heterotopic Ossification.   Heterotopic ossification (HO) is the deposition of bone in major joints, which can potentially cause complete ankylosis of the joint and functional impairment.[322,327] The etiology of HO after brain injury remains unclear. HO is most commonly seen in the hips, elbows, knees, and shoulders. Symptoms of HO include extremity or joint swelling and redness and low-grade fever. Plain x-ray films may be negative in the early inflammatory phase, but HO may be apparent on bone scan. Alkaline phosphate levels may also be increased.[322] Nonsteroidal antiinflammatory drugs (NSAIDs; e.g., indomethacin) may be helpful in reducing the pain and may decrease inflammation associated with HO.[322] Etidronate disodium (Didronel) has been commonly used to prevent or decrease the severity of HO, although its efficacy remains questionable and the exact dosage and when its use is appropriate remain controversial.[322,324] The potential adverse effects of this drug (e.g., osteoporosis, osteomalacia) make it sometimes contraindicated or useful only for a limited time.[324] Surgical resection of the bone deposit may be indicated in severe cases, and low-dose radiation may be provided after excision to help prevent return of ectopic bone deposition.[328]

MANAGEMENT OF BOWEL AND BLADDER FUNCTION.   Patients in a vegetative state may have persistent bowel and bladder incontinence. Female patients with urinary incontinence may require an indwelling catheter, intermittent catheterization, an external urine collection bag, or diapers, whereas male patients can generally be managed using an external condom device for collection of urine. Prevention of urinary tract infection is critical.

Constipation is common in the immobilized patient. A bowel regimen should be initiated once the patient tolerates enteral feedings, and the patient should be checked regularly for bowel impaction. Bowel retraining, typically initiated in the intermediate phase, can be done even when the patient is comatose. The goal is to establish an effective bowel evacuation pattern.

COGNITIVE REHABILITATION.   Some patients who have suffered severe brain injury may continue to have very low levels of cognitive function consistent with Rancho Tool scores of I, II, or III. These patients are typically referred to long-term care facilities or to coma stimulation programs, where attempts are made to illicit a response to environmental stimuli, as described in the critical care phase. Other patients have less cognitive impairment or may demonstrate improvement in their cognitive status, giving them a higher level of cognitive function.

A patient who is confused and agitated, or confused and inappropriate (levels IV and V, respectively, on the Rancho Tool), should have stimulation and informational input drastically reduced. Patients exhibiting these behaviors have impaired ability to process information, and they rapidly reach a point of sensory overload. Short-term memory is also severely impaired, so patients are unable to ground themselves with information about people, places, or events. Bizarre behavior, such as screaming outbursts, aggression, disinhibition, delusions, hallucinations, or incoherent verbalizations, may be evident. Patients have a limited attention span and may confabulate or perseverate.

The nurse must provide a structured environment with

controlled stimulation, order, repetition, and consistency to optimize the patient's cognitive processing.[318,319] A break in routine can increase the patient's confusion or rebellious behavior. This can often be avoided by preparing the patient for change as far in advance as possible and providing frequent reinforcement. Choices must be restricted so that the patient's confusion is not increased. A strict schedule of therapies and activities should be established, accompanied by intermittent rest periods.

These patients have difficulty deciphering stimuli; when bombarded with sensory input, their behavior can become erratic and confused. Stimuli should not be excessive. Music and television may be productive for short periods but may become overwhelming if used excessively. Visitors should be limited to one or two persons, and conversation should involve only one person at a time. A calm, quiet atmosphere supports information processing.

Stimuli should be meaningful, and repetition should be encouraged. When patients need to relearn previous skills, it is most productive to use meaningful objects (e.g., use a cup to teach grasping and grasp release). Patients should be given only one-step commands if that is all they are capable of handling. If more steps are given, confusion results and patients are unable to carry out any of the commands. Simple mnemonics, visual imagery, and association and organizational strategies are helpful to cue patients with memory deficits. Patient teaching should be simple and concrete with positive reinforcement. Considerable time and patience are typically required to assist the patient in achieving the goal of functioning independently.

Disruptive and at times aggressive behavior is common.[318] The nurse needs to be cognizant of the potential for self-injury and injury to others. This type of behavior can be handled by use of distracting tactics, capitalizing on the patient's short-term attention span and impaired processing skills.

It is common for patients to go through a period of agitation during recovery from brain injury. Agitated patients are usually confused and have severe short-term memory impairment.[322] Every effort should be made to rule out other physiologic causes for agitation, such as hypoxia, sleep disturbances, seizures, fluid and electrolyte imbalance, or pain. Unnecessary noxious stimuli should be removed and avoided if possible. Psychomotor activities such as ambulation are encouraged to help decrease agitation. A quiet environment, a room with padding to prevent injury, and reassuring one-to-one supervision may be necessary during periods of extreme agitation. Various pharmacologic agents have been used in attempts to control agitation. Popular agents include lorazepam (Ativan), trazodone (Desyrel), and haloperidol (Haldol). No one agent has been found to work best for all patients.[322]

Patients at Rancho Tool level VI are confused but appropriate and able to accomplish tasks with supervision. Information processing has improved, although memory deficit persists. A daily routine should be established and followed closely. Patients may be given more responsibility for their own activities of daily living and toileting. Feedback should be provided to reinforce appropriate behavior. Behavior modification programs can be used to control uninhibited, disruptive behavior. Cognitive remediation at this point in the patient's recovery addresses five core deficit areas: (1) arousal and attention, (2) skills structures, (3) memory, (4) language and thought processes, and (5) emotion. Cognitive remediation is based on assessment of deficits and strengths, remedial cueing interventions, and the patient's ability to respond to the interventions.

At a level VII on the Rancho Tool, the patient's behavior is automatic and appropriate, with minimal to no confusion, but there may still be some difficulty with socialization, emotions, and returning to work. Structure should be reduced and self-care responsibilities should be increased for the patient at this level of cognitive functioning.[318] It is essential to give the patient positive and constructive feedback. The patient may also require continued follow-up to deal with the emotional difficulties that may persist after TBI.

At a Rancho Tool level VIII, the patient will be purposeful and appropriate, totally oriented, with good recall, but problem solving and reasoning difficulties may continue to be challenging. The patient is typically able to compensate for these persistent difficulties (e.g., with the use of cue cards to compensate for short-term memory impairment).

MANAGEMENT OF PSYCHOLOGIC AND EMOTIONAL DISTURBANCES. Emotional and psychologic disturbances associated with brain injury can increase the patient's disability and inhibit optimal recovery. Depression, mood changes, apathy, mania, and acute stress disorder are a few of the psychologic and emotional disturbances described after brain injury. Depression is particularly common after brain injury and can impede achievement of optimal functional outcomes.[329-331] The advent of sophisticated diagnostic technology has allowed brain anatomy and neurochemical correlates of depression to be identified.[330] Several psychosocial correlates with depression after brain injury have also been identified.[330,331] The physical and psychologic sequelae of brain injury can confound the diagnosis and assessment of depression.[330] Accurate assessment, diagnosis, and treatment of depression are essential. If the patient is taking medications that may cause depression, they should be discontinued if possible. Antidepressants are often used to manage depression in these patients. Cognitive-behavioral therapy, psychotherapy, and support groups may also be helpful for the patient.[330]

FAMILY AND RESOURCES

Trauma affects not only the patient but also the family, which is often unprepared for the sudden onset of brain injury and the long-term rehabilitation it may require. Shock, disbelief, denial, grief, and anger are common initial feelings described by families of patients with a TBI.[332] Caregivers of patients with TBI have said that the patient's neurobehavioral and emotional disturbances, rather than the physical disabilities, have the most significant impact on the family members' quality of life.[333-335] Family members often develop relationship strains, social isolation, substance abuse problems, and financial burden related to caring for the patient and lack of employment. A high incidence of major depression has been reported among caregivers of patients with TBI.[333]

It is extremely important to provide care and support for the family, as well as the patient. Long-term monitoring of caregivers' emotional status is important to identify onset of depression or increased anxiety. The nurse should establish daily communication with the family and assist in identifying other resources that will enable the family to cope more effectively with the catastrophic event. It is important to provide families with information about the patients' quality of life after TBI. The correct information needs to be provided to the family at the right time for the message to have the most beneficial effect. Information about behavioral and emotional changes that may be caused by TBI should be provided to enhance the family's ability to cope with these disabilities.[336] Support and counseling to enhance coping skills are extremely important. It is important to offer frequent reassurance for their positive coping skills and to try to decrease feelings of guilt. The need for respite care should be emphasized to decrease the fatigue and emotional distress that is often felt when caring for the patient with TBI. In addition, support groups or individual therapy may be necessary for some family members.

Families should be made aware of all brain injury support services within the hospital, in the community, and across the nation. Sources of referral within the acute care setting may include social services, nursing psychiatric specialties, pastoral care, neuropsychologic consultations, and an in-house brain injury support group. Community and national support referrals include local brain injury support groups, the Brain Injury Association, and the state chapter of the Brain Injury Association. The family should be informed of possible benefits and sources of financial assistance at the state and federal levels for patients with TBI.

COMMUNITY REINTEGRATION

Complex emotional, psychosocial, behavioral, cognitive, and physical disabilities may persist for years after a TBI. Disposition of patients after brain injury depends on the extent of the neurologic disability. The majority of mildly brain-injured patients without obvious neurologic deficiencies are discharged home with follow-up instructions. Although superficially these patients may have normal neurologic function, after return to work or school, difficulty concentrating, poor memory, fatigue, and other types of symptoms associated with mild TBI may become evident and quite disabling. With resumption of the patient's previous lifestyle, the chronic nature of deficits and the limiting effects of disabilities become apparent. Distress is increased and patients tire easily, are overwhelmed, and may withdraw, resulting in family conflict.

Patients with obvious deficits may be discharged with plans for continued outpatient rehabilitation or to independent living programs or community reentry programs. Patients in a vegetative state or too severely disabled to actively participate in a structured rehabilitation program are typically discharged to extended care facilities or to facilities that have special coma management programs. Other specialized brain-injury programs are also available to meet the needs of brain-injured patients. In addition to acute rehabilitation and coma management programs, other options include behavioral programs, transitional living, independent living, community reentry, and prevocational, vocational, and sheltered work training.[337]

OUTCOME FROM TRAUMATIC BRAIN INJURY

Improved survival after TBI is important but means little without concomitant improvement in quality of life. Epidemiologic and treatment studies done during the past decade have focused on more carefully defining outcomes of both acute and chronic care beyond merely survival.

Neurologic deficits after head injury are referred to as "impairments" in the World Health Organization International Classification of Impairments, Disabilities and Handicaps (ICIDH), whereas "disability" is any restriction or lack of ability to perform an activity within the range considered normal for a human being.[338,339] Even though a brain injury is classified as mild or moderate, with few measurable deficits, the disability resulting from a combination of cognitive, motor, and sensory dysfunction may be extremely troublesome and a source of great anxiety to the individual and the family.[340]

Disability results from motor, sensory, cognitive, and behavioral deficits (impairments). The list is limitless, with the type and degree of deficit depending on the site and severity of the injury, as well as preinjury factors.[329,341,342] Many motor and mild sensory deficits improve over time. Some patients have complete functional recovery, and the majority of those with permanent deficits generally learn to compensate or adapt to their loss. Cognitive and personality deficits, however, tend to persist even after focal deficits have resolved; they are the major cause of chronic disability after head injury.

Short-term memory impairment is the most persistent of all deficits. In patients with severe disability, it may not return to any functional extent. This presents a major problem in recovery because new information cannot be retained sufficiently for relearning to take place.

For research studies describing natural recovery or comparing modes of treatment, outcome is generally assessed 6 months after injury, because maximum recovery occurs in about 90% of patients during this period.[343] This is not to say that no further recovery continues, but the rate is much slower in the years after injury. It appears that physical deficits improve more quickly than cognitive ones, with the latter showing slow improvement over the years.[344] There is growing evidence that formalized rehabilitation

TABLE 19-10 **Characteristics Defining Each Category of the Glasgow Outcome Scale**

Categories	Characteristics
Good recovery (GR)	• Able to participate in normal social activities and return to work
	• Some restrictions in extent of social and leisure participation, or infrequent personality changes that interfere with return to normal life place person in lower GR category
Moderate disability (MD)	• Inability to work in previous capacity
	• Restriction on previous social and leisure activities
	• Frequent or constant posttraumatic personality changes
	• The lower range of MD is characterized by inability to work or ability to work only in sheltered workshop or noncompetitive job, inability to participate in prior social and leisure activities
Severe disability (SD)	• Implies consciousness, but dependence on others for at least some of daily needs
	• Needs assistance in home for some activities of daily living, cannot shop without assistance, cannot travel locally without assistance
	• If person also needs someone to be around home most of the time, he or she qualifies for the lower SD category on GOSE
Vegetative state (VS)	• Have sleep and awake periods, but with no evidence of sentient responsiveness
Death (D)	

programs improve vocational and social function beyond that expected from spontaneous recovery alone.[345,346] Consequently, outcome may be reasonably assessed as early as 6 months and as long as 3 to 5 years after injury.[347]

MEASURES OF OUTCOME

The formal measurement of outcome has become much more extensive in recent years as survival has increased, and there has been more emphasis on outcomes indicating quality of survival. The most commonly used outcome measure is the Glasgow Outcome Scale (GOS). The original Glasgow Outcome Scale has five categories (Table 19-10).[348] A more recent 8-point refinement, called the Extended Glasgow Outcome Scale (GOSE), includes two gradations within each of three categories of functional survival.[349,350] Its structured interview format[350] provides good reproducibility of classification among observers. The Disability Rating Scale (DRS),[351] Functional Independence Measure (FIM),[352] and Community Integration Questionnaire (CIQ)[338,353-355] are other measures of outcome often used in studies of treatment of and recovery from TBI. Two sources of information about specific measures and their use are the *Handbook of Neurologic Rating Scales*[339] and the Traumatic Brain Injury Model Systems Web site (www.tbims.org/combi.html).

PREDICTORS OF OUTCOME

Although some patients with a poor prognosis do well and others who should conceivably do well make poor recoveries, the outcome of most people with severe head injuries in terms of survival and good versus poor recovery can be fairly well predicted from injury and clinical data. The most reliable predictors of outcomes after severe head injury are depth of coma (based on postresuscitation GCS score), pupil reaction, eye movements, motor response, age, and type of head injury.[98,356,357] Factors that contribute to secondary brain injury, such as prehospital oxygenation and

hypotension, are also important predictors of poor versus good recovery outcome in both children and adults.[358,359]

Predicting cognitive recovery and psychosocial functioning from early clinical indicators is more difficult. The GCS score and the length of posttraumatic amnesia are both indicators of the extent of injury and correlate best with cognitive outcomes.[360] In addition, preinjury education, level of function, psychosocial characteristics, and social support also influence psychosocial and cognitive outcome potential in both children and adults.[17,341,361]

Considerable progress has been made in assessing a range of outcomes from traumatic brain injury. These include not only survival but also the quality of recovery and cognitive and psychosocial outcomes.

SUMMARY

Nurses in each phase of trauma care play a pivotal role in ensuring that the patient with TBI achieves optimal outcomes. Equipped with knowledge about TBI pathophysiology, assessment interpretation, and current evidence-based recommendations for treatment, the nurse is able to work collaboratively with the multidisciplinary team to plan and implement the most appropriate care. New developments in defining TBI pathophysiology and innovations in assessment and monitoring techniques for the injured brain open opportunities for nursing research to define the care that will best enable optimal outcomes to be achieved.

REFERENCES

1. Thurman DJ, Alverson C, Dunn KA et al: Traumatic brain injury in the United States: A public health perspective, *J Head Trauma Rehabil* 14:602-615, 1999.
2. Berube JE: A good first step toward nationwide aid to persons with brain injury: the traumatic brain injury act of 1996, *J Head Trauma Rehabil* 13:80-82, 1998.

3. Kraus JF, McArthur DL: Epidemiologic aspects of brain injury, *Neurol Clin* 14:435-450, 1996.

4. Thurman DJ, Sniezek JE, Johnson D et al: *Guidelines for surveillance of central nervous system injury,* Atlanta, 1995, Centers for Disease Control and Prevention.

5. Sosin DM, Sniezek JE, Thurman DJ: Incidence of mild and moderate brain injury in the United States, 1991, *Brain Inj* 10:47-54, 1996.

6. Centers for Disease Control and Prevention: *Epidemiology of traumatic brain injury in the United States,* www.cdc.gov/nipc/dacrrdp/tbi.htm, March 21, 2000.

7. Guerrero JL, Thurman DJ, Sniezek JE: Emergency department visits associated with traumatic brain injury: United States, 1995-1996, *Brain Inj* 14:181-186, 2000.

8. Thurman D, Guerrero J: Trends in hospitalization associated with traumatic brain injury, *JAMA* 282:954-957, 1999.

9. Sosin DM, Sniezek JE, Waxmeiler RJ: Trends in death associated with traumatic brain injury, 1979 through 1992, *JAMA* 273:1778-1780, 1995.

10. Brain Injury Association: *The costs and causes of Traumatic Brain Injury,* www.biause.org/costsand.htm, July 14, 2001.

11. Hickey JV: *The clinical practice of neurological and neurosurgical nursing,* ed 4, Philadelphia, 1997, JB Lippincott.

12. Nikas DL: The neurologic system. In Alspath JG, editor: *Core curriculum for critical care nursing,* ed 5, Philadelphia, 1998, WB Saunders, 339-463.

13. Golding EM, Robertson CS, Bryan RM: The consequences of traumatic brain injury on cerebral blood flow and autoregulation: a review, *Clin Exp Hypertens* 21:299-332, 1999.

14. Obrist WD, Marion DW: Xenon techniques for CBF measurements in clinical head injury. In Narayan RK, Wilberger JE Jr, Povlichock, editors: *Neurotrauma,* New York, 1997, McGraw-Hill, 471-485.

15. Thurman DJ, Jeppson L, Burnett CL et al: Surveillance of traumatic brain injuries in Utah, *West J Med* 165:192-196, 1996.

16. Schootman M, Harlan M, Fuortes L: Use of the capture-recapture method to estimate severe traumatic brain injury rates, *J Trauma* 48:70-75, 2000.

17. Harrison-Felix C, Zafonte R, Mann N et al: Brain injury as a result of violence: preliminary findings from the traumatic brain injury model systems, *Arch Phys Med Rehabil* 79:730-737, 1998.

18. Centers for Disease Control and Prevention: *Preventing bicycle-related injuries,* www.cdc.gov/ncipc/factsheets/bikehel.htm, January 27, 2000.

19. Thompson DC, Patterson MQ: Cycle helmets and the prevention of injuries: recommendations for competitive sport, *Sports Med Apr* 25(4):213-219, 1998.

20. Morrison AL, King TM, Korell MA et al: Acceleration-deceleration injuries to the brain in blunt force trauma, *Am J Forensic Med Pathol* 19:109-112, 1998.

21. Smith DH, Chen X-H, Xu B-N et al: Characterization of diffuse axonal pathology and selective hippocampal damage following inertial brain trauma in the pig, *J Neuropathol Exp Neurol* 56:822-834, 1997.

22. Liker MA, Aarabi B, Levy ML: Missile wounds to the head: Ballistics and Forensics. In Aarabi B, editor: *Missile wounds of the head and neck,* vol 1, 1999, Park Ridge, IL, The American Association of Neurological Surgeons, 35-55.

23. Sabin SL, Lee D, Har-el G: Low velocity gunshot injuries to the temporal bone, *J Laryngol Otol* 112:929-933, 1998.

24. Kraus JF, McAuthur DL, Silverman TA et al: Epidemiology of brain injury. In Narayan RK, Wilberger JE Jr., Povlishock JT, editors: *Neurotrauma,* New York, 1996, McGraw-Hill, 13-30.

25. Graham DI: Neuropathology of head-injury. In Narayan RK, Wilberger JE Jr, Povlishock JT, editors: *Neurotrauma,* New York, 1996, McGraw-Hill, 43-59.

26. Valadka AB, Narayan RK: Emergency room management of the head-injured patient. In Narayan RK, Wilberger JE Jr, Povlishock JT, editors: *Neurotrauma,* New York, 1996, McGraw-Hill, 119-135.

27. Prow HW, Cole JW, Yeakley J et al: Non-invasive neuroimaging in closed head trauma. In Evans RW, editor: *Neurology and trauma,* Philadelphia, 1996, WB Saunders Co, 29-52.

28. Kampfl A, Franz G, Aichner F et al: The persistent vegetative state after closed head injury: clinical and magnetic resonance imaging findings in 42 patients, *J Neurosurg* 88:809-816, 1998.

29. Cook RJ, Dorsch NWC, Fearnside MR et al: Outcome pediction in extradural haematomas, *Acta Neurochir* 95:90-94, 1998.

30. Firsching R, Heimann M, Frowein RA: Early dynamics of acute extradural and subdural hematomas, *Neurol Res* 19:257-260, 1997.

31. Servadei F: Prognostic factors in severely head injured adult patients with acute subdural haematomas, *Acta Neurochir* 139:279-285, 1997.

32. Seelig JM, Becker DP, Miller JD et al: Traumatic acute subdural hematoma: major mortality reduction in comatose patients treated within four hours, *N Engl J Med* 304(25):1511-1518, 1981.

33. Graham DI, McIntosh TK: Neuropathology of brain injury. In Evans RW, editor: *Neurology and trauma,* Philadelphia, 1996, WB Saunders, 53-90.

34. Greene KA, Jacobowitz R, Marciano FF et al: Impact of traumatic subarachnoid hemorrhage on outcome in nonpenetrating head injury. Part II: Relationship to clinical course and outcome variables during acute hospitalization, *J Trauma* 41:964-971, 1996.

35. Kakarieka A, Braakman R, Schakel EH: Clinical significance of the finding of subarachnoid blood on CT scan after head injury, *Acta Neurochir* 129:1-5, 1994.

36. The European Study Group on Nimodipine in Severe Head Injury: A multicenter trial of the efficacy of nimodipine on outcome after severe head injury, *J Neurosurg* 80:797-804, 1994.

37. Teasdale GM, Graham DI: Craniocerebral trauma: protection and retrieval of the neuronal population after injury, *Neurosurgery* 43:723-737, 1998.

38. Gennarelli TA: Cerebral conclusion and diffuse brain injuries. In Cooper PR, editor: *Head injury,* ed 3, Baltimore, 1993, Williams & Wilkins, 137-158.

39. Flanagan S: Physiatric management of mild traumatic brain injury, *Mt Sinai J Med* 66:152-159, 1999.

40. Abu-Judeh HH, Parker R, Singh M et al: SPET brain perfusion imaging in mild traumatic brain injury without loss of consciousness and normal computed tomography, *Nucl Med Comm* 20:505-510, 1999.

41. Abdel-Dayem HM, Abu-Judeh H, Kumar M et al: SPECT brain perfusion abnormalities in mild or moderate traumatic brain injury, *Clin Nucl Med* 23:309-317, 1998.

42. Ross BD, Ernst T, Kreis R et al: ^{1}H MRS in acute traumatic brain injury, *J Magn Reson Imaging* 8:829-840, 1998.

43. Kant R, Smith-Seemiller L, Isaac G et al: Tc-HMPAO SPECT in persistent post-concussion syndrome after mild head injury: comparison with MRI/CT, *Brain Inj* 11:115-124, l997.

44. Bryant RA, Harvey AG: Postconcussive symptoms and post-traumatic stress disorder after mild traumatic brain injury, *J Nerv Ment Dis* 187:302-305, 1999.

45. Kushner D: Mild traumatic brain injury toward understanding manifestations and treatment, *Arch Intern Med* 158:1617-1624, 1998.

46. Gasquoine, PG: Postconcussion symptoms, *Neuropsych Rev* 7:77-85, 1997.

47. Wade DT, King NS, Wenden FJ et al: Routine follow up after head injury: a second randomised controlled trial, *J Neurol Neurosurg Psychiatry* 65:177-183, 1998.

48. Sturmi JE, Smith C, Lombardo JA: Mild brain trauma in sports, *Sports Med* 25:351-358, 1998.

49. Kelly J: From the centers for disease control and prevention: sports related recurrent brain injuries—United States, *JAMA* 277:1190-1191, 1997.

50. Fiser SM, Johnson SB, Fortune JB: Resource utilization in traumatic brain injury: the role of magnetic resonance imaging, *Am Surg* 64(11):1088-1093, 1998.

51. Jennett B: Clinical and pathological features of vegetative survival. In Levin HS, Benton AL, Muizelaar JP et al, editors: *Catastrophic brain injury*, New York, 1996, Oxford University Press, 3-13.

52. Tymianski M, Tator CH: Normal and abnormal calcium homeostasis in neurons: a basis for the pathophysiology of traumatic and ischemic central nervous system injury, *Neurosurgery* 38:1176-1195, 1996.

53. McIntosh TK, Saatman KE, Raghupathi R et al: The molecular and cellular sequelae of experimental traumatic brain injury: pathogenetic mechanisms, *Neuropathol Appl Neurobiol* 24:251-267, 1998.

54. Koura SS, Doppenberg EMR, Marmarou A et al: Relationship between excitatory amino acid release and outcome after severe human head injury, *Acta Neurochir* 71:244-246, 1998.

55. Vespa P, Prins M, Ronne-Engstrom E et al: Increase in extracellular glutamate caused by reduced cerebral perfusion pressure and seizures after human traumatic brain injury: a microdialysis study, *J Neurosurg* 89:971-982, 1998.

56. Bullock R, Zauner A, Woodward JJ et al: Factors affecting excitatory amino acid release following severe human head injury, *J Neurosurg* 89:507-518, 1998.

57. Bullock MR, Lyeth BG, Muizelaar JP: Current status of neuroprotection trials for traumatic brain injury: Lessons from animal models and clinical studies, *Neurosurgery* 45:207-220, 1999.

58. Tasker RC: Pharmacological advance in the treatment of acute brain injury, *Arch Dis Child* 81:90-95,1999.

59. Zafonte R, Muizelaar JP, Peterson PL: The pathophysiology of brain injury: understanding innovative drug therapies, *J Head Trauma Rehabil* 13:1-10, 1998.

60. Marshall LF, Maas AI, Marshall SH et al: A multicenter trial on the efficacy of using tirilazad mesylate in cases of head injury, *J Neurosurg* 89:519-525, 1998.

61. Doppenberg EM, Choi SC, Bullock R: Clinical trials in traumatic brain injury: what can we learn from previous studies? *Ann N Y Acad Sci* 825:305-322, 1997.

62. Kaya SS, Mahmood A, Li Y et al: Apoptosis and expression of p53 response proteins and cyclin D1 after cortical impact in rat brain, *Brain Res* 818:22-33, 1999.

63. Savitz SI, Rosenbaum DM: Apoptosis in neurological disease, *Neurosurgery* 42:555-574, 1998.

64. Ghirnikar RS, Lee YL, Eng LF: Inflammation in traumatic brain injury: role of cytokines and chemokines, *Neurochem Res* 23:329-340, 1998.

65. McKeating EG, Andrews PJD: Cytokines and adhesion molecules in acute brain injury, *Br J Anaesth* 80:77-84, 1998.

66. Stahel PF, Morganti-Kossman MC, Kossmann T: The role of the complement system in traumatic brain injury, *Brain Res Rev* 27:243-256, 1998.

67. Graham DI, Horsburgh K, Nicoll JA et al: Apolipoprotein E and the response of the brain to injury, *Acta Neurochir (Suppl)* 73:89-92, 1999.

68. Smith DH, Chen XH, Nonaka M et al: Accumulation of amyloid beta and tau and the formation of neurofilament inclusions following diffuse brain injury in the pig, *J Neuropathol Exp Neurol* 58:982-992, 1999.

69. Friedman G, Froom P, Sazbon L et al: Apolipoprotien E-ε4 genotype predicts a poor outcome in survivors of traumatic brain injury, *Neurology* 52:244-248, 1999.

70. Teasdale GM, Nicoll JA, Murray G et al: Association of apolipoprotein E polymorphism with outcome after head injury, *Lancet* 350(9084):1069-1071, 1997.

71. Fawcett JW, Asher RA: The glial scar and central nervous system repair, *Brain Res Bull* 49:377-391, 1999.

72. Stichel CC, Muller HW: Experimental strategies to promote axonal regeneration after traumatic central nervous system injury, *Prog Neurobiol* 56:119-148, 1998.

73. Ramirez JJ, Finkelstein SP, Keller J et al: Basic fibroblast growth factor enhances axonal sprouting after cortical injury in rats, *Neuroreport* 10:1201-1204, 1999.

74. Chesnut RM: The management of severe traumatic brain injury, *Emerg Med Clin North Am* 15:581-604, 1997.

75. Cherian L, Robertson CS, Goodman JC: Secondary insults increase injury after controlled cortical impact in rats, *J Neurotrauma* 13:371-383, 1996.

76. DeWitt DS, Jenkins LW, Prough DS: Enhanced vulnerability to secondary ischemic insults after experimental traumatic brain injury, *New Horiz* 3:376-383, 1995.

77. Signorini DF, Andrews PJ, Jones PA et al: Adding insult to injury: the prognostic value of early secondary insults for survival after traumatic brain injury, *J Neurol Neurosurg Psychiatry* 66:26-31, 1999.

78. Chesnut RM: Secondary brain insults after head injury: clinical perspectives, *New Horiz* 3:366-375, 1995.

79. Jones PA, Andrews PJ, Midgley S et al: Measuring the burden of secondary insults in head-injured patients during intensive care, *J Neurosurg Anesthesiol* 6:4-14, 1994.

80. Chesnut RM, Marshall SB, Piek J et al: Early and late systemic hypotension as a frequent and fundamental source of cerebral ischemia following severe brain injury in the traumatic coma data bank, *Acta Neurochir (Suppl)* 59:121-125, 1993.

81. Chesnut RM, Marshall LF, Klauber MR et al: The role of secondary brain injury in determining outcome from severe head injury, *J Trauma* 34:216-222, 1993.

82. Miller JD, Becker DP: Secondary insults to the injured brain, *J R Coll Surg Edinb* 27:292-298, 1982.

83. Juul N, Morris GF, Marshall SB et al: Intracranial hypertension and cerebral perfusion pressure: influence on neurological deterioration and outcome in severe head injury, *J Neurosurg* 92:1-6, 2000.

84. Kelly DF, Kordestani RK, Martin NA et al: Hyperemia following traumatic brain injury: relationship to intracranial hypertension and outcome, *J Neurosurg* 85:762-771, 1996.

85. Douzinas EE, Kostopoulos V, Kypriades E et al: Brain eigenfrequency shifting as a sensitive index of cerebral compliance in an experimental model of epidural hematoma in the rabbit: preliminary study, *Crit Care Med* 27:978-984, 1999.

86. Marmarou A: Monitoring and Treatment: Pathophysiology of intracranial pressure. In Narayan RK, Wilberger JE Jr., Povlishock JT, editors: *Neurotrauma,* New York 1996, McGraw-Hill, 413-444.

87. Kirkness CJ, Mitchell PH, Burr RL et al: Intracranial pressure waveform analysis: clinical and research implications, *J Neurosci Nurs* 32:271-277, 2000.

88. Lubillo S, Bolanos J, Carreira L et al: Prognostic value of early computerized tomography scanning following craniotomy for traumatic hematoma, *J Neurosurg* 9l:581-587, 1999.

89. Junger EC, Newell DW, Grant GA et al: Cerebral autoregulation following minor head injury, *Neurosurgery* 86:425-432, 1997.

90. Strebel S, Lam AM, Matta BF et al: Impaired cerebral autoregulation after mild brain injury, *Surg Neurol* 47:128-131, 1997.

91. Obrist WD, Langfitt TW, Jaggi JL et al: Cerebral blood flow and metabolism in comatose patients with acute head injury. Relationship to intracranial hypertension, *J Neurosurg* 61:241-153, 1984.

92. Bouma GJ, Muizelaar JP, Stringer WA et al: Ultra-early evaluation of regional cerebral blood flow in severely head-injured patients using xenon-enhanced computerized tomography, *J Neurosurg* 77:160-168, 1992.

93. Kelly DF, Martin NA, Kordestani R et al: Cerebral blood flow as a predictor of outcome following traumatic brain injury, *J Neurosurg* 86:633-641, 1997.

94. Bouma GJ, Muizelaar JP, Choi SC et al: Cerebral circulation and metabolism after severe traumatic brain injury: the elusive role of ischemia, *J Neurosurg* 75:685-693, 1991.

95. Marion DW, Darby J, Yonas H: Acute regional cerebral blood flow changes caused by severe head injuries, *J Neurosurg* 74:407-414, 1991.

96. Higashi K: Epidemiology of catastrophic brain injury. In Levin HS, Benton AL, Muizelaar JP et al, editors: *Catastrophic brain injury,* New York, 1996, Oxford University Press, 15-34.

97. Zafonte RD, Lee CY: Kernohan-Woltman notch phenomenon: an unusual cause of ipsilateral motor deficit, *Arch Phys Med Rehabil* 78:543-545, 1997.

98. Signorini DF, Andrews PJ, Jones PA et al: Predicting survival using simple clinical variables: a case study in traumatic brain injury, *J Neurol Neurosurg Psychiatry* 66:20-25, 1999.

99. Levin HS, Gary HE Jr, Eisenberg HM et al: Neurobehavioral outcome 1 year after severe head injury. Experience of the traumatic coma data bank, *Neurosurgery* 73:699-709, 1990.

100. Downey DL, Leigh RJ: Eye movements: pathophysiology, examination and clinical importance, *J Neurosci Nurs* 30:5-24, 1998.

101. Cushing H: The blood-pressure reaction of acute cerebral compression, illustrated by cases of intracranial hemorrhage, *Am J Med Sci* 125:1017-1044, 1903.

102. Teasdale G, Jennett B: Glasgow coma scale, *Lancet* 2:81-84, 1974.

103. Segatore M, Way C: The Glasgow coma scale: time for change, *Heart Lung* 21:548-557, 1992.

104. Price DJ: Factors restricting the use of coma scales, *Acta Neurochir (Suppl)* 36:106-111, 1986.

105. Teasdale G, Murray G, Parker L et al: Adding up the Glasgow coma score, *Acta Neurochir* 28:13-16, 1979.

106. Teasdale G, Safar P, Smyder J et al: Brain resuscitation clinical trial II, 1984-1989 (Glasgow-Pittsburgh coma scoring method). In Safar P, Bircher NG, editors: *Cardiopulmonary cerebral resuscitation,* ed 3, Philadelphia, 1988, WB Saunders, 262.

107. Born JD: The Glasgow-Liege scale: Prognostic value and evolution of motor response and brain stem reflexes after severe head injury, *Acta Neurochir* 91:1-11, 1988.

108. Benzer A, Mitterschiffthaler G, Marosi M et al: Prediction of non-survival after trauma: Innsbruck Coma Scale, *Lancet* 338:1537, 1991.

109. Benzer A, Traweger C, Ofner D et al: Statistical modelling in analysis of outcome after trauma Glasgow Coma-Scale and Innsbruck-Coma Scale, *Anasthesiol Intensivmed Notfallmed Schmerzther* 4:231-235, 1995.

110. Stanczak DF, White III JG, Gouview WD et al: Assessment of level of consciousness following severe neurological insult. A comparison of the psychometric qualities of the Glasgow coma scale and the Comprehensive Level of Consciousness Scale, *J Neurosurg* 60:955-960, 1984.

111. Giacino JT, Kezmarsky MA, DeLuca J et al: Monitoring rate of recovery to predict outcome in minimally responsive patients, *Arch Phys Med Rehabil* 72:897-901, 1991.

112. Crosby L, Parsons LC: Clinical neurologic assessment tool: development and testing of an instrument to index neurologic status, *Heart Lung* 18:121-125, 1989.

113. Suguira K, Muraoka K, Chishiki T et al: The Edinburgh-2 coma scale: a new scale for assessing impaired consciousness, *Neurosurgery* 12:411-415, 1983.

114. Starmark JE, Stalhammar D, Holmgren E: The reaction level scale (RLS 85): manual & guidelines, *Acta Neurochir* 91:12-20, 1988.

115. Tesseris J, Pantazidis N, Routsi CR et al: A comparative study of the reaction level scale (RLS 85) with Glasgow coma scale (GCS) and Edinburgh-2 coma scale (Modified) ($E_2CS(M)$), *Acta Neurochir* 110:65-76, 1991.

116. Hagen C, Malkmus D, Stenderup-Bowman K: Los Amigos Research and Education, Ranchos Los Amigos Hospital, Downey, Calif, 1973. Revised by Hagen CC, 1998.

117. Hannay HJ, Sherer M: Assessment of outcome from head injury. In Narayan RK, Wilberger JE Jr, Povlishock JT, editors: *Neurotrauma,* New York, 1996, McGraw-Hill, 723-747.

118. Bullock MR, Chesnut RM, Clifton GL et al: Guidelines for the management of severe traumatic brain injury. In Brain Trauma Foundation and American Association of Neurological Surgeons: *Management and prognosis of severe traumatic brain injury,* New York, 2000, Brain Trauma Foundation, 7-165.

119. van der Naalt J, Hew JM, van Zomeren AH et al: Computed tomography and magnetic resonance imaging in mild to moderate head injury: early and late imaging related to outcome, *Ann Neurol* 46:70-78, 1999.

120. Hankins L, Taber KH, Yeakley J et al: Magnetic resonance imaging in head injury. In Narayan RK, Wilberger JE Jr, Povlishock JT, editors: *Neurotrauma,* New York, 1996, McGraw-Hill, 151-161.

121. Servadei F, Murray GD, Penny K et al: The value of the "worst" computed tomographic scan in clinical studies of moderate and severe head injury, *Neurosurgery* 46:75-77, 2000.

122. Diaz-Marchan PJ, Hayman LA, Carrier DA et al: Computed tomography of closed head injury. In Narayan RK, Wilberger JE Jr., Povlishock JT, editors: *Neurotrauma,* New York, 1996, McGraw-Hill, 137-147.

123. McQuillan KA: Care of intraventricular devices and care of intraventricular monitoring devices. In *AACN critical care competency checklists,* Philadelphia, 1999, Lippincott Williams & Wilkins.

124. Kunkel J, Webb D, Clancey J et al: *American Association of Neuroscience Nurses clinical guideline series,* Chicago, 1997, American Association of Neuroscience Nurses.

125. Chambers IR, Mendelow AD, Sinar EJ et al: A clinical evaluation of the Camino subdural screw and ventricular monitoring kits, *Neurosurgery* 26(3):421-423, 1990.

126. Gray WP, Palmer JD, Gill J et al: A clinical study of parenchymal and subdural miniature strain-gauge transducers for monitoring intracranial pressure, *Neurosurgery* 39(5): 927-932, 1996.

127. Gopinath SP, Robertson CS, Contant CF et al: Clinical evaluation of a miniature strain-gauge transducer for monitoring intracranial pressure, *Neurosurgery* 36(6):1137-1141, 1995.

128. March K: Intracranial pressure monitoring and assessing intracranial compliance in brain injury, *Crit Care Nurs Clin North Am* 12:429-436, 2000.

129. Feldman Z, Narayan RK: Intracranial pressure monitoring: techniques and pitfalls. In Cooper PR, editor: *Head injury,* ed 3, Baltimore, 1993, Williams & Wilkins.

130. Guyot LL, Dowling C, Diaz FG et al: Cerebral monitoring devices: analysis of complications, *Acta Neurochir (Suppl)* 71:47-49, 1998.

131. Holloway KL, Barnes T, Choi S et al: Ventriculostomy infections: the effect of monitoring duration and catheter exchange in 584 patients, *J Neurosurg* 85:419-424, 1996.

132. Ueno T, Ballard RE, Shuer LM et al: Noninvasive measurement of pulsatile intracranial pressure using ultrasound, *Acta Neurochir (Suppl)* 71:66-69, 1998.

133. Penson RP, Allen R: Intracranial pressure monitoring by time domain analysis, *J R Soc Health* 118:289-294, 1998.

134. Sahuquillo J, Poca M-A, Arribas M et al: Interhemispheric supratentorial intracranial pressure gradients in head-injured patients: are they clinically important? *J Neurosurg* 90:16-26, 1999.

135. Mindermann Th, Gratzl O: Interhemispheric pressure gradients in severe head trauma in humans, *Acta Neurochir (Suppl)* 71:56-58, 1998.

136. Cardoso ER, Rowan JO, Galbraith S: Analysis of the cerebrospinal fluid pulse wave in intracranial pressure, *J Neurosurg* 59:817-821, 1983.

137. Rosner MJ, Rosner SD, Johnson AH: Cerebral perfusion pressure: management protocol and clinical results, *J Neurosurg* 83:949-962, 1995.

138. Robertson CS, Valadka AB, Hannay J et al: Prevention of secondary ischemic insults after severe head injury, *Crit Care Med* 27:2086-2095, 1999.

139. Bouma GJ, Muizelaar JP: Cerebral blood flow in severe clinical head injury, *New Horiz* 3:384-394, 1995.

140. Robertson CS: Nitrous oxide saturation technique for CBF measurement. In Narayan RK, Wilberger JE Jr, Povlishock JT, editors: *Neurotrauma,* New York, 1996, McGraw-Hill, 487-501.

141. Matz PG, Pitts L: Monitoring in traumatic brain injury, *Clin Neurosurg* 44:267-294, 1997.

142. Sioutos PJ, Orozco JA, Carter LP: Regional cerebral blood flow techniques. In Narayan RK, Wilberger JE Jr, Povlishock JT, editors: *Neurotrauma,* New York, 1996, McGraw-Hill, 503-517.

143. Horn P, Vajkoczy P, Thome C et al: Effects of 30% stable xenon on regional cerebral blood flow in patients with intracranial pathology, *Keio J Med* 49(Suppl 1):A161-A163, 2000.

144. Lucke KT, Kerr ME, Chovanes GI: Continuous bedside cerebral blood flow monitoring, *J Neurosci Nurs* 27:164-173, 1995.

145. Lam JMK, Hsiang JNK, Poon WS: Monitoring of autoregulation using laser Doppler flowmetry in patients with head injury, *J Neurosurg* 86:438-445, 1997.

146. Sioutos PJ, Orozco JA, Carter LP et al: Continuous regional cerebral cortical blood flow monitoring in head-injured patients, *Neurosurgery* 36(5):943-950, 1995.

147. Caron MJ: PET/SPECT imaging in head injury. In Narayan RK, Wilberger JE Jr, Povlishock JT, editors: *Neurotrauma,* New York, 1996, McGraw-Hill, 163-168.

148. Ricker JH, Zafonte RD: Functional neuroimaging and quantitative electroencephalography in adult traumatic head injury: clinical applications and interpretive cautions, *J Head Trauma Rehabil* 15:859-868, 2000.

149. Fontaine A, Azouvi P, Remy P et al: Functional anatomy of neuropsychological deficits after severe traumatic brain injury, *Neurology* 53:1963-1968, 1999.

150. Emanuelson IM, von Wendt L, Bjure J et al: Computed tomography and single-photon emission computed tomography as diagnostic tools in acquired brain injury among children and adolescents, *Dev Med Child Neurol* 39:502-507, 1997.

151. Shiina G, Onuma T, Kameyama M et al: Sequential assessment of cerebral blood flow in diffuse brain injury by ^{123}I-Iodoamphetamine single-photon emission CT, *Am J Neuroradiol* 19:297-302, 1998.

152. Corte FD, Giordano A, Pennisi MA et al: Quantitative cerebral blood flow and metabolism determination in the first 48 hours after severe head injury with a new dynamic SPECT device, *Acta Neurochir* 139:636-642, 1997.

153. Diringer MN, Yundt K, Videen TO et al: No reduction in cerebral metabolism as a result of early moderate hyperventilation following severe traumatic brain injury, *J Neurosurg* 92:7-13, 2000.

154. Laatsch L, Pavel D, Jobe T et al: Incorporation of SPECT imaging in a longitudinal cognitive rehabilitation therapy programme, *Brain Inj* 13:555-570, 1999.

155. Yamaki T, Yoshino E, Fujimoto M et al: Chronological positron emission tomographic study of severe diffuse brain injury in the chronic stage, *J Trauma* 40:50-56, 1996.

156. Laatsch L, Jobe T, Sychra J et al: Impact of cognitive rehabilitation therapy on neuropsychological impairments as measured by brain perfusion SPECT: a longitudinal study, *Brain Inj* 11:851-863, 1997.

157. Manno EM: Transcranial Doppler ultrasonography in the neurocritical care unit, *Crit Care Clin* 13:79-104, 1997.

158. Doberstein C, Martin NA: Transcranial Doppler ultrasonography in head injury. In Narayan RK, Wilberger JE Jr, Povlishock JT, editors: *Neurotrauma,* New York, 1996, McGraw-Hill, 539-552.

159. Newell DW: Transcranial Doppler measurements, *New Horiz* 3:423-430, 1995.

160. March K: Application of technology in the treatment of traumatic brain injury, *Crit Care Q* 23:26-37, 2000.

161. Cormio M, Valadka AB, Robertson CS: Elevated jugular venous oxygen saturation after severe head injury, *J Neurosurg* 90:9-15, 1999.

162. Feldman Z, Robertson CS: Monitoring of cerebral hemodynamics with jugular bulb catheters, *Crit Care Clin* 13:51-77, 1997.

163. Gopinath SP, Cormio M, Siegler J et al: Intraoperative jugular desaturation during surgery for traumatic intracranial hematomas, *Anesth Analg* 83:1014-1021, 1996.

164. Sheinberg M, Kanter MJ, Robertson CS et al: Continuous monitoring of jugular venous oxygen saturation in head-injured patients, *J Neurosurg* 76:212-217, 1992.

165. Gopinath SP, Robertson CS, Contant CF et al: Jugular venous desaturation and outcome after head injury, *J Neurol Neurosurg Psychiatry* 57:717-723, 1994.

166. Robertson C: Desaturation episodes after severe head injury: influence on outcome, *Acta Neurochir (Suppl)* 59:98-101, 1993.

167. Robertson CS, Cormio M: Cerebral metabolic management, *New Horiz* 3:410-422, 1995.

168. Clay HD: Validity and reliability of the Sjo_2 catheter in neurologically impaired patients: a critical review of the literature, *J Neurosci Nurs* 32:194-203, 2000.

169. Cruz J: An additional therapeutic effect of adequate hyperventilation in severe acute brain trauma: normalization of cerebral glucose uptake, *J Neurosurg* 82:379-385, 1995.

170. Cruz J: The first decade of continuous monitoring of jugular bulb oxyhemoglobin saturation: management strategies and clinical outcome, *Crit Care Med* 26:344-351, 1998.

171. Coplin WM, O'Keefe GE, Grady MS et al: Thrombotic, infectious, and procedural complications of the jugular bulb catheter in the intensive care unit, *Neurosurgery* 41:101-109, 1997.

172. Coplin WM, O'Keefe GE, Grady MS et al: Accuracy of continuous jugular bulb oximetry in the intensive care unit, *Neurosurgery* 42:533-540, 1998.

173. Metz C, Holzschuh M, Bein T et al: Jugular bulb monitoring of cerebral oxygen metabolism in severe head injury: accuracy of unilateral measurements, *Acta Neurochir (Suppl)* 71: 324-327, 1998.

174. Madsen PL, Secher NH: Near-infrared oximetry of the brain, *Prog Neurobiol* 58:541-560, 1999.

175. Gopinath SP, Chance B, Robertson CS: Near-infrared spectroscopy in head injury. In Narayan RK, Wilberger JE Jr, Povlishock JT, editors: *Neurotrauma,* New York, 1996, McGraw-Hill, 169-183.

176. Van der Brink WA, van Santbrink H, Steyerberg EW et al: Brain oxygen tension in severe head injury, *Neurosurgery* 46:868-878, 2000.

177. Dings J, Meixensberger J, Roosen K: Brain tissue Po_2 monitoring: catheter stability and complications, *Neurol Res* 19:241-245, 1997.

178. Van Santbrink H, Maas AIR, Avezaat CJJ: Continuous monitoring of partial pressure of brain tissue oxygen in patients with severe head injury, *Neurosurgery* 38:21-31, 1996.

179. Bardt TF, Unterberg AW, Hartl R et al: Monitoring of brain tissue Po_2 in traumatic brain injury: effect of cerebral hypoxia on outcome, *Acta Neurochir (Suppl)* 71:153-156, 1998.

180. Valadka AB, Gopinath SP, Contant CF et al: Relationship of brain tissue Po_2 to outcome after severe head injury, *Crit Care Med* 26:1576-1581, 1998.

181. Zauner A, Doppenberg EMR, Woodward JJ et al: Continuous monitoring of cerebral substrate delivery and clearance: initial experience in 24 patients with severe acute brain injuries, *Neurosurgery* 41:1082-1093, 1997.

182. Kiening KL, Hartl R, Unterberg AW et al: Brain tissue Po_2-comatose patients: Implications for therapy, *Neurol Res* 19:233-240, 1997.

183. Gopinath SP, Valadka AB, Uzura M et al: Comparison of jugular venous oxygen saturation and brain tissue Po_2 as monitors of cerebral ischemia after head injury, *Crit Care Med* 27:2337-2345, 1999.

184. Bruzzone P, Dionigi R, Bellinzona G et al: Effects of cerebral perfusion pressure on brain tissue Po_2 in patients with severe head injury, *Acta Neurochir (Suppl)* 71:111-113, 1998.

185. Dings J, Jager A, Meixensberger J et al: Brain tissue Po_2 and outcome after severe head injury, *Neurol Res* 20:S71-S75, 1998.

186. Dings J, Meixensberger J, Amschler J et al: Continuous monitoring of brain tissue Po_2: a new tool to minimize the risk of ischemia caused by hyperventilation therapy, *Zentralbl Neurochir* 57:177-183, 1996.

187. Goodman JC, Simpson Jr. RK: Biochemical monitoring in head injury. In Narayan RK, Wilberger JE Jr, Povlishock JT, editors: *Neurotrauma,* New York, 1996, McGraw-Hill, 577-591.

188. Vazquez MD, Sanchez-Rodriguez F, Osuna F et al: Creatine kinase BB and neuron-specific enolase in cerebrospinal fluid in the diagnosis of brain insult, *Am J Forensic Med Pathol* 16:210-214, 1995.

189. Herrmann M, Curio N, Jost S et al: Release of biochemical markers of damage to neuronal and glial brain tissue is associates with short and long term neuropsychological after traumatic brain injury, *J Neurol Neurosurg Psychiatry* 70: 95-100, 2001.

190. Herrmann M, Jost S, Kutz S et al: Temporal profile of release of neurobiochemical markers of brain damage after traumatic brain injury is associated with intracranial pathology as demonstrated in cranial computerized tomography, *J Neurotrauma* 17:113-122, 2000.

191. McKeating EG, Andrews PJD, Mascia L: Relationship of neuron specific enolase and protein S-1 concentrations in systemic and jugular venous serum to injury severity and outcome after traumatic brain injury, *Acta Neurochir (Suppl)* 71:117-119, 1998.

192. Rothoerl RD, Woertgen C, Holzschuh M et al: S-100 serum levels after minor and major head injury, *J Trauma Inj Infect Crit Care* 45:765-767, 1998.

193. Haselman M, Fox S: Microsensor and microdialysis technology. Advances techniques in the management of severe head injury, *Crit Care Nurs Clin North Am* 12:437-446, 2000.

194. Hamani C, Luer MS, Dujovny M: Microdialysis in the human brain: review of its applications, *Neurol Res* 19:281-288, 1997.

195. Landolt H, Langemann H: Cerebral microdialysis as a diagnostic tool in acute brain injury, *Eur J Anaesthesiol* 13:269-278, 1996.

196. Hillered L, Persson L: Neurochemical monitoring of the acutely injured human brain, *Scand J Clin Lab Invest (Suppl)* 229:9-18, 1999.

197. Cecil KM, Hills EC, Sandel E et al: Proton magnetic resonance spectroscopy for detection of axonal injury in the splenium of the corpus callosum of brain-injured patients, *J Neurosurg* 88:795-801, 1998.

198. Holshouser BA, Ashwal SA, Luh GY et al: Proton MR spectroscopy after acute central nervous system injury: outcome prediction in neonates, infants, and children, *Radiology* 202:487-496, 1997.

199. Friedman SD, Brooks WM, Jung RE et al: Quantitative proton MRS predicts outcome after traumatic brain injury, *Neurology* 52:1384-1391, 1999.

200. Jordan KG: Continuous EEG monitoring in the neuroscience intensive care unit and emergency department, *J Clin Neurophysiol* 16:14-39, 1999.

201. Newlon PG: Electrophysiological monitoring in head injury. In Narayan RK, Wilberger JE Jr, Povlishock JT, editors: *Neurotrauma*, New York, 1996, McGraw-Hill, 563-575.

202. Sloan TB: Electrophysiologic monitoring in head injury, *New Horiz* 3:431-438, 1995.

203. Carter BG, Butt W: Review of the use of somatosensory evoked potentials in the prediction of outcome after severe brain injury, *Crit Care Med* 29:78-186, 2001.

204. Sleigh JW, Havill JH, Frith R et al: Somatosensory evoked potentials in severe traumatic brain injury: a blinded study, *J Neurosurg* 91:577-580, 1999.

205. Ghajar J, Hariri R, Narayan RK et al: Survey of critical care management of comatose, head-injured patients in the United States, *Crit Care Med* 23:560-567, 1995.

206. Marion DW, Spiegel TP: Changes in the management of severe traumatic brain injury: 1991-1997, *Crit Care Med* 28:16-18, 2000.

207. The Cochrane Collaboration: www.cochrane.org/cochrane/crgs.htm, March 15, 2000.

208. Tator CH: Management of associated spine injuries in head-injured patients. In Narayan RK, Wilberger JE Jr, Povlishock JT, editors: *Neurotrauma*, New York, 1996, McGraw-Hill, 263-267.

209. Doyle JA, Davis DP, Hoyt DB: The use of hypertonic saline in the treatment of traumatic brain injury, *J Trauma* 50:367-383, 2001.

210. Qureshi AI, Suarez JI: Use of hypertonic saline solutions in treatment of cerebral edema and intracranial hypertension, *Crit Care Med* 28:3301-3313, 2000.

211. Simma B, Burger R, Falk M et al: A prospective, randomized, and controlled study of fluid management in children with severe head injury: lactated Ringer's solution versus hypertonic saline, *Crit Care Med* 26(7):1265-1270, 1998.

212. Wade CE, Grady JJ, Kramer GC et al: Individual patient cohort analysis of the efficacy of hypertonic saline/dextran in patients with traumatic brain injury and hypotension, *J Trauma* 42(5):S61-S65, 1997.

213. McKhann II GM, Copass MK, Winn HR: Prehospital care of the head-injured patient. In Narayan RK, Wilberger JE Jr, Povlishock JT, editors: *Neurotrauma*, New York, 1996, McGraw-Hill, 103-117.

214. Mirski MA, Muffelman B, Ulatowski JA et al: Sedation for the critically ill neurologic patient, *Neurol Crit Care* 23(12):2038-2053, 1995.

215. Aguilera D: *Crisis intervention: theory and methodology,* ed 8, St. Louis, 1998, Mosby, 26-42.

216. Munro N: Pulmonary challenges in neurotrauma, *Crit Care Nurs Clin North Am* 12:457-464, 2000.

217. Sullivan J: Positioning of patients with severe traumatic brain injury: research-based practice, *J Neurosci Nurs* 32:204-209, 2000.

218. Kerr ME, Weber BB, Sereika SM et al: Effect of endotracheal suctioning on cerebral oxygenation traumatic brain-injured patients, *Crit Care Med* 27:2776-2781, 1999.

219. Brucia J, Rudy E: The effect of suction catheter insertion and tracheal stimulation in adults with severe brain injury, *Heart Lung* 25:295-303, 1996.

220. McQuillan, KA: The effect of the Trendelenburg position for postural drainage on cerebrovascular status in head-injured patients, *Heart Lung* 16:327, 1987.

221. Williams A, Coyne SM: Effects of neck position on intracranial pressure, *Am J Crit Care* 2:68-71, 1993.

222. Kerr ME, Rudy EB, Brucia J et al: Head-injured adults: recommendations for endotracheal suctioning, *J Neurosci Nurs* 25:86-91, 1993.

223. Crosby LJ, Parsons LC: Cerebrovascular response of closed head-injured patients to a standardized endotracheal tube suctioning and manual hyperventilation procedure, *J Neurosci Nurs* 24:40-49, 1992.

224. Rudy EB, Turner BE, Baun M et al: Endotracheal suctioning in adults with head injury, *Heart Lung* 20:667-674, 1991.

225. Parsons LC, Shogun JSO: The effects of the endotracheal tube suctioning/manual hyperventilation procedure on patients with severe closed head injuries, *Heart Lung* 13:372-380, 1984.

226. Ghajar K: Traumatic brain injury, *Lancet* 356:923-929, 2000.

227. Suozo JAC, Maas AIR, van den Brink WA et al: CO_2 reactivity and brain oxygen pressure monitoring in severe head injury, *Crit Care Med* 28:3268-3274, 2000.

228. Yundt KD, Diringer MN: The use of hyperventilation and its impact on cerebral ischemia in the treatment of traumatic brain injury, *Crit Care Clin* 13:163-182, 1997.

229. Muizelaar JP, van der Poel HG: Cerebral vasoconstriction is not maintained with prolonged hyperventilation. In Hoff JT, Betz AI, editors: *Intracranial pressure*, ed 7, Berlin, 1989, Springer-Verlag, 899-903.

230. Muizelaar JP, Marmarou A, Ward JD et al: Adverse effects of prolonged hyperventilation in patients with severe head injury: a randomized clinical trial, *J Neurosurg* 75:731-739, 1991.

231. Skippen P, Seear M, Poskitt K et al: Effect of hyperventilation on regional cerebral blood flow in head-injured children, *Crit Care Med* 25:1402-1409, 1997.

232. Paczynski RP: Osmotherapy, *Crit Care Clin* 13:105-129, 1997.

233. Kirkpatrick PJ, Smielewski P, Piechnik S et al: Early effects of mannitol in patients with head injuries assessed using bedside multimodality monitoring, *Neurosurgery* 39:714-721, 1996.

234. Fortune JB, Feustel PJ, Graca L et al: Effect of hyperventilation, mannitol, and ventriculostomy drainage on cerebral blood flow after head injury, *J Trauma* 39:1091-1099, 1995.

235. Luvisotto TL, Auer RN, Sutherland GR: The effect of mannitol on experimental cerebral ischemia, revisited, *Neurosurgery* 38:131-139, 1996.

236. Roberts PA, Pollay M, Engles C et al: Effect on intracranial pressure of furosemide combined with varying doses and administration rates of mannitol, *J Neurosurg* 66:440-446, 1987.

237. Kaufmann AM, Cardoso ER: Aggravation of vasogenic cerebral edema by multiple-dose mannitol, *J Neurosurg* 77:584-589, 1992.

238. Wilkinson HA, Rosenfield S: Furosemide and mannitol in the treatment of acute experimental intracranial hypertension, *Neurosurgery* 12:405-410, 1983.

239. Pollay M, Fullenwider C, Roberts A et al: Effect of mannitol and furosemide on blood-brain osmotic gradient and intracranial pressure, *J Neurosurg* 59:950-983, 1983.

240. Duhaime A-C: Conventional drug therapies for head injury. In Narayan RK, Wilberger JE Jr, Povlishock JT, editors: *Neurotrauma*, New York, 1996, McGraw-Hill, 365-374.

241. Chesnut RM: Treating raised intracranial pressure head injury. In Narayan RK, Wilberger JE Jr, Povlishock JT, editors: *Neurotrauma*, New York, 1996, McGraw-Hill, 445-469.

242. Qureshi AI, Suarez JI, Bhardwaj A et al: Use of hypertonic (3%) saline/acetate infusion in the treatment of cerebral edema: effect on intracranial pressure and lateral displacement of the brain, *Crit Care Med* 26:440-446, 1998.

243. Peterson B, Khanna S, Fisher B et al: Prolonged hypernatremia controls elevated intracranial pressure in head-injured pediatric patients, *Crit Care Med* 28:1136-1143, 2000.

244. Khanna S, Davis D, Peterson B et al: Use of hypertonic saline in the treatment of severe refractory posttraumatic intracranial hypertension in pediatric traumatic brain injury, *Crit Care Med* 28:1144-1151, 2000.

245. Schatzmann C, Heissler HE, Konig K et al: Treatment of elevated intracranial pressure by infusion of 10% saline in severely head injured patients, *Acta Neurochir (Suppl)* 71:31-33, 1998.

246. Hartl R, Ghajar J, Hochleuthner H et al: Hypertonic/hyperoncotic saline reliably reduces ICP in severely head-injured patients with intracranial hypertension, *Acta Neurochir (Suppl)* 70:126-129, 1997.

247. Bacher A, Wei J, Grafe MR et al: Serial determinations of cerebral water content by magnetic resonance imaging after an infusion of hypertonic saline, *Crit Care Med* 26:108-114, 1998.

248. Alderson P, Roberts I: Corticosteroids in acute traumatic brain injury: systematic review of randomized controlled trials, *Br Med J* 314:1855-1859, 1997.

249. Henker RA, Brown SD, Marion DW: Comparison of brain temperature with bladder and rectal temperatures in adults with severe head injury, *Neurosurgery* 42:1071-1075, 1998.

250. Rumana CS, Gopinath SP, Uzura M et al: Brain temperature exceeds systemic temperature in head-injured patients, *Crit Care Med* 26:562-567, 1998.

251. Slade J, Kerr ME, Marion D: Effect of therapeutic hypothermia on the incidence and treatment of intracranial hypertension, *J Neurosci Nurs* 31:264-269, 1999.

252. Shiozaki T, Sugimoto H, Taneda M et al: Selection of severely head injured patients for mild hypothermia therapy, *J Neurosurg* 89:206-211, 1998.

253. Marion DW, Penrod LE, Kelsey SF et al: Treatment of traumatic brain injury with moderate hypothermia, *N Eng J Med* 336:540-545, 1997.

254. Shiozaki T, Sugimoto H, Taneda M et al: Effect of mild hypothermia on uncontrollable intracranial hypertension after severe head injury, *J Neurosurg* 79:363-368, 1993.

255. Clifton GL, Barrodale AS, Plenger B et al: A phase II study of moderate hypothermia in severe brain injury, *J Neurotrauma* 10:263-271, 1993.

256. Clifton GL, Miller ER, Choi SC et al: Lack of effect of induction of hypothermia after acute brain injury, *N Engl J Med* 344:556-563, 2001.

257. Roberts I: Barbiturates for acute traumatic brain injury (Cochrane Review). In *The Cochrane library*, issue 1, Oxford, 2000, Update Software.

258. Goodman JC, Valadka AB, Gopinath SP et al: Lactate and excitatory amino acids measured by microdialysis are decreased by pentobarbital coma in head-injured patients, *J Neurotrauma* 13:549-556, 1996.

259. Eisenberg HM, Frankowski RF, Contant CF et al: High-dose barbiturate control of elevated intracranial pressure in patients with severe head injury, *J Neurosurg* 69:15-23, 1988.

260. Rea GL, Rockswold GL: Barbiturate therapy in uncontrolled intracranial hypertension, *Neurosurgery* 12:401-404, 1983.

261. Ward JD, Becker DP, Miller JD et al: Failure of prophylactic barbiturate coma in the treatment of severe head injury, *J Neurosurg* 62:383-388, 1985.

262. Winer JW, Rosenwasser RH, Jimenez F: Electroencephalographic activity and serum and cerebrospinal fluid pentobarbital levels in determining the therapeutic end point during barbiturate coma, *Neurosurgery* 29:739-742, 1991.

263. Stover JF, Stocker R: Barbiturate coma may promote reversible bone marrow suppression in patients with severe isolated traumatic brain injury, *Eur J Clin Pharmacol* 54:529-534, 1998.

264. Hsiang JK, Chesnut RM, Crisp CB et al: Early, routine paralysis for intracranial pressure control in severe head injury: is it necessary? *Crit Care Med* 22:1471-1476, 1994.

265. Brucia JJ, Owen DC, Rudy EB: The effects of lidocaine on intracranial hypertension, *J Neurosci Nurs* 24:205-214, 1992.

266. Silber SH: Rapid sequence intubation in adults with elevated intracranial survey of emergency medicine residency programs, *Am J Emerg Med* 15:263-267, 1997.

267. Yano M, Nishiyama H, Yokota H et al: Effect of lidocaine on ICP response to endotracheal suctioning, *Anesthesiology* 64:651-653, 1986.

268. Guerra WK-W, Gaab MR, Dietz H et al: Surgical decompression for traumatic brain swelling: indications and results, *J Neurosurg* 90:187-196, 1999.

269. Kunze E, Meixensberger J, Janka M et al: Decompressive craniectomy in patients with uncontrollable intracranial hypertension, *Acta Neurochir (Suppl)* 71:16-18, 1998.

270. Polin RS, Shaffrey ME, Bogaev CA et al: Decompressive bifrontal craniectomy in the treatment of severe refractory posttraumatic cerebral edema, *Neurosurgery* 41:84-94, 1997.

271. Parsons LC, Wilson MM: Cerebrovascular status on severe closed head injured patients following passive position changes, *Nurs Res* 33:68-75, 1984.

272. Mitchell PH, Ozuna J: Moving the patient in bed: effects on intracranial pressure, *Nurs Res* 30:212-218, 1981.

273. Lipe HP, Mitchell PH: Positioning the patient with intracranial hypertension: how turning and head rotation affect the internal jugular vein, *Heart Lung* 9:1031-1037, 1980.

274. Winkelman C: Effect of backrest position on intracranial and cerebral perfusion pressures in traumatically brain-injured adults, *Am J Crit Care* 9:373-380, 2000.

275. Simmons BJ: Management of intracranial hemodynamics in the adult: a research analysis of head positioning and recommendations for clinical practice and future research, *J Neurosci Nurs* 29:44-49, 1997.

276. Meixensberger J, Baunach S, Amschler J et al: Influence of body position on tissue-Po_2 cerebral perfusion pressure and intracranial pressure in patients with acute brain injury, *Neurol Res* 19:249-253, 1997.

277. Feldman Z, Kanter MJ, Robertson CS et al: Effect on head elevation on intracranial pressure, cerebral perfusion pressure, and cerebral blood flow in head-injured patients, *J Neurosurg* 76:207-211, 1992.

278. Rosner MJ, Coley IB: Cerebral perfusion pressure, intracranial pressure, and head elevation, *J Neurosurg* 65:636-641, 1986.

279. Moraine JJ, Berre J, Melot C et al: Is cerebral perfusion pressure a major determinant of cerebral blood flow during head elevation in comatose patients with severe intracranial lesions? *J Neurosurg* 92:606-614, 2000.

280. Kajs-Wyllie M: Antihypertensive treatment for the neurological patient: A nursing challenge, *J Neurosci Nurs* 31:142-151, 1999.

281. Tietjen CS, Hurn PD, Ulatowski JA et al: Treatment modalities for hypertensive patients with intracranial pathology: options and risks, *Crit Care Med* 24:311-322, 1996.

282. Kordestani RK, Counelis GJ, McBride DQ et al: Cerebral arterial spasm after penetrating craniocerebral gunshot wounds: transcranial Doppler and cerebral blood flow findings, *Neurosurgery* 41:351-360, 1997.

283. Lee JH, Martin NA, Alsina G et al: Hemodynamically significant cerebral vasospasm and outcome after head injury: a prospective study, *J Neurosurg* 87:221-233, 1997.

284. Martin NA, Doberstein C, Zane C et al: Posttraumatic cerebral arterial spasm: transcranial Doppler ultrasound, cerebral blood flow, and angiographic findings, *J Neurosurg* 77:575-583, 1992.

285. Romner B, Bellner J, Kongstad P et al: Elevated transcranial Doppler flow velocities after severe head injury: cerebral vasospasm or hyperemia? *J Neurosurg* 85:90-97, 1996.

286. Weber M, Grolimund P, Seiler RW: Evaluation of posttraumatic cerebral blood flow velocities by transcranial Doppler ultrasonography, *Neurosurgery* 27:106-122, 1990

287. Suwanwela C, Suwanwela N: Intracranial arterial narrowing and spasm in acute head injury, *J Neurosurg* 36:314-323, 1972.

288. Taneda M, Kataoka K, Akai F et al: Traumatic subarachnoid hemorrhage as a predictable indicator of delayed ischemic symptoms, *J Neurosug* 84:762-768, 1996.

289. Langham J, Goldtrad C, Teasdale G et al: Calcium channel blockers for acute traumatic brain injury (Cochrane Review). In *The Cochrane library*, issue 1, Oxford, 2000, Update Software.

290. Annegers JF, Hauser WA, Coan SP et al: A population-base study of seizures after traumatic brain injuries, *N Engl J Med* 338:20-24, 1998.

291. Temkin NR, Haglund M, Winn HR: Post-traumatic seizures. In Narayan RK, Wilberger JE Jr, Povlishock JT, editors: *Neurotrauma*, New York, 1996, McGraw-Hill, 611-619.

292. Asikainen I, Kaste M, Sarna S: Early and late posttraumatic seizures in traumatic brain injury rehabilitation patients: brain injury factors causing late seizures and influence of seizures on long-term outcome, *Epilepsia* 40:584-589, 1999.

293. Brain Injury Special Interest Group of the American Academy of Physical Medicine and Rehabilitation: Practice parameter: antiepileptic drug treatment of posttraumatic seizures, *Arch Phys Med Rehabil* 79:594-597, 1998.

294. Schierhout G, Robert I. Anti-epileptic drugs for preventing seizures following acute traumatic brain injury (Cochrane Review). In *The Cochrane library*, issue 1, Oxford, 2000, Update Software.

295. Temkin NR, Dikmen SS, Wilensky AJ et al: A randomized, double-blind study of phenytoin for the prevention of post-traumatic seizures, *N Engl J Med* 323:497-502, 1990.

296. Glotzner FL, Haubitz I, Miltner F et al: Seizure prevention using carbamazepine following severe brain injuries, *Neurochirurgia (Stuttg)* 26:66-79, 1983.

297. Haltiner AM, Newell DW, Temkin NR et al: Side effects and mortality associated with use of phenytoin for early posttraumatic seizure prophylaxis, *J Neurosurg* 91:588-592, 1999.

298. Temkin NR, Dikmen SS, Anderson GD et al: Valproate therapy for prevention of posttraumatic seizures: a randomized trial, *J Neurosurg* 91:593-600, 1999.

299. Woiciechowsky C, Asadudllah K, Nestler D et al: Sympathetic activation triggers systemic interleukin-10 release immunodepression induced by brain injury, *Nat Med* 4:768-769, 1998.

300. Meert KL, Long M, Kaplan J et al: Alterations in immune function following head injury in children, *Crit Care Med* 23:822-828, 1995.

301. Quattrocchi KB, Frank EH, Miller CH et al: Severe head injury: effect upon cellular immune function, *Neurol Res* 13:13-20, 1991.

302. Taha JM, Haddad FS: Central nervous system infections after craniocerebral missile wounds. In Aarabi B, editor: *Missile wounds of the head and neck*, vol 2, Park Ridge, IL, 1999, The American Association of Neurological Surgeons, 271-279.

303. Wiercisiewski DR, McDeavitt JT: Pulmonary complications in traumatic brain injury, *J Head Trauma Rehabil* 13:28-35, 1998.

304. Bratton SL, Davis RL: Acute lung injury in isolated traumatic brain injury, *Neurosurgery* 40:707-712, 1997.

305. Morris MT: Adult respiratory distress syndrome. In Secor VH, editor: *Multiple organ dysfunction & failure*, ed 2, St. Louis, 1996, Mosby, 167-195.

306. Parobek V, Alaimo I: Fluid and electrolyte management in the neurologically-impaired patient, *J Neurosci Nurs* 28:322-328, 1996.

307. Zafonte RD, Mann NR: Cerebral salt wasting syndrome in brain injury patients: a potential cause of hyponatremia, *Arch Phys Med Rehabil* 78:540-542, 1997.

308. Harrigan MR: Cerebral salt wasting syndrome: a review, *Neurosurgery* 38:152-160, 1996.

309. Kappy MS, Ganong CA: Cerebral salt wasting in children: the role of atrial natriuretic hormone, *Adv Pediatr* 43:271-299, 1996.

310. Hoots WK: Experience with antithrombin concentrates in neurotrauma patients, *Semin Thromb Hemost* 23(Suppl 1): 3-16, 1997.

311. May AK, Young JS, Butler K et al: Coagulopathy in severe closed head injury: is empiric therapy warranted? *Am Surg* 63:233-236, 1997.

312. Stein SC, Young GS, Talucci RC et al: Delayed brain injury after head trauma: significance of coagulopathy, *Neurosurgery* 30:160-165, 1992.

313. Brown TH, Davidson PF, Larson GM: Acute gastritis occurring within 24 hours of severe head injury, *Gastrointest Endosc* 35:37-40, 1989.

314. Venkatesh B, Townsend S, Boots RJ: Does splanchnic ischemia occur in isolated neurotrauma? A prospective observational study, *Crit Care Med* 27:1175-1180, 1999.

315. Sumas ME, Narayan RK. Cardiopulmonary management if the head-injured patient. In Narayan RK, Wilberger JE Jr, Povlishock JT, editors: *Neurotrauma*, New York, 1996, McGraw-Hill, 313-329.

316. Wilson RF, Tyburski JG: Metabolic responses and nutritional therapy in patients with severe head injuries, *J Head Trauma Rehabil* 13:11-27, 1998.

317. Young B, Ott L. Nutritional and metabolic management of the head-injured patient. In Narayan RK, Wilberger JE Jr., Povlishock JT, editors: *Neurotrauma*, New York, 1996, McGraw-Hill, 345-363.

318. Grzankowski JA: Altered thought processes related to traumatic brain injury and their nursing implications, *Rehabil Nurs* 22:24-31, 1997.

319. Hagen C: Planning a therapeutic environment for the communicatively impaired post closed head injury patient. In Shanks SJ, editor: *Nursing & the management of adult communication disorders*, San Diego, 1983, College-Hill Press, 137-169.

320. Schurr MJ, Ebner KA, Maser AL et al: Formal swallowing evaluation and therapy after traumatic brain injury improves dysphagia outcomes, *J Trauma* 46:817-823, 1999.

321. Loubser PG: Spasticity associated with spinal cord injury. In Narayan RK, Wilberger JE Jr, Povlishock JT, editors: *Neurotrauma*, New York, 1996, McGraw-Hill, 1245-1258.

322. Bontke CF, Zasler ND, Boake C: Rehabilitation of the head-injured patient. In Narayan RK, Wilberger JE Jr, Povlishock JT, editors: *Neurotrauma*, New York, 1996, McGraw-Hill, 841-858.

323. Gormley ME, O'Brien CF, Yablon SA: A clinical overview of treatment decisions in the management of spasticity, *Muscle Nerve Suppl* 6:S14-S20, 1997.

324. Wroblewski BA, Glenn MB: Pharmacological treatment for survivors of severe brain injury. In Levin HS, Benton AL, Muizelaar JP et al, editors: *Catastrophic brain injury*, New York, 1996, Oxford University Press, 93-120.

325. Meythaler JM, Guin-Renfroe S, Grabb P et al: Long-term continuously infused intrathecal baclofen for spastic-dystonic hypertonia in traumatic brain injury: 1-year experience, *Arch Phys Med Rehabil* 80:13-19, 1999.

326. Rawlins P: Patient management of cerebral origin spasticity with intrathecal baclofen, *J Neurosci Nurs* 30:32-46, 1998.

327. Johns JS, Cifu DX, Keyser-Marcus L et al: Impact of clinically significant heterotopic ossification on functional outcome after traumatic brain injury, *J Head Trauma Rehabil* 14:269-276, 1999.

328. Sarafis KA, Karatzas GD, Yotis CL: Ankylosed hips caused by heterotopic ossification after traumatic brain injury: a difficult problem, *J Trauma* 46:104-109, 1999.

329. Satz P, Zaucha K, Forney DL et al: Neuropsychological, psychosocial and vocational correlates of the Glasgow Outcome Scale at 6 months post-injury: a study of moderate to severe traumatic brain injury patients, *Brain Inj* 12:555-567, 1998.

330. Rosenthal M, Christensen BK, Ross TP: Depression following traumatic brain injury, *Arch Phys Med Rehabil* 79:90-103, 1998.

331. Gomez-Hernandez R, Max JE, Kosier T et al: Social impairment and depression after traumatic brain injury, *Arch Phys Med Rehabil* 78:1321-1326, 1997.

332. Dell Orto AE, Power PW: *Brain injury and the family: a life and living perspective*, ed 2, Boca Raton, 2000, CRC Press.

333. Gillen R, Tennen H, Affleck G, et al: Distress, depressive symptoms, and depressive disorder among caregivers of patients with brain injury, *J Head Trauma Rehabil* 13:31-43, 1998.

334. Koskinen S: Quality of life 10 years after a very severe traumatic brain injury (TBI): the perspective of the injured and the closest relative, *Brain Inj* 12:631-648, 1998.

335. Knight RG, Devereux R, Godfrey HPD: Caring for a family member with a traumatic brain injury, *Brain Inj* 12:467-481, 1998.

336. Junque C, Bruna O, Mataro M: Information needs of the traumatic brain injury patients' family members regarding the consequences of the injury and associated perception of physical, cognitive, emotional and quality of life changes, *Brain Inj* 11:251-258, 1997.

337. NIH Consensus Development Panel on Rehabilitation of Persons with Traumatic Brain Injury: Rehabilitation of persons with traumatic brain injury, *JAMA* 282:974-983, 1999.

338. World Health Organization: *International classification of impairments, disabilities and handicaps*, Geneva, 1980, World Health Organization.

339. Herndon R: Introduction to clinical neurological scales. In Herndon R, editor: *Handbook of neurologic rating scales*, New York, 1997, Demos Vermande, 1-6.

340. Hellawell DJ Taylor RT Pentland B: Cognitive and psychosocial outcome following moderate or severe traumatic brain injury, *Brain Inj* 13:489-504, 1999.

341. Karzmark P: Prediction of long-term cognitive outcome of brain injury with neuropsychological, severity of injury, and demographic data, *Brain Inj* 6:213-217, 1992.

342. Eisenberg H: Outcome after head injury: general considerations and neurobehavioral recovery. In Becker D, Povlishock J, editors: *Central nervous system trauma: status report 1985*, Publication 1988-520-149/00028, Washington, DC, 1998, U.S. Government Printing Office, 271-299.

343. Jennett B: Outcome after severe head injury. In Reilly P, Bullock R, editors: *Head injury: pathophysiology and management of severe closed injury*, London, 1997, Chapman & Hall Medical.

344. Dikmen S, Machamer J, Temkin N et al: Neuropsychological recovery in patients with moderate to severe head injury: 2 year follow-up, *J Clin Exp Neuropsychol* 12:507-19, 1999.

345. Brooks N: The effectiveness of post–acute rehabilitation. *Brain Inj* 5:103-109, 1991.

346. Cope D Cole J Hall K Barkans H: Brain injury: Analysis of outcome in a post–acute rehabilitation program: I. General analysis. *Brain Inj* 5:111–125, 1991.

347. Colantonio A, Dawson DR, McLellan BA: Head injury in young adults: long-term outcome, *Arch Phys Med Rehabil* 79:550-558, 1998.

348. Jennett B, Bond MR: Assessment of outcome severe brain damage, *Lancet* 1:480, 1975.

349. Teasdale GM, Pettigrew LE, Wilson JT et al: Analyzing outcome of treatment of severe head injury: a review and update on advancing the use of the Glasgow Outcome Scale, *J Neurotrauma* 15:587-597, 1998.

350. Wilson JT, Pettigrew LE, Teasdale GM: Structured interviews for the Glasgow Outcome Scale and the extended Glasgow Outcome Scale: guidelines for their use, *J Neurotrauma* 15:573-585, 1998.

351. Choi SC, Marmarou A, Bullock R et al: Primary end points in phase III clinical trials of severe head trauma: DRS versus GOS. The American Brain Injury Consortium Study Group, *J Neurotrauma* 15:771-776, 1998.

352. Corrigan JD, Smith-Knapp K, Granger CV: Validity of the functional independence measure for persons with traumatic brain injury, *Arch Phys Med Rehabil* 78:828-34, 1997.

353. Sander AM, Fuchs KL, High WM Jr et al: The Community Integration Questionnaire revisited: an assessment of factor structure and validity [published erratum appears in *Arch Phys Med Rehabil* 80(12):1608, 1999], *Arch Phys Med Rehabil* 80:1303-1308, 1999.

354. Willer B, Ottenbacher KJ, Coad ML: The community integration questionnaire. A comparative examination, *Am J Phys Med Rehabil* 73:103-111, 1994.

355. Paniak C, Phillips K, Toller-Lobe G et al: Sensitivity of three recent questionnaires to mild traumatic brain injury-related effects, *J Head Trauma Rehabil* 14:211-219, 1999.

356. Cifu DX, Kreutzer JS, Marwitz JH et al: Functional outcomes of older adults with traumatic brain injury: a prospective, multicenter analysis, *Arch Phys Med Rehabil* 77:883-888, 1996.

357. Mamelak AN, Pitts LH, Damron S: Predicting survival from head trauma 24 hours after injury: a practical method with therapeutic implications, *J Trauma* 41:91-99, 1996.

358. Michaud LJ, Rivara FP, Grady MS et al: Predictors of survival and severity of disability after severe brain injury in children, *Neurosurgery* 31:254-264, 1992.

359. Lang EW, Pitts LH, Damron SL et al: Outcome after severe head injury: an analysis of prediction based upon comparison of neural network versus logistic regression analysis, *Neurol Res* 19:274-280, 1997.

360. Haslam C, Batchelor J, Fearnside MR et al: Post-coma disturbance and post-traumatic amnesia as nonlinear predictors of cognitive outcome following severe closed head injury: findings from the Westmead Head Injury Project, *Brain Inj* 8:519-528, 1994.

361. Max JE, Roberts MA, Koele SL et al: Cognitive outcome in children and adolescents following severe traumatic brain injury: influence of psychosocial, psychiatric, and injury-related variables, *J Int Neuropsychol Soc* 5:58-68, 1999.

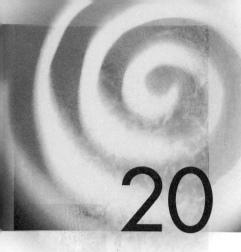

Maxillofacial Trauma

Bradley C. Robertson •
Karen A. McQuillan

Effective management of maxillofacial injuries is indeed complex and challenges virtually every member of a multidisciplinary health care team. It requires not only a profound appreciation of the functional components of the orbit, nose, and oral cavity, but also of subtle interrelationships between the skeletal and soft tissue components that define the individual's physical identity. The patient with facial injuries in conjunction with multisystem injuries requires integrated and coordinated assessment and management by multiple health care team members.

This chapter provides a review of maxillofacial anatomy and describes how to perform an assessment to detect maxillofacial injuries. Specific types of maxillofacial injuries and current recommended treatments are explained. Priorities of care and appropriate nursing interventions are described for each phase of the trauma cycle.

Mechanism of Injury

Despite mandatory seat belt laws, lower speed limits, and air bag systems, the incidence of facial injuries remains high after motor vehicle crashes because the face is exposed and vulnerable to the forces associated with rapid deceleration.[1,2] The magnitude of maxillofacial injury is directly proportionate to the velocity at impact when the face makes contact with an object. In low- and mid-velocity mechanisms of injury such as assaults, athletic mishaps, falls, and low-speed motor vehicle crashes, the source of injury is usually a single-vector force and the injuries are minor, limited to soft tissue contusions, abrasions, and lacerations. However, as the velocity of single-vector injuries increases, there is greater dissipation of energy along with increased soft tissue disruption, and the underlying bone structures begin to fracture along predictable fault lines, as described by Le Fort[3] (Figures 20-1 and 20-2).

In high-speed crashes with unrestrained occupants, the injury forces become exaggerated and quite often multivectored, resulting in even greater soft tissue disruption, bone comminution, and a loss of distinguishable Le Fort fracture patterns. In these extreme injuries the facial structures expand outward, away from the vital orbital and intracranial structures, resulting in a distorted spheric shape.

Less common facial injuries are penetrating wounds resulting from shootings and avulsions resulting from high-speed motorcycle crashes. These represent a unique subset of injuries that do not follow Le Fort's pattern of fractures and have a high potential for tissue devascularization and progressive necrosis. Patients with these injuries frequently require multiple operations during the early phase of hospitalization to debride necrotic tissue, followed by bone and soft tissue reconstruction performed before infection and wound contracture develop.[4,5]

Assessment of Maxillofacial Injuries With Correlative Facial Anatomy

Comprehensive management evolves from an initial thorough clinical examination, which then directs further diagnostic studies and culminates with development of a multidisciplinary plan of care for the patient. Obvious maxillofacial injuries should not distract the trauma team from first stabilizing the patient's airway, breathing, and circulation and then performing a thorough maxillofacial evaluation and a comprehensive assessment of other body systems to rule out associated injuries.[6,7] Comprehensive maxillofacial evaluation starts with a thorough assessment of soft tissue injury followed by examination of the underlying bony elements and evaluation of possible functional disruption. Knowledge of the anatomic location and function of maxillofacial structures provides rationale for strategies used to assess facial injuries and allows appropriate interpretation of assessment findings.

A generalized inspection of contusions, abrasions, and disruptive lacerations provides cues to direct a more thorough assessment of the underlying bony skeleton and functional elements. The ear canal, nose, oral cavity, and pharynx should be assessed thoroughly to identify any occult lacerations. A thorough intraoral examination should account for all teeth and consider the possibility that a tooth is displaced into the alveolar bone (intrusion) or dislodged into the respiratory tract.[8] A seemingly simple abrasion and laceration of the lateral cheek from a low-impact injury may have penetrated deep to injure the parotid gland or its duct or may have injured the facial nerve, affecting facial

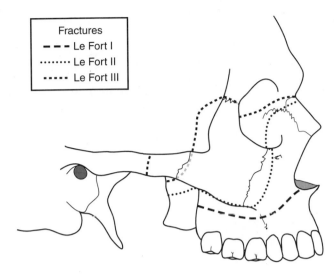

Fractures
- - - Le Fort I
········ Le Fort II
----- Le Fort III

FIGURE 20-1 Le Fort lines of fracture. (From Cohen SR: Craniofacial trauma. In Ruberg RL, Smith DJ, editors: *A core curriculum plastic surgery,* St. Louis, 1994, Mosby, 323.)

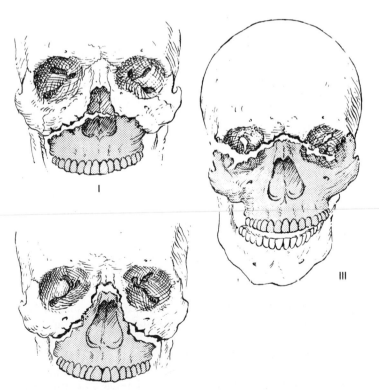

I

II

III

FIGURE 20-2 Le Fort classification of maxillary fractures. (From Schultz RC: Maxillofacial injuries. In Barrett BM, editor: *Patient care in plastic surgery,* ed 2, St. Louis, 1996, Mosby, 319.)

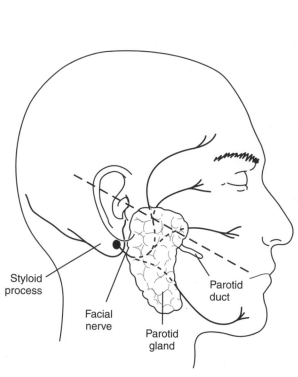

FIGURE 20-3 Lateral cheek injury and topical landmarks for localizing the parotid gland and duct and the facial nerve.

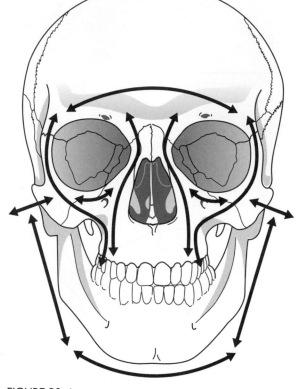

FIGURE 20-4 Craniofacial buttresses (*arrows* indicate buttresses).

animation[9,10] (Figure 20-3). A spectacle hematoma of the orbit is indicative of an anterior cranial base fracture with bleeding into the intracoronal fat compartment of the orbit and mandates a thorough and serial assessment of both ocular and neurologic function.

Facial bones are relatively thin and arranged to allow deformation and displacement away from the associated functional elements of the orbit, airway, and brain. Surrounding each of the craniofacial functional units are dense bony struts organized in a system of vertical, transverse, and horizontal buttresses (Figure 20-4). These buttresses determine the three-dimensional structure of the face and act as energy-absorbing shields around the vital craniofacial structures. When the transmitted energy exceeds the absorptive capacity of these buttresses, facial fractures occur. As Le Fort described in the early 1900s, this excess force results in predictable fractures at the junction of one buttress system with another.[3]

Skeletal structures should be inspected for symmetry, irregularity of bone continuity, and functional imbalance. Palpation should also be performed to identify the abnormal presence of crepitus, tenderness, or bony irregularity. Clinical evaluation techniques are shown in Figure 20-5.

The care provider should anticipate and recognize the functional disturbances associated with each type of facial fracture. Disturbances of vision, smell, nasal breathing, facial sensation, and the perception of bite relationship are the key functional pathways that lead to the diagnosis of specific facial fractures. Maxillofacial clinical assessment, like any other assessment, is an orderly system-related evaluation of structures and their related function.

Functionally the face is most easily divided into thirds (Figure 20-6).[11] The upper third of the face includes the lower portion of the frontal bone, supraorbital ridge, nasal glabellar region, and frontal sinus. In this region the frontal sinus, an air cell with thin surrounding bone, is most vulnerable to injury. Fractures typically pass through its anatomic boundary. As a result, most patients present with epistaxis, absent or abnormal smell, and possible cerebrospinal fluid (CSF) drainage from the nose (rhinorrhea). If the fracture communicates more laterally through the supraorbital ridge, the patient may have decreased sensation in the upper face and forehead area resulting from disruption of the trigeminal nerve branch (V1) innervating this region (Figure 20-7). If the supraorbital ridge is depressed, this fragment may impinge on the orbit, causing inferior displacement (vertical dystopia) and double vision (diplopia). A severe fracture of the orbital roof may communicate posteriorly with the superior orbital fissure (between the greater and lesser sphenoid wings, through which branches of cranial nerves III, IV, V, and VI traverse to the orbit), producing an associated superior orbital fissure syndrome (SOFS). Patients with this syndrome present with absent V1 sensation, pupillary fixation and dilation, loss of extraocular eye muscle movement, a down and out positioning of the eye, and upper eyelid ptosis (drooping).[12,13] Finally, patients

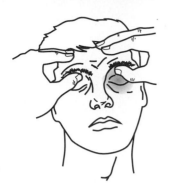

1. Palpate for irregularities of supraorbital ridge

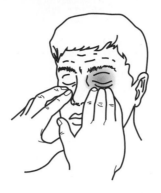

2. Palpate for irregularities of infraorbital ridge and zygoma

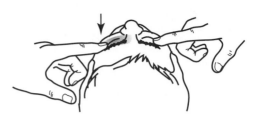

3. Compare height of malar eminences

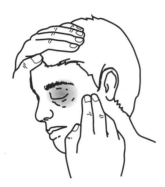

4. Palpate for depression of zygomatic arch

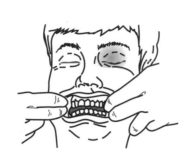

5. Visualize gross dental occlusion

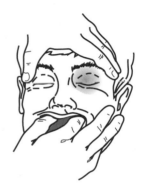

6. Maneuver maxilla to ascertain motion

FIGURE 20-5 Techniques for palpating facial injuries.

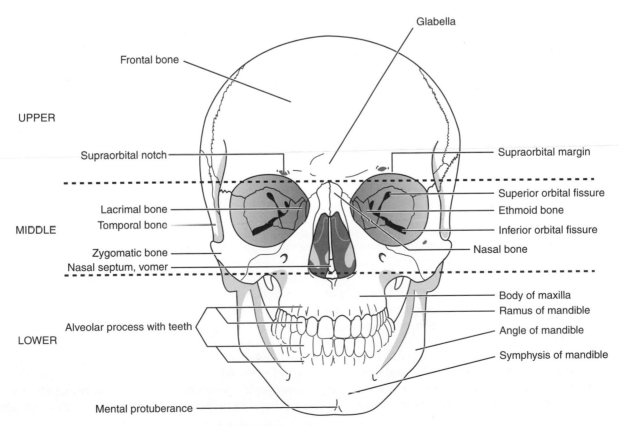

FIGURE 20-6 Functional thirds of the face.

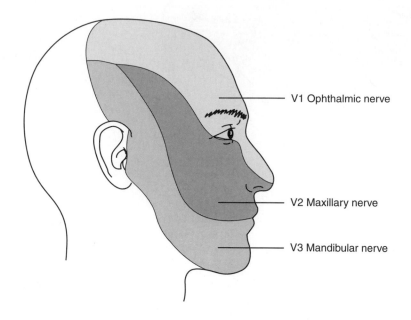

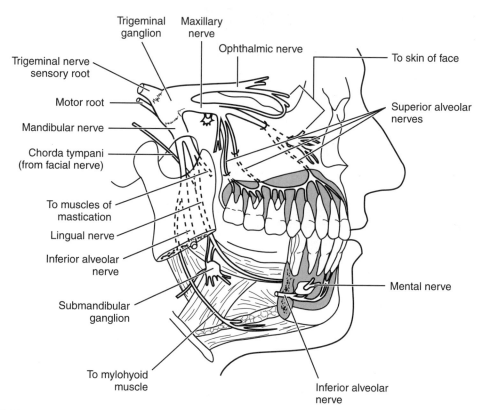

FIGURE 20-7 Trigeminal nerve (cranial nerve V) and its branches. V1 gives sensation from the upper eyelid to the apex of the scalp; V2 supplies the lower eyelid, cheek, upper lip, and lateral nose; V3 innervates the chin and lower lip.

with injuries of this region often have associated injuries of the intracranial vault and an abnormal neurologic assessment. Any abnormal neurologic assessment mandates a complete neurosurgical consultation.

The middle facial third (midface) includes the orbits, maxillary sinuses, nose, zygoma bones, and basal bone of the maxilla. In this region, from a functional standpoint, fractures involve the orbit or nose. The nasal bones are the most prominent structures of the midface and therefore are the facial bones most commonly fractured. Clinically a nasal fracture presents with contour deformity and deviation, epistaxis, subcutaneous emphysema, airway obstruction, and absent or abnormal smell. In all instances the nasal septum should be examined to rule out the presence of a nasal septal hematoma. A nasal septal hematoma must be evacuated to prevent avascular necrosis of the nasal septum and subsequent saddle-nose deformity (markedly depressed nasal bridge) or septal perforation.[14] Sense of smell provided by the olfactory nerve (cranial nerve I) is evaluated simply by determining if the patient can smell an alcohol wipe held approximately 8 inches from the nares.

In his classic paper Le Fort described three basic patterns of midface maxillary fractures, each of which has unique clinical findings[3] (see Figures 20-1 and 20-2). A Le Fort I fracture is the transverse disarticulation of the maxillary dentoalveolar process from the remaining basal bone of the maxilla and midface. Clinically this fracture presents with mobility of the maxillary dentition but stability of the nose, orbit, and midface. A Le Fort II fracture is a pyramidal fracture involving the entire maxilla and nasal complex. Clinically this fracture presents with unified mobility of the maxillary teeth along with the nose but stability of the orbit and remaining midface. A Le Fort III fracture is a complete craniofacial-midface disassociation. With this fracture there is unified mobility of the maxillary dentition, nose, and orbits. Other subtle clinical findings with a fracture of midface structures include an alteration of the horizontal orbital plane resulting from downward displacement of the zygoma and contour deformity of the malar eminence and nasal bony pyramid.

Most remaining midfacial fractures communicate through the orbit; therefore a complete ocular assessment is mandatory.[15] The eyes should be assessed for obvious signs of trauma such as conjunctival hemorrhage or ruptured globe. Vision and visual acuity should be evaluated. Movement of the eyes through the fields of gaze evaluates the ability of the extraocular muscles to move the eyes freely and the integrity of cranial nerves III, IV, and VI, which innervate the extraocular muscles. The patient should be observed closely for conjugate gaze in the horizontal, vertical, and sagittal eye positions. Impaired eye movement may result from edema restricting ocular movement; hemorrhage; direct injury to cranial nerves III, IV, or VI; contusion of the extraocular muscles; or an orbital fracture that causes extraocular muscle entrapment.[16] Diplopia may result from dysconjugate gaze.

All patients with facial fractures, in particular those with periorbital ecchymosis, should be assessed frequently for pupillary response to light. Assessment of the pupillary light reflex evaluates cranial nerve II (optic nerve), which enables the patient to perceive incoming light stimuli, and cranial nerve III (oculomotor nerve), which causes the pupil to constrict in response to the light stimulus. The Marcus Gunn pupil test (swinging light test) should be performed on all patients[17] (Figure 20-8). When the healthy eye is illuminated with a bright light, the pupils constrict bilaterally, but the when the light is moved quickly to the diseased eye, the pupil dilates.[18] This test can be performed even in the unconscious patient and is the single most sensitive test for injury of the visual tract between the retina and optic chiasm.[17] An ophthalmology consultation is indicated whenever ocular injury is suspected by evidence of diplopia, restricted eye movement, altered forehead (V1) or cheek

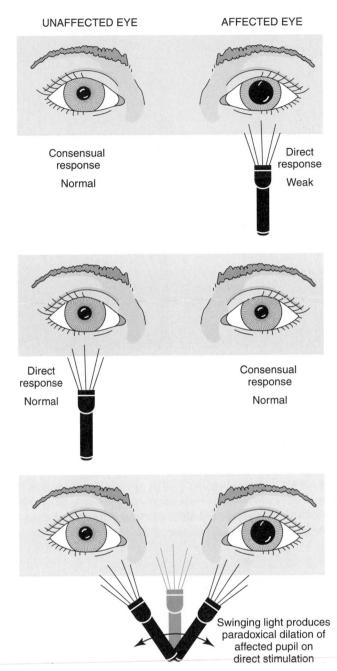

FIGURE 20-8 The Marcus Gunn (swinging light) test. Conduct test in a dark room with the patient's eyes fixed on a distant object. **Top,** Shining the light in the affected eye produces minimal, weak, or no constriction of that pupil. **Center,** Shining a light in the unaffected eye produces normal direct and consensual pupil constriction. **Below,** When the light is moved quickly from the unaffected eye to the affected eye, a paradoxical dilation, rather than constriction, of the affected pupil occurs indicating a positive test.

(V2) sensation, hyphema (anterior chamber ocular hemorrhage), ptosis, or periocular fractures.[19,20] Any abnormality in the visual assessment should be regarded as emergent and warrants an immediate ophthalmology consultation.[20]

The lower third of the face includes the maxillary and mandibular teeth-bearing bone and the basal bone of the mandible. The posterior-superior aspect of the mandible

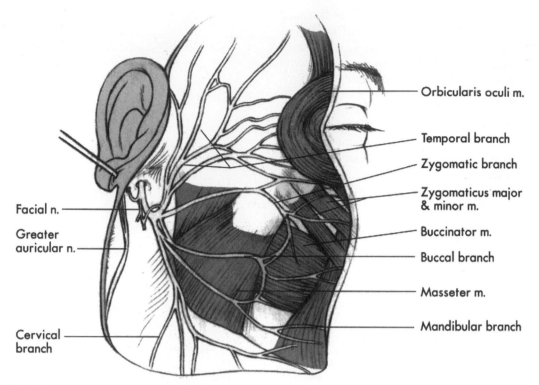

FIGURE 20-9 Facial nerve (cranial nerve VII) and its branches. The temporal, zygomatic, buccal, mandibular, and cervical branches of the facial nerve emerge from superior to inferior along the anterior border of the parotid gland. (From Mathers LH, Chase RA, Dolph J et al: *Clinical anatomy principles,* St. Louis, 1996, Mosby, 180.)

includes the temporomandibular joint and its associated condyle and meniscus. The position of the mandible and its functional relationship with the maxilla are directed by the muscles of mastication as they function through the temporomandibular joint. Therefore a functional assessment of the lower facial structures involves an evaluation of the muscles of mastication and their movement of the mandible through the temporomandibular joint. The patient should be asked to open and close the mandible and move it in all directions. Any fracture of the mandible or maxilla will upset the balance of this musculoskeletal system and manifest with muscular pain, splinting, and an altered bite (malocclusion). An altered bite is often quite subtle and frequently perceived only by the patient; nonetheless, any objective or subjective irregularity of the bite is always abnormal and should alert the practitioner that the maxilla or mandible has been fractured.[7,21]

Other subtle clinical findings associated with facial fractures in any of the three facial regions include altered facial sensation and motor function. Facial sensation should be assessed over the areas of distribution for each of the three branches of the trigeminal nerve (cranial nerve V) (see Figure 20-7). The ophthalmic, or V1, division innervates the upper face; the maxillary, or V2, division innervates the midface; and the mandibular, or V3, division provides sensation to the lower face. Abnormal sensation in any one of these regions indicates an associated fracture coursing through the cranial nerve skeletal foramen. In addition to supraorbital ridge fractures, which can alter V1 sensation,

orbital floor, zygoma, and Le Fort II fractures typically are associated with altered V2 sensation, and a mandible fracture may manifest with diminished V3 sensation.

Any abnormality of facial animation indicates injury to the facial nerve (cranial nerve VII), which innervates the muscles of facial expression and conveys taste for the anterior two thirds of the tongue (Figure 20-9). Facial movement can be assessed by having the patient puff out his or her cheeks, smile, show the teeth, frown, raise the eyebrows, and tightly close the eyes. In the absence of a direct laceration to one of the branches of the facial nerve, a thorough neurologic evaluation should be performed to further evaluate possible traumatic brain injury. If only the lower portion of the face is paretic and the upper face is spared, an upper motor neuron lesion involving the central nervous system should be suspected. If the entire half of the face is paretic, a peripheral nerve injury involving the facial nerve is indicated.[18,22] When the injury is believed to be proximal to the mastoid foramen, a neurosurgery consultation should be obtained in conjunction with a temporal bone and intracranial computed tomography (CT) scan. Even in the comatose patient, the motor function of the facial nerve and the sensory function of the trigeminal nerve can be assessed by testing the corneal reflex. Normally, light touch with a wisp of cotton on the cornea stimulates the trigeminal nerve, which triggers the facial nerve to cause the eye to blink.[18]

Comprehensive assessment then directs specific radiologic examination. A detailed discussion of the indications for specific radiographs is beyond this review, but in general

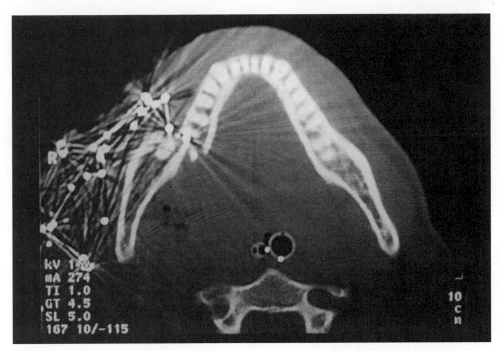

FIGURE 20-10 Computed tomography scan of facial shotgun injury demonstrating the complexity of a mandible fracture as it relates to the surrounding soft tissue envelope. (From: Robertson BC, Manson PN: High-energy ballistic and avulsive injuries: a management protocol for the next millennium, *Surg Clin North Am* 6:1493, 1999.)

the most effective method for quick and thorough radiographic assessment of the face is axial and coronal computed tomography. The advantages of CT assessment over plain radiographs is the ability to more accurately evaluate the complexity of maxillofacial fractures, their comminuted parts, and the relationship of the fractures with the surrounding soft tissue[23,24] (Figure 20-10). In the absence of true coronal CT scans, a reconstructive version can be substituted.

Before formalizing the diagnosis and management plan, added information can be obtained from dental impressions, old dental records, and comparison of the clinical presentation to preinjury facial photographs. Management of complex facial injuries frequently requires nursing coordination among the patient, family, and multiple medical teams (e.g., ophthalmology, neurosurgery, orthopedic surgery, critical care, and general surgery). Therefore it becomes crucial for the nursing staff to be up to date with all diagnoses, individual team plans, and expectations of the patient and family.

SPECIFIC TYPES OF MAXILLOFACIAL INJURIES

SOFT TISSUE WOUNDS

All open facial soft tissue wounds have the potential for contamination; therefore the patient's tetanus immunization status should be verified. If a patient has not been immunized, simultaneous intramuscular injection with 250 U of tetanus immune globulin (Hyper-Tet) and 0.5 ml of tetanus

toxoid is recommended. Two additional tetanus toxoid boosters should be given at monthly intervals to complete the immunization. In general, tetanus toxoid is given to individuals who have been immunized previously to ensure sufficient immunization.[25]

Contusions, abrasions, and lacerations are usually not life threatening, and the timing of their treatment depends on the patient's status and the ability to establish a surgically clean wound. Tissue that is obviously contaminated and crushed is quite susceptible to infection and should be debrided, followed by delayed primary closure or primary repair with serial reexamination ("second-look procedure") every 24 to 36 hours for further debridement of progressive necrosis.[26] This latter form of soft tissue management is most common for facial gunshot wounds and massive avulsive injuries.[4,5]

All wounds should be examined carefully for the presence of foreign material. The presence of foreign material reduces the bacteria required to cause infection. Meticulous hemostasis will reduce the potential for hematoma formation (a perfect medium for bacterial growth) and hence reduce the potential for infection. The use of drains may be indicated in lacerations of the parotid gland or in extensive injuries where fluid may accumulate and produce a dead space, which fosters bacterial colonization and potentiates infection.

Special attention should be devoted to the care of abrasions. Even though these injuries may be superficial, their mismanagement can lead to severe disfigurement.

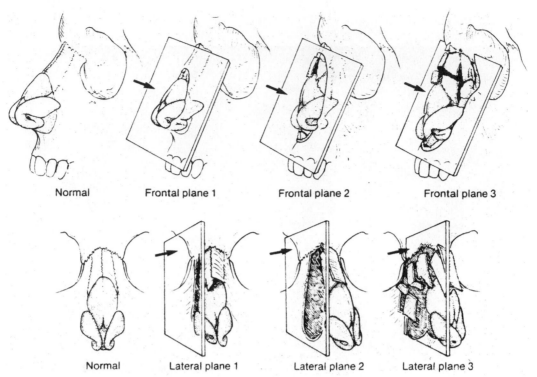

Normal Frontal plane 1 Frontal plane 2 Frontal plane 3

Normal Lateral plane 1 Lateral plane 2 Lateral plane 3

FIGURE 20-11 The concept of forces of impact and levels (planes) of destruction. **A,** With frontal forces, fracture can involve (1) nasal tip; (2) nasal dorsum, septum, and anterior nasal spine; and (3) frontal processes of maxilla, lacrimal, and ethmoid bones. **B,** With laterooblique forces, fractures can involve (1) ipsilateral nasal bone; (2) contralateral nasal bone and septum; and (3) nasal bones, frontal processes of maxilla, and lacrimal bone.

Entrapment of dirt, grease, or other foreign material beneath healed skin will lead to permanent tattooing, a situation extremely difficult to manage secondarily. These wounds should be cleansed aggressively with a brush while the patient is under appropriate anesthesia.

More complex soft tissue injury may require skin grafts or local or remote tissue flaps. Refer to Chapter 27 for more in-depth discussion about soft tissue injury.

NASAL FRACTURES

The nose is a triangular pyramid with both cartilaginous and bony structural support. High-velocity injuries will create more anteroposterior displacement and comminution. Low-velocity fractures typically cause a disjunction of the nasal cartilaginous vault from the nasal bony pyramid. In these cases the patient has an inverted V deformity of the nasal dorsum.

Stranc and Robertson classified nasal fractures according to their anteroposterior displacement and lateral deviation (Figure 20-11).[27] In this classification a plane 1 nasal fracture involves only the end of the nasal bony pyramid, and there is little deformity. This type of nasal fracture usually can be managed with internal reduction and nasal packing. A plane 2 nasal fracture is more extensive, involving the base of the nasal bony pyramid and nasal septum. Typically patients with this type of injury present with a flattened nasal dorsum, obstruction of the nasal passage, and absence of smell. Treatment may require, in addition to

internal reduction, some degree of external splinting and bone grafting. A plane 3 nasal fracture is in reality a nasoethmoidal-orbital fracture. This type of fracture commonly requires wide clinical exposure, bone graft reconstruction, and internal fixation techniques.

ZYGOMA AND ORBITAL FRACTURES

The zygoma is a major buttress of the midface, and its eminence gives prominence to the cheek. Additionally, it forms the lateral portion of the orbit. Almost all fractures of the zygoma involve the orbital floor and the V2 division of the trigeminal nerve. Clinically patients with this type of injury often have an abnormal ocular examination with periorbital ecchymosis, double vision (diplopia), and ocular proptosis secondary to edema. With extreme comminuted fractures, there may be acute enophthalmos (ocular recession within the orbit) secondary to severe loss of skeletal support. The eyes should be assessed for restriction of extraocular eye muscle movement. If there is restriction in any visual field, one must assume that there is bony entrapment of the muscle requiring decompression as soon as possible.[28] Additional findings specific for zygomatic fractures are depression of the malar eminence and zygomatic arch and downward displacement of the lateral canthus (see Figure 20-5). In most instances the zygoma is depressed and displaced downward; hence, the lateral canthus of the eye follows the lateral orbital rim (Figure 20-12). Occasionally the zygomatic arch can be displaced

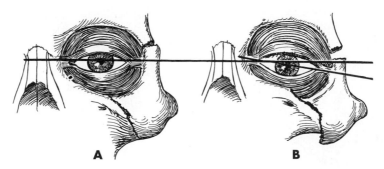

FIGURE 20-12 When the frontal process of the zygoma is depressed downward, the lateral canthal mechanism and the canthus of the eye follow. **A,** Normal position of the lateral canthus and a fracture without displacement. **B,** Downward displacement of the globe and lateral canthus as a result of frontozygomatic separation and downward displacement of the zygoma and the floor of the orbit. (From Manson PN: Facial injuries. In McCarthy JG, editor: *Plastic surgery,* vol 2, The face, part 1, Philadelphia, 1990, WB Saunders, 995.)

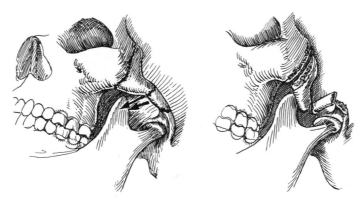

FIGURE 20-13 Fracture of the zygomatic arch with medial displacement against the coronoid process of the mandible, limiting mandibular motion. (From Manson PN: Facial injuries. In McCarthy JG, editor: *Plastic surgery,* vol 2, The face, part 1, Philadelphia, 1990, WB Saunders, 993.)

inward, impinging on the mandibular coronoid process and thereby creating a mechanical block to mandibular opening (Figure 20-13).

Surgical management of zygomatic and orbital floor fractures is directed by the presence of functional ocular impairment (e.g., reduced eye movement caused by entrapment of extraocular muscle, diplopia, enophthalmos), depressed zygoma with deformity, altered V2 sensation, or impingement on maxillary and mandibular musculoskeletal function.[29] The primary goal of treating the orbital floor component is to decompress any entrapped ocular tissue and simultaneously restore proper orbital volume to minimize the potential for secondary diplopia and enophthalmos.[29] With respect to the zygoma itself, the goal is to anatomically reposition the zygoma for proper midface projection and width dimension (Figure 20-14). For accurate anatomic reduction and stabilization of the quadrangular zygoma bone, three points of fixation typically are required: the frontozygomatic buttress, infraorbital rim, and zygomaticomaxillary buttress (Figure 20-15). Access to these buttresses can be obtained through a lower eyelid incision and an intraoral maxillary buccal sulcus incision. Severe high-velocity comminuted zygomatic fractures may also require a posterior approach to reconstruct the zygomatic arch.[30] The orbital floor compo-

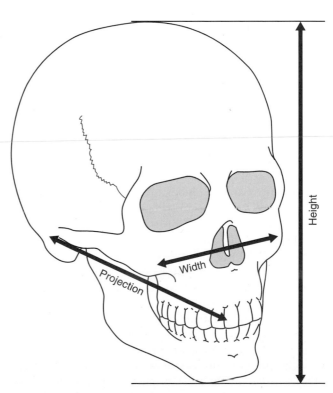

FIGURE 20-14 The goal in midface fracture repair is to reestablish normal facial width, height, and projection.

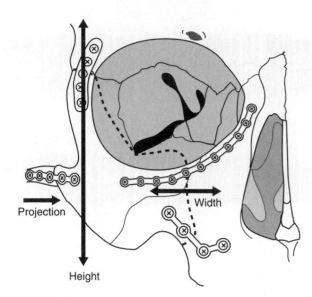

FIGURE 20-15 Technique of open reduction and internal fixation of a zygoma fracture.

nent is explored and reconstructed through the eyelid incision using an alloplastic implant.[29]

MAXILLARY AND MANDIBULAR FRACTURES

Fractures involving the maxilla or mandible are managed functionally to restore the preinjury habitual bite relationship. The bite relationship acts as a template for accurate anatomic reduction of fractures involving the basal bone of the maxilla and mandible. By establishing this relationship the surgeon can determine the proper facial height, width, and projection[4] (see Figure 20-14).

In most instances the preinjury bite relationship can be recognized and established by the wear facets on the teeth. However, in injured patients whose teeth or segments of bone are missing, it may be difficult to determine the normal occlusal relationship. In these instances old photographs, dental records, and dental models are extremely helpful.

The starting point for stabilizing any maxillary or mandibular fracture is placing the patient in maxillary and mandibular fixation. This is most easily accomplished by securing dentoalveolar arch bars to the dentition and wiring the jaws closed. After this the basal bone fractures of the maxilla and mandible are exposed, reduced anatomically, and stabilized with rigid titanium plates and screws.[11,31]

TOOTH FRACTURES

Essentially there are four types of tooth fractures (Figure 20-16). A type I fracture involves only the insensate tooth enamel, and the patient will complain of the sharp fractured edges but not experience significant discomfort. A type II fracture involves the tooth dentin, which contains nerve extensions from the tooth pulp. Patients with this type of fracture have moderate discomfort to hot and cold liquids but generally are comfortable at rest. A type III fracture involves exposed pulp; patients have significant pain at rest. A type IV fracture is through the root and also causes pain at

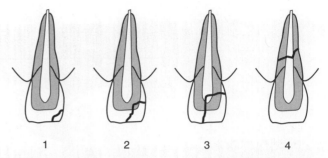

FIGURE 20-16 Types of tooth fractures. **1,** Enamel injuries. **2,** Dentin injuries. **3,** Pulp injuries. **4,** Root injuries.

rest. Most type II and III fractures require urgent dental attention for relief of discomfort and tooth salvage versus extraction.[32]

MANAGEMENT

Interdisciplinary communication of assessment findings and anticipated treatment needs enable the health care team to develop a coordinated comprehensive plan for managing the patient with maxillofacial injury in each phase of the trauma cycle. Management of complex facial injuries demands a thorough appreciation of facial anatomy and an orderly management scheme that will allow anatomic reconstruction of the facial skeletal structures, followed by redraping of the overlying soft tissue elements. Only with a consistent comprehensive approach can the harmonious balance of facial function and restoration of the patient's characteristic identity be achieved. An effective multidisciplinary plan of care considers treatment of the patient's actual injuries, interventions to avoid potential detrimental complications, and the psychologic and emotional aspects of facial injury.

RESUSCITATION PHASE

Priorities of care during the resuscitation phase are the same for all trauma patients and include the need to establish a patent airway and provide adequate ventilation and sufficient circulation.[33] Maxillofacial injuries can cause life-threatening airway obstruction, impaired ventilation, and hemorrhage, mandating immediate attention and nondefinitive treatment.[6] Unless maxillofacial injuries pose a threat to the airway, breathing, or circulation, management generally falls into the urgent category, and definitive treatment is not performed until all other actual or potential life-threatening injuries have been addressed.[6,10] In addition to managing potentially lethal injuries, interventions that recognize and treat neurologic dysfunction and those that manage pain and anxiety should be included in the resuscitation phase plan of care for patients with maxillofacial injuries.

MAINTAIN PATENT AIRWAY AND ENSURE ADEQUATE VENTILATION. In the patient with maxillofacial injury the airway can be obstructed and ventilation compromised as a result of pharyngeal swelling or occlusion of the pharynx by the tongue. Secretions, blood, vomit, unsupported soft tissue, displaced bone, dislodged dental appliances, avulsed teeth, and tooth fragments can also obstruct the airway. Initial attempts to establish a patent airway include use of the chin-lift or jaw-thrust maneuver and suction of secretions and foreign debris from the airway. Airway obstruction caused by tongue edema or loss of mandibular skeletal support may be managed by pulling the tongue forward and, if necessary, securing the tongue with sutures to prevent prolapse back over the airway.[10,21] Care must be taken to maintain head and neck alignment throughout maneuvers to establish an airway until any possible cervical spine injury has been definitely ruled out.[9] If initial attempts fail to establish and maintain a patent airway, early endotracheal intubation is indicated. An oral rather than a nasal route for emergent placement of endotracheal or gastric tubes is preferred to avoid additional midfacial injury and inadvertent insertion of the tube into the brain through possible coexisting cranial base fractures.[34] A cricothyroidotomy or tracheostomy may be preferred in the presence of severe facial injuries when the patient has multiple mandible or maxillary fractures or massive soft tissue damage.

Care is also taken to ensure that the airway remains patent and aspiration is prevented. The patient is at high risk for aspiration of secretions, debris, and blood from the traumatized nasopharynx and oropharynx. Patients with multiple fractures of the mandible that involve the floor of the mouth or with profuse nasal hemorrhage are at particularly high risk for aspiration.[35] Nursing interventions that may help prevent aspiration include suctioning the mouth and oropharynx frequently and positioning the patient in a side-lying position (unless otherwise contraindicated) to promote the removal of blood and secretions from the oral cavity. Placement of an orogastric tube to decompress the stomach also helps prevent aspiration. Risk of aspiration is decreased in the intubated patient by ensuring that the endotracheal or tracheostomy tube cuff remains adequately inflated. Symptoms indicating that aspiration has occurred include audible rales or rhonchi on chest auscultation, decreased blood oxygen saturation (Spo_2) and partial pressure of oxygen (Pao_2), reduced lung compliance, and, eventually, infiltrates visible on chest radiographs. Aggressive pulmonary toilet, namely endotracheal suctioning, is indicated if aspiration is suspected. Bronchoscopy may be necessary to remove aspirated blood or foreign debris (e.g., a tooth) from the patient's airway.

Once a patent airway is established, ensuring adequate ventilation becomes a priority. Nurses should assess the quality and effort of spontaneous respiration, symmetry of chest wall movement, and breath sounds. Noninvasive measures of Spo_2 and end-tidal carbon dioxide levels provide an indication about whether respiratory gas exchange is sufficient. Inadequate ventilation may occur secondary to aspiration, associated injuries, or administration of medications that suppress respiration during resuscitation. Insufficient spontaneous ventilation is treated initially by manually bagging the patient, followed eventually by employing mechanical ventilation. Supplemental oxygen is generally provided to foster adequate oxygenation.

CONTROL HEMORRHAGE AND ENSURE ADEQUATE INTRAVASCULAR VOLUME. Hemorrhage is the next immediate concern. Extensive hemorrhage and significant blood loss can result from injury to one or more of the multiple facial arteries[10] (Figure 20-17). Application of direct pressure on the site of vessel injury is the primary method of hemorrhage control.[7,10] Circumferential pressure bandages can also be used. If these measures fail to control the bleeding and the source of blood loss is visible, clamping and ligation or repair of the vessel may be indicated. Nurses should monitor dressings closely for blood saturation and keep the physician apprised of the estimated blood loss. Surgical hemostats, clamps, and suture material should be readily available. Hemorrhage caused by facial fractures, such as those involving the mandible, maxilla, nose, zygoma, frontal sinus, or nasoethmoid, may be controlled by reduction of the fracture.

Profuse epistaxis (nasal bleeding) can occur with any facial fracture that communicates with the nose (e.g., nasal, maxillary, cranial base, and sinus fractures).[9] Actively bleeding vessels in the nasal region can be compressed by inserting a 30-ml balloon or petroleum gauze into each nares. Nasal packing is removed by the physician under controlled conditions within 24 to 48 hours. Packing that remains in place for longer than 2 days becomes a source of infection and may cause compression necrosis of the mucous membranes. Early maxillary fracture surgical reduction and fixation may be necessary to control profuse nasopharyngeal bleeding. Transvascular embolization of bleeding vessels performed during angiography may be effective in halting intractable oronasal hemorrhage when other conventional treatments have failed.[36]

Restoration of intravascular fluid volume is achieved by intravenous administration of crystalloids, colloids, and, when appropriate, blood products. The patient's hemodynamic status, including measures such as blood pressure, heart rate, and central venous pressure, and assessment parameters that indicate sufficiency of tissue perfusion (e.g., mentation, urine output, lactate levels), guide the necessary volume of fluid replacement. Serial assessment of hemoglobin, hematocrit, and coagulation factors determine the need for blood product administration and alert the practitioner to further bleeding. Other sources of blood loss besides hemorrhage from maxillofacial injury also need to be ruled out or controlled if identified.

RECOGNIZE AND TREAT NEUROLOGIC DYSFUNCTION. Brain injury may accompany maxillofacial trauma.[1,6] Penetrating objects causing maxillofacial injuries (e.g., bullets, knife blades) and maxillofacial fractures themselves can extend into the cranial vault and injure the brain. Acceleration-deceleration forces that result in maxillofacial injury can set the semisolid brain into motion within the

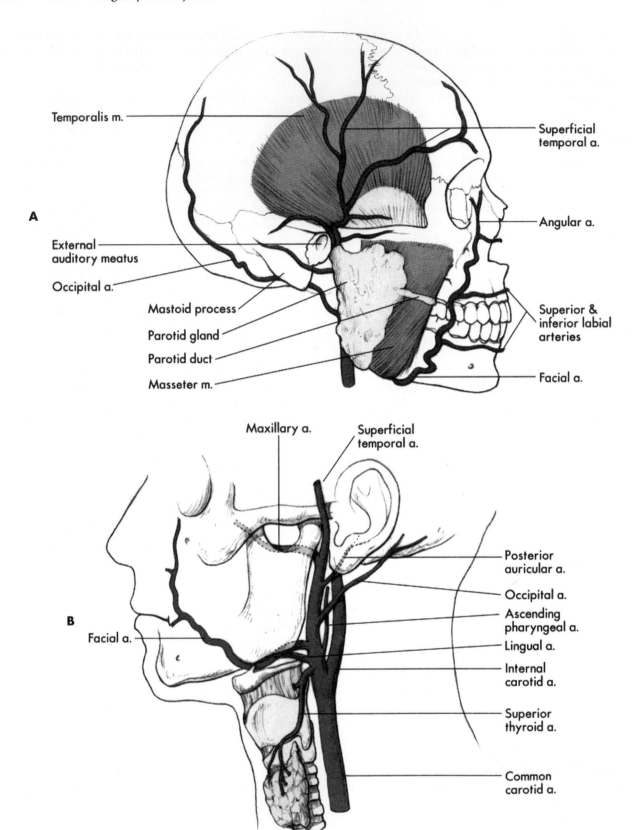

FIGURE 20-17 Vascular supply of the face. **A,** Branches of the external carotid artery. **B,** Further branches of the external carotid and the carotid bifurcation. (From Mathers LH, Chase RA, Dolph J et al: *Clinical anatomy principles,* St. Louis, 1996, Mosby, 182.)

rigid skull, possibly causing the brain to be injured as it comes into contact with the skull surface or by causing stretching, tension, and shearing of involved tissue. Brain and cervical spine injuries should always be suspected until ruled out. Refer to Chapter 19 for more specific information on traumatic brain injuries.

Frequent neurologic assessments are warranted throughout the resuscitation phase. Any changes or abnormal findings should be reported immediately to the physician. Neurosurgical consultation is recommended to completely evaluate any suspected central nervous system injury. Radiographic studies to evaluate the cervical spine and CT scan of the head should be included in the patient's initial workup if alterations in level of consciousness, motor function, sensation, or eye and pupil function are evident during patient assessment.

Intracranial injury with a dural tear and CSF leak should be suspected in any patient with severe nasal, frontal sinus, nasoethmoid, or Le Fort III fractures. CSF rhinorrhea is often difficult to detect when there is blood in the nares. A nasal drip pad (i.e., a folded gauze pad) should be placed loosely under the nares to collect drainage so that its amount and character can be evaluated. When drainage contains CSF, a yellowish "halo ring" typically appears around a stain of blood on the drip pad and the draining fluid will test positive for glucose (blood also contains glucose and will cause a positive test result).[18]

MANAGE PAIN AND ANXIETY.   Maxillofacial and associated injuries may cause substantial patient discomfort. Prescribed analgesia should be administered to achieve an acceptable level of pain control. If possible, a mechanism should be developed with the patient unable to verbalize to communicate pain and pain relief (e.g., holding up 1 to 10 fingers to indicate level of pain severity). A neurologic examination should be obtained and documented before providing analgesia; short-acting or easily reversible agents (e.g., morphine, fentanyl) are preferable to allow ongoing neurologic evaluation of the patient.

Nurses should orient patients to their surroundings and offer appropriate reassurance to help allay anxiety. Clear, concise explanations regarding procedures and reinforcement of physician explanations regarding diagnosis and the treatment plan should also be provided. Nurses should be aware of their own actions and behaviors (e.g., facial expressions, eye contact, and voice) while caring for the patient, taking care not to convey alarm or disgust, which can heighten the patient's anxiety.[37] Medications to reduce or alleviate anxiety may be necessary, and their effect on the neurologic examination should be considered before administration.

OPERATIVE PHASE

During the past 100 years three hallmark developments led to current surgical management of facial injuries. In the early 1900s Le Fort conducted research on the effect of injury on the craniofacial skeleton.[3] He demonstrated that the craniofacial skeleton will fracture predictably along the weak fault lines that lie between the supporting buttresses, which surround and protect the delicate functional elements of the face. Le Fort then classified three basic fracture patterns, as described earlier in this chapter.

During the next 60 years management of facial injuries focused on reducing and controlling the position of these structural buttresses via indirect techniques. Small incisions were used to identify the line of fracture, and the buttresses were stabilized with interosseous wires and external fixators. In the hands of a master surgeon the outcome of these techniques was often exceptional; however, all too often these indirect techniques led to incomplete reduction of skeletal buttresses and distortion of the functional elements and facial appearance. In the late 1970s, with the advent of computed tomography, injury patterns and the interrelationship of the soft tissue and underlying bony construct became more fully understood. Injuries were no longer diagnosed as isolated Le Fort fractures but in addition were classified regarding the level of energy required to produce the specific pattern of injury.[24] This led to the realization that wide exposure and direct visualization of the fractured components was required for accurate anatomic reduction of the craniofacial buttresses. Perfection of diagnostic techniques, adaptation of cosmetic surgical exposure, development of biocompatible materials for rigid stabilization of buttresses, and improved understanding of bone physiology and bone healing have led to the current standards for management of facial skeletal injuries. Today the standard of care requires an accurate three-dimensional reconstruction.

The concept of accurate anatomic reduction and stabilization of the craniofacial buttresses can be applied to all levels of fracture patterns.[31] Even when treating a high-velocity fracture with severe bone comminution and soft tissue disruption, adherence to this principle will allow accurate facial reconstruction. This same basic principle also can be extrapolated to low-velocity facial gunshot wounds. However, in high-velocity facial gunshot wounds and facial avulsive injuries, there is the potential for soft tissue and bone devascularization, which does not necessarily manifest at the time of initial presentation. Typically progressive soft tissue and bone necrosis evolve over several days.[4,26] At the R Adams Cowley Shock Trauma Center between 1977 and 1993, a high potential for complications after immediate reconstruction of missing bony components using nonvascularized bone graft was observed. A review demonstrated a failure to recognize the evolution of this necrosis phenomenon, specifically oral mucosal lining necrosis.[5] As a result, today a rapid sequential protocol is in place that calls for immediate anatomic stabilization of the bony and soft tissue elements, followed by serial take-back procedures for "second-look" debridements of necrotic tissue and definitive vascularized bone and soft tissue reconstruction during the primary phase of wound healing (Figure 20-18A-E). This provides complete vascularized soft tissue reconstruc-

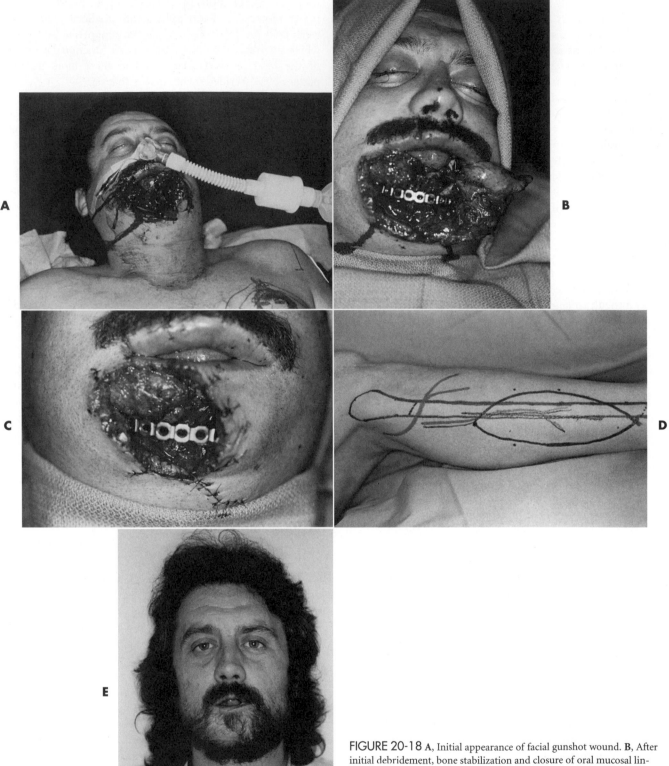

FIGURE 20-18 **A**, Initial appearance of facial gunshot wound. **B**, After initial debridement, bone stabilization and closure of oral mucosal lining. **C**, Hospital day 5, after serial second-look debridement and ready for free microvascular reconstruction. **D**, Site of microvascular fibula osteo-cutaneous flap. **E**, Six months after completed reconstruction. (From Robertson BC, Manson PN: High-energy ballistic and avulsive injuries: a management protocol for the next millennium, *Surg Clin North Am* 6:1489-1502, 1999.)

tion of all missing tissue before the secondary phase of wound contracture, when profound soft tissue distortion can occur. With this modified technique, all craniofacial buttresses are anatomically restored within the primary phase of wound healing, and these buttresses are surrounded with stable vascularized tissue. This results in less secondary wound contraction impinging on the functional elements and less distortion of the surrounding soft tissues. Secondary soft tissue rearrangement using adjacent aesthetic units of the face for an optimal final surgical outcome then is allowed.

Facial reconstruction procedures, whether simple or complex, may take several hours. Intraoperative nursing care is directed toward the anesthetized patient but must also include support of the family or significant others awaiting information about their loved one. One family spokesperson should be identified who will receive brief updates about the progress of the patient's surgery, estimated time remaining, and planned disposition of the patient postoperatively. The operating surgeon should provide specific information about the operative procedure, patient diagnosis, and future treatment plan. Family members should be directed to write down questions regarding these topics and address them with the surgeon after the surgery.

CRITICAL CARE AND INTERMEDIATE CARE PHASES

Postoperatively the patient with maxillofacial injury may require critical care or intermediate care management, depending on the severity of injury, threat to airway, breathing or circulation, associated injuries, and medical history. Airway patency, adequate ventilation, and circulation remain the most important care priorities during these phases. Complications such as inadequate oxygenation, tissue hypoperfusion, infection, and inadequate nutrition can compromise wound and fracture healing and must be avoided. For more specific information on wound healing, refer to Chapter 15. Attention to potential neurologic compromise, pain control, and psychologic well-being must also be included in the plan of care.

ENSURE ADEQUATE RESPIRATORY FUNCTION. Airway patency and adequate ventilation are threatened by a number of factors after maxillofacial fracture repair or soft tissue reconstruction. Upper airway edema caused by trauma, operative manipulation, or prolonged intubation can cause airway occlusion, necessitating endotracheal intubation or tracheostomy until the edema subsides (Figure 20-19). Ineffective clearance of intraoral and pulmonary secretions also can cause airway obstruction. Prolonged time under anesthesia for lengthy facial repair increases the likelihood of atelectasis formation, which compromises respiratory gas exchange.

Indications for early tracheostomy in patients with maxillofacial injuries include complex fractures involving the nose, maxilla, and mandible and fractures associated with significant loss of mandibular or maxillary skeletal

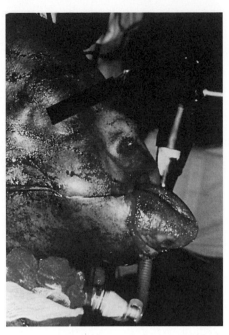

FIGURE 20-19 Postoperative edema of the face and tongue.

support of the surrounding soft tissue. In the latter group the unsupported soft tissues will collapse into the airway (Figure 20-20). Patients with associated severe brain or pulmonary injury, for whom prolonged intubation is likely, are also candidates for early tracheostomy.[29]

Every effort should be made to maintain an established airway by employing measures to avoid premature artificial airway removal, continuing aggressive pulmonary toilet, and taking precautions against aspiration. Patient positioning should ensure that unnecessary tension on an artificial airway is avoided so that the tube is not inadvertently dislodged and further airway irritation and edema formation do not occur. The patient should be kept calm through frequent verbal reassurance and appropriate use of sedation and anxiolytics. Premature self-extubation or inadvertent airway dislodgment can be life threatening for the patient with maxillofacial injury because reintubation may be difficult or impossible because of massive upper airway edema.[36] Appropriate use of physical and chemical restraints should be considered to prevent this from occurring. Patients with intermaxillary fixation should have wire cutters or some other device that allows rapid release of the fixation at the bedside in the event of an airway emergency.[38]

Aggressive pulmonary toilet, including suctioning and chest physiotherapy (CPT), remains important to remove secretions and maintain airway patency. Sometimes the extent of the injury or type of maxillofacial reconstruction prohibits head-down positioning for postural drainage in the early period just after injury or surgical intervention. Nurses should confer with the surgeon who preformed the facial repair to determine what type of patient positioning is permitted. Nonintubated patients should be encouraged to use the incentive spirometer at frequent intervals. Interventions initiated in the resuscitation phase to avoid aspiration,

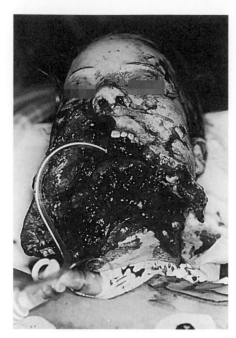

FIGURE 20-20 Unsupported soft tissue collapse.

including ensuring tracheal cuff inflation, frequent removal of intraoral secretions, positioning the patient to enhance outflow of oral drainage, and gastric decompression, remain relevant throughout the critical care and intermediate care phases.

ADEQUATE HYDRATION.   Adequate intravascular volume must be maintained to ensure sufficient perfusion to the site of tissue injury and repair. After a prolonged surgical intervention for maxillofacial repair, the nurse should carefully evaluate the patient's fluid balance and hemodynamic status to determine if hydration is adequate. The physician should be notified immediately if the patient appears dehydrated or hemodynamically unstable so that the problem can be quickly remedied.

ONGOING NEUROLOGIC ASSESSMENT.   It is imperative that the nurse compares the patient's postoperative neurologic assessment with the baseline assessment obtained preoperatively. Serial neurologic assessments, including examination of consciousness, motor function, sensation, eye and pupil reflexes, and other cranial nerve functions, should be performed thereafter to detect possible deterioration. Thorough neurologic assessment provides a systematic evaluation of the craniofacial structure functions. Any deterioration in the patient's neurologic function should be reported immediately to the physician.

During the critical care phase, barriers to assessment of certain neurologic parameters may exist for patients with maxillofacial injuries. Assessment of the patient's orientation, speech, and cognitive abilities is difficult in the intubated patient. Asking simple yes or no questions, which allow the patient to nod or signal the answer, is one strategy that can be used to elicit this information. Periorbital edema

and suturing the eyelids closed make the eyes inaccessible for evaluation. In the cooperative patient able to acknowledge simple questions, assessment of light perception by shining a light directly over the closed or covered eye is recommended every 2 to 4 hours for the first 24 hours after zygoma and orbit repair.

Nasal drainage should continue to be monitored for the presence of CSF. The nasal drip pad should be checked frequently to determine the amount, consistency, color, and odor of drainage. Any change in these characteristics should be reported immediately to the physician.

PAIN MANAGEMENT.   Pain generally persists postoperatively and requires use of prescribed analgesics for control. Dressing changes or wound irrigations may increase pain intensity, increasing the need for analgesia and possibly sedation just before these procedures. Application of ice to the face for the first 24 hours after surgical intervention may help reduce facial swelling and discomfort. Refer to Chapter 17 for more specific information on pain and sedation management.

WOUND CARE.   Skin integrity likely is altered in patients with maxillofacial injury from traumatic lacerations, degloving, abrasions, and surgical incisions. Suture lines and facial abrasions should be cleansed at the prescribed frequency using the method requested by the surgeon. If prescribed, a thin layer of antibiotic ointment (e.g., bacitracin) is applied over the cleaned incision or wound site.[7,9] A pH-corrected ointment for ophthalmic use is applied to incisions in the periorbital region. Operative incisions are often left open to air once any significant drainage from the site has ceased.[9] Skin flaps or grafts will require unique, specialized care, which is described in Chapter 27, Soft Tissue Injuries.

The operating surgeon should provide specific instructions about oral care required for the patient with intraoral lacerations or incisions. Dental hygiene is essential even when intraoral devices such as arch bars or elastics are in place. A prescribed oral rinse (e.g., chlorhexidine gluconate [Peridex], 50:50 mixture of normal saline and 3% hydrogen peroxide) generally is used to irrigate the mouth at regular intervals.[7] A mixture of 10% betadine, 40% peroxide, and 50% saline may be prescribed as the mouthwash solution for patients with intraoral infections. Oral lavage is usually done at least four to six times a day until serosanginous secretions subside (which can be a minimum of 2 to 3 days). A large syringe with a flexible peripheral intravenous catheter sheath attached can be used to inject the rinse solution into spaces that are difficult to reach within the mouth. As the oral cavity is irrigated, a suction catheter is used to remove the rinse and secretions. Patients with a decreased level of consciousness will need to be positioned on their side to prevent aspiration during the lavage. A toothbrush or commercial toothpaste should not be used until approved by the physician. Orthodontic wax may be applied over metal arch bars to prevent irritation to the oral mucosa but should be removed daily to allow thorough cleansing of the mouth.

NUTRITION. Adequate hydration and nutrition are essential to allow fractures and soft tissue to heal and to reduce the risk of infection. Wound healing depends on the intake of adequate protein, carbohydrates, and fat and sufficient vitamins and minerals.[39,40] Consultation with a registered dietitian is helpful for determining the patient's individualized nutritional requirements. Refer to Chapter 16 for a complete review of metabolic and nutritional management of the trauma patient.

If bowel sounds are absent or enteral feeding is contraindicated for any other reason, total parenteral nutrition should be considered. As soon as the gastrointestinal tract is functional, enteral feedings can be started. A patient with intermaxillary fixation or with some other restriction to mastication may require an orogastric or intestinal feeding tube to deliver commercially prepared tube feedings. The head of the bed should be elevated at least 30 degrees (unless contraindicated) while the patient is receiving enteral feedings to promote gastric emptying and discourage reflux, thereby reducing risk of aspiration. The nurse should remain vigilant for symptoms that indicate intolerance to the enteral feedings (e.g., nausea, vomiting, diarrhea, excessive gastric residual, abdominal distention). Suction apparatus should be kept readily available to assist with removal of any vomitus, and patients should be positioned on their side to reduce risk of aspiration if vomiting occurs. Wire cutters must be readily accessible for patients with intermaxillary fixation so that the fixation can be released if vomiting occurs and the emesis cannot be removed with suction and positioning.[7,38] The physician should be notified immediately if fixation is released. The patient in this situation should not be left unattended.

Once oral feedings are permitted, the prescribed diet is initiated. Generally, clear liquids are introduced, with advancement to full and pureed liquids and foods as tolerated by the patient. A pureed or soft diet can be continued until mastication becomes more comfortable for the patient. Care should be taken to ensure that food fibers from blended foods are removed to avoid the particles becoming trapped between dentition or between fixation devices. A dietician can assist in finding attractive and creative ways to enhance necessary caloric intake.

POTENTIAL FOR INFECTION. Maxillofacial injuries, with or without penetrating wounds, usually are considered contaminated because the fractures pass through the perinasal sinuses and communicate with teeth and the oral cavity. Despite this hostile environment, the actual incidence of infection is remarkably low unless there has been incomplete debridement of devascularized tissue and foreign material, incomplete evacuation of hematoma, failure to obliterate dead space, incomplete establishment of oral lining closure, or obstruction of glandular ducts. The incidence of infection is highest in penetrating gunshot wounds and high-speed

avulsive injuries that involve the mandible.[41] In these instances the potential for progressive soft tissue and bone necrosis over the first several days is high; therefore serial second-look operative washout and debridement procedures are advised until the wound becomes stable (Figure 20-18, *A-C*). At this point all missing tissue, including lining, bone, and overlying skin envelope, should be reconstructed with vascularized tissue.[4,26] (Figure 20-18, *D-E*).

Antibiotics are usually administered during the perioperative period. Ongoing prophylactic antibiotic coverage may be considered for patients with an open brain injury (i.e., cerebrospinal fluid leak or pneumocephalus), fractures opening into the mouth, fractures communicating with the teeth or adjacent to tooth roots, lacerations into the oral cavity, animal bites, sinus fractures, or orbital emphysema. A great deal of controversy surrounds the indiscriminate use of antibiotic prophylaxis because it may place the patient at risk for infections caused by antibiotic-resistant organisms. More important than antibiotics is timely intervention to decontaminate the maxillofacial wound. When a clean wound cannot be established, prophylactic antibiotics are usually indicated and should be administered as prescribed.[9] Antibiotics provided for prophylaxis are typically discontinued after 2 to 3 days.

Early signs of infection unique to maxillofacial injuries include disproportionate edema and pain in the region of the parotid and submandibular glands, a persistent foul breath odor despite good oral hygiene, persistent serous or seropurulent drainage from incision lines, rapidly spreading erythema, and increasing discomfort when moving the eyes or tongue. Early detection of infection is critical because the causative organisms are usually anaerobic and spread rapidly through the head and neck tissue planes. As with any infection, early evacuation of the source, along with operative debridement of devascularized tissue and initiation of appropriate antibiotics based on organism sensitivity, is required. The surgeon must reinspect and ensure adequate drainage of the perinasal sinuses and parotid and submandibular glands, reevaluate the fracture sites that communicate through tooth sockets, remove teeth that have become mobile, and ensure a water-tight closure of the oral mucosal lining.

Facial fractures often increase the risk of sinusitis. To prevent this infectious process, long-term placement of nasal packing and nasogastric or nasal endotracheal tubes should be avoided. The nasal cavity should be cleansed daily with normal saline nose drops to prevent obstruction of the perinasal sinuses and ensure a patent nasal airway. Decongestants may also be prescribed to help maintain the nasal airway and clear the sinuses, but administration of these agents should be limited to 3 to 5 days. Presence of fever, halitosis, and purulent nasal drainage should alert the practitioner to the possibility of a sinus infection. Sinusitis can be verified with radiographs demonstrating opacification of the sinuses. Needle aspiration or surgical drainage is indicated to drain the infected sinuses, and appropriate antibiotics should be initiated. Follow-up sinus x-ray films may be indicated in 2 to 3 weeks to determine if sinus opacification has resolved.

Le Fort II and Le Fort III fractures and nasoorbital-ethmoidal and frontobasilar fractures frequently communicate with the anterior cranial base through the cribriform plate and are associated with dural lacerations and CSF leakage (CSF rhinorrhea). Anatomic reduction and stabilization of these fractures usually will allow the dural injury to seal within 24 to 36 hours. If the CSF leak does not stop spontaneously, surgical intervention to repair the dura may be necessary. Measures should be taken to avoid retrograde migration of bacteria into the cranial vault and thus decrease the risk of meningitis. Nasal packing, nasal intubation with gastric or endotracheal tubes, and blowing of the nose should be avoided.[29] Patients with these injuries should be examined frequently for changes in their neurologic status, which may indicate intracranial infection.[42] When meningitis is confirmed or highly suspected, the patient is treated with an antibiotic that crosses the blood-brain barrier and is effective in treating the known or likely infectious organisms.

EYE CARE.   When injuries occur in or near the orbital region, special attention should be given to care of the eye. Prescribed ophthalmic drops or ointment should be applied to the eye at regular intervals to maintain lubrication and prevent corneal abrasions. Eyelids may also be sutured by the surgeon or taped closed to protect the eyes. Use of ophthalmic lubricant and special protective interventions for the eye are particularly important if eyelid closure is impaired, eyelid injuries are present, the corneal reflex is absent, or natural tear formation is insufficient. Refer to Chapter 21 for more information on ocular injuries.

Early double vision after management of periorbital fractures is common but should gradually improve as edema resolves.[15] Ocular function should be compared with the findings from the preoperative baseline evaluation. Any variance should be brought to the attention of the physician. If there is a change in light perception or pupillary response, optic nerve compression from a retrobulbar hematoma[20] or displaced bone fragment must be suspected and an emergent ophthalmology consultation obtained.

ALTERED BODY IMAGE.   Any type of facial trauma threatens the concept of self. Each patient's reaction to sudden disfigurement is different, whether the injury involves a small laceration or massive tissue loss. Human interaction usually occurs face to face, and if the appearance of the face is altered, the interaction process also changes. Altered body image caused by maxillofacial injury can have a profound impact on the patient's self-esteem, interpersonal interactions, and role performance. Individuals with such alterations in body image often respond by grieving and some experience depression.[37]

Encouraging the patient to express feelings about the injury and communicating to the patient with a caring, empathetic approach are strategies that may be helpful. Al-

ternative modes of communication need to be established with the patient who is unable to verbalize (e.g., an intubated patient). Nurses must remain conscientious about their nonverbal communication, which should focus on maintaining eye contact and relaying an accepting and positive attitude when caring for the wound. Reinforcing positive qualities can also help enhance self-worth. Referral to a psychiatric liaison or crisis counselor may assist the patient in coping with the injury and altered body image. Refer to Chapter 18 for more information on the psychologic impact of trauma and appropriate nursing interventions.

Altered body image caused by facial wounds may prompt the patient to cope by use of denial, withdrawal, repression, suppression, or regression.[37] The patient may refuse wound care or prefer to isolate himself or herself from interactions with others. Adequate pain and anxiety relief should always be provided when caring for the wound site. Discussion about possible negative reactions to the facial disfigurement should be encouraged. The patient should not be forced into unwanted social interaction, but a supportive significant other may prove helpful in decreasing anxiety and apprehension about the wound and socialization.

REINTEGRATION INTO THE COMMUNITY

Although the hospital course for patients with maxillofacial trauma will vary depending on the type and severity of injuries they sustained, the final desired outcome for all patients is reintegration into society. After discharge from the hospital, most patients with maxillofacial injury need continued care for the physical and psychologic aspects of their injury. A great deal of clear and comprehensible patient and family education and adequate home health care resources are required for successful reintegration of the patient back into society.

PATIENT AND FAMILY EDUCATION.   A clear plan of care and realistic outlook for the patient's facial restoration need to be clearly communicated to the patient and family by the physician. Anticipated follow-up surgeries and expected outcomes of reconstruction should be explained to the patient and family by the surgeon. The nurse should reinforce this information. Offering false reassurances and reinforcing unrealistic hopes for a new facial appearance is strongly discouraged.

Wound care should be explained and demonstrated to the patient and family, and then a return demonstration by the individual who will be performing the care at home should be observed. Instruction and demonstration of suture line care may be best done with the patient in front of a mirror. Patients should be instructed to wash their hands frequently, to keep their hair clean and styled away from the operative incision, and to avoid air pollutants (e.g., cigarette smoke and excessive dust). Patients should be advised to avoid direct hand contact with wound sites. Education should also be provided on symptoms of potential localized, systemic, or intracranial infections and actions to take if such symptoms are recognized.

Direct exposure of incisions or wounds to sunlight or ultraviolet rays should also be avoided to prevent the wound from becoming deeper in color. Patients should be taught that if sunlight exposure is anticipated, strong sunscreen should be applied over and around the facial scar.[7] Incisions will appear red and elevated for approximately 6 months after repair.

Intraoral irrigations and rinses after meals are usually continued after hospitalization and must be stressed as part of discharge instructions. The patient should be taught when and if a bristled toothbrush or toothpaste can be used. A water-jet appliance can be recommended for removal of retained food residue in hard-to-reach areas of the mouth. Appropriate use of orthodontic wax is reviewed if relevant for the patient.

Patients requiring long-term tracheostomy need education about care and safety measures concerning the artificial airway device. Patients and their families should be instructed on airway clearance techniques and tracheostomy site care. Emergency care to be taken if the airway becomes occluded or dislodged should be described and demonstrated thoroughly.

After surgical intervention for mandibular fractures, particularly condylar and subcondylar fractures, an exercise regimen may be prescribed to enhance mandibular range of motion. The surgeon determines the timing for introduction of these exercises. The patient should be encouraged to perform these exercises in front of a mirror to allow observation of progress. Other measures that may be used to increase mandibular motion include heat application and muscle relaxants.

Patients and families should be informed that psychologic adjustment and adaptation to facial injury might take several weeks or months. Posttraumatic stress disorder may develop in individuals who suffer facial trauma.[43] Patients and families should be aware that frequent reactions to such injury may include altered mood patterns, depression, increased anxiety, and nightmares or flashbacks about the injury event. Follow-up counseling or therapy is an option that the patient should consider if these or other psychologic symptoms become evident.

Other late complications of maxillofacial injuries include issues related to musculoskeletal scar formation and scar contracture, persistent double vision, enophthalmos, glandular obstruction, fracture nonunion or malunion, devitalization of teeth, and malocclusion. These late complications are generally not present at the time of release from the primary acute care hospital; however, the physician, nurse, and therapist need to review symptoms of these potential problems with the patient and family at the time of discharge. Scars and scar contracture can cause unacceptable alterations in appearance and function and thus require intervention. Techniques used to treat scars and scar contracture are described in Chapter 27, Soft Tissue Injuries.

Persistent double vision from eye muscle injury may continue after edema subsides in 6 to 8 weeks.[15] This may require treatment by an ophthalmologist with prisms or ocular muscle surgery to readjust functional movement of the eye. Postinjury enophthalmos may occur secondary to malreduction of orbital fractures with increased orbital volume, reduced ocular volume secondary to intraocular fat atrophy, retroocular scar retraction, or some combination thereof. Postinjury enophthalmos is generally corrected by surgically releasing the scar tissue or correcting the volume of the orbit by reconstructing the involved malpositioned orbital walls.[15,29] This late form of enophthalmos usually takes several months to reach its final position, and correction is deferred until scar maturation has occurred at 6 to 12 months.

Occasionally parotid and submandibular glandular dysfunction does not manifest during the primary phase of hospitalization. Patients with this condition will complain of persistent glandular swelling and marked pain when eating. Glandular function is checked by evaluating for clear salivary flow from the parotid duct (located on the buccal mucosa opposite the maxillary second molar) or the mandibular duct (located on the floor of the mouth just behind the mandibular central incisors). If there is no flow or if pain and a cloudy discharge are present, further investigation for glandular dysfunction is indicated. A sialogram or CT scan may be warranted.

The primary focus of follow-up evaluation during the convalescent phase of recovery from maxillofacial fractures is to determine fracture union and to maintain a stable, balanced, functional occlusion. Occasionally fracture nonunion or malunion (bony malalignment) may occur. In these cases patients may experience persistent pain at the fracture site, mobility, and if the maxilla or mandible are involved, malocclusion. Further surgery may be required to restore the proper bite relationship and to realign the bony components.[44,45] A bone graft may be necessary to ensure bone union.

HOME HEALTH CARE RESOURCES. Home health care may be needed if facial reconstruction is extensive, complex dressing changes are required, intravenous medications must be continued, or a tracheostomy remains in place. A home health care nurse may be needed to supervise initial wound or tracheostomy care after discharge from the hospital. Adequate supplies and resources should be arranged for the patient before discharge.

COSMETICS. A patient may be interested in using cosmetics to conceal prominent facial scars. A plastic or oral maxillofacial surgeon should be consulted to verify the types of makeup that can be used during scar healing and maturation. Referral to a cosmetologist with experience in scar coverage and concealment may also be offered to the patient. The cosmetologist can educate the patient on techniques to achieve symmetry of color and contour between scarred areas and natural pigmentation. Through use of color and outline, scars and other defects can be made to appear less prominent.

SUMMARY

In the future more biocompatible materials that are resorbable will be adapted for use in facial repair, and specific tissue structures will be engineered for improved tissue reconstruction without the morbidity currently associated with autogenous tissue transfer. Work with automobile manufacturers may enable development of improved protective devices that could further reduce the incidence of facial injuries. Research to define nursing therapeutics that best promote wound and fracture healing, relieve pain, and deal effectively with the psychologic effects of facial trauma will continue to be important for improving care to patients with maxillofacial injuries.

With a comprehensive approach to managing complex facial injuries, one can achieve harmonious balance of facial function and restoration of the patient's individual characteristic identity. Nursing plays a critical role in providing the physical and psychologic care necessary for patients with maxillofacial trauma. Knowledge of facial anatomy and assessment strategies to recognize maxillofacial injury prepares the nurse to anticipate and deliver the care required for specific types of maxillofacial trauma. Together with the rest of the multidisciplinary health care team, the nurse who is knowledgeable about maxillofacial injuries is able to plan and implement care in each phase of the trauma cycle to optimize outcomes for patients with these injuries.

REFERENCES

1. Hogg NJV, Stewart TC, Armstrong JEA et al: Epidemiology of maxillofacial injuries at trauma hospitals in Ontario, Canada, between 1992 and 1997, *J Trauma* 49:425-432, 2000.
2. Major MS, MacGregor A, Bumpous JM: Patterns of maxillofacial injuries as a function of automobile restraint use, *Laryngoscope* 110:608-611, 2000.
3. Le Fort R: Etude experimentale sur les fractures de la machoire supreieure, *Rev Chir Paris* 23:208, 360, 479, 1901.
4. Robertson BC, Manson PN: High-energy ballistic and avulsive injuries: a management protocol for the next millennium, *Surg Clin North Am* 6:1489-1502, 1999.
5. Clark N, Birely B, Manson PN et al: High-energy ballistic and avulsive facial injuries: classification, patterns, and an algorithm for primary reconstruction, *Plast Reconstr Surg* 98: 583-601, 1996.
6. Tung TC, Tseng WS, Chen CT et al: Acute life-threatening injuries in facial fracture patients: a review of 1,025 patients, *J Trauma* 49:420-424, 2000.
7. Sadrian R, Rappaport NH: An overview of maxillofacial trauma for nurses, *Plast Surg Nurs* 18:177-181, 1998.
8. Tung TC, Chen YR, Chen CT et al: Full intrusion of a tooth after facial trauma, *J Trauma* 43:357-359, 1997.
9. Seyfer AE, Hansen JE: Facial trauma. In Mattox KL, Feliciano DV, Moore EE, editors: *Trauma,* New York, 2000, McGraw-Hill, 415-433.
10. Shenaq SM, Dinh T: Maxillofacial and scalp injury in neurotrauma. In Narayan RK, Wilberger JE, Povlishock JT, editors: *Neurotrauma,* New York, 1996, McGraw-Hill, 225-237.
11. Kelly KJ, Manson PN, Vanderkolk CA et al: Sequency Le Fort fracture treatment (organization of treatment for a panfacial fracture), *J Craniofac Surg* 1:168-178, 1990
12. Bun RJ, Vissink A, Bos RRM: Traumatic superior orbital fissure syndrome: report of two cases, *J Oral Maxillofac Surg* 54:758-761, 1996.
13. Campiglio GL, Signorini M, Candiani P: Superior orbital fissure syndrome complicating zygomatic fractures: pathogenesis and report of a case, *Scand J Plast Reconstr Hand Surg* 29:69-72, 1995.
14. Kastenbaure ER: Management of hematoma of the septum in abscesses of the nasal septum, *Laryngo Rhino Otolaryngol* 76:A1-A5, 1997.
15. Amrith S, Saw SM, Lim TC et al: Ophthalmic involvement in cranio-facial trauma, *J Cranio-Maxillofac Surg* 28:140-147, 2000.
16. Iliff N, Manson PN, Katz J et al: Mechanisms of extraocular muscle injury in orbital fractures, *Plast Reconstr Surg* 103: 787-799, 1999.
17. Jabaley ME, Lerman M, and Sanders HJ: Ocular injuries in orbital fractures. A review of 119 cases, *Plast Reconstr Surg* 56:410-418, 1975.
18. Hickey JV: *The clinical practice of neurological and neurosurgical nursing,* ed 4, Philadelphia, 1997, JB Lippincott.
19. Pelletier CR, Jordan DR, Braga R et al: Assessment of ocular trauma associated with head and neck injuries, *J Trauma* 44:350-354, 1998.
20. Zachariades N, Papavassiliou D, Christopoulos P et al: Blindness after facial trauma, *Oral Surg Oral Med Oral Pathol Oral Radiol Endod* 81:34-37, 1996.
21. Carithers JS, Koch BB: Evaluation and management of facial fractures, *Am Family Physician* 55:2675-2682, 1997.
22. Francis HW: Facial nerve emergencies. In Eisele DW, McQuone SJ, editors: *Emergencies of the head and neck,* St. Louis, 2000, Mosby, 337-365.
23. Mirvis SE, Hastings G, Scalea TM: Diagnostic imaging, angiography and interventional radiology. In Mattox KL, Feliciano DV, Moore EE, editors: *Trauma,* New York, 2000, McGraw-Hill, 261-310.
24. Manson PN, Markowitz B, Mirvis S et al: Toward CT-based facial fracture treatment, *Plast Reconstr Surg* 85:202-212, 1990.
25. Graham JR, Scott TM: Notes on the treatment of tetanus, *N Engl J Med* 235:846-852, 1946.
26. Robertson BC, Manson PN: The importance of serial debridement and "second look" procedures in high-energy ballistic and avulsive facial injuries, *Operative Tech Plast Reconstr Surg* 5:236-245, 1998.
27. Stranc MF, Robertson GA: A classification of injuries of the nasal skeleton, *Ann Plast Surg* 2:468-474, 1979.
28. Manson PN, Iliff N: Management of blow-out fractures of the orbital floor. II. Early repair for selected injuries, *Surv Ophthalmol* 35:280-292, 1991.
29. Manson PN: Facial Injuries. In McCarthy JG, editor: *Plastic surgery,* vol 2, Philadelphia, 1990, WB Saunders, 867-1141.
30. Gruss JS, Van Wyck L, Phillips JH et al: The importance of the zygomatic arch in complex midfacial fracture repair and correction of posttraumatic orbitozygomatic deformities, *Plast Reconstr Surg* 85:878-890, 1990.
31. Manson PN, Hoopes JE, Su CT: Structural pillars of the facial skeleton: an approach to the management of Le Fort fractures, *Plast Reconstr Surg* 66:54-61, 1980.

32. Shetty V, Freymiller E: Teeth in the line of fracture: a review, *J Oral Maxillofac Surg* 47:1303-1306, 1989.

33. American College of Surgeons' Committee on Trauma: *Advanced trauma life support doctors' student course manual,* ed 6, Chicago, 1997, The College.

34. Marlow TJ, Goltra DD, Schabel SI: Intracranial placement of a nasotracheal tube after facial fracture: a rare complication, *J Emerg Med* 15:187-191, 1997.

35. Robinson RJS, Mulder DS: Airway control. In Mattox KL, Feliciano DV, Moore EE, editors: *Trauma,* New York, 2000, McGraw-Hill, 171-194.

36. Komiyama M, Nishikawa M, Kan M et al: Endovascular treatment of intractable oronasal bleeding associated with severe craniofacial injury, *J Trauma* 44:330-334, 1998.

37. Magnan MA: Psychological considerations for patients with acute wounds, *Crit Care Nurs Clin North Am* 8:183-193, 1996.

38. Hayes KM, Combs NL: Perioperative nursing care of patients with craniofacial injuries, *AORN J* 64:385-406, 1996.

39. Flanigan KH: Nutritional aspects of wound healing, *Adv Wound Care* 10:48-52, 1997.

40. Bagley SM: Nutritional needs of the acutely ill with acute wounds, *Crit Care Nurs Clin North Am* 8:159-167, 1996.

41. Greene D, Raven R, Carvalho G et al: Epidemiology of facial injury in blunt assault: determinants of incidence and outcome in 802 patients, *Arch Otolaryngol Head Neck Surg* 123:923-928, 1997.

42. Clemenza JW, Kaltman SI, Diamond DL: Craniofacial trauma and cerebrospinal fluid leakage: a retrospective clinical study, *J Oral Maxillofac Surg* 53:1004-1007, 1995.

43. Bisson JI, Shepherd JP, Dhutia M: Psychological sequelae of facial trauma, *J Trauma* 43:496-500, 1997.

44. Mathog RH, Toma V, Clayman L et al: Nonunion of the mandible: an analysis of contributing factors, *J Oral Maxillofac Surg* 58:746-752, 2000.

45. Blanchaert R, Shafer DM: Surgical-orthodontic correction of adult facial deformities, *Dental Clin North Am* 40:945-959, 1996.

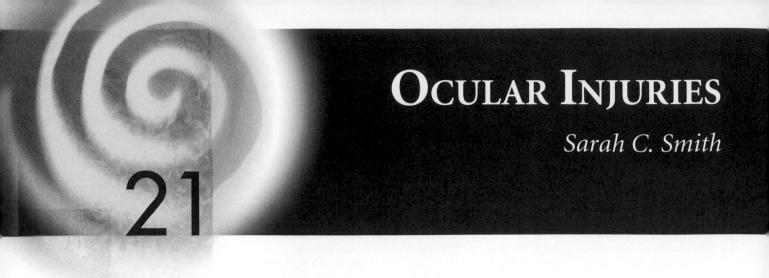

OCULAR INJURIES

Sarah C. Smith

21

The United States Eye Injury Registry (USEIR) collects, analyzes, and reports data on serious eye injuries by type and location from 38 states. Actual numbers of injuries are higher than reported because participation in the registry is voluntary at this time. The USEIR is able to quantify and qualify where, when, how, and to whom ocular injuries occur. With the long-range goal of reducing and preventing injury, this is meaningful information. As of July 1998 the USEIR database reported that motor vehicle crashes are the number one cause of bilateral injuries, but this cause represents only 9% of total eye injuries. The highest number of injuries (41%) occurs in the home. Injuries to males outpace injuries to females by at least 3:1 and up to 7:1 from infancy until age 70, when the incidence equals out. Most injuries occur in the summer; baseball and softball account for the highest number of sports-related injuries.[1,2] (Table 21-1).

The immediate goals in managing ocular injury are (1) protection of the intact portions of the visual system and avoidance of further damage to ocular structures, (2) accurate assessment of the extent of injury and referral of the patient for immediate repair of injured tissue, and (3) institution of therapeutic measures that will achieve optimal functional outcomes and maximal cosmetic results.[3,4]

Recently a standardized system for classifying mechanical ocular injuries was proposed by the Ocular Trauma Classification Group; it is endorsed by the USEIR, the American Academy of Ophthalmology, and other organizations. The system is designed to classify ocular injuries at the time of initial examination and assist caregivers in better predicting final visual outcomes. The system classifies both open globe and closed globe injuries according to four variables: type of injury, pupil function, zone of injury, and extent of injury[5] (Table 21-2).

To minimize the incidence of permanent visual loss associated with ocular trauma, it is important that those who care for patients with such injuries understand ocular anatomy and function, examination techniques, and treatment methods. With this in mind, this chapter explains anatomy and physiology of the eye, prevention of ocular injuries, ocular examination, management of a variety of traumatic eye injuries, and referral sources for patients with visual loss after trauma. Nursing care provided to the patient with ocular injury in each phase of the trauma cycle is also described. This care has a tremendous impact on the patient's entire recovery process.

ANATOMY AND PHYSIOLOGY

During embryonic development, the ocular and periocular tissues are derived from surface ectoderm, neuroectoderm, and mesoderm. The optic nerve, retina, and portions of the iris and ciliary body are all neuroectodermal structures, as are all components of the central nervous system. Important features of these structures are their inability to regenerate when damaged and their need for a continuous supply of nutrients and oxygen. If that supply is compromised for even minutes, cells will be damaged irreversibly. Injury to these neuroectodermal structures, particularly the optic nerve and retina, is primarily responsible for permanent visual loss in cases of trauma.

The conjunctiva, lens, corneal epithelium, and eyelid skin all are derived from surface ectoderm. The cells of these tissues are able to regenerate and repair themselves after injury and can survive a relatively long time without a constant supply of blood and oxygen.

Mesodermal structures include the bony orbit, extraocular muscles, sclera, corneal stroma, ocular and periocular connective tissue, blood vessels, and internal eyelid structures. These tissues are also able to regenerate to varying extents after damage.[6]

INTRAOCULAR STRUCTURES

The eye and its adnexal structures are as complex anatomically and functionally as they are in embryonic development. Light rays enter the eye through the cornea, pupil, and lens and fall on the diaphanous retina (Figure 21-1), thereby activating the retinal photoreceptor elements and the rods and cones. Rods function best in dim lighting and are responsible for night vision. Cones (of which there are three types: red, blue, and green) function best in bright illumination and are responsible for color and detailed vision. Cones

TABLE 21-1 United States Eye Injury Registry Selected Data 1988-1999

This analysis reflects USEIR's database, October 1999 (N = 10,309) and contains reports of serious eye injuries from AL, AR, CA, CT, FL, GA, HI, IA, ID, IL, IN, KS, KY, MA, MD, ME, MN, MO, MT, NC, ND, NE, NJ, NM, OH, OR, PA, RI, SC, SD, TN, TX, UT, US Military, VA, WA and WI.

Place of Injury

Home 40%
Unknown 9%
Recreation or Sport 13%
Other 12%
Work 13%
Street or Highway 13%

Source of Injury

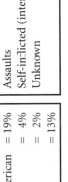

Blunt Objects 31%
Unknown 1%
Falls 4%
Fireworks 5%
Nails/Hammer on Metal 10%
BB/Pellet Guns 6%
Sharp Objects 18%
Gunshots 5%
Other 11%
Vehicle Crashes 9%

Age

Range: 0-103 years
Mean: 29 years Median: 26 years
57% were less than 30 years old

Age	Percentage	Male:Female Ratio
0-9	13%	3:1
10-19	23%	5:1
20-29	22%	5:1
30-39	18.5%	6:1
40-49	10%	5:1
50-59	6%	7:1
60-69	3.5%	4:1
≥70	4%	1:1
	100%	4:1 OVERALL

Race

Caucasian	= 61%
African American	= 19%
Hispanic	= 4%
Other	= 2%
Unknown	= 13%

Intention

Unintentional injuries	= 77%
Assaults	= 16%
Self-inflicted (intentional)	= 1%
Unknown	= 6%

When Injured

Winter	= 22%
Spring	= 27%
Summer	= 30%
Fall	= 21%

Eye Protection

None	= 78%
Regular Rx Gls	= 3%
Safety glasses	= 2%
Unknown/Other	= 17%

- Bystanders = 20% (M:F) 3:1
- Reported alcohol use when injured = 10%
- Bilateral injuries = 3.6%
- Leading source of bilateral injury = motor vehicle crash
- Open globe injuries = 42%
- Injured eye: OD = 49% OS = 51%

Work-Related Injuries = 20%

Leading reported occupation: Construction workers
Leading reported injury sources: Hammer on metal & nails

Sports Injuries = 8%

Baseball/Softball = 38%	Racquetball = 6%	Golf = 5%	
Fishing = 18%	Football = 5%	Tennis = 4%	
Basketball = 11%	Soccer = 5%	Other = 8%	

TABLE 21-2 Ocular Trauma Classification System

Open-Globe Injury Classification

Type

A. Rupture
B. Penetrating
C. Intraocular foreign body
D. Perforating
E. Mixed

Grade

Visual acuity[*]:

1. 20/40 or greater
2. 20/50-20/100
3. 19/100-5/200
4. 4/200-light perception
5. No light perception[†]

Pupil

Positive: Relative afferent pupillary defect present in affected eye
Negative: Relative afferent pupillary defect absent in affected eye

Zone

   I. Isolated to cornea (including corneoscleral limbus)
  II. Corneoscleral limbus to a point 5 mm posterior into the sclera
 III. Posterior to the anterior 5 mm of sclera

Closed-Globe Injury Classification

Type

A. Contusion
B. Lamellar laceration
C. Superficial foreign body
D. Mixed

Grade

Visual acuity[*]:

1. 20/40 or greater
2. 20/50-20/100
3. 19/100-5/200
4. 4/200-light perception
5. No light perception[†]

Pupil

Positive: Relative afferent pupillary defect present in affected eye
Negative: Relative afferent pupillary defect absent in affected eye

Zone[‡]

   I. External (limited to bulbar conjunctiva, sclera, and cornea)
  II. Anterior segment (involving structures internal to the cornea and including the posterior lens capsule; pars plicata but not pars plana)
 III. Posterior segment (all internal structures posterior to the posterior lens capsule)

Piermaici DJ, Sternberg P Jr, Aaberg TM et al: A system for classifying mechanical injuries of the eye (globe). The Ocular Trauma Classification Group, *Am J Ophthalmol* 123(6):820-831, 1997.
[*]Measured at distance (20 ft, 6 m) using Snellen chart or Rosenbaum near card with pinhole when appropriate.
[†]Confirmed with bright light source and fellow eye well occluded.
[‡]Requires B-scan ultrasonography when media opacity precludes assessment of more posterior structures.

predominate in the macula, which is the only site capable of 20/20 vision. Through complex synaptic interconnections among a variety of cell types, the rods and cones transmit the light messages they receive to the 1 million retinal ganglion cells, whose axons are gathered together at the optic disk and form the optic nerve. The optic disk (Figure 21-2) measures 1.5 mm in diameter and contains a central depression, or cup, which averages one third the disk diameter. As the axons leave the globe, they travel for approximately 1 mm through the sclera. They are then covered by dura and arachnoid while extending 25 to 30 mm through the orbit, 4 to 9 mm through the optic canal, and 10 mm intracranially before forming the optic chiasm and finally terminating deep in the brain substance.

Anterior to the retina is the vitreous, a gelatinous substance constituting two thirds of the volume of the eye. External to the retina is the choroid, a layer of vascular channels. Surrounding the choroid is the sclera, a tough connective tissue layer that both protects the internal ocular structures and acts as the structural skeleton for the globe.

Anterior to the vitreous lies the lens. This structure is approximately 9 mm in diameter and 4 mm thick. It is suspended just behind the iris by fibers that connect it to the wedge-shaped ciliary body, which consists of muscular, vascular, and epithelial elements. The ciliary body is responsible both for producing aqueous humor and for changing the shape of the lens, which becomes more biconvex for near vision and flattens for distance vision. The iris is an anterior extension of the ciliary body. This flat structure lies just anterior to the lens and contains a central round aperture, the pupil. Contraction of the iris sphincter muscle, innervated by the parasympathetic nervous system, reduces pupil diameter; contraction of the iris dilator fibers, innervated by the sympathetic nervous system, enlarges the size of the pupil. These actions control the amount of light entering the eye.

In front of the iris lies the anterior chamber, which contains the aqueous fluid produced by the ciliary body. Aqueous humor is continuously produced by the ciliary body. It moves forward through the posterior chamber and pupil into the anterior chamber, where it drains out via the trabecular meshwork and Schlemm's canal. These structures are located in the angle created by the junction of the iris, cornea, and sclera. The sclera blends into the cornea, an avascular, crystal-clear, convex disklike structure that is much like the crystal of a watch. It is covered by a layer of epithelium five to six cells thick, which can regenerate in 24 to 48 hours when scratched or abraded. The cornea becomes continuous with the epithelium of the conjunctiva, the mucous membrane that lines the posterior surface of the eyelids and the anterior portion of the sclera. Overlying the cornea is the tear film, which is composed of lacrimal, mucinous, and lipid gland secretions. These secretions are produced by the lacrimal and accessory lacrimal glands, conjunctiva goblet cells, and meibomian glands. An adequate tear film evenly distributed across the cornea and an

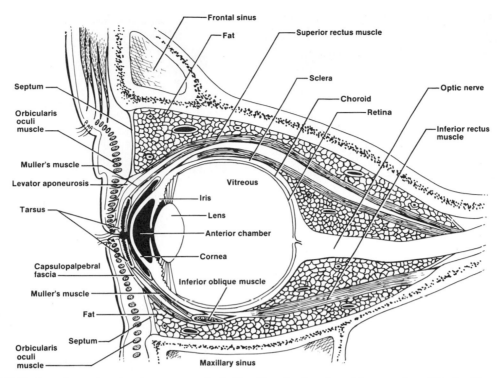

FIGURE 21-1 **Ocular and Periocular Anatomy, Including Vascular Supply and Innervation of Ocular Structures.**

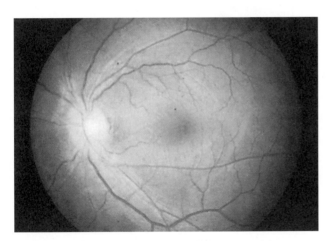

FIGURE 21-2 **Normal Ocular Fundus With Optic Disk, Retina, Macula, and Vessels.**

intact corneal epithelium are essential factors for achieving clear vision.

PERIOCULAR AND ORBITAL STRUCTURES

The eyelids cover and protect the globe. They also distribute the tear film evenly across the cornea and aid in the removal of excess tears and tear film debris. The eyelids can be divided into five layers. Most posterior is the conjunctiva. Anterior to this in the upper lid is Müller's muscle, a structure that is partially responsible for eyelid elevation. When Müller's muscle loses its sympathetic innervation, the eyelid may develop ptosis (droop). Müller's muscle is attached to the tarsus, a dense, fibrous connective tissue structure containing the meibomian glands. The superior

and inferior tarsus are the structural support elements for the upper and lower eyelids, respectively. Anterior to Müller's muscle and tarsus are the levator muscle complex in the upper eyelid. An analogous structure, the capsulopalpebral fascia, attaches to the inferior border of the tarsus in the lower eyelid. The third cranial nerve innervates the levator muscle, which is responsible for elevating the eyelid. For this reason, ptosis (Figure 21-3) may be present with third nerve paresis. Because the parasympathetic fibers to the iris sphincter muscle also travel in the third nerve, a dilated (mydriatic) pupil may be associated with third nerve paresis. Anterior to the levator muscle complex is the orbicularis muscle, a structure innervated by the seventh cranial nerve. When this nerve is paretic, as in Bell's palsy (Figure 21-4), the eyelids cannot close, resulting in tear film evaporation and corneal epithelial damage. If this is not treated vigorously, the cornea can perforate. Skin is the final structure covering the eyelid. A component of the eyelid that cannot be overlooked is the orbital septum, which is a continuation of the periosteum covering the bony orbit. This structure extends from the orbital rim and attaches to either the levator muscle complex or the capsulopalpebral fascia and represents the boundary between the orbital and periorbital structures. Violation of this protective barrier exposes the orbital contents to external forces, specifically infectious agents. Infection can easily involve the entire orbit, causing subsequent visual loss and possible intracranial spread, resulting in meningitis and abscess formation.

The globe lies within the bony orbit, which consists of the maxillary, lacrimal, ethmoid, greater and lesser sphenoid, frontal, palatine, and zygomatic bones. These bones are

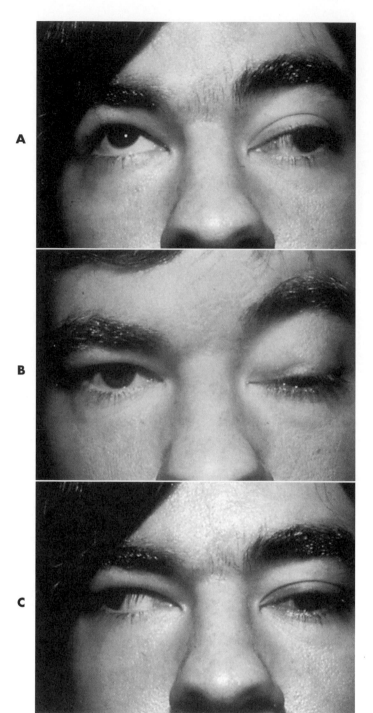

FIGURE 21-3 **Ptosis Associated With Left Third Nerve Paresis.**
A, Upgaze. B, Primary gaze. C, Right gaze.

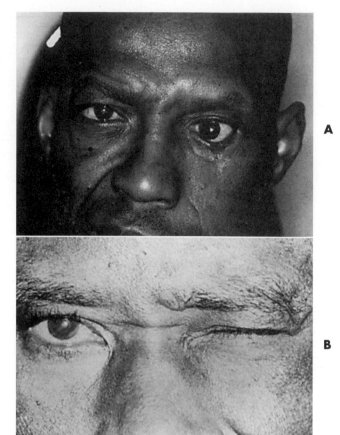

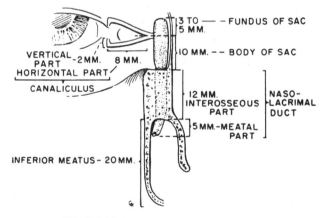

FIGURE 21-4 **A,** Left-sided Bell's palsy causing facial paralysis and lower eyelid sag. **B,** Right-sided Bell's palsy causing inability to close right eye.

FIGURE 21-5 **Lacrimal Drainage System.**

joined to form a quadrilateral pyramid with its apex placed posteriorly. The anterior opening of the adult orbit measures approximately 35 mm in height and 40 mm in width. The orbit is 40 to 45 mm deep. Superior to the orbit are the frontal sinus anteriorly and the anterior cranial fossa posteriorly. Medial to the orbit are the ethmoid and sphenoid sinuses and the nasal cavity. Inferiorly is the maxillary sinus. Laterally are the temporalis fossa anteriorly and the middle cranial fossa, temporal fossa, and pterygopalatine fossa posteriorly. Posterior to the orbital apex are the clinoid processes, pituitary, cavernous sinus, carotid arteries, middle cranial fossa, and optic chiasm. Because the globe and orbit are close to many important nonocular structures, serious ocular injury is often seen concomitantly with serious nonocular injury.

In addition to many other structures, the orbit contains the extraocular muscles that are responsible for coordinated eye movements. Disruption of the third, fourth, or sixth cranial nerves that innervate the extraocular muscles may result in various abnormal alignments of the eyes.

Tear secretions exit through the lacrimal drainage system (Figure 21-5). Any damage to this system may result in epiphora (excessive tearing) and infection. Puncta (orifices leading to the lacrimal drainage system) are present in the upper and lower eyelids. These lead to the canaliculi, which connect to the lacrimal sac. This latter structure lies within the lacrimal fossa and beneath the medial canthal tendon. Tear secretions flow from the lacrimal sac into the bony nasolacrimal duct within the maxillary bone before entering the nose under the inferior meatus approximately 4 cm from the nasal vestibule.

The arterial supply to the globe and orbit is derived almost entirely from the ophthalmic artery and its branches. This vessel is the first branch from the internal carotid artery after it enters the cranial cavity. This important factor explains the tendency for emboli flowing through the internal carotid artery to enter the ophthalmic artery, resulting in visual symptoms and deficits. The facial and maxillary arteries, which are branches of the external carotid artery, provide additional blood supply to the lower eyelid, medial canthus, and inferior orbit. The venous drainage of the eye and orbit occurs via the inferior and superior ophthalmic veins to the cavernous sinus. This is an important route for the intracranial spread of infection. There are no lymphatics within the orbit. However, the eyelids have a rich lymphatic system draining into the preauricular and submaxillary nodes.

Sensory innervation to the ocular structures is provided by the fifth cranial (trigeminal) nerve. The ophthalmic division of this nerve supplies the forehead, upper eyelid, nose, and cornea. The maxillary division of the fifth cranial nerve supplies the lower eyelid, cheek, medial aspect of the nose, upper lip, gums, and lateral forehead. Portions of this nerve travel beneath the orbital floor. This explains the loss of sensation involving the cheek, lips, and gums after inferior orbital rim and floor fractures.

PREVENTION

Prevention of ocular injuries is as important as their management. Use of protective eyewear, safety helmets, and seat belts and avoidance of driving while intoxicated prevent much serious facial and ocular trauma.[7] Recent literature points to air bags as possible culprits of ocular injury. Although there are reported injuries from air bag deployment, they protect rather than harm the eyes in the vast majority of cases.[8] The likelihood of sustaining an ocular injury increases 256% in cars without a deploying airbag.[9,10]

Safety glasses are essential for certain athletic and occupational activities.[11] Neither regular glasses nor contact lenses alone provide adequate protection for environments involving projectile objects, chemicals, particulate matter, intense heat, or radiation energy. Ocular protection ranges from full-face protection (wire mesh, polycarbonate, or both) attached to a helmet for sports such as football and hockey to one-piece molded eye protectors with polycarbonate lenses backed by a posterior lip that is part of the molded front for use in racquet sports. Protective requirements for specific sports have been defined by the American Society of Testing Materials (ASTM), the American National Standards Institute (ANSI), the Canadian Standards Association (CSA), and the British Standards Institution (BSI).[11]

A variety of ocular safety protectors are available for occupational uses, depending on the job requirements. The ANSI Z87.1-1979 Standard Practice for Occupational and Educational Eye and Face Protection defines three types of safety spectacles: Style A has no side shields; style B has orbital-fitting cup-type side shields of wire mesh or perforated or nonperforated plastic; and style C has semi- or flat-fold plastic side shields. All have polycarbonate or CR-39 lenses. Style B glasses provide the best protection against hazardous material coming from all angles. Additional protection is required for specific occupations involving radiation and light (welding goggles) or chemical splashes and dust (eye cups or rigid-cover goggles). Polycarbonate goggles are very useful when a spectacle correction is required. These protectors fit over spectacles and are convenient for use at home and on the job.[7]

When vision is 20/200 or less in one eye with the best spectacle correction, or when unilateral anophthalmos is present, a person is considered to have monocular sight. These individuals should not wear contact lenses even when engaging in recreational activities because no protection is afforded their only sighted eye. It must be emphasized that in such cases polycarbonate lenses provide the best ocular protection and should be used at all times during both leisure and occupational activities. In addition, these individuals cannot be employed in occupations requiring stereopsis or binocular vision (e.g., airline pilots, police officers). They also may have restrictions on their driving licenses, such as requiring bilateral outside mirrors or, for people in whom the better eye also has a visual deficit, being limited to daytime driving only. The motor vehicle administration of each state should be consulted for specific restrictions.

TRAUMA MANAGEMENT

When managing a trauma patient, it is essential to set priorities for the treatment of injuries. Establishing an airway, breathing, and circulation are the management priorities during resuscitation; however, this prioritization of interventions may have implications for treating ocular trauma. Examining, diagnosing, and treating ocular trauma may need to be delayed until emergency and life-threatening injuries are treated and the patient has been adequately stabilized to allow further evaluation.[12] The priorities established for treating each trauma patient require individualization based on the nature and severity of each injury.

Trauma patients may not be capable of assisting in an examination. Administration of paralytic agents, heavy sedation or anesthesia, intubation (which compromises communication), confusion, disorientation or combativeness secondary to a brain injury, hypoxia, or hemodynamic instability are some of the variables inhibiting assistance by a patient. Physical examination in such instances may be limited or incomplete. Repeated examinations may be required before complete knowledge of any ocular pathology is possible.

Assessment

The ocular trauma examination begins with an ocular history. Patient-reported symptoms of vision loss or blurred vision that does not improve with blinking, double vision, sectorial visual loss (Figure 21-6), or ocular pain are important findings and require immediate referral to an ophthalmologist. The mechanism of injury and course of events, symptoms, and any therapeutic interventions provided must be determined. It is important to ascertain whether ocular disease or visual loss was present before the traumatic event and whether the patient is currently receiving any chronic ocular therapy that needs to be continued. When the patient cannot provide an accurate history, it may be necessary to obtain an ocular history from other sources, when available, such as family, friends, or personal ophthalmologist.

A few simple instruments are required to examine the patient with ocular trauma. A near-vision chart and pinhole occluder are useful in assessing visual acuity. A penlight with a cobalt blue filter, tonometer, Hertel exophthalmometer, and ophthalmoscope will help in other parts of the examination. A slit-lamp biomicroscope, if accessible, will greatly aid in the evaluation of the conjunctiva, cornea, anterior chamber, iris, lens, and anterior vitreous cavity. Topical anesthetic agents such as tetracaine or proparacaine will help in examining patients who are unable to open their eyes because of corneal abrasions or erosions. A lid retractor or bent paper clip retractors (Figure 21-7) may be required for patients with corneal injury or for evaluating infants. Sodium fluorescein test strips are needed to evaluate the extent of corneal epithelial loss. These are used with a cobalt blue filter covering a penlight. Short-acting dilating drops such as 2.5% phenylephrine or 1% tropicamide, both of which have a duration of action lasting 3 to 6 hours, are essential for an adequate examination of the ocular fundus in patients with ocular trauma. However, these agents prevent evaluation of the pupils and must be either avoided or used with great caution in any patient with intracranial trauma. Finally, it is important to have the name and phone number of an easily accessible and available ophthalmologist for emergency consultation and management.

VISUAL ACUITY. The most essential aspect of the ocular examination is determination of visual acuity. This is preferably performed with the patient using his or her spectacle correction for distance and near acuity. If a patient does not have spectacle correction or if there is a question

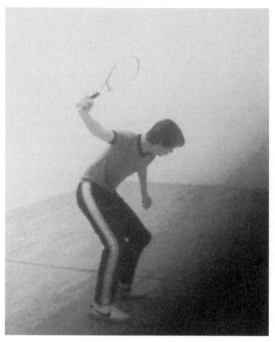

FIGURE 21-6 **Sectorial Vision.** (From American Academy of Ophthalmology: *The athlete's eye*, San Francisco, 1984, The Academy.)

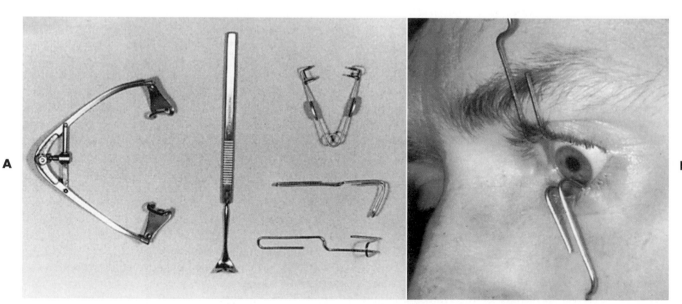

FIGURE 21-7 **A,** Eyelid retractors. **B,** Paper clip retractors.

concerning the adequacy of a particular correction, a pinhole occluder allows the measurement of visual acuity to within one or two lines of the patient's expected best corrected vision. In a presbyopic patient who does not have a spectacle correction available, a loose +2.50 spherical lens can be used to aid near vision. (Presbyopia is the age-related reduced ability to focus on near objects, which requires reading glasses or a bifocal lens). If a standardized distance or near visual acuity chart is not available, a newspaper or some other printed material can be used. Visual acuity can then be recorded as the size of print (large, medium, or small) the patient sees at a specified distance, usually 14 inches. If the patient is a child or is unable to read, a picture chart such as an Allen chart or the E game (determination of which way the letter E points at specific distances) can be used. If the patient is unable to see any of these, the ability to count fingers or ascertain hand motions at a specific distance is determined. If the patient performs inadequately on the visual acuity tests, the ability to perceive light with or without the ability to determine the direction from which the light is projecting must be ascertained. If no light perception is present, this is recorded as NLP. Vision is always measured for each eye separately, with the opposite eye covered. In general, any patient with a best corrected visual acuity of 20/40 or worse needs to be evaluated by an ophthalmologist.

PUPILS.   The next aspect of the visual examination is evaluation of the pupils. First, the patient is asked to look at a distant object. This prevents the pupillary constriction that normally occurs when viewing a near object. Second, the pupil is observed for size and shape bilaterally in a moderately lit room. The patient's pupils should be similar in size, round, and equally reactive to light and accommodation (PERRLA). Approximately 20% to 25% of people naturally have unequal pupil size, but this variation normally does not exceed 1 mm. Third, the pupil's reaction to light stimuli is noted. The pupillary light reflex evaluates the optic nerve, which must be intact to perceive the light, and the oculomotor nerve integrity, which allows the pupil to constrict. To evaluate this reflex the examiner should stand in front of the patient. The patient is asked to look at a distant object while the examiner shines the light into one eye, moving the light from the side onto the eye so that the pupillary reaction can be observed. Constriction of the pupil should occur within 1 second after presentation of the light stimulus. This is repeated for the other eye to evaluate each pupil's response to direct light stimulus. Fourth, one eye is examined while shining the light onto the opposite eye. The examiner should see constriction in the observed eye while shining a light in the opposite eye. This is called the *consensual response*. Normally the pupils are linked together in response to light stimulus, each constricting an equal amount to the stimulus. If both oculomotor nerves and one optic nerve are intact and the opposite optic nerve is damaged, the pupils both constrict equally when a light stimulus is presented to the intact side. When the light is presented to the damaged optic nerve, the stimulus will not be perceived, and the pupils will not constrict.

Last, the response to the "swinging flashlight" test is observed. In a dimly lit room, light is shined on one eye for 3 seconds. The light is then quickly moved in a swinging motion across the bridge of the nose and into the opposite eye while pupil response is noted. In patients without visual pathway disturbances and normal iris function, the eye will not constrict or dilate to the swinging light. This is because direct and consensual responses are equal in the normal patient. The opposite eye is then tested. If the swinging flashlight produces dilation in the second eye, the eye has a relative afferent pupillary defect, sometimes known as a Marcus Gunn pupil. The eye exhibiting dilation upon direct light stimulation is said to have the defect. In trauma patients, if the retina or optic nerve back to the chiasm is damaged or the eye is filled with blood so that less light is perceived, the pupil on that side will paradoxically dilate.

Unequal or nonreactive pupils can be seen in many different conditions besides ocular trauma, including brain lesions affecting the midbrain, optic nerve or oculomotor nerve, acute glaucoma, interruption of the pupillary sympathetic innervation, and previous eye surgery. Trauma patients with pupil abnormalities should be seen by a neurosurgeon to rule out brain injury. If pupil abnormalities are noted in a patient with an otherwise normal neurologic exam and trauma to the eye, ocular injury is a suspected cause for pupil dysfunction and an ophthalmologist should be consulted.

OCULAR MOTILITY.   Evaluation of ocular motility is the next step in the examination process. The patient is asked to fixate on a penlight, which is moved to the right, left, up, and down. The eyes are linked in tandem and should move an equal amount at the same speed in each gaze direction. There are nine cardinal gaze positions: straight ahead, directly up, up and to the right, directly lateral, lateral and down, directly down, down and laterally left, directly left, and up and to the left. However, in most clinical situations, measuring straight ahead, directly up, left, right, and down provides enough information to assess for the presence of a deviation. In an unconscious patient with an uninjured cervical spine, the "doll's eye" maneuver, or oculocephalic reflex can be tested to evaluate ocular motility. Rapid, passive side-to-side head turning is performed; the normal oculocephalic response is movement of the eyes in the direction opposite the head movement. When there is a suspicion that a restrictive component is contributing to impaired ocular motility, as in cases of orbital floor fractures, forced duction testing needs to be performed (Figure 21-8). This involves anesthetizing the eye with topical anesthesia, grasping the limbal conjunctiva and sclera with toothed forceps, and rotating the globe up and down to test the vertical rectus muscles and right and left to test the horizontal rectus muscles while noting any restriction to free movement of the globe. Common causes of abnormal ocular movements include orbital edema; extraocular muscle

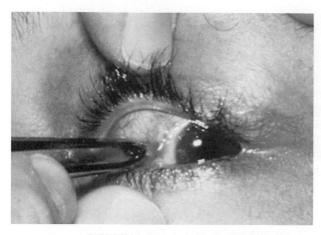

FIGURE 21-8 **Forced Duction.**

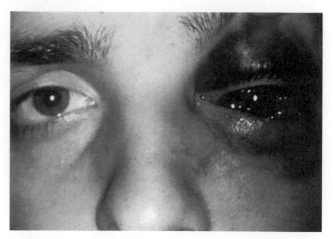

FIGURE 21-10 **Acute Orbital Fracture With Periorbital Edema, Ecchymosis, and Hypoophthalmos.** (From American Academy of Ophthalmology: *The athlete's eye,* San Francisco, 1984, The Academy.)

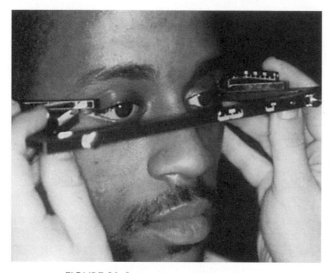

FIGURE 21-9 **Hertel Exophthalmometry.**

entrapment; and damage to cranial nerves III, IV, or VI. Any patient with a disturbance of ocular motility requires a thorough evaluation by an ophthalmologist.

ORBIT. As part of the ophthalmic examination, it is important to assess the periorbital and orbital structures and the relationship of the globe to these structures. Evaluating the position of the globe within the orbit and comparing the ocular structures of both eyes are important to diagnose such conditions as orbital fractures, the presence of foreign bodies, retrobulbar hemorrhage, and orbital cellulitis or abscess. Normally a comparison of the two globes by Hertel exophthalmometry (Figure 21-9) shows less than a 2-mm difference between opposite sides in the distance from the lateral orbital rim to the corneal apex. The normal measurement for this distance is approximately 17 to 20 mm. When the difference is 2 mm or greater and the globe is pushed out of the orbit (exophthalmos), orbital edema, a retained foreign body, retrobulbar hemorrhage, orbital abscess or cellulitis, dysthyroid ophthalmopathy, or an orbital tumor should be considered. When the difference is 2 mm or

greater and the globe is sunken back into the orbit (enophthalmos), orbital fractures must be considered. If a straight edge is held horizontally to bisect the pupil, the center of each pupil should be on the same horizontal plane. When one eye is lower than the other, an orbital floor fracture may be present (Figure 21-10). The horizontal distance from the medial canthus to the middle of the nasal bones is approximately 16 mm. When this is widened or when there is inequality between opposite sides, telecanthus (a wider than normal distance between the eyes) associated with a midfacial fracture may be present. The orbital rim should be smooth, without any breaks or irregularities that might indicate an orbital rim fracture. Crepitus on palpation of the eyelids is another sign associated with fractures of the orbital bones. Periorbital edema and ecchymosis commonly accompany many types of orbital, head, and facial trauma and, although not specific signs, do indicate the possibility of severe ocular injury. Where there is the possibility of orbital fracture, retrobulbar hemorrhage, or orbital infection or foreign bodies, an ophthalmologist should be consulted to fully evaluate and appropriately manage the patient.

INTRAOCULAR PRESSURE. Assessment of intraocular pressure is another important aspect of the examination following ocular trauma. This should not be performed when there is any question concerning the integrity of the globe because any pressure on a perforated eye could result in extrusion of the ocular contents and permanent loss of vision. To measure intraocular pressure, a topical anesthetic is instilled into the ocular cul-de-sacs. A Schiøtz tonometer with a 5.5-g weight is used to measure the pressure. To do this the patient's head is placed so that the face is toward the ceiling. The patient is asked to look straight up, and the footplate of the tonometer is placed on the central portion of the cornea. The scale value indicated by the tonometer needle is read and then translated into the appropriate intraocular pressure reading using a special table. Normal

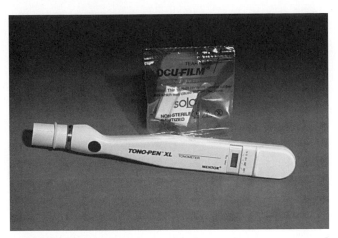

FIGURE 21-11 **Tono-pen.** (Courtesy University of Iowa Health Care, Department of Ophthalmology & Visual Sciences, Iowa City, Iowa.)

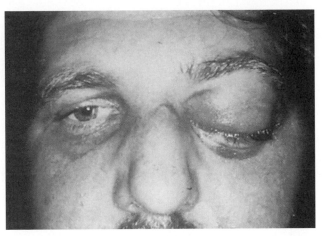

FIGURE 21-12 **Traumatic Ptosis.**

intraocular pressure is 10 to 22 mm Hg. Alternately, a Tono-pen may be used to measure intraocular pressure. With the patient looking straight ahead, the tip of the Tono-pen is lightly bounced on the center of the cornea, perpendicular to the face (Figure 21-11).

Patients with high intraocular pressure (>30 mm Hg) may have angle closure glaucoma, pupillary block glaucoma, or a retrobulbar hemorrhage. Urgent treatment is needed to lower elevated pressure and prevent permanent loss of vision caused by optic nerve damage. Patients with low intraocular pressure (<10 mm Hg) may have a perforated globe or severe intraocular trauma and may require immediate evaluation by an ophthalmologist.

EYELIDS. The eyelids protect the globe, remove excess tear secretions and debris, and facilitate complete and adequate corneal wetting. They are frequently injured when ocular trauma occurs. Ptosis (Figure 21-12) often accompanies periorbital edema and ecchymosis. Ptosis may also result from direct damage to the levator complex or Müller capsule or may be seen with enophthalmos associated with an orbital fracture. Inability to adequately close the eyelids is a more serious problem associated with damage to the seventh cranial nerve. It also may be seen with scarring after repair of eyelid lacerations. Decreased corneal sensation from damage to the fifth cranial nerve can result in a weak or absent corneal reflex and inadequate surfacing of the pericorneal tear film. Misdirected lashes can result in severe corneal damage. Patients with conditions that result in damage to the cornea, such as those caused by an inability to close the eye, inadequate blinking, poor corneal wetting, or misdirected lashes, need immediate referral to an ophthalmologist to prevent visual loss.

Lacerations of the eyelids are usually deep and may have concomitant prolapse of orbital fat. These injuries require a thorough ocular evaluation to eliminate the possibility of severe injury to the globe (Figure 21-13). When lacerations involve the eyelid margin or canalicular system or when they are deep or complicated, repair by an experienced ophthal-

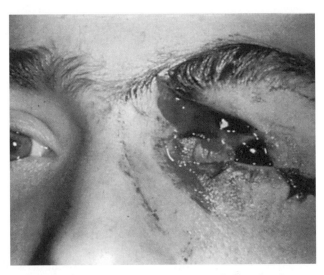

FIGURE 21-13 **Severe Eyelid Laceration With Associated Penetrating Trauma to Globe.** (From American Academy of Ophthalmology: *Eye trauma and emergencies,* San Francisco, 1985, The Academy.)

mologist is essential to prevent permanent functional and cosmetic deficits.

CONJUNCTIVA. Examination of the conjunctiva, tear film, cornea, anterior chamber, iris, lens, and anterior vitreous cavity is best performed with a slit-lamp biomicroscope. Because this instrument is usually available only to ophthalmologists, a penlight can be used. The eyelids must be everted (a cotton-tipped applicator facilitates this maneuver) to examine their conjunctival surface thoroughly for foreign bodies or embedded material. It is also important to examine the anterior conjunctiva for injection, lacerations, foreign bodies, chemosis (edema of the conjunctiva), or hemorrhage. The presence of any of these signs may indicate a perforated globe. In addition, conjunctival injection is often present after trauma that causes ocular inflammation and in cases of infectious and noninfectious conjunctivitis, corneal abrasions, and acute glaucoma. Perilimbal (the area where cornea and sclera blend together) dilated blood

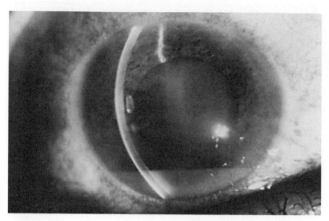

FIGURE 21-14 **Hyphema Involving 15% of the Inferior Anterior Chamber.**

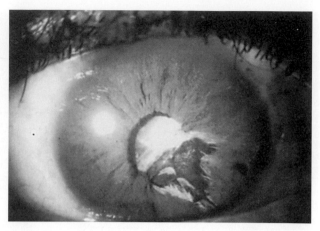

FIGURE 21-15 **Traumatic Pupillary Irregularities With Posterior Synechiae and Cataract Formation.**

vessels often associated with proptosis can be a manifestation of a posttraumatic intracranial arteriovenous fistula. If there is any uncertainty regarding ocular integrity or the presence of severe ocular injury, an ophthalmologist should be consulted.

CORNEA. Normally the cornea is crystal clear and glistening. A penlight can easily demonstrate corneal lacerations, foreign bodies, abrasions, and irregularities. Instillation of sodium fluorescein, which stains areas denuded of epithelium, and use of a cobalt blue filter over a penlight will facilitate evaluation of the cornea. A cloudy cornea may indicate acute glaucoma, edema from trauma, a foreign body in the anterior chamber, or an infectious process. Many cases of conjunctivitis, corneal foreign bodies, and abrasion can be safely managed without an ophthalmologist, but if there is any uncertainty about the seriousness of the disease process, an ophthalmologist should be consulted.

ANTERIOR CHAMBER. On penlight examination the anterior chamber should be clear and deep, with the iris well separated from the posterior corneal surface. When blood (hyphema) (Figure 21-14) or white cells (hypopyon) are present, serious ocular injury, inflammation, or infection has occurred, and immediate ophthalmologic consultation is required. Shallowing of the anterior chamber can be demonstrated by shining the beam from a penlight across the chamber from the temporal side of the globe. The beam should highlight the entire chamber without impediment. When the chamber is shallowed, the beam will fall on the iris, creating shadows, and will not illuminate the chamber. Acute angle closure glaucoma is a consideration in such cases, especially if there is an associated rise in intraocular pressure; clouding of the cornea; complaints of visual loss, halos around objects, eye pain, or nausea; or vomiting. Urgent ophthalmic consultation is needed if these symptoms are present.

IRIS. Examination of the iris in cases of ocular trauma may reveal tears and holes. These may cause pupillary irregularities (Figure 21-15) or, more importantly, may be associated with hyphema (from damage to iris blood vessels) (see Figure 21-14) or chronic glaucoma (from damage to the trabecular meshwork and aqueous drainage system). Iris tears and hyphema can be associated with penetrating foreign bodies. When tears are seen, the globe is considered perforated, and immediate evaluation by an ophthalmologist is required. Sometimes small foreign bodies will be embedded on the iris surface or may bounce off the iris and fall into the anterior chamber angle. Small, colored foreign bodies may be confused with small, pigmented nevi, which are normally present on the surface of the iris.

LENS. The normal lens is a crystalline structure. It is not uncommon for the lens to develop opacities and become cataractous after ocular trauma. These defects are often visible on penlight examination. If severe inflammation is associated with ocular injury, adhesions (posterior synechiae) (see Figure 21-15) between the iris and the lens may develop. These may lead to an elevation of intraocular pressure and subsequent optic nerve damage. When a force of sufficient intensity is delivered to the globe, the lens can be torn from its moorings to the ciliary body. In some cases the lens may be dislocated to float free in the vitreous or settle on the retina. Rarely, it may become positioned in the anterior chamber, blocking aqueous outflow and resulting in acute glaucoma. Proper evaluation and management of these serious conditions require prompt ophthalmic consultation. In many situations the cataractous lens can be removed and replaced with an artificial lens (intraocular lens [IOL]) at the time of injury repair or as a secondary procedure weeks to months later.

FUNDUS. The fundus examination is the final aspect of the ocular evaluation. Normally the vitreous is a clear structure that allows an unimpeded view of the retina. Hemorrhage (Figure 21-16A) within the vitreous occasionally occurs in association with intracranial hemorrhage. It also may occur when a retinal vessel is torn and may indicate

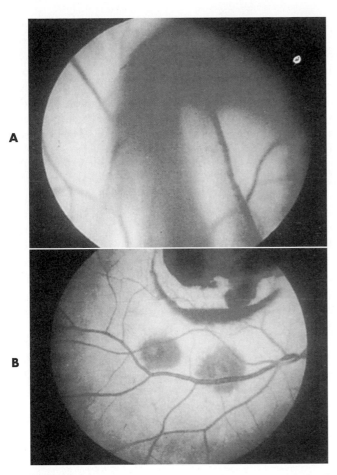

A

B

FIGURE 21-16 A, Vitreous hemorrhage. B, Traumatic intraretinal and periretinal hemorrhages.

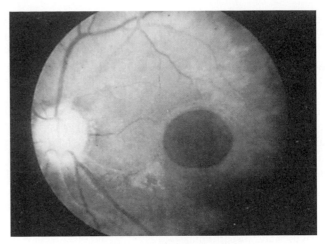

FIGURE 21-17 **Macular Hole.**

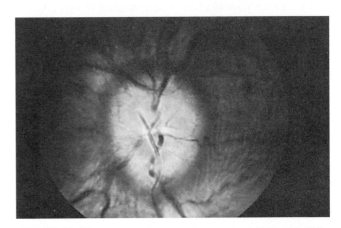

FIGURE 21-18 **Edema of the Optic Nerve Head (Disk Edema).**

damage from a penetrating foreign body or a retinal detachment. The normal retina is thin, relatively clear, and colorless. The orange color imparted to it on fundus examination is caused by to the underlying retinal pigment epithelium and vascular choroid. Retinal edema (Berlin's edema, commotio retinae) is common after blunt ocular trauma. In such cases the retina appears milky white and a pseudo-cherry red spot may be present. Although this condition usually subsides spontaneously, resulting in a return of vision, some patients with macular involvement (Figure 21-17) suffer permanent loss of the central visual field. Traumatic hemorrhages (Figure 21-16B) can occur on, within, or beneath the retina or choroid when the retinal or choroidal vessels are damaged. These may be associated with retinal tears and holes, retinal detachment, and choroidal layer ruptures. Hard exudates also may be associated with retinal trauma. Proliferation of glial tissue may cause neovascular fronds (abnormal new blood vessels) to occur after retinal trauma, resulting in retinal detachment or hemorrhage. Choroidal layer ruptures are another posttraumatic cause of visual loss and fibrovascular proliferation. All these pathologic processes can cause severe and in many cases permanent visual loss and therefore necessitate careful ophthalmologic evaluation.

OPTIC NERVE.   The optic nerve head usually appears somewhat yellow, with sharply defined margins, when an ophthalmoscopic exam is performed. Its central cup constitutes approximately one third of its substance and has a single branching central retinal artery and vein. Blurring of the disk margin caused by edema of the nerve fibers is seen with an increase in intracranial pressure (papilledema) or pressure on the optic nerve (disk edema) (Figure 21-18). Atrophy of the optic nerve after contusion or transsection injuries results in a loss of disk substance and a whitening of the nerve head.

DIAGNOSTIC STUDIES

In addition to the ophthalmic examination, several other modalities can further aid in the evaluation of the eye and its adnexal structures after trauma. Computed tomography (CT) scanning (Figure 21-19) and magnetic resonance imaging (MRI) are essential to delineate completely the extent of orbital and optic canal fractures and to identify and locate intraocular and orbital foreign bodies. If foreign bodies are metallic, MRI is contraindicated. Coronal and anteroposterior cuts of 3 mm thickness overlapped by 2 mm are required to obtain the most complete data concerning both the exact location of a foreign body and the extent of any orbital fractures. Thinner sections of 1.5 mm are needed to evaluate the optic canal and foreign bodies within the globe itself. Formal visual field examination with Goldmann or Humphrey perimetry is essential for delineating damage to the optic nerve, chiasm, and tract. This provides additional important localizing information about intracranial pathology. Orbital and intraocular ultrasonography greatly aids in the evaluation of retinal and choroidal detachments, intraocular and intraorbital foreign bodies, vitreous hemorrhage, dislocation of the lens, and lacerations of the globe. It can be performed at the bedside and is advantageous to use when an unstable patient cannot be moved or when the eye cannot be fully examined because of anterior segment opacities and disruption.

PREHOSPITAL MANAGEMENT

Prehospital management of ocular trauma is very limited. The most important aspect is the protection of an injured eye, which is achieved by shielding it (Figure 21-20). To decrease anxiety, it must be explained to the patient why this is being done. No ocular medicine should be given during this phase except in cases of chemical injury, when immediate, in-the-field irrigation must be performed, or with severe facial burns, when the eyes must be lubricated vigorously with artificial tear ointments. It is best to keep the patient quiet and still. If any active bleeding is noted, a dressing can be applied; however, any pressure to the eye itself needs to be avoided.

The introduction of acidic or alkaline substances into the eye constitutes a medical emergency requiring attention within minutes of injury. Chemical injuries can occur at home (e.g., oven cleaners), at schools (e.g., chemicals from chemistry laboratories), or in the workplace (e.g., industrial toxins). Chemical and thermal burns of the eye are less common than those of the eyelids because the protective blink response shields the eye with the eyelids. In cases of chemical injury the eye should be irrigated immediately with water or saline for at least 15 to 20 minutes. A loose, moist saline dressing can be applied until the patient arrives at a hospital if irrigation is not possible at the scene because of other life-threatening injuries.

RESUSCITATION

When ocular trauma occurs in conjunction with other injuries, management needs to be prioritized. The treatment of an ocular injury may be delayed until more serious, life-threatening injuries are addressed and the patient is stabilized. During this period a shield should be maintained over any eye suspected of having sustained injury (see Figure 21-20). Immediate ophthalmologic consultation should be obtained as soon as possible when any ocular injury is suspected.

When managing a patient's nonocular injuries, it is essential to remember that if there is any suspicion that a globe may be perforated, the eyelids, ocular adnexa, orbit, and facial structures must not be manipulated in any way. In some cases it may be necessary to immobilize the head and administer pain medication and sedation while awaiting ophthalmologic consultation. Periorbital lacerations must

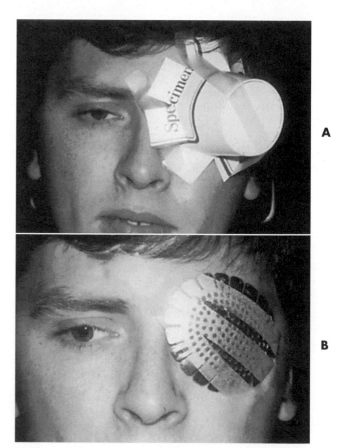

FIGURE 21-20 **A**, Cup shield. **B**, Metal shield.

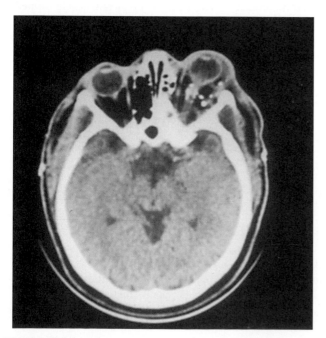

FIGURE 21-19 **CT Scan of Bullet Fragments in Orbit and Around Optic Nerve.**

not be sutured and orbital fractures must not be palpated until the perforating ocular injuries are repaired. Generally, bleeding associated with eyelid lacerations and penetrating orbital trauma is minimal and will stop spontaneously. Pressure should never be put on the eyelids, eyeball, or periorbit to stop bleeding if there is any suspicion that the globe is not intact. Any increased pressure on an open eye may result in loss of the intraocular contents and irreparable damage to the eye (Figure 21-21).

Access to a variety of items is necessary for the successful treatment of ocular injury before ophthalmologic consultation. At least 2 L of normal saline are needed for irrigation after chemical injuries. Intravenous (IV) acetazolamide (Diamox) and mannitol, 0.5% timolol maleate and 2% pilocarpine eye drops, and either 50% oral glycerin or 45% isosorbide are needed for pressure reduction in cases of acute glaucoma. A short-acting mydriatic/cycloplegic, such as 1% tropicamide, 1% cyclopentolate hydrochloride, or 5% homatropine hydrobromide, and antibiotic eye drops, such as ofloxacin, tobramycin, sulfacetamide sodium, or ciprofloxacin, are needed to treat corneal abrasions and bacterial conjunctivitis. A long-acting mydriatic and cycloplegic such as 0.25% scopolamine or 1% atropine sulfate and topical steroid drops (1% prednisolone acetate) are needed to treat severe intraocular inflammations. Artificial teardrops and ointments are essential for managing patients with inadequate blinking or poor eyelid closure. Eye pads and tape are needed to treat corneal abrasions.

Anesthetic ointments should never be used in cases of eye trauma because their prolonged effect may result in inadvertent self-mutilation. For a similar reason, anesthetic drops should not be used on a long-term basis or prescribed for patient use after discharge. Ocular ointments of any type should not be used when examination of the fundus is necessary (they obscure visualization of the fundus) or when

penetrating ocular trauma is present (they may enter the globe). In rare cases of eyelid avulsion or severe thermal injury, it may be necessary to apply artificial tear ointment to the cornea to protect it. Corticosteroid eye drops should never be used if there are any diagnostic uncertainties or if infection with herpes simplex virus or any fungus is a possibility because they can elevate intraocular pressure and mask preexisting infection. Atropine eye drops are not for routine use. Atropine's mydriatic effect is too long lasting, and it can cause chemical and allergic reactions.

Acute management of ocular injuries also requires extensive emotional support. If there is any visual impairment (secondary to either patching or injury), the patient must be assured that the injury is being assessed thoroughly and treated appropriately and expertly. Explanation of what has happened and what is being done for the patient is essential to help alleviate fears of the unknown.

MANAGEMENT OF SPECIFIC OCULAR INJURIES

CHEMICAL INJURY. Chemical injuries are treated by immediate and copious irrigation of the eye with the most readily available source of water. The longer the period between injury and lavage, the worse the prognosis. The lids must be held apart so that the injured globe can be irrigated copiously (Figure 21-22). A cloth will help in holding the eyelids apart. In addition to the brief ocular irrigation performed in the prehospital setting, lavage should be continued in the emergency center until the pH of the tear film in the cul-de-sac is neutral (approximately 7.0). An intravenous infusion set for irrigation, eyelid retractors to hold the eyelids apart, and topical anesthetic drops to reduce the blepharospasm caused by corneal damage will all greatly help in carrying out adequate lavage. The eyelids need to be everted to ensure removal of any particulate matter clinging to the conjunctiva.

After lavage a cycloplegic/mydriatic such as 0.25% scopolamine or 1% atropine should be instilled to reduce pain from ciliary spasm and to prevent synechiae (Table 21-3).

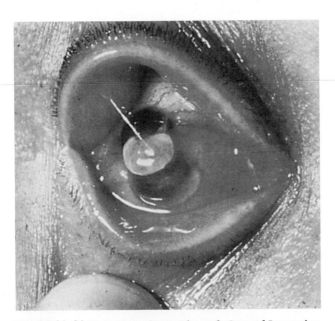

FIGURE 21-21 **Extrusion of Lens Through Corneal Laceration.**

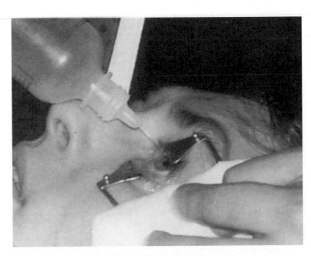

FIGURE 21-22 **Ocular Lavage.**

TABLE 21-3   Eyedrop Instillation Procedure

Overview

Ophthalmic medications may be used as:

1. Diagnostic agents.
2. Treatment agents of ocular conditions.
3. Adjuncts to surgical interventions.

Ointments are used for their lubricant property and to increase contact time of medication to the ocular surface. Ointments tend to blur the vision when first applied and therefore are often used at bedtime.

Objective

To deliver medication to the eye by way of ophthalmic drops or ointments.

Equipment

Eye drops or ointment as ordered
Tissue

Action	Rationale
1. Check physician's order.	1. Note correct medication, time, eye, and patient; and expiration date on label.
2. Wash hands.	2. Good hygiene.
3. Explain procedure to patient.	3. Patient cooperation.
4. Have patient in sitting or supine position.	4. Patient comfort and ease in instilling drops.
5. Instruct patient to tilt head backward, if in sitting position, open eyes and look up.	5. Reduces blepharospasm.

6. Pull down on the lower lid to expose the cul-de-sac.
   a. For infants and small children, separate lids by placing thumb on bony prominence below lid, and index finger on bony prominence above lid. Gently pull lids apart. Do not apply pressure on eye.
	6.
	   a. For infants and small children, if it is contraindicated or difficult to separate the lids, place the drop of medication in the inner canthus and have the patient remain supine until opening the eye.

7. Gently squeeze the dropper between your thumb and forefinger of opposite hand to instill correct amount of medication.
   a. If using ointment, hold applicator end of tube close to the eye and squeeze out a ¼ to ½ inch ribbon.
   b. Do not touch the lid, lashes or surface of the eye with the dropper or ointment tip to avoid contamination.
	7. If not sure drop went in, use another drop. The eye only holds one drop, so overdosing will not occur.
	   a. If contaminated discard; do not use on multiple patients. Use separate medication bottles perioperatively and for patients with a known infection.

8. Punctal occlusion:
   a. Ask patient to close both eyes gently without squeezing.
 	
   b. Alternately, place your finger over the patient's lacrimal sac and apply light pressure for one minute or more (or instruct patient to do this if able).
	8.
	   a. *Squeezing* increases the lacrimal pump shunting the medication away from the eye. In most cases *closing* the eyelids provides enough pressure to temporarily occlude the punctal drain.
	   b. Digital punctal occlusion is indicated when (1) systemic absorption of medication may prove harmful to the patient (i.e. atropine, phospholine iodide, beta-blockers such as timolol or betaxolol, or antineoplastic agents such as mitomycin or thiotepa used in treatment of pterygia, (2) prolonged corneal-drug contact is desired, or (3) tasting or feeling of ocular medication in the nasopharyngeal mucosa is distressing to the patient.

9. If using ointment, hold lower lid down while ointment melts; then ask patient to blink gently several times.	9. If patient blinks immediately, much of the ointment is expressed out of the cul-de-sac. Blinking gently distributes the melted ointment over the cornea.
10. Gently wipe away tears and/or excess medication with tissue.	10. Do not apply direct pressure to eyelid or rub eye.

From Hill J, editor: *Ophthalmic procedures: a nursing perspective*, San Francisco, 1999, American Society of Ophthalmic Registered Nurses.

TABLE 21-3	**Eyedrop Instillation Procedure—cont'd**
Action	Rationale
11. If administering more than one medication to the eye wait 2 to 5 minutes between medications. Administer drops before ointment.	11. The conjunctival sac cannot hold more than one drop at a time. Allow time for absorption.
12. Date newly opened bottle or tube of ointment.	12. Policy to establish length of time to use drops or ointment after being opened should be approved by local institution Infection Control Committee.
13. Wash hands.	
14. Document on medical record.	

Standard

All personnel responsible for the instillation of eye drops for the ophthalmic patient will be given proper instruction on the correct method of instilling eye drops and ointments.

Outcome

All patients receiving eye drops or ointments will have the procedure performed by trained personnel in a safe and effective manner.

Topical antibiotics may also be considered for prophylaxis against infection. Increases in intraocular pressure frequently accompany serious alkali injuries; therefore evaluation of intraocular pressure is important. If the pressure is highly elevated, it should be treated with 500 mg intramuscular or intravenous acetazolamide, intravenous mannitol, and topical antiglaucoma drops (e.g., timolol maleate). Pain control with analgesic administration is also an important aspect of therapy. While this initial treatment is carried out, ophthalmologic consultation must be sought for further management.

HYPHEMA. Hyphema (blood in the anterior chamber) often accompanies severe blunt and perforating ocular trauma. Until proven otherwise, the globe should be considered perforated in the presence of a hyphema and therefore should be protected with a shield. An ophthalmologist should be consulted for further management. If the globe is intact, the involved eye should be dilated and kept dilated with a mydriatic/cycloplegic to prevent synechiae formation and to better view the fundus. Both the visual acuity and the intraocular pressure should be evaluated. In general, all patients with hyphema need to be examined daily for the first week to monitor intraocular pressure and watch for re-bleeding. Re-bleeding has its maximal incidence 3 to 5 days after the initial trauma and can result in additional ocular pathology. Aminocaproic acid in a dose of 50 mg/kg orally every 4 hours (maximal dose 30 g/24 hr) may be used to prevent re-bleeding. Although this does not improve resorption of blood, it inhibits fibrinolysis of the clot at the site of the injured vessel. Patients are advised to avoid use of anticoagulants, to rest with their head elevated, and to have minimal activity so that the possibility of re-bleed is reduced and the hemorrhage will settle to the bottom of the anterior chamber. This permits better visualization of the internal ocular contents, particularly the retina and optic nerve. When enough blood is present to cause high intraocular pressure, paracentesis or anterior chamber washout of the hyphema may be performed to evacuate blood and lower intraocular pressure.[13]

SECONDARY GLAUCOMA RELATED TO HYPHEMA. Many traumatic hyphema will resolve spontaneously with time. The red blood cells are broken down and washed from the eye through the same channels (trabecular network and canal of Schlemm) that normally route aqueous humor.

Sometimes cells or cell remnants can clog the trabecular meshwork, causing a rise in intraocular pressure and secondary glaucoma. Topical antiglaucoma drops, which act by either constricting the pupil, thereby stretching open the trabecular drainage canal, or reducing the production of aqueous humor, may be prescribed to normalize the pressure until reabsorption of all the cell remnants has occurred.

PENETRATING AND PERFORATING INJURIES. Penetrating and perforating injuries of the ocular structures are a major cause of traumatic visual loss. Such injuries may occur in isolation or in association with severe injuries, including lacerations and fractures of facial structures. Failure to aggressively manage lacerations of the cornea and sclera will almost assuredly result in visual loss.

When it is suspected that an injured patient has a ruptured globe, an eye shield or paper cup should be taped over the injured eye before any further manipulation of the patient is carried out. This prevents the application of any pressure on the periocular structures or the globe itself, which can result in the extrusion of the ocular contents, causing severe and irreparable ocular damage. Treatment of all non-life-threatening injuries of the face and head should

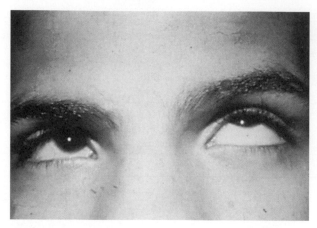

FIGURE 21-23 **Orbital Fracture With Decreased Upward Mobility.**

be deferred until an ophthalmologist can evaluate the extent of the ocular injuries. Surgical repair of penetrating or perforating ocular trauma generally can be delayed until all specialized ophthalmic surgical equipment, such as an ophthalmic operating microscope and vitrectomy instrumentation, and skilled operating room staff are available. In the interim, appropriate radiologic evaluation, CT scan, or MRI for the visualization of intraocular foreign bodies, laboratory tests, cultures, and administration of antibiotics and tetanus prophylaxis can be carried out.

ORBITAL FRACTURES.   Management of orbital fractures must be considered in the context of both functional and cosmetic deficits. Patients usually present with periorbital swelling (see Figure 21-10), ecchymosis, crepitus, proptosis, chemosis, subconjunctival hemorrhage, ophthalmoplegia (decreased movement of the globe) (Figure 21-23), infraorbital and buccal anesthesia, and palpable defects in the bony orbital rims. Orbital fractures can be associated with optic nerve trauma and globe perforation. These associated injuries must be managed as described elsewhere in this chapter. Radiologic studies are essential for determining the extent of any orbital fractures. Immediate repair of these fractures is not necessary; treatment of other injuries, especially those to the globe and optic nerve, may take precedence. As previously mentioned, if the globe is perforated, there should be no manipulation of the orbital bones or eyelids. Nose blowing should be discouraged because this may lead to the development of intraorbital and intraeyelid air, which can cause proptosis, pressure on the globe, and pressure on the optic nerve, with possible loss of vision. Both swelling and muscle entrapment can be causes of ophthalmoplegia. Forced duction testing (see Figure 21-8) and CT examination can help to determine whether either of these is present or whether there is nerve damage or muscle contusion. Indications for surgery include clinical or CT evidence of muscle entrapment, acute enophthalmos, or hypophthalmos (see Figure 21-10). Rim fractures with a 2-mm or greater displacement of the bony fragments and flattening of the malar eminence are indications for open

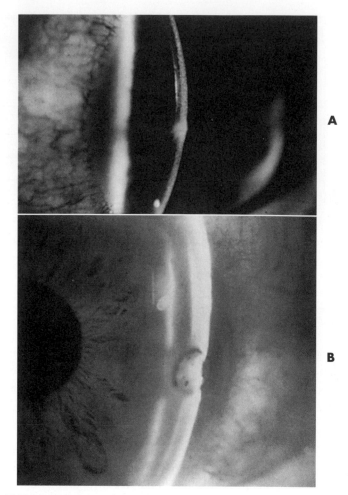

FIGURE 21-24 **A,** Foreign body (rose thorn) embedded in cornea. **B,** Rust ring after removal of foreign body.

reduction and wiring. Midfacial telecanthus and Le Fort fractures generally require repair. Complications of orbital fracture repair include permanent loss of vision, persistent enophthalmos and diplopia, scarring, eyelid retraction, and implant extrusion. Some patients may feel that the cosmetic deficit does not justify surgery and its possible complications.[14]

CORNEAL INJURIES AND FOREIGN BODIES.   The management of corneal foreign bodies (Figure 21-24), corneal abrasions, and radiation injuries to the cornea (e.g., from welding arcs or sun lamps) is similar in certain aspects. Anesthetic drops and fluorescein staining facilitate corneal examination. Short-acting cycloplegic drops, antibiotic drops with good gram-negative coverage, and lubricating ointments are the mainstays of management for these injuries. Pressure patching may increase comfort during healing and is often used for the first 24 hours.[15] However, as a precaution against fungal growth, patching should be avoided if the abrasive agent was vegetative matter or a fingernail. A soft contact lens (a bandage lens) may be used in place of patching, along with topical ophthalmic nonsteroidal antiinflammatory drug (NSAID) drops such as ketorolac (Acular) or diclofenac (Voltaren).

If a foreign body is suspected or seen, it must be removed. Topical anesthetic drops can be very helpful for the removal of foreign bodies. Both the upper and lower eyelids need to be everted, and any clinging particulate matter must be removed. A cotton-tipped applicator can be used to remove superficial conjunctival foreign bodies and some corneal foreign bodies. More often, a 23- or 25-gauge needle on the end of a tuberculin syringe is needed to pry the foreign body from the cornea. To facilitate this maneuver and prevent perforation of the cornea, a slit lamp or high-powered loupe should be used. A small, handheld, battery-driven burr can be used to remove rust rings associated with metallic foreign bodies. Deeply embedded foreign bodies should be removed by an ophthalmologist.

Contact lenses are another type of foreign body often requiring removal. As part of a trauma patient's management, even in the absence of ocular trauma, it is important to determine whether contact lenses are being worn. Corneal abrasion can occur when contacts are worn for extended periods, especially during prolonged surgical procedures. Often it is necessary to examine the eye closely for contact lenses because not all lenses are tinted. Clear ones are more difficult to locate. After trauma, lenses frequently become dislodged from the cornea and can be found in the superior or inferior ocular cul-de-sacs. A bulb contact lens remover (Figure 21-25A) uses suction to lift hard contact lenses from the cornea or sclera. Soft contact lenses can be removed by finger manipulation or by irrigating the eye with balanced salt solution or normal saline, which allows the lens to "float" off the globe (Figure 21-25B). Once removed, lenses should be placed in the appropriate storage solution and stored in a contact lens case that delineates the right from left lens. Contact lenses may be worn 2 or 3 days after a corneal abrasion has healed.

SUBCONJUNCTIVAL HEMORRHAGE. Subconjunctival hemorrhage and chemosis frequently occur after trauma. Although these may herald serious intraocular and orbital trauma, they often occur as isolated signs. The management of these problems in the absence of more serious trauma involves waiting and watching. Generally, both subconjunctival hemorrhages and chemosis will spontaneously resolve over a 1- to 3-week period. In extreme instances of conjunctival prolapse and drying, ocular ointments may be helpful in maintaining an intact conjunctiva.

OPTIC NERVE INJURIES. Severe penetrating orbital injury can result in optic nerve damage and sudden visual loss. This type of injury is most frequently caused by a handgun, shotgun, or knife.[16] Trauma to the optic nerve also can occur in association with blunt orbital trauma and orbital fractures. Loss of vision can be caused by transsection or avulsion of the optic nerve, optic nerve sheath hemorrhage, pressure on the optic nerve from bone fragments or orbital hemorrhage, direct contusion of the nerve, or disruption of the blood supply to the nerve and globe. Often such injuries are irreversible. However, every effort must be made to try to

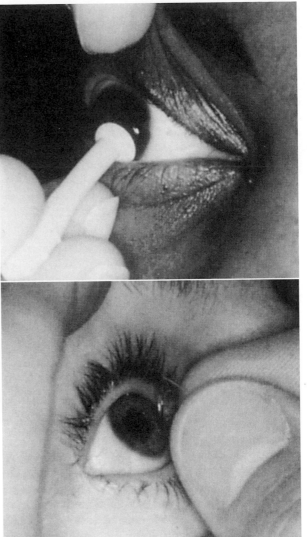

FIGURE 21-25 **A,** Bulb contact remover for hard contacts. **B,** Removal of soft contact lens.

restore vision. Evaluation of such injuries should include a visual acuity assessment, if possible, and examination of the pupils for an afferent defect. Thin-cut CT or MRI scans of the optic nerve and canal are important for evaluating the extent of optic nerve injury. Surgical intervention, such as unroofing the optic canal or opening the optic nerve sheath, may be required in those cases in which there is nerve sheath hemorrhage or edema or fracture of the optic canal. Intravenous high-dose steroids are essential for managing optic nerve injuries to reduce inflammation and prevent further injury secondary to the inflammatory response. The usual dosage in these cases is the same as for spinal cord injury: methylprednisolone, 30 mg/kg intravenously infused over a 20- to 30-minute period, followed by IV infusion of 5.4 mg/kg/hr for each of the next 23 hours. No further treatment is given after this 24 hours of infusion. An alternative to this regimen is an initial 30 mg/kg intravenous infusion followed by 15 mg/kg 2 hours later and at 6-hour intervals. Improvement in visual function has been seen even if therapy is begun several days after injury. However, initiation of treatment within the first 12 to 24 hours after injury provides the best chance for visual recovery.

OPERATIVE CARE

Immediate surgical repair after accurate evaluation of the ocular damage is almost always required. A conservative wait-and-see approach often results in permanent scarring, atrophy, loss of tissue, or permanent visual disability. Unlike other systems, the function of the eye depends on exact maintenance of anatomic relationships between its structures, including the eyelids, cornea, anterior chamber, lens, retina, extraocular muscles, and nerves.

EXPLORATION AND REPAIR OF GLOBE.
If there is any question concerning the presence of a penetrating ocular injury, the globe should be explored thoroughly and, if possible, repaired while the patient is under general anesthesia. Generally, every attempt should be made to salvage or repair any lacerated globe. Such surgery is often complex and can require several hours to perform. Few patients with ruptured globes need to undergo primary enucleation because of the extent of the injuries they have sustained.

CRITICAL CARE/INTERMEDIATE CARE

After the two initial phases (prehospital management and resuscitation), patients in the critical care and intermediate care phases of trauma continue to require physical care, patient and family education, and a significant emphasis on psychologic and emotional support. As with any injury, reactions to ocular injury and its sequelae will be individual, but an awareness of potential patient reactions by the health care team facilitates more effective care planning. It is essential to closely monitor the patient for signs of infection, further visual loss, increasing pain, hemorrhage, or other complications. These changes must be reported promptly to the ophthalmologist so that proper therapy can be instituted and further visual loss prevented.

PAIN MANAGEMENT.
Pain management is an important aspect of care for the patient with ocular injury. Although there is usually minimal or moderate pain after ocular surgery and trauma, pain medications and sedation may be helpful in many cases. Continuous ice compresses for the first 24 hours after eyelid or orbital surgery decrease swelling and its associated pain. Warm compresses over the next 48 hours also may be helpful in reducing swelling. Keeping the head elevated to 30 degrees during rest or sleep also may aid in promoting patient comfort.[17] Unrelieved or increasing pain should be considered an indication for further ophthalmologic evaluation.

SKIN/WOUND MANAGEMENT.
Patients who have had ocular surgery are at risk for disruption of the surgical repair as a result of elevated intraocular pressure and inadvertent blunt trauma to the operative site. It is important for any eye on which intraocular surgery has been performed to be protected at all times with either a metal or plastic eye shield to prevent additional trauma to the globe.

Elevated intraocular pressure may result from hemorrhage or edema after surgical repair. As previously stated, prolonged or sudden increases in intraocular pressure may lead to partial or total visual loss. Therefore nursing measures must focus on the prevention of increased pressure and accurate assessment for early detection. Activities that increase intraocular pressure include coughing, gagging, lying flat or in Trendelenburg's position, straining for bowel movements, bending over, and lifting heavy objects. Sedation or antiemetics may be necessary to prevent persistent coughing or vomiting. Chest physiotherapy, which might normally be a routine intervention to prevent atelectasis and clear secretions, may be contraindicated for the patient who sustains an ocular injury. Ambulatory patients must be cautioned not to lift heavy objects or to bend over to pick up objects. Stooping to retrieve objects is an acceptable alternative. Unnecessary coughing and sneezing should be avoided. Laxatives or stool softeners may be necessary to prevent straining for bowel elimination.

Wound care should be performed as prescribed. The injury or surgical site should be assessed regularly for healing progression and evidence of infection. Purulent discharge, erythema, increased tenderness, pain, and inflammation at the wound or surgical site are symptoms of possible wound infection. The presence of these symptoms should be reported to the ophthalmologist.

POTENTIAL FOR IRITIS.
A mild inflammatory reaction involving the iris and ciliary body frequently occurs after blunt trauma. It causes various amounts of photophobia, aching pain, minimally decreased vision, and either increased or decreased intraocular pressure. After serious ocular injury is eliminated by a thorough ocular examination, symptomatic relief can be achieved through the use of short-acting cycloplegic/mydriatic drops and topical steroid drops two to four times daily for 7 to 10 days. A follow-up examination is always indicated.[18]

POTENTIAL FOR CELLULITIS.
Preseptal or periorbital cellulitis (Figure 21-26A) is commonly associated with breaks in the periorbital or eyelid skin occurring with both blunt and penetrating trauma. Several days may elapse between the time of injury and the occurrence of cellulitis. Commonly there is marked eyelid edema and skin erythema. Usually there is some degree of skin tautness and inflammation. Edema may extend to the opposite lid and cheek and may be so severe as to prevent elevation of the eyelid in order to examine the globe. Associated with these suppurative changes are purulent drainage and superficial abscess formation. Despite the apparent severity of the adnexal signs, the globe is usually normal unless it is perforated. Proptosis, loss of vision, and pain on eye motion are usually absent in contrast to orbital cellulitis. The patient usually does not appear ill. Staphylococci, streptococci, and

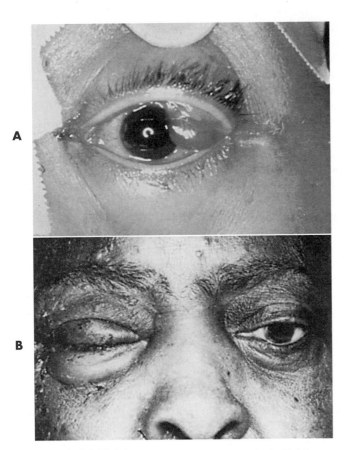

FIGURE 21-26 **A**, Periorbital cellulitis. **B**, Orbital cellulitis.

hemophili are the most common pathogens. Treatment consists of oral antibiotics and incision and drainage of any suppurative area. In severe cases or when the patient is unable to take medications orally, intravenous antibiotics may be required.

Orbital cellulitis (Figure 21-26B) is a serious disease associated with severe ocular, intracranial, and systemic morbidity, including loss of vision from optic nerve damage, glaucoma, corneal or retinal damage, brain abscess, cavernous sinus thrombosis, and sepsis. Patients appear ill and have a fever and leukocytosis. Although the periorbital structures may appear normal, conjunctival hyperemia and chemosis, pain on eye movement, proptosis, resistance to globe retropulsion, increased intraocular pressure, and visual loss are typically evident with orbital cellulitis. There may be an associated orbital or subperiosteal abscess. Penetrating ocular trauma or eye surgery may cause this severe infective process, or, more frequently, it may occur secondary to a paranasal sinusitis or oral infection. CT or MRI scan and orbital ultrasonography are important diagnostic modalities for determining the extent of the orbital disease process. CT scan is essential for assessing sinus and intracranial disease. It is important to obtain the aid of an otolaryngologist and an ophthalmologist to manage orbital cellulitis adequately. Intravenous antibiotics and removal or drainage of any infectious source are the mainstays of therapy.

Cavernous sinus thrombosis may result from orbital cellulitis; it also may occur independently and be difficult to distinguish from orbital cellulitis. Patients with cavernous sinus thrombosis appear severely ill and have fever, nausea, vomiting, headache, and an altered level of consciousness in addition to signs of orbital cellulitis. Orbital pain is absent and cranial nerves III, IV, and VI are impaired as a result of their compression within the cavernous sinus.

POTENTIAL FOR CORNEAL EROSION. A corneal erosion can be caused by abnormal eyelid positions such as: ectropion or lid retraction, abnormal eyelashes (trichiasis), poorly fitted contact lenses, abnormalities of the eyelid margin, inadequate tear film, inability to close the eyelids, poor closure of the eyelids during blinking, or infrequent blinking. Traumatic facial nerve damage that impairs eyelid closure is frequently associated with corneal abnormalities, as are eyelid and conjunctival scarring and injury. Traumatic ptosis, eyelid closure, and blinking may improve spontaneously during the subsequent 6 to 12 months. In the interim, vigorous use of artificial tears and ointments, as frequently as every hour, is essential. A bandage contact lens is often helpful in healing chronic erosions. Surgical correction of eyelid abnormalities may be required in some cases. If drops and ointments are inadequate to prevent continued exposure keratopathy (corneal noninflammatory dystrophy), it may be necessary to tape the eyelids shut, apply a cellophane vapor barrier, or use various types of suture tarsorrhaphy (temporary or permanent closure of part or all of the eyelid). It is essential that patients with corneal pathology caused by exposure be managed vigorously to prevent ocular discomfort, blepharospasm, permanent scarring, corneal ulcers, and corneal perforation.

POTENTIAL FOR SYMPATHETIC OPHTHALMIA. The prevention of sympathetic ophthalmia (SO) is the major indication for enucleation of a severely injured, nonreparable perforated globe or a globe that has been initially repaired. Sympathetic ophthalmia is a rare condition characterized by a severe, bilateral, granulomatous uveitis (inflammation of the uveal tract of the eye, which includes the iris, ciliary body, and choroid). It manifests as early as 5 days after penetrating ocular injury or as late as years after the injury. If untreated, the inflammatory response may result in loss of vision in the uninjured eye. The incidence of SO has declined sharply with advanced microsurgical techniques and the appropriate early enucleation of eyes without hope of recovering useful vision. When SO does occur, aggressive therapy using systemic and topical corticosteroids is initiated. This is often successful in eliminating the sympathetic response.

PATIENT AND FAMILY EDUCATION. Patient and family teaching during the critical care and intermediate care phases should include information regarding the injury, the symptoms the patient may expect, and therapeutic interventions. Education regarding pressure patching, ocular medication, pain, wound care, and restrictions on mobility and activities is especially important. Patients undergoing surgical intervention for ocular repair should also receive information about the procedure and their anticipated preoperative and postoperative management. Patients usually have no ambulating restrictions and are often discharged to home the same day or within 1 to 2 days after surgical repair of isolated traumatic ocular injuries. Potential complications and their symptomatology should also be well explained to the patient and family.

COPING ASSISTANCE.   Visual loss has long been considered by many to be the ultimate catastrophe. Psychologic and emotional support from health care providers, family, and friends is essential for the temporarily or permanently, partially or totally visually impaired person. The impact of blindness may be so severe that professional counseling is required to adjust to this unfamiliar situation. The emotional effects of shock, denial, anger, and depression that a patient experiences in order to adapt to a permanent visual loss are similar to the grieving process that is experienced with the loss of a loved one (see Chapter 18 on Psychosocial Impact of Trauma).

The partially or totally blinded individual has lost the major sense through which information is processed from the environment. The individual is faced with learning new ways to retrieve and process this information. Activities of daily living and all social interactions are altered drastically. Expressing pity and being overly solicitous are counterproductive in allowing a visually impaired person to adapt to the new situation. Families of the newly blind may encounter serious financial burdens if the disabled individual is the primary wage earner. They must adjust their lifestyles and activities of daily living to accommodate the patient with a visual disability within the home environment.

As the trauma patient becomes less acutely ill, the patient and family members become more aware of the full impact that a permanent visual deficit will have on their lives. The family and patient must be allowed time and support to grieve and deal with this devastating injury. They should be encouraged to verbalize their feelings and concerns within an accepting atmosphere and should be assisted in finding resources to help with transitions. It must be acknowledged that the patient's self-image will be altered dramatically. A father and husband may no longer be the provider for the family; a mother may no longer be able to care for her children without assistance.

Because of continuous interaction with the patient, the nurse plays a significant role during the initial period after visual impairment is sustained. Providing quality nursing care for the temporarily or permanently visually impaired is challenging and yet rewarding. Understanding the patient's fears, concerns, and anxieties is imperative to enable the nurse to individualize the care given to each patient.

Frequent orientation to date, time, place, and the unfamiliar environment (including noises and smells) assists in alleviating fears of the unknown. It is essential that all interventions be described before carrying them out. Each person entering the patient's immediate environment should introduce himself or herself. The patient with unilateral visual impairment should be approached from the sighted side.

"Long-distance" information is conveyed to a person through the sensory modality of vision. Normally, size, dimension, color, shape, and density of objects all are quickly processed visually. With loss of vision, this input and assessment of the environment and the people within it are lost. Only "short-distance" information receptors are available to analyze the environment. The patient must now use other senses to bring in long-distance information. This relearning takes time and requires thought, sensitivity, and, above all, patience from the care providers. The patient should be allowed to feel and smell objects. The color of objects should be described to the patient. Nurses and other health team members interacting with the patient should describe themselves (e.g., color of eyes, hair, height, weight) if the patient desires because the blind patient now can visualize people and the environment only through description. The patient should be allowed to feel your face if this is helpful. Environmental stimulation is provided through conversation, radio, television, or audio tapes.

Whether the visual loss is temporary or permanent, the absence of this vital and major sense is frightening and devastating. Visual loss combined with the presence of other systemic injuries, the circumstances of the trauma event, pain, and potential morbidity contribute to anxiety and fear, compounding the feelings of complete powerlessness felt by the patient. Use of touch is extremely important and helpful in managing such feelings. A gentle touch conveys many messages to a frightened patient, including care, concern, and a desire to help. It is reassuring and comforting to a patient to be able to identify a voice and gentle touch together. Anxiety, fear, and apprehension can be diminished, making the experience less terrifying for the patient and making the recovery process easier.

It is important to promote the patient's sense of independence, which may be difficult to do in the acute phase of hospitalization. Within the limitations imposed by other injuries and the patient's general condition, the patient should be encouraged to assist with tasks, even things as simple as hand washing, so that a sense of accomplishment and self-control is fostered. Occupational therapists can help a patient learn new ways to perform activities of daily living (ADL). The patient also may be taught how to perform simple tasks related to ocular therapy and management such as the instillation of ocular medication or patching an eye. When possible, the patient should be offered choices about how and when care should be delivered.

Psychiatrists, psychologists, social workers, and clergy can be extremely helpful in assisting the patient and the family as they adapt. Referral to rehabilitative services (e.g., occupational therapy, physical therapy, vocational rehabilitation, and community agencies providing services for the visually impaired) should be initiated. The multidisciplinary health care team can incorporate recommendations of these referral services into an individualized plan of care that best meets the needs of the patient. Interventions that assist the patient in coping with the visual impairment remain important throughout hospitalization.

SAFETY RISK MANAGEMENT.   The environment must be safe, stable, organized, and consistent for the person who is visually impaired and cannot see impending dangers. The mobile patient must be protected from sharp-edged furniture and equipment, small objects easily tripped over, objects that can be broken easily and cause injury, and objects protruding from walls or hanging from the ceiling. The nurse should instruct the patient on the content and confines of the room. Because vision provides many clues relating to distance, simply explaining how far away something is may not be sufficient. Counting off the number of steps to the bathroom with the patient will be more meaningful. Consistency in the placement of objects in the room (e.g., phone on left side of bed stand, tissues on right, fork at left of plate) facilitates the patient's independence. For a sense of security, a call bell or other means of attracting assistance is important.

REHABILITATION AND COMMUNITY INTEGRATION

Rehabilitation efforts actually begin in the critical care phase, when planning should be started, and takes special prominence in the intermediate phase as the patient prepares for discharge. Decisions regarding care are determined by the individual requirements of each patient. Discharge placement depends on information and advice from the many persons involved, including the patient, family, nurse, physician, social worker, and therapists. Some visually impaired persons may be discharged directly home, using support services, whereas others may benefit from admission to a rehabilitation facility. Another consideration is the type of services and facilities offered in the region where the patient resides. Programs vary in the type of services offered. Day programs, halfway houses, and intensive overnight facilities are examples of rehabilitation services that may be available.

The goal during this phase of recovery is to prepare the visually impaired person for a life of independence within the limitation of his or her disability. The patient must be encouraged and motivated to attain maximal potential independent functioning. Promotion of self-esteem, personal value, and self-confidence and learning to master living in a sightless world are essential for maximal recovery. Learning Braille, independent household management, and new modes of ambulating with a visual impairment (possibly using a seeing-eye dog or cane) are examples of priorities during this phase. Rehabilitation is carried out closely in conjunction with community integration.

Community integration must be planned and initiated

TABLE 21-4	**Resource Organizations for the Visually Impaired**

American Foundation for the Blind
15 W 16th Street
New York, NY 10011
(800)232-5463

American Council of the Blind
1010 Vermont Ave NW, Suite 100
Washington, DC, 20005
(202)393-3666

American Printing House for the Blind
PO Box 60851839, Frankfort Ave
Louisville, KY, 40206
(502)895-2485

Association for the Education and Rehabilitation of the Blind
    and Visually Impaired
206 N Washington Street, Suite 320
Alexandria, VA 22314
(703)548-1884

National Association for the Visually Handicapped
22 West 21st Street
New York, NY 10010
(212)889-3141

Prevent Blindness America
500 Remmington Road
Schaumburg, IL 60173
(215)843-2020

American Academy of Ophthalmology
655 Beach Street
San Francisco, CA 94119
(415)561-8500

American Society of Ophthalmic Registered Nurses (ASORN)
PO Box 193030
San Francisco, CA 94119
(415)561-8513

Social Security Administration
6401 Security Boulevard
Baltimore, MD 21235-0001
(800)772-1213
www.ssa.gov

U.S. Department of Health and Human Services
200 Independence Avenue SW
Washington, DC 20201
(877)696-6775
www.hhs.gov

State Department of Rehabilitation Services
Contact information varies by state.

well before the patient is ready to go home, either from the hospital or rehabilitation facility. Appropriate housing and home care for the patient must be arranged. Supplies, equipment, and medications required for wound or injury management must be procured for the patient. Some patients may benefit from a visiting nurse to assess their progress and some may need the temporary assistance of a meal delivery program. Each patient's needs require individualized evaluation for safe discharge planning. The nurse needs to use fully community resources for optimal patient care at home. The patient, the family, and the involved health care providers should have a thorough understanding of the care required, including medications, wound management, activity restrictions, necessary safety precautions, signs and symptoms of complications, physician follow-up appointments, and actions to take in an emergency.

Patients and families need to be educated about state and federal tax relief, Social Security and Medicare benefits, travel discounts (both local and national), and vocational rehabilitation. Health care providers who care for patients with ocular injuries should be knowledgeable about community agencies and services available for the visually disabled. Visiting nurse agencies can assist the patient in using the assistance available from community and national organizations (Table 21-4). Introductions to other patients with visual loss who have adapted to their disability and are functioning as productive members of society may greatly help the newly blind. Social workers can be a great help by providing financial, vocational, and social resources for the patient.

SUMMARY

Familiarity with ocular anatomy and function and ocular examination form the basis for evaluating and managing ocular trauma. Appropriate interpretation of ocular assessment findings allows recognition of eye injuries and their possible complications. The prevention of permanent damage from trauma depends on the use of appropriate management techniques. More importantly, ocular trauma may be avoided if proper safety measures are taken in the workplace, at home, and during recreational activities. If permanent visual disability occurs despite appropriate protective measures and trauma management, a variety of individuals and groups are available to aid in the patient's adjustment to a severe disability and reintegration into society.

Although nursing management of patients with ocular injuries has advanced significantly, there are still many unknowns in this field. How do nurses identify the patient's priorities for rehabilitation? What are the most effective methods for promoting independence for the visually impaired? How do nursing measures affect intraocular pressure and, ultimately, healing of the eye? Research in this area of injury is relatively limited compared with other areas

(e.g., shock, sepsis, pulmonary insufficiency). With further research in both medical and nursing management of ocular injury, there is hope that patients increasingly will be less likely to develop complications and more likely to retain normal vision after ocular trauma.

REFERENCES

1. United States Eye Injury Registry (USEIR): *Reports of serious eye injury data 1988-1998,* Birmingham, Ala, 1998, USEIR.
2. Baker RS, Wilson MR, Flowers CW Jr et al: Demographic factors in a population-based, work-related, ocular injury, *Am J Ophthalmol* 122(2):213-9, 1996.
3. Marsden J: Systemic eye examination in the A&E, *Emerg Nurs* 6(6):16-9, 1998.
4. Marsden J: Care of patients with minor eye trauma, *Emerg Nurs* 6(7):10-3, 1998.
5. Piermaici DJ, Sternberg P Jr, Aaberg TM et al: A system for classifying mechanical injuries of the eye (globe). The Ocular Trauma Classification Group, *Am J Ophthalmol* 123(6):820-31, 1997.
6. Sires BS, Lemke BN, Kincaid MC: Orbital and ocular anatomy. In Wright KW, editor: *Textbook of ophthalmology,* Baltimore, 1997, Williams & Wilkins.
7. Venger PF: Injury protection: where do we go from here? *J Am Optom Assoc* 70(2):87-98, 1999.
8. Duhn F, Mester V, Witherspoon CD et al: Epidemiology and socioeconomic impact of ocular trauma. In Alfaro DV, Liggett PE, editors: *Vitreoretinal surgery of the injured eye,* Philadelphia, 1999, Lippincott-Raven.
9. Singer HW: Potential air bag-related injuries require special ER attention, *J Ophthalmol Nurs Tech* 17(1):21-22, 1998.
10. Mohamed AA, Banerjee A: Patterns of injury associated with automobile airbag use, *Postgrad Med J* 74(874):455-458, 1998.
11. Zagelbaum BM: *Sports ophthalmology,* London, 1996, Blackwell Scienctific.
12. Poor A, McClusky PJ, Hill DA: Eye injuries in patients with major trauma, *J Trauma* 46(3):494-499, 1999.
13. Crouch ER Jr., Crouch ER: Management of traumatic hyphema and therapeutic options, *J Pediatr Opthhalmol Strabismus* 36(5):238-250, 1999.
14. Patel BC, Hoffman J: Management of complex orbital fractures, *Fac Plastic Surg* 14(1):83-104, 1998.
15. Wingate S: Treating corneal abrasions, *Nurse Pract* 24(6):53-4, 57, 60, 1999.
16. Spoor TC: *An atlas of ophthalmic trauma,* St. Louis, 1997, Mosby.
17. Mason G: Ocular trauma. In Goldblum K, editor: *Core curriculum for ophthalmic nursing,* Dubuque, 1997, Kendall Hunt.
18. MacCumber MW, editor: *Management of ocular injuries and emergencies,* Philadelphia, 1997, Lippincott-Raven.

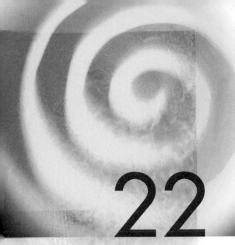

SPINAL CORD INJURIES

Tammy A. Russo-McCourt

22

Spinal cord injury (SCI) was described in the literature as early as 2500 BC by the Egyptian surgeons as "an ailment not to be treated."[1] A combination of many events in the late 1960s and early 1970s led the way in changing the approach to the management of acute spinal injury. Introduction of the military model for triaging and rapid transport of trauma victims and the understanding of the multisystem effects of SCI enabled many more paralyzed veterans to survive their injury.[2] This demonstrated not only the ability to successfully treat such injuries but highlighted the need for appropriate SCI rehabilitation. The pioneering work of Sir Ludwig Guttmann identified the need to provide comprehensive multidisciplinary care from the onset of SCI through rehabilitation so that individuals can return as productive members of society.[3] Guttmann's holistic approach to care serves as the basis for the modern model of SCI care.

In the early 1900s Dr. Alfred Reginald Allen hypothesized that the response of the body to spinal cord trauma was twofold: (1) direct injury to the axons at the time of impact and (2) the nervous tissues' response to the injury over time. Research has consistently supported the concept of primary and secondary injury. The potential to interrupt this secondary response and prevent worsening outcome has prompted early, aggressive treatment of SCI.[3,4]

Spinal cord injury, with its multisystem sequelae, creates a ripple effect on every facet of the patient's life, the family's life, and society at large. There are enormous burdens placed on resources to provide the necessary care for the paralyzed person; until recently, very little support existed. The United States Veterans Administration and the National Institute on Disability and Rehabilitation Research have made significant contributions in this area.

The primary goal of this chapter is to provide a thorough description of SCI and its effects. A brief review of neuroanatomy facilitates greater understanding of the mechanisms of injury and the multisystem impact of the injury. Assessment and management of SCI will be presented in a "cycle of trauma" format to highlight the importance of interventions within each phase of trauma care on patient outcomes.

EPIDEMIOLOGY

It is estimated that there are 30 to 40 new cases of SCI per million U.S. citizens each year. This translates to 7600 to 10,000 new cases per year.[5] Researchers estimate that an additional 4800 victims of SCI die before reaching the hospital.[5] Although this is considered a relatively low incidence, it is considered a high-cost disability. It is currently estimated that 250,000 individuals in the United States are living today with spinal cord injury or dysfunction.[5] The average lifetime direct cost is estimated at $1.9 million for ventilator-dependent quadriplegics, $1.1 million for quadriplegics, and $700,000 for paraplegics. A conservative estimate of the economic burden of SCI in the United States is $4.5 billion per year.[5-7] This does not reflect indirect costs such as loss of wages, fringe benefits, and productivity, which represent an additional $2.6 billion dollars annually.[6,7]

In 1973 the National Spinal Cord Injury Database was established at the University of Alabama at Birmingham. This registry captures approximately 15% of new SCI cases per year. Because this group is representative of the SCI population at large, it has contributed significantly to our ability to compile incidence, prevalence, and demographic information on SCI. The typical SCI patient is a single white male under the age of 30 who was involved in a motor vehicle crash and sustained complete paraplegia. He was employed at the time of injury and has a 36% chance of remaining employed after 1 year.[4] Demographics are beginning to show shifts in several areas: (1) an increase in the proportion of those injured over age 61, matching a rise in the median age of the general population; (2) a rise in the proportion of injuries in the African-American population (increasing from 13% in the 1970s to 29% in the 1990s); and (3) a sharp rise in violent events as the cause of injury.[4]

In years past the average life expectancy of a person sustaining a spinal cord injury was less than 1 year. With the improvements made in prehospital care, critical care, and the prevention of complications, SCI patients can expect a near normal life expectancy.[8,9] Because patients are living longer, more of them will receive Medicare and disability income. We can expect a dramatic increase in the annual expenditure for related health care.[6,7] There also has been a dramatic shift in the leading causes of death for SCI patients. Historically, the leading cause of death was renal failure. With significant advances in urologic management, the most common causes of death have become pneumonia, pulmonary emboli, and septicemia.[8,9] It is of vital importance that care during the cycle of trauma be focused on limiting complications to achieve maximal recovery.

PREVENTION

The key to preventing injuries is to assess epidemiologic data and develop programs targeted at high-risk groups and behaviors. The group at greatest risk of sustaining a spinal cord injury consists of males under the age of 25. This is the group most associated with risk-taking behaviors. One merely needs to look at the increasing popularity of "extreme sports" for evidence of this fact. There are three general strategies to prevent injuries: persuasion, legal requirements, and provision of automatic protection. Persuasion is the most difficult strategy to apply effectively. The Think First Foundation, developed and supported by the American Association of Neurologic Surgeons and the Congress of Neurological Surgeons, is one group that assists communities in providing programs to educate children and adolescents about prevention of brain and spinal injuries. Changes in laws creating safer vehicles and more effect restraint systems and enforcement of these laws can help protect the public. Aggressive campaigns, such as those sponsored by Mothers Against Drunk Drivers (MADD), provide media attention, public education regarding the dangers of high-risk behaviors, and social reform, which can be effective in reducing SCIs. The fourth leading cause of SCI today is diving accidents.[4,5,10] Studies by DeVivo et al investigating the circumstances surrounding these injuries have provided pertinent information for pool safety guidelines and for the development of educational programs.[10] One such program developed in Florida, "Feet First, First Time," focuses on prevention of diving in shallow water and has demonstrated a significant reduction in the number of SCIs. Raising public awareness, providing education, employing passive protective mechanisms, and enacting social and legal reform can be effective prevention methods.

BASIC SPINAL ANATOMY

Gross spinal anatomy can be divided into three categories: (1) the vertebral bony column, intervertebral disks, ligaments, and muscles; (2) the spinal cord and associated nerves and membranes; and (3) the spinal cord vasculature. The spinal, or vertebral, column consists of 33 vertebrae (Figure 22-1) separated and cushioned by fibrocartilaginous pads called intervertebral disks. The vertebrae and disks are joined by ligaments.

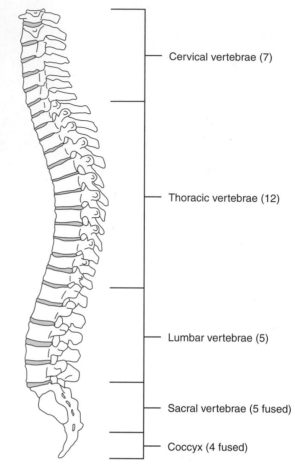

Cervical vertebrae (7)

Thoracic vertebrae (12)

Lumbar vertebrae (5)

Sacral vertebrae (5 fused)

Coccyx (4 fused)

FIGURE 22-1 **Lateral View of the Vertebral Column.**

THE BONY STRUCTURES

The majority of the vertebrae have similar anatomic features. Each vertebrae can be divided into two sections: an anterior body, the segment that faces toward the front of a person, and the posterior arch (Figure 22-2). The opening created between the body and the arch is the vertebral foramen, where the spinal cord, its coverings, and blood vessels pass. The arch is a series of fused bony parts. Starting at the midpoint is the spinous process. These are the points that can be seen or felt protruding along the midline of the back. Moving laterally in either direction are more distinct bony prominences called the transverse processes with superior and inferior articular processes or facets. These are joined to the spinous process by the lamina. The transverse processes are connected to the vertebral body by the pedicles. When the vertebrae are aligned in a column, the inferior articular processes, which deflect downward, meet the inflected superior articular processes of the vertebrae directly below. Between these processes and the bodies and disks an opening exists, the intervertebral foramen, through which peripheral nerves pass.

Of special interest are the C1 (atlas) and C2 (axis) vertebrae (Figure 22-3). The first cervical vertebra is called

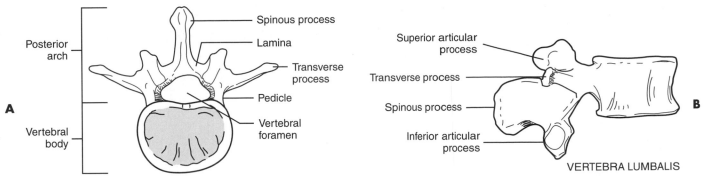

FIGURE 22-2 **A** and **B,** Structural view of the vertebrae.

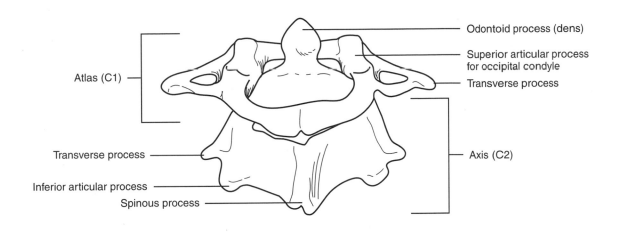

C1-2 ARTICULATION

FIGURE 22-3 **Articulated View of the C1-2 Structure.**

the atlas because it literally supports the "globe" of the head. By articulating with the skull, C1 provides 50% of the normal motion of the neck. It is unusual in that it lacks a vertebral body. The odontoid, a bony projection jutting upward from the C2 vertebral body, protrudes through the anterior arch of C1. The odontoid process forms the pivot on which the atlas and skull rotate (hence the term *axis*). The sacrum and coccyx are also unique because the vertebral bodies of these areas are fused together.

The intervertebral disks confer a degree of flexibility to the spine. They act as shock absorbers by temporarily flattening and bulging from between the vertebrae when they are compressed. Under an extreme load the central nucleus can burst through the surrounding cartilaginous fibers, the annulus fibrosus, producing a herniated disk. The vertebrae and disks are held in alignment by ligaments (Figure 22-4). The ligaments prevent extreme flexion and extension of the spine. The anterior and posterior longitudinal ligaments join the bodies of adjacent vertebrae whereas the strong ligamenta flava join the lamina. The ligamentum nuchae extends from the skull through the spinous process of the seventh cervical vertebra. Below this level, supraspinal ligaments join the spinous processes. Adjacent spinous

processes are joined from their roots to their ends by interspinal ligaments.

THE SPINAL CORD

The spinal cord, a gelatinous bundle of nerve tracts covered by meninges, is housed inside the vertebral column. The spinal cord, essentially an extension of the medulla oblongata, begins at the foramen magnum and terminates around the first or second lumbar vertebrae. This conical termination point is called the conus medullaris.

Spinal nerve roots exit from the cord at each intervertebral foramen. There are a total of 31 pairs of spinal nerves: 8 cervical, 12 thoracic, 5 lumbar, 5 sacral, and 1 coccygeal. Each spinal nerve has a dorsal root (posterior part of the cord) and a ventral root (anterior part of the cord). The dorsal root consists of sensory or afferent fibers, which carry impulses from the body to the cord. The dorsal root contains a spinal ganglion, which is located outside the cord but within the intervertebral foramen. The ganglion contains the cell bodies of the sensory neurons. The ventral root consists of the motor, or efferent, fibers. The cell bodies of the motor neurons are located within the gray matter of the cord. These fibers

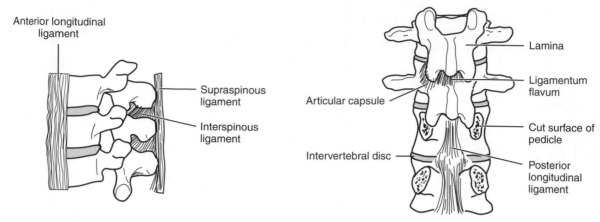

FIGURE 22-4 The Chief Ligaments of the Vertebral Column. (From Jenkins DB: *Hollinshead's Functional anatomy of the limbs and back,* ed 7, Philadelphia, 1998, WB Saunders.)

carry the impulses from the cord to the appropriate effector site.

The spinal cord is surrounded by three meninges: the dura mater, the arachnoid, and the pia mater. The meninges are continuations of the meninges covering the brain. Above the pia mater is the subarachnoid space. The subarachnoid space is filled with cerebrospinal fluid (CSF), as is the central canal that pierces the central gray matter of the cord. The central canal is continuous with the fourth ventricle. The spinal cord is tethered to the meninges via the dentate (or denticulate) ligaments.

GRAY AND WHITE MATTER

The substance of the spinal cord is divided into two types: gray matter and white matter.

The gray matter is centrally located in an H or butterfly-shaped pattern. It is composed of cell bodies and their axons and dendrites. It can be divided into three areas or horns: the anterior, the intermediolateral, and the posterior. The anterior horn provides the motor component of the spinal nerves, often referred to as the final common pathway. The intermediolateral horn contains cell bodies, which give rise to the preganglionic sympathetic fibers of T1-L2 and the preganglionic parasympathetic fibers of the sacral spine. The posterior horn contains axons from peripheral sensory neurons. These may terminate there or ascend or descend into the white matter.

The white matter surrounds the gray matter of the cord and is divided into large fiber bundles called columns. There are three columns: the posterior, the lateral, and the anterior. Each column contains ascending sensory tracts and descending motor tracts (Figure 22-5).

The major ascending tracts include the posterior columns, the spinocerebellar tracts, and the spinothalamic tracts. The posterior column mediates proprioception, vibration, two-point discrimination, deep pressure, and touch. These columns ascend on the ipsilateral side of the spinal cord, where they enter and decussate in the medulla and ascend through the thalamus to the cerebral cortex. There are eight well-identified ascending tracts of the lateral

column. The most significant of these are the spinocerebellar tracts and the spinothalamic tracts. The spinocerebellar tracts carry information on position sense and body movement necessary for coordination of body movement from the extremities and trunk to the cerebellum. The spinothalamic tracts carry information from the periphery to the thalamus. The anterior spinothalamic tracts transmit light touch and pressure impulses, whereas the lateral spinothalamic tract mediates most pain and temperature sensations. The spinothalamic tracts decussate almost at the level of entrance into the spinal cord and ascend in the contralateral anterolateral system to the thalamus. The anterior column tracts are primarily involved with motor function, posture reflexes, light touch, and pressure.

The major descending pathways are the corticospinal, reticulospinal, vestibulospinal, rubrospinal, and tectospinal tracts. The largest and the one of greatest clinical concern is the lateral corticospinal, or pyramidal, tract. Fibers originate in the motor cortex, and the majority cross to the opposite side in the medulla and descend the spinal cord as the lateral corticospinal tract delivering voluntary motor function. Fibers of the lateral corticospinal tract are arranged in the spinal cord; the motor fibers controlling the lower extremities are located peripherally, and the fibers controlling the upper extremities are located medially.

The descending tracts or motor pathways can be divided into two categories: upper motor neurons (UMNs) and lower motor neurons (LMNs). UMNs originate and terminate within the central nervous system (CNS) and include all neurons or nerve cells, which modulate the motor output of the anterior horn cell of the spinal cord. The four major motor modulators that constitute the majority of the UMNs are the cerebral cortex, the cerebellum, the basal ganglia, and the reticular neurons. Any lesion or trauma that disrupts these areas and their modulation of the LMNs will create an upper motor neuron deficit. This deficit is characterized by paralysis, hypertonicity in affected muscle groups, and hyperreflexia.

The LMNs constitute the anterior horn cells and their

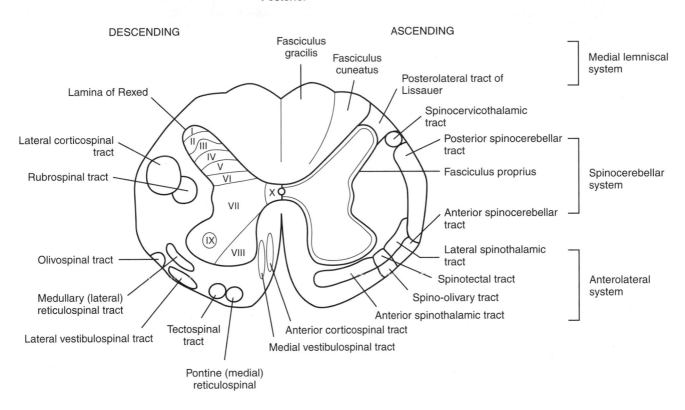

FIGURE 22-5 **Cross-Section of Spinal Cord Detailing Major Descending (Motor) and Ascending (Sensory) Tracts.**

efferent motor neurons—the final common pathway. They originate in the CNS and terminate in the muscle fibers. All nerves that influence the final common pathway are UMNs. Destruction of the LMNs results in loss of muscle tone, muscle atrophy, hyporeflexia (absent reflexes), muscle flaccidity, and fasciculations.

In summary, the primary motor tracts are located in the anterior and anterolateral portion of the spinal cord and the primary sensory tracts are located in the posterior and posterolateral section of the cord (Figure 22-5). This generalization helps provide an understanding of incomplete spinal cord syndromes.

SPINAL BLOOD SUPPLY

Branches from the terminal portion of the vertebral artery unite at the level of the foramen magnum to form the anterior spinal artery (Figure 22-6). The artery descends down the median ventral aspect of the spinal cord, supplying blood to its anterior two thirds. The remaining blood supply is provided by the two posterior spinal arteries, which descend down the posterolateral aspect of the spinal cord from their vertebral artery source. As these three vessels descend the cord, they receive additional perfusion from branches of the cervical, intercostal, lumbar, and sacral arteries. Although the venous drainage of the spinal cord may be variable, the network parallels the arterial system.[11,12]

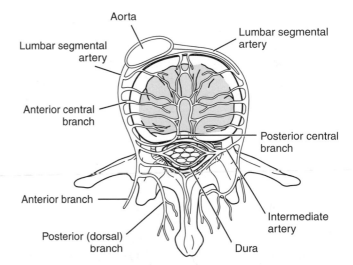

FIGURE 22-6 **Cross-Section of the Spinal Cord Demonstrating Arterial Supply.** (From Levine AM, Eismont FJ, Garfin SR et al, editors: *Spine trauma*, Philadelphia, 1998, WB Saunders, 61.)

THE AUTONOMIC NERVOUS SYSTEM

The autonomic nervous system (ANS) controls and regulates the functioning of the involuntary muscles and glands of the major body systems. It is regulated by the hypothalamus, which is located at the crossroads of the ascending and descending spinal tracts in the diencephalon. The ANS is

TABLE 22-1 Autonomic Nervous System: Effects on Various Effector Sites		
Effector Organ	Sympathetic Influence	Parasympathetic Influence
Eye		
Pupil	Dilation (mydriasis)	Constriction (miosis)
Glands		
Lacrimal	Decreased	Increased
Nasal	Decreased	Increased
Salivary	Decreased	Increased
Sweat	Increased	None
Heart	Increased rate	Decreased rate
	Increased conduction velocity	
	Increased contractility	Decreased contractility
Blood vessels		
Coronary	Vasodilation	Minimal dilation
Skeletal	Vasodilation	None
Abdominal viscera	Vasoconstriction	None
Cutaneous	Vasoconstriction	None
Blood pressure	Increased	Decreased
Lungs	Bronchodilation	Bronchoconstriction
Gastrointestinal		
Motility	Decreased peristalsis	Increased peristalsis
Sphincter	Increased tone	Relaxation
Secretions	Inhibition	Stimulation
Bladder	Decreased detrusor tone	Increased detrusor tone
Sex organs	Ejaculation	Erection
Skin		
Pilomotor muscles	Excited (contraction)	None

Modified from Guyton AC, Hall JE: *Textbook of medical physiology,* ed 9, Philadelphia, 1996, WB Saunders.

divided into two antagonistic branches: the sympathetic branch and the parasympathetic branch.

The sympathetic branch controls functions commonly referred to as the "fight or flight" response. It exits the spine in the thoracolumbar area and prepares the body to respond to stressful situations. The parasympathetic branch is responsible for energy conservation and system relaxation. The parasympathetic system, including the third, seventh, ninth, and tenth cranial nerves, exits the spine at the cervicosacral level. This information is important in understanding the systemic consequences of a spinal cord injury (Table 22-1).

MECHANISM OF INJURY

The primary mechanisms that result in spinal injury are hyperflexion, hyperextension, axial loading (vertical compression), rotation, and penetrating trauma (Figure 22-7). These can occur in isolation or in combination.

HYPERFLEXION

Hyperflexion injury occurs when a portion of the spine receives a force, direct or indirect, exerted toward the anterior surface of the vertebral body, causing flexion beyond the normal range of motion. This is often associated with head-on collisions. On impact the driver's head continues forward, and with sufficient speed and force, the weight of the head forces the chin to the chest, causing a hyperflexion injury. In hyperflexion injuries the most

flexible levels of the spine absorb this energy and act as fulcrums. This extreme force and stretch can cause a vertebral compression (wedge) fracture or intervertebral disk herniation. Ligaments also may tear, which allows the vertebrae to sublux. Subluxation of the vertebral column disrupts the continuity of the vertebral foramen, stretching and impinging on the spinal cord and altering spinal cord blood flow. Disk matter can also extrude into the vertebral foramen toward the cord.[13-16]

HYPEREXTENSION

Hyperextension injury results when there is extreme extension of the spinal column, such as in a fall, when the chin strikes an immovable object, or in a rear-end collision. Whiplash is a mild form of this mechanism. Once again the extreme force is absorbed by the flexible points of the spine, producing a stretch or tear of the anterior longitudinal ligaments, possible fracture, and subluxation of the vertebrae and rupture of the disks. If the integrity of the spinal canal is compromised, the spinal cord may be damaged. Injury also occurs when the hyperextended spinal cord is stretched excessively because of the wide arch between the posterior aspect of the head and back, causing cord contusion and ischemia.[13,15,16] Persons with preexisting conditions such as degenerative cervical stenosis are at greater risk for developing spinal cord injury as the result of hyperextension because of the presence of osteophytes and narrowing of the vertebral foramina.

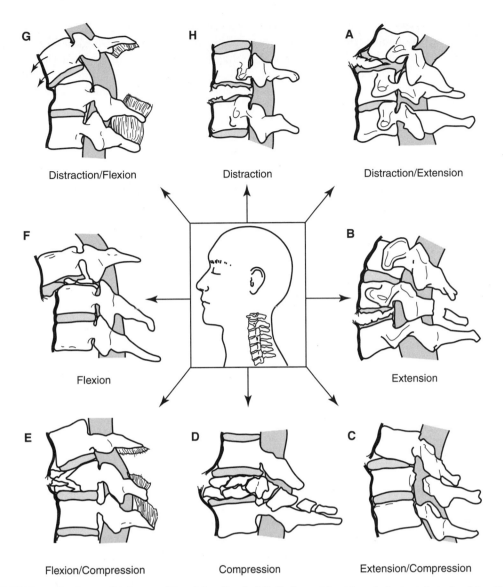

G Distraction/Flexion

H Distraction

A Distraction/Extension

F Flexion

B Extension

E Flexion/Compression

D Compression

C Extension/Compression

FIGURE 22-7 Mechanisms of Injury and Resulting Cervical Pathology. Subaxial cervical spine injuries involving C3 through C7 commonly follow a pattern. These injury patterns were developed at the University of Maryland Shock Trauma Center and incorporate the work of Allen and Ferguson. **A,** Extension injuries in the midcervical spine can cause disruption of the anterior longitudinal ligament with some posterior displacement of the superior or cephalad vertebrae on the more caudal vertebrae. **B,** When there is more forced extension, there may be fracture of the spinous process and even the lamina. This is different from the clay-shoveler's fracture, which occurs at the C7 spinous process and is thought to be an avulsion injury. **C,** A forced extension injury in which some form of fracture occurs through the facet region like an incomplete spondylolysis which is seen in a lumbar spine. Injuries represented in **A, B,** and **C,** can occur in the elderly with preexisting cervical spondylolytic stenosis. **D,** With further compression injuries, the patient typically suffers a burst fracture. **E,** A combination of flexion and compression. The vertebral body will fracture anteriorly, and there may be posterior disruption of the interspinous ligaments. Without significant canal compromise, a neurologic deficit may be absent. (Modified from Clark CR, editor: *The cervical spine,* ed 3, Philadelphia, 1998, Lippincott-Raven, 458.)

AXIAL LOADING

Axial loading, also referred to as vertical compression, occurs when sufficient force is exerted vertically through the spinal column. The vertebral bodies and intervertebral disks attempt to absorb the energy and literally burst. This is referred to as a compression or burst fracture. The concussive energy created by imploding bone sends shearing forces through the spinal cord, which it surrounds. Bone fragments and disk matter are sent in all directions, including into the spinal canal.[13,16] This injury often occurs with shallow diving and generally results in significant spinal cord injury.

ROTATIONAL INJURIES

Rotational injuries are the result of extreme lateral flexion of the head and neck. Rotational forces stretch and rupture the posterior ligaments, dislocate the facets, and often cause compression fracture of the bony structure.[13]

PENETRATING INJURIES

Penetrating injuries are classified as low velocity or high velocity. Stabbings or shootings with low-caliber handguns that actually pierce or transect the spinal cord cause low-velocity wounds. They rarely disrupt spinal column integrity and therefore are typically considered "stable" injuries. Foreign objects, such as a bullet from a high-caliber gun or shrapnel from an explosion that enters the body at great force, cause high-velocity injuries. Bony injury may or may not be present. However, the concussive forces alone are sufficient to cause spinal cord damage.[13,17]

SPINAL COLUMN INJURIES

SOFT TISSUE INJURIES

Injuries can affect the soft tissues that surround and support the spine, including the muscles, disks, and ligaments. Disk injury can compress and injure the spinal cord or nerve roots. Disruption of spinal ligaments can threaten vertebral column stability, allowing vertebrae to dislocate and injure the underlying spinal cord. *Whiplash* is a common term used to describe a hyperextension injury of the neck that causes stress and strain injury to neck ligaments and muscles.[13,18,19] Symptoms, including headache, stiff neck, neck and shoulder pain, muscle spasm, and limitation of movement, are thought to be caused by the stretching, microhemorrhage, and edema incurred by the neck muscles. The results of physical examination are usually normal except for the above symptoms, and radiologic findings are negative. Palliative treatment measures generally include mild analgesics, nonsteroidal antiinflammatory drugs (NSAIDs), heat therapy, muscle relaxants, and bedrest. In more severe cases cervical collars and traction may be employed.[13,18]

VERTEBRAL INJURIES

An easy method for understanding injuries to the vertebrae is to classify them by fracture type and location within the vertebral column. Fractures can occur in any part of the vertebrae. The fracture site and type are generally a result of the traumatic mechanism and forces sustained by the vertebral column.

SIMPLE FRACTURE.   A simple fracture is a singular break that usually occurs to the spinous or transverse process, pedicles, or facets of the vertebral arch. They are stable fractures and usually do not produce neurologic compromise. Simple fractures are usually managed conservatively.[13]

COMPRESSION FRACTURE.   Compression (wedge) fracture occurs when the anterior portion of the vertebral body becomes compressed by the force exerted on it by adjacent vertebrae. If the posterior elements remain intact, the fracture is stable. The spinal cord may or may not be spared. It is most often associated with axial loading and hyperflexion injury.[13,14]

BURST FRACTURE.   Burst fracture results from vertical forces directed onto the spinal column, which shatter the vertebral body and are frequently associated with intervertebral disk rupture. Bone fragments and disk material may be driven into the vertebral foramen, producing serious spinal cord compromise.[13,16]

TEARDROP FRACTURE.   Teardrop fracture, usually associated with a compression-flexion force, occurs when a small fragment of bone from the anterior edge of the vertebra breaks off; the fragment may be displaced into the spinal canal.[14] The bone fragment can cause spinal cord contusion or partially severed neural elements. The vertebral body may also be dislocated posteriorly. Surgical intervention is required to remove the fragment and stabilize the spine.

DISLOCATION.   Dislocation injury, a result of extreme flexion force, occurs when one vertebrae subluxates over another, often resulting in unilateral or bilateral facet dislocation. The injury is staged based on the degree of vertebral involvement (fracture and displacement) and ligamentous disruption.[14] Accompanying ligamentous injury ranges from stretch or strain to complete rupture of the stabilizing ligature.

FRACTURE-DISLOCATION.   *Fracture-dislocation* is a term used to convey the presence of a vertebral break in combination with displacement of the vertebral body. This injury is the result of shearing force in combination with another injury mechanism.[14] Fracture-dislocation injury is complex and unstable and usually involves spinal cord injury. It requires surgical fixation for stabilization.

HIGH CERVICAL FRACTURE.   The unique properties of the C1 and C2 vertebrae necessitate that separate attention be focused on injury to this area. The majority of head and neck movement is derived from the atlantoaxial relationship to the occiput. The wide range of motion in this area makes it highly susceptible to injury secondary to excessive rotation. Several unique patterns of injury and fracture have been identified.

Atlantooccipital dislocation (AOD) results when the occiput is avulsed from the atlas. Injury to the spinal cord and brainstem occur, causing this injury to be fatal in most cases. In addition to bony disruption and neural damage, impingement of the vertebral artery may occur. Surviving patients may have variable motor and sensory deficits, cranial nerve defects, and cardiopulmonary instability. Management of these injuries is directed toward immediate stabilization and reduction of the spine. Application of a halo apparatus and early fusion are recommended.[15,20]

A Jefferson fracture is the result of vertical compression of the atlas. As the vertebra absorbs the force, it is split into several parts. The fractures permit widening of the vertebral foramen, and therefore the spinal cord usually remains undamaged. However, any movement of the head can displace a fragment and sever the cord, which often results in death.

An odontoid or dens fracture (C2) is a rather common traumatic cervical injury.[14,21] It usually results from multiple mechanisms, including compression, hyperextension, extreme rotation, hyperflexion, lateral flexion, and shear forces.[21] These fractures can be classified according to location of the dens fracture (Figure 22-8). The majority of these fractures are not associated with neurologic deficit. Odontoid fractures are best visualized radiographically with lateral or open-mouth views of the cervical spine. Management is dictated by the type of fracture.

Traumatic spondylolisthesis of the axis, commonly referred to as Hangman's fracture, is characterized by fractures through the neural arch and pedicles of the axis (C2) with possible displacement of C2 on C3. Given the large vertebral foramen of the high cervical spine and because the anterior

and posterior elements generally separate, the majority of these fractures are without neurologic impingement. Treatment will vary depending on the severity of vertebral angulation, distraction, and facet dislocation. Most fractures can be treated conservatively.[22]

Spinal Cord Injuries

Injury to the spinal cord results from direct or indirect insult. When direct insult occurs, such as when a missile or bone fragment impacts the cord, the physical severing of neural elements is clear. However, in many spinal injuries the damage results from the normal physiologic response to the concussive forces.

The concept of primary and secondary injuries, first proposed more than 80 years ago, has emerged as an explanation for the phenomenon of delayed neural injury.[23-25] A primary injury is the mechanical disruption that occurs to the spinal cord substance at the time of injury whereas the progressive pathologic responses that occur subsequently are known as secondary injury. Although there is little that can be done to change the circumstances of the initial trauma, the outcome of the secondary injury may be amenable to therapeutic intervention. The intrinsic responses occurring during SCI have been well documented.[23-27] Understanding the cascade of events that ultimately lead to cellular death is key to understanding the use of investigational agents to interrupt the sequence of biochemical events and improve neurologic outcomes (Figure 22-9).

CLASSIFICATION BY TYPE OF INJURY. Types of spinal cord injury include concussion, contusion, laceration, transection, hemorrhage, and vascular disruption. A concussion

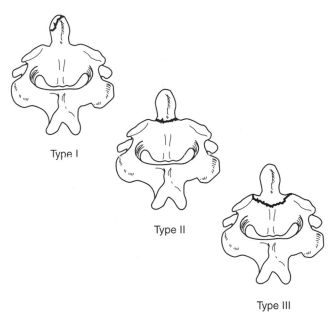

FIGURE 22-8 **Anderson and DeLonzo Classification of Odontoid Fractures.** *Type I:* fracture results from avulsion of the alar ligament. *Type II:* fractures are through the base of the odontoid separating it from the vertebral body. *Type III:* fractures occur through the C2 body.

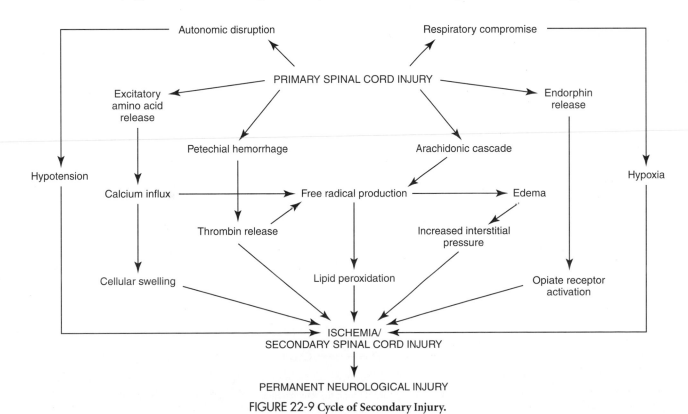

FIGURE 22-9 **Cycle of Secondary Injury.**

of the spinal cord causes a temporary loss of function lasting no more than 24 to 48 hours. It produces a transient dysfunction of the spinal cord from jarring forces. A contusion of the spinal cord is actual bruising of the neural substance. It includes the intrinsic responses to bleeding, including edema, compression, ischemia, and possibly infarction. The severity of this injury depends on its size, location, and the physiologic response to the bleeding. A laceration is an actual tear in the cord, which results in permanent injury. Surrounding contusion and the normal physiologic response to injury accompany a tear. A transection is a complete severing of the neural elements. Complete transection results in the spinal cord being physically separated into two distinct pieces; this is a rare finding. However, in functional terms, a complete transection is frequently the result of significant injury. Hemorrhage into or around the spinal cord can compress the neural substance and initiate the intrinsic cascade. This may produce ischemia and neurologic deficits. Vascular disruption to the spinal cord causes a loss of blood flow to the neural substance and results in ischemic changes. The duration of ischemia is directly related to the neurologic outcome.

CLASSIFICATION BY FUNCTION. Spinal cord injury can be classified as either complete or incomplete, according to functional outcome. In complete SCI there is loss of all voluntary muscle control and sensation at and below the level of the lesion. Clinical implications depend on the level of injury. Injuries to the cervical spine, especially at and above C4, are typically the most life threatening secondary to the potential loss of diaphragmatic innervation and respiratory failure (Figure 22-10). Functional

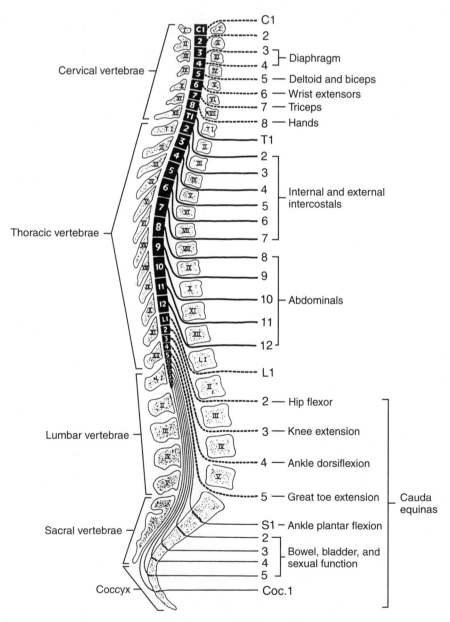

FIGURE 22-10 Spinal nerves emerging from the spinal cord through the intervertebral foramina and muscle movements that evaluate specific levels of spinal nerve function.

outcomes are covered in greater detail in the rehabilitation phase.

CLASSIFICATION BY INCOMPLETE SPINAL CORD INJURY SYNDROME.

Incomplete spinal cord injuries are distinguished by partial preservation of neurologic function below the level of the lesion. Incomplete injuries can be grouped into several recognizable syndromes.

Anterior Cord Syndrome. Anterior cord syndrome is usually associated with flexion injuries and may be associated with acute disk herniation. An injury to the anterior part of the spinal cord or interruption of blood supplied by the anterior spinal artery results in ischemia to the anterior gray horn and the anterolateral columns of the white matter. There is usually complete motor loss accompanied by a loss of pain, temperature, and touch sensation at and below the level of the lesion. There is preservation of the light touch, proprioception, and vibration senses. This syndrome is rare (Figure 22-11A).[28,29]

Central Cord Syndrome. The cardinal feature of central cord syndrome is a disproportionate loss of upper extremity motor function, especially fine motor movement, compared with to the lower extremities. This usually occurs as the result of a hyperextension injury often seen in elderly persons who have experienced degenerative changes of the cervical spine (a natural result of aging). Injury and edema occur in the center of the spinal cord. Anatomically the corticospinal tracts are arranged in such a way that the sacral fibers are most peripheral and the cervical fibers are most central. Hence when contusion occurs, there is a decrease or loss of upper motor function and a preservation of lower function[28-30] (Figure 22-11B). Varied degrees of sensory loss may accompany this syndrome.[29]

Brown-Séquard Syndrome. Brown-Séquard syndrome results from a unilateral cord lesion. Ipsilateral motor deficit and loss of light touch, proprioception, and vibration sensations occur at and below the level of the lesion. On the opposite side, below the level of injury, there is nearly complete loss of pain and temperature sensations with preserved posterior column and motor function. This injury classically is caused by penetrating trauma that partially severs the spinal cord but may also result from nonpenetrating mechanisms such as disk herniation, hyperextension injury, or unilateral articular process fracture-dislocation.[29] Partial Brown-Séquard syndrome can occur. In general, this label is applied to anyone presenting with preserved motor function and decreased sensation on one side and reduced or lost motor function and abnormal sensation on the opposite side (Figure 22-11C).

Posterior Cord Syndrome. Posterior cord syndrome is an extremely rare finding. It is associated with hyperextension injury. In its purest form only the posterior column sensory functions are lost. Patients with this syndrome generally have excellent functional recovery.

Conus Medullaris. In most people almost all of the lumbar cord segments are anatomically located opposite the T12 vertebral body. The majority of the sacral cord segments are opposite the L1 vertebral body.[29] Injuries at the T11-12 and T12-L1 levels are relatively common because of the great degree of mechanical flexibility that exists at these vertebral junctions. As a result, injuries to the conus medullaris are frequent.[29] These injuries usually produce a combination of LMN deficits, including flaccid paralysis and muscle atrophy; in the chronic phase, spasticity and hyperreflexia may occur. The sensory involvement can be variable. In severe cases bowel and bladder deficits can be significant. Patients with this type of LMN syndrome do not have a good prognosis for recovery.

Cauda Equina Lesions. Cauda equina lesions involve injuries to the spinal nerve roots, usually resulting from direct fracture-dislocation trauma. The cauda equina is composed of LMNs, which originate from the spinal cord around the L1-2 disk space. Injuries at or below this level involve the cauda equina nerve roots although spinal origins of some roots may be affected by injuries one to two levels above L1-2. Nerve roots can be involved unilaterally or bilaterally. Motor and sensory loss may occur independently or together. Because this injury involves LMN axons, which are capable of regeneration if the root is not completely transected, there exists a potential for recovery.[29]

PREHOSPITAL/RESUSCITATION PHASE

Resuscitation of the patient with a spinal cord injury begins with prehospital care and continues until the patient is diagnosed and medically stabilized and a treatment plan has been devised. The initial treatment priorities for the patient suspected of having SCI are the same as with all injured patients: (1) prevention of further injury to the patient and emergency personnel through rapid assessment of the scene and the patient; (2) initial spinal stabilization with an extrication collar; (3) extrication of the patient if necessary; (4) full systems assessment, including airway patency, ventilation, and circulation; (5) further stabilization of the spine and splinting of other fractures; and (6) transport to the nearest appropriate facility.[19,31,32]

Examination of the scene provides rescue workers with important clues about the mechanism and pattern of suspected injury. Initial assessment of the patient may be hampered by physical limitations, but a brief initial assessment of airway patency, ability to breathe, pulse, and level of consciousness and a brief gross motor exam help determine how extrication should proceed. Simply because a patient appears neurologically intact does not mean a spinal injury does not exist. Any patient who has received a force to the head should be considered at high risk for a SCI.[32]

Once the patient has been moved to a secure area, a detailed systems assessment should be performed with strict attention given first to airway patency, effectiveness of breathing, and adequacy of circulation. Evidence of airway

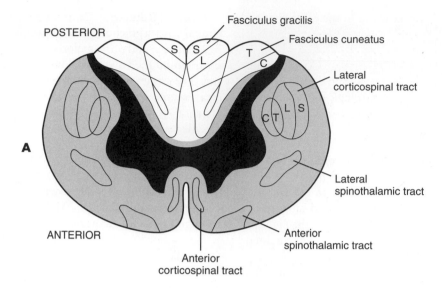

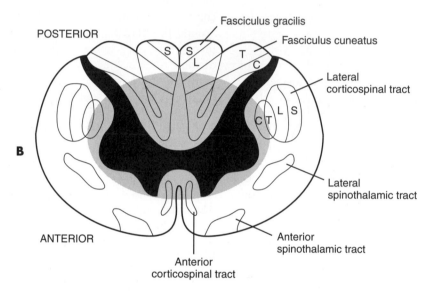

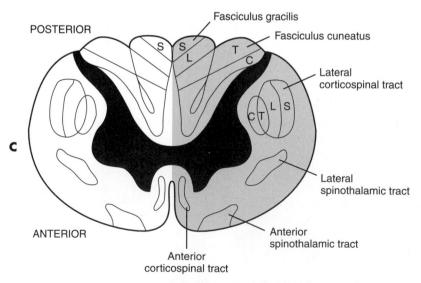

FIGURE 22-11 **Cross-Sectional Representation of the Spinal Cord Syndromes. A,** Anterior cord syndrome. **B,** Central cord syndrome. **C,** Brown-Séquard syndrome. (From Browner BD, Levine AM, Jupiter JB et al, editors: *Skeletal trauma: fractures, dislocations, ligamentous injuries,* ed 2, vol 1, Philadelphia, 1992, WB Saunders, 588.)

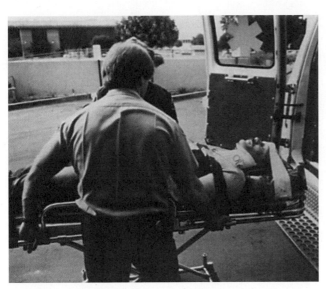

FIGURE 22-12 **Combined Use of Sandbags, Tape, and a Cervical Hard Collar for Transport.**

compromise, ineffective respiration, or inadequate circulation should be remedied immediately to prevent hypoxia, hypercapnia, or hypoperfusion, which can precipitate systemic complications and exacerbate a SCI. A brief assessment of the patient's neurologic status, including sensory and motor function, can then follow. If the suspicion of SCI is high based on examination findings or on mechanism of injury, the patient should be properly immobilized on a backboard with a hard collar, head blocks, and forehead and chin straps or taping (Figure 22-12). Finally, other body systems are evaluated carefully for evidence of injury.

Once the patient is assessed and initial stabilization is performed, the patient should be monitored closely and transported rapidly to the nearest appropriate hospital. On arrival at the hospital or trauma center, a physical systems assessment is made with attention again focusing on the airway, breathing, and circulation. Careful consideration is given to avoiding disruption of spinal alignment, which could further injure the spinal cord.

EXAMINATION OF THE SPINE AND NEUROLOGIC ASSESSMENT

Once airway patency, effective ventilation, and adequate circulation are ensured, the focus of assessment shifts to evaluation of the patient's spine and neurologic function. The patient's clothing is removed carefully and he or she is inspected for penetrating wounds or evidence of spinal injury. The patient should be log-rolled and the spinal column inspected for contusion, bulging, or obvious deformity and palpated for tenderness and malalignment.

A formal evaluation of neurologic function is performed. This examination includes motor, sensory, and reflex testing. In the unconscious or uncooperative patient, observation of movement and response to noxious sensory stimuli are the only means of ascertaining spinal cord function on physical examination. A more thorough evaluation of motor and sensory function is done if the patient is able to follow

commands reliably and can communicate sensory perceptions. A comprehensive motor and sensory evaluation should evaluate three nerve tracts: the lateral corticospinal, lateral spinothalamic, and dorsal column tracts. The lateral corticospinal (motor) tract is evaluated by having the patient move all major muscle groups on both sides of the body, beginning with the deltoids and moving downward. The strength of each movement should be graded using a 5-point scale (5 is normal and 1 is trace movement) (Figure 22-13). Assessment of proprioception, the ability to determine body position in space, evaluates dorsal column function. Proprioception is assessed by having the patient communicate if a limb or digit is being moved up or down. The lateral spinothalamic tract is evaluated by using a sterile needle to apply sharp and dull stimuli and determining if the patient can distinguish stimuli in each sensory dermatome (Figures 22-13 and 22-14). Frequent examination with the use of a consistent grading system and documentation provides practitioners with an ability to monitor improvement or deterioration of function.

Reflex function is evaluated to determine sensory or motor sparing and approximate the level of SCI. Specific nerve roots innervate each reflex. The major deep tendon reflexes (DTR) assessed are the biceps (C5-6), brachioradialis (C5-6), triceps (C7-8), quadriceps (knee jerk) (L3-4), and Achilles (S1-2). The following superficial or cutaneous reflexes should also be assessed: abdominal, cremasteric, bulbocavernosus, and superficial anal. Rectal tone should be evaluated to determine if rectal sparing is present. Priapism, a reflexive penile erection, may be noted initially in male patients with complete SCI.

Neurologic deficits and vital sign alterations caused by SCI can mask other systemic injuries. Intrathoracic, intraabdominal, and skeletal injuries may be present without the typical clinical findings of muscle rigidity or patient-reported pain. A thorough assessment, including physical assessment, x-ray examination, computed tomography (CT) scan, and other necessary diagnostic studies, should be performed as soon as possible to rule out associated injuries.[33] Hypotension and bradycardia associated with high SCI may mask signs of hemorrhagic shock. All potential sites of hemorrhage should be investigated.

DIAGNOSTICS

The most common radiologic studies performed on patients with suspected spinal trauma are plain x-ray films. The lateral view, which visualizes from the base of the occiput to the top of T1, remains the most important study for cervical spine trauma.[34-36] Trauma protocols also typically recommend obtaining anteroposterior (AP) and odontoid views to enhance the likelihood that cervical spine injury will be diagnosed. AP and lateral films are also done for the thoracic and lumbar spine. These pictures provide information about fractures, alignment, and soft tissue swelling. X-ray films can be obtained quickly at the patient's bedside, eliminating the need to transport the patient with suspected spinal injury. There are technical limitations with these films; therefore

UNIVERSITY OF MARYLAND MEDICAL SYSTEM

SPINAL CORD INJURY FLOW SHEET

Muscle Strength

5 Normal
4 Active movement through range of motion
   against resistance
3 Active movement through range of motion
   against gravity
2 Active movement through range of motion
   with gravity eliminated
1 Palpable or visible contraction
0 Total paralysis
U Unable to test strength of extremity

Rectal Tone, Proprioception, Diaphragm
P–Present   A–Absent   U–Untestable

Medication	Sensation
S—Sedation	N—Normal
PL—Paralytic	ABN—Abnormal
T—Tranquilizer	A—Absent
P—Pain	U—Untestable

MOTOR LEVEL   *Circled entry means to refer to nurses note*

Level of bony/ligamentous injury	
Anatomical Classification	
Date	
Time	
Medications	
Diaphragm (R/L)	C4
Deltoid (raise arms) (R/L)	C5
Biceps (elbow flexion) (R/L)	C5.6
Wrist extensors (R/L)	C6
Triceps (elbow extension) (R/L)	C7
Flexer digitorum profundus (finger flexion) (R/L)	C8
Hand intrinsics (finger abduction) (R/L)	T1
Iliopsoas (hip flexion) (R/L)	L2
Quadriceps (knee extension) (R/L)	L3
Tibialis anterior (dorsiflex foot) (R/L)	L4
Extensor hallucis longus (great toe extension) (R/L)	L5
Gastrocnemius (ankle plantar flexion) (R/L)	S1
Function	Level
Proprioception (finger) (R/L)	
Proprioception (toe) (R/L)	
Rectal Tone (P/A)	
Initials	
Initials/signature	

Medical Records No.

FIGURE 22-13 Spinal Cord Injury Assessment Tool.

SENSATION

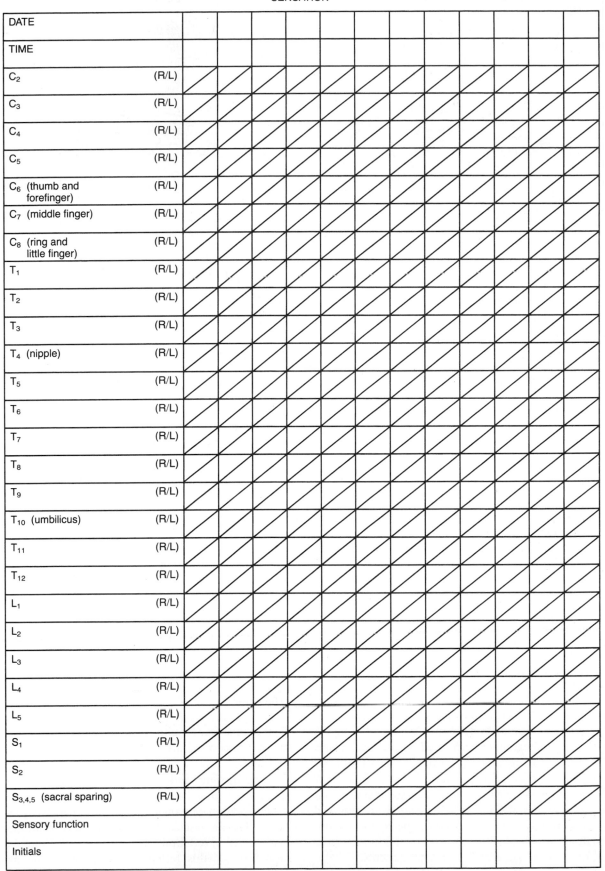

FIGURE 22-13—cont'd **For legend see previous page.**

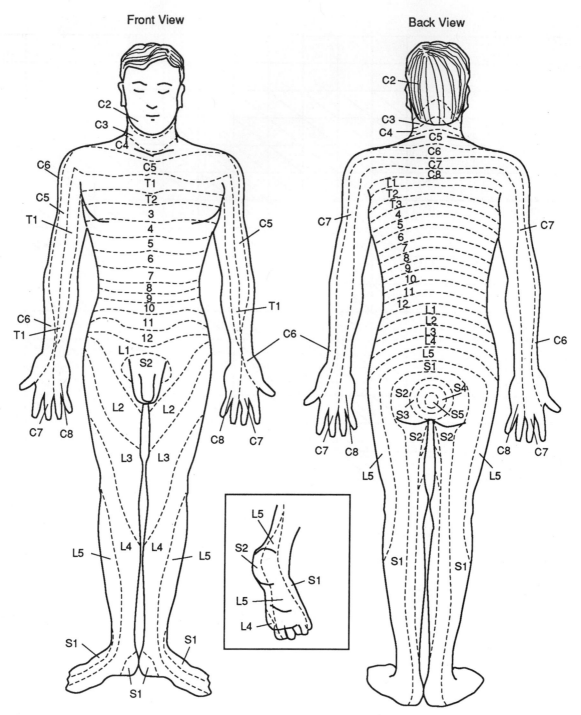

Front View

Back View

FIGURE 22-14 **Dermatomes.**

they are rarely used alone to determine the extent of injury.

Computed tomography, performed in an axial plane, provides successive horizontal views or slices at set intervals along the spinal column to provide a close look at bony structures and disk integrity. Fractures are easily visualized. The newer spiral CT scan allows rapid imaging and reconstruction into multiple planes. The speed of this examination, combined with newer portable scanning technology, has made it accessible for unstable patients.

Magnetic resonance imaging (MRI) provides clear, distinct images without the use of radiation. MRI can visual-

ize the spine from multiple planes, providing clean pictures of bony anatomy, disks, ligaments, epidural masses and hematomas, and, most importantly, the spinal cord. Changes in signal intensity provide the ability to see cord contusion, hemorrhage, or transection. The development of magnetic resonance angiography (MRA) enables physicians to visualize any vascular impingement or disruption, particularly possible vertebral artery occlusion.[36] There are many limitations of this technology. Because of the magnetic fields, many pumps and ventilators cannot be used in the scanning room. Any patient with metallic implants may not be able to enter the MRI field. Other disadvantages of MRI include high cost, longer study time, relative inaccessibility, and the inability to monitor the patient adequately within the bore of the magnet.[34,36-38] Most patients require a mild sedative to assist with overcoming the confines and noise of the scanner; any movement creates distortion of the images. If MRI is not available and vascular injury is suspected, angiography may be performed.[35] Once definitive diagnosis has been made, a plan for stabilization and management can be formulated.

Somatosensory evoked potential (SSEP) is used to assess and monitor the integrity of the somatosensory pathway from the site of peripheral nerve stimulation to the cerebral cortex. Most often the ulnar or median nerve and the posterior tibial nerve are selected for stimulation, and cortical and subcortical responses are monitored readily via noninvasive scalp electrodes. SSEP is often used for intraoperative physiologic monitoring of the spinal cord, providing "real-time" information for surgeons regarding impending neurologic damage. Baseline studies are obtained preoperatively, and monitoring continues throughout the perioperative event. Sustained reductions in values alert the surgical team to possible ischemia within the spinal cord, providing an opportunity to evaluate the patient immediately and, when possible, to take corrective action to reverse processes that may lead to permanent neurologic deficit.[39,40] SSEP monitoring is limited in that SSEPs only evaluate ascending sensory tracts, predominantly located in the dorsal columns. Selective injury to the anterior parts of the spinal cord can occur without detection.[39]

SYSTEMS MANAGEMENT

RESPIRATORY INSUFFICIENCY. If the patient is unable to maintain the airway or to breathe adequately, there is an increased risk of secondary hypoxic injury, particularly to the damaged cord. The chin-lift or jaw-thrust maneuver should be used in attempting to establish an airway in the unconscious patient with airway compromise. When possible, patients unable to maintain an airway or ventilate adequately should be intubated emergently in the field by trained emergency medical services (EMS) personnel. Every effort should be made to avoid neck movement, especially hyperextension or flexion, during intubation. Nasal intubation is often preferred for patients with unstable cervical spine injuries to avoid movement of the neck.[19,32,33] However, nasal intubation can be traumatic and technically difficult. Bleeding from traumatic intubation can further obstruct the patient's airway and lead to aspiration of blood. If oral intubation is opted for, manual traction should be applied to minimize neck motion.

When a spinal cord injury occurs at the high thoracic or cervical level, there may be paralysis of the intercostal muscles, abdominal muscles, and diaphragm, which may lead to respiratory failure. The patient should be monitored for rate, depth, and pattern of breathing (use of accessory muscles or paradoxical breathing), strength and effectiveness of cough, and the ability to oxygenate and ventilate. A chest film should be obtained to assess for underlying thoracic trauma such as rib fractures, hemothorax, pneumothorax, or pulmonary contusion, as well as aspiration or atelectasis.[32,33] Arterial blood gases (ABGs) and pulse oximetry should be monitored. In addition to these studies, tidal volume (TV) can be assessed via incentive spirometry. In most patients with a tidal volume less than 1 L, respiratory fatigue and failure can be anticipated.[41,42] In patients with poor respiratory parameters, intubation and mechanical ventilation should be implemented to prevent hypoxia and further spinal cord insult. Patients with complete injuries at C4 and above require mechanical ventilation; most of these patients will remain ventilator dependent for life.

SPINAL SHOCK. Spinal shock occurs when there is a loss of continuous tonic impulses from the brain, causing a transient suppression of reflexes below the SCI. Spinal shock is manifested as follows: (1) flaccid paralysis, (2) absence of cutaneous/proprioceptive sensation, (3) loss of autonomic function, and (4) cessation of all reflex activity below the site of injury. The degree of severity is often associated with the level of injury. Onset of spinal shock typically occurs at or near the time of injury and generally lasts a few days to weeks, depending on injury severity.[13] Spinal shock gradually resolves, which is evidenced by return of reflexes and development of spasticity below the level of SCI.

NEUROGENIC SHOCK. Neurogenic shock can be loosely defined as the cardiovascular component of spinal shock. In the acute phase of shock an abrupt loss of sympathetic innervation caused by a high thoracic or cervical SCI produces loss of vasomotor reflexes. Loss of vascular tone causes vasodilation, reducing systemic vascular resistance and lowering blood pressure. Hypotension and decreased venous return lower cardiac output and reduce tissue perfusion. Increasing IV fluid administration rarely results in a rise in central venous pressure and may lead to hypervolemia, pulmonary edema, and increased swelling of the injured spinal cord. Blood pressure is managed with judicious use of crystalloids and introduction of alpha agents, such as dopamine, to help restore vascular tone. A systolic blood pressure of 80 to 90 mm Hg is usually adequate for transport.[31] Maintaining normotension in the SCI patient, usually a mean arterial pressure of 80 mm Hg, helps provide adequate blood flow to the injured spinal cord and ensures end-organ perfusion. Placement of a central venous catheter or a pulmonary artery catheter is desirable to gain intravascular volume information and facilitate administration of vasoactive agents. A noninvasive blood pressure monitor or an arterial line should be used to provide continuous information on the patient's response to therapy.

Bradycardia, seen with high thoracic or cervical lesions, results from the inhibition of the sympathetic cardiac accelerator response and unopposed parasympathetic vagal outflow. This bradycardia may not be harmful to the patient because cardiac output is maintained through increased stroke volume secondary to decreased systemic vascular resistance (SVR). When the heart rate declines below a level sufficient to maintain adequate tissue perfusion, the patient becomes symptomatic. The patient's heart rate and rhythm should be monitored continuously. The use of alpha agents to restore vascular tone facilitates the maintenance of venous return and may provide some support for the heart rate. In cases of symptomatic bradycardia, administration of a positive chronotropic drug, such as atropine, may be necessary. In lower injuries tachycardia may develop.

TEMPERATURE REGULATION. Maintenance of normal body temperature is imperative for spinal cord-injured patients. Poikilothermia, a condition in which body temperature varies with the environment around it, is a result of the loss of sympathetic function below the level of injury. The lack of sympathetic function produces vasodilation, which promotes loss of body heat, eliminates shivering or muscle contractions to generate heat, and inactivates the sweat glands that cool the body. Many patients arrive at the hospital with hypothermia. This may further depress heart rate and cardiac function. Frequent or continuous monitoring of the patient's body temperature is advised. Gentle warming with a hyperthermia blanket and warmed intravenous fluids will help restore core body temperature. Care must be taken to prevent overwarming.

URINARY RETENTION. The abrupt disruption of the spinal cord and the onset of spinal shock renders the bladder atonic. Acute urinary retention develops. Placement of an indwelling catheter permits drainage of the bladder and monitoring of urinary output. Intermittent catheterization is generally avoided at this time because of the high urinary output that results from volume resuscitation.

SKIN INTEGRITY. Patients with suspected spinal cord injuries are transported on a rigid backboard to support the spinal elements. While conferring the desired immobility of the spine, it also produces pressure to multiple points along the spine, most specifically the sacral area. Extrication collars, designed to be an inexpensive, easily applied means for cervical immobilization, also present significant risk to skin integrity. The constant pressure coupled with the hypotensive state after injury reduces blood flow to the tissues, putting the patient at high risk for skin breakdown. Most SCI patients are insensate and unable to perceive pain and pressure below the SCI. Significant pressure sores can delay surgery if they develop in the area of surgical approach or if they become infected. It is prudent to remove the patient from the backboard as soon as possible.

PAIN AND ANXIETY. Fear may be the greatest problem for the conscious patient. Frequent verbal and physical contact with the patient to provide information and offer reassurance can reduce feelings of anxiety, fear, and helplessness. He or she should be touched in areas where sensation remains. Patient-family contact should occur as soon as feasible. Cautious use of sedation is advised to prevent impairment of sensorimotor exam, reduction of blood pressure, and depression of respiratory drive. Anxiety also heightens the pain experience.

Spinal cord-injured patients may experience bony pain from fractures, muscle and soft tissue pain, or neurogenic pain. Appropriate pain management should be implemented with the same precautions as for sedation. The use of short-acting, reversible medications is generally recommended in the emergent phase of care.

PHARMACOLOGIC INTERVENTION TO REDUCE SECONDARY SCI AND OPTIMIZE OUTCOME

Medical management of a patient with spinal cord injury is aimed at limiting secondary spinal cord injury by reducing and stabilizing the bony injury and maintaining tissue perfusion and oxygenation. Much of the treatment to optimize perfusion and oxygenation is focused on the support of other body systems. Despite much research, few drugs have been proven effective in limiting secondary injury and improving outcomes of SCI patients.

The use of methylprednisolone in acute nonpenetrating spinal cord injury has been shown to improve neurologic outcomes at 6 weeks and at 6 months after injury if administered within 8 hours of injury.[43] A later clinical trial investigating the use of methylprednisolone demonstrated that patients initiated on the steroid protocol within 3 hours of injury should receive 24 hours of therapy. Patients initiated on therapy 3 to 8 hours after injury should receive steroids for 48 hours. Patients who receive 48-hour treatment and who start treatment 3 to 8 hours after injury are more likely to improve one full neurologic grade at 6 weeks and at 6 months. It is also important to note that these same patients experience more severe sepsis and pneumonia than patients who receive methylprednisolone for only 24 hours.[44] (Table 22-2 describes guidelines for this protocol.) Glucocorticoids such as methylprednisolone have multiple theoretic effects, including suppression of vasogenic edema, enhancement of spinal cord blood flow, stabilization of lysosomal membranes, inhibition of pituitary endorphin release, alteration of electrolyte concentrations in injured tissue, and attenuation of the inflammatory response.[23,24,26,27,44] It is postulated that most of their beneficial effects are derived from the antioxidant capacity of these agents, which inhibit lipid peroxidation and cell membrane destruction.[23,24,26,27]

Other pharmacologic agents targeting various points in the cycle of secondary injury/ischemia have also been investigated to determine their effectiveness for treatment of SCI. One class of drugs showing promise is the 21-aminosteroids, or lazeroids. One lazeroid, tirilazad, has been studied extensively. It scavenges lipid peroxyl and superoxide radicals and inhibits lipid peroxidation. In clinical evaluation tirilazad was given for 48 hours in conjunction with a bolus of methylprednisolone. Results

TABLE 22-2 Guidelines for Methylprednisolone Treatment

Loading dose:

$$\frac{30 \text{ mg/kg} \times (\text{pt weight in kg})}{(\text{mg/ml based on drip concentration})} = \text{Total bolus dosage (ml)}$$

Set infusion pump to deliver total bolus in 15 minutes, followed by a maintenance infusion of normal saline for 45 minutes. Then proceed with maintenance infusion.

Maintenance dose:

$$\frac{5.4 \text{ mg/kg} \times (\text{pt weight in kg})}{(\text{mg/ml based on drip concentration})} = \frac{\text{Maintenance dosage}}{\text{per hour (ml)}^*}$$

Set infusion pump to deliver hourly maintenance dose for 23 to 47 hours.†

NOTE: Reconstitute methylprednisolone in sterile water to a concentration of 50 mg/ml.

*If drug infusion is inadvertently stopped, new flow rates are calculated so that the remaining drug can be administered within the remaining time of the originally planned infusion schedule.

†Treatment initiated within 3 hours of injury delivers a total of 24 hours of therapy; treatment initiated within 3 to 8 hours postinjury delivers a total of 48 hours of therapy.

demonstrated similar outcomes to the group treated with only methylprednisolone for 24 hours. However, because an initial bolus of methylprednisolone was given, it is not possible to make conclusive statements about the role of tirilazad in the treatment of SCI.[44] Other agents under investigation that may interrupt the cycle of secondary injury are opiate antagonists, excitatory amino acid (EAA) receptor antagonists, calcium channel blockers, antioxidants and free radical scavengers, and arachidonic acid inhibitors. Although these agents provide theoretic benefit, there is no clinical evidence that they improve neurologic outcomes in humans with SCI.

Research also has been focused on attempting to identify pharmacologic agents that promote neurologic regeneration. GM-1 ganglioside, which augments and promotes neural outgrowth, plasticity, and synaptic transmission, has demonstrated enhanced recovery of white matter tracts to the lower extremities. This finding suggests that the agent improved the function of axons traversing the injury site but had no effect on the gray matter at the level of injury.[23,26,45] To date, there is no research that support routine use of ganglioside in the management of SCI.

In addition to gangliosides, other drugs have been studied in regard to neural regeneration. Historically, it has been held that injured CNS tissue did not possess the ability to regenerate. It now appears that many therapeutic interventions can promote crucial aspects of outgrowth, guidance, target recognition, and synaptic stabilization in the laboratory setting. Research is currently focused on Schwann cell, stem cell, and astrocyte transplantation and the application of exogenous growth factors. Although these approaches have not been effective in humans, they demonstrate that neural regrowth is a realistic goal for the future.[23-25]

SPINAL COLUMN ALIGNMENT AND STABILIZATION

A plan for spinal realignment, decompression, and stabilization is established as soon as possible once the diagnostic evaluation of the spinal column and cord is complete. Injuries may require surgical or nonsurgical intervention to decompress, realign, and stabilize the spine. The choice of surgical intervention versus conservative nonoperative management is controversial and is determined in part by physician preference. Most physicians base their treatment decision on the mechanism of injury, the neurologic status, the structural dysfunction of the spine, and the patient's medical history and current condition.

The "hard" neck collar is usually maintained on patients throughout resuscitation and until a cervical spine injury is ruled out or stabilized in another way. In patients with an unstable cervical spine injury, cervical traction may be applied to assist in immobilizing the spine, realigning the vertebrae, and relieving spinal cord compression. This can be accomplished with application of Crutchfield or Gardner-Wells Tongs (Figure 22-15) or a halo ring. Weight is added gently and steadily, in 5-lb increments, to the in-line traction with sequential neurologic exam and radiologic evaluation. Radiologic evaluation may be performed either by lateral radiography after each manipulation or with the use of the C-arm fluoroscope to prevent overdistraction or worsening of alignment.[22,32] Once reduction and alignment are achieved, the weights are reduced to the minimal amount necessary to maintain alignment and stability. A wedge turning frame (Figure 22-16) or kinetic bed (Figure 22-17) may be employed to permit pressure relief and prevent pulmonary complications while maintaining spinal immobility. Care must be taken to maintain the cervical traction by keeping the weights hanging freely and the traction rope knot away from the traction pulley. If necessary, the patient can be pulled down in bed by several people but can never be pulled up because traction would be lost.

For lower injuries, various types of braces can be used eventually. Until the brace is applied, the patient is typically maintained on bedrest with the head of the bed flat. If the patient cannot be log rolled, a specialty bed such as a wedge turning frame or a kinetic bed should be considered for mobilization.

Patients can be transported while maintaining spinal alignment by using the scoop or breakaway stretcher. This device separates into two halves that can be slid beneath the patient being log rolled side to side. The two sides connect at the head and feet to form a complete lifting device. Patients in cervical traction can be transported by having the

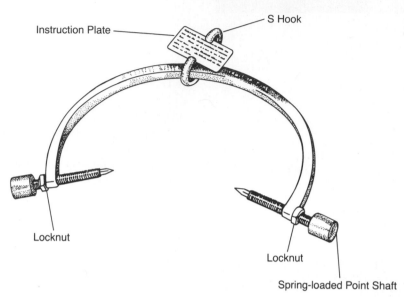

FIGURE 22-15 **Gardner-Wells Tongs.**

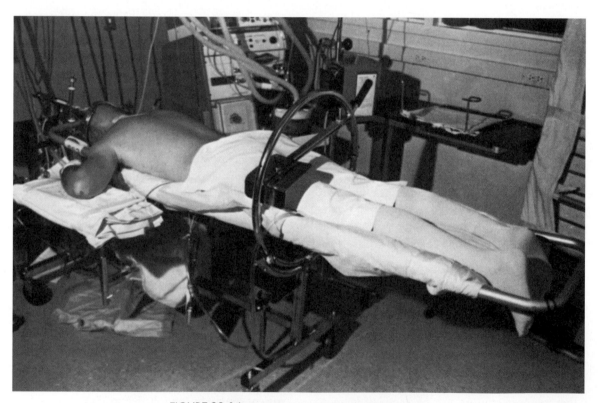

FIGURE 22-16 **The Stryker® Wedge Turning Frame.**

physician maintain manual traction while log rolling the patient onto an in-line traction board and connecting him or her to the traction weights or a traction wheel.

The timing of surgical intervention is controversial.[46-50] When it is not possible to reduce the spine with traction, further intervention is required to realign the spinal column and restore blood flow to the injured cord. There exists a window of opportunity to safely reduce a patient within the first 72 hours after injury. After this period, the window closes because the spinal cord is extremely refractory to any manipulation because of edema and circulatory changes. The window opens again after 7 days. Early intervention (within the first 72 hours) might improve neurologic recovery, facilitate early mobilization to reduce complication

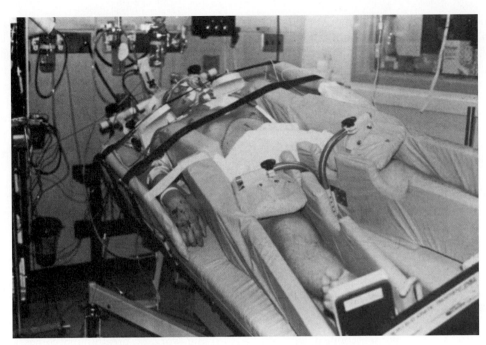

FIGURE 22-17 The Rotorest® Kinetic Therapy Bed.

rates, decrease hospitalization time, and lower overall costs.[47,48] A clear candidate for emergent surgical intervention is the patient with neurologic deterioration who displays evidence of spinal cord compression from bone or disk fragments, vertebral malalignment, or hematoma.[16,32,48] Advocates of delayed surgery argue that early operative intervention may increase the risk of neurologic deterioration or cause cardiopulmonary instability that compromises recovery. They also point out that early fixation failed to demonstrate improved overall outcomes in initial trials and may be prohibited by the lack of necessary resources at the admitting hospital.[46,49,50]

THE OPERATIVE PHASE

The goals of surgical intervention are to decompress the spinal cord, align and stabilize the bony column, and promote early mobilization. This may be accomplished through the removal of bone fragments, hematoma, or extruded disk matter; vertebral realignment; and spinal fusion. Placement of a bone graft to maintain disk spacing in conjunction with the use of instrumentation such as plates, screws, wires, cables, or rods may be necessary to maintain alignment and stability until the vertebral column fuses. External orthotic devices such as a collar, halo vest, or thoracolumbar jacket may be employed as adjunctive treatment to promote increased fusion rates.

Care of the spinal cord-injured patient in the operative phase is the same as for any patient. Strict attention is given to respiratory, hemodynamic, body temperature, and neurologic responses. Adequate respiratory gas exchange must be ensured throughout the operative phase. Hemoglobin and hematocrit levels should be monitored during and after surgery. This is especially true for patients undergoing thoracic and lumbar procedures that are likely to involve large volumes of blood loss. Succinylcholine is avoided as part of balanced anesthesia in SCI patients because it may cause dangerous elevations in serum potassium levels.[51] Postoperative sensorimotor evaluations and follow-up x-ray films are performed to detect any changes from the preoperative assessment findings.

THE CRITICAL CARE PHASE

Once the injury has been diagnosed and stabilized and a plan of care has been developed, the patient is transferred to the intensive care unit for further systems management. The patient with acute SCI should be approached as a multi-trauma patient because injury to the central nervous system affects all body systems. The goal of care is to prevent further secondary injury and neurologic deterioration. Prevention, prompt recognition, and appropriate treatment of systemic complications reduce the risk of secondary SCI and help optimize patient outcomes. These goals are best met with the use of a multidisciplinary team approach that includes physicians; nurses; respiratory, physical, occupational, and speech therapists; nutritionists; and social workers.

RESPIRATORY IMPLICATIONS

Injuries to the cervical or thoracic spinal cord may affect innervation of the diaphragm (C3-5), the internal intercostals (T1-11), the external intercostals (T1-11), and the abdominal muscles (T7-12).[42,52] In normal respiration the inspiratory phase is an active process in which the diaphragm contracts and descends, increasing the vertical diameter of the thoracic cavity. The external intercostals elevate the ribs, causing an increase in the lateral and anteroposterior diameter. These events produce a negative pressure gradient, drawing air into the lungs. Expiration is usually passive unless a defensive process such as a cough or sneeze is required. During forced expiration the abdominal muscles contract, driving the diaphragm upward and causing the internal intercostals to contract. In a spinal cord-injured patient paralysis of these muscles dramatically alters the mechanics of respiration, reducing inspiratory and expiratory flow. If the intercostals are involved, chest wall mobility is impaired. The loss of abdominal muscle innervation eliminates function of the major "defense" muscles needed for coughing or sneezing. Lack of abdominal muscle function also alters the position of the diaphragm because of the loss of viscera support. The dropping of the diaphragm produced by a loss of abdominal tone lowers the diaphragm, reducing diaphragmatic excursion and decreasing the patient's inspiratory capacity. Forced exhalation and cough are reduced dramatically. Once spinal shock has resolved, spasticity develops in the abdominal and thoracic muscles. This increased tone helps stabilize respiratory mechanics although forced expiration and cough remain weak.[41,53] The reduction in ventilatory volumes coupled with the increased work of breathing predispose the SCI patient to significant pulmonary complications. These complications—atelectasis, pneumonia, and respiratory failure—remain the leading causes of mortality and morbidity after acute SCI.[8,41,53,54] Promoting optimal respiratory function and preventing pulmonary complications are primary goals for the patient with acute SCI.

COMPLICATIONS. The acutely injured individual is at risk for many pulmonary complications. At the time of injury the patient is at risk for aspiration and subsequent pneumonia. Placement of an artificial airway and secretion retention further increases risk for pneumonia. The use of steroid therapy to reduce spinal edema can worsen the resulting pneumonia. Swelling of injured paraspinal soft tissues may threaten airway patency. Pulmonary edema from excessive fluid infusion is always a threat during resuscitation. The presence of neurogenic shock, pneumonia, or aspiration may trigger the onset of adult respiratory distress syndrome (ARDS). Alterations in respiratory mechanics and immobility put SCI patients at high risk for the development of significant atelectasis. Immobility and decreased venous return also put them at risk of a deep venous thrombosis (DVT) and pulmonary embolism (PE). The critical care nurse must make pulmonary management a top priority to prevent life-threatening complications that can impair respiratory gas exchange and exacerbate secondary SCI. Respiratory complications also can delay surgery for spinal fixation, prolonging immobilization and increasing the length of hospitalization.

Patients should be monitored vigilantly by paying strict attention to respiratory rate and pattern, work of breathing, evidence of fatigue, respiratory gas exchange, and breath sounds. Patients with cervical and high thoracic injuries exhibit a paradoxic breathing pattern as a result of the loss of intercostal muscle function. On inspiration, as the diaphragm descends, the paralyzed muscles of the rib cage passively collapse; they reexpand as the diaphragm rises on exhalation. The use of accessory muscles is commonplace. Resting respiratory rates and work of breathing tend to be higher in patients with SCI. Serial pulmonary function tests, which may include measures of vital capacity, inspiratory and expiratory reserve volumes, functional residual capacity, residual volume, tidal volume, and negative inspiratory pressure, that demonstrate worsening trends provide evidence of respiratory muscle fatigue or an ascending spinal cord lesion. In the patient with a natural airway vital capacity can be measured through incentive spirometry. If the vital capacity is less than 800 ml, mechanical ventilation may be necessary. Pulse oximetry and routine assessment of arterial blood gases should be performed to monitor Pao_2 and Pco_2. Patients with cervical and high thoracic injuries are prone to develop mild hypercarbia. Auscultation of all lung fields can detect secretion retention and early signs of atelectasis, pneumonia, or consolidation. Routine chest films can provide additional evidence of pathologic pulmonary conditions.

If the work of breathing becomes laborious and the patient demonstrates fatigue, intubation and mechanical ventilation may be required. Patients with cervical or high thoracic SCI have very little respiratory reserve. Expending a large amount of energy to breathe means that a great deal of energy also is required to clear secretions. If the energy for breathing cannot be redirected for use in respiratory defense, the patient tires, suggesting a need for mechanical ventilation. In one study the use of biphasic positive airway pressure (BiPAP) was investigated as an alternative to intubation and was found to be an effective means of assisting the SCI patient in recruiting alveoli, reducing the work of breathing, and improving oxygen saturation.[55]

Aggressive pulmonary toilet is essential to prevent and treat pulmonary complications.[41,43] Studies done using a spinal cord-injured population have demonstrated that postural drainage and percussion are effective methods to clear secretions, resolve atelectasis, and increase oxygenation.[41] Endotracheal suctioning can effectively remove secretions from intubated patients. Bronchoscopy may be necessary to remove retained secretions and open atelectatic airways when routine suctioning, postural drainage, and chest physiotherapy (CPT) prove to be insufficient. Patients with a weak cough and who have a natural airway or are intubated but stable enough to participate in pulmonary toilet should use an assistive cough technique. The patient is instructed to take three breaths; on the expiratory phase of the third breath, the nurse places the heel of the hand halfway between the patient's umbilicus and xiphoid process and thrusts in and upward while the patient coughs. Performed correctly, this can be an effective means of clearing secretions. Many patients can be instructed to perform this procedure on themselves. Increasing mobility reduces the patient's risk for posterior pooling of secretions and the development of lower lobe atelectasis and pneumonia. Whenever possible, patients should be repositioned at least once every 2 hours. Use of a Stryker or wedge turning frame (see Figure 22-16) or kinetic therapy bed (see Figure

22-17) provides greater mobility for the patient in cervical traction or with lower spine instability.

When a person with SCI sits in an upright position, the weakened or paralyzed abdominal muscles permit the abdominal contents to relax forward, pulling the diaphragm downward. Use of an abdominal binder to support the viscera can assist the patient's breathing by bringing the diaphragm into a better resting position.[41,43,52] Proper placement of the binder is important to prevent impingement of chest movement. The binder should be placed below the costal margin and extend over the iliac crests bilaterally. The lower portion of the binder should be tighter than the section running along the floating ribs.

Many patients with cervical spine injuries require mechanical ventilation. Patients with complete injuries at C3 and higher will likely remain ventilator dependent. Other patients may require prolonged mechanical ventilation until respiratory muscles can be strengthened and pulmonary complications resolve. Early tracheostomy is desirable for these patients to reduce anatomic dead space, decrease the discomfort of prolonged intubation, and facilitate communication. A weaning strategy should be devised by the multidisciplinary team caring for the patient to promote strengthening of the respiratory muscles and provide time for psychologic separation from the ventilator. Many different methods of weaning have been used, most of which are based on a work-rest principle.[41,43] The ventilator is placed on a setting that requires a phase of active respiration, during which time the patient experiences increased breathing work and then is permitted a rest period to garner energy and prevent diaphragmatic fatigue. The work phase is slowly lengthened until the patient is off the ventilator completely. Weaning can be a long process, often extending into the intermediate cycle of care. When the tracheostomy is no longer required, the patient can be decannulated.

CARDIOVASCULAR IMPLICATIONS

HYPOTENSION. Decreased systemic blood pressure caused by loss of sympathetic outflow typically remains problematic in the critical care phase. Continued use of vasopressor agents such as dopamine or phenylephrine hydrochloride (neosynephrine) produces vasoconstriction of the vessels, improving venous return and augmenting blood pressure. Although controversial, a "hemodynamic push," maintaining a mean blood pressure of 75 to 85 mm Hg, often is continued for 3 to 5 days to ensure adequate perfusion of the spinal cord and other body organs.[56-58] If not placed during resuscitation, invasive hemodynamic monitoring lines may be inserted during the critical care phase to assist with ongoing assessment and treatment of neurogenic shock. A central venous pressure (CVP) or pulmonary artery catheter can help guide vasoactive administration and fluid replacement. Placement of an arterial line provides constant blood pressure assessment to guide titration of vasopressors and an ability to easily access serum for laboratory analysis. A SCI patient is always at risk for orthostatic hypotension, but ultimately the body resets its internal parameters to perfuse at a lower pressure.

As with any critically injured patient, maintenance of cardiovascular function to ensure adequate tissue perfusion is of utmost importance. Close monitoring of the patient's hemodynamic parameters provides information helpful in guiding management decisions. Ensuring adequate filling pressures, heart rate and rhythm, blood pressure, and cardiac output promotes optimal end-organ perfusion. Monitoring intake, output, and laboratory values to ensure fluid and electrolyte balance assists in the maintenance of proper intravascular volume and cardiac function.

Venous pooling and dependent edema are other consequences of altered vascular tone. Application of pneumatic calf pumps promotes venous return and reduces the risk of deep vein thrombosis. Introduction of prophylactic heparin or low-molecular-weight heparin is appropriate once risk of any hemorrhage has been ruled out.

BRADYCARDIA. Bradycardia resulting from sympathetic blockade can also persist into the critical care phase. In addition to bradycardia, other arrhythmias may occur, such as junctional escape beats, atrioventricular blocks, and premature atrial or ventricular complexes.[59] It is also important to remain cognizant of the effects of hypothermia and hypoxia on heart rate and rhythm. For patients with symptomatic bradycardia, atropine should be given as needed. Vasopressor agents also provide some heart rate support. In profound cases temporary pacing may be necessary.

VASOVAGAL RESPONSE. In addition to baseline bradycardia, many patients experience a vasovagal response. The unopposed parasympathetic flow causes cardiac arrest. This response can be stimulated by a number of patient or nursing actions, including sudden position changes, coughing, gagging, and suctioning. Strategies to reduce the occurrence of this response are to change the patient's position slowly and to induce hyperoxygenation before suctioning. Symptomatic events can be treated by administration of atropine or, in some cases, use of a temporary pacer.

GASTROINTESTINAL IMPLICATIONS

The gastrointestinal system is disrupted by loss of sympathetic nervous system innervation, resulting in autonomic nervous system imbalance. Initially, most patients experience a loss of intestinal motility (adynamic ileus). Acute abdominal distention resulting from the paralytic ileus may harbor a large volume of third space fluid and can further inhibit respiratory function. This condition rarely lasts longer than 2 to 5 days. A gastric tube should be placed for decompression, and displaced intravascular volume should be replaced as necessary.[60,61]

Gastritis, esophagitis, and gastrointestinal ulcers with associated hemorrhage can occur secondary to stress, unopposed vagal outflow, steroid administration, and relative intestinal ischemia.[60-62] Patients should receive routine gastric prophylaxis with histamine blockers, antacids, mucosal protective agents (sulcrafate), or proton pump inhibitors. A gastric tube should be placed for stomach decompression and gastric aspirate should be monitored for presence of occult blood or abnormal pH. Hemoglobin, hematocrit, blood urea nitrogen (BUN), and creatinine should also be monitored.

Pancreatic dysfunction can occur in the SCI patient.[61] Serum amylase should be monitored, especially with the start of low-dose enteral feedings. If the amylase concentration rises as feedings are increased, the patient's oral intake should be restricted (NPO) and hyperalimentation provided until serum amylase levels return to normal.

Every effort should be made to meet the nutritional requirements of the patient with appropriate parenteral or enteral nutrition. Initiation of early enteral feeding is important to maintain gastrointestinal integrity and provide nutritional support. Early enteral feeding also may help reduce septic complications, decrease the hypermetabolic response to critical injury, improve wound healing, and maintain intestinal immunologic defenses.[63-65] Patients with cervical spine injuries may experience a delay in gastric emptying. Placement of a transpyloric tube is recommended to facilitate enteral feeding if gastric intolerance occurs.[60] Before initiating oral feedings for a patient with a high SCI, a swallowing evaluation is often recommended.

Constipation can occur as a result of reduced gastrointes-tinal motility, narcotic and sedative use, and immobility. Occasionally this may create a bowel obstruction. A bowel routine including stool softeners and stimulant cathartic suppositories (e.g., bisacodyl [Dulcolax]) should be implemented as soon as possible to assist with regular bowel emptying.[60,61]

STABILIZATION DEVICES

Spinal orthoses are used to protect the injured or unstable spine by controlling the position and limiting the mobility of the spine or segment of the spine. Spinal motion can be loosely categorized as flexion-extension, lateral bending, or rotation and is quantified by degrees.[66] Different orthoses restrict spinal motions in different ways and to varying degrees.[67] A brace is chosen according to location of injury, desired function, and specific treatment goals. Braces are categorized by the spinal segments involved. These categories are cervical orthoses (CO), head cervical orthoses (HCO), cervical thoracic orthoses (CTO), thoracolumbosacral orthoses (TLSO), lumbosacral orthoses (LSO), and cervical thoracolumbosacral orthoses (CTLSO). Construct (rigid, semirigid, or flexible) and indication (corrective or supportive) can further stratify these categories (Figure 22-18).

Skin breakdown, loss of spinal alignment, pain, weaken-

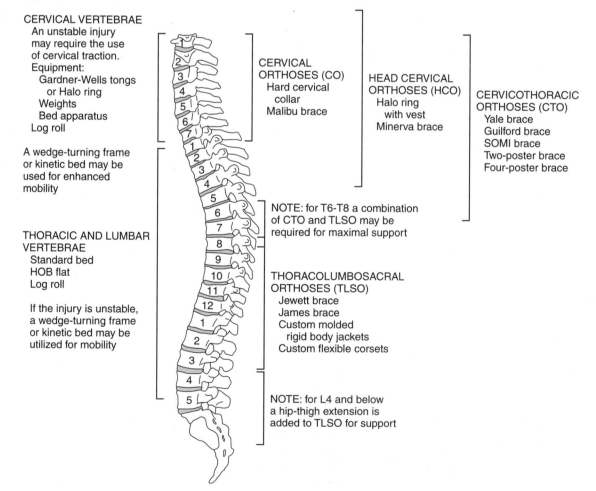

FIGURE 22-18 **Spinal Immobilization Devices.**

ing of immobilized muscles, soft tissue contractures, restriction of pulmonary excursion, and increased lower extremity venous pressure, which can produce varicosities and dependent edema, are all potential complications of spinal orthoses.[66] Proper brace fit and meticulous skin care beneath the brace are essential to maintain skin integrity. Two people are required to perform skin care. The patient is placed flat while the anterior portion of the brace is removed. The patient should be instructed to avoid movement while the brace is open. Skin is cleansed with soap and water and dried thoroughly. A light dusting of powder or cornstarch is applied. Lotion, which creates a moisture layer, is avoided. The skin is inspected for redness or breakdown. To perform back care, the anterior shell is reapplied, the patient is log rolled, and care is performed with one person stabilizing the patient and the anterior shell. Patients and their families must be educated on the proper application and fit of a brace, cleaning the brace, skin care, proper body mechanics, and appropriate exercises for reducing the deconditioning effects of the brace.

Care of the patient in a halo vest (Figure 22-19) demands special focus. The halo vest is opened at the thoracic belts only, one side at a time. Skin beneath the vest should be well cleaned and dried while the thoracic straps are open. Replacement pads or sheepskins are available, which can be

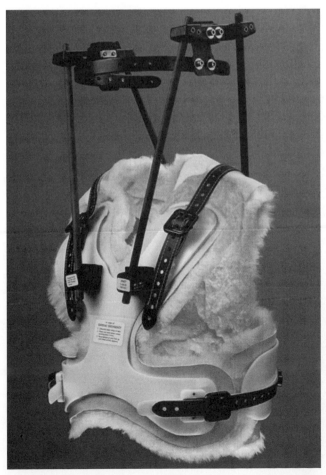

FIGURE 22-19 **Halo Vest.** (Courtesy PMT Corporation, Chanhassen, Minn)

rolled into and out of the vest for washing. A wrench should be kept secured to the chest plate of the vest for emergency vest removal. The skeletal traction pin insertion sites should be regularly cleansed and monitored closely for symptoms of infection. Grabbing or pulling on the support rods to position the patient or to adjust the brace fit must be avoided.

PAIN

Pain is also an issue in the acute phase of injury, and for many patients it remains a chronic issue. Individuals may experience bony pain associated with fracture or use of skeletal traction, soft tissue and muscular pain associated with acute injury, and neurogenic pain associated with CNS trauma. Associated injuries involving areas where sensation is intact also contribute to the pain experienced by the patient. The nurse must assess carefully the patient's pain and collaborate with the physician to determine the appropriate pharmacologic intervention. If available, consultation with a pain management service to assess and coordinate pain control facilitates care.

PSYCHOSOCIAL IMPLICATIONS

Acute spinal cord injury is devastating and overwhelming for the patient and the family. Because of the sudden nature of the injury, there is no time for the patient to prepare for the event. Fear and anxiety are the primary emotions seen in the critical phase of care. Interventions should be aimed at providing reassurance and assisting patients to reassert control over their situation and environment. Initially, many patients are too ill to comprehend the long-term consequences of their injury; they exist in a state of denial, functioning only in the present. Immediate gratification of needs is desired. Early implementation of a daily schedule and development of a stable team of care providers can help to establish trust. A means of communication should be established as soon as possible so that the patient can relay needs and ventilate feelings. This can be accomplished with a blink board, a picture board, an artificial larynx, a Passy-Muir valve, or other strategies. Specialized call bells should be available for the patient to use to summon the nurse. If no other alert mechanism is established, the patient may resort to "clicking" (moving the tongue and mouth to create a clicking sound) to draw the attention of caregivers. Nurses must set limits on the patient to prevent excessive clicking. The nurse should reach an agreement with the patient on when clicking is appropriate. It is imperative that when a patient uses the call bell or clicks, someone responds. This develops trust in the caregivers and decreases the patient's fears and anxiety, which ultimately reduces the frequency of calling or clicking.

It is not unreasonable to use pharmacologic interventions in the initial stages of injury to calm the patient and prevent panic attacks. Excessive anxiety resulting in flailing can cause patients to accidentally disrupt their spinal alignment. Hyperventilation caused by anxiety can hamper the patient's pulmonary status.

It is also important to regulate the patient's sleep cycle.

TABLE 22-3   Functional Goals for Spinal Cord–Injured Patients

Spinal Cord Level	Muscle Function	Functional Goals
C3-4	Neck control Scapular elevators	Manipulate electric wheelchair with mouth stick Limited self-feedings with ball bearing feeders Dress upper trunk Turn self in bed with arm slings Dependent bowel and bladder
C5	Fair to good shoulder control Good elbow flexion	Propel wheelchair with handrim projections Self-feeding with handsplint Assist getting to and from bed Dependent bowel and bladder
C6	Good shoulder control Wrist extension Supinators	Transfer from wheelchair to bed and car with or without minimal assistance Self-feeding with tenodesis hands Assist getting to and from commode chair Assistance with bladder Driving with adapted van
C7	Weak shoulder depression Weak elbow extension Some hand function	Independent in transfer to bed, car, and toilet Total dressing independence Wheelchair without handrim projections Self-feeding with no assistance devices Independent with bowel and bladder Driving car with hand controls or adapted van
C8-T4	Good to normal upper extremity muscle function	Wheelchair to floor and return Wheelchair up and down curb Wheelchair to tub and return
T5-L2	Partial to good trunk stability	Total wheelchair independence Limited ambulation with bilateral long leg braces and crutches
L3-L4	All trunk-pelvic stabilizers intact Hip flexors Adductors Quadriceps	Ambulation with short leg braces with or without crutches, depending on level
L5	Hip extensors, abductors, knee flexors, ankle control	No equipment needs if plantar flexion is enough for push off at end of stance

Modified from Boston University School of Nursing.

Sleep deprivation is a constant threat in the critical care environment. Measures should be taken to maintain a day-night cycle for patients and to allow for REM sleep. Sleep deprivation can make the patient's pain management more difficult and reduce the patient's ability to cope with the stress caused by the injury.

Families also must be involved with patients' care from the beginning. Patient and family education about SCI begins on admission and continues through rehabilitation. It is often necessary to share information repeatedly for the patient and family to assimilate it. Health care providers should also assist the patient and family in identifying and using support systems and appropriate coping mechanisms.

INTERMEDIATE CARE AND REHABILITATION PHASES

After definitive spinal treatment has been rendered and body systems are stabilized, the patient enters the intermediate and rehabilitation phases of care. During this time the patient is at risk for late complications of SCI related to alterations in body functions caused by interruption of sympathetic outflow and immobility. The goals of intermediate and rehabilitation care are to prevent complications,

enhance physical strength, relearn activities of daily living (ADLs) (Table 22-3), and regain emotional stability. When these goals are met, the outcome potential of the patient with an SCI is optimized, and return to the "outside" world is more likely to be successful.

Patient goals are achieved best through a multidisciplinary team approach. The care team evaluates patients to determine the best means to achieve these goals. The SCI patient is often evaluated using the American Spinal Injury Association (ASIA) standards to determine level and completeness of injury which assists in setting realistic functional goals (Table 22-4). The functional independence measure (FIM) is useful in evaluating the patient's functional outcome (Table 22-5).[68]

CARDIOVASCULAR IMPLICATIONS

AUTONOMIC DYSREFLEXIA.   Once spinal shock has resolved, patients sustaining an SCI at the T6 level or above are at risk for autonomic dysreflexia (AD). AD is an uncontrolled, massive sympathetic reflex response to noxious stimuli below the level of the lesion. Common stimuli precipitating AD include a full bladder, distended bowel, or skin irritation (e.g., decubitus ulcer). The irritant stimulates

TABLE 22-4 ASIA Impairment Scale Used in Grading Degree of Sensory and Motor Impairment

Grade		Description	
☐	A	Complete	No sensory or motor function is preserved in sacral segments S4-S5.
☐	B	Incomplete	Sensory but not motor function is preserved below the neurologic level and includes sacral segments S4-S5.
☐	C	Incomplete	Motor function is preserved below the neurologic level, and more than half of key muscles below the neurologic level have a muscle grade less than 3.
☐	D	Incomplete	Motor function is preserved below the neurologic level, and at least half of key muscles below the neurologic level have a muscle grade greater than or equal to 3.
☐	E	Normal	Sensory and motor functions are normal.

Clinical Syndromes

- ☐ Central cord
- ☐ Brown-Séquard
- ☐ Anterior cord
- ☐ Conus medullaris
- ☐ Cauda equina

From American Spinal Injury Association: *International standards for neurological classification of spinal cord injury*, Chicago, 1992, American Spinal Injury Association.

TABLE 22-5 Functional Independence Measure Scale

Independent

7 Complete independence. The activity is typically performed safely, without modification, assistive devices or aids, and within reasonable time.

6 Modified independence. The activity requires an assistive device, more than reasonable time, or is not performed safely.

Modified Dependence

5 Supervision or setup. No physical assistance is needed, but cuing, coaxing, or setup is required.

4 Minimal contact assistance. Subject requires no more than touching and expends 75% or more of the effort required in the activity.

3 Moderate assistance. Subject requires more than touching and expends 50%-75% of the effort required in the activity.

Dependent

2 Maximal assistance. Subject expends 25%-50% of the effort required in the activity.

1 Total assistance. Subject expends 0%-25% of the effort required in the activity.

The functional independence measure (FIM) focuses on six areas of function: self-care, sphincter control, mobility, locomotion, communication, and social cognition. The FIM total score (summed across all items) estimates the cost of disability in terms of safety issues and of dependence on others and on technical devices. (From State University of New York at Buffalo, the Center for Functional Assessment Research: *Guide for the uniform data set for medical rehabilitation (adult FIM)*, version 4.0, Buffalo, NY, 1993, Uniform Data System for Medical Rehabilitation.)

the sympathetic nervous system below the injury, resulting in severe vasoconstriction below the level of the SCI lesion. Pallor, chills, goosebumps, and cool skin are evident below the injury level. Blood volume is shunted into the nonconstricted vessels above the lesion, causing hypertension. Baroreceptors in the carotid arteries and aortic arch respond to the hypertension by sending a message to the higher vasomotor centers in the brain. These centers send messages to the heart, causing reflexive slowing, and to the blood vessels, resulting in vasodilation. Unfortunately, these messages cannot go beyond the level of the lesion; thus vasodilation occurs only above the level of injury, producing facial flushing, nasal congestion, and a pounding headache. If left untreated, hypertension can lead to myocardial infarction or cerebrovascular accident. This syndrome is potentially life threatening to the SCI patient.[67,69,70]

Nursing interventions should be aimed at preventing stimuli that might trigger the onset of AD. If AD does occur, the first step in care is to sit the patient upright to cause orthostatic hypotension. The patient's blood pressure should be monitored every 5 minutes during the crisis. The next step is to identify and remove the offensive stimulus. The bladder should be palpated for distention and immediate catheterization performed. If a catheter is in place, any obstruction of urine outflow should be alleviated immediately. Next, a digital rectal examination should be performed, using an anesthetic ointment, to assess for

impaction. If the abdomen is distended and no impaction is noted in the rectum, a laxative should be administered. Clothing should be loosened and any adaptive splints removed. If these measures fail to resolve the problem, hypertensive management (e.g., hydralazine hydrochloride, diazoxide) should be initiated.[67,69] The use of α-adrenergic blockers such as terazosin has successfully prevented symptoms in patients who experience recurrent AD in the absence of acute predisposing factors.[71] Although AD is likely to be most severe in the first 6 to 12 months after SCI, it remains a lifelong potential complication. Patients and families must be educated about the symptoms and treatment of AD.

DEEP VENOUS THROMBOSIS. Any immobilized patient is at risk for deep venous thrombosis (DVT) formation. The SCI population may be at slightly higher risk as a result of venous pooling, decreased venous return, hypercoagulability from injury-induced stimulation of thrombogenic factors, and possible presence of a vessel injury.[72-74] The greatest risk to the patient appears to be within the first 2 weeks after injury.[54,72,73] Clinical features of DVT, such as extremity swelling, pain, or mottling when dependent, can be obscured by the normal physical response to spinal injury. The nurse should remain vigilant for signs of increased lower extremity girth, redness or warmth, and elevation in body temperature, which may indicate DVT. Diagnosis can be made with duplex ultrasonography of the lower extremities. Lower extremity DVT and pelvic thrombosis also can be detected with a venogram.

Prevention is the key to DVT management. Current clinical practice guidelines for prophylaxis recommended by the Consortium for Spinal Cord Medicine include the use of pneumatic compression devices for the first 2 weeks after injury and prophylactic anticoagulation with heparin or low-molecular-weight (LMW) heparin until discharge from a rehabilitation center. Patients with clinical contraindications for anticoagulation or those who have failed prophylaxis should have a vena cava filter placed.[72,75,76] Range-of-motion exercises, early mobilization, and adequate hydration also may reduce the risk of DVT formation. If DVT is detected, full anticoagulation is initiated unless contraindicated. Patients and their families should receive education on the signs, symptoms, risk factors, and prevention of DVT.

ORTHOSTATIC HYPOTENSION.   Orthostasis or postural hypotension occurs as a result of venous pooling in the lower extremities. Patients with SCI above T7 are particularly vulnerable to this complication. Symptoms include a decrease in blood pressure, possibly an increased heart rate, dizziness or lightheadedness, blurred vision, and even loss of consciousness when the patient assumes an upright position. Treatment of orthostasis is generally successful with conservative measures. Gradual elevation of the head of the bed, application of an abdominal binder, compression of the lower extremities with antiembolism stockings or ace wraps when out of bed, and maintenance of hydration are interventions that can reduce postural hypotension.[54,67,77] If these measures fail, administration of salt tablets to promote volume expansion may be helpful. In severe cases administration of a mineralocorticoid, such as fludrocortisone (Florinef), to promote salt and water retention may be effective.[78] The use of sympathomimetics such as pseudoephedrine or ephedrine may elevate blood pressure and reduce postural hypotension.[54,67] A recent study by Sampson et al[79] employing functional electrical stimulation to the lower extremities demonstrated an increase in blood pressure, which may be useful in treating orthostatic hypotension.

GASTROINTESTINAL IMPLICATIONS

Altered bowel elimination is an issue for most spinal cord-injured individuals throughout the course of their lives. The level of injury dictates the type of alteration in bowel elimination the patient experiences. Cervical or thoracic injury is associated with spastic paralysis and an inability to feel the urge to defecate, although the reflex activity for defecation remains intact. With an injury to the sacral cord segments in the conus medullaris or cauda equina, the reflex center for defecation is destroyed, and

there is a loss of anal tone. Fecal retention and oozing of stool through the flaccid anal sphincter are associated with this type of lower motor neuron injury.

Constipation and impaction are common complications for patients with SCI. Constipation and fecal impaction are also linked to abdominal distention, pain, and the precipitation of autonomic dysreflexia.[80-82] It is important to initiate bowel training as soon as possible. Consistency is the cornerstone to a successful program. A fiber-rich diet, adequate fluid intake, exercise, and a combination of medications (stool softeners, stimulant cathartic suppositories, and small-volume enemas) all aid in bowel evacuation.[61,83] Harsh laxatives are avoided to prevent unpredictable time of defecation and diarrhea leading to incontinence. Digital stimulation is helpful to initiate defecation in patients with cervical or thoracic injury. It is ineffective in patients with a lesion of the sacral cord segments that has resulted in loss of the anorectal reflex. If patients with a cervical or thoracic injury become impacted, they are at significant risk for autonomic dysreflexia. An anesthetic lubricant should be used to reduce initiation of dysreflexia if manual disimpaction is necessary.

Gall bladder disease is another complication that has an increased incidence after spinal cord injury. The most frequent cause of emergency abdominal surgery in spinal cord-injured persons is cholecystitis or cholelithiasis. It is postulated that the causes may be abnormal gall bladder motility, abnormal enterohepatic circulation, and altered intestinal motility leading to abnormal biliary secretion.[61] Classic clinical signs of gall bladder disease such as a rigid abdomen, tenderness, and peritoneal rebound are often absent in patients with midthoracic and higher spinal cord lesions, leading to a delayed diagnosis. Referred shoulder tip pain, anorexia, nausea, vomiting, increased spasticity, and autonomic dysreflexia are the most important indications of gall bladder disease in patients with high SCI.[84]

GENITOURINARY IMPLICATIONS

Voiding results from a series of events that culminate in the micturition reflex. Normal micturition involves coordination among the bladder, the internal and external sphincters, micturition control centers in the brain, and the autonomic nervous system. Sympathetic innervation to the bladder, carried by the hypogastric nerves, whose cell bodies lie in the T11-12 cord segments, produces relaxation of the bladder body and narrowing of the bladder neck. Parasympathetic nervous system innervation occurs via the pelvic nerves, which enter and exit the spine at the S2-4 spinal segments. The parasympathetic nervous system facilitates bladder emptying through contraction of the detrusor muscle and relaxation of the internal sphincter. The external sphincter is innervated by the somatic nervous system via the pudendal nerves, whose cell bodies arise from the sacral cord segments (S2-4). Stimulation of the pudendal nerves produces tightening of the external sphincter. This permits bladder filling and inhibition of urination.[67,85]

Stretch receptors in the urethra and bladder walls are

stimulated when the bladder is full. Afferent fibers conduct signals via the pelvic nerves to the sacral area of the spinal cord, and an efferent response is sent back via the parasympathetic nervous system to the bladder. This causes contractions of the detrusor muscles of the bladder and concomitant relaxation of the internal and external sphincters. The pelvic musculature begins to relax, the abdominal muscles and diaphragm contract as the glottis closes to increase intraabdominal pressure, urine flows into the urethra, and voiding begins. When voiding is complete, reflexive and voluntary closure of the sphincters occurs and the bladder relaxes.[67]

SCI above the level of the conus causes uninhibited, involuntary contraction of the detrusor muscle, resulting in spontaneous voiding, which can occur at abnormally low bladder volumes (reflexive neurogenic bladder). If the SCI occurs in the area of the sacral plexus (conus medullaris or cauda equina), the bladder and sphincter are denervated and urinary retention with overflow voiding occurs (areflexic neurogenic bladder).

The bladder and lower urinary tract are rendered flaccid by the state of spinal shock. Initial bladder management during spinal shock requires an indwelling catheter. After the critical phase and when systems have stabilized and spinal shock has resolved, the patient is ready for a bladder program. Major management considerations should include gender, functional level of injury, age, body habitus, motivation, and lifestyle.[86] Intermittent catheterization, associated with fewer complications than indwelling catheterization, is generally the best method for long-term management.[67,85-88] To begin bladder training, the patient is placed on a 2000 to 2400 ml/day fluid restriction in an attempt to limit the volume of urine produced to approximately 500 to 600 ml every 4 to 6 hours. This volume should be adequate to maintain hydration and bladder flushing while preventing repetitive distention, which can damage the bladder wall.[87] Patients are taught to perform regular palpation of the suprapubic area to assess for bladder fullness. In male patients with reflexive voiding, an external condom catheter can be used. As spontaneous reflexive voiding develops, it is important to perform intermittent catheterizations to assess postvoid residuals. Urodynamic studies also help to assess intravesical pressures. If postvoid residual bladder volumes exceed 75 to 100 ml or intravesical pressures are high (>60 cm H_2O in males and >30 cm H_2O in females), intermittent catheterizations should continue to be employed.[86,88] Suprapubic tapping can be employed to elicit reflexive voiding. Reflexive voiding is often considered an inadequate means of management for females because there is a lack of appropriate external appliances. If an indwelling catheter is selected for long-term drainage, a suprapubic catheter is placed to avoid the complications associated with transurethral placement. Suprapubic catheters are associated with infection, leakage, and recurrent bladder stones.[85,87,88] Patients with a suprapubic catheter are encouraged to increase their fluid intake to up to 4 L/day to maintain bladder flushing. Many new surgical procedures have been developed to assist patients in obtaining continence. Continent conduits, augmentation cystoplasty, and sphincter prostheses are options that are gaining favor.[67,85,86]

A long-term complication of reflexive bladder is detrusor sphincter dyssynergia (DSD). DSD is the result of a loss of coordination between the bladder and the external sphincter. As the bladder reflexively contracts in response to fullness, the external sphincter also contracts, prohibiting release of urine. DSD is associated with elevated voiding pressures, which can cause vesicourethral reflux and hydronephrosis. Annual urodynamic evaluation should be performed to monitor for high bladder pressures and sequelae. Pharmaceutical management includes the use of α_1-adrenergic blockers (e.g., prazosin, terazosin) to reduce bladder outlet resistance, antispasmodic agents (e.g., dantrolene, baclofen) to reduce external sphincter spasticity, and anticholinergic agents (e.g., propantheline bromide) to relax the detrusor muscle and lower bladder pressures. Historically, oxybutynin (Ditropan) was used to balance bladder function. Recent studies have shown this drug to be ineffective, and it may even aggravate the dyssynergia by facilitating neurotransmission to the sphincter.[87] Surgical intervention (sphincterotomy) for external sphincter spasticity is usually delayed for at least a year to evaluate for spontaneous recovery of bladder contraction and external sphincter coordination and is used only when conservative treatment fails.[86,88]

Conus and cauda equina injuries result in the bladder being insensate and hypocontractile or noncontractile (areflexic). Patients may void by using Valsalva's maneuver or manual bladder compression (Credé's maneuver). Loss of reflexive muscle tone can produce urinary incontinence. External collection devices such as condom catheters for males or incontinence pads for women are employed. Maintenance of skin integrity is important with the use of these products. Condom catheters must be changed at least once a day to prevent a buildup of bacteria and promote airflow to the penile tissues. Intermittent catheterization is usually reserved for patients with elevated postvoid residuals. Female patients present unique problems. They frequently experience breakdown of perineal tissue from incontinence, and intermittent catheterization can be technically difficult. Many women are managed with indwelling catheters. Surgical procedures such as the continent conduit provide women with more options for urinary management.

URINARY TRACT INFECTION. Urinary tract infections (UTIs) are the most common complication for SCI patients in the first year after injury. Every effort should be made to prevent UTIs by removing indwelling bladder catheters as soon as possible and ensuring adequate bladder emptying. Patients must be educated about the signs and symptoms of an acute UTI, which include fever; spontaneous voiding between catheterizations; autonomic dysreflexia; hematuria; cloudy, foul-smelling urine; vague abdominal discomfort; and pyuria. It is important to recognize that patients with neurogenic bladder dysfunction usually present with persistent bacteriuria. Bacteriuria in absence of clinical symptoms represents colonization. To reduce the risks of suprainfection and antibiotic-resistant bacteria, antibiotic treatment is typically not indicated in the asymptomatic patient.[86,88,89] UTI implies microbial invasion of any tissues of the urinary tract.[89] UTIs are treated with appropriate antibiotics and increased fluids. Repetitive infections may indicate other urologic problems such as renal calculi or improper lower urinary tract management. Further evaluation through renal ultrasound and urodynamic studies is recommended if other urologic problems are suspected.[86]

URINARY TRACT CALCULI.   The presence of urine bacteria and sediment, long-term indwelling catheters, urinary stasis, and chronic calcium loss that occurs after SCI predispose patients to the formation of urinary tract calculi. Approximately 8% to 15% of SCI patients develop renal calculi.[61,88] Calculi should be suspected in the presence of persistent UTI, hematuria, or unexplained AD. A definitive diagnosis is reached through diagnostic studies (e.g., kidney/ureter/bladder [KUB] x-ray films, intravenous pyelogram [IVP], or cystogram) or with passage of a stone. Treatment modalities are based on the size and location of the stone. Patients prone to develop stones should modify their diet and increase their fluid intake to dilute and flush the urinary tract.

SKIN IMPLICATIONS

Immobility, loss of sensation, incontinence of stool and urine, spasticity, use of adaptive splints and braces, edema, hypotension, and poor nutrition are factors that contribute to the development of skin breakdown in SCI patients.[90,91] A pressure sore can delay surgery, prolong immobilization, increase hospital stay, and increase the risk of AD. The most common site for pressure sore development is the sacrum. Other common locations are the heels, trochanteric areas, occiput (especially when cervical collars are worn), and ischium.[91,92] The best treatment for pressure sores is prevention. Use of a pressure-relieving mattress in conjunction with log rolling every 2 hours during bedrest will help reduce skin breakdown risk. Ensuring proper fit of braces or splints and providing good skin care beneath these devices help preserve skin integrity. The nurse should routinely inspect bony prominences and skin under splints and braces. Nutritional support to maintain healthy tissues is essential. Once the patient can be mobilized, it is imperative that the right chair (i.e., a high-back wheelchair) be used with a pressure-relieving cushion. While the patient is in the chair, weight-shifting or pressure release maneuvers should be performed every 20 minutes by the patient or nurse. Pressure release maneuvers consist of tilting the wheelchair back for 5 minutes, leaning sideways, and lifting the hip for a few minutes or performing a pushup on the arms of the wheelchair. Patients and family members should be instructed how to perform these maneuvers.

Once a pressure sore occurs, treatment is based on its location, size, and depth. The stage and measurement of the wound should be assessed routinely and documented.[90] Consulting wound care specialists, such as enterostomal therapists, assists in developing a program of wound and skin care. Frequent inspection, pressure relief, cleansing, debridement, and protection of the wound should continue during healing.[90] If the wound has significant depth, surgical intervention may be required. In cases that require significant surgical intervention the patient requires full pressure relief from the area involved. A fluid therapy bed can provide this relief if the physician determines that the patient's spinal stability can tolerate the lack of support offered by this type of bed. If this option is employed, nurses must be vigilant in performing range-of-motion exercises to prevent contractures. The nurse must recognize the emotional impact of prolonged immobilization and hospitalization. Various therapies and family members should be involved in assisting the patient to attain some rehabilitation goals while waiting for breakdown to heal.

MUSCULOSKELETAL IMPLICATIONS

Spinal cord injury has significant ramifications for the musculoskeletal system. Depending on the type and level of injury to the spinal cord, flaccidity, paresis, or spasticity may result. In severe injury, as spinal shock resolves, reflexes return and spasticity develops below the level of injury. A loss of muscle innervation, leading to a shortening of muscle fibers, imbalance of opposing muscle group strength, and immobility of joints, predisposes patients to the development of contractures. Also complicating matters is the potential development of heterotopic ossification.

SPASTICITY.   The pathophysiology of spasticity is not clearly understood. The "gamma release" hypothesis states that descending inhibitory influences on gamma motor neurons are interrupted and, in turn, become highly sensitive to local and supraspinal facilitory influences (vestibulospinal, reticulospinal, corticorubrospinal, and pyramidal corticospinal tract facilitation). Delwaide's "presynaptic inhibition" hypothesis states that Ia interneurons (responsible for changes in muscle length) are the prime source of inhibition and that spasticity is produced by removing facilitation of Ia interneurons. Over time, increased spinal reflex excitability can be attributed to intrinsic changes in the cord.[93-95]

Two distinct patterns of muscle spasm often occur: flexor patterning and extensor patterning. In flexor pattern the major limb flexors contract, drawing the limb toward the body. In extensor pattern the extensor muscles contract, resulting in rigid extension of the limbs. The pattern of spasm a patient experiences may be related to the stimulus received and the position of the limb at the time of stimulation. The patterns may also alternate.

Spasticity can have positive and negative effects. Increased muscle tone can reduce venous pooling, stabilize the thoracic musculature used in respiration, and assist patients in dressing and stand-pivot transfers.[94,95] Detrimental effects of spasticity have been linked to chronic pain syndrome, joint contracture, heterotopic ossification, and skin breakdown.[94,95] Assessing resistance to passive motion of an

TABLE 22-6	**Modified Ashworth Scale***
Grade	Description
0	No increase in tone
1	Slight increase in tone, giving a "catch" and release or minimal resistance at the end of the range-of-motion (ROM) when the affected part is moved in flexion or extension
1+	Slight increase in tone, giving a "catch" followed by minimal resistance throughout the remaining ROM
2	More marked increase in tone, but limb easily flexed
3	Considerable increase in tone, passive movement difficult
4	Limb rigid in flexion or extension

*Modified from Bohannon RW, Smith MB: Interrater reliability of a modified Ashworth Scale of Muscle Spasticity, *Phys Ther* 67(2):206-207, 1987.

affected extremity evaluates spasticity. The Modified Ashworth Scale is one of several methods that have been developed to quantify spasticity in terms of degree of tone and frequency of event (Table 22-6). Most important to the evaluation of spasticity is the patient's perception of its impact on quality of life.[96]

The goals of spasticity management are to decrease muscle tone that interferes with function, retain joint range of motion, and relieve associated pain. These goals are best achieved with a multidisciplinary approach. Treatment of spasticity usually begins with range-of-motion exercises, positioning techniques, weight-bearing exercises, and orthoses or splinting.[94,95] If these conservative interventions fail to provide adequate relief, pharmacologic agents can be introduced. The major inhibitory neurotransmitter in the spinal cord is believed to be γ-aminobutyric acid (GABA). Agents such as baclofen and benzodiazepines are able to potentiate GABA and have been used successfully to reduce spasticity. Recent trials with two α_2-adrenergic agonists, clonidine and tizanidine, have demonstrated their potential to reduce spasticity, especially when used in conjunction with baclofen.[97,98] There also has been some limited success with the use of gabapentin.[96] Intrathecal delivery of antispasmodic medications via implantable pump has revolutionized the management of severe SCI spasticity. This route maximizes CSF concentrations of antispasmodics, reducing the required dosage and side effects.[98-100] Injection therapy using Botulism toxin and phenol has demonstrated promising results for regional control of spasticity.[94] In severe cases that fail to respond to conservative physical and pharmacologic intervention, surgical interventions are considered. Surgical interventions tend to be drastic measures that involve severing of neural elements to prevent spasm. Given the direction of neural regeneration research, surgery should be used only for the most desperate cases.

HETEROTOPIC OSSIFICATION. Heterotopic ossification (HO) is the deposition of ectopic bone within connective tissue. The cause of this complication is unclear. It occurs below the level of spinal cord injury, the most common site being the anterior aspect of the hips.[101,102] The incidence is higher in patients with neurologically complete injuries, especially those with spasticity. The classic clinical presentation of HO includes swelling, warmth, redness and painful or reduced range of motion of the affected area, and fever.[101,102] Differential diagnosis is made by bone scan. Treatment of HO in the early phases consists of aggressive range-of-motion exercises and mobilization of the patient. Treatment to reduce spasticity may be of value. Pharmacologic management consists of etidronate disodium (Didronel) to reduce ectopic bone formation.[101,103] Etidronate disodium is contraindicated in patients with actively healing fractures because it prevents ossification of the fractured bone. Nonsteroidal antiinflammatory agents may help alleviate inflammation and pain.[104] In extreme cases surgical intervention to restore joint mobility may be required once the area of ectopic bone formation has matured.[101,104,105]

CONTRACTURES. Joint contractures can occur within 1 week of injury. Imbalance of muscle innervation that occurs with paralysis causes certain muscle groups to become stronger than their opposing muscle group. This produces a shortening of the stronger, contracted muscle fibers. Additional risk factors for the development of joint contractures include high level of spine injury, presence of a pressure ulcer, concomitant head injury, spasticity, HO, and extremity fracture.[106] Aggressive range-of-motion exercises assist in preservation of joint movement. Antispasmodic medications to reduce tone may facilitate maintenance of joint range. Early introduction of physical and occupational therapy in conjunction with patient and family education on range-of-motion exercises, positioning, and the use of splints can combat the development of contractures.[106,107] Serial casting with weekly removal for skin assessment and further limb mobility may help reverse a contracting joint. Caution must be taken to avoid forcing joint range of motion so that bone fracture does not occur.

IMPROVING MOBILITY

Loss of upper extremity function is a severe problem for tetraplegic patients because it threatens their ability to be independent. Orthoses and surgical reconstruction play an important role in the rehabilitation of the upper extremity. New techniques in functional electrical stimulation (FES) have shown tremendous promise in restoration of function.

The goals of surgical reconstruction are to restore active elbow extension and single handgrip. This is accomplished by muscle tendon transfer. Selection for surgical reconstruction is dependent on existing motor and sensory function. Surgical intervention is usually not performed for at least 1 year after injury. This provides adequate time for neurologic recovery to plateau, for spasticity of the extremity to become static, and for the patient to progress in adjustment to the psychologic ramifications of injury.[108]

FES is the electrical stimulation of a muscle to provide a specific movement or function of the extremity. The muscles can be stimulated by surface electrodes placed on the skin or by surgically-implanted electrodes. Prerequisites for successful use of FES include control of spasticity, adequate seated balance, nearly full range of motion of the affected extremity, and intact LMN.[109] FES systems can be used to facilitate upright positioning, augment walking, and allow finger movement. Surface systems can be difficult to apply and remove, cumbersome for the patient to wear, and cosmetically unattractive. Surgically implantable systems may be superior for long-term use.[109]

SEXUAL FUNCTION

Spinal cord-injured patients have the same sexual desires as any other person. The goal of sexual rehabilitation in the SCI patient is the same as any other rehabilitative goal—to assess residual capacity and attempt to maximize posttraumatic potential. Perhaps the greatest obstacle to achieving this goal lies in the myths that society has created surrounding sex and sexual fulfillment. Phrases such as "able-bodied" or "less of a man or woman" embody the attitude that permeates society, equating physical capabilities with the ability to attain sexual satisfaction. Sexual intimacy has become synonymous with the physical act of intercourse.[110] With the overwhelming changes in body image and self-concept coupled with the fear of rejection, it is not surprising for patients with SCI to experience an initial reduction in libido.[111] Sexual counseling to explore attitudes, history, experience, and options should be offered early in rehabilitation. Sexual experimentation is necessary to discover new ways for the individual to please and be pleasured.[110,112]

The normal physiologic response centers that control sexual behavior and the conscious experience of pleasure are located in the brain. These higher centers integrate afferent input from the genitals; skin; auditory, visual, and gustatory centers; and psychogenic or fantasy information.[111] In people with SCI there is a break in afferent information from below the level of injury to the brain; however, sensory input from above the injury remains intact. The physical act of intercourse remains possible for most individuals. Female patients, though they lack innervation of the pelvic floor muscles, maintain reflex lubrication and congestion.[112-114] For men the ability to have and maintain an erection and to ejaculate is a significant issue. Both sympathetic innervation and parasympathetic innervation are involved in these processes. Erection is a function of the parasympathetic nervous system. In men with intact sacral reflexes, obtaining an erection is possible.[112,115] The problem is that the duration tends to be short. The treatment of erectile dysfunction can be managed with technical aides (rings or vacuum pumps), pharmacologic agents (intracavernous injection), or penile prosthesis.[111,112,115-117] Ejaculation, a function of the sympathetic nervous system, is an issue when fertility is considered. Most spinal cord-injured men will not experience reflex ejaculation. At present, three methods for artificial ejaculation are available: intrathecal drug injection, electroejaculation, and vibroejaculation. Caution must be used to prevent eliciting AD when stimulating the genitals. Spinal cord-injured men tend to have poor sperm quality; serial ejaculation may improve sperm motility.[117] In vitro fertilization has been a very successful method for spinal cord-injured men to father a child. For women fertility is generally not an issue and conception is possible. Pregnancy and delivery may be complicated by increases in blood pressure, inability to sense contractions, and possible precipitation of AD during labor.[118] Close monitoring and good prenatal care and planning help prevent these complications.

CHRONIC PAIN AND DEPRESSION

Chronic pain is a significant issue for SCI patients. Multiple studies investigating the prevalence of chronic pain in SCI have found rates of 40% to 46%.[119-121] Chronic pain limits patients' ability to perform activities of daily living (ADLs), which diminishes quality of life and increases depression. Pain can be separated loosely into two categories: nonneurologic and neurogenic.[119,122,123] Nonneurologic or nociceptive pain is caused by noxious stimuli to the normally innervated body parts. Neurogenic pain is related to injury of the nerve tissue in the central or peripheral nervous system. The perception of pain and its severity is influenced by many factors, particularly depression and adjustment disorders.[120] In patients with cervical injury, there is a high incidence of shoulder pain. This chronic shoulder pain is exacerbated by excessive use in ADLs and wheelchair locomotion. Range-of-motion exercises, shoulder strengthening exercises, massage, local application of heat or cold, and the use of muscle relaxants and analgesics generally help to manage this pain. Electrical stimulation (transcutaneous electrical nerve stimulator [TENS] and functional electrical stimulator [FES]) may effectively reduce nociceptive pain.[122,123]

Neurogenic pain can be more difficult to treat. Rarely can a specific cause be pinpointed other than the trauma to nerve tissue. Anticonvulsants such as carbamazepine (Tegretol) and gabapentin and antidepressant/tricyclic compounds such as amitriptyline have been used with varying success. In extreme cases implantable intrathecal pumps with narcotic infusion have been used. Destructive surgical procedures to control chronic pain after SCI have largely been abandoned.[122,123]

In cases where depression is a precipitating factor, counseling or cognitive behavior therapy can be of value. Studies by Summers[124] and Lundqvist[125] demonstrate that pain causes psychologic distress and reduces quality of life. Pain also reduces the ability to cope with severe impairment, producing even greater emotional distress and depression. Given the life-altering nature of SCI, individuals are at risk of developing feelings of powerlessness. This despondency can easily develop into clinical depression. The Consortium for Spinal Cord Medicine has developed clinical practice guidelines to assist primary providers in screening and treating this disorder. Routine screening done by the physician interviewing the patient and family focuses on identifying the general risk factors; specific risk factors; and biologic, social, and psychologic risk factors.[126] Once this information is compiled and depression is suspected, the patient should be referred to an appropriate mental health provider. A comprehensive treatment plan that delineates the responsibility of the primary care provider and mental health provider should be developed and articulated. This plan should provide patient and family education and counseling, appropriate pharmacologic intervention, and development of a supportive environment and social system.[126] The treatment plan should be evaluated with a focus on revitalizing the patient and restoring him or her to an optimal level of well-being and functioning. It is also important to monitor the coping ability of the family. Often family members are also the primary caretakers and are just as vulnerable to feelings of inadequacy and helplessness.

NEUROLOGIC IMPLICATIONS

POSTTRAUMATIC SYRINGOMYELIA. Posttraumatic syringomyelia (PTS) is a relatively late-occurring complication of SCI. A syrinx, a fluid-filled cavity within the spinal cord, may develop within a few months to decades after SCI.[128] It has been detected clinically in 0.3% to 3.4% of patients and on MRI in up to 22% of patients. This complication is seen more often in paraplegics than in tetraplegics.[127-130] The etiology of PTS development is not well understood. Common to all theories of pathogenesis is the loss of spinal cord substance and subsequent formation of a cystic cavity within the parenchyma of the spinal cord. The most common symptom of PTS is pain, usually described as a dull ache that increases with straining, coughing, or sneezing.[130] Additional symptoms include ascending sensory loss, motor weakness, and changes in spasticity.[67,70,127-129] Autonomic symptoms such as increased sweating and hypertension may also occur. The earliest clinical sign is loss of deep tendon reflexes.[67,70,127-130] Definitive diagnosis is made through clinical exam and MRI.

Management of PTS is as controversial as the theories surrounding its development. The advent of MRI technology has increased the accuracy of imaging, permitting surgeons to detect cavitation within the cord, measure size and length, monitor progression over time, and monitor surgical decompression.[128-130] The goal of surgical intervention is to reduce pain and to prevent further neurologic deterioration. Surgical intervention to drain the cavity has had unreliable success rates and exposes patients to the risk of further neurologic insult.[129]

Decompression techniques include laminectomy with subarachnoid space reconstruction, primary drainage, and use of shunts. In most patients surgery decreases pain and reduces motor deficit, but there is little effect on sensory deficits or spasticity.[128-130] There are patients who continue to deteriorate despite surgical intervention. Despite the controversy and need for continued study, PTS remains a threat to all SCI patients. It is important to consider the presence of PTS whenever intractable upper extremity, shoulder, or scapular pain is a presenting symptom. Early diagnosis may minimize the potentially devastating neurologic losses caused by PTS.

SUMMARY

Although the incidence of SCI is relatively small, the effects on the individual, the family, and society are staggering.

Although prevention of SCI is a daunting task, the ability to prevent just one case per year is a tremendous cost savings, especially over time. For many years it appeared that an injured spinal cord could not be repaired or regenerated. However, exciting progress has been made in neural regeneration and pharmacologic intervention that may interrupt the cycle of secondary injury. The burgeoning field of biomedical technology is creating many options to assist patients in becoming more independent in their daily lives. Spinal cord injury is a fertile area for nursing research. The nurse is challenged in providing care, preventing complications, and facilitating the patient's reintegration into society. Social reform and legislation to protect the rights of handicapped individuals and provide accessibility has improved the quality of life for the individual with SCI. As our evolving body of knowledge on the care of patients with acute SCI grows, our ability to limit complications and enhance outcomes improves.

REFERENCES

1. Bearsted JH: *The Edwin Smith surgical papyrus*, Chicago, 1930, University of Chicago.
2. Guttmann L: *Spinal cord injuries: comprehensive management and research*, London, 1976, Blackwell Scientific, 9-21.
3. Collins WF: Historical perspectives on spinal cord injury. In Narayan RK, Wilberger JE, Povlishock JT et al: *Neurotrauma*, New York, 1996, McGraw-Hill, 1041-1047.
4. Go BK, DeVivo MJ, Richards JS: The epidemiology of spinal cord injury. In Stover SL, DeLisa JA, Whiteneck GG, editors: *Spinal cord injury: clinical outcomes from the model systems*, Gaithersburg, Md, 1995, Aspen, 21-55.
5. DeVivo MJ: Causes and costs of spinal cord injury in the United States, *Spinal Cord* 35:809-813, 1997.
6. DeVivo MJ, Whiteneck GG, Charles ED: The economic impact of spinal cord injury. In Stover SL, DeLisa JA, Whiteneck GG, editors: *Spinal cord injury: clinical outcomes from the model systems*, Gaithersburg, Md, 1995, Aspen, 34-269.
7. Berkowitz M, Harvey C, Greene CG et al: *The economic consequences of traumatic spinal cord injury*, New York, 1992, Demos.
8. DeVivo MJ, Stover SL: Long-term survival and causes of death. In Stover SL, DeLisa JA, Whiteneck GG, editors: *Spinal cord injury: clinical outcomes from the model systems*, Gaithersburg, Md, 1995, Aspen, 289-316.
9. Frankel HL, Coll JR, Charlifue SW et al: Long term survival in spinal cord injury: a fifty year investigation, *Spinal Cord* 36:266-274, 1998.
10. DeVivo MJ, Sekar P: Prevention of spinal cord injuries that occur in swimming pools, *Spinal Cord* 35:509-515, 1997.
11. Snell R: *Basic information in clinical neuroanatomy for medical students*, ed 4, Philadelphia, 1997, Lippincott-Raven, 160-167.
12. Amundson G, Garfin SR, Parke WW: Vascular anatomy of the spine. In Levine AM, Eismont FJ, Garfin SR et al, editors: *Spine trauma*, Philadelphia, 1998, WB Saunders, 75-86.
13. Hickey JV: *The clinical practice of neurological and neurosurgical nursing*, ed 4, Philadelphia, 1996, JB Lippincott.
14. Levine A: Classification of spinal injury. In Levine AM, Eismont FJ, Garfin SR et al, editors: *Spine trauma*, Philadelphia, 1998, WB Saunders, 113-132.

15. Nelson R: Nonsurgical management of cervical spine instability. In Capen D, Haye W, editors: *Comprehensive management of spine trauma,* St. Louis, 1998, Mosby, 144-184.

16. Finkelstein JA, Anderson PA: Surgical management of cervical instability. In Capen D, Haye W, editors: *Comprehensive management of spine trauma,* St. Louis, 1998, Mosby, 134-143.

17. Neuberger CO, Yoshida GM: Penetrating spinal trauma. In Capen D, Haye W, editors: *Comprehensive management of spine trauma,* St. Louis, 1998, Mosby, 298-309.

18. Capen D: Soft tissue injuries to the spine acceleration-deceleration trauma. In Capen D, Hayes W, editors: *Comprehensive management of spine trauma,* St. Louis, 1998, Mosby, 96-103.

19. Mattera C: Spinal trauma: New guidelines for assessment and management in the out-of-hospital environment, *J Emerg Nurs* 24(6):523-534, 1998.

20. Eismont FJ, Frazier DD: Craniocervical trauma. In Levine AM, Eismont FJ, Garfin SR et al, editors: *Spine trauma,* Philadelphia, 1998, WB Saunders, 196-208.

21. Carlson GD, Heller JG, Abitbol JJ et al: Odontoid fractures. In Levine AM, Eismont FJ, Garfin SR et al, editors: *Spine trauma,* Philadelphia, 1998, WB Saunders, 227-248.

22. Levine AM: Traumatic spondylolisthesis of the axis (Hangman's fracture). In Levine AM, Eismont FJ, Garfin SR et al, editors: *Spine trauma,* Philadelphia, 1998, WB Saunders, 276-299.

23. Amar AP, Levy ML: Pathogenesis and pharmacological strategies for mitigating secondary damage in acute spinal cord injury, *Neurosurgery* 44(5):1027-1037, 1999.

24. Wilberger JE: Pharmacological resuscitation for spinal cord injury. In Narayan RK, Wilberger JE, Povlishock JT, editors: *Neurotrauma,* New York, 1996, McGraw-Hill, 1219-1228.

25. Tator CH: Biology of neurological recovery and functional restoration after spinal cord injury, *Neurosurgery* 42(4):696-705, 1998.

26. Rhoney D, Luer M, Hughes M et al: New pharmacologic approaches to acute spinal cord injury, *Pharmacotherapy* 16(3):382-393, 1996.

27. Faden AI: Pharmacological treatment approaches for brain and spinal cord trauma. In Narayan RK, Wilberger JE, Povlishock JT, editors: *Neurotrauma,* New York, 1996, McGraw-Hill, 1479-1490.

28. Sullivan J: Incomplete spinal cord injuries-nursing diagnosis, *Dimen Crit Care Nurs* 8(6):338-346, 1989.

29. Tator C: Classification of spinal cord injury based on neurological presentation. In Narayan RK, Wilberger JE, Povlishock JT, editors: *Neurotrauma,* New York, 1996, McGraw-Hill, 1059-1073

30. Tow AM P-E, Kong KH: Central cord syndrome: functional outcome after rehabilitation, *Spinal Cord* 16:156-160, 1998.

31. Shaw TC, Wardrope J, Frost E: Initial care of the spinal cord injury. In Lee B, Ostrander L, Cochran G, Shaw W, editors: *The spinal cord injured patient: comprehensive management,* Philadelphia, 1990, WB Saunders, 20-44.

32. Capen D: Emergency management of spine trauma. In Capen D, Haye W, editors: *Comprehensive management of spine trauma,* St. Louis, 1998, Mosby, 33-37.

33. Shackford S: Spine injury in the polytrauma patient: general surgical and orthopaedic considerations. In Levine AM, Eismont FJ, Garfin SR et al, editors: *Spine trauma,* Philadelphia, 1998, WB Saunders, 9-15.

34. An H: Cervical spine trauma, *Spine* 23(24):2713-2727, 1998.

35. Andersen B, Stringer W: Imaging after spinal injury. In Narayan RK, Wilberger JE, Povlishock JT, editors: *Neurotrauma,* New York, 1996, McGraw-Hill, 1149-1165.

36. Kaiser JA, Holland BA: Imaging of the cervical spine, *Spine* 23(24):2701-2710, 1998.

37. Nichols JS, Elger C, Heminger L et al: Magnetic resonance imaging: utilization in the management of central nervous system trauma, *J Trauma* 42(3):520-524, 1997.

38. Young JWR, Cure JK: Radiologic evaluation of the spine-injured patient. In Levine AM, Eismont FJ, Garfin SR et al, editors: *Spine trauma,* St. Louis, 1998, Mosby, 28-60.

39. Kalkman CJ, Drummond JC: Intraoperative evaluation: somatosensory evoked potentials and motor evoked potentials. In Levine AM, Eismont FJ, Garfin SR et al, editors: *Spine trauma,* Philadelphia, 1998, WB Saunders, 156-170.

40. Harbaugh RD, Henry RE: Role of spinal cord monitoring in spine surgery. In Capen D, Haye W, editors: *Comprehensive management of spine trauma,* St. Louis, 1998, Mosby, 119-133.

41. Lucke KT: Pulmonary management following acute SCI, *J Neurosci Nurs* 30(2):91-104, 1998.

42. Kocan MJ: Pulmonary considerations in the critical care phase, *Crit Care Nurs Clin North Am* 2(3):369-374, 1990.

43. Bracken D, Shepard M, Collins W et al: A randomized controlled trial of methylprednisolone or naloxone in the treatment of acute spinal cord injury, *N Engl J Med* 322(20):1405-1411, 1990.

44. Bracken MB, Shepard MJ, Holford TR et al: Administration of methylprednisolone for 24 or 48 hours or tirilazad mesylate for 48 hours in the treatment of acute spinal cord injury. Results of the third national acute spinal cord injury randomized controlled trial. National acute spinal cord injury study, *JAMA* 277(20):1597-1604, 1997.

45. Geisler FH, Dorsey FC, Coleman WP: Recovery of motor function after spinal cord injury—a randomized, placebo controlled trial with GM-1 ganglioside, *N Engl J Med* 326:1829-1838.

46. Amar AP, Levy ML: Surgical controversies in the management of spinal cord injury, *J Am Coll Surg* 188(5):550-564, 1999.

47. Mizra SK, Krengel WF 3rd, Chapman JR et al: Early versus delayed surgery for acute cervical spinal cord injury, *Clin Orthopaedics* Feb(359):104-114, 1999.

48. Wolf A, Wilberger JE: Timing of surgical intervention after spinal cord injury. In Narayan RK, Wilberger JE Jr, Povlishock JT, editors: *Neurotrauma,* New York, 1996, McGraw-Hill, 1193-1199.

49. Fehlings M, Tator CH: An evidence-based review of decompressive surgery in acute spinal cord injury: rationale, indications, and timing based on experimental and clinical studies, *J Neurosurg* 91(1 suppl):1-11, 1999.

50. Tator CH, Fehlings MG, Thorpe K et al: Current use and timing of spinal surgery for management of acute spinal cord injury in North America: results of a retrospective multicenter study, *J Neurosurg* 91(1 suppl):12-18, 1999.

51. Teeple E, Heres EK: Anesthesia management of spinal trauma. In Narayan RK, Wilberger JE, Povlishock JT, editors: *Neurotrauma,* New York, 1996, McGraw-Hill, 1167-1177.

52. Epstein SK: An overview of respiratory muscle function, *Clin Chest Med* 15(4):619-639, 1994.

53. Lemmons VR, Wagner FC: Respiratory complications after cervical spinal cord injury, *Spine* 19(20):2315-232, 1994.

54. Ragnarsson KT, Hall KM, Wilmot CB et al: Management of pulmonary, cardiovascular, and metabolic conditions after spinal cord injury. In Stover SL, DeLisa JA, Whiteneck GG, editors: *Spinal cord injury: clinical outcomes from the model systems,* Gaithersburg, Md, 1995, Aspen, 79-99.

55. Tromans AM, Mecci M, Barrett FH, et al: The use of the BiPAP biphasic positive airway pressure system in acute spinal cord injury, *Spinal Cord* 36(7):481-484, 1998.

56. Guha A, Tator CH, Rochon J: Spinal cord blood flow and systemic blood pressure after experimental spinal cord injury in rats, *Stroke* 20(3):372-377, 1989.

57. Dolan EJ, Tator CH: The effect of blood transfusion, dopamine, and gamma hydroxybutyrate on post-traumatic ischemia of the spinal cord, *J Neurosurg* 56:350-358, 1982.

58. McBride DQ, Rodts GE: Intensive care of patients with spinal trauma, *Neurosurg Clin North Am* 5(4):755-766, 1994.

59. Schwenker D: Cardiovascular considerations in the critical care phase. In Sullivan J: *Spinal cord injury: critical care nursing clinics of North America,* Philadelphia, 1990, WB Saunders, 363-367.

60. Rodts GE, Haid RW: Intensive care management of spinal cord injury. In Narayan RK, Wilberger JE, Povlishock JT, editors: *Neurotrauma,* New York, 1996, McGraw-Hill, 1201-1212.

61. Cardenas DD, Farrell-Roberts L, Sipski ML et al: Management of gastrointestinal, genitourinary, and sexual function. In Stover SL, DeLisa JA, Whiteneck GG, editors: *Spinal cord injury: clinical outcomes from the model systems,* Gaithersburg, Md, 1995, Aspen, 120-143.

62. Lu WY, Rhoney D, Boling WB et al: A review of stress ulcer prophylaxis in the neurosurgical intensive care unit, *Neurosurgery* 41(2):416-422, 1997.

63. Krenitsky J: Nutrition and the immune system, *AACN Clin Issues* 7(3):359-369, 1996.

64. Romito RA: Early administration of enteral nutrients in critically ill patients, *AACN Clin Issues* 6(2):242-225, 1995.

65. Moore FA, Moore EE, Haenel JB: Clinical benefits of early post-injury enteral feeding, *Clin Intensive Care* 6(1):21-27, 1995.

66. Vaccaro AR, Lavernia CJ, Botte M et al: Spinal orthoses in the management of spine trauma. In Levine AM, Eismont FJ, Garfin SR et al, editors: *Spine trauma,* St. Louis, 1998, Mosby, 171-194.

67. Ragnarsson KT, Stein AB, Kirshblum S: Rehabilitation and comprehensive care of the person with spinal cord injury. In Capen D, Haye W, editors: *Comprehensive management of spine trauma,* St. Louis, 1998, Mosby, 365-413.

68. Maynard FM, Bracken MB, Creasey G et al: International standards for neurological and functional classification of spinal cord injury, *Spinal Cord* 35:266-274, 1997.

69. Consortium for Spinal Cord Medicine: *Acute management of autonomic dysreflexia: adults with spinal cord injury presenting to health care facilities,* Washington, DC, 1997, Paralyzed Veterans of America.

70. Baskin DS: Spinal cord injury. In Evans RW: *Neurology and trauma,* Philadelphia, 1996, WB Saunders, 276-299.

71. Vaidanathan S, Soni BM, Sett P et al.: Pathophysiology of autonomic dysreflexia: long-term treatment with terazosin in adult and paediatric spinal cord injury patients manifesting recurrent dysreflexic episodes, *Spinal Cord* 36(11):761-770, 1998.

72. Consortium for Spinal Cord Medicine: *Prevention of thromboembolism in spinal cord injury,* Washington, DC, 1997, Paralyzed Veterans of America.

73. Fowler SB: Deep vein thrombosis and pulmonary emboli in neuroscience patients, *J Neurosci Nurs* 27:224-228, 1995.

74. Merli GJ, Crabbe S, Paluzzi RG et al: Etiology, incidence, and prevention of deep vein thrombosis in acute spinal cord injury, *Arch Phys Med Rehabil* 69:661, 1993.

75. Green D, Anderson FA, Heit J et al: Prophylaxis of thromboembolism in spinal cord-injured patients, *Chest* 102:S649-S651, 1994.

76. Wilson JT, Rogers FB, Wald SL et al: Prophylactic vena cava filter insertion in patients with traumatic spinal cord injury: preliminary results, *Neurosurgery* 34(2):234-239, 1994.

77. Maury M: About orthostatic hypotension in tetraplegic individuals reflections and experience, *Spinal Cord* 36:87-90, 1998.

78. Groomes TE, Huang CT: Orthostatic hypotension after spinal cord injury: treatment with fludrocortisone and ergotamine, *Arch Phys Med Rehabil* 1(72):56-58.

79. Sampson EE, Burnham RS, Andrews BJ: Functional electrical stimulation effect on orthostatic hypotension after spinal cord injury, *Arch Phys Med Rehabil* 2(81):139-143, 2000.

80. Han TR, Kim JH, Kwon BS: Chronic gastrointestinal problems and bowel dysfunction in patients with spinal cord injury, *Spinal Cord* 36:485-490, 1998.

81. Harari D, Sarkarat IM, Gurwitz JH et al: Constipation-related symptoms and bowel program concerning individuals with spinal cord injury, *Spinal Cord* 35:394-401, 1997.

82. Glickman S, Kamm M: Bowel dysfunction in spinal cord injury patients, *Lancet* 347:1651-1653, 1996.

83. Stiens S, Bergman SB, Goetz LL: Neurogenic bowel dysfunction after spinal cord injury: clinical evaluation and rehabilitative management, *Arch Phys Med Rehabil* 78:S86-S99, 1997.

84. Bar-On Z, Ihry A: The acute abdomen in spinal cord injury individuals, *Paraplegia* 33:704-707, 1995.

85. Nygaard IE, Kreder KJ: Urological management in patients with spinal cord injuries, *Spine* 21(1):128-131, 1996.

86. The urinary bladder in spinal cord disease. In Young RR, Woolsey RM, editors: *Diagnosis and management of disorders of the spinal cord,* Philadelphia, 1995, WB Saunders.

87. Wheeler JS, Walter JW: Acute urologic management of the patient with spinal cord injury. Initial hospitalization, *Urol Clin North Am* 20(3):403-411, 1993.

88. Selzman AA, Hampel N: Urologic complications of spinal cord injury, *Urol Clin North Am* 20(3):453-461, 1993.

89. National Institute for Disability Rehabilitation Research Consensus Statement: The prevention and management of urinary tract infections among people with spinal cord injuries, *J Am Paraplegia Soc* 15:194, 1992.

90. Andrychuk MA: Pressure ulcers: causes, risk factors, assessment, and intervention, *Orthop Nurs* 17(4):65-81, 1998.

91. Silveri CP, Cotler JM: Recovery and functional outcome in spinal trauma. In Capen D, Hayes W, editors: *Comprehensive management of spine trauma,* St. Louis, 1998, Mosby, 350-364.

92. Yarkony GM, Heinemann AW: Pressure ulcers. In Stover SL, DeLisa JA, Whiteneck GG, editors: *Spinal cord injury: clinical outcomes from the model systems,* Gaithersburg, Md, 1995, Aspen, 100-119.

93. Young RR: Spasticity: a review, *Neurology* 44(9):S12-S20, 1994.

94. Young RR: Spastic paresis. In Young RR, Woolsey RM, editors: *Diagnosis and management of disorders of the spinal cord,* Philadelphia, 1995, WB Saunders, 363-375.

95. Loubser PG: Spasticity associated with spinal cord injury. In Narayan RK, Wilberger JE, Povlishock JT, editors: *Neurotrauma,* New York, 1996, McGraw-Hill, 1245-1258.

96. Nance PW, Bugaresti J, Shellenberger K et al: Efficacy and safety of tizanidine in the treatment of spasticity in patients with spinal cord injury, *Neurology* 44(9):S44-S52, 1994.

97. Priebe MM, Sherwood AM, Graves DE et al: Effectiveness of gabapentin in controlling spasticity: a quantitative study, *Spinal Cord* 35:171-175, 1997.

98. Middleton JW et al: Intrathecal clonidine and baclofen in the management of spasticity and neuropathic pain following spinal cord injury: a case study, *Arch Phys Med Rehabil* 77(8):824-826, 1996

99. Penn RD: Intrathecal baclofen for spasticity of spinal origin: 7 years of experience, *J Neurosurg* 77:236, 1992.

100. Loubser PG: Continuous infusion of intrathecal baclofen: long-term effects on spasticity in spinal cord injury, *Paraplegia* 29:48, 1991.

101. Banovac K, Gonzalez F: Evaluation and management of heterotopic ossification in patients with spinal cord injury, *Spinal Cord* 35:158-162, 1997.

102. Bravo-Payno P, Esclarin A, Arzoz T et al: Incidence and risk factors in the appearance of heterotopic ossification in spinal cord injury, *Paraplegia* 30:740-745, 1992.

103. Banovac K, Gonzalez F, Wade N et al: Intravenous disodium etidronate therapy in spinal cord injury patients, *Paraplegia* 31(10):660-666, 1993.

104. Freebourn TM, Barber DB, Able AC: The treatment of immature heterotopic ossification in spinal cord injury with combination surgery, radiation therapy and NSAID, *Spinal Cord* 37:50-53, 1999.

105. Garland DE: Resection of heterotopic ossification in patients with spinal cord injuries, *Arch Phys Med Rehabil* 242:169-176, 1987.

106. Dalyan M, Sherman A, Cardenas DD: Factors associated with contractures in acute spinal cord injury, *Spinal Cord* 36:405-408, 1998.

107. Yarkony GM, Chen D: Rehabilitation of patients with spinal cord injuries. In Braddon RL, editor: *Physical medicine and rehabilitation,* Philadelphia, 1996, WB Saunders, 1149-1179.

108. Freehafer A: Tendon transfers in tetraplegic patients: the Cleveland experience, *Spinal Cord* 36:315-319, 1998.

109. Botte M: Complications of the musculoskeletal system following spinal cord injury. In Levine AM, Eismont FJ, Garfin SR et al, editors: *Spine trauma,* Philadelphia, 1998, WB Saunders, 639-661.

110. Althoff SE, Levine SB: Clinical approach to the sexuality of patients with spinal cord injury, *Urol Clin North Am* 20(3):527-533, 1993.

111. Stien R: Sexual dysfunctions in the spinal cord injured, *Paraplegia* 30:54-57, 1992.

112. Smith E, Bodner DR: Sexual dysfunction after spinal cord injury, *Urol Clin North Am* 20(3):535-543, 1993.

113. Harrison J, Glass CA, Owens RG et al: Factors associated with sexual functioning in women following spinal cord injury, *Paraplegia* 33:687-692, 1995.

114. Whipple B, Koisaruk BR: Sexuality and women with complete spinal cord injury, *Spinal Cord* 35:136-138, 1997.

115. Courtois FJ, Charvier KF, Leriche A et al: Sexual function in spinal cord injury men. I. Assessing sexual capability, *Paraplegia* 31(12):771-784, 1993.

116. Courtois FJ, Charvier KF, Leriche A et al: Clinical approach to erectile dysfunction in spinal cord injured men. A review of clinical and experimental data, *Paraplegia* 33(11):628-635, 1995.

117. Le Chapelain L, Nguyen Van Tam Ph, Dehail P et al: Ejaculatory stimulation, quality of semen and reproductive aspects in spinal cord injured men, *Spinal Cord* 36:132-136, 1998.

118. Atterbury JL, Groome LJ: Pregnancy in women with spinal cord injuries, *Nurs Clin North Am* 33(4):603-613, 1998.

119. Siddall PJ, Taylor DA, Cousins MJ: Classification of pain following spinal cord injury, *Spinal Cord* 35:69-75, 1997.

120. Kennedy P, Frankel H, Gardner B et al: Factors associated with acute and chronic pain following traumatic spinal cord injuries, *Spinal Cord* 35:814-817, 1997.

121. Anke AGW, Stenehjem AE, Stanghelle JK: Pain and life quality within 2 years of spinal cord injury, *Parapegia* 33:555-559, 1995.

122. Ragnarsson KT: Management of pain in persons with spinal cord injury, *J Spinal Cord Med* 20(2):186-199, 1997.

123. Loubser PG, Donovan WH: Chronic pain associated with spinal cord injury. In Narayan RK, Wilberger JE, Povlishock JT, editors: *Neurotrauma,* New York, 1996, McGraw-Hill, 1311-1322.

124. Summers JD, Rapoff MA, Varghese G et al: Psychosocial factors in chronic spinal cord injury pain, *Pain* 47(2):183-189, 1991.

125. Lundqvist C, Siosteen A, Blomstrand C et al: Spinal cord injuries. Clinical, functional and emotional status, *Spine* 16(1):78-83, 1991.

126. Consortium for Spinal Cord Medicine: *Depression following spinal cord injury: clinical practice guidelines for primary care physicians,* Washington, DC, 1997, Paralyzed Veterans Administration.

127. Nielson OA, Biering-Sorenson F, Botel F et al: Post-traumatic syringomyelia, *Spinal Cord* 37: 680-684, 1999.

128. Perrouin B, Lenne-Aurier K, Robert R et al: Post-traumatic syringomyelia and post-traumatic spinal canal stenosis: a direct relationship: a review of 75 patients with a spinal cord injury, *Spinal Cord* 36:137-143, 1998.

129. Sgouros S, Williams B: Management and outcome of post-traumatic syringomyelia, *J Neurosurg* 85:197-205, 1996.

130. Umbach I, Heilporn A: Post-spinal cord injury syringomyelia, *Paraplegia* 29:219-221, 1991.

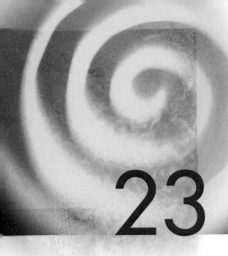

THORACIC INJURIES

Suzanne F. Sherwood •
Robbi Lynn Hartsock

23

Thoracic injuries are diverse, yet they account for much of the immediate life-threatening trauma encountered in the field or in the hospital setting. These injuries usually require rapid and skilled responses by nurses and considerable clinical judgment. They are frequently the "glamorous," frightening injuries to which the public is exposed via the press and visual media. Trauma patients occasionally have some knowledge, and many misconceptions, about chest injuries and how they are treated. Yet the pervasive chest pains, inability to breathe, and growing weakness from hypovolemic shock are unexpected. Such a situation is terrifying and different for each person.

Chest injuries and their effect on patients is the subject of this chapter. The purpose is to educate the nurse about the most common injuries sustained in the thoracic region and about complications of these injuries throughout the phases of trauma recovery. This chapter describes specific organ injuries of the heart, lungs, lower airways, major vascular structures, and bony thorax itself. Each of these organs is a part of the cardiopulmonary system or the thoracic cardiovascular system. Thoracic trauma encompasses both the anatomic injury and an alteration in physiologic function. Therefore injuries and posttraumatic thoracic complications are presented in sequence throughout the chapter. Also presented is airway management because this topic is traditionally included in a review of thoracic injuries. The remainder of this chapter deals with general problems that all thoracic trauma patients experience and is organized according to the phase of trauma recovery in which the patient is most likely to have the problem.

This injury-based approach is used to organize and simplify a great volume of detailed information. The discussion of each injury begins with a description not only of the injury's symptoms, pathophysiology, diagnosis, and treatment but also of the patient's pain and fear of treatment and death. The analysis of each intervention begins with the nurse's action in explaining the procedure, treating the pain and fear, and supporting the patient and family through medical and nursing therapies. The reader will not find these statements written over and over again but must understand that they are implied in each injury, each complication, and

each outcome. There is time to assist in treating the pneumothorax *and* to change the uncomfortable position *and* to explain what a chest tube will be like as a constant companion for several days. Each of these three therapeutic actions is done in the appropriate order of priority as assessed for the individual patient.

EPIDEMIOLOGY OF THORACIC INJURIES

Thoracic injuries are responsible for 25% of all trauma-related deaths[1-3] and are second only to central nervous system injuries as the leading cause of all trauma deaths. At least half of all fatalities, regardless of primary cause, involve significant chest trauma. An estimated 70% of motor vehicular crashes result in thoracic injury.[3] Fortunately, sophisticated prehospital care and expeditious air transportation have improved the detection and treatment of injuries that were previously found only on postmortem examinations. Of those patients admitted to a hospital, 15% require a thoracotomy as definitive management. These patients have sustained severe, life-threatening injuries that necessitate complex postoperative care, and they experience numerous complications. However, the remaining 85% are treated successfully with general resuscitative measures and ventilatory management.[4] The epidemic of societal violence has changed the patterns of chest injuries that dominated previous decades. One seventh of all deaths by injury now involve violent interpersonal exchanges. A significant number of these interactions result in penetrating chest trauma from shootings or stabbings.[5] Likewise, growth in the elderly segment of the population has an impact on the changing pattern of thoracic injury. Approximately 10% of all blunt chest trauma patients are now 65 years of age or older. Significant morbidity, specifically pneumonia and respiratory distress syndrome, is associated with 50% of aging patients who sustain thoracic injury.[6]

THORACIC ASSESSMENT IN TRAUMA

The assessment of patients with thoracic injury is based, as in any type of trauma examination, on a series of diagnostic clues obtained from directed data collection. Initially the data are used to form a diagnostic set known as the *index of suspicion*. In other words, given the specific details of the incident and the initial, rapid assessment, what injuries are most likely to be present? The total assessment is frequently completed after the initial resuscitation but always includes the initial datebase.[7]

INJURY DATABASE

The injury database is the most immediate part of the patient history and helps to identify patterns of thoracic injury. It is the first component of the thoracic assessment process. There are at least four major areas of essential information:

1. *Type of incident.* Information about the type of incident or injury provides clues as to the cause of injury. Was the patient involved in a motor vehicle crash? Was the injured person wearing a seat belt or shoulder harness? Did the vehicle have an air bag? Was the person a driver or passenger? Was the person riding a motorcycle or was he or she a pedestrian? Was the patient shot or stabbed?

2. *Events of the incident.* Field care providers, police, or witnesses may provide information about what occurred during the incident. In patients with penetrating chest trauma, highly useful details include the type of weapon used, the design and range of the weapon, and an estimate of missile velocity. In the case of a car crash, how fast was the vehicle traveling on impact? Did the person travel within the car? What types of deceleration forces were involved?

3. *Mechanism of injury.* Mechanism information is critically important to obtain as part of the injury history. No detail is unimportant. Is the injury a result of blunt force? What part of the thorax received the initial impact? Did the anterior chest hit the steering wheel, or was the patient thrown forward against a shoulder harness? Did the patient fall and, if so, how far; how did the patient land and on what type of surface? Was the patient kicked by an animal? Or is injury the result of penetrating force such as a stabbing or shooting? Does the apparent mechanism correlate with the findings on initial examination and resuscitation?

4. *Events of the extrication or transport.* How long did it take the rescuers to extricate the person from the car? Were there special problems in freeing the torso from surrounding metal? What were the events of transporting the patient from the field? How long did it require? Were there airway problems? What were the vital signs?

PREVIOUS HEALTH HISTORY

In addition to the injury history, the personal health history gives insight into the individual's unique response to shock and thoracic injury. Whether the historian is the patient or, more likely, a family member, the nurse attempts to determine the patient's previous respiratory, cardiac, and vascular status. Previous cardiopulmonary problems are uncovered through the usual review-of-systems approach and selective and directed questioning. The injured person is frequently young and presents an unremarkable cardiopulmonary or vascular history. Nevertheless, questions should be asked specifically about the presence of persistent upper or lower respiratory infections, asthma, or chronic sinus problems; smoking, alcohol, and drug abuse history should also be investigated. Any of these problems may affect the patient's tolerance of nasal or oral endotracheal tubes or the response to mechanical ventilation. Is there a history of chest pain, heart disease, cardiac surgery, or vascular implantation? It is particularly important to ask if there have been any previous incidents or injuries.

PHYSICAL EXAMINATION

The physical assessment always begins with a primary survey of the ABCs: airway status with cervical spine control, breathing, and circulation. This basic principle holds for all trauma patients from resuscitation to rehabilitation. For example, during the resuscitation phase, airway status assessment includes evaluation of tongue position and examination for the presence of blood, vomitus, foreign bodies, and edema in the upper or lower airway. In later phases of the patient's trauma course the examination may focus on evaluating maxillofacial restraining devices that affect airway status, tracheostomy cuff pressure, or simply the patient's ability to manage oral secretions. The ABCs imply that the nurse must always know at any point whether a patient's cervical spine has been cleared radiographically. Breathing, whether spontaneous or mechanically assisted, and circulation are rapidly evaluated to complete the primary survey. Only at this point does the detailed examination begin.

THORACIC ANATOMY

Correlation of underlying anatomy and surface landmarks is imperative in the trauma examination. The examiner must be able to identify key structures in the true thorax, the cervicothoracic inlet, and the boundaries of the thoracoabdominal cavity (Figure 23-1). Key structures include the trachea, carotid arteries, carina, lung fields, diaphragm, cardiac borders, aorta, subclavian arteries, and pulmonary artery (Table 23-1). External landmarks and knowledge of the relationships between internal structures assist in identifying injuries (Figures 23-2 and 23-3).

SECONDARY AND DETAILED EXAMINATIONS

The traditional physical examination techniques (inspection, palpation, percussion, and auscultation) are used in the thoracic assessment of the trauma patient, usually in an adapted form. The key word is *adapted,* not *deleted.* Visual inspection of the thorax requires a clean field for examination. The removal of debris and blood wherever possible helps to avoid overlooking wounds or subtle signs of trauma. Hair-covered areas are inspected carefully. The examiner must be particularly alert to contusions, steering

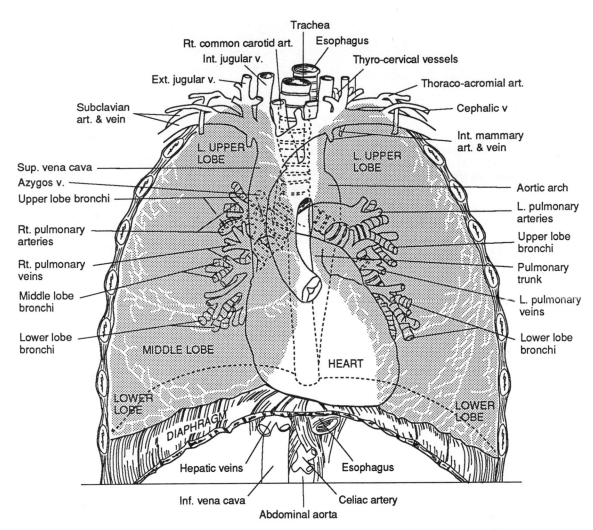

FIGURE 23-1 **Anatomy of the Thorax and Its Contents.** (From Shires GT: *Care of the trauma patient,* New York, 1985, McGraw-Hill.)

TABLE 23-1	**Thoracic Surface Anatomy**
Structure	**Landmarks**
Aorta	
Root	Angle of Louis, midsternal line
Arch	First rib, sternal border
Pulmonary artery	Within and below aortic arch
Subclavian artery	First rib, clavicle
Cardiac borders	
Apex	Fifth left ICS, midclavicular line
Base	Second left ICS, substernal
Carina	Angle of Louis
Diaphragm	Right dome superior to left
Full inspiration	Tenth-eleventh rib posteriorly, sixth-eighth rib anteriorly
Full expiration	Tenth thoracic vertebra posteriorly, fourth-fifth rib anteriorly

ICS, Intercostal space.

wheel marks, seat belt marks, and sites of a penetrating wound's entrance and exit.[8] Palpation and percussion are difficult to perform in the patient with numerous tubes, dressings, and traction, yet each anatomic area must be palpated for crepitus, hematomas, and unstable bone frag-

ments. Percussion is used to locate blood and air by identifying inappropriately dull or tympanic notes over the chest wall. Chest auscultation may be difficult over the noise of a ventilator or bubbling chest tubes. However, each of these techniques can and must be used in examining the thoracic region.

During the initial evaluation and resuscitation phase of care, each technique is applied rapidly and specifically. Treatment may precede diagnostic examination when life-threatening injuries such as tension pneumothorax or cardiac tamponade are present. In the critical care phase the examination may be much more detailed and is assisted by a variety of invasive technologies. The focus of the assessment is slightly different, centering on occult injuries, overlooked injuries, and later complications of serious injury and shock. A great deal of additional data is available through electromechanical monitoring and extensive laboratory and radiographic procedures. These additional data are always correlated with the history and physical examination. As the patient progresses through each phase of care, the thoracic assessment builds on the findings of the preceding phase. What is learned during resuscitation must be communi-

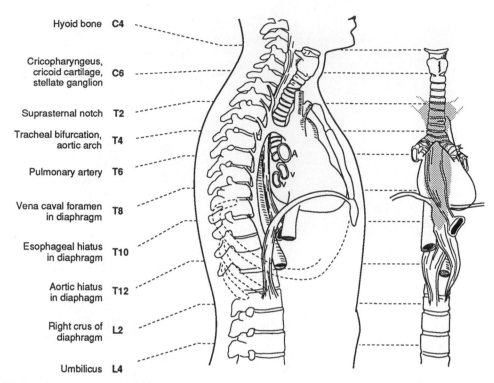

Hyoid bone **C4**

Cricopharyngeus,
cricoid cartilage, **C6**
stellate ganglion

Suprasternal notch **T2**

Tracheal bifurcation, **T4**
aortic arch

Pulmonary artery **T6**

Vena caval foramen **T8**
in diaphragm

Esophageal hiatus **T10**
in diaphragm

Aortic hiatus **T12**
in diaphagm

Right crus of **L2**
diaphragm

Umbilicus **L4**

FIGURE 23-2 The cervical, thoracic, and lumbar vertebrae correspond with specific anatomic structures. These landmarks are helpful in determining different thoracic levels. Palpation of the spinous processes proves helpful in ascertaining the level of the wound and the structures that may be involved. (From Naclerio EA: *Chest injuries,* Orlando, 1971, Grune & Stratton.)

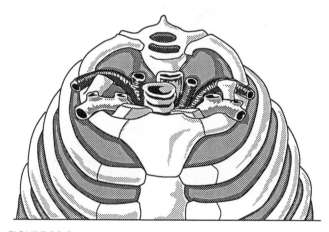

FIGURE 23-3 The root of the neck is actually the cervicothoracic region, which forms a boundary between the neck and the thorax. It is occupied by a number of vital structures that enter or leave the thoracic cavity. As shown, the apex of the lung rises above the level of the anterior part of the first rib. The subclavian artery lateral to the subclavian vein is separated from the lung by the membranous cervical diaphragm and the pleura. (From Naclerio EA: *Chest injuries,* Orlando, 1971, Grune & Stratton.)

cated and reassessed during critical, intermediate, and rehabilitative care.

ANATOMIC APPROACH TO THORACIC EXAMINATION

The anatomic examination component in thoracic trauma assessment includes the neck, cervicothoracic region, upper abdomen, and the true thorax. Each area is examined for injuries and abnormalities. Focal points in the neck examination include the trachea, neck veins, and carotid arteries.

The trachea is inspected and palpated to identify any deviation in position from the midline that is indicative of mediastinal shifting. Neck veins are examined for distention or flatness as an indication of intrathoracic pressure. The carotid arteries are palpated separately for decrease or loss of pulse and then are auscultated for bruits (Figure 23-4).

The overall size and shape of the patient's true thorax should be noted. The thoracic cavity size provides clues as to underlying lung disease and how well a specific injury may be tolerated. For example, a large male will tolerate a considerably greater volume of intrathoracic bleeding without signs of lung or mediastinal compression than will the patient with a small or inflexible chest. The difference may be as much as 4000 ml of air and fluid.

The entire surface of the chest is inspected for signs of trauma. The bony points of the thorax and intercostal spaces provide references for localizing internal thoracic structures (Figure 23-5). All supporting structures (clavicles, sternum, ribs, and the thoracic spine) are palpated for fractures and observed for symmetry. Percussion of the chest begins at the apices and moves downward across both the lateral and anterior aspects. Examination of the back must not be delayed although it is frequently limited to palpation until the patient can be safely moved for a more complete assessment. The examiner searches for changes in normal resonance on percussion or loss of normal diaphragmatic excursion. Breath sounds are auscultated over the anterior and lateral chest wall in order to identify air entry in each lobe of the lung. Heart sounds are evaluated for overall loudness or distance of the sounds and for the presence of murmurs across the right ventricle and septum.

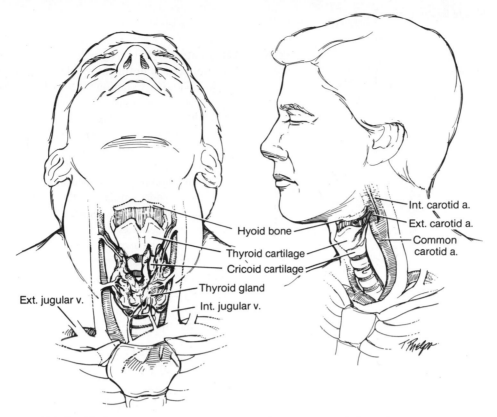

FIGURE 23-4 Important Structures in the Neck Component of Thoracic Assessment.

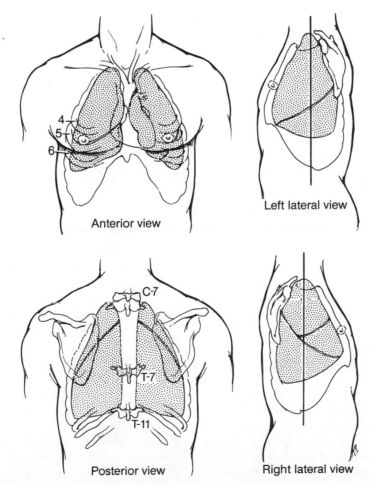

FIGURE 23-5 Correlation of Surface to Underlying Thoracic Anatomy. Anterior view, Note the relationship of the heart, great vessels, and lungs to bony thorax. **Posterior** and **right lateral views,** Major and minor interlobar fissures. **Left lateral view,** Note single interlobar fissure.

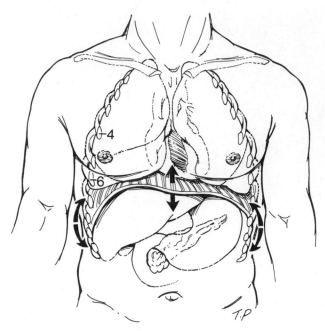

FIGURE 23-6 **The Thoracoabdominal Region in Thoracic Assessment.** Note the variation in diaphragm and lung position during respiration.

Finally the thoracoabdominal area is examined carefully for evidence of trauma. This is particularly of concern in patients with penetrating injuries, which may have had an upward trajectory with possible diaphragmatic tears and involvement of the pleural space. The position of the diaphragm is located on inspiration and expiration (Figure 23-6).

PHYSIOLOGIC APPROACH

Clinical monitoring of blood pressure, cardiac rate and rhythm, respirations, urine output, and arterial blood gases is always considered part of the thoracic assessment process. However, it is generally recognized that blood pressure is frequently unaffected until a 15% to 20% loss in blood volume has been sustained. Although invasive monitoring of central venous pressure may be helpful, it is not routinely initiated during the initial fluid replacement and management of significant thoracic injuries. The time required to insert a central venous catheter cannot be afforded during initial resuscitation; therefore large-bore (14-gauge) peripheral intravenous catheters are preferable for volume repletion. If the patient has limited intravenous access, a no. 7 or 8 French cordis can be used.

Definitive management in the operative and critical care phases requires a practical yet comprehensive approach to systemic cardiopulmonary monitoring. The nurse must be familiar with an extensive array of cardiopulmonary variables and accompanying monitoring technology to be able to assess patients who present with thoracic trauma. The patient-ventilator system is monitored as a unit and is an important source of data about the patient's pulmonary status. For example, one important mechanical parameter, static pulmonary compliance, can be monitored in intu-

bated patients via the ventilator system. Measurements are accomplished by noting tidal volume, airway pressure at end inspiration after inflation of the lung has stopped, and end-expiratory pressure. Static compliance is the ratio of tidal volume to the change in pressure from end inspiration to end expiration. Normal values are approximately 60 to 80 ml/cm H_2O; however, in patients with respiratory distress syndrome the value commonly drops to 30 ml/cm H_2O.

The insertion of peripheral arterial and pulmonary artery catheters provides much of the information needed for assessment of extensive injuries, their complications, and the effect of therapies such as mechanical ventilation and positive end-expiratory pressure (PEEP). When available, mixed venous oxygen tension (Pvo_2) and saturation (Svo_2) monitoring are useful tools in determining circulatory sufficiency and tissue oxygenation. Table 23-2 is a summary of physiologic parameters that are often obtained via invasive monitoring.

NONINVASIVE MONITORING

The oxygenation status of the patient can be assessed using noninvasive monitoring via pulse oximeters and transcutaneous, conjunctival, or tissue oxygen tension monitors. Pulse oximetry is well accepted as a convenient, portable, and cost-effective monitor of peripheral arterial oxygen saturation. In general, oximetry estimates fractional hemoglobin saturation by determining the maximal light absorbances of the different hemoglobin species. In pulse oximetry, multiple arteriolar beds may be used (e.g., fingers, toes, nasal septum). Accuracy is approximately 3% to 5% at true saturations greater than 70%, assuming that the only hemoglobin species present are reduced hemoglobin and oxyhemoglobin. Accuracy falls in the presence of significant amounts of carboxyhemoglobin, hypothermia, severe anemia, and hypovolemia with mean arterial blood pressure less than 50 mm Hg.[9] Because the technique depends on pulse transmission, intense peripheral vasoconstriction also may be associated with lost or inaccurate readings.

Noninvasive assessment of carbon dioxide (CO_2) is more difficult, especially in critically ill patients with significant ventilation-perfusion (V/Q) abnormalities, increased physiologic dead space, and hemodynamic instability. When these confounding factors are stable, changes in end-tidal CO_2 can be assumed to reflect changes in alveolar ventilation and arterial CO_2 tension ($Paco_2$). End-tidal CO_2 monitoring using mass spectrometry or infrared analyzer correlates reasonably well with $Paco_2$ in normal patients and is used in a variety of environments, including the resuscitation, operating, recovery, and critical care areas.[10] Analysis of trends over time rather than individual values is most useful because there is considerable breath-to-breath variability in all patients.

PATIENT-VENTILATOR SYSTEM

The integrity and effectiveness of the ventilator equipment is part of the thoracic assessment. There is no one preferred ventilator system or mode. Volume-cycled ventilators are by

TABLE 23-2   Cardiopulmonary Parameters in Thoracic Assessment

Variable	Abbrev.	Measurements or Calculation	Normal Range Low	Normal Range High	Units
Heart rate	HR	Direct measurement	70	90	beats/min
Mean arterial pressure	MAP	Direct measurement	80	100	mm Hg
Central venous pressure	CVP	Central venous catheter Direct measurement	1	9	mm Hg
Pulmonary capillary wedge pressure	PCWP	Pulmonary artery catheter Direct measurement	4	12	mm Hg
Mean pulmonary artery pressure	$\overline{PA}$	Pulmonary artery catheter Direct measurement	11	16	mm Hg
Cardiac output	Q_T	Fick method or thermodilution Direct measurement	\multicolumn{2}{c} Varies with size	
Cardiac index	CI	Q_T/body surface area	2.8	3.6	$L/min/m^2$
Stroke index	SI	CI/HR	30	50	ml/m^2
Left ventricuiar stroke work	LVSW	$SI \times MAP \times 0.0144$	44	68	$g\text{-}m/m^2$
Right ventricular stroke work	RVSW	$SI \times \overline{PA} \times 0.0144$	4	8	$g\text{-}m/m^2$
Systemic vascular resistance	SVR	$79.92 \times (MAP - CVP)/CI$	1700	2600	$dyne\text{-}sec\text{-}cm^5 m^2$
Pulmonary vascular resistance	PVR	$79.92 \times (\overline{PA} - PCWP)/CI$	45	225	$dyne\text{-}sec\text{-}cm^5 m^2$
Arterial blood gases	ABGs	Direct measurement			
Pao_2			80	100	mm Hg
$Paco_2$			35	45	mm Hg
pH			7.35	7.45	
HCO_1			22	26	mEqL
Oxygen saturation	Sao_2		\multicolumn{2}{c}{>95}		%
Base excess			−2	2	
Mixed venous blood gases	MVBGs	Direct measurement			
Pvo_2			35	40	mm Hg
$Pvco_2$			41	51	mm Hg
pH			7.31	7.41	
HCO_3			22	26	mEq/L
Oxygen saturation	Svo_2		70	75	%
Base excess			−2	2	
Arterial O_2 content	Cao_2	$Sao_2 \times (1.39 \times Hgb) + 0.003 \times Pao_2$	\multicolumn{2}{c}{20 ml O_2/100 ml}		
Mixed venous O_2 content	Cvo_2	$Svo_2 \times (1.39 \times Hgb) + 0.003 \times Pvo_2$	\multicolumn{2}{c}{15 ml O_2/100 ml}		
Arterial-mixed venous O_2 content	$Ca\text{-}vo_2$	$Cao_2 - Cvo_2$	4	5.5	ml/dl
Oxygen delivery	O_2 del	$Cao_2 \times CI \times 10$	500	700	$ml/min\text{-}m^2$
Oxygen consumption	$\dot{V}o_2$	$Ca\text{-}vo_2 \times CI \times 10$	100	180	$ml/min\text{-}m^2$
Respiratory rate	RR	Direct measurement	12	20	breath/min
Tidal volume	V_T	Spirometry	\multicolumn{2}{c}{Varies with size}		
			200	550	ml
End inspiratory pressure	P_i	Direct measurement	\multicolumn{2}{c}{Volume-dependent e.g., 7 cm H_2O for $V_T = 600$ ml}		
Vital capacity	VC	Spirometry	65	75	ml/kg
Inspiratory force	IF	Direct measurement	−100	−75	cm H_2O
Dead space/tidal volume ratio	$\dot{V}_D/\dot{V}_T$	$(Paco_2 - Peco_2 /Paco_2)$	0.2	0.4	
Respiratory compliance	C	$V_T/(P_i - PEEP)$	60	100	ml/cm H_2O
Physiologic shunt fraction	Q_s/Q_t	$(C_{end\text{-}cap}o_2 - Cao_2)/ (C_{end\text{-}cap}o_2 - Cvo_2)$	3	5	%

Modified from Shoemaker WC: Pathophysiology and therapy of shock states. In Berk J, Sampliner J, editors: *Handbook of critical care*, Boston, 1982, Little Brown.

far the most commonly used because the minute volume, flow, and resultant airway pressure can be manipulated. Specialized methods of ventilation such as high-frequency ventilation may be useful in specific types of airway or chest trauma. In addition, several modes of conventional mechanical ventilation are used:

1. *Control mode (CMV).* CMV allows total control of the patient's rate and tidal volume. It is generally used for short-term ventilation when no inspiratory effort is desired or in multiply injured patients without spontaneous ventilatory efforts because of accompanying neurologic injury or drug overdose.

2. *Assist/control.* This mode is also known as *continuous mandatory ventilation* on newer generation ventilators. The patient can initiate spontaneous ventilation, and each breath is assisted by the ventilator to a preset volume. Infrequently used in thoracic trauma or multiply injured patients, assist/control can allow an inappropriately high minute ventilation and increase the work of breathing.

3. *Intermittent mandatory ventilation (IMV).* IMV allows the patient to receive a baseline minute volume but also breathe spontaneously at a fast or slow rate and variable tidal volume. *Synchronized intermittent mandatory ventilation* (SIMV) provides the additional advantage that the IMV mandatory breaths are triggered when the ventilator senses inspiratory effort by the patient. SIMV is generally well tolerated in most patients and diminishes the risk of barotrauma because there is less chance of ventilator breaths imposed over spontaneous inspiration (stacking). All IMV modes provide several key advantages: the individual patient's respiratory efforts are used, weaning begins at the outset of ventilation, and mean intrathoracic pressure is decreased (and therefore venous return and cardiac filling are increased). The last advantage is particularly important in hypovolemic patients and in those with myocardial injury.

4. *Continuous positive airway pressure (CPAP).* This mode generally refers to a patient breathing spontaneously at an elevated baseline airway pressure. The objective, as with PEEP, is to increase functional residual capacity (FRC) and therefore the surface area available for gas exchange. During inspiration the ventilator provides gas flow as a function of the patient's inspiratory effort. Exhalation is passive to the level of the preset baseline pressure. CPAP can be used to support the patient during weaning and allows ventilation at a lower inspired oxygen concentration. Conversely, CPAP does not provide mandatory breaths via positive-pressure mechanical ventilation; it only supports the patient's FRC while the patient maintains spontaneous alveolar ventilation.

5. *Pressure support ventilation.* Pressure support ventilation facilitates spontaneous breathing to a set airway pressure; however, the pressure is provided only during inspiration, not continuously. The patient initiates a breath, and the ventilator delivers gas flow to the patient while maintaining a preset inspiratory pressure. In theory, pressure support increases the pressure gradient across the airway, therefore reducing resistance.[11] The effect can be useful in patients with high airway resistance related to underlying pulmonary pathology or a small artificial airway. Pressure support decreases the work of breathing and can prevent fatigue when combined with IMV. These factors can be critical in solving weaning difficulties. However, pressure support alone does not ensure an adequate minute ventilation because neither rate nor tidal volume is guaranteed.

6. *Pressure control (PC) and pressure control with inverse ratio ventilation (PC-IRV).* PC is a pressure mode of ventilation with a rapid, decelerating gas flow pattern that allows more time for alveolar ventilation and oxygenation. The PC-IRV mode uses PC ventilation with an inverse ratio of inspiration to expiration. This process is an exaggerated form of PC and is used for patients at risk for barotrauma.

7. *Airway pressure release ventilation (APRV).* In Europe, APRV is known as *BIPAP.* This is a timed triggered mode using CPAP with regular episodes of pressure release intervals. Lung volume is maintained by near continuous airway pressure, and oxygenation can be maintained with lower peak pressures. Patients require less sedation because they can breath spontaneously and easily throughout the respiratory cycle as a result of the "floating" exhalation valve.[12]

8. Ventilatory modes may be used singly or in combination (i.e., IMV with pressure support). It is impossible to overemphasize the importance of a thorough understanding of ventilatory modalities and their physiologic and psychologic effects.[13]

INTEGRATING OTHER DATA SOURCES

Laboratory and radiographic data provide the final components of the total thoracic trauma assessment. Essentials include arterial blood gases, hematocrit and hemoglobin, complete blood count, clotting studies, serum electrolytes, osmolality, lactate, and a recent sputum or transtracheal aspirate culture.

Thoracic evaluation includes, at minimum, a chest roentgenogram in order to visualize any significant bone, vascular, or pulmonary injuries (Figure 23-7).

The angle of the film (supine, upright, or lateral) is used for best exposure of specific structures yet must consider any restrictions in positioning the patient. A supine anteroposterior film is selected for the patient who is being evaluated for cervical spine injury or whose hemodynamic instability makes an upright position impossible.[14]

One of the most valuable assessment tools in thoracic trauma is a clear, true upright chest radiograph. The patient

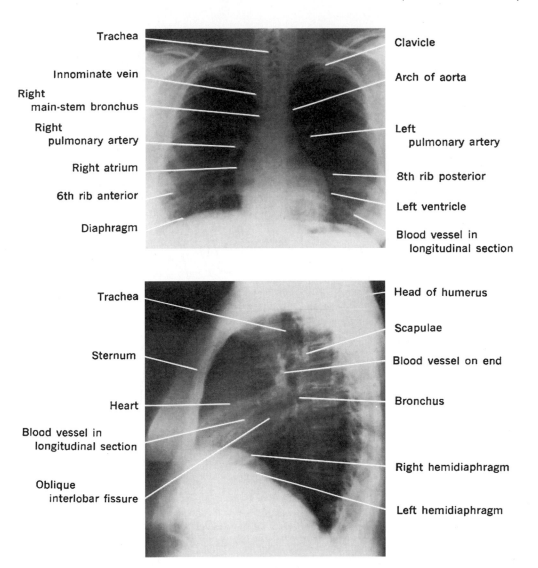

Trachea

Innominate vein

Right
main-stem bronchus

Right
pulmonary artery

Right atrium

6th rib anterior

Diaphragm

Clavicle

Arch of aorta

Left
pulmonary artery

8th rib posterior

Left ventricle

Blood vessel in
longitudinal section

Trachea

Sternum

Heart

Blood vessel in
longitudinal section

Oblique
interlobar fissure

Head of humerus

Scapulae

Blood vessel on end

Bronchus

Right hemidiaphragm

Left hemidiaphragm

FIGURE 23-7 Normal Posteroanterior and Lateral Films of the Chest. (From Naclerio EA: *Chest injuries,* Orlando, 1971, Grune & Stratton.)

faces the radiograph beam at a 110-degree angle so as to avoid unnecessary distortion of underlying structures on the radiograph (Figure 23-8). The true upright film allows better visualization of vascular injuries within the chest and some estimation of the amount of blood or fluid in the chest cavity. Cardiac and aortic borders are also less distorted. Research has shown that an early diagnosis using thoracic computed tomography (TCT) has a "positive influence on the therapeutic management" of patients with thoracic injuries.[14] Before obtaining an upright film, cervical spine injury must be ruled out. Radiographs of the cervical and thoracic spine must be completed and visualized before the backboard is removed. If the patient is intubated, suctioning may be necessary before the procedure. When the patient is pharmacologically paralyzed and sedated, support of the head and neck is necessary. The agitated patient must be protected from inadvertent dislodgment of an endotracheal tube or vascular catheters.

Additional diagnostic information is provided through thoracic computed axial tomography (CT scan). The CT scan is more sensitive in detecting air and fluid in the pleural space than is the radiograph. Evaluation of underlying lung, cardiac, and mediastinal structures is also enhanced by the use of CT scans.[14]

The use of magnetic resonance imaging (MRI) provides detailed visualization of blood vessels with rapid flow rates. Contrast dye is not required. Although its accuracy makes MRI a valuable diagnostic tool, its use in the acutely injured patient is somewhat limited by the difficulties encountered in hemodynamic monitoring and ventilatory support within the field around the magnet.[14]

REASSESSMENT AND EARLY THORACOTOMY

Repeated thoracic assessment is the key to determining missed or progressive injuries. Should the patient's condition deteriorate or result in cardiac arrest, immediate exploratory thoracotomy may be performed. Indications for the procedure have been the subject of considerable controversy. Dunham and Cowley[11] maintain that the point at which a youthful myocardium arrests usually represents an

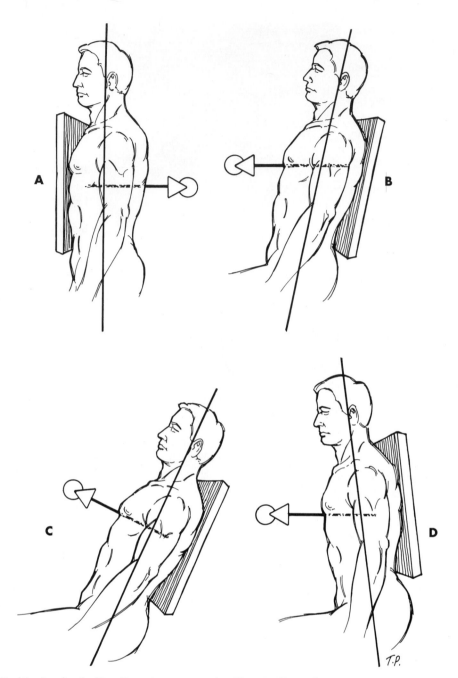

FIGURE 23-8 **Positioning for the True Erect Anteroposterior Chest Radiograph. A,** Normal position for posteroanterior film. **B,** Most common position for portable anteroposterior chest film. **C,** Unacceptable position for erect anteroposterior film. **D,** True erect position.

irreversible insult and recommend specific indications for emergency thoracotomy. These include arrest in a young patient, an arrest time of less than 5 minutes duration, and positive neurologic signs such as reactive pupils and spontaneous movement of the extremities. Questionable outcomes, risk to health care providers, and cost also drive the controversy of immediate exploratory thoracotomy. Current research supports the use of thoracoscopy in limited situations. This procedure may be used on stable patients presenting with penetrating chest injuries, as a diagnostic evaluation, or to control bleeding and remove blood clots.[15]

THE INJURIES

OBSTRUCTION

Every injured patient is at risk for developing some form of airway problem. Airway obstruction occurs frequently in trauma as a primary problem or as the result of some other injury. The source of an obstruction and the therapeutic approach are slightly different in the patient with a natural airway or one with an artificial airway already in place. However, the principles of basic and advanced life support are fundamental in management of all obstructions.

THE PATIENT WITH A NATURAL AIRWAY. The most common sources of obstruction are the tongue and foreign bodies such as teeth, blood clots, and bone fragments. The unconscious patient in shock or one with central nervous system, maxillofacial, or neck injuries is particularly at risk. Assessment begins with rapid determination of level of consciousness and mental status, followed by observation of rate and pattern of respiration. Air movement through the airway, if any, is noisy. Respiratory distress may or may not be immediately evident, and arterial blood gases are measured as the most certain method of assessing oxygenation and ventilation. Continuous pulse oximetry monitoring can detect reductions in the oxygen saturation of hemoglobin.

Initially the airway is opened by a chin-lift or jaw-thrust maneuver, and the oropharynx is cleared by suction and digital exploration. Each step is performed with great care to maintain immobility of the cervical spine unless injury to the spine has been ruled out clinically and radiographically. Initial airway maneuvers may be inadequate or only temporary solutions; therefore more definitive airway control is often required.

The simplest adjuncts are placement of an oral or nasal airway. Both are generally for short-term use in trauma and have restricted use in patients with facial trauma such as nasal fractures, cribriform plate fractures, or oropharyngeal injury. When positioning does not relieve the obstruction, endotracheal intubation is the management technique of choice in most types of trauma. An esophageal obturator airway (EOA) or esophageal gastric tube airway (EGTA) are ineffective and should not be used in maintaining the airway.[11] However, they may still be encountered in patients received from the prehospital setting. Complications such as inadvertent tracheal intubation, esophageal trauma from excessive cuff inflation, and vomiting with aspiration on removal are common with EOAs and EGTAs.

In general, oral endotracheal intubation with rapid-sequence induction is the preferred method for securing an airway. This may be done safely after cervical spine injury has been ruled out or even in cases of unknown cervical spine status provided the neck does not require aggressive manipulation to visualize the vocal cords. Cricoid pressure is applied routinely during the procedure. The rationale is that the trauma patient is likely to have a full stomach and is therefore at risk for aspiration of gastric contents.[11]

Oral-tracheal intubation constitutes the preferred airway management, with several caveats. However, if the patient is unstable but breathing and the urgency of airway management does not allow preliminary cervical spine clearance, blind nasotracheal intubation may be attempted (Figure 23-9). Conversely, an oral-tracheal route is used if the patient is apneic and the cervical spine is immobilized manually in a neutral position. Lastly, fiberoptic bronchoscope may be useful to facilitate difficult intubations in stable patients, particularly in those individuals with maxillofacial or cervical spine trauma and in patients with short necks.[16]

If the patient cannot be intubated successfully, emergency cricothyroidotomy is recommended.[16] There are two crico-

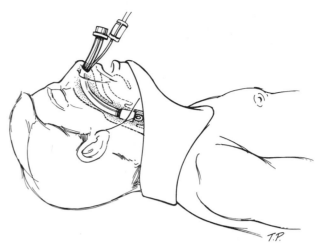

FIGURE 23-9 **Blind Nasotracheal Intubation in a Patient With Potential Cervical Spine Injury.**

thyroidotomy procedures currently in use. The first is a surgical technique in which a transverse incision is made through the skin and the cricothyroid membrane, located below the thyroid prominence of the neck, is opened. A standard tracheotomy tube is inserted into the exposed airway (Figure 23-10). A second approach, needle cricothyroidotomy or percutaneous transtracheal ventilation, is initiated by insertion of a 14-gauge needle into the trachea at the cricothyroid membrane below the level of obstruction. Pressurized oxygen is insufflated intermittently through the needle into the trachea. Which method is used depends on the injury, available equipment, and capability of the resuscitating health professional.

The choice of appropriate airway requires consideration not only of available equipment and personnel but factors specific to the patient, the injury, and the short- and long-term management. For example, early intubation may be indicated not only for airway management but also for intraoperative or critical care management of patients with thoracic injuries. Table 23-3 summarizes the advantages of the different artificial airways, their restrictions, and their potential complications.

THE PATIENT WITH AN ARTIFICIAL AIRWAY. In trauma patients with an artificial airway in place (routinely an endotracheal or tracheostomy tube), obstructions or partial obstructions can occur, usually in an insidious and subtle fashion. Assessment of airway patency and effectiveness includes an ongoing evaluation. Is the reasoning behind originally placing this airway still valid? Is this still the right airway for the patient? The following factors should be considered as part of the assessment:

1. The level of consciousness at this phase of trauma care. What is the patient's ability to guard his or her own airway and manage oral and nasal secretions?
2. The prophylactic aspects of the airway. Is there a future risk of obstruction, as in glottic edema from airway burns or maxillofacial trauma?

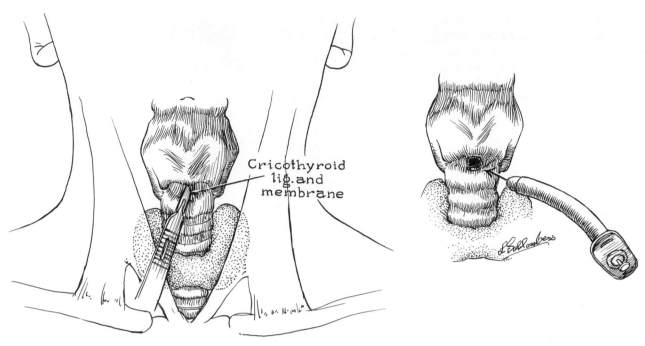

FIGURE 23-10 **Cricothyroidotomy Technique.** (From Zuidema GD, Rutherford RB, Ballinger WF: *Management of trauma,* ed 4, Philadelphia, 1985, WB Saunders.)

TABLE 23-3   Airway Adjuncts in Trauma

Oropharyngeal Airway

Indications	Unconscious patients without gag reflex; short-term use
Advantages	Holds tongue away from posterior pharynx
Restrictions	Oropharyngeal injuries
Complications	Intraoral injury; induction of vomiting and aspiration; increased obstruction if positioned incorrectly by pushing the tongue back into pharynx

Nasopharyngeal Airway

Indications	Semicomatose or arousable patients with decreased control of upper airway; prevention of tissue trauma during frequent nasotracheal suctioning
Advantages	Better tolerated in awake patients than oral airway; easily secured
Restrictions	Maxillofacial trauma such as nasal, nasoethmoid fractures
Complications	Nasopharyngeal injury; nasal bleeding

Esophageal Obturator Airway (EOA), Combitube, Pharyno-Tracheal Lumen (PTL) Airway, Laryngeal Mask Airway (LMA)

Indications	When unable to successfully place ETT
Advantages	Can be positioned quickly without direct visualization, with minimal manipulation of cervical spine
Restrictions	Cannot be used in awake or semiconscious patients
Complications	Induction of vomiting and aspiration; esophageal tears; post-pharyngeal bleeding; unrecognized incorrect placement

TABLE 23-3 **Airway Adjuncts in Trauma—cont'd**	
Endotracheal Tube (ETT)	
Indications	Preferred method of airway control
Advantages	Stable airway; provides protection from aspiration; permits mechanical ventilation to be used; decreases gastric distention associated with bag-mask ventilation; nasal intubation preferred in awake patient or when cervical spine integrity is unknown
Restrictions	Used with caution in presence of laryngotracheal injuries (glottis, subglottis, and upper trachea)
Complications	Esophageal intubation leading to hypoxia; right main-stem bronchus intubation; induction of vomiting and aspiration; vocal cord injury; pharyngeal injury; tracheal lacerations; conversion of cervical spine injury without neurologic deficit to injury with deficit; dislodged tube
Cricothyroidotomy	
Indications	When intubation does not relieve obstruction or trachea cannot be intubated
Advantages	More rapid, greater ease of accessibility, and lower incidence of bleeding than tracheostomy
Restrictions	Children under 12 years; laryngeal injury or inflammation
Complications	Subglottic stenosis; vocal cord injury; aspiration; hemorrhage; tracheal or esophageal laceration; mediastinal emphysema; dislodged tube
Standard Tracheostomy	
Indications	When intubation does not relieve obstruction or in significant laryngeal or tracheal trauma; used for prolonged ventilatory support
Advantages	Bypasses upper airway and glottis; stable airway with low resistance to airflow; easily suctioned
Restrictions	Limited use as an emergency procedure because of time requirements and potential for bleeding
Complications	Early or delayed hemorrhage; aspiration; mediastinal emphysema with or without pneumothorax; tracheoesophageal fistula; tracheal stenosis; tracheomalacia; tracheoarterial fistula; dislodged tube

3. Complications apparent from the present airway. If the intubation time will be longer than 2 weeks, is tracheotomy a better alternative? Is there purulent nasal drainage caused by developing sinusitis while a nasal tube is in place? Does a previously overlooked injury such as an intraoral laceration or tracheal tear change the choice in airway management?

4. The patient's response to the airway. Are head and neck movements rapid and agitated, endangering tube position or creating further airway damage? What is the probability of self-extubation?

Assessment for partial or impending obstruction is ongoing. Frequent signs include increasing level of agitation, increasing airway pressures during mechanical ventilation, difficulty in advancement of a suction catheter, and frequent evacuation of bloody clots or mucous plugs. Proper airway position and cuff pressure are determined by clinical and radiographic examinations.

General nursing management begins by documentation of airway tolerance, complications, length of intubation, and date of tracheostomy. The specific plan of care is based on such factors as a history of any airway problems, difficulty in intubation, and patient behavior, such as attempts at self-extubation or bronchospasm on suctioning. An identical spare airway and a manual resuscitator bag with face mask should be located at the bedside for rapid management of obstruction. Airway hygiene is implemented on the basis of assessment findings. Tracheostomy care is patient specific depending on the newness of the stoma, type of secretions or peritracheal drainage, and signs of infection. A record is maintained at the bedside of all tube changes, tube size, and any difficulties encountered in tube placement. The need for long-term airway management is apparent in the intermediate care setting, if not before. Substitution of a fenestrated or "talking" tracheostomy will help communication, and speech therapy consultation is required for patients recovering from laryngeal or vocal cord injury. As soon as the patient and family indicate readiness, a teaching plan is begun that covers long-term and home management of secretions and tracheostomy care.

TRACHEOBRONCHIAL TRAUMA

DESCRIPTION. The tracheobronchial tree may be injured at any level; most commonly, injury involves the main-stem bronchi within an inch of the carina (Figure 23-11). Injuries may be complete or incomplete, and total separation of the tracheobronchial tree can occur. However, continuity of the airway may be maintained by the fascia surrounding the trachea and bronchi.[11] The lower airway injuries are of interest to nurses in all phases of trauma care because injury discovery may occur dramatically during intubation and ventilation or surprisingly late in the patient's posttrauma course. The injuries are usually caused by blunt forces, the common denominator being violent injury. Examples are a frontal crush injury, a vertical stretching of the trachea or bronchus, and any impact that suddenly increases pressure within the airway against a closed glottis. Tracheobronchial tears caused by penetrating injury also occur, frequently in association with esophageal, carotid artery, or jugular vein trauma.

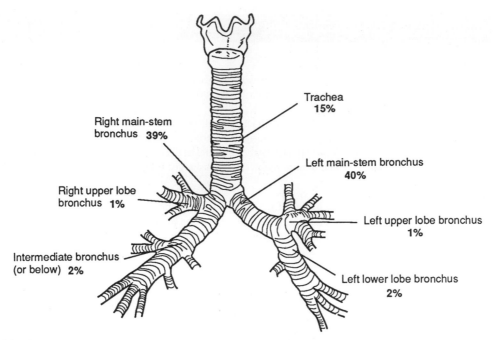

FIGURE 23-11 **Tracheobronchial Ruptures: General Localizations Based on Literature Review.** (From Besson A, Saegesser F: *Chest trauma and associated injuries,* Oradell, NJ, 1983, Medical Economics.)

RESUSCITATION/CRITICAL CARE ASSESSMENT. The index of suspicion is heightened by a history of violent trauma, particularly in patients with fractures of the upper five ribs. The rupture may be immediately symptomatic through dyspnea, hemoptysis, or difficulty in intubation. Severe injuries are frequently fatal. A tear may be suspected in the patient with mediastinal and subcutaneous emphysema accompanied by a persistent pneumothorax that resists reexpansion. More commonly the rupture develops in two stages. The patient shows almost no symptoms until 3 or 4 days after admission, when pneumothorax or subcutaneous emphysema develops. Should the patient already have chest tubes in place, a persistent pleural air leak is evident, possibly with continued extravasation of air into tissues. An additional clinical picture may develop, one that is particularly difficult to diagnose and requires the correlation of nursing and medical observations. Early atelectasis appears and persists as a result of occlusion of the bronchus with blood and secretions. Bloody secretions are evident on coughing or during suctioning as pleural fluid is drawn back through the damaged airway.

In assessing for tracheobronchial tears, possible location, size, and involvement of bronchial vessels or the mediastinal pleura must be considered. The patient may demonstrate significant hemoptysis, airway obstruction, pneumothorax, tension pneumothorax, massive atelectasis, or extensive subcutaneous emphysema. Any one of these characteristic findings raises the possibility of tracheobronchial injury. The diagnosis is confirmed through tracheobronchoscopy.

MANAGEMENT. Initial management is dependent on the severity of the symptoms described above. An airway is secured in the patient with significant hemoptysis and airway obstruction either by insertion of an endotracheal tube or by tracheostomy. If present, pneumothorax, tension pneumothorax, and any mediastinal compression are treated by tube thoracostomy and evacuation of pleural air by suction. The rate and amount of air evacuated by the chest tube are monitored continuously, as is the adequacy of air intake into the lungs. Immediate thoracotomy is indicated in the presence of massive air leak that prevents adequate air intake.

More commonly the initial tube thoracostomy is followed by definitive diagnostic bronchoscopy and plans for injury repair. If the tear is large and irregular or is a complete rupture, early surgical repair is accomplished by a cervical or thoracic approach. The tear is resected and closed by end-to-end anastomosis. A small tear may be treated conservatively solely through airway management. The airway chosen for management depends on the location and leaking effect of the tear. A standard endotracheal tube or tracheostomy may be used. Selective endobronchial intubation with a double-lumen tube also can be accomplished if there is a need for independent lung ventilation; this technique is discussed within the critical care therapeutics section of this chapter. As the inflammation and edema caused by injury subside, the area can heal.

SPECIFIC NURSING MANAGEMENT. The nurse must know the location of the tear and repair status to create an appropriate plan of care. In all cases the existing airway must be secured carefully and protected from dislodgment or inadvertent repositioning. It may be technically difficult to reposition a dislodged tube, exposing the patient to needless risk of hypoxia, asphyxia, or extension of the tear. If surgical repair has been completed, airway protection remains

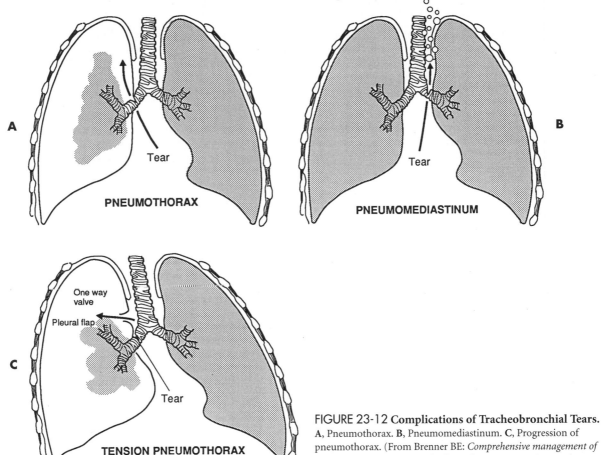

FIGURE 23-12 Complications of Tracheobronchial Tears.
A, Pneumothorax. **B**, Pneumomediastinum. **C**, Progression of
pneumothorax. (From Brenner BE: *Comprehensive management of
respiratory emergencies*, Rockville, Md, 1985, Aspen Systems.)

critical while the suture line heals. Careful suctioning and
neck positioning to avoid increased suture tension protect
the area of surgical repair.

An additional management focus is measurement of the
quantity and effect of any air leak on ventilation and
oxygenation. Pleural drainage is inspected regularly for
sudden air evacuation and increases in a known leak.
Thoracic examination is repeated to appreciate changes in
subcutaneous air and the development of pneumomediastinum or pneumothorax (Figure 23-12). Nursing care is
directed toward avoiding sudden rises in the patient's airway
pressure, which will delay healing of the injury.

Bronchial injury may be accompanied by lung injury
with tears in surrounding small blood vessels, allowing air to
enter the pulmonary venous circulation. Monitoring for
signs of air embolism is important, particularly before repair
or for the patient who is managed conservatively without
repair. A sudden cardiovascular deterioration after endotracheal intubation without signs of bleeding may be indicative of air embolism. Focal neurologic signs in the
non-head-injured patient are also significant. Placing the
patient in the head-down Trendelenburg's position is presumably optimal to trap air in the apex of the left
ventricle. Immediate cardiocentesis may be indicated to
evacuate the air, and thoracotomy may be required to
control the air leak.[11,16]

INTERMEDIATE CARE ASSESSMENT AND MANAGEMENT.
Tracheobronchial tears are often diagnosed late in the
assessment for occult or missed injury. An additional focus
of the assessment is the identification of posttraumatic
complications such as bronchial stenosis. The initial tracheobronchial tear results in a stenosed airway obstructed by
granulation tissue and prone to repeated inflammation and
infection. Delayed atelectasis appears as granulation tissue
obstructs the bronchus. Resection of the area of stricture
and reanastomosis may be required to prevent repeated
infections and heightened scar tissue formation below the
level of the stenosis. Laser ablation of stenotic lesions and
endobronchial stents are also used.[17] Nursing management
is directed toward specific chest physiotherapy for the
affected areas and airway clearance. The patient's vital
capacity, chest film, and secretions are monitored. Assistance in coughing is a priority because the injury frequently
leaves a residual decrease in bronchial sensitivity and a
diminished cough reflex.[17]

Tracheal injury or, less commonly, tracheostomy may
result in tracheal stenosis, which is made apparent by a
hoarse, unproductive cough; wheezing; and periodic dyspnea on exertion. Occasionally assessment may reveal signs
of tracheomalacia, which is a softened tracheal wall. This is
the outcome of damage and loss of tracheal cartilage from
tissue ischemia, necrosis, infection, and long exposure to an

overinflated cuff. The patient's trachea expands and collapses during respiration (truncated loop sign). Repairs of both types of complications are achieved by surgical resection and anastomosis or graft insertion.

POSTTRAUMATIC TRACHEAL FISTULA

DESCRIPTION AND ETIOLOGY. Tracheoarterial or esophageal fistula may be the result of blunt injury in much the same fashion as tracheobronchial tears. More commonly it is a form of "tube trauma." Although the association between high pressure or overdistended cuffs and tracheal fistulas is well known, cuff pressures and positions can be difficult to manage and require special consideration and cooperation from the trauma team. Significant airway pathology can occur after as little as 6 hours of intubation and mechanical ventilation.[16] Tube trauma can be a sequela of a difficult intubation or tracheostomy.[17] During these procedures a retropharyngeal or tracheal wall nick or tear can occur. The area becomes infected with upper airway secretions, erodes, and becomes a fistula. Successful repair of tracheoarterial (TA) and tracheoesophageal (TE) fistulas is reported with increased frequency. Discussion of surgical repair and its complications is found elsewhere.[11]

TRACHEOARTERIAL FISTULA. The vessel involved may be the innominate, right carotid, or a lower thyroid artery that has been exposed to pressure from an overinflated cuff or a poorly positioned airway. As the tracheal wall erodes, the vessel is perforated and suddenly bleeds into the airway. The patient may die immediately from hemorrhage through the tracheostomy. Figure 23-13 shows how poor tube positioning and cuff over inflation cause a hemorrhage.

Prevention. Physiologic cuff pressure is maintained at less than mean mucosal capillary pressure of 20 to 25 mm Hg. The different commercially available tracheostomy

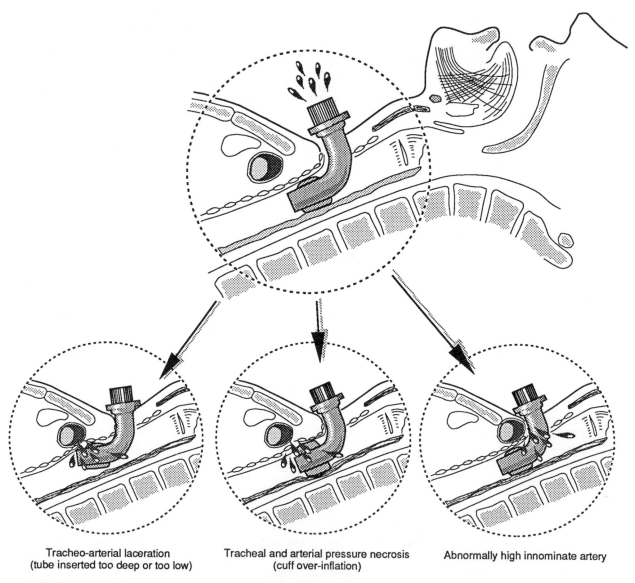

Tracheo-arterial laceration
(tube inserted too deep or too low)

Tracheal and arterial pressure necrosis
(cuff over-inflation)

Abnormally high innominate artery

FIGURE 23-13 **Tracheoarterial Fistula.** (From Besson A, Saegesser F: *Chest trauma and associated injuries*, Oradell, NJ, 1983, Medical Economics.)

and endotracheal tubes all exert varying tracheal wall pressures, including the soft, large-volume cuffs and foam cuffs, which are autoregulated by air valve. Proper inflation of the cuff according to product recommendations is useful; however, the actual cuff pressure must be measured. Measurement is made by a special cuff pressure gauge or, if necessary, by a simple stopcock and manometer apparatus. The current standard of continuous inflation to a minimal leak or minimal occlusion is discussed in the nursing research literature.[18] If there is reason to believe that the patient is at risk for TA fistula, a shorter or longer tube of appropriate diameter may be inserted to relieve the immediate pressure. A pulsating tracheostomy tube is evidence of such risk but does not confirm fistulization. Any patient at high risk can be examined by tracheoscopy for evidence of fistula formation.[18,19]

Immediate Management of the Disaster.   An attempt is made by immediate maximal cuff inflation to stem the bleeding. If cuff overinflation fails, the tracheostomy tube is removed, and a translaryngeal tube is inserted. The cuff is again inflated at the level of the fistula to control the bleeding, or the tube may be positioned to allow direct finger pressure and control. The finger is inserted along the anterior trachea and compresses the blood vessel against the sternum.[11] The patient is ventilated and prepared for immediate transport to the operating room. If transport is not possible, the surgical equipment necessary for artery ligation is readied. A standard thoracotomy tray or a complete cutdown preparation tray contains the needed equipment. Suction must be immediately at hand.

Definitive Management.   Should the patient survive the initial hemorrhage and artery ligation, ventilation is provided by a long transtracheal tube with the cuff positioned below the necrotic area. Delayed repair of the trachea and arterial reconstruction is accomplished once the risk of infection is lessened. The repair includes resection and anastomosis or grafting if necessary. Every effort should be made to wean the patient from the ventilator and remove the tracheostomy tube as soon as possible.

TRACHEOESOPHAGEAL FISTULA.   A tracheoesophageal fistula also can be life threatening although not as rapidly as a vascular fistula. It is not an emergency, yet it threatens life through respiratory insufficiency and infection. The injury is a pressure necrosis of the trachea and the anterior esophageal wall. Rarely is it a primary injury from blunt trauma. Figure 23-14 shows how fistulas occur from tube placement and cuff inflation.

Prevention.   The techniques described for prevention of vascular fistulas are also appropriate in this case. The most likely pressure site is between the airway cuff and nasogastric tube. Frequent evaluation of the need for and use of these tubes is a primary preventive action. Each tube is viewed as a risk factor and is eliminated as soon as possible. For example, a gastrostomy tube can be placed for long-term gastric decompression and permit the removal of a nasogastric tube. The risk of a fistula continues into the rehabilitative phase for the trauma patient who requires long-term tracheostomy.

Assessment.   Most symptoms are usually identified by the observing nurse. The patient coughs on swallowing, or pulmonary secretions appear contaminated by gastric contents. The usual amount of tracheal secretions increases, and gastric distention may be evident consistently. The appearance of swallowed methylene blue dye in tracheal aspirate is a classic bedside test. Visualization of the fistula is accomplished by endoscopy or bronchoscopy. Contrast studies are associated with a high risk of aspiration and are not recommended.

Management.   The fistula must be closed surgically, generally through a cervical incision, but the timing of surgical repair depends on the patient's general condition. The patient may require considerable pulmonary care and nutritional support via parenteral nutrition and jejunostomy before repair is attempted. A large-volume, low-pressure cuff airway is used during the period of supportive preoperative therapy and after the surgical repair. The airway cuff is positioned at a different site within the trachea if possible.

BONY THORAX FRACTURES

DESCRIPTION AND FRACTURES SITES.   The triad of pain, ineffective ventilation, and secretion retention is observed consistently in patients with rib fractures, sternal fractures, or flail chest. It is from this perspective that the patient with thoracic cage fractures presents the greatest demand for creative and effective nursing care. The first two ribs are generally protected by the surrounding muscles, clavicle, scapula, and humerus. Fractures of these ribs signal high-impact trauma and are generally accompanied by injury to the lungs, aortic arch, or vertebral column. Ribs 3 through 9 are most commonly fractured in blunt trauma and are frequently associated with underlying lung injury. The lower rib has a similar anatomic association with liver tears or other abdominal injuries. Sternal fractures are also generally associated with considerable blunt trauma. (Table 23-4).

FLAIL CHEST.   Flail chest is an injury of multifocal fractures, whether anterior, lateral, or posterior. Generally multiple rib fractures and a sternal fracture are present. The continuity of the thorax is destroyed, and the rib cage no longer moves evenly and in unison. The injured parts of the bony thorax do not respond to the action of the respiratory muscles but move according to changes in intrapleural pressure. The flail segments move paradoxically, and from this appearance the term *paradoxical breathing* has been used to describe the patient's respiratory efforts. Gas flow within the lungs may or may not move paradoxically, but it is significantly diminished. The bellows effect of the chest is lost, intrapleural pressure is less negative than normal, and

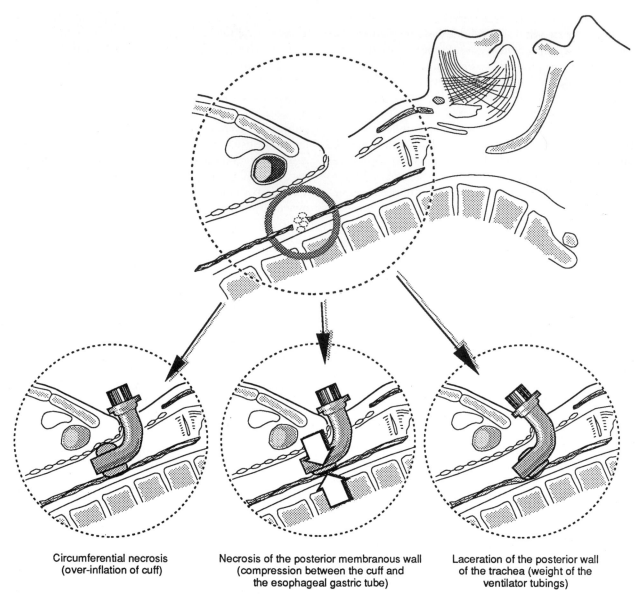

Circumferential necrosis
(over-inflation of cuff)

Necrosis of the posterior membranous wall
(compression between the cuff and
the esophageal gastric tube)

Laceration of the posterior wall
of the trachea (weight of the
ventilator tubings)

FIGURE 23-14 Causes of tracheoesophageal fistula in patients with tracheostomy. (From Besson A, Seagesser F: *Chest trauma and associated injuries,* Oradell, NJ, 1983, Medical Economics.)

ventilation is compromised. The decreased gas flow and increased respiratory dead space are evident in lowered patient tidal volume, increased respiratory effort, and varying degrees of hypoxia.

Resuscitation Assessment of Flail Chest. The best assessment is simply to carefully observe the patient's breathing and chest wall movement. Breathing is rapid and labored, and the chest wall moves in an asymmetric and uncoordinated manner. The flail will be evident by inspection and by palpation of crepitus from bony fragments although it may not be seen while the patient is on full ventilatory support. The amount of dyspnea and initial hypoxia depends on the size of the flail, associated pulmonary parenchymal injuries, and the patient's ability to exert the needed respiratory effort in compensation for the flail.

The injury causes great chest wall pain and patient fatigue. The initial chest film identifies the general extent of the flail and additional thoracic injuries.

It is difficult to characterize a specific profile for patients with flail chest because their injury is so often accompanied by either a pneumothorax or some degree of pulmonary contusion. Both conditions are discussed in detail later in this chapter. It is essential to associate flailing thoracic injuries with a high probability of underlying parenchymal damage. Serial blood gases, continuous pulse oximetry monitoring, and continuous observation of the patient's tidal volume and respiratory effort should be initiated, particularly in the patient who is not immediately intubated and mechanically ventilated. Flail chest and associated injuries frequently also produce upper and lower airway obstruction from blood, mucus, or vomit.

TABLE 23-4	**Classification of Rib Fractures**
Injury	**Major Manifestations, Related Injuries, and Common Complications**
Fractures of one rib	
Simple	Pain aggravated by deep breathing, coughing
	Localized tenderness
	Roentgenograms may or may not demonstrate fracture
Complicated	Pneumothorax, hemothorax
	Pulmonary infection or atelectasis
Multiple rib fractures	
With stable chest wall	Severe chest wall pain
	Underlying lung contusion or contusion of opposite lung
	Decreased cough and accumulation of secretions
	Acute gastric dilation
	Hemothorax, pneumomediastinum, and pneumothorax
With instability of chest wall	Generally involves fracture of each rib in two sites
	Panel of chest wall moves independently of thoracic cage (paradoxical respiration)
	Severely impaired cough and airway clearance
	Contusion of underlying lung
	Hemothorax and pneumothorax
Fractures of first rib	Usually associated with fractures of clavicle and upper ribs
	May involve neurovascular structures of neck
	Intrathoracic injuries
Fractures of lower ribs	Injuries to liver and spleen
(seventh to twelfth)	Acute gastric dilation

From Guenter CA, Welch MH: *Pulmonary medicine,* ed 2, Philadelphia, 1982, JB Lippincott.

Initial Management.   Most patients with flail chest injury will require appropriate airway management, some type of analgesia, and oxygen therapy to maintain the Pa_{O_2} at levels of 80 to 100 mm Hg. The flail must be stabilized so as to reestablish the thoracic bellows effect and promote air exchange.[16] Positioning the patient with the injured side down may improve oxygenation, but it is generally precluded by the need for immobilization of the spine and supine positioning for transport. In-hospital management includes internal "splinting" through positive-pressure ventilation.[20] Surgical internal stabilization of rib and sternal fragments also has been recommended, especially if thoracotomy is required for some other reason. Internal fixation significantly improves patient outcomes and avoids the complications associated with prolonged ventilatory support.[4,16]

Ventilatory Therapy.   There are several ways to support ventilation in patients with significant flail chest. Nonventilator support with oxygen therapy may be successful with patients who can follow commands and do not have underlying parenchymal damage. In other patients mechanical ventilation offers specific advantages, including airway and ventilatory control for pulmonary hygiene, functional positioning of flail segments, decreased muscular work, and a decrease in painful, paradoxic chest wall motion. Specific patients who benefit from mechanical ventilation in some mode include nonambulatory or disoriented patients, those with significant lung pathology, and those with consistently diminished tidal volume (i.e., <15 ml/kg) as a result of fatigue and other injuries. Critics of mechanical ventilation cite disadvantages such as increased risk of barotrauma,

pulmonary contamination, and a potentially longer need for therapy. A reasonable approach to ventilatory therapy in flail chest injuries is to individualize ventilatory support for the patient. The choice of therapy depends on the size of the flail; immediate degree of pulmonary dysfunction; work of breathing and fatigue; the presence of other thoracic injuries, particularly underlying pulmonary contusion; the need for general anesthesia and surgical procedures related to associated traumatic injuries; and the risk of posttraumatic respiratory insufficiency. Intubation/tracheostomy and mechanical ventilation are indicated if the respiratory rate is faster than 35 breaths/min, if Pa_{O_2} is below 60 mm Hg on supplemental oxygen, or if Pa_{CO_2} is acutely above 50 mm Hg.[4,16]

Critical Care Assessment and Management.   The choice of intubation and ventilator therapy may not be made until admission to the critical care unit. In addition to the preceding criteria, the choice may depend on equipment and available nursing management. The patient with significant flail and underlying lung contusion frequently has a long-term stay in the intensive care unit. Management of the injuries and weaning from ventilator support may require as many as 10 to 25 days. Appropriate equipment and effective nursing management must be available throughout the period. As stated earlier, the common triad in flail chest is ineffective ventilation, accumulation of secretions, and chest pain. Specific nursing care includes management of the patient-ventilator unit, pulmonary care, and pain control.

Managing the Patient-Ventilator Unit.   Whichever ventilator therapy is selected, the patient must be monitored closely through pulse oximetry, blood gases, and pulmonary function studies such as vital capacity, inspiratory force, tidal volume, and a measure of the work of breathing in order to determine therapy results. Most frequently the patient is treated and later weaned by IMV or SIMV with pressure support with rate, pressures, tidal volume, and oxygen concentration adjusted to maintain acceptable blood gases. Repeated clinical examinations and daily chest films reveal trends in respiratory complications such as respiratory distress syndrome or atelectasis and progress toward chest wall stability. Chest wall rigidity is apparent at approximately 3 weeks, and a full 6 weeks are usually required before the fractures are consolidated.

Pulmonary Care. As ventilation becomes stabilized, pulmonary care begins to clear the airways and lung fields. Aggressive chest physiotherapy consisting of postural drainage, gentle percussion, vibration, and suctioning are used at varying intervals, depending on the patient's pulmonary status. The quality and quantity of secretions are monitored for infection. A plan for patient position change is based on observation of which position provides greatest chest wall stability (such as lying on the flail segment) and best ventilation/oxygenation. These treatments are discussed in more detail in the section on critical care therapeutics.

Pain Control. Pain control is critically important and may be the primary problem for patients with bony thorax fractures. A variety of useful treatments have been reported for thoracic pain; they include intercostal nerve blocks, intrapleural administration of narcotics, and patient-controlled analgesia (PCA), both intravenous and epidural (EPCA). These methods are supported by nursing research as safe and effective modalities for pain control.[21-23] Continuous intravenous narcotics, which can be titrated by the nurse to the patient's respiratory status, level of consciousness, and level of pain, also constitute a well-accepted method of pain control, especially with patients not candidates for epidural or intravenous PCA. Research now supports the use of epidural over intravenous PCA for optimal pain relief and better outcomes for patients with thoracic injuries. However, not all patients will be candidates for EPCA.[21] Regardless of the method or route of administration, appropriate dosage ranges are established for the patient and then are monitored by nursing observation and management. Nonpharmacologically, the application of a transcutaneous electrical nerve stimulator (TENS) may relieve the pain associated with thoracic injuries. Relaxation, distraction, and guided imagery are also part of the nonpharmacologic armamentarium to help control the pain resulting from thoracic trauma.[24]

INTERMEDIATE/REHABILITATION CARE ASSESSMENT AND MANAGEMENT. At this point in the trauma recovery, new complications of bony thorax fractures become evident. The normal healing of the fractures may be altered, and deformities may be noticeable to the patient and family.

Some deformities, from flail chest in particular, are permanent, unattractive, and difficult for the individual to accept. Others may create ventilatory impairment, leading to chronic disability and changes in lifestyle. Attempts at surgical reconstruction may dominate the patient's recovery experience.

The plan of care for the patient is built around assessment of the emerging complications and disability, previously described needs for pulmonary care, control of retained secretions and infection, and relief of chest pain. The goal of pulmonary care is support of spontaneous ventilation and weaning from oxygen therapy. Chest physiotherapy and incentive spirometry are continued in order to clear problem areas in the lungs and improve respiratory mechanics such as thoracic muscle strength. The patient continues to experience chest pain to some degree: some individuals endure intractable intercostal pain or neuralgia. Chest pain can be managed pharmacologically. However, other methods must be initiated if they are not already in progress because pain relief is frequently a lengthy and complex problem. TENS, massage, and positioning are only a few of the possibilities.

COMPLICATIONS OF FRACTURE HEALING. Rib fractures usually heal within 6 weeks. Occasionally, malunion or a failure to consolidate fractures, even an entire flail segment, does occur. Inspection and palpation, as previously described, will identify the unstable chest segment and can be confirmed radiographically. Internal fixation can be achieved by the wiring of bone fragments or insertion of a metal plate.

Abnormal healing also results in excessive or hypertrophic callus formation, which may be gradually reabsorbed or surgically excised. The callus rubs on surrounding tissue and muscle, creating considerable pain. An abnormal union of adjacent ribs, intercostal synostosis, may proceed during the months after injury. Clinical and radiographic examinations identify abnormal healing in a patient who continually experiences pain and restricted chest wall movement.[25]

Surgical intervention may be needed for definitive management of these healing abnormalities. As with any surgical patient, preoperative teaching is required, with detailed discussion of the procedure, anticipated experiences, and outcomes. The initial trauma did not allow for such preoperative preparation, and the current surgery may have a unique and special meaning for the patient.

POSTTRAUMATIC RESPIRATORY DISABILITY. Observation and interviewing help to identify dyspnea, shortness of breath, and a feeling of chest tightness in some patients. Blood gas analysis and chest film findings are frequently unchanged. The long-term sequelae of significant bony thorax trauma are unclear, and published case reports are few. Restrictive defects in ventilation have been identified in patients with flail chest and accompanying pleural or lung injury, as evidenced by moderate or severe dyspnea, abnormal spirometry, and lessened overall activity levels. The current nursing approach includes tracking the patient's unique problems, instituting measures that provide comfort, ensuring appropriate physical therapy referrals, and providing a great deal of psychologic support.

PLEURAL SPACE INJURIES

All pleural space injuries have both blunt and penetrating causes. The force of injury, whether from blunt impact against the steering column or from a knife wound, produces laceration or perforation of an intrathoracic structure, usually a lung or blood vessel. Blood and air collect between the pleural layers, and the normal negative intrathoracic pressure is lost. All or part of the lung on the affected side collapses because of its unopposed elasticity. The result may be a pneumothorax (intrapleural air collection), hemothorax (intrapleural blood collection), or, very commonly in trauma, hemopneumothorax (mix of both air and blood). If intrapleural air or blood continues to increase within the constraints of the closed intrathoracic cavity, internal structures are compressed and tension builds. The result is a tension pneumothorax or hemothorax. In all cases the pleural space injury may be unilateral or bilateral.

ASSESSMENT OF PLEURAL SPACE INJURY.   Examination for any type of pleural space injury follows the thoracic assessment procedure described earlier. It is useful to remember that the clinical findings are determined by the severity of all thoracic injuries as a whole and the severity of the pleural space injury. In addition, the signs of injury may change over the period of examination and resuscitation. A small hemothorax may become massive if bleeding resumes at some point after the patient's admission. An apparently small pneumothorax can evolve into a tension pneumothorax.[25]

Several classic assessment findings are seen in all significant pleural space injuries. Some degree of respiratory difficulty or dyspnea is evident. Because the primary problem is altered ventilation, there is evidence of poor gas exchange. There is frequently a loss of breath sounds on the affected side or sides. Diminished or absent breath sounds are evident with a collapsed lung and when blood loss into the thoracic cavity is significant (generally >350 ml). There is a loss of normal resonance on percussion of the affected side. Dullness is audible in hemothorax, and there is hyperresonance when significant pneumothorax is present.

Early analysis of blood gases is useful only in the context of the patient's clinical examination and response to trauma. The patient who is breathing rapidly because of shock and pain may have relatively normal initial blood gases levels. Alternatively, there may be the "expected" rise in $Paco_2$ and fall in Pao_2 that is normally associated with poor ventilation.[25]

Chest film findings assist in documenting the injury and must be obtained as rapidly as possible. Small amounts of blood may not be visible, but in an average-sized chest, blood filling the costophrenic angle on an upright film is usually more than 300 ml. An air-fluid level that extends

5 cm above the diaphragm contains at least 1000 ml whereas the volume of air in the chest can only be estimated. The film may reveal not only blood in the intrathoracic cavity but also a segment of spleen or liver that has been displaced through a ruptured diaphragm.[14,25]

CLOSED PNEUMOTHORAX OR HEMOTHORAX.   A simple, closed pneumothorax is usually the result of a lung laceration caused by a fractured rib or penetrating wound (Figure 23-15). In more complex injuries a diaphragmatic tear allows abdominal contents to protrude into the chest cavity, causing a compressive pneumothorax or hemopneumothorax. In many instances the intrapleural air leak is self-limiting in that the progressive collapse and decreasing ventilation of the affected lung seal the leak. In other cases, depending on the size and location of the injury, the lung may collapse completely.

Common sources of bleeding in hemothorax include systemic chest wall vessels, internal mammary arteries, and intercostal arteries and accompanying veins. Penetrating wounds may involve major pulmonary vessels, any of the mediastinal structures, or the diaphragm. Although the pulmonary parenchyma is a common source of bleeding, major blood loss is generally not from parenchymal vessels. The lung is a low-pressure vascular system capable of tamponading sources of bleeding[4] (Figure 23-16).

Resuscitation Management.   As always, appropriate airway, ventilatory, and oxygen therapy begins the management process. Occult pneumothoraces resulting from blunt trauma may not require chest tube placement; however, careful pulmonary assessment is paramount in preventing further injury.[25] Moderate pneumothorax or hemothorax requires the correct placement of a chest tube for the purposes of lung reexpansion and drainage of air, blood, and clots from the pleural space. Inadequate drainage creates short- and long-term complications, including intrapleural infections and adhesions. Insertion of a chest tube also reduces the risk of tension pneumothorax, which may develop as blood or air fill the chest cavity. Explanations of the injury and treatment are offered to the patient in a manner most appropriate for his or her emotional state and level of consciousness. The patient's pain must be recognized and treated.

A large-bore chest tube, such as a no. 40 French, is inserted, usually in the fourth or fifth intercostal space in the midaxillary line, to drain both air and blood. Alternatively, but less optimal in traumatic injuries, a tube may be placed in the second intercostal space in the midclavicular line to drain a simple pneumothorax. As soon as the tube is connected to the underwater seal system and suction drainage, the effects of the treatment are assessed by analysis of blood gases, chest x-ray, and physical examination. The bleeding is frequently self-limited, and estimated blood loss is replaced at a rate consistent with the patient's overall status. Small to moderate air leaks will usually seal over in the first few days after trauma. Occasionally a major air leak

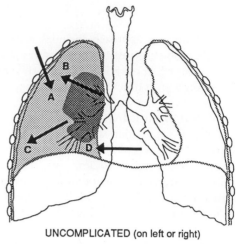

FIGURE 23-15 **Orgins of Pneumothorax.** (From Besson A, Saegesser F: *Chest trauma and associated injuries,* Oradell, NJ, 1983, Medical Economics.)

	UNDER TENSION (on left or right)				UNCOMPLICATED (on left or right)
A	7%	Perforating or penetrating wound			20%
B	13%	Tracheobronchial injury (including barotrauma)			5%
C		Pulmonary laceration			
	71%	27% probable	36%	}	73%
		44% documented	37%	}	
D	9%	Oesophageal injury			3%
	33%	Accompanied by haemothorax			54%
	26%	Accompanied by subcutaneous emphysema			33%

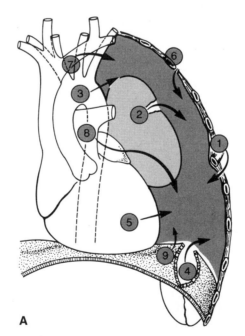

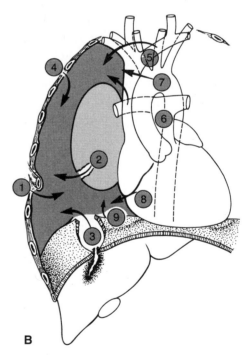

FIGURE 23-16 **Sources of Bleeding in Hemothorax.** (From Besson A, Saegesser F: *Chest trauma and associated injuries,* Oradell, NJ, 1983, Medical Economics.)

A

Source of bleeding in left hemothorax (moderate or massive)

1.	Rib fracture	36%
2.	Pulmonary parenchyma	35%
3.	Aortic isthmus	15%
4.	Spleen	5%
5.	Heart chamber	5%
6.	Intercostal or internal mammary artery	5%
7.	Supraaortic vessel	3%
8.	Major pulmonary vessel	2%
9.	Diaphragm	0%

There are several sources of bleeding in 6 percent of cases.

B

Source of bleeding in right hemothorax (moderate or massive)

1.	Rib fracture	51%
2.	Pulmonary parenchyma	27%
3.	Liver	10%
4.	Intercostal or internal mammary artery	5%
5.	Supraaortic vessel	4%
6.	Pulmonary vessel	3%
7.	Aortic isthmus	1%
8.	Heart chamber	1%
9.	Diaphragm	0%

There are several sources of bleeding in 2 percent of cases.

persists, requiring more negative pressure in the suction drainage system or an additional chest tube. Bronchoscopy and open thoracotomy may be required to determine if major bronchial injury is responsible for the continued air leak.

Critical Care/Intermediate Care Management. A simple pneumothorax or moderate hemothorax will not necessarily require critical care for the patient. However, this type of injury may be one of several thoracic injuries and is frequently a symptom of more life-threatening injuries.

Monitoring the Injury and Drainage. The nurse evaluates the functioning of the chest tube system and the progress of the injury. Repeated physical assessment and follow-up chest films determine if the lung has reexpanded and ventilation has returned to the patient's normal baseline. Pulse oximetry and blood gases are used, and a chest film is obtained whenever problems arise or the clinical status changes. Blood loss through or around the chest tube is measured and evaluated for further progression of bleeding. Drainage of more than 200 ml/hr for 2 successive hours may indicate additional or missed injuries and the need for exploratory thoracotomy.[16] Trends in the patient's tidal volume and air evacuation through the chest tube system are monitored for significant air leaks and loss of ventilatory volume. Nursing management of pleural drainage is discussed in more detail later in this chapter.

MASSIVE HEMOTHORAX. Massive hemothorax, defined as a 1.5 to 4 L of intrathoracic blood loss, is truly a life-threatening injury. Frequently there are severe associated thoracic injuries, and the source of bleeding is a large systemic blood vessel or mediastinal structure. Because the chest cavity is large enough to contain most of the patient's circulating blood volume, the bleeding slows only when the pressure within the pleural cavity is equal to or greater than the pressure within the damaged vessel. A left massive hemothorax is more common than a right one and is often associated with aortic rupture.[16]

Resuscitation Assessment and Management. Thoracic assessment is initiated after basic life support needs are managed. The patient may arrive in cardiopulmonary arrest and in need of immediate thoracotomy to control bleeding. Assessment findings in massive hemothorax differ from the moderate pleural injuries in degree. The immediate clinical picture includes signs of hypovolemic shock, dyspnea, tachypnea, and cyanosis. Shock is the predominant picture evident before or concomitantly with impaired ventilation. Ventilation problems are caused by lung compression and collapse, and signs of mediastinal shift with cardiac compression also may be evident. The initial chest film identifies the extent of the massive hemothorax which appears as a predominantly opaque chest cavity.

Hypovolemic shock is managed by immediate insertion of a large-bore intravenous line and administration of resuscitation fluids. The response to fluid resuscitation in hemorrhagic shock seems to depend on whether the hemorrhage is controlled or uncontrolled.[16,26] Large amounts of fluid resuscitation in patients with uncontrolled bleeding can actually increase bleeding from the injured site, resulting in a poor outcome.[26] The next step is dependent on the amount of anticipated or apparent intrathoracic bleeding. The truly massive injury requires emergent exploratory thoracotomy with rapid control of bleeding. Delay of thoracotomy and initial insertion of a chest tube may provide an avenue for exsanguination by eliminating any tamponade effect from a closed chest injury (Figure 23-17). Assuming that one or more chest tubes are in place and signs

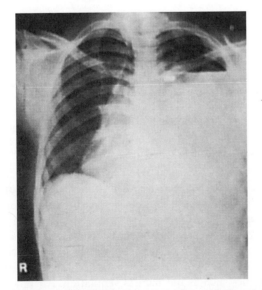

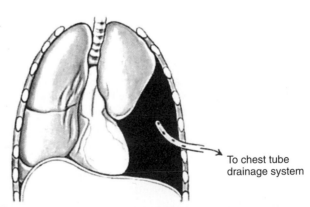

To chest tube drainage system

FIGURE 23-17 Radiograph of a young man in profound shock from a gunshot wound to the chest. Bullet entry was in the sixth intercostal space in the midaxillary line. Hemothorax and shock were treated by chest tube drainage and fluid administration. Film (R) shows the central position of the bullet. The patient was transported to the operating room but died there as a result of continuing hemorrhage from injury to the pulmonary hilar vessels. In massive hemothorax, exsanguination may occur after chest tube drainage. (From Naclerio EA: *Chest injuries,* Orlando, 1971, Grune & Stratton.)

of exsanguination occur, the chest tube is clamped as an interim measure pending emergency thoracotomy. In general, urgent thoracotomy is performed if there are the following indications:

1. More than 1500 ml of blood evacuated on initial chest tube insertion
2. Continued bleeding of more than 200 ml/hr for 3 consecutive hours
3. Bleeding of more than 150 ml/hr for 3 consecutive hours in an elderly patient
4. Any of the preceding in the face of hemodynamic instability[16]

Autotransfusion. Autotransfusion is useful in the management of hemothorax and intrathoracic sources of bleeding. The reinfusion of blood aspirated from the chest as a thoracic trauma management method was reported by military surgeons as early as 1916.[27] A variety of techniques and commercially available autotransfusion devices are available for resuscitation of the injured patient.

The increasing use of autotransfusion in resuscitative, operative, and critical care attests to the numerous advantages of autologous blood administration. These include the following:

1. The blood is readily available and particularly useful in the patient with massive hemorrhage that exhausts or severely taxes the bank blood availability.
2. Autologous blood requires no cross-matching and should be free of pyrogens, avoiding allergic and febrile reactions.
3. Autotransfusion avoids the risk of hepatitis, AIDS, or exposure to homologous antigens.
4. Platelet counts and 2,3-diphosphoglycerate (2,3-DPG) levels essential to normal oxygen delivery to tissues are reported to be near normal in rapidly autotransfused blood. No warming is required.
5. Autologous blood may be acceptable to patients, such as Jehovah's Witnesses, who would normally refuse bank blood.
6. Cost savings generally are appreciated, depending on institutional pricing of equipment, operation, and packaging.[28]

Current autotransfusion devices range in cost, sophistication of function, and requirements for special technical assistance. One system separates out red cells and washes and resuspends them before patient infusion as a means of removing any plasma contaminants or debris while retaining red blood cells. Simpler techniques can be employed rapidly in patients with blunt and penetrating chest trauma. A thoracostomy tube inserted by standard technique and connected to suction provides an avenue for retrieval of shed intrathoracic blood. The blood is aspirated through sterile tubing, collected in a lined plastic reservoir, filtered, and returned to the patient intravenously. The retrieval bag may contain citrate phosphate dextrose (CPD), other types of anticoagulants, or no anticoagulant.

Specific contraindications to autotransfusion include known malignancy; inadequate renal or hepatic function; wounds more than 3 hours old; and significant contamination caused by bowel, stomach, or esophageal disruption. Clinical judgment is required as to the degree of contamination and risk of septic complications.

Precautions and implications for nursing management center on the procedure's effect on the blood and the risk of coagulopathy and microembolism. The primary effect on the blood is hemolysis leading to reduced hematocrit and increased urine and serum hemoglobin levels. Typical falls in hematocrit of 10% to 15% and increases in serum hemoglobin of 5 to 10 times normal have been reported. The hemolysis appears to occur at the blood-tissue and blood-plastic interfaces if roller pumps are used during collection and infusion.[28,29] Autologous blood from serosal cavities such as the thorax lacks fibrinogen, contains elevated levels of fibrin split products, and shows prolonged prothrombin (PT) and partial thromboplastin (PTT) times. Microembolism on infusion of shed blood is of concern because of hemolytic cell debris or platelet aggregation. Filters are used during the collection of autologous blood and a 40 micron filter is used as part of the blood administration protocol to reduce risk of emboli infusion. Air embolism is also a concern, especially when the shed blood is reinfused using a surrounding pressure bag. Extraordinary care must be used to expel all the air within the reservoir bag before application of the pressure bag.

In view of these concerns the patient who is or has recently been autotransfused is monitored through coagulation profiles, including complete blood count and urine hemoglobin. Platelets and fresh-frozen plasma are given if clotting factors need to be replaced. If an anticoagulant accompanied the autotransfused blood, the same concerns are present as for banked blood. The serum calcium level is measured to assess the chelating effect of citrate on calcium. If contaminated shed blood is reinfused, the patient is monitored for symptoms of emerging sepsis.

Use of an autotransfusion system may be episodic in many hospital units. The entire team, particularly nurses who assume responsibility for the use of equipment and monitoring the patient's response to treatment, must maintain their knowledge and skills. Methods and equipment need to be the subject of periodic inservice training, with the goal that all trauma team members can initiate autotransfusion rapidly, safely, and without complications.[28,30]

TENSION PNEUMOTHORAX. Immediate recognition of this life-threatening condition is required of nurses who manage patients in any phase of trauma care. Tension pneumothorax may be the immediate result of the primary traumatic injury, a delayed complication of an occult injury such as bronchial tear, or the undesirable result of necessary therapies such as mechanical ventilation. Air (and possibly blood) that has entered the pleural space is trapped without exit, creating a one-way-valve closed system (Figure 23-18). One or more internal thoracic structures (most notably the trachea, lung, heart, and great vessels) are compressed

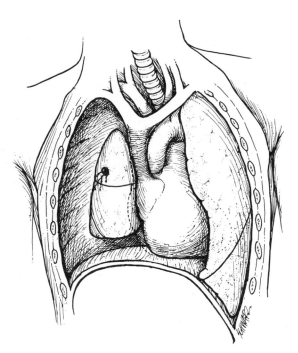

FIGURE 23-18 Tension Pneumothorax. A bullet or knife wound to the lung can create a check-valve perforation, resulting in a tension pneumothorax. Pressure builds in the right hemithorax, impeding venous return, shifting the mediastinum to the left, and depressing the diaphragm. The great vessels become twisted and distorted. This decreases cardiac output and leads to shock with cyanosis, dyspnea, and neck distension. Atelectasis of an entire lobe leads to shunting, with cyanosis and tachypnea. Insertion of a venting needle or chest tube can be lifesaving. (From Weiner SL, Barrett J: *Trauma management for civilian and military physicians,* Philadelphia, 1986, WB Saunders.)

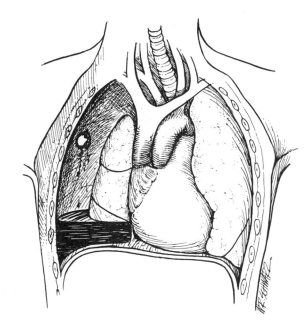

FIGURE 23-19 Open Chest Wound and Resulting Hemothorax. (From Weiner SL, Barrett J: *Trauma management for civilian and military physicians,* Philadelphia, 1986, WB Saunders.)

progressively and fail to function adequately. The compression/failure mechanism may affect one or both sides of the chest cavity simply because pressure is transmitted through the chest as a whole. The patient outcome is a failure in ventilation, venous return, and eventually cardiac output. Assessment and treatment deal with the problem in ventilation and cardiovascular performance.

Initial Assessment. Systematic assessment and diagnosis are not always simple in the trauma patient. Classic signs of tension pneumothorax may be obscured by shock and other injuries or treatments until the patient is badly compromised. Under these circumstances the initial assessment begins by identifying the high-risk patient, such as one with an inadequately resolved pneumothorax, bronchial tear, lung contusion, or pulmonary cyst. The use of moderate to high levels of PEEP also creates a risk of tension pneumothorax. The injury may not be discovered until the patient experiences a rapid and steep fall in oxygenation. The patient is difficult to ventilate yet appears to have an open airway.[16,25]

The patient is examined carefully and rapidly for clues to the reason for failure in ventilation or cardiac output. One focus of the assessment is signs of increased intrathoracic pressure, the compression/failure effect. Chest wall movement is observed for asymmetry, and the chest wall is percussed for the characteristic hypertympanic note of trapped air. Tracheal shift is a classic finding but may be difficult to

determine in the intubated patient except by chest radiograph. Unless the patient is severely hypovolemic, neck veins may be distended, reflecting downstream intrathoracic pressure. Breath sounds are compared carefully from one side to the other and are diminished. Pulse oximetry measures decline and blood gases, if available, show a sudden drop in Pao_2. Finally, cardiac output is assessed quickly through decreases in blood pressure, tachycardia, or a general shock state that is unexplained by other injuries.

Immediate Management. Supplemental oxygen is provided, and then the chest must be decompressed by release of the trapped air. Decompression is achieved in three phases. Initial relief can be accomplished by inserting a 14- or 16-gauge needle into the pleural space, usually at the second to fourth anterior intercostal space. The needle is inserted over the rib and only 1 cm beyond to avoid puncturing the lung or injuring intercostal nerves and vessels.[11,16] As air is released, ventilation should improve. The pleural space equilibrates with atmospheric pressure, and the tension pneumothorax is converted temporarily to an open pneumothorax. The next phase of treatment occurs as one or more chest tubes are inserted both to reexpand the lung (or both lungs in bilateral tension pneumothoraces) and as prophylaxis for any repeated episodes. Third, the cause of the injury must be explored and managed appropriately. The chest film, blood gases, hemodynamic measurements, and clinical examination are repeated to reassess the patient's posttreatment state.

OPEN PNEUMOTHORAX. Penetrating chest trauma caused by a pleural space open to the atmosphere creates an open pneumothorax or sucking chest wound (Figure 23-19).

Described as early as the thirteenth century, the open pneumothorax is a common combat injury. It is most likely seen in civilian life as the result of penetrating injury or impalement. A number of factors have been proposed to explain the ventilatory difficulty presented by open pneumothorax. If the size of the chest wall defect is approximately two thirds the tracheal diameter, air will preferentially enter the chest wall during respiration. This "false airway" allows intrathoracic and atmospheric pressures to equalize, losing the essential pressure gradient required for normal ventilation.[16,25] Loss of normal intrathoracic negative pressure reduces venous return and cardiac performance, which is aggravated by mediastinal shift and compression of the vena cava and heart.

Resuscitation Assessment and Management.   The first step is locating the wound. Careful inspection of the entire thorax, including the patient's back, reveals the injury. Once the wound has been found, the sucking action is readily apparent. Frequently there are gas bubbles at the wound site, and abnormal gas exchange may be audible. Not all penetrating chest wounds create an open pneumothorax; some are superficial although menacing in appearance. Conversely, a small and unassuming wound may be responsible for the pneumothorax and other threatening injuries.

The management objectives are to restore ventilation and to debride and close the wound. Ventilation is, as always, the priority. Extensive open wounds, such as from a close-range shotgun blast, require intubation and mechanical ventilation. In all cases the false airway must be sealed and the lung allowed to reexpand. A sterile semiocclusive dressing is applied immediately over the entire wound, the effects of which are reassessed repeatedly. An old but still useful method is three-sided taping of dressing materials to the chest wall. This creates a flutter effect as the dressing is sucked down to the chest wall on inspiration yet allows air to escape on expiration.[13] Should the occlusive dressing seal off the wound without a means of escape for the trapped air, barotrauma and tension pneumothorax are possible. Therefore the effect of the dressing on ventilation is observed over time, particularly while waiting for effective placement of the chest tube. After the dressing is applied, a chest tube is inserted at another site to treat the pneumothorax. The treatment effect is monitored without removing the dressing by noting changes in breath sounds and signs of intrathoracic pressure.

After ventilation has been managed adequately, the wound requires cleansing and debridement. The need for definitive surgical exploration and closure depends on the wound and on the presence of additional injuries requiring high-priority treatment.

PULMONARY CONTUSION
MECHANISM AND PATHOPHYSIOLOGY.   Essentially a compression/decompression injury, lung contusion occurs as the chest wall hits an object such as a steering wheel or is acted on by an outside force such as an explosion. The force

against the chest wall is transmitted to the lung, rupturing tissue, small airways, and alveoli. The pressure wave abates, and the chest wall springs back, pulling the lung with it and causing additional injury. It is a bruising process possibly accompanied by pulmonary tear or laceration. This injury occurs most often in young people because the chest wall is more flexible than in older individuals. Whereas the older person might sustain multiple rib fractures, the young person might sustain more contusions.[31] Individuals with thin chests sustain greater contusions because there is less protection provided by muscle and adipose tissue.

Contusions may be mild and go unnoticed in the treatment of associated injuries such as flail chest or hemopneumothorax. However, unilateral or bilateral contusion can be severe, even life threatening, and can seriously interfere with gas exchange. The contusion process is hemorrhagic and is accompanied by interstitial and alveolar edema as a response to injury. Hemorrhage and edema occur within the area of contusion and gradually involve surrounding tissue in general inflammation. Damaged or closed alveolar-capillary units produce ventilation and perfusion abnormalities and shunt. If no further lung injury occurs, the areas of infiltrate begin to clear and healing occurs. More commonly, however, the injured area evolves into areas of atelectasis as a result of secretion retention and infection. Blunt trauma that produces significant lung contusion is frequently associated with pulmonary hematoma or laceration. Severe lacerations that bleed into the pleural space or airway require thoracotomy and pulmonary resection.

RESUSCITATION ASSESSMENT.   During initial resuscitation, respiratory distress may be evident. Accompanying rib fractures are common but not universal. If the contusion is clinically significant, the Pao_2 is frequently less than 60 mm Hg on room air. Lung infiltrates may be seen on the admission chest film. The sputum may be bloody.[32]

CRITICAL CARE ASSESSMENT.   Predicting the outcomes of patients who present with pulmonary contusions is difficult at best. In the first 24 hours the patient shows progressive clinical and radiographic changes that correlate with underlying alveolar capillary injury. Patchy infiltrates persist on subsequent chest films. Bloody sputum continues to be evident on suctioning either as fresh blood or as old blood and clots in the mature contusion. Local areas of wheezing are a common finding. Patients with significant contusions show progressive evidence of stiff, wet lungs and increased work of breathing. Measured pulmonary compliance falls. Peak airway pressure increases. The degree of deterioration in Pao_2 and pH is usually a function of failure to recognize the extent of the contusion and to institute early ventilatory support and pulmonary hygiene. The presence of associated injuries, including shock, produces secondary changes within the lung. Posttraumatic respiratory distress syndrome may be superimposed on the evolving lung contusion.

CRITICAL CARE MANAGEMENT

Managing Gas Exchange. Supportive oxygen therapy and pulmonary care to mobilize and clear bloody secretions are required in every patient as the contusion resolves during the first few days after trauma. The need for early intubation and mechanical ventilation of patients with blunt chest trauma remains a controversy, as discussed in the section on flail chest injuries. Support of spontaneous ventilation with supplemental oxygen may be adequate for some patients. Others require mechanical ventilation support. Criteria for instituting mechanical ventilation are available.[32] Ventilatory management can be effective for individual patients provided the benefits and risks of that therapy are monitored. In all cases adequate gas exchange is observed over time by continuous pulse oximetry monitoring when possible, capnography, frequent blood gas analysis, and calculating parameters such as Q_s/Q_t, Pao_2/Fio_2 ratio, and compliance.[33,34]

Managing the Patient-Ventilator Unit. Massive contusions may require pharmacologic paralysis and controlled mandatory ventilation or high-frequency ventilation in an effort to aerate the poorly compliant, damaged lungs. This poses considerable risk of pneumothorax or tension pneumothorax if chest tubes are not in place and positioned adequately. The risk of barotrauma can be reduced by maintaining adequate sedation and analgesia levels. Further discussion of barotrauma is found in the section on critical care therapeutics.

Airway Management. Airway management is problematic and requires careful monitoring for obstruction. Many patients with pulmonary contusions have an endotracheal or tracheostomy tube in place. The airway lumen may become partially obstructed with bloody mucus, clots, and pieces of dead tissue. Frequent suctioning may be required to avoid obstruction. Meticulous sterile suction technique is essential because these procedures always increase the risk of contamination and infection. Keeping a spare airway at the bedside is an essential precaution because airway obstruction may occur even with apparently adequate irrigation and suction.

Pulmonary Hygiene. This is particularly important in managing patients with significant lung contusion. Early institution of chest physiotherapy, postural drainage, and percussion assists in avoiding or treating postcontusion atelectasis. The treatment should be specific to the lung segment involved. Monitoring the quality of pulmonary secretions provides an important outcome criteria. Within 48 to 72 hours the bloody mucus should become thinner and darken, eventually clearing to normal appearance. If symptoms of infection become evident, sputum cultures and chest films are required.

Fluid Administration. There remains considerable debate over the therapeutic range for fluid administration. Some investigators have found that aggressive crystalloid administration is associated with pulmonary insufficiency and interstitial edema after pulmonary injury.[31,32] Conversely, others propose that crystalloid infusion in volumes necessary to restore and maintain preload and hemodynamic stability is not detrimental.[33] Regardless of the controversy, volume administration is guided by monitoring clinical indicators of tissue perfusion sufficiency (e.g., urine output, mentation, lactate levels) and invasive hemodynamic parameters. Typically the contusion begins to clear radiographically within 72 hours of injury. The presence of one or more persistent infiltrates suggests a pulmonary complication such as pneumonia, aspiration, or posttraumatic respiratory distress syndrome.[33]

INTERMEDIATE CARE/REHABILITATION MANAGEMENT. The focus of nursing management continues to be pulmonary hygiene and restoration of respiratory reserve. Weeks after injury the patient may develop a traumatic cyst, a further concern for pulmonary infectious sequelae. Most patients appear to recover from significant lung contusion with minimal respiratory disability.[34]

ACUTE RESPIRATORY DISTRESS SYNDROME

Severe respiratory insufficiency was observed after trauma as early as World War II, and during the Vietnam era it came to be viewed as the point beyond which severely injured patients did not survive. Although originally known as "wet" or "shock" lung, it has become apparent over the years that hypotensive shock per se is not the sole cause or mechanism of the syndrome. Numerous traumatic and biochemical insults produce apparently similar responses in the lung and a characteristic clinical picture. Mortality from posttraumatic respiratory insufficiency remains high despite prolific research that has identified specific risk factors, described the pathology, and evaluated clinical management strategies.[35]

Terminology used to describe posttraumatic respiratory distress can be confusing. In addition to older literature centered on "shock" lung, one encounters references to "traumatic respiratory insufficiency," "wet" lung, and the ubiquitous "adult respiratory distress syndrome," which has been renamed *acute* respiratory distress syndrome (ARDS). ARDS was formerly described by Ashbaugh, Bigelow, and Petty[36] in 1967 as a cluster of clinical features with apparent similarities in pathology and pathophysiology. Of the dozens of causes or related factors, ARDS is clearly linked with severe traumatic injury, sepsis, and shock.

DESCRIPTION AND RISK FACTORS. ARDS is not a primary disease. It is a syndrome that is always secondary to some other insult or combination of injuries. Major risk factors or conditions associated with the development of ARDS in trauma include shock of any type (septic, hemorrhagic, cardiogenic, neurogenic, or anaphylactic), multisystem trauma with extensive tissue destruction, direct pulmonary contusion, multiple orthopedic injuries (particularly long bone or pelvic fractures), massive transfusions, thoracic trauma (such as pulmonary contusions, bacterial pneumonia, sepsis, near drowning, and gastric aspiration), and major head injuries.[37] There is a higher incidence of the syndrome in those patients with multiple risk factors than in those with a single risk factor.[35,37] ARDS is a sequela of hemorrhagic shock and hypotension and develops in hypovolemic patients with other insults or predisposing problems. The presence of sepsis is a key factor leading to ARDS, usually from a nonpulmonary source. Newer research describes two different forms of ARDS: early and late ARDS. Early ARDS is identified by capillary leak resulting from hemorrhage; late ARDS follows pneumonia and is associated with multiple system injury.[38]

The varied insults result in a final common pathway of lung response that is clinically evident 2 to 48 hours after injury. The major problem is respiratory insufficiency, evidenced by hypoxemia, noncardiogenic pulmonary edema, pulmonary hypertension, and intrapulmonary shunting. A description of the major clinical features helps to define the syndrome[35,37] (Table 23-5). There is a need to exclude other pulmonary or cardiac conditions and use four broad but statistically powerful components in describing the syndrome: (1) the presence of a severe defect in oxygenation, (2) the presence of new, diffuse bilateral infiltrates on chest film, (3) the presence of a pulmonary wedge pressure less than 18 mm Hg, and (4) the absence of other clinical explanations for these findings.[39]

PATHOPHYSIOLOGY.　Whatever the precipitating insults, the central pathophysiologic component is damage to the alveolar-capillary interface, both endothelial and epithelial. The architecture and degree of alveolar-capillary disruption varies. Studies with CT scans demonstrate considerable regional variability within the lung fields; normal areas are adjacent to areas of severely injured tissue.[40] Early stages of the syndrome's pathophysiology are explained by this primary loss of microvascular and alveolar membrane integrity, resulting in noncardiac pulmonary edema, hypoxemia, pulmonary hypertension, V/Q mismatching, and decreased pulmonary compliance. Progressive alveolitis and

fibrosis occur in later stages of ARDS, accompanied by respiratory infection and pneumonia.[38]

ARDS has often been described as "high-permeability" pulmonary edema; however, the characteristic edema is due in part to increased capillary permeability and in part to increased hydrostatic pressure secondary to pulmonary hypertension. The effect within the lung includes formation of interstitial and then alveolar edema, abnormal surfactant action, and nonuniform collapse of functional lung units. The lung edema may not necessarily correlate well with the clinical findings, particularly with the severity of the early oxygenation deficit.[36] The apparent lack of correlation is related to the ability of the pulmonary lymphatics to compensate for increases in microvessel permeability. It is also related to the concept that edema, although a hallmark of ARDS, is a consequence of lung injury, not a causative agent.[40]

One of the most significant problems is hypoxemia, which is relatively resistant to supplemental oxygen. The increased work of breathing associated with the underlying inflammatory process and edema may rapidly consume a large portion of available oxygen and energy stores.[35,37] Eventually the inflammatory exudate overwhelms lymphatic drainage, and the lung interstitium can no longer act as a reservoir, leading to alveolar flooding. Compensatory hypoxic pulmonary vasoconstriction is lost, and pulmonary hypertension occurs. There is significant intrapulmonary shunting and a lack of response to oxygen.[41]

ARDS produces stiff lungs, resulting in reduced functional residual capacity and high airway pressures required to inflate the lungs. Pulmonary compliance is decreased initially as a result of interstitial and alveolar edema and cellular infiltration and then because of fibrosis later in the patient's course. The efficacy of surfactant is decreased, perhaps as a result of metabolic abnormalities in the alveolar type II cells, which retain the capability to produce surfactant.[42] Peribronchial edema can lead to airway constriction with wheezing, decreased V/Q ratio, and increased airway pressures (Tables 23-6 and 23-7).

The cause of the underlying alveolar-capillary lesion is unclear. It is the subject of extensive research, primarily through several animal models of lung injury that employ biochemical agents, microembolism, acid aspiration, and

---

TABLE 23-5　Clinical Features of Posttraumatic Respiratory Distress Syndrome

History compatible with known risk factors
Respiratory distress
　Tachypnea (>30 breaths per minute)
　Dyspnea
Hypoxemia
　Pao_2 <50 mm Hg when Fio_2 >0.6)
　Pao_2/Fio_2 <200 mm Hg with mechanical ventilation
Increased shunt fraction (Q_V/Q_T >15-20%)
Increased dead space ventilation ($\dot{V}_D$/$\dot{V}_T$ >0.6)
Decreased static compliance (<30 ml/cm H_2O)
Pulmonary hypertension ($PAP_{systolic}$ >30 mm Hg)
Diffuse pulmonary infiltrates on chest film (interstitial then alveolar)

From Maier RV, Mendez C: Respiratory insufficiency. In Feliciano DV, Moore EE, Mattox KL, editors: *Trauma*, Stamford, Conn, 1996, Appleton and Lange.

TABLE 23-6　ARDS: Diagnostic

- Clinical respiratory distress
　Tachypnea, dyspnea
- Hypoxemia refractory to supplemental O_2
- Decreased Pao_2/Fio_2 ratio <150 or <200 with PEEP
- Diffuse peripheral infiltrates on chest radiograph
- Exclusion of cardiogenic pulmonary edema; PCWP appropriate for level of PEEP
- Decrease in pulmonary compliance

From Maier RV, Mendez C: Respiratory insufficiency. In Feliciano DV, Moore EE, Mattox KL, editors: *Trauma*, Stamford, Conn, 1996, Appleton and Lange.
PCWP, Pulmonary capillary wedge pressure.

hemorrhagic or septic insults. A single injury mechanism or pathophysiologic cascade has not been identified; however, numerous substances have been implicated (Table 23-8). In general, leukocyte aggregation is an important factor in producing lung injury, potentially involving several types of phagocytic cells (e.g., neutrophils, eosinophils, monocytes, and macrophages). Neutrophils are present in large numbers within the lungs of patients with ARDS[43] and are well known as a source of toxic oxygen radicals and proteolytic enzymes. A number of studies have indicated that activation of the complement system creates lung injury by leukocyte stimulation and chemotaxis. More recent data suggest that although complement activation may initiate injury in some forms of lung pathology, it is not a necessary or sufficient condition in trauma-related ARDS.[44]

However, a large body of experimental evidence supports the hypothesis that white cells elaborate mediators that contribute to alveolar and capillary pathology and pulmonary edema. The importance of understanding these mediators lies in the future potential for pharmacologic therapies and interventions to interrupt the pathophysiologic cascade and improve patient outcomes. Leukocyte products include oxygen free radicals (e.g., superoxide anion, hydrogen peroxide, and hydroxyl radicals), proteases that can destroy the vascular basement membrane (e.g., elastase, cathepsin G, and collagenase), and arachidonic acid metabolites.[43] Phagocytic cells such as pulmonary alveolar macrophages are able to synthesize various products of endogenous and exogenous arachidonic acid via the cyclooxygenase or lipoxygenase pathways. Which metabolites are released at what point in ARDS pathology is not known. Nevertheless, these lipid mediators have potent effects on the pulmonary vascular and airway smooth muscle and on cell membrane permeability. For example, prostaglandin I_2 or

TABLE 23-7 ARDS Stages

Stage 1 (acute)	Dyspnea, tachypnea, respiratory alkalosis
Stage 2 (~24 hr)	Cyanosis, hypoxemia (refractory to $\uparrow F_{IO_2}$), pulmonary hypertension $\downarrow$ FRC and compliance, scattered lung infiltrates
Stage 3 (24-96 hr)	Respiratory failure, severe hypoxemia requiring ventilator plus PEEP, microvascular thrombosis increases dead space with CO_2 retention, diffuse pulmonary infiltrates
Stage 4 (progressive, days to weeks)	Progressive refractory hypoxemia, increasing hypercapnea, metabolic acidosis, interstitial fibrosis ("pulmonary hepatization") with decreasing compliance, increasing pulmonary hypertension, right heart failure, dense pulmonary consolidation

From Maier RV, Mendez C: Respiratory insufficiency. In Feliciano DV, Moore EE, Mattox KL, editors: *Trauma*, Stamford, Conn, 1996, Appleton and Lange.
FRC: Functional residual capacity.

TABLE 23-8 Mediators in ARDS

Mediator	Source	Function
Complement	Plasma, macrophage	Neutrophil chemotaxis, capillary permeability
Proteases	Neutrophil, macrophage	Cellular/basement membrane damage, complement activation
Reactive oxygen intermediates	Neutrophil, macrophage	Cell membrane peroxidation
TNF-α	Monocyte, macrophage, neutrophil	Macrophage secretion IL-1, IL-6, IL-8, IL-1, TXA_2, PGE_2, LTB, PAF, PCA Activates neutrophil and endothelial cells Fever, shock $\uparrow$ Vascular permeability
IL-1β	Monocyte, macrophage	Macrophage secretion of TNF, IL-6, PAF; neutrophil release and adherence Activates endothelial cells Fever, shock Hypermetabolism
IL-8	Monocyte, macrophage	PMN chemotaxis, activation, retention
TXA_2	Macrophage, platelets	Platelet aggregation, pulmonary vasoconstriction, bronchoconstriction
PGE_2	Macrophage, endothelial cell	Inhibits macrophage cytokine release
PGI_2	Macrophage, endothelial cell	Vasodilation, vascular permeability
LTB_4	Macrophage, endothelial cell	Neutrophil chemotaxis
PAF	Monocyte, macrophage, neutrophil, endothelial cell, platelets, pneumocyte	Macrophage priming, neutrophil priming, chemotaxis and activation, platelet histamine and serotonin release
PCA (TF)	Macrophage, endothelial cell	Coagulation, thrombosis

From Maier RV, Mendez C: Respiratory insufficiency. In Feliciano DV, Moore EE, Mattox KL, editors: *Trauma*, Stamford, Conn, 1996, Appleton and Lange.
IL-1, Interleukin-1; *IL-1β*, Interleukin-1β; *IL-6*, Interleukin-6; *IL-8*, Interleukin 8; *LTB₄*, Leukotriene B₄; *TXA₂*, Thromboxane A₂; *PAF*, Platelet-activating factor; *PCA (TF)*, Procoagulant activity tissue factor; *PGE₂*, Prostaglandin E₂; *PGI₂*, Prostacyclin; *TNF-α*, Tumor necrosis factor α.

prostacyclin (PGI$_2$) is a potent pulmonary vasodilator that may affect inflammatory cell function. Prostaglandin F$_2$ (PGF$_2$) and thromboxane are vasoconstrictors with effects on both microvascular and large-vessel smooth muscle. Thromboxane (TXA) also enhances platelet aggregation. Some experimental models have shown that platelets play an important role in ARDS pathology.[40]

Much of the clinical evidence for the role of neutrophils is dependent on their presence and that of their products in the lungs of patients with differing forms of the disease process. A cause-and-effect relationship has not been established, and it is possible that leukocyte activation only aggravates a pathologic condition from some other mechanism. Furthermore, it was suggested recently that it is the failure of neutrophilic defense mechanisms that is important in ARDS pathology. Neutrophils have key protective and reparative functions such as the production of oxidant scavengers and bactericidal agents. Loss of these functions may have important consequences in these patients, particularly in preventing pulmonary infections.[43]

Other factors may act as mediators or markers of injury. Platelet activating factor (PAF) is a phospholipid mediator produced by numerous cell types such as platelets, vascular endothelium, and leukocytes. PAF is associated with a variety of important effects on pulmonary and systemic vascular tone, vessel permeability, and other ARDS-linked mediators such as cyclooxygenase and lipoxygenase products. Its role in ARDS, if any, is inconclusive. Monokines, protein mediators of inflammation released by macrophages and monocytes, are currently under investigation in late-stage ARDS and multiple organ failure.[38,44] Interleukin-1 (IL-1) may be important in attracting phagocytic cells and lymphocytes and in promoting cell adherence to injured endothelium. A second monokine, tumor necrosis factor (TNF), produces acute lung inflammation in a manner similar to that of endotoxin when injected into animals, and it also increases capillary protein leakage.[39,44]

RESUSCITATION ASSESSMENT.   Clinical evidence of the syndrome is not apparent during the initial resuscitation period. A major requirement is to assess and document the risk of posttraumatic respiratory insufficiency for each patient. It remains unclear if the type and volume of resuscitation fluids have implications for the pulmonary edema of posttraumatic ARDS. However, fluids are administered and documented carefully with pulmonary sequelae in mind.[41]

CRITICAL CARE ASSESSMENT.   Patients who are at risk for ARDS after major trauma should be observed closely for signs of respiratory difficulty. There are three clinical phases based on clinical findings and pathophysiologic changes: impending insufficiency, clinical insufficiency, severe failure, and resolution.[38]

Impending Insufficiency.   The physical examination may be essentially normal. Lungs are dry to auscultation, and secretions are minimal or explained by other injuries.

However, the patient is dyspneic, even though Pao$_2$ is relatively normal. Arterial blood gases also reveal decreased Paco$_2$ and respiratory alkalosis, either as a new finding or as a continuation of the tachypnea observed during initial resuscitation. Changes in the chest film that are characteristic of ARDS are rarely evident. Lung pathology is poorly defined in this early phase, except that neutrophil sequestration and some degree of interstitial edema are apparent. Knowledge of the patient's risk factors and these early assessment findings form the basis for supportive oxygen therapy and pulmonary care.

Clinical Insufficiency.   Within the first 24 hours there are both clinical and pathologic signs of acute lung inflammation. Oxygenation is markedly depressed in relation to the delivered concentration. The patient is dyspneic and in respiratory distress with hypoxemia. Increases in physiologic dead space and pulmonary vascular resistance are measurable. Patchy lung infiltrates are evident on the chest film, particularly in dependent areas. With appropriate ventilatory management and control of underlying infection or unresolved trauma, the ARDS process can be resolved at this point.

Some patients continue to experience progressive respiratory failure over the next 2 to 3 days and require progressive ventilatory and hemodynamic support. Physiologic dead space continues to increase, and the shunt fraction is high. The patient requires a high concentration of inspired oxygen despite PEEP. Characteristic bilateral infiltrates are recognizable on the chest radiograph. The lungs are heavy and wet, with continued white cell infiltration, alveolar edema, and microvascular congestion. Many individuals are in a hyperdynamic state with elevated cardiac index, regional perfusion shifts, and peripheral defects in oxygen use.[38] The hyperdynamic state may be caused by the same processes, trauma and sepsis, that originally produced the respiratory dysfunction.

Severe Failure.   Frequently irreversible, pathologic respiratory conditions include fibrosis, atelectasis, and recurrent pneumonia. Hypoxemia is refractory to continued increases in delivered oxygen concentration. Despite careful ventilator adjustments, impaired gas exchange and a progressive decrease in compliance are accompanied by impaired peripheral O$_2$ extraction and acidosis.

Despite advances in ventilatory support, posttraumatic ARDS mortality remains high. Mortality has been reported at 41% in blunt trauma and 65% in a mixed critically ill population.[35] Deaths associated with ARDS can occur within 72 hours of the initial insult; however, early deaths are not as common as delayed mortality secondary to sepsis.[37] Typically the patient dies within 2 weeks of the onset of the syndrome, not because of hypoxemia or complications of respiratory support but because of an inability to eliminate the underlying disease or infectious process. Multiple organ failure is associated with high patient mortality.[35,36]

Resolution. Some patients do not progress to the severe failure stage. If complications such as infection are contained and the functional lung tissue is supported appropriately over time, the alveolar-capillary injury heals and clinical abnormalities abate. Most studies indicate that there is little or no permanent respiratory disability in survivors of ARDS. It is toward this end that nursing management is directed.

CRITICAL CARE MANAGEMENT. Despite early identification of patients at high risk for ARDS and knowledge of the progressive disease pattern, there are no clearly preventative agents or procedures. Similarly, there is no one cure for the syndrome. Therapies designed to intervene in the process of mediator activation may ultimately be useful in ameliorating the disease process. Studies of ARDS pathophysiology have led to trials of numerous therapeutic agents, including methylprednisolone, prostaglandin E_1 (PGE_1), ibuprofen, indomethacin, prostacyclin, free-radical scavengers, antifungal drugs, and fibronectin. These agents are being evaluated for clinical use. Meduri and associates studied the use of methylprednisolone in ARDS patients and obtained promising results. They conclude, "Prolonged administration of methylprednisolone in patients with unresolving ARDS was associated with improvement in lung injury and MODS [multiple organ dysfunction syndrome] scores and reduced mortality."[45] More clinical trials are needed to verify these positive patient outcomes. Early and effective ventilatory and hemodynamic support remains the foundation of critical care management. Equally important is the treatment of underlying trauma, infection, or other inciting factor. The patient with ARDS requires sedation and analgesia that balance both comfort and desired ventilatory status, consistent emotional support, and planned periods of rest and sleep. Explanation of the patient's injury and expected outcomes of ventilatory therapy are needed not once but many times throughout the changing events.

Ventilatory Support. Patients with known risk factors are monitored closely for signs of respiratory deterioration. Alternative causes of respiratory dysfunction, such as atelectasis or pulmonary contusion, should be considered and treated appropriately. Most patients require mechanical ventilation once dyspnea, tachypnea, and hypoxemia are evident. Numerous criteria must be analyzed when selecting the right ventilatory method and equipment, including work of breathing, compliance, airway resistance, and possible complications of the therapies. The ventilatory mode chosen for the patient should be one that provides adequate mean airway pressure to promote alveolar recruitment while avoiding injurious high peak airway pressures.[46] Newer studies indicate that it may be safer to accept a higher $PaCO_2$ (permissive hypercapnia) rather than subject the lungs to damaging high tidal volumes (e.g., 5-7 ml/kg body weight).[47] The inspired oxygen concentration is chosen to establish a sufficient physiologic PaO_2 at a nontoxic FiO_2. An initial inspiratory-to-expiratory time (I/E) ratio of 1:2 is commonly used. However, as respiratory failure progresses, longer inspiratory times can improve V/Q mismatching by recruiting alveolar segments.[18,48] A number of techniques have been recommended, including control mode, IMV or SIMV with or without pressure support, inverse I/E ratio ventilation, airway pressure release ventilation, and, in selected cases, simultaneous independent lung ventilation or high-frequency ventilation.[49]

Use of CMV with PEEP. Controlled ventilation can be used for patients with marked compliance problems and difficulty in achieving adequate gas exchange by other ventilatory methods. A common example in trauma is the individual with severe pulmonary contusion and progressive respiratory distress syndrome. One goal of nursing management is to synchronize patient-ventilator interaction so as to avoid barotrauma and further lung injury. This is a much greater problem for the patient with CMV and significant PEEP levels than with IMV or SIMV therapy. Pharmacologic paralysis is usually required for total control of patient ventilation. Intravenous pancuronium or vecuronium can be administered at regular intervals or by continuous infusion. Both sedation and analgesia must accompany paralytic agents. Heavy sedation may be used alone for ventilatory control but is not as effective as therapeutic paralysis. The nurse assesses for the desired level of paralysis and ventilatory control.

Supported Ventilation. There is ongoing controversy concerning the advantages of IMV or SIMV modes versus CMV in ARDS patients. At the least, these modes are commonly used to wean the patient from ventilatory support.[50] Advantages include decreased need for sedation or muscle relaxants to promote ventilator synchrony and decreased barotrauma. Pressure-support ventilation also has been employed and is reportedly more comfortable than IMV for the semialert patient.[50] However, pressure-support ventilation alone will not generate mean airway pressure adequate to support patients with severe respiratory failure.

Appropriate Application of PEEP. One of the most essential treatment components is PEEP, when positive airway pressure is applied at end expiration. One obvious benefit of appropriate PEEP in posttraumatic ARDS patients is an increased PaO_2 at lower inspired oxygen concentrations. The mechanisms of improved PaO_2 are increased functional residual capacity, prevention of alveolar collapse, and recruitment of closed alveoli. PEEP can be applied regardless of the mode of ventilation selected for the patient. Low- or moderate-level PEEP (<15 cm H_2O) is used widely; however, higher levels may be required in patients with refractory hypoxemia.

PEEP has no prophylactic value in ARDS, has well-recognized adverse effects on cardiovascular function (specifically cardiac output), and may contribute to selected alveolar overdistention and physical lung injury.[47,48] Unfortunately, the adverse effects of PEEP are neither uniform nor predictable. Compliance may be increased or decreased by PEEP, and effects on dead-space volume are also variable. In view of the benefits and negative effects of PEEP, it is essential to define the optimal level for the individual patient and the time to initiate the therapy. A rational management approach includes the use of PEEP trials, a series of systematic assessments of changes in cardiopulmonary parameters as PEEP is increased in small increments (2.5-5 cm H_2O or less). Changes can be made rapidly, allowing 15 to 20 minutes for evaluation of the effect of the new PEEP level. All parameters related to tissue oxygen delivery should be assessed when PEEP levels are adjusted.[46,47]

Nonconventional Ventilatory Techniques. Conventional methods of ventilation with generalized PEEP may worsen ventilation-perfusion relationships in patients with severe ARDS.[50] Consequently, several modified ventilation modes can be useful. Simultaneous independent lung ventilation can be used in patients with asymmetric lung disease. High-frequency ventilation may improve gas exchange with lower peak airway pressures and less barotrauma in patients with ARDS than conventional ventilation. In addition, inverse-ratio ventilation has been used in both infants and adults with severe respiratory dysfunction. This technique employs conventional volume or pressure-cycled ventilation with I/E ratios of up to 4:1.[49] The maneuver extends inspiratory time, which theoretically can improve gas exchange at lower PEEP levels and airway pressures. Patients must be monitored for adverse hemodynamic effects of the therapy because venous return and cardiac filling can be altered. In addition, most patients require sedation because the long inspiratory time can produce discomfort and anxiety.[24,49]

Airway pressure release ventilation (APRV) is an evolution of pressure-controlled ventilation with inverse-ratio ventilation that can enable an adequate PaO_2 with lower tidal volumes and peak airway pressures. This is a pressure mode developed with a rapid and then decelerating gas flow pattern. There is infinite ability to control inspiratory and expiratory times, which allows very precise titration of the ventilatory pattern to the patient. With the innovation of a "floating" exhalation valve, patients can remain comfortably awake or minimally sedated while on high ventilatory support, and the use of paralytics can be virtually eliminated.[51]

Permissive hypercapnia is a newer treatment for patients with ARDS that is gaining recognition. Because ventilation at high volumes and pressures is deleterious to the lungs, patients who can tolerate higher than normal CO_2 levels may benefit from this therapy. Research on this therapy developed from patients with severe asthma. Attempts to normalize patients' CO_2 level with an increase in volume and pressure led to the development of barotrauma. Patients may tolerate an increase in CO_2 and a low pH for a time. Continued research is being done to prove that permissive hypercapnia does in fact avoid lung injury and improve lung compliance and weaning success.[48]

Partial Liquid Ventilation. Partial liquid ventilation has been studied recently in humans to reduce lung damage. Animal trials have shown an increase in oxygenation and lung compliance with reduced alveolar damage. The lung is partially filled via the endotracheal tube with perfluorocarbons, chemicals with a reduced surface tension and increased solubility for O_2 and CO_2; the usual ventilation is then superimposed.[52]

Extracorporeal Lung Assist. Extracorporeal lung assist (ECLA) is a therapeutic alternative to current mechanical ventilation when a patient is hypoxic and unresponsive to conventional therapy. Oxygen is supplemented and CO_2 removed via the venovenous bypass. Concurrently, gas exchange through the natural lungs is maintained using low respiratory rates, volumes, and pressures while allowing the patient's lungs to rest.[53] Highly specialized practitioners are required to care for the patient on ECLA and to maintain the extremely technical equipment. ECLA presents great risks to the patient, is extremely invasive, and is a very costly treatment. Continued controversy remains regarding the use of ECLA for the treatment of ARDS.[54]

There has been no definitive, controlled study evaluating the efficacy of extracorporeal therapy. Application of ECLA should be limited to experienced centers.

Positioning.   In many cases the interstitial and alveolar infiltrates of ARDS appear to be distributed uniformly throughout the lung fields on chest radiograph. However, CT scans emphasize that the pathologic condition is irregular in nature, and the most involved segments of the lung are those in dependent positions.[55,56] Changes in body position affect blood gases by altering V/Q matching within the lung. Therefore it is clearly important that no one segment of the lung remain constantly in a dependent position. In addition, oxygenation can be manipulated by therapeutic positioning such as positioning the patient so as to achieve an improved PaO_2. If the patient is monitored with pulse or transcutaneous oximetry, arterial oxygen saturation is used as the therapeutic endpoint when the patient is moved from the supine to the lateral decubitus position.[57,58] The prone position also has been advocated for patients with acute ARDS; the Stryker frame or a proning device may be used to facilitate this form of therapy.[56,57]

Cardiovascular Therapies.   Patients with posttraumatic ARDS may have premorbid or injury-related myocardial dysfunction or develop cardiovascular dysfunction because of pulmonary hypertension induced by ARDS. Underlying hypovolemia may also be present. Frequently the patient's physiologic reserve is insufficient to maintain cardiac output when the additional stress of the hemodynamic consequences of mechanical ventilation and PEEP are added. In addition, the net surface area for gas exchange is reduced because of the alveolar-capillary lesion of ARDS. Optimizing cardiac function and ventricular output supports pulmonary perfusion and therefore gas exchange. Preload, contractility, and afterload can be manipulated to support hemodynamic performance while respiratory failure is treated.

Appropriate fluid management is directed toward (1) decreasing the intrapulmonary edema that is a great part of the syndrome's pathology without compromising intravascular volume and cardiac performance and (2) maximizing the blood's oxygen-carrying capacity. Actual or effective intravascular volume depletion is corrected with the fluid of choice, whether balanced electrolyte solutions, colloids, or blood, and is titrated to the desired ventricular filling pressure. The type of fluid to be administered remains a subject of debate, and reports are conflicting in regard to pulmonary function. Hypotonic solutions are generally avoided to discourage extravasation of intravascular fluid, which can exacerbate edema. Periodic transfusion of red cells may be required to support oxygen delivery. Response to therapy must be monitored to avoid overhydration and increased pulmonary lung water. Sequential measurements of pulmonary artery pressure, wedge pressure, and cardiac output and construction of ventricular function curves are useful in guiding fluid management. In all cases accurate fluid balance, recording of intake and output, and daily weight measurement, whenever possible, help to monitor fluid needs.[39]

Pharmacologic agents also can be used; specific vasodilator therapy with low-dose isoproterenol has been reported to be helpful in reducing right-sided heart afterload; and dobutamine provides inotropic support. Afterload-reducing agents such as nitroprusside are at times included in the therapy to improve stroke volume and left ventricular filling pressure. However, vasodilators such as nitroprusside can worsen pulmonary shunt and oxygenation. The goal of using such agents is to improve cardiac output and pulmonary blood flow without greatly increasing pulmonary shunt fraction or myocardial work.

INTERMEDIATE/REHABILITATION CARE. Published reports of respiratory abnormalities in recovering patients differ in the patterns and severity of dysfunction. These differences may be partially explained by the variability in ARDS etiology, in the patient's previous health history, and in the length of time over which patients were studied. Measurable aberrations in vital capacity and FRC, respiratory mechanics, and arterial oxygenation, particularly during exercise, have been described in patients recovering from ARDS. There is general agreement that lung function is restored in most survivors by 1 year after onset of symptoms.[41] Most interestingly, there is no apparent correlation between severity of the syndrome, duration of ventilatory support, and degree of residual respiratory impairment.

Nursing management is directed toward weaning the patient from ventilatory support and protecting the patient from further respiratory complications, particularly retained secretions and infection. Weaning from mechanical ventila-

tion may begin at varying points in the patient's recovery course. In general, weaning is initiated once the patient is alert, with a stable hemodynamic status, and when respiratory drive and muscle strength are sufficient for spontaneous ventilation. Withdrawal of support is unsuccessful if there is a persistent septic focus or major organ insufficiency. Most patients are successfully weaned. However, it has been reported that up to 19% of spontaneously breathing patients require reinstitution of mechanical support during recovery from ARDS.[39,59] Weaning strategies are discussed in both the critical and intermediate care therapeutics sections.

Once the patient no longer requires ventilatory support, blood gases and pulmonary function are evaluated as needed. The patient is observed for dyspnea and shortness of breath both at rest and during exercise, and the plan of care is modified accordingly. The survivor of posttraumatic ARDS needs considerable support and information to integrate the events of his or her recovery and to understand any current limitations in respiratory function and exercise tolerance.[60]

CARDIAC TAMPONADE

DESCRIPTION.   Both a symptom and an injury, cardiac tamponade is life threatening and requires immediate treatment. Injury to the pericardium or heart results from a penetrating wound or from blunt anterior chest wall trauma. Hemopericardium, bleeding into the pericardial sac, or a small pericardial rupture may or may not be accompanied by cardiac tamponade, depending on intrapericardial pressure.[61] The pericardial sac, a tough and nondistensible structure, normally holds approximately 25 ml of fluid that cushions and protects the heart. Usually the addition of small amounts (50-100 ml) of blood or air from traumatic injury into the sac produces only a small rise in intrapericardial pressure. Continued bleeding increases this pressure sharply and produces the symptoms of cardiogenic shock. Cardiac output falls as the increased intrapericardial pressure interferes with venous return into the right atrium (Figure 23-20). Decline in cardiac performance is directly related to the speed with which the pericardial sac must accommodate blood and fluid. The slower the leak, the longer the increased pressure can be tolerated. This characteristic is important because injury recognition and treatment may not occur immediately on the patient's admission to the emergency department or critical care unit.[62]

RESUSCITATION ASSESSMENT AND MANAGEMENT.   Diagnosis can be difficult because some of the classic symptoms may be obscured by hypovolemic shock. The index of suspicion is used in discovery of the injury. The patient with an inappropriately low cardiac performance in relationship to his or her injuries falls within the index. Evidence of precordial trauma, such as a wound along the lateral sternal border from the second to seventh intercostal space or a history that indicates the possibility of myocardial injury, also leads to the diagnosis. The patient experiences midthoracic pain and dyspnea.

Classic symptoms include the presence of Beck's triad: systemic hypotension, muffled heart tones, and elevated venous pressure reflected in neck vein distention.[16] The latter may not be evident in the injured patient who is already hypotensive and volume depleted. Distant or muffled heart tones are difficult to assess in noisy patient care areas. Pulsus paradoxus higher than 15 mm Hg during inspiration is significant but difficult to measure reliably unless an arterial line is in place. Useful parameters include elevated central venous pressure (CVP), narrowed pulse

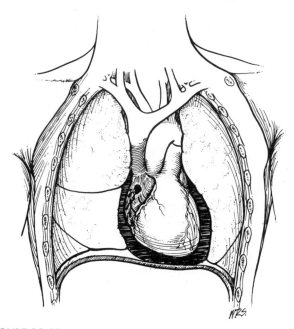

FIGURE 23-20 Cardiac Tamponade Resulting From a Knife Wound. Such wounds may bleed slowly enough to permit survival for several hours. The heart becomes compressed by blood, and cardiac output decreases, resulting in shock. Removal of blood by pericardiocentesis can restore cardiac output and allow time for definitive repair. (From Weiner SL, Barrett J: *Trauma management for civilian and military physicians,* Philadelphia, 1986, WB Saunders.)

pressure, and precipitously falling cardiac output. The electrocardiogram (EKG or ECG) may demonstrate low-voltage complexes, particularly in the precordial leads.

Diagnosis and immediate treatment may occur simultaneously through pericardiocentesis or a pericardial tap (Figure 23-21). One method is as follows: a long (6-inch), 18-gauge over-the-needle catheter attached to a stopcock is inserted below or along the left side of the xiphoid process into the pericardial sac. The fluid present in the sac is aspirated, usually with some immediate improvement in cardiac performance. Because the pericardium is self-sealing, the tamponade may recur. Therefore the catheter is left in place and secured for possible repeated aspiration.

Pericardiocentesis may be falsely negative, often because the needle becomes obstructed by tissue or clots during the procedure. The correctly performed procedure aspirates the pericardium without cardiac puncture. One indication that the heart has been entered is rapid clotting of aspirated blood. Pericardial blood should not clot because it is defibrinated by cardiac motion within the pericardium.

Cardiac tamponade is an injury but also a symptom. The underlying cause of the cardiac tamponade must be determined, and thoracotomy may be required to identify and repair the source of bleeding. The choice of management by pericardiocentesis alone or by thoracotomy is an area of historical debate among resuscitating physicians. Factors that influence management include the mechanism of injury (ice pick wound versus gunshot wound), hemodynamic status, and response to pericardiocentesis. The resuscitation nurse needs to be aware of these factors, monitor the patient's response to pericardiocentesis, and make preparations for rapid thoracotomy should it be required.[63]

MYOCARDIAL CONTUSION

DESCRIPTION.   Blunt cardiac injuries include cardiac wall rupture, valvular disruption, coronary artery dissection, and ventricular contusions. Cardiac contusions are the most

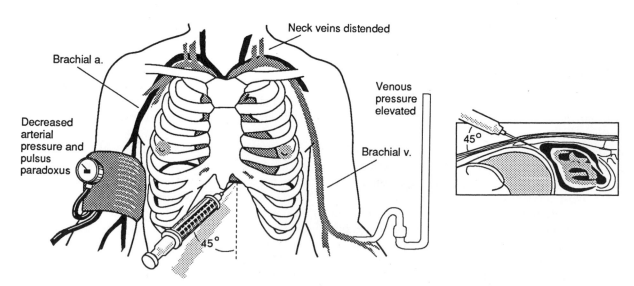

FIGURE 23-21 Technique of paraxyphoid pericardiocentesis for diagnosis and temporary treatment of cardiac tamponade. (From Daughtry D: *Thoracic trauma,* Boston, 1980, Little Brown.)

common result of injury, with arrhythmias being of greatest concern. The contusion itself is rarely fatal, except in relationship to other traumatic injuries.

IDENTIFICATION DURING RESUSCITATION.   The index of suspicion is established in the patient with chest wall contusions, severe anterior blunt trauma, and fractures of sternum and ribs. A standard 12-lead ECG is obtained because nearly half the patients suspected of having myocardial contusion have ECG abnormalities on admission. Continuous ECG monitoring is initiated, and blood is analyzed for cardiac isoenzymes or troponin. Of special interest is an elevation in the myocardial band of the creatine kinase (CK-MB) or of troponin I. Standard antiarrhythmic agents are administered if ECG changes become clinically significant.[61]

CRITICAL CARE ASSESSMENT.   Current literature contains an exhaustive debate over the standard of care for patients with myocardial contusion.[64] There is no diagnostic method that is universally accepted; therefore the postresuscitative management is equally controversial. The patient is surveyed continuously for symptomatic arrhythmias, specifically ventricular irritability and conduction defects. Two-dimensional echocardiography and multigated angiography (MUGA) may be useful in determining abnormalities in ventricular wall movement and ejection fraction.[65] Serial monitoring of cardiac isoenzymes is supported by some authors. However, current treatments include assessing troponin I levels. Studies demonstrate that increased troponin levels are more specific to cardiac damage from blunt trauma than CK-MB. MBs also are elevated when patients present with skeletal muscle trauma, making it difficult to diagnose cardiac contusion using CK-MB alone.[64]

CRITICAL CARE MANAGEMENT.   The patient with a clinically significant contusion chiefly requires nursing observation. Myocardial oxygenation is maintained through appropriate ventilatory support. Continuous ECG and hemodynamic monitoring is needed to detect and manage arrhythmias. Intravenous fluid administration is guided by hemodynamic parameters. Low stroke volume and ejection fraction are treated pharmacologically with inotropic agents such as dopamine, dobutamine, and digitalis. Cardiovascular data are correlated with the effect of drugs, fluids, and any treatments the patient receives for associated injuries. Chest pain that mimics angina but does not respond to nitrates is managed by other pain control modalities.

Nurses are caring for the equivalent of a cardiac patient in the busy environment of a surgical intensive care unit or general medical-surgical floor. This implies that nursing care should be targeted toward eliminating unnecessary stressors and preventing needless myocardial work or increases in oxygen consumption until the injury has healed. However, few studies have been done that help to direct the nursing care of these patients or that compare patient outcomes with those of patients with primary cardiac disease.[7]

AORTIC DISRUPTION

Disruption of the thoracic aorta as a result of blunt trauma is a leading cause of immediate death in patients involved in motor vehicle crashes, pedestrian/vehicular collisions, and falls.[3] A recent comprehensive study within a sophisticated trauma system revealed that 22% of patients who sustained a ruptured aorta died before reaching the trauma center, and another 37% died during initial resuscitation or in the operating room. An additional 14% died postoperatively. Of the remaining survivors, 19% developed paraplegia or paresis.[66] Its lethal nature demands that nurses be familiar with the injury and its difficulties in diagnosis, operative repair, and postoperative care.

DESCRIPTION.   In survivors of blunt trauma there are three common locations of vessel rupture. The thoracic aorta is relatively mobile, and the tears occur at points of anatomic fixation. The most common is at the aortic isthmus, just distal to the left subclavian artery, where the vessel is attached to the chest wall by the ligamentum arteriosum. Two other sites of rupture are in the ascending aorta, where the aorta leaves the pericardial sac, and at the entry to the diaphragm (Figure 23-22). On deceleration from impact, the inner layers of the vessel (intima and media) tear. Only the outer layer, the adventitia, remains

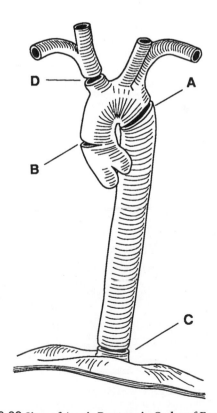

FIGURE 23-22 **Sites of Aortic Rupture in Order of Frequency.** **A,** Distal to left subclavian artery at the level of the ligamentum arteriosum. **B,** Ascending aorta. **C,** Lower thoracic aorta above diaphragm. **D,** Avulsion of innominate artery from aortic arch. (From Frey C: *Initial management of the trauma patient,* Philadelphia, 1976, Lea & Febiger.)

intact and balloons out into a pseudoaneurysm. Alternatively, a partial circumferential hematoma may be tamponaded by surrounding tissue (Figure 23-23). Either mechanism prolongs the survival of the patient, but it is clearly a time-limited effect.

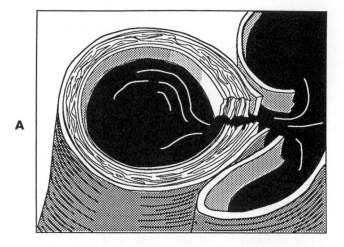

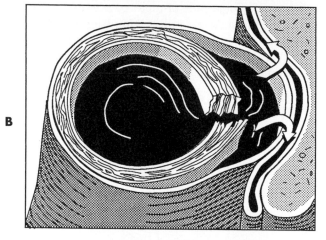

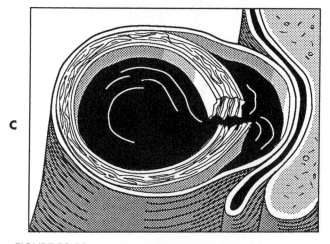

FIGURE 23-23 **Pathogenesis of Aortic Rupture. A,** Complete rupture and death. Transection of all layers of the thoracic aorta and mediastinal pleura; death occurs within minutes. **B,** Lethal delayed rupture. Hematoma is tamponaded temporarily by adventitia or aorta and mediastinal pleura. These structures are torn completely, usually within the first 24 to 48 hours. **C,** Chronic aneurysm formation. A chronic aneurysm results when the adventitial layers remain intact. (From Naclerio EM: *Chest injuries,* Orlando, 1971, Grune & Stratton.)

RESUSCITATION ASSESSMENT.   The injury or assault history and associated injuries raise the question of aortic disruption. Penetrating mediastinal injuries or thoracic injuries sustained by the car occupant wearing a shoulder harness are reasons to heighten the index of suspicion.[7,8] First or second rib fractures, high sternal fracture, left clavicular fracture at the sternal margin, and massive left-sided hemothorax are associated with aortic injury.

The underlying physiologic problem is loss of effective blood transport as a result of major vessel disruption. The goal of assessment is to seek evidence of poor perfusion beyond the aortic lesion. Although many patients are surprisingly free of symptoms, certain findings are associated with the injury:

1. Pulse deficit in any area, particularly lower extremities or left arm
2. Hypotension unexplained by other injuries
3. Upper extremity hypertension relative to lower extremities
4. Sternal pain or interscapular pain
5. Precordial or interscapular systolic murmur caused by turbulence across the disrupted area
6. Hoarseness caused by hematoma pressure around the aortic arch
7. Dyspnea or respiratory distress
8. Lower extremity neuromuscular or sensory deficit

The initial chest film is done with the patient in the supine position for reasons related to spine immobilization and hemodynamic instability. A widened mediastinum or obscured aortic knob is highly suggestive of aortic disruption and demands further evaluation. As soon as it is safe to do so, a true upright (110-degree erect) chest film is obtained. This position greatly enhances radiographic power to reveal the characteristic findings of great vessel disruption. However, up to a 50% error rate has been reported on the basis of chest film findings. A supine or semierect chest film distorts the mediastinum and makes it appear widened.[66,67]

Unless the patient is deteriorating rapidly, the definitive diagnosis is made by aortography, a retrograde dye study performed via the femoral artery, which allows visualization of the aneurysm or hematoma. Although this study is essential for identifying the site or sites of the life-threatening rupture, there is risk of aneurysm rupture during transport to the angiography suite or during the procedure. The risk of rupture is greatest on catheter insertion and dye injection. More data have emerged regarding the accuracy of the dynamic helical and multi-slice computerized chest tomogram for aortic disruption, which carries less risk and is less invasive.[68,69]

TRANSPORT.   Transport of the patient must be approached by preparing for adverse affects, including full cardiopulmonary arrest. An emergency cart must accompany the patient and transport team. All equipment and supplies required to care for an arrest, including a thoracotomy tray, chest tube apparatus, and additional resuscitation fluids, must be available immediately. Vital signs and baseline physical findings are monitored intensively during transport and throughout the aortogram procedure. Aortography is a priority procedure. Any needless delays in transport or during the procedure must be anticipated and eliminated.[7]

RESUSCITATION MANAGEMENT. The rupture will require surgical resection and repair. The initial resuscitation includes establishing an appropriate airway (frequently endotracheal intubation), securing large-bore intravenous access, and treating other immediately life-threatening injuries. Other injuries may be treated in the operating room or be assigned a lower priority than the disrupted aorta. Should delay in repair occur (e.g., awaiting transport to a trauma center), the resuscitation nurse must keep the patient as quiet and comfortable as possible. A major focus of care is directed toward maintaining the blood pressure within a specified range. Patients with aortic isthmus lesions are usually hypertensive as a result of baroreceptor stimulation within the cardiac plexus at the isthmus. Because vessel stress must be minimized, mean blood pressure is maintained under 90 mm Hg with antihypertensive agents. An indwelling arterial catheter is essential in monitoring pressures. Blood is typed and crossmatched, and 10 units of packed red blood cells are made available.

OPERATIVE MANAGEMENT. The operative procedure is determined by the site or sites of rupture and the choice of the surgical team. Cardiopulmonary bypass is used although the need for anticoagulation presents difficulties in the multiply injured patient. A shunt bypass technique maybe used, allowing perfusion of the distal aorta while resection and repair are completed (Figure 23-24). A left thoracotomy incision is made for best visualization of the aorta, and the vessel is cross-clamped to control bleeding. A heparinized shunt is placed proximally and distally, the rupture site is resected, and a Dacron graft is inserted with anastomosis to the vessel edges. Flow through the grafted vessel is observed, the shunt is removed, and insertion sites are closed with patch grafts. Chest tubes are placed for drainage, and the chest is closed.

One disadvantage of the shunt technique is the time needed for insertion before repair. This may be an additional 1.5 hours before effective aortic blood flow is restored. An alternative and faster approach is a cross-clamp repair without shunt. The aorta is clamped proximally and distally to the tear, the rupture site is resected, and the graft is inserted as previously described. Cross-clamp time must be as short as possible, generally less than 30 minutes, because flow to the distal aorta is occluded. The concept of a "safe" cross-clamp time is difficult to define because of individual variation in tolerance. Long cross-clamp times are associated with markedly increased postoperative complications resulting from poor perfusion of the spinal cord, kidneys, and mesentery. All repair techniques described hold the risk of perfusion-related complications.[7]

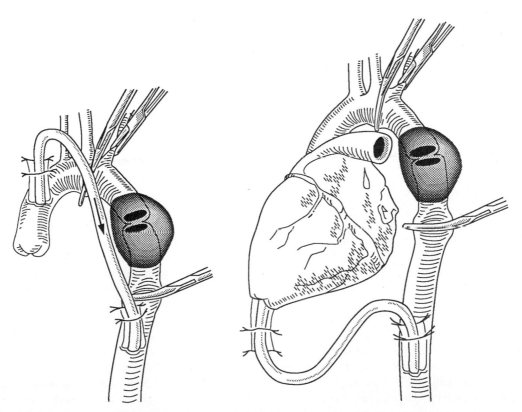

FIGURE 23-24 **Shunt Bypass Technique in Aortic Repair.** (From FW Blaisdell, DD Trunkey: *Cervicothoracic trauma*, New York, 1986, Thieme Medical.)

INTRAOPERATIVE PROBLEMS.   Blood pressure control remains a focal point of concern. An antihypertensive agent is administered by continuous intravenous infusion, if not already in progress, to regulate mean arterial pressure. Reducing vessel and graft anastomosis stress is the primary objective. An additional intraoperative objective is replacement of blood loss with blood, colloids, and crystalloids. Autotransfusion, as previously described, is highly useful in fluid management.[28]

CRITICAL CARE ASSESSMENT AND MANAGEMENT.   Many of the individuals who survive the operative period die within the first week after injury. Repair of the thoracic aorta requires similar postoperative monitoring and management as for any patient recovering from major chest surgery. Systematic assessment for residual injury effects and complications of tissue hypoperfusion is an additional and primary concern for these patients. Any organ system below the level of aortic tear may be damaged during the period of hypoperfusion. This period extends from the time of injury until reestablishment of adequate blood transport through the vessel. It is important for the nurse to determine the hypoperfusion time, particularly the length of cross-clamp time, in order to predict postoperative problems. The patient's age, previous cardiovascular status, preexisting diabetes or pulmonary or renal disease, and additional injuries are factors that influence the incidence of postoperative problems.[66] The most serious postoperative problems are transient or permanent hypertension, paraplegia, bowel infarction, renal failure, graft leaks, and infection.[25]

Hypertension.   Patients with aortic isthmus repairs frequently remain hypertensive postoperatively. Continuous hemodynamic monitoring is essential to track systemic and pulmonary pressures. After clear postoperative parameters for acceptable systolic, diastolic, and mean blood pressure have been established with the surgeon, antihypertensives are titrated to those parameters. The nurse correlates the effect of the drugs not only with mean arterial pressure but also with tissue perfusion. Dosages are balanced carefully to protect the integrity of the fresh graft and the tissue needs of the brain, spinal cord, kidneys, and other organs.

Postoperative Paraplegia.   Evidence of paraplegia caused by interruption of spinal cord blood supply may have been apparent during the initial resuscitation. More often, critical care assessment reveals the effect of spinal cord hypoperfusion. Lower extremity weakness, loss of reflexes, spasticity, or overt paralysis may be evident. Spinal cord perfusion can be compromised by preoperative hypotension or lengthy cross-clamp time. The anterior spinal arteries and intercostal vessels are significant sources of spinal cord blood supply and can be damaged as a consequence of the injury or the reparative surgery. The use of antihypertensives as described previously can maintain mean arterial blood pressure at a level incompatible with spinal cord perfusion. Once the paraplegia has been identified, every effort is made to maximize possible recovery of function.

Bowel Ischemia.   The bowel is at risk for ischemia and infarction if mesenteric arterial perfusion is compromised. Older patients with primary vascular disease are particularly at risk. The nurse assesses for delayed return of bowel sounds, fever, abdominal pain, and distention. Surgical removal of dead or diseased bowel segments is required for definitive management.

Renal Failure.   Hypoperfusion of the kidneys may result in poor renal function or outright failure.

Graft Leaks and Infection.   Graft leaks are possible because there is little permanent bonding of the graft to the aorta. Chest tube drainage is monitored carefully for signs of re-bleeding as long as the tubes are in place because delayed leakage is possible. Intermittent leakage and fever of unknown origin are particular concern because these are some of the first signs of graft infection. Prophylactic antibiotics and rigorous precautions are employed to prevent bacteremia, which could seed the graft site.

INTERMEDIATE/REHABILITATION PHASE CONCERNS.   The patient's specific plan of care will depend on the resulting disabilities. For example, if postinjury paraplegia persists, spinal cord injury care and rehabilitation protocols are implemented. Frequently these patients are able to regain a great deal of lower extremity function with the help of exercise and physical therapy. Postoperative hypertension also may be encountered in the long-term survivor of a ruptured aorta. It can persist for months after aortic repair and is treated with standard antihypertensive agents if necessary.[25]

There are also a number of general considerations for the patient during the intermediate and rehabilitative stages. Surveillance for graft leaks and infection continues throughout this part of the trauma recovery. Intermittent, small leaks may occur at the graft-vessel anastomosis, resulting in chronic aneurysm formation that is dangerous because of the risk of delayed hemorrhage into the pleural cavity or pericardium. Additionally, thrombus formation within the aneurysm presents a risk of embolism.

The patient must always be protected from bacteremias. Continuing assessment includes systematic inspection of all wounds, old chest tube sites, and incisions. Temperature, white cell count, and fluid and electrolyte status are all monitored for signs of infection and sepsis. The patient and family become part of an instructional plan regarding the vascular prosthesis, the risk of infection, concern for long-term aneurysm formation, and the need for long-term follow-up care in a thoracic clinic.

The degree of continued chest pain is individual and is related to any additional thoracic injuries. Pulmonary care is directed toward the goal of preventing retained secretions and atelectasis. More detailed discussion of this area is contained in the section on intermediate care therapeutics.

Nursing Therapeutics in the Critical Care Phase

The previous survey of thoracic injury management includes actions and strategies specific to a given injury and highlights therapeutics common to all chest trauma and its complications. The following sections are intended to provide greater detail concerning these therapies as used in critically ill patients.

The Patient-Ventilator Unit

Many patients with significant chest trauma require mechanical ventilation during their critical care hospital stay and, less commonly, into the intermediate care phase. The rationale for initiating some form of mechanical ventilation may be either as definitive management, as in the case of flail chest, or as a supportive therapy, as in posttraumatic ARDS. It is useful to keep the well-known goals for ventilatory therapy in mind: to improve oxygenation, correct hypoventilation and acidosis, and ease the work of breathing. Although the decision to commit the trauma patient to any given form of ventilatory therapy is based on individual history, type of injury, and injury complications such as sepsis, some general criteria for initiating mechanical ventilation can be applied (Table 23-9).[70]

Common ventilator techniques used in managing thoracic injuries are summarized in the section on thoracic assessment. The nurse must be familiar with the benefits, disadvantages, complications of several ventilator modes and settings, and unique system features. IMV or SIMV is most commonly used in the acute injury phase because they allow the patient to stabilize while preserving respiratory muscle function.

Close communication among nurse, physician, and respiratory therapist is essential in determining which specific equipment and therapies are to be used. This communication is particularly important when a complicated technique such as independent lung ventilation or some form of high-frequency ventilation is in progress. Whatever the type of ventilator or mode chosen, the nurse monitors not only the patient's responses to therapy but also the functional status of the patient-ventilator unit. Disconnections or leaks within the breathing circuit may or may not be obvious and must be included as part of continuous monitoring. Checking to see that all alarms are functional at all times is one of the simplest and most essential nursing actions. The bedside nurse and respiratory therapist are the most likely persons to note high resistance or obstruction in the endotracheal tube, increased resistance in the inspiratory and expiratory circuits, or improper function of the exhalation valve. Changes in equipment or ventilator technique are explained to the semialert patient, who may panic at sudden changes in airflow or work of breathing.

In addition to the common types of ventilation, nurses may be required to develop a plan of care for the thoracic trauma patient who requires more unusual respiratory therapy.

Independent Lung Ventilation (ILV). In limited instances a patient with a tracheobronchial tear or asymmetric pulmonary contusion with massive air leak may not respond well to conventional mechanical ventilation and PEEP. Volume delivered by the ventilator will go to the more compliant lung, particularly when there are large differences in compliance between lungs. The good lung can then be at risk of hyperinflation and barotrauma, while the stiffer lung receives inadequate volume. Under such circumstances, intubation of each bronchus with a double-lumen tube and ILV provides an alternative ventilatory therapy. The endotracheal tubes are connected to (1) separate, synchronized ventilators, (2) a modified circuit allowing independent but synchronized ventilation, or (3) separate ventilators without synchronization.[25] ILV is used most frequently to manage the patient with high peak inspiratory pressures and a persistent large air leak.[70]

Nursing management can be unusually demanding depending on the complexity of ventilator setup and the cardiopulmonary stability of the patient. Blood gases, ventilatory parameters (including end-tidal CO_2 monitoring), and hemodynamic status are closely observed. Air leak through the chest tubes is monitored. The patient may have large amounts of pulmonary or bloody secretions requiring careful airway hygiene and suctioning. It is rarely necessary to remove the patient from the ventilator system for suctioning or changing body position, but it is useful to have two manual resuscitation bags and spare double-lumen endotracheal tubes at the bedside. Pharmacologic paralysis is generally required, accompanied by sedatives and analgesia. Family members need some explanation of the therapy before entering the patient care area because it may appear complex and frightening.

TABLE 23-9	Criteria for Initiation of Mechanical Ventilation	
	Normal Range	**Failing Function**
Respiratory rate	12-20/min	>35/min
Vital capacity	65-75 ml/kg	<15 ml/kg
Tidal volume	10-15 ml/kg	<7 ml/kg
Inspiratory force	−75 to −100 cm H_2O	>−25 cm H_2O
$Paco_2$	35-45 mm Hg	>50 mm Hg
$\dot{V}_D/\dot{V}_T$	0.2-0.4	>0.6
Pao_2	80-100 mm Hg	<70 mm Hg (on oxygen therapy)
A − aDo_2	50-75 mm Hg	>300 mm Hg (on 100% O_2)
$\dfrac{Pao_2}{Fio_2}$ (P/F ratio)	>280	<200

HIGH-FREQUENCY VENTILATION. High-frequency ventilation (HFV) is identified by the use of high respiratory rates and small tidal volume, which is less than the patient's anatomic dead space volume. *High-frequency ventilation* is a general term used to include different types of mechanical systems, specifically high-frequency oscillation (HFO) and high-frequency jet ventilation (HFJV). HFJV is the most commonly used and delivers small pulses of gas through a cannula in either an endotracheal tube or tracheostomy tube or via a specialized jet endotracheal tube. The pulses can be delivered under high pressure at rates of 30 to 1000 per minute. In practice the rate is limited to less than 150 per minute because of current regulations from the Food and Drug Administration.[70] The major advantage of HFJV for trauma patients is that ventilation can be accomplished effectively at reduced peak airway pressures.

HFV has been used successfully during bronchoscopy, laryngoscopy, and tracheal reconstruction; as a weaning procedure; and in the treatment of bronchopleural fistula, acute ARDS, and flail chest.[70] It also has demonstrated use in a variety of thoracic surgical procedures.

Because HFV is used with patients who also may suffer multiple injuries and system failure, intensive patient monitoring is essential and complex. Tidal volume, system pressures, inspired oxygen concentration, and ventilator frequency are difficult to measure accurately unless specialized equipment is available. Bilateral breath sounds and chest wall movements are carefully assessed to identify potential cannula dislodgment and barotrauma. In some systems the lack of conventional ventilator safety features such as alarms requires constant nursing vigilance and the immediate availability of a respiratory therapist. Humidification is problematic and has not been uniformly successful in HFV. Increased mobilization of pulmonary secretions may be evident and may require increased suctioning and airway care. To avoid decreases in Pa_{O_2}, the patient is not disconnected from the ventilatory system during suctioning. Decreased sedation needs have been reported during HFV as opposed to conventional ventilation; however, the need for analgesia and sedation in trauma patients is difficult to predict and should be determined by individual evaluation.[25]

VENTILATOR-ASSOCIATED LUNG INJURY. Injuries include barotrauma, volutrauma, atelectrauma, and biotrauma. Barotrauma caused by high airway pressures during positive pressure ventilation has been recognized for decades. Research continues toward identifying the pressure most crucial to assess (peak, mean, PEEP) and the levels at which these pressures become injurious to lung tissue. Volutrauma is a more subtle injury that occurs with overdistention of alveoli associated with high peak airway pressures and may lead to diffuse alveolar damage, increased fluid filtration, pulmonary edema, and epithelial or microvascular permeability. Atelectrauma may be caused by high or low lung volumes resulting from repetitive opening and collapse of distal airways. Biotrauma related to mechanical factors may lead to "injury that is cell and inflammatory mediator based."[46] More clinical trials are needed so that the incidence of these associated injuries can be reduced.

Barotrauma. Defined broadly as injury resulting from alveolar overdistention and rupture, barotrauma is a complication of conventional mechanical ventilation and PEEP. Because controlled mechanical ventilation has been replaced in most hospitals by the widespread use of SIMV, pressure support, and APRV, barotrauma is less common and usually less severe. However, patients with significant lung damage are particularly susceptible to the effects of pressure-induced injury regardless of the type of mechanical ventilation used in the management of respiratory sequelae.[46]

A variety of mechanisms produce barotrauma. Secretions trapped in the lower airways may produce a ball-valve obstruction effect when, on inspiration, the ventilator cycles gas past the partial obstruction into the alveoli. When expiration of the gas is blocked, the lung unit remains inflated. As the cycle is repeated, the alveolus ruptures. Air escapes through the ruptured area into surrounding structures.

Regional hyperinflation also may cause alveolar rupture. Unstable lung units resulting from contusion, ARDS, or necrotizing pneumonia are unable to tolerate high pressure and appear to "blow out," leaking air into surrounding tissue or potential space. The end result is subcutaneous emphysema, pneumomediastinum, pneumothorax, or tension pneumothorax. The patient most likely to experience the complication has poor total lung compliance, high airway pressures, or requires high levels of PEEP and tidal volumes. The patient with lung injury is also at risk because the injured areas vary in level of damage and healing. Regional hyperinflation or obstruction may occur within the injured region. Patients require monitoring for a sudden increase in airway pressure, a change in air leak through or around chest tubes, subcutaneous emphysema, and any change in their vital signs or oxygenation level.[70] Changes in breath sounds may be difficult to appreciate because referred breath sounds from ventilated areas may be audible across lung fields.

Nursing management is directed toward controlling events that increase intrathoracic pressure. Pulmonary care may reduce an accumulation of secretions, which leads to extensive coughing, fighting the ventilator, and periods of preventable bronchospasm. Sedation and analgesia are not administered randomly but given in early response to a rising level of patient discomfort or agitation. The source of discomfort or agitation is controlled or eliminated by appropriate positioning, massage, or distraction.

VENTILATOR DEPENDENCE. Ventilator dependence has not been studied extensively in patients with single or multiple system injuries. The trauma patient may be difficult to wean from ventilatory support for many of the same reasons present in any group of critically ill individuals. Previous respiratory disease complicates the recovery from injury and can be anticipated from the patient's health history. Psychophysiologic factors have a profound effect on weaning success and are discussed extensively in the literature.[59,62,71]

Ventilator dependence can arise from direct thoracic injury, or it can be a function of central nervous system injury, ARDS, or the enormous metabolic demand of sepsis or healing. The patient may be unable to protect his or her airway and may sustain numerous, yet difficult to detect, episodes of aspiration.

Weaning Methods. Weaning plans are established by the primary nurse, trauma surgeon, or intensivist and respiratory therapist. At least four weaning techniques are currently in use: (1) T-piece weaning, (2) IMV protocols, (3) CPAP weaning, and (4) pressure support or PSV. T-piece weaning alternates periods of full ventilator support with progressively prolonged periods of spontaneous ventilation.[72] IMV protocols employ a gradual reduction in the mechanical breaths delivered per minute while allowing the patient to breathe spontaneously. CPAP weaning allows the patient to breathe entirely without machine-delivered breaths but with continuous positive airway pressure. Lastly, PSV allows the patient to control the length, depth, and frequency of inspiration while augmenting each breath with a predetermined positive pressure from the ventilator. Weaning criteria and desired endpoints are adapted to the unique demands of the patient's injuries, previous delivered oxygen concentration, and level of ventilator support. Each change in ventilatory support or oxygen therapy is evaluated by repeated clinical examinations, end-tidal CO_2 monitoring or capnography, and blood gas analyses. Continuous online evaluation of peripheral oxygen saturation is particularly helpful. Explanations of the weaning process and daily progress should be reviewed with the patient and family members. Table 23-10 provides examples of weaning criteria.[72,73]

Weaning criteria have limited value under some circumstances, particularly in the trauma patient with preexisting pulmonary disease. A patient who does not meet the usual criteria may be extubated successfully. Such a patient must be reevaluated repeatedly and all equipment must be readied for rapid reintubation and continued ventilatory support if needed. Another patient may not progress beyond a given level of support. This type of weaning failure is likely due to incomplete resolution of underlying trauma or an emerging sepsis. Clearly there are no general solutions for weaning difficulties. One or more strategies may be required, such as changing the patient from T-piece weaning to an alternative such as pressure support.[74]

Pulmonary Therapeutics

Procedures that effectively clear the airways at all anatomic levels and remove retained secretions are the foundation of thoracic injury management. Pulmonary care is frequently a difficult and time-consuming process in trauma patients. How can the repetitive clogging of the endotracheal tube or tracheostomy with bloody secretions and tissue clots be

TABLE 23-10 **Weaning Criteria in Trauma**
Underlying trauma and septic complications are resolved.
Oxygenation:
P/F ratio is >250 at all times
Q_s/Q_t is <15%
Ventilatory mechanics:
VC is >15 ml/kg
Total compliance is >35 ml/cm H_2O
Ventilatory drive is sufficient:
Sedation and analgesia are tapered
Evidence of electrolyte balance
No evidence of over ventilation, pH >7.35
Work of breathing is not excessive:
Appropriate size airway is in place
Bony thorax is intact or stabilized
Adequate pain management is in progress
Muscle strength is adequate:
Nutritional deficits are eliminated
Maximal inspiratory force is <−20 cm H_2O
Ventilatory demand is reasonable:
Pa_{CO_2} is <45-50 mm Hg
CO_2 production through carbohydrate intake is not excessive
Maximal temperature is reasonable
$\dot{V}_D/\dot{V}_T$ is <0.5
Spontaneous respiratory rate is <30 per minute
Airway remains intact and protected.
Plan for psychologic and family support is in place.

P/F, Peak/flow; *VC*, Vital capacity.

avoided? How can a piece of tooth be removed from the posterior lung segment? How does one maximize overall oxygenation and ventilation in a patient with edematous or hemorrhagic lung segments? Problems such as these are encountered frequently in patients with traumatic injuries and are treated with chest physiotherapy (CPT), suctioning, and injury-specific positioning.

CHEST PHYSIOTHERAPY. A plan for CPT includes selection and evaluation of several treatment components. Postural drainage, percussion, and vibration are used to mobilize intrapulmonary secretions, accompanied by suctioning or coughing to clear the larger airways. Effective postural drainage, such as positioning the patient so that the affected segmental bronchus is uppermost, assists movement of secretions from the lung by gravity and requires knowledge of which lung segments are abnormal.[75] Percussion (rhythmic clapping with a cupped hand) is performed directly on the chest wall throughout the respiratory cycle. Vibration intermittently compresses the involved area during expiration. Percussion can be used carefully and gently over fractures or painful areas.

Each selected component, its frequency, and the length of a therapeutic session are planned in relation to the patient's total injuries and specific respiratory abnormalities. The frequency of treatment, usually every 4 hours in critically ill patients, is evaluated every 12 to 24 hours on the basis of desired endpoints such as the appearance of the daily chest film, trends in total lung compliance, stability of blood gases, and clinical examination. Patients with copious secretions or high-risk injuries, such as flail chest with significant lung contusion, may require more frequent or longer treatments. The length of treatment is determined by clinical parameters such as improved breath sounds and changes in airway pressures and lung volumes. The amount of sputum or suctioning aspirate is rarely an indicator of the therapy's effectiveness and does not serve as the sole criterion for ending a therapy session. The duration of a treatment also may be determined by adverse effects on intracranial pressure or hemodynamic stability.[25]

CPT may be performed by the nurse, physical therapist, or respiratory therapist. Frequently, positioning for therapy requires several assistants to avoid inadvertent extubation, disconnection of intravenous or arterial lines, and physical trauma to the patient. Plans for appropriate positioning and use of restraints need to be in place when treating agitated patients. The therapy session is coordinated with the patient's analgesia and sedation requirements. In all cases the nurse's role includes planning the treatment schedule and evaluating both desirable and undesirable effects during and after treatment. Desired effects include improvement in sequential chest films, blood gases, total compliance, and airway resistance. Undesired effects on arterial oxygenation and hemodynamic parameters occur but are difficult to predict. The use of prone, head-down, or lateral positions during CPT may be responsible for the adverse effects and the benefits.[57]

SUCTIONING.   Optimal methods of endotracheal suctioning have been the subject of considerable nursing research and clinical review.[76] Controversy remains regarding the use and amount of hyperinflation and hyperoxygenation before and after suctioning.[77] The value of instilling sterile saline into the endotracheal tube also has been debated but has not proven to be effective. Current research does not support the use of saline before suctioning.[78] Because mucus and water are immiscible, instilling saline down the endotracheal tube is of little or no value. A study conducted by Kinlock measured the time it took a patient's oxygen saturation to return to baseline after endotracheal suctioning with and without instillation of saline before suctioning.[79] Patients who received saline required a longer time for their saturation to return to baseline compared with patients who did not receive saline. Research also has shown that patients have an increased risk of infection if they receive saline before suctioning.[79] There needs to be consistency among practitioners of all disciplines to apply research and follow a common practice related to suctioning; until consensus is reached, the controversy will continue.[80] However, it is well accepted that there are risks associated with suctioning, including hypoxemia, aspiration, hypertension, and serious arrhythmias. Suctioning in the multiply injured individual has not been well studied, particularly in patients with preexisting lung disease or significant physiologic instability. The need for suctioning and the technique used is best determined by the patient's injuries, clinical presentation, and assessment findings.[76,78,81]

POSITIONING.   Altering body position can be used to improve arterial oxygenation in some patients.[56] Another form of pulmonary therapy is therapeutic positioning, the use of specific body positions to maximize oxygenation and ventilation despite lung abnormalities. Turning the patient has long been accepted as treatment for the complications of immobility, and the effect of position on gas exchange must be considered in clinical management. The usefulness of positioning techniques is based on the effect of gravity on the lung fields, specifically on gravity-dependent ventilation-perfusion matching in particular respiratory segments. Recognizing that perfusion is greatest in the dependent lung or dependent portions of the lung, it is possible to position the patient so that specific lung areas receive a greater or lesser proportion of blood flow. Position is manipulated so that the healthy portion of the lung is dependent and therefore receives greatest perfusion.[82] In a similar way, lung areas that are compromised by injury and poor ventilation are positioned uppermost, thus receiving a gravity-dependent reduction in blood flow. The result is increased blood flow to areas of best ventilation, decreased flow to poorly ventilated areas, and overall improved matching of perfusion and ventilation. The prone position is an important therapy with ARDS patients because pulmonary infiltrates are gravity dependent. Repeated clinical trials have demonstrated an improvement in PaO_2 with patients who are prone.[56] Stryker frames and proning device are being used to facilitate prone positioning.

Positioning becomes part of pulmonary care in many patients with respiratory abnormalities and significant thoracic trauma. Thoracic assessment and knowledge of the most recent chest film are used to choose positions: sitting, prone, and, most commonly, lateral decubitus. Immediate effects of the position are noted, such as change in airway position, respiratory rate, chest excursion, airway pressures, and hemodynamic and continuously monitored respiratory gas parameters. The effect of body position is also evaluated after 30 minutes to determine changes in respiratory gases, hemodynamic parameters, and subsequent oxygen transport to tissues. In all cases body alignment, support of head and neck, and comfort are evaluated. Part of the positioning protocol is planning for pain relief and removing secretions mobilized by turning. Frequency of position change is determined by the results of this ongoing evaluation, not by an arbitrary recommendation for turning every 2 hours.

PLEURAL SPACE DRAINAGE

Most thoracic injuries are treated by the insertion of one or more chest tubes, often under emergent conditions. Although the management of pleural space drainage systems is common to all types of critical care nursing, there are some special concerns for the thoracic trauma patient. For example, how can nursing management decrease the persistently high incidence of chest tube-related infections? A chest tube may be inserted in close proximity to fractures, wounds, and large skin abrasions. What can be done to prevent chest tubes from aggravating other injuries? Fragile, damaged lung tissue may be in close proximity to the lumen of the tube. What is the best way to milk the chest tube of drainage without causing further damage? Major considerations for nursing are maintaining an effective and infection-free chest tube system, protecting associated injury sites, and avoiding damage to underlying lung tissue.[25]

CHOICE OF DRAINS.   The chest tube chosen for trauma management is large bore, such as a no. 40 French, so as to evacuate a mixture of air, blood, and tissue fragments. The usual insertion site is the fourth intercostal space at the midaxillary line. Multiple tube insertion sites may be necessary to capture drainage and evacuate air.

REMOVAL OF THE DRAINAGE TUBE.   Daily chest radiograph and physical examination assist in determining the need to reposition the chest tube or to insert additional drains. The decision to remove the tube is frequently a matter of balancing the risk of infection and the possibility of a secondary pleural space injury.[17] Generally a chest tube that drains liquid exudate is removed 3 or 4 days after insertion. Chest tubes that drain primarily air are removed 2 to 10 days after insertion, depending on the amount of continued air evacuation and the degree of lung reexpansion. Partial lung reexpansion does not necessarily imply that a previous leak has sealed. The gradual absence of air in the tube or water seal and clinical and radiographic examination for subcutaneous or mediastinal air provide assurance that the leak has sealed.

ADEQUATE SUCTION.   Suction through the drainage system is generally maintained at 20 cm H_2O. The suction must be adequate to facilitate drainage of air and blood but not high enough to entrap tissue or delay healing of the injury. Occasionally the suction level is inadequate to properly evacuate air and seal an existing air leak. Additional suction may be provided. The new level of suction is evaluated clinically and radiographically.

Conversely, low suction levels may be required in selected patients managed with controlled mechanical ventilation to avoid increasing the gradient between positive airway pressure and negative intrapleural suction. The increased gradient may delay healing, create additional air leak, and potentiate a bronchopleural fistula.

EXAMINING THE DRAINAGE.   The pleural drainage system must be checked regularly to determine if it is fully functional. This is generally determined by fluctuation or bubbling of the water seal as negative pressure is transmitted during inspiration. A seemingly obstructed drain that

continues to evacuate large amounts of fluid or air is likely to still be functional. Liquid drainage through the system is easily measured and is correlated with the patient's injury and recovery. The amount of blood initially evacuated from the pleural cavity is a criterion for estimation of blood loss and replacement need. The hourly blood loss is useful as an indicator of the need for thoracotomy. The trend of drainage over time, both air and fluid, provides information about the resolution of underlying injury. For example, bleeding visibly slows from a small pulmonary laceration as the lung reexpands, sealing off the injury.

MAINTAINING PATENCY.   The drainage system is positioned below the level of the chest to facilitate the flow of bloody fluid, and the drainage tubing is milked in small segments to remove clots. Patency of the drain is always a concern because a residual intrathoracic clot will require thoracotomy for removal and not a simple chest tube reinsertion. High intrathoracic pressures can be generated by compressing or pulling on the chest tube to the point of collapse (stripping), and should not be done. To minimize the stress on underlying tissue, a sequential short-segment squeezing motion is used instead.

PROTECTING AGAINST INFECTION.   A pleural-space injury may become infected by a break in the drainage system or by inadequate dressing techniques. Several therapeutic nursing measures can minimize this risk or prevent infection. As always, careful hand washing and skillful and careful assistance during insertion or removal of the drainage system are essential. Even under emergent conditions, the skin must be disinfected. Surveillance for aseptic technique is required on the part of all individuals during insertion, repositioning, or removal of the chest tube. All parts of the drainage system that connect to the pleural space must be sterile. Every connection is taped or secured with chest tube bands. Collection containers are replaced when contaminated. It is important to date the drainage system and to document when it was initiated or changed. Many patients have large amounts of drainage and require several changes of the collection system. Under these circumstances, disposable systems that allow replacement of only the collecting canister are particularly useful.

The chest tube is sutured in place, dressed, and carefully secured to the chest wall. The objective is to avoid slippage of the tube back and forth, which increases local injury and the possibility of infection. Cloth adhesive tape is used for greatest security. Underlying skin can be protected by commercial skin preparation or by the use of sterile-stoma care materials.

The dressing procedure is sterile, requiring a small sterile field, mask, and gloves. It can be done economically and quickly without compromising sterile technique. The site and the surrounding skin are cleansed with separate sponges and antiseptic solution. The use of an antibiotic ointment at the site has not been shown to decrease infection. The final dressing is closed to the environment by adhesive tape and changed whenever it is wet or contaminated. It is useful to establish a standard for routine changing and to systematically document the date of dressing change, the appearance of the site, and the drainage apparent on the dressing.

Wounds around the chest tube site are dressed separately whenever possible. These wounds may require frequent dressing changes to avoid contamination of the chest tube site.

NURSING THERAPEUTICS IN THE INTERMEDIATE AND REHABILITATION CARE PHASES

Not all patients with thoracic injuries require critical care nursing. Many need subacute postresuscitation or postoperative care, progression into rehabilitation, and return to the community. Alternatively, numerous patient problems identified and initially managed in the critical care phase persist into intermediate care and rehabilitation. The following sections focus on such specific nursing therapeutics.

VENTILATOR DEPENDENCE

In some instances a patient remains dependent on mechanical ventilation even though the causes of weaning failure have been considered and considerable management has already been directed toward the problem. The causes of extended ventilatory dependence are not usually complications of thoracic injury per se but are related to central nervous system injury or previous chronic respiratory disease. Under these circumstances, weaning therapies are continued into the patient's intermediate trauma phase, and the problem of ventilator dependence is incorporated into the plan of care. If continued dependence on some form of mechanical ventilation is preventing the patient from hospital discharge, home respiratory therapy may be considered.[74]

Table 23-10 lists criteria for weaning based on experience with trauma patients. The most valid predictors of successful weaning have not been determined in the multiply injured population. It seems reasonable to use well-studied predictors obtained in general surgical patients to evaluate readiness for spontaneous breathing with supplemental oxygen: tidal volume greater than 5 ml/kg, forced vital capacity greater than 10 to 15 ml/kg, maximal inspiratory pressure less than 20 cm H_2O, and an acceptable Pao_2/Fio_2 ratio. However, a large survey of weaning practices indicated that clinical assessment rather than pulmonary function tests forms the basis for weaning decisions.[72] Furthermore, there is no clear consensus on the value of measurements or predictors in ventilator dependence.

More is known about the mechanisms of ventilator dependence. One principal factor is respiratory muscle failure after terminating mechanical ventilation. Muscle contractility is diminished in the presence of low plasma phosphate, magnesium, and calcium levels and hypercapnia and acidosis. Respiratory performance is decreased by infections. For example, muscle performance as measured by maximal inspiratory and expiratory mouth pressures falls by approximately 30% of control values during an upper respiratory infection. Atrophy has been demonstrated to be associated with septic processes, and weaning failure has been reported to occur in the presence of positive blood cultures.[71]

Once causative factors have been corrected, ventilator dependence may be reversed. At this point an appropriate weaning protocol is used to gradually strengthen respiratory muscles through exercise. The basic strategy is to allow the patient to breath spontaneously for gradually longer periods with interspersed rest. The means by which this strategy is put into operation are similar to those described in the critical care therapeutics section. Traditional methods include (1) the familiar T-piece technique with or without CPAP, in which the patient breathes spontaneously for periods of increasing duration and is mechanically ventilated between periods, and (2) IMV, in which the mechanical breaths are progressively reduced in number. Numerous studies have explored the relative efficacy of T-piece or IMV; however, the data do not support the superiority of either technique. A recent review summarizes the data and appropriately emphasizes that the merits of a weaning technique must be suited to the individual patient's circumstances.[71,72] For example, the patient with exercise dyspnea can be supported during ambulation with ventilation via a self-inflating bag. The sleep-deprived patient can receive SIMV during rest periods and night hours. The SIMV periods are gradually shortened and eliminated as the patient gains strength and vitality. Newer techniques have been advocated for weaning such as pressure-support ventilation or airway pressure-release ventilation. Both techniques deliver positive pressure when needed, reportedly without causing excess patient discomfort or increased mean airway pressure and work of breathing.[71,72]

Weaning is a great burden both physically and mentally for the patient who has been ventilated for many days or weeks. Anxiety and fear can prolong ventilator dependence in some patients.[59,71] A number of studies in medical-surgical patients have demonstrated that biofeedback, relaxation, and imagery can reduce negative emotional responses to weaning.[59] These therapies have not been well studied in the multiply injured.

PLEURAL SPACE INFECTIONS

The previous discussion of critical care nursing management of pleural space drainage is pertinent to intermediate care settings. The risk of posttraumatic empyema remains high, and empyema is frequently a product of initial treatment and stabilization.

MANAGEMENT OF EMPYEMA.
Once the pathogens have been identified, specific antibiotic treatment is initiated based on the results of the Gram stain. The contents of the infected pleural space are drained, and the underlying lung is allowed to reexpand. Closed or open drainage techniques can be used, depending on the number of infectious pockets

and organization of the infected material. Each requires lengthy and persistent medical and nursing management. Decortication may be chosen as definitive management as opposed to prolonged drainage or as a method to remove thickened pleura that entraps the lung and prevents healing.

In closed techniques a chest tube is inserted or an existing thoracostomy tube is converted to an "empyema tube." Although the general management of the closed system is as previously described, frequent cultures of drainage fluid are needed. The nurse avoids milking the chest tube or positioning the drainage collection container in a manner that allows reflux of contaminated material back into the pleural space. The drainage initially appears as a purulent fluid but may change to a thicker, more fibrous material. After 2 or 3 weeks the closed system may be converted into open drainage of the most dependent part of the cavity. Should open drainage be required, nursing care includes a specific protocol for irrigation, absorbent wound dressing, and protection of surrounding skin. As the infection clears and healing begins, the drainage tube is withdrawn slowly and then removed as the cavity closes behind it.[25]

PARAPLEGIA

Spinal cord injury is the most serious complication encountered in patients who survive the critical care phase of ruptured thoracic aorta. Whether the paraplegia results from cord ischemia during aortic cross-clamping or from direct injury to the spinal arteries, spinal cord injury is a devastating condition that has been reported in as many as 20% of survivors.[66]

PERICARDITIS

Posttraumatic pericarditis may become symptomatic weeks or months after myocardial contusion. Bleeding into the pericardial sac irritates the epicardium and pericardium, producing inflammation and edema. Three types of pathology have been associated with blunt chest trauma. These include pericarditis with or without effusion and constrictive pericarditis. Individuals with effusion slowly develop signs of cardiac tamponade whereas those without effusion demonstrate a significant pericardial rub, fever, and retrosternal pain. The patient with constrictive pericarditis shows signs that mimic right-sided heart failure. Heart sounds are diminished, and a third heart sound may be heard. Nursing care includes careful physical examination, including auscultation of heart sounds. Identification of a friction rub and a change in the quality and quantity of chest pain are important findings.

PERSISTENT PAIN

Chronic chest wall pain has been described in nearly half of all long-term survivors of flail injuries. Likewise, the same percentage of patients are unable to return to full-time employment after 5 years as a result of continued and significant pain.[23] The nurse must be able to differentiate between acute and chronic pain in order to provide appropriate therapy.

NUTRITIONAL DEFICIENCIES

Restoration of optimal nutritional status is a common problem in trauma patients. The individual with insufficient or excessive caloric and protein intake is likely to experience respiratory disability and difficulty in weaning from supplemental oxygen. Consultation with nutritional support services and education of the patient's family are essential to ensure appropriate nutritional intake.

DELAYED WOUND HEALING

Healing difficulties are not common in chest tube sites or thoracic soft tissue wounds because of their muscular blood supply. Deformities, diminished sensation caused by intercostal nerve damage, and soft tissue defects are more common and may be associated with higher morbidity and longer hospital stays for the trauma patient. Although some chest wall and related musculoskeletal deformities may require surgical intervention, others can be prevented or treated by exercise.

PULMONARY THERAPEUTICS

All trauma patients, particularly those with thoracic injuries, require care directed toward removal of retained pulmonary secretions from the airways and protection from aspiration and associated pneumonia. CPT is used extensively, as described in the section on critical care therapeutics. Airway clearance may be accomplished by suctioning through an existing airway such as a tracheostomy, by a nasotracheal route, or by directed coughing. Breathing exercises are added to the plan of care, particularly in postoperative patients and those with neuromuscular or chronic pulmonary disease. Providing a clear rationale for therapy and simple-to-follow instructions is particularly important because the patient may not remember therapies employed early in the recovery course.

DIRECTED COUGHING. Coughing remains the most rapid and effective method for clearing the larger airways. It is generally a reflex under control of the afferent vagus nerve triggered by mechanical stimulation of laryngeal and bronchial receptors. However, both involuntary and voluntary cough suppression occurs in trauma patients as a result of decreased inspiratory or expiratory effort, poor glottic function, or fear and pain.

Directed coughing techniques are accompanied by monitoring for cough suppression and treating its cause. For example, the unhealed stoma left after tracheostomy tube removal can reduce the effectiveness of coughing and should be sealed with an airtight dressing. The patient is taught to put light pressure on the dressing during coughing. If the patient has difficulty mobilizing secretions toward the primary bronchi, coughing is less effective as a means of removing mucus. In this case directed coughing is preceded by postural drainage, percussion, or vibration as one way of centralizing secretions and increasing the cough's effectiveness. Effective pain relief must be in progress before the majority of patients can even attempt to breathe deeply and cough. Although many patients naturally "splint" injured or postoperative areas during coughing, the majority benefit from a demonstration of effective splinting that does not impair chest wall movement.

Several methods can be used to stimulate coughing. "Huff coughing" is a single, large inspiration followed by short, forceful exhalations producing rapid changes in airflow and an improved cough. External tracheal stimulation by gentle pressure above the sternal notch can stimulate coughing. Gentle oropharyngeal stimulation with the end of a suction catheter or direct suction aspiration may be necessary when the patient has difficulty clearing secretions in this area. Directed coughing takes place over short periods, alternating with rest. Repetitive and strained coughing is tiring and can precipitate bronchospasm.

BREATHING EXERCISES.   The main goals of breathing exercises are improved tidal volume, chest wall mobility, mobilization of secretions, and relaxation. Muscle training may increase respiratory strength and endurance. Specific exercises include diaphragmatic breathing, pursed-lip breathing, forced expiration, costal excursion exercises, and summed breathing.

ADJUNCTS USED TO IMPROVE LUNG EXPANSION.   Numerous devices are available to augment CPT, directed coughing, and breathing exercises. Most are types of incentive spirometry. Blow bottles are expiratory incentive devices; most commercial equipment packages are inspiratory incentive spirometers. Although published reports of the relative benefits and complications of these devices are abundant, the effectiveness of these adjuncts in reducing postoperative or posttraumatic pulmonary complications remains in question.[83]

Should such devices be incorporated into the plan of care, they are considered an addition to, not a substitute for, the pulmonary therapeutics described earlier. How frequently and for what length of time the patient uses a device are determined by its effectiveness in improving lung volumes and respiratory status. The patient should be instructed and supervised periodically to determine if the device is being used properly and if benefits or problems are present. If incentive spirometry is a consistent part of the patient's pulmonary care, the nurse or respiratory therapist monitors the achieved volumes and maintains a record of volume change over time.

ACTIVE EXERCISE PROGRAMS

Muscular exercise and range-of-motion programs are appropriate for the thoracic trauma patient even in unusual situations when other injuries restrict the patient to bed. In consultation with a physical therapist, an exercise program for involved joints or muscles is included in the plan of care. Patients are likely to avoid moving the trunk and upper extremities after thoracotomy or significant chest wall injury. As a result, they can develop deformities, most commonly frozen shoulder syndrome. Range-of-motion

exercises include passive stretch of the affected area or active contraction of opposing muscle groups. Repeated exercises with weights can improve strength and endurance.

The presence of chest tubes and even ventilatory or oxygen delivery equipment does not commit the patient to bedrest. After reviewing all tubes, drains, and oxygen requirements with the trauma physician, progressive ambulation is planned as part of the exercise program. Chest tube drainage systems can be disconnected temporarily from suction, and oxygen tanks, if needed, are attached to a rolling pole or walker.

SUMMARY

This chapter outlines nursing knowledge of chest trauma, yet it must be emphasized that a great deal is unknown about the physiologic and psychologic effects of our nursing therapies. In solving these unknowns, we do the greatest service for our patients.

Thoracic injuries can be highly lethal, and nursing management must be rapid, technically flawless, and comprehensive. Many chest injuries do not threaten life or create permanent disability, again in large part because of nursing expertise. The trauma nurse's expert care is based on a thorough understanding of thoracic anatomy, respiratory physiology, injury mechanics, and the techniques of cardiopulmonary assessment. Management of chest injuries revolves around individualized ventilator support, exquisite airway care, objective pain control strategies, and intensive pulmonary hygiene.

Trauma nursing care is built from experience, consultation with nursing specialists and other disciplines, and research. We have much to offer the patient with thoracic injuries. We offer relief from the pervasive chest pain, the inability to breathe, and the growing weakness of hypovolemic shock. We also offer the patient support in tolerating chest tubes and the endless days until it is possible to be discharged home.

REFERENCES

1. Fulda G, Brathwaite CEM, Rodriguez A et al: Blunt traumatic rupture of the heart and pericardium: a ten-year experience, *J Trauma* 31(2):167-173, 1991.
2. Rodriguez A: Initial patient evaluation and indications for thoracotomy. In Turney SZ, Rodriguez A, Cowley RA, editors: *Management of cardiothoracic trauma*, Baltimore, 1990, Williams & Wilkins.
3. Flynn MB, Bonini S: Blunt chest trauma: a case report, *Crit Care Nurse* 19(5):68-77, 1999.
4. Rodriguez A: Injuries of the chest wall, the lungs, and the pleura. In Turney SZ, Rodriguez A, Cowley RA, editors: *Management of cardiothoracic trauma*, Baltimore, 1990, Williams & Wilkins.
5. Moschella JM, Wilson D: The cycle of violence: important considerations for EMS providers, *J Emerg Med Serv* 24(6): 46-56, 1999.

6. Shorr RM: Blunt chest trauma in the elderly: the MIEMSS experience. In Turney SZ, Rodriguez A, Cowley RA, editors: *Management of cardiothoracic trauma,* Baltimore, 1990, Williams & Wilkins.

7. Greenburg MD, Rosen CL: Evaluation of the patient with blunt chest trauma: an evidence based approach, *Emerg Med Clin North Am* 17(1):41-62, 1999.

8. Velmahos GC, Tatevossian R, Demetriades D: "The seat belt mark" sign: a call for increased vigilance among physicians treating victims of motor vehicle accidents, *Am Surg* 65(2): 181-185, 1999.

9. Ralston AC, Webb RK, Runciman WB: Potential errors in pulse oximetry: I. pulse oximeter evaluation, *Anesthesia* 46:202-206, 1991.

10. Schuster DP: Bedside evaluation of respiratory function. In Parrillo JE, editor: *Current therapy in critical care medicine,* Philadelphia, 1991, BC Decker.

11. Dunham CM, Cowley RA: *Shock trauma/critical care manual,* Gaithersburg, Md, 1991, Aspen.

12. Pradermacher EC: Airway pressure release ventilation and biphasic positive airway pressure. A 10-year literature review, *Clin Intensive Care* 10(5):296-301, 1997.

13. Richless CI: Current trends in mechanical ventilation, *Crit Care Nurs* 11:41-50, 1991.

14. Mirvis SE: Imaging of thoracic trauma. In Turney SZ, Rodriguez A, Cowley RA, editors: *Management of cardiothoracic trauma,* Baltimore, 1990, Williams & Wilkins.

15. Mineo TC, Ambrogi V, Pompeo E: Changing indications for thoracotomy in blunt chest trauma after the advent of video thoracoscopy, *J Trauma* 47(6):1088-1091, 1999.

16. Committee on Trauma, American College of Surgeons: *Advanced trauma life support care course,* Chicago, 1998, American College of Surgeons.

17. Doyle RL: Assessing and modifying the risk of postoperative pulmonary complications, *Chest* 115(5):77-81, 1999.

18. Sandur S, Stoller JK: Pulmonary complications of mechanical ventilation, *Clin Chest Med* 20(2):223-234, 1999.

19. Ruschult H, Osthaus A, Heine J: Tracheal injury as a sequence of multiple attempts of endotracheal intubation in the course of a preclinical cardiopulmonary resuscitation, *Resuscitation* 43(2):147-150, 2000.

20. Smith TR, Ramzy AI: Prehospital care of thoracic trauma. In Turney SZ, Rodriguez A, Cowley RA, editors: *Management of cardiothoracic trauma,* Baltimore, 1990, Williams & Wilkins.

21. Wu CL, Jani ND, Perkins FM et al: Thoracic epidural analgesia versus intravenous patient-controlled analgesia for the treatment of rib fracture pain after motor vehicle crash, *J Trauma* 47(3):564-567, 1999.

22. Puntillo KA: Pain experiences of intensive care patients, *Heart Lung* 19(5):526-533, 1990.

23. Peeters C, Gupta S: Choices in pain management following thoracotomy, *Chest* 115(5):122-124, 1999.

24. Carroll KC, Atkins PJ, Herold GR et al: Pain assessment and management in critically ill postoperative and trauma patients: a multi-site study, *Am J Crit Care* 8(2):105-117, 1999.

25. Aensio JA, Hanpeter D et al: Thoracic injuries. In Waxman K, Shoemaker WC, editors: *Textbook of critical care,* Philadelphia, 2000, WB Saunders.

26. Velmahos GC, Chan L, Cornwall EE: Is there a limit to massive blood transfusion after severe trauma? *Arch Surg* 133(9): 947-952, 1998.

27. Henry H, Elliott T: The morbid anatomy of wounds of the thorax, *J Army Med Corps* 27:520-555, 1916.

28. Ullman K: Demystifying autotransfusion, *Cardiovasc Nurs* 1:8-9, 1991.

29. Dutton RP: Shock and trauma anesthesia, *Clin North Am* 17(1):83-95, 1999.

30. Dunham CM, Belzberg H, Lyles R et al: The rapid infusion system: a superior method for the resuscitation of hypovolemic trauma patients, *Resuscitation* 21(2-3):207-227, 1991.

31. Ruth-Sahd LA: Pulmonary contusion: the hidden danger in blunt chest trauma, *Crit Care Nurs* 11(6):46-57, 1991.

32. Luchtefeld WB: Pulmonary contusion, *Focus Crit Care* 17(6): 482-488, 1990.

33. Cohn SM: Pulmonary contusion: review of the clinical entity, *J Trauma* 42(5):973-979, 1997.

34. Ruth-Shad LA: Pulmonary contusions: management and implications for trauma nurses, *J Trauma Nursing* 4(4):90-98, 1997.

35. Sutchyta MR, Grissom CK, Morris AH et al: Epidemiology in ARDS, *Intensive Care Med* 25(5):538-539, 1999.

36. Ashbaugh DG, Bigelow DB, Petty TL et al: Acute respiratory distress in adults, *Lancet* 2:319-323, 1967.

37. Hudson LD, Steinberg KP: Epidemiology of acute lung injury and ARDS, *Chest* 116(1):74S-82S, 1999.

38. Croce MA, Fabian TC, Davis KA et al: Early and late acute respiratory distress syndrome: two distinct clinical entities, *J Trauma* 46(3):361-357, 1998.

39. Sair M, Evans TW: ARDS: are we winning at last? *Anaesthesia* 53(9):831-832, 1998.

40. Parsley EL: Acute respiratory distress syndrome. Cellular biology and pathology, *Respir Care Clin N Am* 4(4):583-609, 1998.

41. Lesur O, Berthiaume Y, Blaise G et al: Acute respiratory distress syndrome: 30 years later, *Can Resp J* 6(1):71-86, 1999.

42. Aufmkolk M, Fisher R, Voggenreiter G et al: Local effect of lung contusion on lung surfactant composition in multiple trauma patients, *Crit Care Med* 27(8):1441-1446, 1999

43. Matute-Bello G, Liles WC, Radella F II et al: Modulation of neutrophil apoptosis by granulocyte colony-stimulating factor and granulocyte/macrophage colony-stimulating factor during the course of acute respiratory distress syndrome, *Crit Care Med* 28(1):1-7, 2000.

44. Melton SM, Moomey CB, Fabian TC et al: Mediator-dependent secondary injury after unilateral blunt thoracic trauma, *Shock* 11(6):396-402, 1999.

45. Meduri GM, Headley AS, Golden E et al: Effect of prolonged methylprednisolone therapy in unresolving acute respiratory distress syndrome, *JAMA* 280(2):159-165, 1998.

46. Papadakos PJ, Apostolaakos MJ: High-inflation pressure and positive end-expiratory pressure. Injurious to the lung? Yes. *Crit Care Clin* 12(3):627-634, 1996.

47. Fahy BG, Barnas GM, Flowers JL et al: Effects of PEEP on respiratory mechanics are tidal volume and frequency dependent, *Respir Physiol* 109(1):53-64, 1997.

48. Hirvela ER: Advances in the management of acute respiratory distress syndrome: protective ventilation, *Arch Surg* 135(2): 126-135, 2000.

49. McCarthy MC, Cline AL, Lemmon GW et al: Pressure control inverse ratio ventilation in the treatment of adult respiratory distress syndrome in patients with blunt chest trauma, *Am Surg* 65(11):1027-1030, 1999.

50. Sessler CN: Mechanical ventilation of patients with acute lung injury, *Crit Care Clin* 14(4):707-729, 1998.

51. Smith RA, Smith DB: Does airway pressure release ventilation alter lung function after acute lung injury? *Chest* 107(3):805-808, 1995.

52. Hirschl RB, Parent AC, Tooley R et al: Liquid ventilation improves pulmonary function, gas exchange, and lung injury in a model of respiratory failure, *Ann Surg* 221:79-88, 1995.

53. Cottingham CA, Habashi NM: Extracorporeal lung assist in the adult trauma patient, *AACN Clin Issues* 6(2):2179-2188, 1995.

54. Peek GJ, Moore HM, Moore N et al: Extracorporeal lung assist in the adult respiratory failure, *Chest* 112(3):759-764, 1997.

55. Schmitz TM: The semi-prone position in ARDS: five case studies, *Crit Care Nurse* 11:22-33, 1991.

56. Klein DG: Prone positioning in-patients with acute respiratory distress syndrome: the Vollman Prone Positioner, *Crit Care Nurse* 19(4):66-71, 1999.

57. Rappert D, Rossaint K, Slama K et al: Influence of positioning on ventilation perfusion relationships in severe adult respiratory distress syndrome, *Chest* 206:1511-1516, 1994.

58. Stocker R, Neff T, Stein S et al: Prone positioning and low-volume pressure limited ventilation improves survival in-patients with severe ARDS, *Chest* 111(4):1008-1017, 1997.

59. Wunderlich RJ, Perry A, Lavin MA et al: Patient's perceptions of uncertainty and stress during weaning from mechanical ventilation, *Dimens Crit Care Nurs* 18(8):8-12, 1999.

60. Burns SM: Mechanical ventilation and weaning. In Kinney MR, Dunbar SB, Brunn JA, editors: *AACN clinical reference for critical care nursing,* St. Louis, 1998, Mosby.

61. Moomey CB Jr, Fabian TC, Croce MA et al: Determinant of myocardial performance after blunt chest trauma, *J Trauma* 45(6):988-996, 1998.

62. Hayden AM: Thoracic surgery. In Kinney MR, Dunbar SB, Brunn et al, editors: *AACN clinical reference for critical care nursing,* St. Louis, 1998, Mosby.

63. Wahl WL, Michaels AJ, Wang SC et al: Blunt thoracic aortic injury: delayed or early repair? *J Trauma* 47(2):259-260, 1999.

64. Adams JE, Roman VG, Bessey PQ et al: Improved detection of cardiac contusion with cardiac troponin I, *Am Heart* 131(2):308-312, 1996.

65. Chan D: Echocardiography in thoracic trauma, *Emerg Med Clin North Am* 16(1):191-207, 1998.

66. Morgan PB, Buechter KJ: Blunt thoracic aortic injuries: initial evaluation and management, *South Med J* 93(2):173-175, 2000.

67. Blackmore CC, Zweibel A, Mann FA: Determining risk of traumatic aortic injury: how to optimize imaging strategy, *Am J Roentgenol* 174(2):343-347, 2000.

68. Wicky S, Capasso P, Meuli R et al: Spiral CT aortography: an efficient technique for the diagnosis of traumatic aortic injury, *Eur Radiol* 8(5):828-833, 1998.

69. Demetriades D, Gomez H, Velmahos GC: Routine helical computed tomographic evaluation of the mediastinum in high-risk blunt trauma patients, *Arch Surg* 133(10):1084-1088, 1998.

70. Battistella FD: Ventilation in the trauma and surgical patient, *Crit Care Clin* 14(4):731-742, 1998.

71. Cull C, Inwood H: Weaning patients from mechanical ventilation, *Prof Nurse* 14(8):535-538, 1999.

72. Dries DJ: Weaning from mechanical ventilation, *J Trauma* 43(2):372-384, 1997.

73. Winslow EH, Guzzetta C, Ahrens T: Nursing and mechanical ventilation weaning, *Crit Care Med* 24(9):1606-1607, 1998.

74. Burns SM: The long-term mechanically ventilated patient. An outcome management approach. *Crit Care Nurs North Am* 10(1):87-99, 1998.

75. Ciesla ND: Chest physical therapy for patients in the intensive care unit, *Phys Ther* 76(6):609-625, 1996.

76. Brooks D, Solway S, Graham I et al: A survey of suctioning practices among physical therapists, respiratory therapists and nurses, *Can Resp J* 6(6):513-520, 1999.

77. Ackerman CH: The effect of saline lavage prior to suctioning, *Am J Crit Care* 2:326-330, 1993.

78. Blackwood B: Normal saline instillation with endotracheal suctioning: primum non nocere (first do no harm), *J Adv Nurs* 29(4):928-934, 1999.

79. Kinloch D: Instillation of normal saline during endotracheal suctioning: effects on mixed venous oxygen saturation, *Am J Crit Care* 8(4):231-240, 1999.

80. Schwenker D, Ferrin M, Gift AG: A survey of endotracheal suctioning with instillation of normal saline, *Am J Crit Care* 7(4):255-260, 1998.

81. Baraka AS, Taha SK, Aouad MT et al: Preoxygenation: comparison of maximal breathing and tidal volume breathing techniques, *Anesthesiology* 91(3):612-616, 1999.

82. Dries DJ: Prone positioning in acute lung injury, *J Trauma* 45(4):849-852, 1998.

83. Grove JM, Bradley CA: The effectiveness of IS with physical therapy for high-risk patients after coronary arterial bypass surgery, *Phys Ther* 77(3):260-268, 1997.

ABDOMINAL INJURIES

24

Jean M. Montonye

Trauma is the third leading cause of death for all age groups in the United States.[1] Abdominal injuries rank third among the causes of traumatic death, preceded only by head and chest injuries.[2] Abdominal injuries account for 13% to 15% of trauma deaths, primarily as a result of hemorrhage; causes of death occurring more than 48 hours after injury are sepsis and its complications.[3] Death and disability from traumatic injury have become a significant health and social problem. Whether the injury is single system or multisystem, trauma significantly affects the morbidity and mortality associated with abdominal injury. Numerous authors have noted a higher rate of morbidity and mortality associated with an increased length of time from initial injury to treatment and the number of injured systems.[3-6] Intraabdominal trauma is seldom a single organ injury or single system injury; therefore a concomitant rise in morbidity and mortality is evident.

There are two injury mechanisms for abdominal trauma: blunt and penetrating. The most common mechanism of blunt injury is a motor vehicle crash. The diagnosis of blunt abdominal injury can be complex and challenging, especially in patients with multisystem injury. Multiple organ involvement, with or without central nervous system depression, can present a complex series of symptoms that cloud normal assessment parameters, making definitive diagnosis more difficult. The presence of abdominal tenderness or guarding, circulatory instability, lumbar spine injury, pelvic fracture, retroperitoneal or intraperitoneal air, or unilateral loss of the psoas shadow on radiographic examination should raise the question of visceral damage.

Abdominal trauma challenges even the most experienced nurse. The manifestations of abdominal injury are often subtle, requiring continual assessment and care modification as the patient progresses from the initial assessment to the critical care phase. Frequent assessments and ongoing evaluations are essential components of the nursing process for detection of changes in the patient's condition. Unrecognized abdominal trauma is a frequent cause of preventable death.[7] An organized, methodical approach to assessment, diagnosis, and intervention is necessary for the management of the patient with suspected abdominal injury. Knowledge of the mechanism of injury, patient complaints, serial physical assessments, and quick diagnostic testing are the nurse's resources for identifying potentially life-threatening abdominal injuries.

THE ABDOMEN: ANATOMY AND PHYSIOLOGY

The abdomen is formally thought of as containing structures bordered by the diaphragm, inferiorly by the pelvis, posteriorly by the vertebral column, and anteriorly by the abdominal and iliac muscles (Figure 24-1). For this discussion of abdominal trauma, the esophagus, which passes through the diaphragm and connects with the stomach, has been added to this chapter.

The peritoneal cavity contains the stomach, small intestine, liver, gallbladder, spleen, transverse colon, sigmoid colon, upper third of the rectum, and, in women, the uterus. Retroperitoneal structures include the ascending and descending colon, kidneys, pancreas, adrenal glands, aorta, vena cava, part of the duodenum, and other major vessels.

For purposes of examination, the abdomen is divided into four quadrants: right upper quadrant (RUQ), left upper quadrant (LUQ), right lower quadrant (RLQ), and left lower quadrant (LLQ). General characteristics of each major organ are highlighted in Figure 24-2.

ESOPHAGUS

The esophagus, the first segment of the digestive process, carries food from the pharynx to the stomach. The presence of food within the esophagus stimulates peristaltic action and causes food to move into the stomach. Mucosal glands of the esophagus secrete mucus to lubricate and facilitate passage of the food bolus.[8]

The esophagus traverses the posterior mediastinum of the thorax through the esophageal hiatus in the central tendon of the diaphragm to join the stomach at the level of the tenth thoracic vertebra. The posterior surface of the intraabdominal esophagus overlies the aorta, and the anterior surface is covered by peritoneum. The anterior and posterior vagus nerves pass through the esophageal hiatus. There are three areas of narrowing that predispose the

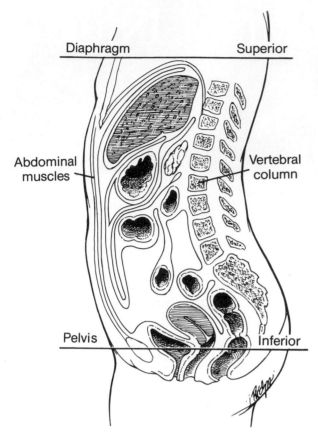

FIGURE 24-1 **The Abdominal Boundaries.**

esophagus to injury: at the cricoid cartilage, at the arch of the aorta, and as it passes through the diaphragm. The esophageal wall lacks a serosal layer, which may affect the integrity of anastomoses, increasing the chance for leaking after surgical repair.

DIAPHRAGM

The diaphragm assists with inspiration and expiration by changing the thoracic volume during respiration. Flattening and contraction of the diaphragm lengthen the thoracic cavity, increasing thoracic volume during inspiration.[9] During expiration the diaphragm relaxes, returning to its original dome shape and reducing thoracic volume.[9] This process is aided by the accessory intercostal muscles. The diaphragm also separates the thoracic and abdominal cavities, preventing herniation of organs.

The diaphragm is a musculotendinous, dome-shaped structure attached posteriorly to the first, second, and third lumbar vertebrae; anteriorly to the lower sternum; and laterally to the costal margins dividing the thoracic and abdominal regions. There are three foramina. The aorta passes through the diaphragm at the T12 level, the esophagus passes through at the T10 level, and the vena cava foramen is at T8. The phrenic nerve, which innervates the diaphragm, passes through the thorax along the posterolateral aspect of the pericardium on both sides and divides into anterior and posterior branches. Any damage to the spinal cord between the third and fifth cervical vertebrae may paralyze the phrenic nerve and therefore the diaphragm.

STOMACH

The stomach has multiple digestive functions, including (1) serving as a reservoir to store food; (2) secreting gastric juice containing acids and enzymes to aid in the digestion of food; (3) secreting intrinsic factor; (4) carrying on a limited amount of absorption of certain drugs, alcohol, some water, and some short-chained fatty acids; and (5) producing the hormone gastrin, which helps regulate digestive functions.[10]

The stomach joins the esophagus approximately 3 cm below the diaphragm. It is located in the LUQ and suspended superiorly by the gastrohepatic ligament, inferiorly by the gastrocolic ligament, and laterally by the gastrosplenic ligament. The stomach resides within the peritoneal cavity. It is divided into the fundus, body, and pylorus (Figure 24-3). The stomach wall contains glands that secrete mucus, hydrochloric acid (HCl), intrinsic factor, and pepsinogen (type I); serotonin is secreted in the fundus and body; and mucus and pepsinogen II are secreted in the pylorus. Perforating gastric injury causes the release of these digestive contents into the peritoneal cavity. These same gastric secretions cause stress ulceration's in the stomach.

The stomach has a rich blood supply. Arterial supply is provided by the splenic artery, gastric arteries, gastroepiploic arteries, and short gastric arteries (Figure 24-4). Venous drainage occurs through the hepatic portal system, which branches out to include the gastric and the gastroepiploic veins, which drain into the splenic vein. Gastric emptying is facilitated by peristaltic movement from the pylorus and stimulated by stretch receptors. An inhibiting function is controlled in the duodenum.

LIVER

The liver, the largest gland in the body, performs many vital, life-sustaining functions, including those listed below[11]:

- Detoxification of various substances, such as drugs and alcohol
- Synthesis of plasma proteins, important in maintaining blood volume and controlling blood coagulation
- Storage of iron and vitamins A, D, E, K, and B_{12} in liver cells
- Metabolism of carbohydrates, which has a role in regulating blood glucose levels
- Metabolism of protein, which can synthesize amino acids and converts nitrogen to urea for excretion by the kidneys
- Metabolism of fats, which breaks down fatty acids, synthesizes cholesterol and phospholipids, and converts excess dietary protein and carbohydrates to fat
- Phagocytization of bacteria via Kupffer cells

The liver is the largest intraabdominal organ, weighing approximately 3 to 4 pounds. It is an extremely vascular organ and lies in the RUQ, extending transversely across the midline. The right margin lies at the sixth to tenth ribs and the left margin at the seventh and eighth ribs (Figure 24-5). It is divided into two lobes, right and left. Fissures on the inferior surface separate them. Between these two lobes is

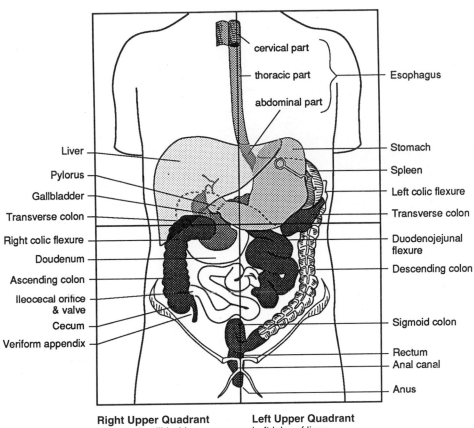

Liver
Pylorus
Gallbladder
Transverse colon
Right colic flexure
Doudenum
Ascending colon
Ileocecal orifice
& valve
Cecum
Veriform appendix

cervical part
thoracic part
abdominal part

Esophagus
Stomach
Spleen
Left colic flexure
Transverse colon
Duodenojejunal
flexure
Descending colon

Sigmoid colon

Rectum
Anal canal

Anus

**FIGURE 24-2 Contents of the
Four Abdominal Quadrants.**
(Modified from *GI series—physical examination of the abdomen*, Richmond, Va, 1975, AH Robins Inc, 6.)

Right Upper Quadrant
Liver and gallbladder
Pylorus
Duodenum
Head of pancreas
Right adrenal gland
Portion of right kidney
Hepatic flexure of colon
Portions of ascending and
    transverse colon

Left Upper Quadrant
Left lobe of liver
Spleen
Stomach
Body of pancreas
Left adrenal gland
Portion of left kidney
Splenic flexure of colon
Portions of transverse and
    descending colon

Right Lower Quadrant
Lower pole of right kidney
Cecum and appendix
Portion of ascending colon
Bladder (if distended)
Ovary and salpinx
Uterus (if enlarged)
Right spermatic cord
Right ureter

Left Lower Quadrant
Lower pole of left kidney
Sigmoid colon
Portion of descending colon
Bladder (if distended)
Ovary and salpinx
Uterus (if enlarged)
Left spermatic cord
Left ureter

Loops of small bowel are found in all quadrants

the porta hepatis, where veins, arteries, nerves, lymphatic vessels, and bile ducts enter or leave the liver.

Approximately three fourths of the blood to the liver is delivered by the portal vein, which carries a rich supply of nutrients after draining the gastrointestinal tract. The rest of the arterial blood supply is rich in oxygen and enters through the hepatic artery. Each lobule (Figure 24-6) has a central vein, which collects the mixture of blood from the portal vein and hepatic artery and channels blood to the lobular veins, which empty into the hepatic vein and then into the inferior vena cava. This rich vascular supply can hemorrhage after injury, which can complicate surgical repair. Uncontrolled hemorrhage is the primary cause of early mortality after liver trauma.

Hepatocytes produce bile, which is essential to the digestion of fats. Bile flows from the hepatic cells into bile canaliculi between the cells toward the periphery of the lobule and empties into the interlobular bile ducts of the hepatic triad. The ducts join, forming the common hepatic duct, which allows bile to flow into the gallbladder. The gallbladder lies on the inferior surface of the liver. Its duct, the cystic duct, meets with the hepatic duct to form the common bile duct, which drains through the head of the pancreas into the duodenum (see Figure 24-6).

SPLEEN
The spleen is a lymphoid organ with various functions including defense, hematopoiesis, and red blood cell

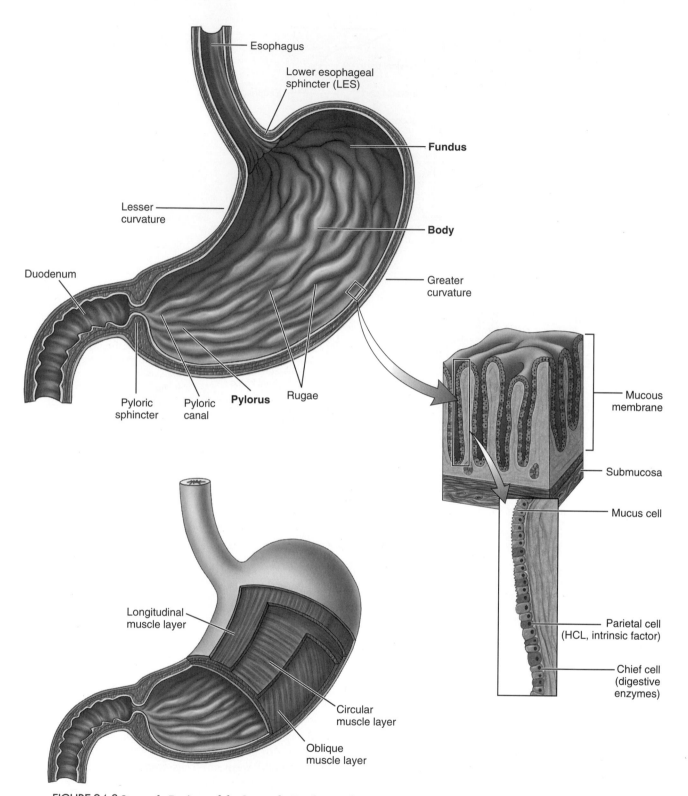

FIGURE 24-3 **Stomach: Regions of the Stomach: Fundus, Body, and Pylorus.** (From Herlihy B, Maebius NK: *The human body in health and illness,* Philadelphia, 2000, WB Saunders, 394.)

(RBC) and platelet destruction; it also and serves as a reservoir for blood. Macrophages line the spleen and break apart hemoglobin molecules from the destroyed RBCs, salvaging the iron and globin content and returning them to the bloodstream for storage in the bone marrow and liver.[12]

The total circulation of the spleen is estimated at 250 ml/min, with a normal volume of approximately 350 ml.[13,14] This is an impressive blood volume considering that the average weight of the spleen is 150 g. The spleen's volume can be reduced to 200 ml very quickly after sympathetic stimulation, which causes constriction of the smooth muscle capsule. This response to stress can be a result of hemorrhage.[13]

The spleen is an elongated ovoid body located in the LUQ

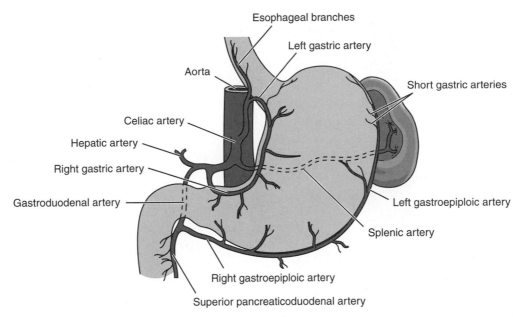

FIGURE 24-4 Arterial Supply to the Stomach. All the arteries are derived from branches of the celiac artery. (From Snell RS, Smith MS: *Clinical anatomy for emergency medicine*, St. Louis, 1993, Mosby, 419.)

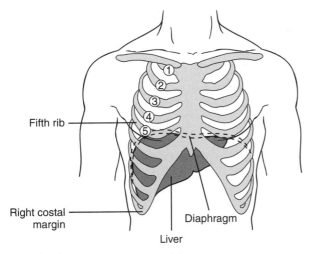

FIGURE 24-5 Anatomic Location of the Liver. The upper border normally lies at the level of the fourth intercostal space or fifth rib, and the lower border does not normally extend more than 1 to 2 cm below the right costal margin. (From Clochesy JM, Breu C, Cardin S et al: *Critical care nursing*, ed 2, Philadelphia, 1996, WB Saunders, 1048.)

of the abdomen. It lies beneath the diaphragm; to the left of the stomach; and in immediate proximity to the tail of the pancreas, the colon, and the left kidney. It is in close proximity to ribs 7 through 10, which makes it vulnerable to injury when ribs are fractured.

The spleen's blood supply is from the splenic artery, which enters at the hilum and divides into five or six branches before entering splenic pulp (Figure 24-7). The splenic vein originates outside the hilum and courses along the dorsal pancreatic surface to join the superior mesenteric vein, forming the portal vein. The vascular nature of the spleen makes it a ready source for profuse bleeding into the peritoneal cavity after injury.

The splenic capsule, 1 to 2 mm thick, encloses the splenic pulp. Lymphoid tissue lies throughout the pulp and is responsible for filtration. The blood supply to the pulp is from arterioles off a central artery. The blood collects in a venous sinus, then moves to trabecular veins coursing to the main splenic veins and finally to the portal circulation (Figure 24-7B). Arterial blood travels to venous sinuses through splenic cords (connective tissue between sinuses) and "sieves" red cells, destroying many in the process. The spleen's sieving process promotes it as a primary defense organ to remove microorganisms from the blood and destroy them by phagocytosis. Approximately 90% of the splenic blood flow participates in this filtering process.

PANCREAS

The pancreas is composed of both exocrine and endocrine glandular tissue. The exocrine pancreas secretes enzymes that digest protein, carbohydrates, and fats. These enzymes include trypsin, chymotrypsin, carboxypeptidase, α-amylase, and lipase. The endocrine pancreas produces two hormones: glucagon from the alpha cells and insulin from the beta cells (Figure 24-8). These hormones facilitate the formation and cellular uptake of glucose.

The pancreas lies at the level of the first lumbar vertebra against the posterior abdominal wall. It extends from the C-loop of the duodenum to the hilum of the spleen. A blunt trauma episode can force the pancreas against the vertebral column and may rupture it. The pancreas is divided into lobules that empty into the main pancreatic duct, which passes through the tail, body, neck, and head of the pancreas, emptying into the duodenum at the ampulla of Vater in conjunction with the common bile duct (see Figure 24-8A). An accessory duct empties into the duodenum from the head of the pancreas. Rupture of the pancreas frequently tears its ductal system, allowing pancreatic juice (rich in

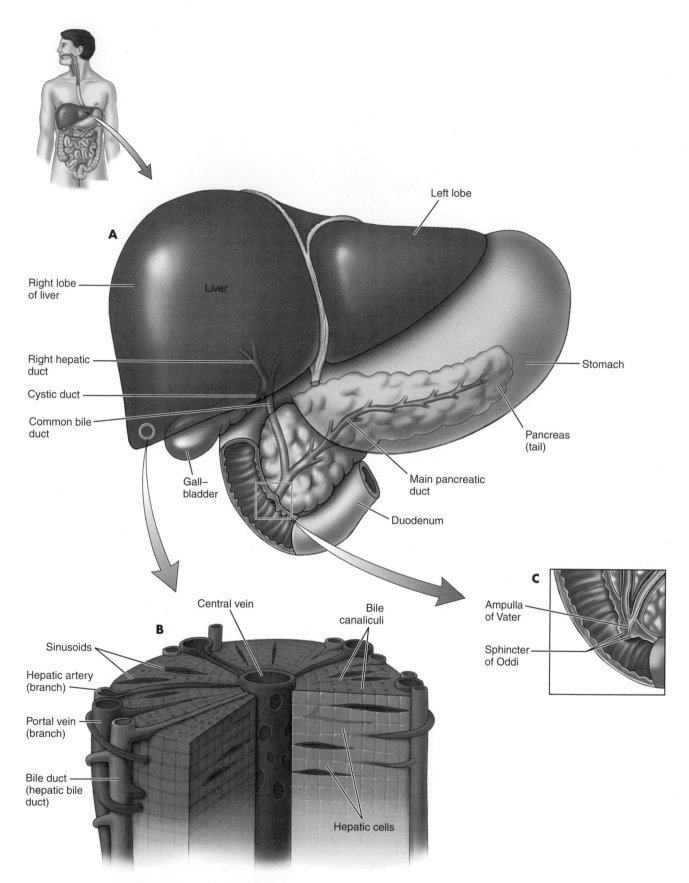

FIGURE 24-6 A, Relationship of liver, gallbladder, and pancreas to the duodenum. **B,** Liver lobule, the functional unit of the liver. Note the blood flow into the liver via the portal vein and hepatic artery. **C,** Ampulla of Vater. (From Herlihy B, Maebius NK: *The human body in health and illness,* Philadelphia, 2000, WB Saunders, 402.)

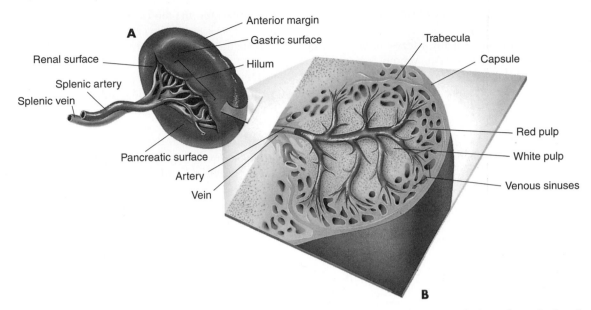

FIGURE 24-7 The Vascular Supply of the Spleen. A, Medial aspect of the spleen. **B,** Section showing the internal organization of the spleen. (From Thibodeau GA, Patton KT: *Anatomy & physiology,* ed 4, St. Louis, 1999, Mosby, 635.)

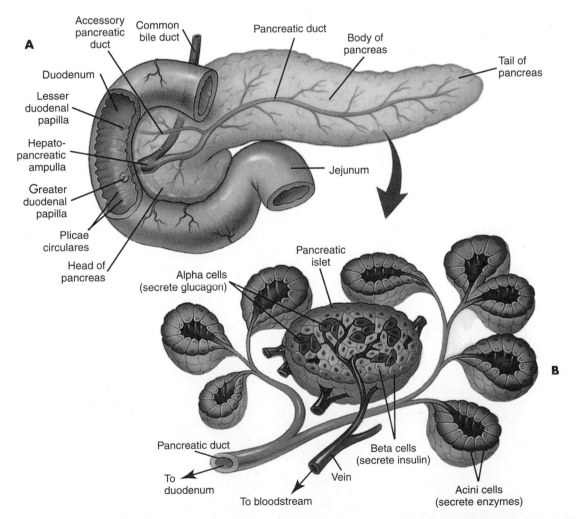

FIGURE 24-8 Pancreas. A, Pancreas dissected to show main and accessory ducts. **B,** Exocrine glandular cells (around small pancreatic ducts) and endocrine glandular cells of pancreatic islets (adjacent to blood capillaries). Exocrine pancreatic cells secrete pancreatic juice, alpha endocrine cells secrete glucagon, and beta cells secrete insulin. (From Thibodeau GA, Patton KT: *Anatomy & physiology,* ed 4, St. Louis, 1999, Mosby, 755.)

digestive enzymes) to invade pancreatic tissue and the peritoneum.

Blood is supplied by the splenic artery and vein and the superior mesenteric artery and vein. Venous drainage from the body and tail of the pancreas occurs through the splenic vein to the portal vein; the head empties directly into the portal vein.

SMALL INTESTINE

The 21 to 23 feet of small intestine are divided into duodenum, jejunum, and ileum (Figure 24-9). The major functions are digestion of food and absorption of nutrients

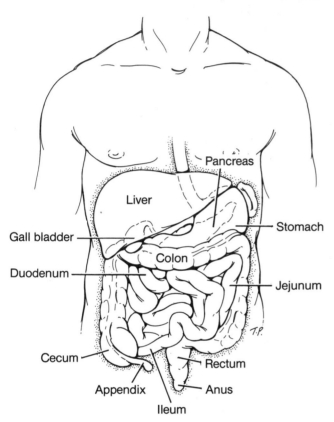

FIGURE 24-9 The small intestine: duodenum, jejunum, and ilium in relationship to other abdominal structures.

and water for the body. The blood supply is from the superior mesenteric artery. Venous drainage is to the portal vein via the superior mesenteric vein.

DUODENUM. Most digestion and absorption occur within the duodenum. The duodenum, the first part of the small intestine, is a C-shaped loop approximately 25 cm long, molded around the head of the pancreas (Figure 24-10). Beginning at the pyloric valve junction, the duodenum receives the highly acidic chyme from the stomach and fluids, enzymes, and electrolytes from the biliary and pancreatic ducts.

The duodenum is divided into four segments, with only the superior portion residing within the peritoneal cavity. The remaining segments, descending, transverse, and ascending, are located in the retroperitoneum. Rapid deceleration injuries may lead to rupture between the anchored and free segments of the duodenum. Three fourths of this organ lies over the vertebral column, which renders it vulnerable to compression injuries.

Blood supply to the duodenum is shared with the pancreas through the superior and inferior pancreaticoduodenal artery. After injury this makes removal of the entire pancreas impossible without devascularizing the duodenum. Drainage occurs via the superior mesenteric veins, which drain into the portal veins and gastrocolic trunk.

JEJUNUM AND ILEUM. From the duodenal jejunal flexure (ligament of Treitz) to the ileocecal junction, the jejunum and ileum are responsible for nutrient absorption and fluid and electrolyte shifts. Peristalsis originating in the duodenum continues through the jejunum and ileum. Some absorption takes place in the jejunum; bile salts and vitamin B_{12} are absorbed in the terminal ileum. Intestinal fluid shifts from the gastrointestinal lumen to the vascular system. All but 0.5 to 1 L of fluid is absorbed in the small intestine, and the remaining fluid passes through to the large intestine.

Most of the jejunum lies in the umbilical region of the abdomen, and the ileum is in the hypogastric and pelvic regions. This expansive placement makes the small intestine vulnerable to seat belt injury (from lap belts) when the

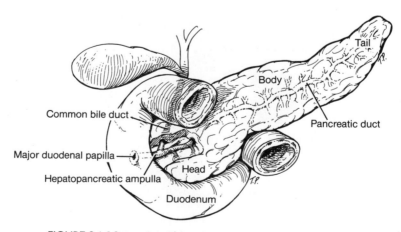

FIGURE 24-10 **Duodenal Location in Relation to the Pancreas.**

bowel is crushed between vertebrae and a solid object such as a steering wheel.

LARGE INTESTINE

The large intestine's digestive functions include (1) absorption of water and electrolytes; (2) synthesis of certain vitamins by the intestinal bacterial, especially vitamin K and the B vitamins; (3) temporary storage of intestinal waste; and (4) elimination of body waste. Peristaltic waves move intestinal material from cecum through the entire colon to the rectum. Substances that increase intestinal motility cause a decrease in water absorption, resulting in diarrhea. Consequently, substances administered to decrease motility cause an increase in water absorption, leading to constipation.

The bacterial content of feces is high, but bacterial species in the intestinal tract are natural. One of these bacteria is *Escherichia coli*. These bacteria are important in the synthesis, for example, of vitamins K and B complex. They cause serious problems if they enter the bloodstream or urinary system, but they are not detrimental when contained within the intestinal tract.

The cecum, colon, and rectum constitute the large intestine. The colon is divided into ascending, transverse, descending, and sigmoid segments (Figure 24-11). The ileum joins the large intestine at the junction of the cecum and ascending colon. The ileocecal valve permits slow movement of intestinal contents through the cecum and colon. The cecum and ascending colon are continuous from the ileum and rise to the undersurface of the right lobe of the liver, bending to the left at the hepatic flexure and becoming the transverse segment. This segment continues across to the splenic flexure (anterior to the left kidney) and then turns downward to become the descending colon. The sigmoid colon, the S-shaped segment, courses from the left iliac fossa to the pelvic cavity, becoming the rectum and terminating at the anal canal. The rectum forms the last 17 to 20 cm of the intestinal structures. The final inch is called the anal canal, and its opening is the anus. The anus is controlled by two sphincter muscles, which are closed except during defecation.

Blood supply to the colon and rectum is predominantly from the superior and inferior mesenteric arteries arising from the abdominal aorta (Figure 24-12). The large intestine drains through the portal vein to sinusoids in the liver.

ABDOMINAL VASCULAR SYSTEM

ARTERIAL SUPPLY. The descending aorta passes through the diaphragm at the T12-L1 level to become the abdominal aorta. At the L4 level the aorta bifurcates into the two common iliac arteries. It further divides into external and internal iliac arteries. Finally the external iliac becomes the common femoral artery (Figure 24-13).

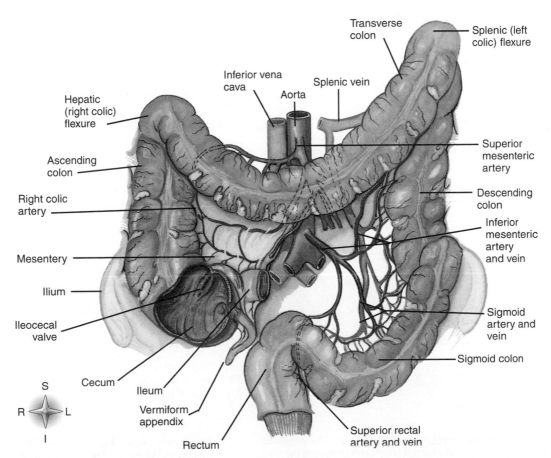

FIGURE 24-11 **Divisions of the Large Intestine.** (From Thibodeau GA, Patton KT: *Anatomy & physiology,* ed 4, St. Louis, 1999, Mosby, 747.)

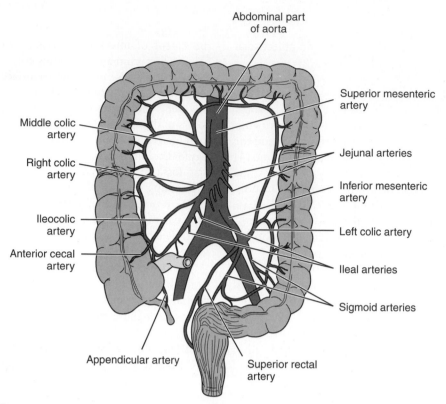

FIGURE 24-12. Arterial Supply to the Small and Large Intestines. Note the branches of the superior and inferior mesenteric arteries. (From Snell RS, Smith MS: *Clinical anatomy for emergency medicine,* St. Louis, 1993, Mosby, 423.)

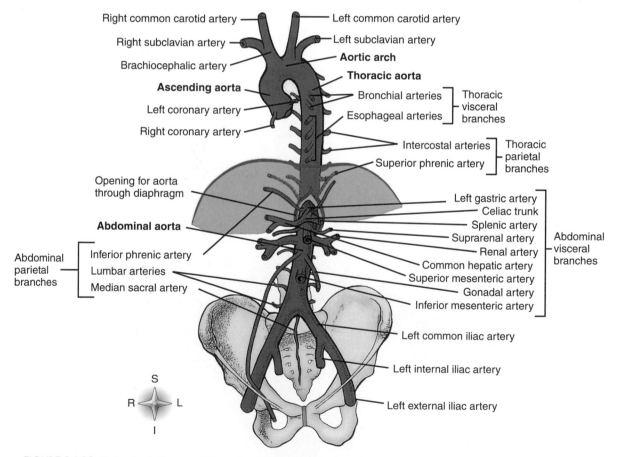

FIGURE 24-13 Abdominal Aorta and Branches. The aorta is the main systemic artery, serving as a trunk from which other arteries branch. Blood is conducted from the heart first through the ascending aorta, then the arch of the aorta, then through the thoracic and abdominal segments of the descending aorta. (From Thibodeau GA, Patton KT: *Anatomy & physiology,* ed 4, St. Louis, 1999, Mosby, 569.)

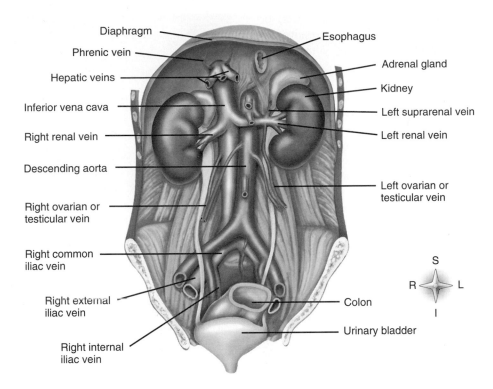

FIGURE 24-14 **Inferior Vena Cava and Abdominal Blood Supply.** (From Thibodeau GA, Patton KT: *Anatomy & physiology,* ed 4, St. Louis, 1999, Mosby, 576.)

Major branches of the aorta include (1) the celiac axis at the T12 level, which divides into the left gastric artery, splenic artery, and common hepatic artery; (2) the superior mesenteric artery at the L1 level, dividing into the middle colic artery and inferior ileocolic artery; (3) the renal arteries at the L2 level, which supply the kidneys directly; and (4) the inferior mesenteric artery at the L3-4 level, dividing into the left colic artery and the superior hemorrhoidal artery. Because of this rich blood supply, any injury to the lower chest or abdomen may induce vascular trauma with widespread effects.

VENOUS DRAINAGE. Venous drainage of the abdomen is more complex than the arterial supply. Blood is drained from the small intestines, stomach, spleen, and pancreas through the superior mesenteric and splenic veins and their tributaries, which join to form the portal vein. This blood then passes through liver sinusoids, supplying nutrients to hepatocytes before emptying into lobular veins and then into the hepatic veins, which empty into the inferior vena cava.

Other abdominal venous flow (Figure 24-14) originates in the external iliac veins in the inguinal ligament, which are joined by internal iliac veins to form the common iliac veins, which become the inferior vena cava at the sacral promontory. The renal veins join the inferior vena cava at the L2 level. Other smaller veins join the inferior vena cava as it passes to the superior margin of the liver. Much of the inferior vena cava lies in close proximity to the aorta, making injury to one vessel likely to affect the other.

MECHANISM OF INJURY

Mechanism of injury refers to the mechanisms by which energy is transferred from the environment to a person. Energy sources may be mechanical, thermal, electrical, or chemical. Examples include mechanical energy from a motor vehicle crash, electrical energy from contact with a high-voltage wire, and chemical energy from contact with hydrofluoric acid. Mechanical energy is the most common mechanism of injury in motor vehicle crashes, auto-pedestrian collisions, falls, stabbings, and gunshot wounds. Knowledge of the mechanism of injury is paramount to rapid and efficient diagnosis and treatment of traumatic injuries.

The mechanism of injury and forces involved direct attention toward certain organ involvement and should heighten a clinician's suspicion regarding certain injuries. Blunt injury from a motor vehicle crash results from a compression or crushing mechanism and involves three collisions. In the first collision the motor vehicle hits a stationary object. A frontal impact may crush the driver's compartment, causing direct injury to the driver or passengers. The second collision occurs when the victim hits internal parts of the vehicle, including the windshield, steering wheel, or dashboard. The third collision involves the supporting structures of the body (e.g., skull, ribs, spine, pelvis) and movable organs (e.g., brain, heart, liver, intestines). As energy is loaded on to the body, internal forces (e.g., stress and strain) are exerted within the body as the dimensions of body tissues change. These forces can be further classified as tensile (stretch), shearing (opposing forces across an object), or compressive (crush). The types of injuries that result from these forces include spleen or liver rupture, comminuted bone fractures, and tearing of the aorta.

The types of forces involved (rotational, crushing, shearing, acceleration or deceleration, or blast) should be investigated. A pedestrian struck by a motor vehicle can suffer acceleration forces and shearing forces, resulting in a closed head injury or degloving injury as layers of tissue are torn away from attachments. The descending thoracic aorta and the duodenum are two anatomic locations susceptible to injury from this type of force. A direct blow to the abdomen may transmit forces sufficient to rupture an organ.

The increased use of restraint devices, such as safety belts and air bags, has reduced fatal outcomes and serious injury, but they certainly cannot prevent injury entirely. Seat belts have been associated with blunt cervical, thoracic, abdominal, and extremity injuries. The addition of the shoulder harness to the lap belt has decreased craniofacial, thoracic, and abdominal injuries; however, classic seat belt injuries include abdominal wall disruption, hollow viscus injury, and flexion-distraction fracture of the lumbar vertebrae (Chance fracture). Some abdominal wall injuries (ecchymosis) arise from direct seat belt injury. Small bowel and colon injuries occur most frequently from a sudden increase intraluminal pressure or shearing forces caused by rapid deceleration. Liver, spleen, and pancreatic injuries are reported as well, but with less frequency.

Penetrating trauma may occur from a stab, impalement, or missile event. The size, shape, and length of the stabbing instrument help to estimate intraabdominal damage. The management is frequently dictated by the degree of penetration into the peritoneal cavity. Impalement injuries are a dirty form of stab wound that result in high mortality as a result of bacterial contamination and multiple organ involvement (Figure 24-15).

Missile injuries are more difficult to evaluate. Mortality depends on major vessel disruption and multiple organ involvement. The terminal velocity, or the amount of energy imparted to the tissue by the missile, often determines the extent of injury. It is reported that 80% to 90% of gunshot wounds cause significant injury.[15,16] The magnitude of entrance and exit wounds may bear little relationship to the degree of damage or course of destruction caused by a bullet. Bullets may ricochet off organs or bones, roll or move throughout the body, or embolize through the vessels. Organs in proximity to the gunshot wound may be injured by a blast effect. Quick evaluation of the situation is necessary because hemorrhage and hollow viscus perforation resulting in chemical and bacterial peritonitis are major problems in this type of abdominal trauma. The extent of tissue destruction varies depending on velocity, type of weapon or bullet, and individual tissue characteristics; therefore, abdominal wounds and their complications have a wide range of presentations.

The mechanism of injury involved in blunt and penetrating trauma provides the nurse with valuable information necessary for quick diagnostic interventions and treatment

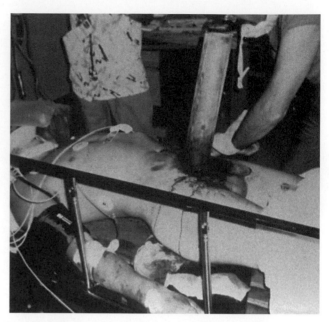

FIGURE 24-15 Impalement Event. Young male impaled by wooden fence rail, which entered the abdomen through the peritoneum.

of patients presenting with potential abdominal injury. A clean versus dirty or open versus closed injury often dictates medical management and subsequent nursing care. The nurse can anticipate what diagnostic modalities will be used, the need for antibiotics, and the potential for emergency surgery.

ABDOMINAL ASSESSMENT

Abdominal injury may be insidious, requiring close, systematic assessment by all team members to promote early diagnosis and intervention. Multiple pieces of data are collected during patient assessment; each has little value when considered alone. However, monitoring these data and correlating the findings with information from the mechanism of injury, diagnostic test results, and the patient's physical findings assist in directing the patient's medical care.

A primary survey addressing the airway (A), breathing (B), circulation (C), and disabilities (D) of resuscitation is initiated upon the patient's arrival in the emergency department (ED). A quick assessment to identify and treat life-threatening conditions is crucial to good trauma patient outcomes. The ABCDs are evaluated constantly throughout all phases of care to determine the effectiveness of treatment. Oxygen administration, vascular access, intravenous fluid administration, cardiac monitoring, and pulse oximetry are required for all trauma patients during the resuscitation phase.

A brief systematic secondary survey is the next step in the resuscitation phase. A head-to-toe assessment is completed to identify all injuries. During this process the nurse and various other team members are simultaneously assessing, providing interventions, and reassessing the patient. The secondary survey includes getting a complete set of vital signs, ordering laboratory studies, placing a nasogastric

(NG) tube and urinary catheter, performing a complete neurologic examination, and obtaining more information about the patient. Diagnostic testing can occur simultaneously during the primary and secondary survey, including bedside ultrasound, diagnostic peritoneal lavage (DPL), and chest radiograph (CXR).

Although an abdominal assessment is not part of the primary survey, an abdominal injury necessitating immediate surgical intervention must be identified early. Continual assessment of the abdomen as part of the secondary survey can occur only after life-threatening events have been managed. This allows the nurse to move on to a continuous, complete reevaluation and subsequent care.

The process for gathering patient information begins as soon as the patient arrives in the emergency department. Prehospital personnel should provide information regarding the circumstances of the traumatic event. Such information should include mechanism of injury, injuries sustained, vital signs, and treatment initiated, along with patient response. Nursing assessment includes patient-generated information such as the patient's complaints upon arrival in the ED, medical and surgical history, medications, allergies, time of last meal, and use of drugs or alcohol.

The physical examination is systematic and continues through all phases of care. Repeated examination by the same nurse or physician provides the consistency necessary to evaluate changes. The physical examination should be adapted to the patient's hemodynamic status. Certainly an unstable patient with a penetrating abdominal wound does not need a prolonged, detailed physical examination; rather, prompt, appropriate intervention is indicated.

Complaint of abdominal pain from an alert patient is a key indicator of abdominal injury. Peritoneal irritation is described as sharp, localized pain. Referred pain complaints signal damage to the spleen (left shoulder pain), liver (right shoulder pain), or retroperitoneal structures (back or testicular pain).

Many patients who sustain abdominal injuries may not be able to participate in the physical examination because of alterations in level of consciousness or spinal cord injury; therefore the four-step abdominal examination, consisting of inspection, auscultation, percussion, and palpation, is essential.

INSPECTION

Inspection begins with noting lower chest wall integrity. Because the last six ribs lie over abdominal structures, disruption to this area may signal organ damage, specifically to the liver, spleen, or diaphragm.

The appearance of the abdomen should be described. The presence of abrasions, contusions, lacerations, and surgical scars and the location, size, description, and number of wounds should be documented. In patients who have been shot, an odd number of wounds indicates the presence of a foreign object within the body. The nurse should resist the temptation to categorize wounds as entrance and exit.

The abdominal contour, normally flat or slightly rounded (or convex in a heavy patient), may be distended, which is indicative of an accumulation of blood, other fluid, or gas secondary to perforation of hollow viscus, rupture of organs (e.g., liver or spleen), or reduced vascular supply to the abdomen. Repeated inspection by the nurse may reveal subtle signs of distention, which, combined with absence of bowel sounds, may be indicative of ileus, peritonitis, or intraabdominal bleeding.

Involuntary guarding indicates injury to underlying structures. This may be less obvious or not present in patients with retroperitoneal injury. The presence of discoloration, protuberances, peristaltic movement, pulsations, abrasions, and old surgical scars should be noted. Repeated inspection alerts the nurse to new discolorations or other changes indicative of underlying injury. Dissection of blood into the abdominal wall from retroperitoneal tissue (Grey Turner's sign) may occur several hours after the initial injury. Proper inspection includes examining the patient's back and flank area and the anterior surface for the signs mentioned. Obvious wounds or ecchymosis of the lumbar or flank areas may indicate damage to retroperitoneal or abdominal organs.

AUSCULTATION

Auscultation is often the most difficult part of the abdominal examination during resuscitative or critical care efforts simply because of the noise created by team members performing lifesaving procedures. The presence or absence of bowel sounds on initial examination is nonspecific information in patients with suspected abdominal injury.[17] While auscultating in all four quadrants, the nurse should be alert for the presence of bowel sounds in unlikely locations, such as the chest cavity, which may indicate a diaphragmatic tear. In serial auscultation, diminished or absent bowel sounds may indicate an ileus or peritonitis. The nurse should listen for bruits, especially over the renal arteries, abdominal aorta, and iliac arteries, which may indicate partially obstructed arterial blood flow.

PERCUSSION

Percussion identifies the presence of air, fluid, or tissue. Tympanic sounds indicate air-filled spaces such as stomach or gut, and a dull sound is present over organ structures such as the liver or spleen.

Dullness throughout the four quadrants indicates free fluid in the abdomen. Fixed areas of dullness (Ballance's sign) in the LUQ may suggest a subcapsular or extracapsular hematoma of the spleen or flank. Dullness that does not change with position suggests the presence of retroperitoneal hematoma. Tympanic percussion may represent air in the abdominal cavity, indicative of perforated viscus. A diaphragmatic tear or hemothorax may be suspected if a dull sound is elicited over the otherwise tympanic thoracic space.

PALPATION

Abdominal tenderness is evaluated by using the whole hand over all four quadrants and progressing from light to deep palpation. Tenderness is the most frequent and reliable sign of intraabdominal injury. Gentle palpation may elicit areas of increased tone or tenderness, suggesting underlying injury. Abdominal wall injury produces focal tenderness, which increases on exertion (tensing muscles). Deep palpation is used to elicit tenderness, guarding, and rebound symptoms associated with peritoneal irritation.

A tender abdomen with guarding, distention, and signs of peritoneal irritation can indicate organ rupture. RUQ tenderness and guarding or tenderness over the right lower six ribs may indicate liver damage. RUQ abdominal tenderness may also be a sign of duodenal or gallbladder injury. Pain elicited in the LUQ may indicate injury to the spleen, stomach, or pancreas. Low abdominal or suprapubic discomfort may signal a potential for colon, bladder, or urethral injuries and may be associated with pelvic fractures.

The patient may experience referred pain. Most common among these is Kehr's sign, pain in the left shoulder secondary to diaphragmatic irritation by blood after splenic rupture. Right shoulder pain is often indicative of liver injury. The patient must be lying flat or in Trendelenburg's position to elicit this type of shoulder pain.

Rectal examination includes testing for gross blood and anterior tenderness, which can indicate bleeding or peritoneal irritation. Positive results may indicate lower gastrointestinal injury.

Diminished or absent pulses in the femoral arteries may indicate common iliac artery thrombosis, dissecting aortic aneurysm, or chronic vascular disease. Information about the quality and rate of pulses during the initial assessment provides the clinician with good baseline information.

ONGOING ASSESSMENT

The four-step systematic physical examination continues during all phases of care. Inspection includes the same assessment techniques; however, changes detected in the examination may be secondary to the operative event, late signs of traumatic injury, or sepsis. A chemical ileus secondary to late pancreatic rupture or gastric repair leakage distends the bowel and therefore the abdomen. Either the bowel sounds are obliterated or a hypertympanic sound is appreciated.

Careful serial examination of the patient is frequently the key to early diagnosis of intraabdominal injuries and prevention of complications. Discolorations around a repair site may indicate vessel re-bleeding into an area. A wound may appear dark or collect excess cloudy exudate and imply an infection.

Small diaphragmatic tears may be missed during the original operative procedure or simply not manifest until days or weeks after the original injury. Therefore auscultation of the chest and abdomen should continue periodically for the presence of bowel sounds.

Physiologic and psychologic stress from the trauma may induce gastric mucosal erosion over time, leading to gastrointestinal bleeding. Abdominal distention, pain, and tenderness are noticed as the erosion progresses. However, no physical symptoms may be appreciated until bleeding is evident. This event can occur at any time throughout the phases of trauma care. Therefore vigilant, systematic physical assessment is required as the patient advances from admission through rehabilitation.

DIAGNOSTIC STUDIES

There are many diagnostic modalities that can be used to evaluate the patient with abdominal trauma, including diagnostic peritoneal lavage (DPL), computed tomography (CT), and ultrasonography (US). Each tool has its own particular advantages. To optimize evaluation of the trauma patient, these tools should be considered complementary rather than mutually exclusive. Accuracy, speed, and safety should be the factors that drive the clinician's decision regarding the most appropriate diagnostic modality.

DIAGNOSTIC PERITONEAL LAVAGE

DPL is a quick diagnostic procedure that is used frequently in the resuscitation phase of care to diagnose intraabdominal bleeding in the hemodynamically unstable trauma patient. Other indications for use include (1) unexplained hypotension, decreased hematocrit, or shock; (2) equivocal results of abdominal examination; (3) altered mental status caused by closed head injury or alcohol or drug intoxication; (4) spinal cord injury; and (5) distracting injuries such as major orthopedic fractures or chest trauma.[18,19] DPL is a simple, low-cost, safe test for quick and accurate determination of intraabdominal hemorrhage.[20,21] Although sensitive and relatively accurate, it is not specific for type or extent of organ damage. In the patient who is hemodynamically unstable, a grossly positive lavage mandates an exploratory laparotomy without further diagnostic workup.

Despite its advantages, DPL has several limitations: It is difficult to perform in patients who are morbidly obese, in those who have had numerous laparotomies, and in women in the third trimester of pregnancy. It is an invasive procedure that poses a risk of omental laceration and visceral or vascular perforation during trocar insertion. DPL can miss certain abdominal injuries, such as those of the bowel, diaphragm, or retroperitoneal structures. Injury may elude detection because there is little bleeding, insufficient fluid is retrieved, the injury is isolated by adhesions, or the DPL is performed early in the resuscitative phase and injury has not yet declared itself, such as with bowel or pancreatic injury.

The use of DPL for some penetrating injuries, specifically stab wounds, is advocated by several authors, but more research is needed to determine its role in the evaluation of gunshot wounds (GSW).[18,19] The current management practice for most patients with an abdominal GSW is immediate surgical intervention.

Interpretation of DPL results is based on whether the mechanism is blunt or penetrating. Criteria for a positive DPL in blunt trauma are 10 ml or more of gross blood on aspiration; a red blood cell (RBC) count of 100,000/mm^3 or more; a white blood cell (WBC) count of 500/mm^3 or more

TABLE 24-1	Peritoneal Lavage Results for Blunt Trauma	
	Result	**Indication**
Aspirant	Gross blood >10 ml	Positive
	Pink fluid	Intermediate*
	Clean	Negative
Lavage fluid	Bloody	Positive
	Clear	Negative
RBC	>100,000 cells/mm³	Positive
	50-100,000 cells/mm³	Intermediate*
WBC	>500 cells/mm³	Positive
	100-500 cells/mm³	Intermediate*
Amylase	>175 U/100 ml	Positive
	75-175 U/100 ml	Intermediate*
	<75 U/100 ml	Negative
Bacteria	Present	Positive
Fecal material	Present	Positive
Bile	Present	Positive
Food particles	Present	Positive

*Intermediate lavage results require further observation of the patient, possibly repeated lavage, and intervention based on clinical presentation.

after the intraabdominal infusion of 1 L of crystalloid; and the presence of bile or fibers[22] (Table 24-1).

DPL is used in the evaluation of stab wounds when local exploration reveals penetration of the peritoneal cavity. The RBC criterion for a positive sign of injury remains controversial. Some surgeons have lowered the limit to 5000 to 1000/mm³ to enhance sensitivity to injury.

Before any DPL procedure a Foley catheter should be placed to empty the bladder and a nasogastric tube inserted to decompress the stomach. This reduces the risk of accidental gastric or bladder perforation when the DPL catheter is inserted. After catheter insertion, and if less than 10 ml of gross blood is aspirated, 1 L of crystalloid (lactated Ringer's solution or 0.9% normal saline) is infused into the peritoneal space. Warmed crystalloid should be infused to prevent hypothermia and decrease peritoneal irritation. After completion of the infusion, the intravenous (IV) bag is placed in a dependent position to allow fluid return by gravity. A sample of the effluent is sent to the laboratory for analysis.

COMPUTED TOMOGRAPHY

Computed tomography (CT) has been used in the assessment of patients with blunt abdominal trauma for almost two decades. It is gradually replacing DPL as a routine screening tool for the hemodynamically stable trauma patient.

This noninvasive procedure provides information about multiple abdominal organs, including intraabdominal and retroperitoneal structures, and furnishes a rough estimate of the amount of blood in the peritoneal, retroperitoneal, and pelvic spaces. Surgeons can use abdominal CT information to grade solid organ lacerations, such as those of the liver and spleen, thus aiding them in the decision regarding operative or nonoperative management. It has limited diagnostic value in patients with penetrating abdominal trauma.

The limitations of CT can restrict its usefulness. Those limitations include cost, time involved in conducting the test, transport of the patient out of the resuscitation area, and inability to diagnosis certain injuries, such as those in the bowel or diaphragm. Most importantly, the patient must be hemodynamically stable and able to cooperate for the examination.

CT has varying degrees of sensitivity, specificity, and accuracy with various intraabdominal and retroperitoneal organs, making it unreliable in diagnosing bowel, pancreatic, and diaphragmatic injuries.[23-26] Diagnostic sensitivity and accuracy may be related to the experience of the technician performing the scan, quality of the imaging equipment, and experience of the radiologist.[27]

Instillation of oral contrast adds additional time to the CT procedure and puts the patient at risk of aspiration or allergic reaction. Several authors suggest that oral contrast is not necessary for diagnostic accuracy; they point out that its use only delays CT scanning and therefore may contribute to morbidity or mortality.[28,29]

CT is an adjunct to serial clinical examinations and monitoring of the patterns of laboratory data in the assessment of the patient with suspected abdominal trauma.

ULTRASONOGRAPHY

Ultrasonography (US) for the evaluation of abdominal trauma has been used in Europe and Japan for more than a decade. It is becoming increasingly popular in the United States as a diagnostic tool in abdominal evaluation of the trauma patient.

Numerous studies report it to be a reliable, fast, and safe modality with a high degree of sensitivity and specificity in detecting peritoneal free fluid or hemoperitoneum.[30-34] Advantages of US include ready access to the necessary equipment, portability, noninvasiveness, ability to perform, cost effectiveness, and the ability to do serial examinations; in addition, it does not require patient transport out of the resuscitation area. It can be performed simultaneously with physical examination, resuscitation, and stabilization within minutes of the patient's arrival in the trauma suite.

The benefits of US have been so compelling that the American College of Surgeons' Committee on Trauma has included US in their algorithm for the assessment of patients with blunt abdominal trauma.[35] Bennett and Jehle (1997) reported the sensitivity of US for identification of free fluid as 82% to 98%, its specificity as 88% to 100%, and its accuracy as 90%.[36] In a study of war casualties, authors cited US sensitivity of 86% to 88%, specificity of 100%, accuracy of 95% to 97%, positive predictive value of 100%, and negative predictive value of 91% to 96%.[37]

Although advocated as a screening tool for potential abdominal injuries, US is not intended to replace DPL or CT. Limitations of US include unreliable results in obese patients and in patients with ascites or subcutaneous emphysema.[38] As with DPL and CT, US is limited in its ability to detect diaphragmatic, intestinal, and pancreatic injury. Interpretation and accuracy of US results are

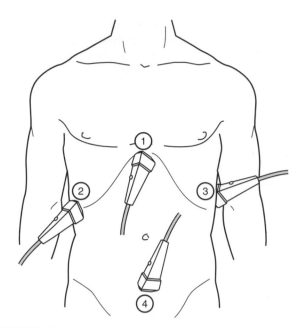

FIGURE 24-16 Ultrasound Evaluation and Sequence. *1,* pericardial (subxiphoid); *2,* Morison's pouch (RUQ); *3,* splenorenal (LUQ); *4,* pelvis (Douglas' pouch). (Modified from Rozycki GS, Ballard RB, Feliciano DV et al: Surgeon-performed ultrasound for the assessment of truncal injuries, *Ann Surg* 228(4):557, 1998.)

dependent on the clinician's experience in using the US machine.

Focused assessment with sonography for trauma (FAST) is recommended for evaluation of hemoperitoneum in patients who have sustained blunt abdominal trauma.[31,32] Identification of hemoperitoneum or fluid in the abdomen by ultrasound entails examination of the following areas: Morison's pouch (RUQ), pericardial sac, splenorenal (LUQ), and pelvis (Douglas' pouch) (Figure 24-16).

Visualization of the RUQ allows evaluation of the right liver lobe, right kidney, and retroperitoneal space. LUQ examination allows visualization of the spleen and perisplenic fluid, intrathoracic fluid, left kidney, and retroperitoneal space. Examination of the epigastrium area can detect abnormalities of the pancreas or left liver lobe and pericardial fluid. Anterior pelvis examination allows visualization of the prostate, uterus, bladder, and lateral pelvic walls. Ultrasonography can identify hemoperitoneum from liver injuries in Morison's pouch and splenic injuries in the pericolic gutter, two areas where fluid accumulates from injuries to these organs.[32]

Ultrasonography should be recognized as one tool in the evaluation of abdominal trauma and not the sole determinant for management. US findings can aid in defining diagnostic and management priorities during resuscitation and evaluation of the trauma patient.

DIAGNOSTIC LAPAROSCOPY

Diagnostic laparoscopy (DL) is emerging as a screening or diagnostic tool in the evaluation of trauma patients. It can be used to detect or exclude findings of hemoperitoneum, organ injury, intestinal spillage, or peritoneal penetration that may require a laparotomy. It has no advantages

over DPL, CT, or US but can be used in addition to these diagnostic interventions to further investigate findings.[39] Direct visualization of intraperitoneal structures such as the diaphragm to rule out rupture may reduce the rate of laparotomies resulting in negative findings.

This invasive procedure has several limitations, most notably its unproven accuracy and high cost. DL cannot be used to visualize the extent or depth of a liver or splenic injury and does not allow visualization of the retroperitoneal space, thus providing only limited information for diagnosing injuries.

Several studies have reported limited usefulness of DL in the evaluation of penetrating abdominal trauma.[40,41] Further studies are required to determine its full applicability in diagnosis and treatment during trauma resuscitation.

RADIOGRAPHIC FILMS

In general, plain film radiographs have a limited role in the diagnosis of abdominal injuries. Chest radiography is used as a primary screening tool and serves to identify concomitant pulmonary or cardiac injuries and abdominal organ displacement. It can also indicate if the pleural cavity is an obvious source of major blood loss and serves as an aid in establishing a baseline for respiratory care. Thoracic injuries are frequently associated with abdominal injuries, particularly in patients with gunshot wounds or multisystem injuries.

Anteroposterior supine abdominal films and left lateral decubitus films may reveal the presence of intraperitoneal fluid, air, or alteration in visceral contours. The examiner may note the presence of a foreign body or determine the trajectory of missiles. On an upright film, inspection for free air may disclose a ruptured hollow viscus. Skeletal structure damage should increase suspicion of damage to certain organs (e.g., liver and splenic injuries often occur with fractures of the lower ribs). Distortion of the outlines of intraabdominal organs may indicate subcapsular hematoma or hemorrhage or may be due to fluid or gas collections.

Use of plain films in diagnosing abdominal injuries is at best equivocal. Normal or negative abdominal films do not exclude significant intraabdominal injury. The minimal volume of intraperitoneal blood that can be detected radiographically is 800 ml. Radiographic films should be used in conjunction with physical examination and other diagnostic tools, such as CT, DPL, or US, in making an accurate diagnosis.

OTHER DIAGNOSTIC STUDIES

Angiography is used infrequently in evaluating abdominal injuries. It is most helpful in patients who are actively bleeding as a result of vascular trauma. In patients who have sustained penetrating injury it can be used to detect arteriovenous fistulas, false aneurysms, and arteriobiliary fistulas. Interventional radiology is particularly useful for embolization of vasculature and in patients with unstable pelvic fractures with unrelenting hemorrhage.

Gastrointestinal studies using meglumine diatrizoate (Gastrografin) or barium are helpful in diagnosing injury to the esophagus, stomach, bowel, or diaphragm. Contrast enemas are used to diagnose rectal or colonic injury secondary to penetrating trauma.

Endoscopic retrograde cholangiopancreatography (ERCP) may be indicated in the stable trauma patient with suspected biliary tract or pancreatic duct injury. It can be used to determine the exact site of ductal injury and the need for surgical intervention. This is the most accurate test to determine injury in the patient with hyperamylasemia who is being observed and in the patient with abdominal complaints after pancreatic surgery.

Retrograde urethrograms or cystograms are used when a patient is suspected of having injury to the bladder or urethra. A quick, one-shot intravenous pyelogram (IVP) may be indicated in the unstable patient requiring emergent surgical intervention; however, CT scan of the abdomen provides a much clearer delineation of renal anatomy and injuries. IVP is also recommended if CT is not available.

NURSING MANAGEMENT DURING RADIOGRAPHIC STUDIES

Most radiographic studies use some form of contrast, and the nurse should be alert to signs and symptoms of allergic reaction. With the first signs of rash, hives, flushing of the skin, or itching, the nurse should contact the physician immediately. A number of multisystem trauma patients require multiple radiologic studies during the resuscitative phase and thus receive large doses of IV radiographic contrast. The nurse should monitor the patient's hydration status, urine output, and creatinine level as the kidneys clear the IV contrast. The physician may order a bolus of IV fluid to ensure clearance of the IV contrast, thus decreasing the risk of renal insult.

LABORATORY DATA

Laboratory results may not be of value in the early phase of resuscitation but may have more utility when used in conjunction with the patient's clinical findings. Laboratory testing should be individualized to each patient's clinical presentation.

HEMOGLOBIN AND HEMATOCRIT

The initial hemoglobin (Hb) and hematocrit (HCT) determinations do not usually reflect the amount of hemorrhage, but they serve as a baseline value during the resuscitative phase. The frequency of Hb and HCT measurements is usually dictated by the patient's hemodynamic stability. Serial values offer valuable data for assessing ongoing bleeding and are used with other assessment parameters through all phases of care.

LEUKOCYTE COUNTS

Elevated white blood cell counts are part of the body's normal response to trauma; therefore this value is of little significance early in the trauma cycle. However, detection of neutrophilia based on serial evaluations may indicate an inflammatory process in the peritoneal cavity. An increase in the WBC count may indicate peritonitis secondary to hollow viscus injury or splenic injury, but this elevation may occur later in the resuscitative phase or critical care phase. During the critical care and intermediate phases of care, an elevation in the WBC count can be indicative of a wound infection, pulmonary infection, or sepsis.

AMYLASE AND LIPASE LEVELS

An elevated amylase level may indicate injury but is not necessarily diagnostic. Serum amylase may become elevated as a result of parotid gland, pancreatic, duodenal, or genitourinary injury. However, some patients sustain no rise in amylase level despite injury to these organs. Routine amylase testing in every trauma patient is not indicated and should be used selectively by the clinician in accordance with the patient's assessment and medical history.

Many patients with pancreatic injuries do not have a rise in serum amylase in the initial phase of resuscitation. The positive predictive value of an elevated amylase level for pancreatic injury in blunt trauma is only 10%.[42] A serum lipase level should be obtained if the amylase is elevated and there is suspicion of pancreatic injury. Serum lipase, an indicator of pancreatic function, is more specific to the inflammatory process of the pancreas. The utility of serum amylase and lipase determinations in the resuscitation phase is questionable. An increasing amylase or lipase level in the critical care or intermediate phase may indicate a missed pancreatic or duodenal injury. These tests can be most useful in conjunction with physical findings and other diagnostic measures to rule out pancreatic or duodenal injury.

BLOOD CHEMISTRY

Serum electrolytes, blood urea nitrogen (BUN), and creatinine levels are obtained many times as baseline values for patients sustaining abdominal trauma. They are indicated in the patient with a history of hypertension, diabetes, or renal disease or who is taking medications such as diuretics. Patients requiring contrast radiographic studies will need a creatinine level to assess renal excretion function. Other blood chemistry tests may be indicated based on the patient's medical history or medications. Evaluation of liver enzymes are indicated in the patient with a history of substance abuse or liver disease.

CLOTTING STUDIES

Prothrombin time (PT), partial thromboplastin time (PTT), and international normalized ratio tests are indicated in the trauma patient with a history of coagulopathy or cirrhosis or who is taking anticoagulants. Baseline PT and PTT are also indicated in the trauma patient who is hemodynamically unstable and when hemorrhage is suspected.

The patient receiving massive blood transfusion requires frequent monitoring of clotting factors. Packed red blood cells do not contain clotting factors and platelets, so the patient may require fresh frozen plasma, platelets, or other clotting factors to prevent coagulopathy.[43] PT and PTT are required before any abdominal surgery.

MONITORING

Unrecognized abdominal injuries continue to be a cause of preventable deaths in trauma patients.[7] A systematic process for initial assessment of the trauma patient is essential for recognizing life-threatening conditions, identifying injuries, and determining priorities of care. Once the initial assessment, which includes primary and secondary assessments, is completed, the nurse plays an instrumental role in the resuscitation and critical care phases. Ongoing evaluation and frequent assessments are vital in detecting changes in the patient's condition. Patients with abdominal injuries may not present with obvious signs and symptoms of hemorrhage. Nurses have always been astute in recognizing subtle changes such as a slight rise in pulse rate, decrease in blood pressure, or waning level of consciousness. It is extremely important to look at trends of vital signs and serial examinations in order to detect injuries early.

RESUSCITATION AND CRITICAL CARE PHASES

The potential for bleeding and hemorrhage is present in all patients who have sustained abdominal trauma. The patient is at risk for fluid volume deficit secondary to hypovolemia and consequently to altered tissue perfusion. Medical management is aimed at maintaining or improving circulating volume and correcting blood loss. There must be continuous monitoring for signs and symptoms of hemorrhage, such as tachycardia, hypotension, pallor of skin, altered level of consciousness, increasing abdominal pain or distention, oliguria, and hypoxia. Fluid volume can be monitored by frequent assessment of vital signs and level of consciousness, repeated hemoglobin and hematocrit levels, and hourly urinary output measurements in addition to serial physical examinations.

Warm isotonic crystalloid solution is used initially for massive volume resuscitation, but administration of blood should be considered after the initial 2 to 3 L of crystalloid if the patient is requiring large amounts of fluid to maintain blood pressure. All fluid, including blood, should be infused using warming devices if available. The preferred replacement blood during resuscitation is type specific until crossmatched blood is available. Universal donor blood can be administered without waiting for type-specific or crossmatched blood. Males should be given Rh-positive blood, whereas girls and women of childbearing age should receive type O, Rh-negative blood to avoid sensitization that would complicate future pregnancies. Warming techniques to avert hypothermia include the use of heating blankets, lights, and heated respiratory gas applications via the ventilator in addition to warmed IV fluids.

The level of hemodynamic monitoring depends on the physiologic and clinical needs of the patient. Monitoring may include a variety of noninvasive and invasive devices to aid in the assessment of circulatory status and tissue oxygenation. Use of cardiac monitoring, pulse oximetry, central venous pressure (CVP) monitoring, and arterial blood monitoring may be sufficient for the stable, uncomplicated trauma patient. Patients needing more intensive surveillance require the addition of a pulmonary artery (PA) catheter.

CENTRAL VENOUS PRESSURE. CVP monitoring is indicated whenever a patient has significant alterations in fluid volume. CVP measurements can be used as a guide to fluid volume resuscitation associated with hypovolemia. CVP monitoring is best used when monitoring trends in serial readings during fluid therapy. CVP measurements provide an excellent early indication of changes in the patient's fluid volume status caused by bleeding. The CVP will drop before a significant decrease in the mean arterial pressure (MAP) becomes evident.

Normal CVP is 5 to 10 mm Hg. A low CVP suggests insufficient blood or fluid volume. Elevated CVP can be related to fluid overload or cardiac compromise suggestive of thoracic injury or cardiac disease.

ARTERIAL PRESSURE MONITORING. An arterial line is indicated when patients require continuous assessment of arterial perfusion. MAP is the clinical parameter most frequently used to assess perfusion. In the trauma patient, arterial pressure monitoring is indicated in conditions that compromise fluid volume status (hemorrhage), cardiac output (hypovolemia), or tissue perfusion (hypoxia). An MAP higher than 60 mm Hg is necessary to perfuse the coronary arteries, brain, and kidneys. Direct arterial access is also helpful in the management of ventilated patients, who require frequent arterial blood gas measurements, and for the hemodynamically unstable patient who requires inotropic drugs for pressure support.

PULMONARY ARTERY PRESSURE MONITORING (PA). A PA catheter is used for diagnosis and evaluation of heart disease, shock, and other conditions that compromise cardiac output or fluid volume. Indications for use in the trauma population include shock, sepsis, multiple organ dysfunction syndrome (MODS), and acute respiratory distress syndrome (ARDS).

Pulmonary artery pressures, pulmonary capillary wedge pressure, and cardiac output measurements are useful in determining volume replacement need and drug therapy and for monitoring response to treatment.

MIXED VENOUS OXYGENATION SATURATION (Svo_2). Svo_2 monitoring is indicated in the patient who has the potential to develop an imbalance between oxygen supply and metabolic tissue demand. This includes the trauma patient in shock with or without severe respiratory dysfunction such as ARDS.

Normal Svo_2 is 75%. For many critical care patients an Svo_2 value between 60% to 80% is evidence of an adequate balance between oxygen supply and demand. An Svo_2 value change of more than 10% that persists for more than 10 minutes should prompt the nurse to determine the causative factor. Changes in Sao_2, cardiac output, hemoglobin, and oxygen consumption (V_{O_2}) can affect the S_{VO_2}. Nursing measures to verify the accuracy of the change in S_{VO_2} include measuring hemoglobin and cardiac output level and checking the oxygen supply delivery system.

Invasive and noninvasive hemodynamic monitoring, interpretation of laboratory data, and serial physical assessments continue through the critical care phase. The critical care phase requires close observation for both clinical and physical changes. Assessment of the abdomen may reveal bruising around the umbilicus (Cullen's sign), which is indicative of blood in the abdominal wall. Flank ecchymosis (Grey Turner's sign) may indicate a retroperitoneal bleed or suggest a renal injury. A distended abdomen may indicate the accumulation of blood, fluid, or gas secondary to a perforated organ or blood vessel, or it may be a sign of postoperative ileus. Serial measurement of abdominal girth may be indicated to evaluate the degree of distention. Wound or incision evaluation includes monitoring for tenderness, induration, erythema, and wound exudates, all of which are possible indications of wound infection or abscess.

The critical care nurse must be suspicious of subtle changes in pulse, blood pressure, respiratory rate, and pulse oximetry. Changes in an intensive care unit (ICU) trauma patient admitted for nonoperative management of a liver or spleen injury indicate the need for another abdominal CT or surgical intervention. Priorities of care include ongoing physical assessment and monitoring of hemodynamic status, including the patient's response to medical therapies. Frequent nursing evaluations and the detection of changes can facilitate timely diagnostic and therapeutic interventions and thus prevent complications.

ABDOMINAL ORGAN INJURY

The initial assessment process has been presented, including a directed history, mechanism of injury, abdominal assessment, diagnostic studies, laboratory data, and monitoring. Specific organ injuries are now presented, including discussion of trauma team management.

THORACOABDOMINAL INJURY

The thoracoabdominal region encompasses the abdominal and thoracic cavities. All patients with penetrating injuries should be suspected of having involvement of both cavities.

DIAPHRAGM INJURY

Isolated diaphragmatic injuries are uncommon and seldom fatal. Typically diaphragmatic injuries occur in conjunction with other organ injuries. They are most commonly associated with penetrating wounds. The incidence of diaphragmatic injuries from blunt trauma is difficult to ascertain from the literature; however, its incidence in patients with penetrating thoracoabdominal trauma is 42% to 44%.[44,45] Diaphragmatic injuries as a result of blunt trauma are caused by a drastic and sudden rise in intraabdominal pressure. The forces necessary to create such an injury are so great that other intraabdominal, orthopedic, and neurologic

injuries are often present. The incidence of left hemidiaphragm injury is higher because of the protective effect of the liver on the right hemidiaphragm.[46-48] A right hemidiaphragm injury resulting from blunt trauma may include a large defect and significant liver involvement.

Physical assessment of the thoracoabdominal structures focuses on auscultation for the presence of peristaltic sounds in the chest and percussion to elicit dull tones indicating a diaphragm rupture. However, if the patient is splinting the area, even normal sounds may not be appreciated. With gross herniation of visceral contents into the chest cavity, the patient may have a shift of mediastinal structures, resulting in respiratory distress and circulatory instability. Difficulty passing a nasogastric tube also may signal that the abdominal contents have herniated into the thorax. Penetrating trauma can produce a small tear not recognized during the acute stage. A rise in intraabdominal pressure may cause a small defect to become larger, with the consequent danger of herniation and intestinal strangulation. Throughout the phases of care, unexplained chest pain and increased respiratory rate suggest the possibility of acute herniation.

TEAM MANAGEMENT. The most definitive diagnostic procedure is exploratory laparotomy or celiotomy. Diagnostic laparoscopy may have a role in diagnosing diaphragm injuries in the patient who has sustained penetrating trauma.[41,44,45] Operative repair is necessary because visceral herniation can occur through small defects. Laparotomy is preferred for acute traumatic diaphragmatic tears. In penetrating trauma, when the entrance wound is in the chest and there is a high suspicion of intrathoracic injury with significant chest bleeding, a thoracic approach may be used to repair the diaphragm.

ESOPHAGEAL INJURY

The incidence of injury to the small portion of the esophagus within the abdominal cavity is low compared with the incidence of esophageal injury in the cervical and thoracic regions. Most esophageal injuries are caused by penetrating trauma and most involve the cervical esophagus. Blunt esophageal injuries are rare. Early diagnosis is paramount because damage results from the corrosion of tissue by digestive juices and bacterial contamination surrounding the site of tissue injury. Fluid losses may be massive and affect the thorax and the abdomen, leading to respiratory compromise. Mediastinitis, paraesophageal abscess, empyema, esophageal fistula, or peritonitis may occur. These injuries, although uncommon, are significant because of the high mortality and morbidity that occurs if definitive treatment is delayed. Mortality is generally related to paraesophageal contamination and infection. The mortality rate increases as time from injury to treatment lengthens.

Signs and symptoms vary according to the site of the injury and the degree of contamination. Symptoms of perforation include pain at the site of injury, fever, and dysphagia. The pain may radiate to the neck, chest, or shoulders or throughout the abdomen.

A tear of the abdominal esophagus may present with the sign of peritoneal irritation from release of gastric contents into the peritoneal cavity. As gastric contents efflux into the pleural space, more fluid than air may be appreciated, producing dyspnea accompanied by pleuritic pain.

TEAM MANAGEMENT.   Initial assessment is complicated because esophageal injuries are rare and are seldom single-system events. Medical management is directed toward quick assessment and intervention to deter the effects of bacterial contamination and enzyme erosion. Gastric decompression by passing a nasogastric tube, antibiotic therapy, and drainage of the wound site are combined with surgical interventions to treat an esophageal tear. Operative therapy is required for all trauma-related esophageal tears. Direct layered closure with drainage of the mediastinum is necessary. However, the extent of injury may dictate defunctionalization, closure of esophagogastric junction, gastrostomy, and drainage of the repair area. The process may be reversed later, after healing has occurred.

Because esophageal injury is difficult to diagnose, complications can occur at any time during the recovery phase. Continuous monitoring for signs of peritoneal irritation, respiratory compromise, or fistula formation is necessary from critical care through rehabilitation. Peritonitis, mediastinitis, intraabdominal abscess formation, esophageal stricture, and esophageal fistula are potential complications after esophageal injury and subsequent repair.

GASTRIC INJURY

The location and relative mobility of the stomach protects it from blunt injury. Blunt injuries to the stomach are rare and appear to be more common in children because of the greater elasticity of their anterior abdominal wall.[49] Most stomach trauma is penetrating, and the prognosis depends on severity of associated injuries, especially vascular wounds. Although gastric perforation secondary to injury can cause severe peritonitis, the initial inflammatory response is caused by chemical irritation and not bacterial contamination.[50] The normal stomach has a relatively high acidic environment and thus is relatively free of bacteria and other microorganisms.

Symptoms of gastric injury can be variable and nonspecific and may include severe epigastric or abdominal pain, tenderness, and signs of peritonitis secondary to release of gastric contents. This clinical presentation may be clouded by associated injuries. Blood from the nasogastric tube and the presence of free air on abdominal radiograph may support the diagnosis.

TEAM MANAGEMENT.   Medical management includes gastric decompression through placement of a nasogastric tube and surgical intervention, which includes simple debridement, primary closure, and diligent irrigation of the peritoneal cavity to remove contaminants. Bleeding from the gastric injury itself is occasionally an emergent problem and is managed with the use of a traumatic clamp or suturing. Removal of gastric particles followed by judicious

irrigation are required to prevent postoperative intraabdominal abscesses, particularly subphrenic, subhepatic, and pelvic abscesses, and abscesses of the lesser sac.[50] Gastric decompression is generally continued until gastric emptying returns to normal. Prolonged courses of antibiotics are of no proven benefit in patients with gastric injuries; instead, copious peritoneal irrigation during surgery and delayed primary closure of the incision are recommended in cases of significant contamination.[51]

Postoperative complications after gastric injury are rare and are usually related to associated injuries.[51] Complications such as peritonitis, intraabdominal abscess formation, and gastric fistulas may occur immediately or during the intermediate care phase of the trauma cycle.

LIVER INJURY

The liver's size and location make it particularly susceptible to injury. It is one of the most commonly injured organs in abdominal trauma from both blunt and penetrating sources. Motor vehicle crashes are the most common cause of blunt hepatic injury.[52] Blunt liver trauma is most often seen at suburban trauma centers, whereas penetrating liver injury has a higher incidence in urban areas. Associated injuries (e.g., head or chest), the length of time from injury to treatment, and the patient's overall premorbid condition all affect mortality. The single greatest danger after liver injury is severe hemorrhage.[53]

Blunt liver injury should be suspected in any patient with a lower chest or abdominal injury, especially on the right side of the abdomen. Motor vehicle crashes cause crushing of the liver between ribs and vertebrae and are responsible for most liver injuries. Stab wounds of the liver and low-velocity gunshots produce lacerations that are relatively minor, and hemorrhage is easily controlled. High-velocity gunshot wounds, however, are likely to produce widespread parenchymal damage, creating massive hemorrhage.

Liver injury can be graded on a scale of I to VI,[54] with type I representing the least severe damage (Table 24-2). This scale creates a classification for comparison of liver injuries. The grading system may be used preoperatively and intraoperatively.

TEAM MANAGEMENT.   Team management includes deciding whether the patient is a candidate for nonoperative or operative treatment. Pachter et al note that success in nonoperative treatment of liver injury in children has spurred an interest in nonoperative treatment in adults.[52] The success of nonoperative management depends on strict patient selection. Patients with grade I, II, or III hepatic injury without active bleeding or expanding hematoma may be considered for nonoperative management.[55] Although the selection criteria may vary from surgeon to surgeon, patients usually considered for nonoperative management are cooperative, alert, hemodynamically stable, neurologically intact, and able to participate in follow-up care. Nonoperative management requires repeated CT scans at approximately 11 weeks, 1 month, and 3 months to evaluate resolution of the injury. The majority (70%-90%) of hepatic

TABLE 24-2 Liver Injury Scale

Grade[a]		Injury Description	ICD-9[b]	AIS 90[c]
I.	Hematoma:	Subcapsular, nonexpanding, <10% surface area	864.01 864.11	2
	Laceration:	Capsular tear, nonbleeding, <1 cm parenchymal depth	864.02 864.12	2
II.	Hematoma:	Subcapsular, nonexpanding, 10-50% surface area: intraparenchymal, nonexpanding, <10 cm in diameter	864.01 864.11	2
	Laceration:	Capsular tear, active bleeding; 1-3 cm parenchymal depth, <10 cm in length	864.03 864.13	2
III.	Hematoma:	Subcapsular, >50% surface area or expanding; ruptured subcapsular hematoma with active bleeding; intraparenchymal hematoma >10 cm or expanding		3
	Laceration:	>3 cm parenchymal depth	864.04 864.14	3
IV.	Hematoma:	Ruptured intraparenchymal hematoma with active bleeding		4
	Laceration:	Parenchymal disruption involving 25-75% of hepatic lobe or 1-3 Couinaud's segments within a single lobe	864.04 864.14	4
V.	Laceration:	Parenchymal disruption involving >75% of hepatic lobe or >3 Couinaud's segments within a single lobe		5
	Vascular:	Juxtahepatic venous injuries, i.e., retrohepatic vena cava/central major hepatic veins		5
VI.	Vascular:	Hepatic avulsion		6

From Moore EE, Cogbill TH, Jurkovich GJ: Organ injury scaling: spleen and liver (1994 revision), *J Trauma* 38:323, 1995.
[a]Advance one grade for multiple injuries, up to grade III.
[b]International Classification of Diseases, ninth revision.
[c]Abbreviated Injury Scale, 1990.

injuries are minor (grades I-II) and require simple suturing, electrocautery, or topical hemostatic agents.[56]

Patients with complex hepatic injuries (grades IV-VI) usually present with hemodynamic instability as a result of hemorrhage; immediate laparotomy is necessary. Deep liver lacerations require various interventions to control bleeding, support viable tissue, and prevent postoperative infection. Regardless of the surgical intervention required for liver repair, drainage of wound exudate via a closed-suction system is necessary.

Complex liver injuries may have vascular involvement, which further complicates surgical intervention to control hemorrhage. Manual compression of the liver may be required to tamponade the bleeding after initial opening of the peritoneum. Patients with this type of injury often require aggressive intraoperative resuscitation simultaneously with hemorrhage control to prevent hypothermia and coagulopathy and maintain hemodynamic stability.

Packing may be required if bleeding persists after successful debridement of nonviable tissue and ligation of severed blood vessels or bile ducts. Additional surgical intervention is aborted, and the patient is taken to the ICU for continued resuscitation and stabilization. The patient will be taken back to the operating room in 24 to 36 hours for removal of the packing and definitive treatment of the liver injury. Patients with liver packing can be at risk for development of abdominal compartment syndrome, and the nurse must be alert to changes in abdominal girth, increasing abdominal distention, increasing peak inspiratory pressures in the mechanically ventilated patient, and decreasing urine output.

A number of surgical interventions can be instituted for complex liver lacerations. The location of the injury, vascular involvement, and surgeon preference may determine the technique to be used. Deep liver suturing, perihepatic packing, hepatic resection, or hepatorrhaphy is used to salvage the liver.

Overall mortality from hepatic trauma continues to be 10% to 15%.[57] Blunt trauma to the liver causes extensive hepatic parenchymal injury in the form of stellate lacerations or major fractures, which are generally more lethal and more difficult to manage than penetrating injuries.[53] Most deaths result immediately from exsanguination and, in the late postoperative period, from sepsis.[54] Complications from hepatic injury include recurrent bleeding, hemobilia, hyperpyrexia, intraabdominal abscess, sepsis, biliary fistula, arterial-portal venous fistula, and liver failure.

Gallbladder and biliary tract injuries are associated with other intraperitoneal injuries, commonly of the liver or major intraabdominal blood vessels.[57] Injury to the extrahepatic biliary tract is most often the result of penetrating mechanisms and accounts for only a small percentage of abdominal trauma.[57] Cholecystectomy is the recommended treatment for all gallbladder injuries.[58] Bile duct injuries are classified as simple or complex, and this classification dictates the surgical intervention required. Simple bile duct injuries require primary suture repair and external drainage. Anatomic involvement dictates the procedure of choice for complex bile duct injuries. Cholecystectomy, construction of a biliary-enteric anastomosis, and external drainage constitute the treatment regimen for these injuries. The team should continue to assess the patient for biliary fistulas or stricture.

SPLENIC INJURY

Among patients with blunt abdominal trauma, the spleen is the most commonly injured organ and is associated with greater severity of injury.[59,60] Its anatomic location makes it a frequent victim of penetrating trauma to the LUQ. Although the lower ribs in the LUQ provide some protection, the spleen is vulnerable to injury secondary to intrusion associated with fracture of these ribs. The patient with suspected splenic injury is assessed for LUQ abdominal pain, Kehr's sign, Ballance's sign, and local tenderness.

The mortality rate from splenic injury depends on the type of trauma (blunt versus penetrating) and the presence of associated injuries. Isolated splenic trauma has little to no mortality associated with it; however, this single-system injury accounts for less than 20% of all splenic trauma.[14] Mortality is related to uncontrolled hemorrhage or to delayed rupture and sepsis.

TEAM MANAGEMENT. Nonoperative versus operative management of splenic injury must be addressed individually with each patient. The patient's age, physiologic stability, associated injuries, and type of splenic injury are evaluated when making management decisions. Splenic injury is graded on a scale from I to V perioperatively and intraoperatively.

Medical management of splenic injury has changed over the years as the role of the spleen in maintaining immunocompetence has been appreciated. Splenorrhaphy and partial splenectomy are the recommended operative procedures for patients with splenic injury.[59,60] The degree of splenic injury is the primary guide to operative treatment selection. Splenectomy is usually indicated for the patient with associated life-threatening injuries, shock, or grade IV or V splenic disruption.[61]

Postoperative complications include bleeding, thrombocytosis, gastric distention, pancreatitis, and infection.[14,62] Overwhelming postsplenectomy infections (OPSI) can occur from 1 to 5 years after the operation. The illness presents with flulike symptoms such as nausea and vomiting, progressing rapidly to confusion, high fever, and shock from sepsis, leading to disseminated intravascular coagulation and death. The mortality rate associated with OPSI is approximately 50%. Causative organisms include *Streptococcus pneumoniae*, *Meningococcus* spp., *Escherichia coli*, *Haemophilus influenzae,* and *Staphylococcus* spp. Preventive measures include vaccination with polyvalent pneumococcal vaccine, and possibly the H. influenza and Meningococcal vaccines, as well as patient education regarding recognition of the early symptoms of infection and the need for early treatment.

PANCREATIC AND DUODENAL INJURIES

Pancreatic injuries are uncommon; the majority are caused by penetrating mechanisms.[63] Pancreatic injury from blunt trauma results from a direct blow to the epigastric area, such as impact with a steering wheel. Morbidity and mortality rates are variable and depend on the mechanism of injury, associated injuries, time to initial diagnosis, and presence or absence of major ductal injury.[64]

Because the pancreas is a retroperitoneal structure, symptoms of injury may not be evident for 24 to 72 hours after a traumatic incident. In addition, the location of the pancreas and proximity to other organs and vessels make multiorgan injury a frequent occurrence, thereby masking symptoms of pancreatic injury. Injuries to the liver, stomach, spleen, and major arteries and veins usually accompany pancreatic injury.

Duodenal injuries frequently occur in association with pancreatic, bile duct, or vena caval trauma. Injury to the duodenum, a predominantly retroperitoneal structure, presents a diagnostic challenge because peritoneal symptoms may not be immediately evident. Blunt injury to the duodenum can produce an intramural hematoma, which may partially or completely obstruct the lumen. Perforation causes contamination of the retroperitoneal and peritoneal spaces with bile, pancreatic enzymes, and gastric sections. Morbidity and mortality increase significantly with delayed treatment.

TEAM MANAGEMENT. Medical management of pancreatic injury depends on its extent, which may range from simple lacerations to transections. Treatment options are dictated by the site and severity of the pancreatic injury. Duct injury complicates repair procedures. Treatment may consist of simple external closed drainage, distal pancreatectomy, or, for major injuries, a pancreatic duodenectomy. The goals of surgery are to control hemorrhage, debride devitalized tissue, and provide adequate drainage.

Surgical management of a duodenal injury usually involves debridement and primary repair. The selection of a surgical procedure depends on the patient's hemodynamic stability and the presence of pancreatic or bile duct involvement. Nonoperative management of duodenal hematomas requires close observation for signs and symptoms of expanding or ruptured hematomas causing bleeding or peritoneal contamination.

The primary cause of initial death from pancreatic injury is hemorrhage; late deaths are attributed to sepsis, ARDS, and multiple organ failure.[65] Complications include fistulas, pseudocyst formation, pancreatic abscess, recurrent hemorrhage, and pancreatitis.

SMALL BOWEL INJURY

The small bowel, a hollow viscus structure, is most frequently injured by penetrating trauma, particularly gunshot. Blunt injury to the small bowel is relatively uncommon; when this type of injury is sustained it typically occurs near the ligament of Treitz and the ileocecal valve.[66] Mechanisms of injury include direct blows, shearing forces, and pseudo-closed loop obstruction. Direct blows crush the intestine between the external force and the spinal column. Shearing forces are imposed by rapid deceleration, as in a motor vehicle crash. Pseudo-closed loop obstruction occurs when a segment of bowel, partially filled with food or gas, becomes trapped between an external force and a firm anatomic object, creating a closed loop. The presence of pancreatic and any solid viscus injuries are predictive of a higher risk of hollow viscus injury in patients with blunt abdominal trauma.[67]

The ileum and jejunum have a neutral pH and harbor few bacteria. Therefore, clinical signs of injury may not be present on initial examination. As bacterial growth occurs, signs of peritonitis become evident. The lack of specific initial symptoms in patients with small bowel injury directs the nurse to carefully evaluate the information presented as the patient is admitted from the scene of the injury. Any blow to the abdomen or penetrating wound of the lower chest or abdomen should raise the index of suspicion regarding possible bowel injury. Spinal injury frequently occurs in conjunction with small bowel trauma and may mask presenting symptoms.

Team Management. Hemoperitoneum can be associated with injuries to the mesentery of the small bowel. Bleeding should be controlled before exploration for small bowel injury. The site of injury, mechanism of injury, and any associated mesentery injury direct surgical management. Debridement followed by primary closure and ligation of mesenteric bleeders constitute the surgical approach for injuries to the small bowel. Bowel resection is recommended if multiple defects are in close proximity to each other, if a segment of bowel has sustained massive destruction, or if significant mesentery injury is causing ischemia in a segment of the bowel.

Postoperative care is quite simple if only the small bowel is involved, but many times other peritoneal injuries complicate the patient's recovery. Gastric decompression and parenteral nutrition are not usually required in the patient with an isolated small bowel injury. Several postoperative doses of antibiotics are recommended to reduce the incidence of postoperative infections after contamination of the peritoneal cavity with contents of the small bowel.

Complications such as wound infection and abscess are related to the extent of contamination and the site of injury. In addition, fistula formation, small bowel obstruction, ischemic bowel, suture line leakage, and short-gut syndrome have been reported.[68]

LARGE BOWEL INJURY

Trauma to the large bowel is one of the most lethal forms of abdominal injury because of the probability of sepsis related to fecal contamination of the abdomen. Five percent of all abdominal injuries include the colon and rectum, and mortality and morbidity statistics are strongly affected by associated injuries.

Ninety-six percent of all trauma to the colon and rectum is the result of penetrating mechanisms of injury. The transverse colon is most often involved. Blunt trauma frequently affects the mobile transverse and sigmoid segments because their anatomic location makes them most vulnerable. The majority of blunt injuries manifest as contusions.

Team Management. Medical intervention is based on early recognition of injury and control of fecal contamination. A laparotomy is performed if colon or rectal perforation is suspected. Preoperative antibiotic therapy is ordered to decrease the probability of sepsis from enteric contamination.

Operative management includes control of hemorrhage and fecal leakage and irrigation to remove fecal material from the abdominal cavity. Surgical options for the treatment of colonic injuries include primary repair (resection and anastomosis) and colostomy. Primary repair is now established as the optimal and most common procedure for traumatic colonic injuries.[69] Operative technique is selected based on the extent and location of injury, the presence of shock, the extent of peritoneal spoilage, the presence of associated injuries, and the length of delay in surgical intervention. Extraperitoneal rectal injuries require the use of drainage and copious irrigation to remove fecal material and debridement and diverting colostomy.

Incisional infection is a recognized complication of colon and rectal injury. Delayed skin closure is advocated in patients with major fecal contamination. Intraabdominal abscess is the most frequent complication, occurring in 5% to 15% of patients with colonic injury.[70] Other complications include wound infections, fecal fistula, and difficulties with the colostomy stoma.

ABDOMINAL VASCULAR INJURY

Until recently, major vessel injuries were not seen in resuscitation areas or emergency departments because patients exsanguinated before transport. With an increase in skilled technicians and emergency resuscitation measures provided at the scene, more patients with vascular injury are surviving long enough to be treated in medical facilities. *Abdominal vascular injury* refers to vessels located in the midline retroperitoneum (zone 1), upper lateral retroperitoneum (zone 2), pelvic retroperitoneum (zone 3), and portal-retrohepatic area[71] (Table 24-3).

Vessels sustain contusions, lacerations, transections, or avulsion injuries. These occur as a result of penetrating or blunt injury, although the majority of severe damage to the vascular system occurs with penetrating trauma. Blunt injury to blood vessels is caused by deceleration, shearing, or crushing forces. Rapid deceleration in a motor vehicle crash causes avulsion of the small branches of the major vessels or intimal tears, resulting in secondary thrombosis.[72,73] Direct crush forces cause intimal tears or flaps, leading to secondary thrombosis of a vessel, or complete disruption of exposed vessels, resulting in intraperitoneal hemorrhage.[72] Vascular injuries are divided into arterial and venous trauma. Although combination injuries may exist and complications such as arteriovenous fistulas may occur, understanding each system separately helps to direct assessment and intervention strategies. The primary goal in management of patients with abdominal vascular injuries should be aggressive resuscitation and early control of hemorrhage.[74-76]

TABLE 24-3 Abdominal Vascular Regions

Zone 1: Midline Retroperitoneum	Zone 2: Upper Lateral Retroperitoneum
Supramesocolic Area	
Suprarenal abdominal aorta, celiac axis, proximal superior mesenteric artery, proximal renal artery, and superior mesenteric vein (either supramesocolic or retromesocolic)	Renal artery and renal vein
Inframesocolic Area	
Infrarenal abdominal aorta and infrahepatic inferior vena cava	
Zone 3: Pelvic Retroperitoneum	**Zone 4: Portal-Retrohepatic Area**
Iliac artery and iliac vein	Portal vein, hepatic artery, and retrohepatic vena cava

ARTERIAL INJURY. The artery, as a result of its elastic quality, may stop bleeding spontaneously after a clean transection occurs secondary to penetrating trauma. The transected intimae curls inward, and the divided media contract and pull the adventitia over the ends of the vessel. Partially transected vessels are unable to activate this process, and thus bleeding continues. In a partial laceration or transection, hematoma formation may occur, stopping further bleeding or leading to a false aneurysm that may rupture at a later date.

Arterial contusions are usually secondary to blunt traumatic force or stretching. Damage may initiate minor bleeding or progress to thrombus formation, occluding the vessel or embolizing distal vessels. Avulsion injury usually occurs with a deceleration event that pulls the artery from its base. In the abdomen this most frequently occurs at the renal pedicle or the root of the mesentery.

Abdominal arterial injuries are sustained frequently in combination with pelvic, thoracic, or visceral injury. This complicates initial assessment because specific signs of vascular injury may be obscured. For example, retroperitoneal hematoma, usually found in conjunction with pelvic or spine injury, may cause up to 4 L of blood to collect in the retroperitoneal space. The presenting symptoms are similar to those of visceral rupture and hemorrhage: abdominal pain, back pain, hypoactive bowel sounds, or tender abdominal mass. Only later will flank discoloration become evident.

Patients presenting in rapid-onset shock without an obvious source of blood loss should be suspected of having a major intraabdominal arterial injury. Patients with abdominal aortic injuries sustained through penetrating trauma present in profound shock and require immediate operative intervention. The presence of a large retroperitoneal hematoma indicates aortic injury.

Team Management. Volume replacement is a priority, but in catastrophic hemorrhage immediate surgery may be indicated because restoration of hemodynamic stability may be impossible without quick surgical intervention. Postoperative care focuses on maintaining an adequate volume status and monitoring for signs of hemorrhage.

Surgical repair depends on the type and extent of injury. Most major abdominal arterial injuries require lateral repair, end-to-end anastomosis, or a graft if the artery would be narrowed by primary repair. Autogenous tissue grafting, as opposed to use of prosthetic material, is preferred because many abdominal injuries are contaminated. Many major abdominal arteries can be ligated, which often becomes necessary when the site of repair lies within a contaminated field.

VENOUS INJURY. The venous system is a low-pressure system capable of realizing a tamponade effect from the pressure of surrounding tissues. Thus profuse bleeding (hemorrhage) must occur into a space at lower pressure, such as an external opening, a body cavity, or a cavity created after injury.

The severity of the vascular injury may not permit multiple diagnostic tests. Patients who appear in the resuscitation area in shock are usually moved quickly to the operating room for definitive diagnosis and treatment. However, for patients who are more stable, time is available for certain diagnostic tests, such as angiography, that help to define the extent of injury. Abdominal vascular injury is most frequently diagnosed during laparotomy for severe hemorrhagic shock. Severe hypotension unresponsive to rapid fluid administration (2-3 L in 10-15 minutes) in a patient with obvious abdominal trauma should lead to suspicion of a major intraabdominal vascular injury.[77]

Team Management. Venous injury requires the use of pressure and packing until the extent of injury is identified. Lateral repair, ligation, and venous grafting are used to treat venous injuries. Historically, complicated repairs led to stenosis of the vessel and increased risk of thrombosis or embolism; therefore, ligation was used as a treatment of choice, except to repair suprarenal or intrahepatic vena cava injuries.

The extent of vascular injury may demand quick assessment, massive fluid resuscitation, and transport to the operating room for definitive diagnosis and treatment. Patient response to fluid resuscitation indicates the amount of time available for further diagnostic testing. If the patient becomes alert and exhibits signs of adequate perfusion, further testing, including arteriography, may be ordered.

Complications of vascular repair in the abdomen include thrombosis, dehiscence of the suture line, and infection.

Bleeding after vascular repair may occur anytime in the postoperative period. Medical management is focused on the source of bleeding, coagulopathy, infection, and vascular repair disruption.

Intermediate and Rehabilitation Phases of Care

Once the critical physiologic abnormalities are stabilized, the patient transitions from critical care to the intermediate phase of care. Not every patient will go through every phase of care; many will not enter the critical care phase but will immediately enter the intermediate phase.

Nursing assessment, treatment implementation, and evaluation in the intermediate phase are directed at assisting the patient toward his or her premorbid functional state. Nutrition, elimination, mobility, pain control, and psychologic state are monitored continuously. At this stage both patient and family are active participants. Abdominal wound assessment, drain management, and dressing changes all involve evaluation for potential wound infection. Educating the patient and family about signs of infection, the role of nutrition in wound healing, and pain control during procedures are important in getting the patient closer to self-care.

The patient goes through many treatment changes during this phase, such as progressing from tube feedings to an oral diet, changing intravenous pain medication to oral, and moving from bedrest to independent mobility. In today's health care environment that progression is quick and may leave the patient feeling without control. Psychologic support through rational explanations for therapy and reassurance to promote comfort should be incorporated into the patient's care plan to ease the transition from critical care to the intermediate phase.

The patient's ability to regain control and independence leading to self-care can depend on his or her premorbid physical state, age, severity of traumatic injury, and family support. Generally, elderly patients require more time to progress to their premorbid state than do younger patients.

Rehabilitation actually starts in the critical care phase, with stabilization of injuries and prevention of secondary disabilities. Early involvement of the rehabilitation team assists with prevention of excessive muscle atrophy and maintenance of the patient's functional state. Early mobilization can be instrumental in preventing atelectasis, pneumonia, ileus, footdrop, and skin breakdown.

The degree of physical or neurologic disability or impairment determines the extent of rehabilitation a patient requires. Some patients need only several weeks to regain endurance and strength before returning to their home, whereas others require months to learn self-care skills such as feeding, personal hygiene, dressing, and basic communication skills in addition to mobility and psychologic therapies. Rehabilitation requires the active participation of the patient and family in preparing the patient for his or her return to a functional role within the family and the community.

Today patients spend even shorter periods in each phase, and it becomes increasingly important for the health care provider to identify a patient's functional deficits as soon as possible so that rehabilitation begins before the day of discharge. Health care is directed at less inpatient hospital care and more in-home nursing services and therapies when possible. The ultimate goal in any circumstance is a safe discharge to home with the appropriate resources.

Complications of Abdominal Trauma

Many individuals who have experienced abdominal trauma move through the phases from resuscitation to rehabilitation with little to no variance from the usual postoperative surgical patient. However, the extent of organ involvement, level of injury, and time from injury until treatment greatly affect the morbidity of these individuals. Injury to any organ or vessel in the abdomen can lead to certain generalized posttraumatic complications. For example, the critical care phase may evidence development of an ileus, peritonitis, cholecystitis, or stress ulcerations. In the intermediate care phase, abscesses may form and wound complications develop. The rehabilitation phase may be the first time that body image alteration, alteration in family coping, or chronic pain control becomes an issue.

After successful resuscitation the effects of injury, hemorrhage, shock, and treatment begin to affect the physical and psychologic adaptation of the patient. These complications are not specific to a single abdominal organ injury but occur by virtue of damage to the abdominal contents, whether it is single-organ or multiorgan involvement or single-system or multisystem injury. The potential for these complications to occur makes it imperative for nursing assessment to continue throughout the phases of care.

Abdominal Compartment Syndrome

Abdominal compartment syndrome (ACS), also referred to as intraabdominal hypertension, is a condition in which abdominal organ dysfunction is caused by increased intraabdominal pressure. ACS can occur in the trauma patient as a result of abdominal distention secondary to resuscitation edema, ileus, bowel obstruction, bowel edema, postoperative hemorrhage, or abdominal packing.[78]

Increased abdominal pressure primarily affects the cardiovascular, pulmonary, and renal systems. Cardiovascular effects manifest as a decrease in cardiac output and hypotension. Renal effects from a lack of perfusion of the renal arteries result in decreased urine output. Pulmonary effects produce a decrease in tidal volume, poor lung compliance, hypercarbia, and increased intrathoracic pressure.

Normal intraabdominal pressure (IAP) is 0 mm Hg. IAP greater than 20 mm Hg produces adverse physiologic effects on various organ systems.[79] If the measured IAP is higher than 20 mm Hg and the patient has oliguria despite good blood pressure and cardiac output, the abdomen should be reexplored.[80] Decompression can be performed either in the ICU or in the operating room.

It is imperative that the nurse be aware of possible causes of ACS and its presenting signs and symptoms. Close monitoring for increases in abdominal girth should alert the nurse to early signs of rising abdominal pressure. Increasing tenseness of the abdomen can be determined by palpation and indicates rising intraabdominal pressure. Monitoring intake and output can help identify decreasing urine output. Increased peak inspiratory pressures and worsening lung compliance should alert the nurse to the possibility of ACS. Early identification and effective management are key to preventing adverse effects of the syndrome. Untreated ACS can progress to anuria, hypoxia, hypercapnia, and death.[79]

After decompression, the greatest nursing priority is wound management. Patients with open abdominal wounds are susceptible to heat and fluid loss. Continuous hemodynamic monitoring is essential in the critical care phase. Monitoring drainage, changing dressings, and protecting the skin to avoid breakdown continue through the critical care and intermediate phases.

Acute Acalculous Cholecystitis (AAC)

AAC is an acute inflammation of the gallbladder in the absence of gallstones. It is also referred to as *acute posttraumatic cholecystitis* or *acute postoperative cholecystitis*. The disease most often occurs in association with other conditions such as burns, major trauma, or operations. Affected patients are often critically ill, requiring extensive monitoring and life-support measures. The cause of AAC is still uncertain and may be multifactorial. Contributing factors include lack of oral intake, administration of total parenteral nutrition, and the administration of narcotics.[81,82] Gallbladder ischemia has also been implicated in patients who have sustained prolonged periods of hypotension or low blood flow during operations after trauma and burn injury.[81]

AAC does not differ from the calculous type, except that the incidence of gangrene and perforation is higher. Symptoms are nonspecific but may include fever, nausea, vomiting, and RUQ tenderness. AAC poses a diagnostic challenge in the critically ill trauma patient with abdominal injuries and subsequent surgical intervention. Symptoms of AAC may be masked because of narcotic administration, incisional abdominal pain from recent surgery, concomitant injuries, or other disease processes.

Imaging of the gallbladder by ultrasonography and cholescintigraphy in conjunction with laboratory and clinical findings will assist in the diagnosis. Inflammation produces an elevated WBC in about 70% of patients and an increased alkaline phosphatase or aspartate aminotransferase (AST) in about 50% of patients.[81] Treatment depends on the patient's underlying disease and hemodynamic state, but ACC requires surgical intervention. The gallbladder can be removed via cholecystectomy or laparoscopic cholecystotomy.

Nursing Research Issues

The incidence of trauma in the United States is a major health care and economic issue. Many young people who have sustained traumatic injuries have long-term disabilities. Nurses have a responsibility to promote safety and education to prevent traumatic injuries in all age groups. Nurses must promote a triad of prevention, education, and research if positive patient outcomes are going to be effected. Nursing research is necessary to refine the art and science of trauma care.

Prevention issues that deserve our attention include proper use of restraint devices and effects of alcohol and drugs when combined with driving. Can we begin safety programs in the elementary schools? Do drinking and driving programs influence a teenager's decision to drive responsibly? Can senior citizens self-assess their ability to drive safely?

Physicians and nurses work together to diagnosis life-threatening injuries to reduce morbidity and mortality. The development of critical clinical pathways has streamlined care of the trauma patient in many institutions in order to reduce unnecessary laboratory testing, length of stay, and cost. What are the consequences, if any, of these protocol-driven treatment plans? What is the incidence of missed abdominal injuries? What is the complication rate? And, of equal importance, what is the level of patient satisfaction?

Through all phases of care the nurse serves as an advocate for the patient and his or her needs. Identification and adequate treatment of pain continues to be a dilemma for even the most seasoned nurse. What alternative healing modalities can be used to reduce or alleviate the pain of the trauma patient? Can massage therapy be helpful in reducing discomfort in critically ill patients? What physiologic parameters can be used to assess pain intensity in the comatose patient? Pain will continue to be an issue in the research literature, and nurses can be instrumental in finding the answers to pain-related questions.

Trauma strikes many young people. Body image is an aspect that should be addressed throughout all phases of care. The patient may feel disfigured after abdominal surgery that creates open wounds or stomas. Patients and their families should be given psychologic support throughout all phases of care, continuing after discharge into the community. Can a nurse's assessment of psychologic and psychosocial needs assist in the development of a patient's discharge interventions? Does the patient's participation in care promote coping behaviors and positively affect recovery?

Advances in trauma care will continue as long as there are complex, challenging issues to be addressed. Many advances have positively affected the outcome of the trauma patient: improved safety restraint devices; sophisticated emergency medicine services; improvements in diagnostic and treatments; devices such as CT scanners, ventilators, and feeding tubes; and new treatment modalities for ARDS and renal failure. Nursing research should continue to address the many questions related to the care and support of trauma patients.

Summary

Although each abdominal organ system has been reviewed singularly, the nurse is much more likely to be confronted with a patient who has sustained multiorgan or multisystem trauma. Certain patterns such as pancreaticoduodenal injury and the resultant confusing diagnostic presentation have been described. Quick multisystem assessment is necessary initially, with an emphasis on identifying the life-threatening injuries first. Airway, ventilation, and circulation are initial priorities, with recognition that ventilatory and circulatory control may be affected by the extent of the abdominal injury. The index of diagnostic suspicion cues the nursing assessment and permits early recognition of insidious abdominal injury in each phase. Delayed rupture or hemorrhage can occur in patients with abdominal trauma. Other consequences of the injury, such as pancreatitis, abscess formation, or wound infection, may become apparent during the intermediate care or rehabilitation phases. Morbidity and mortality are directly related to the failure to diagnose and treat early. Thus the demand remains for knowledgeable, swift nursing assessment in each phase of the cycle, focusing on flexible patient care planning to meet the multiple changing needs of abdominal trauma patients and their families.

REFERENCES

1. MacKenzie EJ, Fowler CJ: Epidemiology. In Mattox K, Feliciano D, Moore E, editors: *Trauma*, ed 4, New York, 2000, McGraw-Hill, 22.

2. Tumbarello C: Ultrasound evaluation of abdominal trauma in the emergency department, *J Trauma* 5(3):67, 1998.

3. Wilson RF, Walt AJ: General considerations in abdominal trauma. In Wilson RF, Walt AJ, editors: *Management of trauma: pitfalls and practice*, ed 2, Baltimore, 1996, Williams & Wilkins, 412.

4. Elliott DC, Militello P: Pitfalls in the diagnosis of abdominal trauma. In Maull K, Rodriguez A, Wiles C, editors: *Complications in trauma and critical care*, Philadelphia, 1996, WB Saunders, 146.

5. Neugebauer G, Wallenboeck E, Hungerford M: Seventy cases of injuries of small intestine caused by blunt abdominal trauma: a retrospective study from 1970 to 1994, *J Trauma* 46(1):116, 1999.

6. Harris HW, Morabito DJ, Mackersie RC et al: Leukocytosis and free fluid are important indications of isolated intestinal injury after blunt trauma, *J Trauma* 46(4):656, 1999.

7. American College of Surgeons' Committee on Trauma: Abdominal Trauma. In *Advanced trauma life support*, ed 6, Chicago, 1997, The College, 159.

8. Herlihy B, Maebius NK: *The human body in health and illness*, Philadelphia, 2000, WB Saunders, 392-393.

9. Thibodeau GA, Patton KT: *Anatomy & physiology*, ed 4, St. Louis, 1999, Mosby, 694-695.

10. Thibodeau GA, Patton KT: *Anatomy & physiology*, ed 4, St. Louis, 1999, Mosby, 744.

11. Herlihy B, Maebius NK: *The human body in health and illness*, Philadelphia, 2000, WB Saunders, 403.

12. Thibodeau GA, Patton KT: *Anatomy & physiology*, ed 4, St. Louis, 1999, Mosby, 635.

13. Thibodeau GA, Patton KT: *Anatomy & physiology*, ed 4, St. Louis, 1999, Mosby, 636.

14. Wilson RF, Steffes CP, Tyburski J: Injury to the spleen. In Wilson RF, Walt AJ, editors: *Management of trauma: pitfalls and practices*, ed 2, Baltimore, 1996, Williams & Wilkins, 474.

15. Fabian TC, Croce MA: Abdominal trauma, including indications for celiotomy. In Mattox K, Feliciano D, Moore E, editors: *Trauma*, ed 4, New York, 2000, McGraw-Hill, 596.

16. Nagy KK, Krosner SM, Joseph KT et al: A method of determining peritoneal penetration in gunshot wounds to the abdomen, *J Trauma* 43(2):242, 1997.

17. Bell RM, Krantz BE: Initial assessment. In Mattox K, Feliciano D, Moore E, editors: *Trauma*, ed 4, New York, 2000, McGraw-Hill, 163.

18. Wilson RF, Walt AJ: General considerations in abdominal trauma. In Wilson RF, Walt AJ, editors: *Management of trauma: pitfalls and practice*, ed 2, Baltimore, 1996, Williams & Wilkins, 418.

19. Bell RM, Krantz BE: Initial assessment. In Mattox K, Feliciano D, Moore E, editors: *Trauma*, ed 4, New York, 2000, McGraw-Hill, 163.

20. Blow O, Bassam D, Butler K et al: Speed and efficiency in the resuscitation of blunt trauma patients with multiple injuries: the advantage of diagnostic peritoneal lavage over abdominal computerized tomography, *J Trauma* 44(2):287, 1998.

21. Mele TS, Stewart K, Marokus B et al: Evaluation of a diagnostic protocol using screening diagnostic peritoneal lavage with selective use of abdominal CT in blunt abdominal trauma, *J Trauma* 46(5):847, 1999.

22. Fabian TC, Croce MA: Abdominal trauma, including indications for celiotomy. In Mattox K, Feliciano K, Moore E, editors: *Trauma*, ed 4, New York, 2000, McGraw-Hill, 587.

23. Porter JM, Singh Y: Value of computed tomography in the evaluation of retroperitoneal organ injury in blunt abdominal trauma, *Am J Emerg Med* 16(3):225, 1998.

24. Akhrass R, Kim K, Brandt C: Computed tomography: an unreliable indicator of pancreatic trauma, *Am Surg* 62(8):647, 1996.

25. Emmick RH, Petersen SR: Evaluation of pancreatic injury after blunt abdominal trauma, *Ann Emerg Med* 27(5):658, 1996.

26. Janzen DL, Zwirewich CV, Breen DJ et al: Diagnostic accuracy of helical CT for detection of blunt bowel and mesenteric injuries, *Clin Radiol* 53:193, 1998.

27. Wilson RF, Walt AJ: General considerations in abdominal trauma. In Wilson RF, Walt AJ, editors: *Management of trauma: pitfalls and practices*, ed 2, Baltimore, 1996, Williams, & Wilkins, 421.

28. Shreve WS, Knotts FB, Siders RW et al: Retrospective analysis of the adequacy of oral contrast material for computed tomography scans in trauma patients, *Am J Surg* 178(1):14, 1999.

29. Stafford RE, McGonigal MD, Weigelt JA et al: Oral contrast solution and computed tomography for blunt abdominal trauma: a randomized study, *Arch Surg* 134(6):622, 1999.

30. Arrillaga A, Graham R, York J et al: Increased efficiency and cost-effectiveness in the evaluation of the blunt abdominal trauma patient with the use of ultrasound, *Am Surg* 65(1):31, 1999.

31. Branney SW, Moore EE, Cantril SV et al: Ultrasound based key clinical pathway reduces the use of hospital resources for the evaluation of blunt abdominal trauma, *J Trauma* 42(6):1086, 1997.

32. Rozycki GS, Ballard RB, Feliciano DV et al: Surgeon-performed ultrasound for the assessment of truncal injuries, *Ann Surg* 228:557, 1998.

33. Yoshii H, Sato M, Yamamoto S et al: Usefulness and limitations of ultrasonography in the initial evaluation of blunt abdominal trauma, *J Trauma* 45(1):45, 1998.

34. Boulanger BR, McLellan BA, Brenneman FD et al: Prospective evidence of the superiority of a sonography-based algorithm in the assessment of blunt abdominal trauma, *J Trauma* 47(4): 632, 1999.

35. American College of Surgeons' Committee on Trauma: Abdominal trauma. In *Advanced trauma life support*, ed 6, Chicago, 1997, The College, 171.

36. Bennett MK, Jehle D: Ultrasonography in blunt abdominal trauma, *Emerg Med Clin North Am* 15(4):763, 1997.

37. Miletic D, Fuckar Z, Mraovic B et al: Ultrasound in the evaluation of hemoperitoneum in war casualties, *Mil Med* 164(8):600, 1999.

38. Nordenholz K, Rubin M, Gularte G et al: Ultrasound in the evaluation and management of blunt abdominal trauma, *Ann Emerg Med* 29:357, 1996.

39. Fabian TC, Croce MA: Abdominal trauma, including indications for celiotomy. In Mattox K, Feliciano K, Moore E, editors: *Trauma*, ed 4, New York, 2000, McGraw-Hill, 588-589

40. Villanvicencio RT, Aucar JA: Analysis of laparoscopy in trauma. *J Am Col Surg* 189(1):11, 1999.

41. Zantut LF, Ivatury RR, Smith RS et al: Diagnostic and therapeutic laparoscopy for penetrating abdominal trauma: a multicenter experience, *J Trauma* 42(5):825, 1997.

42. Purtill MA, Stabile BE: Duodenal and pancreatic trauma. In Naude GP, Bongard FS, Demetriades D, editors: *Trauma secrets*, Philadelphia, 1999, Hanley & Belfus, 126.

43. Carrico CJ, Mileski WJ, Kaplan HS: Transfusions, autotransfusion, and blood substitutes. In Mattox K, Feliciano D, Moore E, editors: *Trauma*, ed 4, New York, 2000, McGraw-Hill, 234.

44. Murray JA, Demetriades D, Cornwell EE et al: Penetrating left thoracoabdominal trauma: The incidence and clinical presentation of diaphragm injuries, *J Trauma* 43:624, 1997.

45. Murray JA, Bernes J, Asensio JA: Penetrating thoracoabdominal trauma, *Emerg Med Clin North Am* 16(1):107, 1998.

46. Murray JA, Demetriades D, Asensio JA: Diaphragm injuries. In Naude GP, Bongard FS, Demetriades D, editors: *Trauma secrets*, Philadelphia, 1999, Hanley & Belfus, 94.

47. Asensio JA, Demetriades D, Rodriguez A: Injury to the diaphragm. In Mattox K, Feliciano D, Moore E, editors: *Trauma*, ed 4, New York, 2000, McGraw-Hill, 610.

48. Wilson RF, Bender J: Diaphragmatic injuries. In Wilson RF, Walt AJ, editors: *Management of trauma: pitfalls and practice*, ed 2, Baltimore, 1996, Williams & Wilkins, 435.

49. Wisner DH: Injury to the stomach and small bowel. In Mattox K, Feliciano D, Moore E, editors: *Trauma*, ed 4, New York, 2000, McGraw-Hill, 716.

50. Wilson RF, Walt AJ: Injury to the stomach and small bowel. In Wilson RF, Walt AJ, editors: *Management of trauma: pitfalls and practice*, ed 2, Baltimore, 1996, Williams & Wilkins, 500.

51. Wisner DH: Injury to the stomach and small bowel. In Mattox K, Feliciano D, Moore E, editors: *Trauma*, ed 4, New York, 2000, McGraw-Hill, 730.

52. Pachter HL, Liang HG, Hofstetter SR: Liver and biliary tract trauma. In Mattox K, Feliciano D, Moore E, editors: *Trauma*, ed 4, New York, 2000, McGraw-Hill, 640.

53. Wilson RF, Walt AJ: Injuries to the liver and biliary tract. In Wilson DF, Walt AJ, editors: *Management of trauma: pitfalls and practice*, ed 2, Baltimore, 1996, Williams & Wilkins, 451.

54. Moore EE, Shackford SR, Pachter HL et al: Organ injury scaling: spleen, liver, & kidney, *J Trauma* 29:1664, 1989.

55. Wilson RF, Walt AJ: Injuries to the liver and biliary tract. In Wilson DF, Walt AJ, editors: *Management of trauma: pitfalls and practice*, ed 2, Baltimore, 1996, Williams & Wilkins, 455.

56. Wilson RF, Walt AJ: Injuries to the liver and biliary tract. In Wilson DF, Walt AJ, editors: *Management of trauma: pitfalls and practice*, ed 2, Baltimore, 1996, Williams & Wilkins, 457.

57. Pachter HL, Liang HG, Hofstetter SR: Liver and biliary tract trauma. In Mattox K, Feliciano D, Moore E, editors: *Trauma*, ed 4, New York, 2000, McGraw-Hill, 670.

58. Pachter HL, Liang HG, Hofstetter SR: Liver and biliary tract trauma. In Mattox K, Feliciano D, Moore E, editors: *Trauma*, ed 4, New York, 2000, McGraw-Hill, 672.

59. Cathey KL, Brady WJ, Butler K et al: Blunt splenic trauma: characteristics of patients requiring urgent laparotomy, *Am Surg* 64(5):450, 1998.

60. Bianchi JD, Collin GR: Management of splenic trauma at a rural level I trauma center, *Am Surg* 63(6):490, 1997.

61. Esposito TJ, Gamelli RL: Injury to the spleen. In Mattox K, Feliciano D, Moore E, editors: *Trauma*, ed 4, New York, 2000, McGraw-Hill, 694.

62. Malangoni, MA: Spleen. In Maull K, Rodriguez A, Wiles C, editors: *Complications in trauma and critical care*, Philadelphia, 1996, WB Saunders, 416-417.

63. Jurkovich GJ: Injury to duodenum and pancreas. In Mattox K, Feliciano D, Moore E, editors: *Trauma*, ed 4, New York, 2000, McGraw-Hill, 740.

64. Wilson RF: Injury to pancreas and duodenum. In Wilson RF, Walt AJ, editors: *Management of trauma: pitfalls and practice*, ed 2, Baltimore, 1996, Williams & Wilkins, 513.

65. Ferrada R, Gomez E: Pancreas. In Maull K, Rodriguez A, Wiles C, editors: *Complications in trauma and critical care*, Philadelphia, 1996, WB Saunders, 380.

66. Wisner DH: Injury to the stomach and small bowel. In Mattox K, Feliciano D, Moore E, editors: *Trauma*, ed 4, New York, 2000, McGraw-Hill, 718.

67. Nance ML, Peden GW, Shapiro MD et al: Solid viscus injury predicts major hollow viscus injury in blunt abdominal trauma, *J Trauma* 43:618, 1997.

68. Wisner DH: Injury to the stomach and small bowel. In Mattox K, Feliciano D, Moore E, editors: *Trauma*, ed 4, New York, 2000, McGraw-Hill, 731.

69. Burch JM: Injury to the colon and rectum. In Mattox K, Feliciano D, Moore E, editors: *Trauma*, ed 4, New York, 2000, McGraw-Hill, 770.

70. Burch JM: Injury to the colon and rectum. In Mattox K, Feliciano D, Moore E, editors: *Trauma*, ed 4, New York, 2000, McGraw-Hill, 771.

71. Feliciano DV, Burch JM, Graham JM: Abdominal vascular injury. In Mattox K, Feliciano D, Moore E, editors: *Trauma*, ed 4, New York, 2000, McGraw-Hill, 783.

72. Feliciano DV, Burch JM, Graham JM: Abdominal vascular injury. In Mattox K, Feliciano D, Moore E, editors: *Trauma*, ed 4, New York, 2000, McGraw-Hill, 784.

73. Wilson RF, Dulchavsky S: Abdominal vascular trauma. In Wilson RF, Walt AJ, editors: *Management of trauma: pitfalls and practice*, ed 2, Baltimore, 1996, Williams & Wilkins, 554.

74. Coimbra R, Hoyt D, Winchell R et al: The ongoing challenge of retroperitoneal vascular injuries, *Am J Surg* 172:541, 1996.

75. Carrillo EH, Bergamini TM, Miller FB et al: Abdominal vascular injuries, *J Trauma* 43(1):164, 1997.

76. Carrillo EH, Spain DA, Wilson MA et al: Alternatives in the management of penetrating injuries to the iliac vessels, *J Trauma* 44(6):1024, 1998.

77. Wilson RF, Dulchavsky S: Abdominal vascular trauma. In Wilson RF, Walt AJ, editors: *Management of trauma: pitfalls and practice,* ed 2, Baltimore, 1996, Williams & Wilkins, 556.

78. Chandler CF, Blinman T, Cryer HG: Acute renal failure. In Mattox K, Feliciano D, Moore E, editors: *Trauma,* ed 4, New York, 2000, McGraw-Hill, 1349.

79. Nayduck DA, Sullivan K, Reed RL: Abdominal compartment syndrome, *J Trauma Nurse* 4(1):5, 1997.

80. Wilson RF, Georgiadis GM: Compartment Syndrome. In Wilson RF, Walt AJ, editors: *Management of trauma: pitfalls and practices,* ed 2, Baltimore, 1996, Williams & Wilkins, 693.

81. Nahrwold DL: Acute cholecystitis. In Sabiston DC, editor: *Textbook of surgery: the biological bases of modern surgical practice,* ed 5, Philadelphia, 1997, WB Saunders, 1130.

82. Hadata T, Kobayashi H, Tanigawa A et al: Acute acalculous cholecystitis in a patient on total parenteral nutrition: case report and review of the Japanese literature, *Hepato-Gastroenterol* 46(28):2208, 1999.

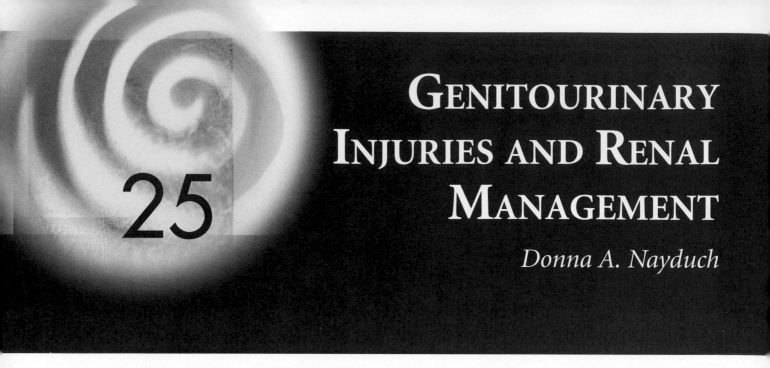

25

GENITOURINARY INJURIES AND RENAL MANAGEMENT

Donna A. Nayduch

Rapid diagnosis and treatment of genitourinary (GU) trauma can be difficult. The trauma victim's most immediate requirement is the establishment of a patent airway and an adequate circulating volume. Assessment of the GU system often begins with the insertion of a Foley catheter to monitor urine output (as a reflection of fluid balance and shock state). This chapter addresses the assessment, treatment, and care of the patient experiencing genitourinary trauma; potential complications; and the impact of GU trauma on the recovering trauma patient.

Genitourinary trauma may be defined as any injury to the kidneys, the kidneys' collecting system, or the reproductive system. The kidneys are generally not susceptible to direct trauma because they are protected by the twelfth ribs. They are anchored in place by Gerota's fascia, surrounded by fat pads, and capped by the adrenal glands. The left kidney is further protected by the spleen, chest wall, diaphragm, pancreatic tail, and descending colon. The right kidney is 1 to 2 cm lower than the left and is surrounded by the diaphragm, liver, and duodenum. The ureters are cushioned bilaterally by abdominal contents and surrounded by the pelvic bones. The urinary bladder is protected anteriorly and laterally by the pubic arch. The pelvic diaphragm supports the bladder inferiorly; the peritoneum covers the bladder superiorly and posteriorly. These anatomic guardians are consistent in both sexes.

The female urethra is protected by the symphysis pubis, as is the vagina. The uterus lies midpelvis, halfway between the sacrum and the symphysis pubis. It rests on the pelvic diaphragm, supported by six ligaments, and is cushioned by bowels and bladder. This same anatomic protection is afforded the ovaries and fallopian tubes on either side of the uterus. The female urethra is shorter than the male urethra and is relatively mobile.

The longer male urethra consists of two segments: the anterior segment, which is distal to the urogenital diaphragm, and the posterior segment, which passes through the urogenital diaphragm and includes the prostatic and membranous segments. The bladder neck is continuous with the prostatic segment of the urethra. The male urethra is approximately 20 cm in length and is fixed at the symphysis. Comparatively little anatomic protection is afforded the male urethra, penis, and scrotal sac. These anatomic considerations are important factors in the occurrence of distal GU trauma in men.

In children under 6 years of age the bladder is an abdominal organ. The kidneys of children have less perirenal fat, are large in comparison with the abdomen as a whole, and have a thinner capsule for protection than those of adults. Children also have a weaker abdominal musculature and a less ossified thoracic rib cage, which offers less kidney protection.

EPIDEMIOLOGY

Injuries to the GU tract account for 8% to 10% of all abdominal trauma.[1] The most commonly injured organs are the kidneys, followed by the bladder and the urethra.[2] Renal injury occurs more frequently in children than in adults and more frequently than any other abdominal injury.[3,4] Injury to the urethra is more common in men than in women.[5] Trauma to the ureters is rarely seen and most often has iatrogenic causes such as obstetric-gynecologic surgery.[6]

Genitourinary trauma is rarely an isolated injury. Approximately 60% to 80% of patients with blunt renal trauma have associated major injuries to other organs.[7] Injuries that occur most frequently with GU trauma include fracture of the pelvis, lower rib fractures, gunshot wounds to the abdomen, and fracture of the transverse process of the lumbar spine. Pelvic fractures are affiliated with a 5% to 10% incidence of bladder injury and an 1% to 11% incidence of posterior urethra injury.[5,8] In contrast, 80% or more of patients with bladder injuries have concomitant pelvic fractures.[5,8] Injury to the right kidney is most often seen with injury to the liver, whereas injury to the left kidney and the spleen tend to occur together.

Genitourinary trauma can contribute to significant morbidity and mortality. Mortality of up to 44% is usually attributed to injuries other than the GU trauma.[5] Morbidity is usually associated with missed or delayed diagnosis of the GU injury, as will be discussed later.

MECHANISM OF INJURY

Blunt trauma causes approximately 80% to 95% of all GU trauma.[2] Blunt forces can be either direct impact or rapid deceleration. Rapid deceleration injury is produced when a body in motion is halted abruptly. This situation can occur during a fall from a height or in a motor vehicle collision (MVC) when the occupant makes contact with the dashboard, lap belt, or steering wheel of the vehicle. The kidney is set in motion on its pedicle in relation to the more stationary aorta. The rotation around the pedicle may tear the intima of the renal artery, resulting in renal artery thrombosis, or may injure the renal vein.[3] Other consequences of this type of blunt injury include disruption of the ureteropelvic junction (UPJ) and contusion of the renal parenchyma (Figure 25-1). UPJ injuries occur mostly in children.[9]

Motor vehicle collisions account for a majority of genitourinary injuries, especially in children.[6] During an MVC an unbelted victim slides forward, the femur is compacted into the pelvis, and the abdomen strikes the steering wheel (Figure 25-2). The stress on the kidney is a combination of forces applied to a fluid-filled inner compartment.[10] Hydrostatic pressure results in injury. The increased intrapelvic pressure associated with hydronephrotic kidneys and renal cysts results in increased susceptibility to injury, particularly at the periphery. In trauma the most common blunt cause of ureter injury occurs when the kidney is compressed against the lower rib cage and upper lumbar transverse processes, thereby stretching the ureter in lateral flexion.[9]

The use of three-point restraint seat belts can decrease the incidence of organ injury by holding the occupant firmly against the seat and allowing the vehicle to absorb the impact of the collision. A lap belt alone or an impact against the steering wheel can result in bladder injury caused by the sudden increase in intraabdominal/intravesicular pressure on a fluid-filled organ.[11]

Smith and Klein reported a case of a child seated sideways on the lap of an adult in the front seat of a vehicle with an air bag.[12] During the crash the air bag came into direct contact with the child's left flank, resulting in GU trauma. The unbelted child suffered an avulsion of the left kidney and subsequently required a nephrectomy as a result of devitalized tissue. The incidence of abdominal trauma with unbelted passengers colliding with air bags will likely increase because all vehicles manufactured since September 1997 are required to have air bags.[13] The velocity of an air bag as it is deployed is between 160 and 320 km/hr, resulting in a significant transfer of kinetic energy. Unbelted passengers and children riding on the laps of adults in the front seat

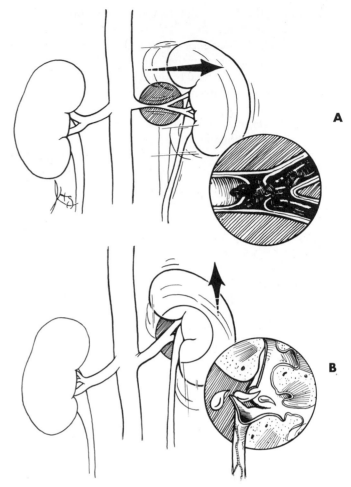

FIGURE 25-1 Acceleration-deceleration injury may produce disruption of the renal artery (**A**) and the ureteropelvic junction (**B**).

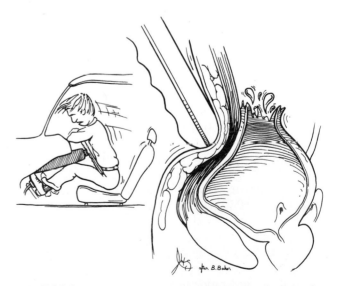

FIGURE 25-2 Compression injuries of the abdomen that do not produce fracture may produce intraperitoneal bladder rupture. (From Guerriero WG, Devine CJ: *Urologic injuries*, Norwalk, Conn, 1984, Appleton-Century-Crofts, 113.)

experience the transfer of kinetic energy directly to the abdomen and flank.

Although the incidence of trauma to the ureters is rising with the increase in gunshot wounds (GSWs), the most common cause of ureteral trauma remains iatrogenic injury during surgery.[6] Iatrogenic injuries to the small ureters are most likely to occur during difficult pelvic procedures in which normal anatomic landmarks are obscured by obstruction, neoplasm, inflammation, congenital anomalies, traumatic displacement, or the effects of radiation. A high index of suspicion must be established to detect and appropriately treat iatrogenic genitourinary trauma.

Penetrating injury is the most common traumatic cause of ureter injury.[6] Causes of penetrating trauma include gunshot, stabbing, and impalement. The ureter accounts for approximately 4% of injuries caused by abdominal gunshot wounds.[14] Of these ureteric injuries, 95% have associated intraabdominal injuries.[14-16] Of all patients with gunshot wounds to the abdomen, 5% to 15% have concomitant genitourinary injury.[17]

In addition to the increasing rate of penetrating injuries, another new mechanism that causes genitourinary injuries is the Jet Ski type of personal watercraft. These injuries range from external perineal injury to rectal and vaginal tears.[18-20] The Jet Ski most commonly collides with another watercraft.[21] These watercraft are propelled by pressurized water thrust through the Jet Ski, without an exposed propeller.[21] The wash from the Jet Ski propels high-pressure water into the perineal area after the passenger falls off. The method of propulsion does avoid propeller injuries, but the impact of the high-pressure water can also result in renal contusions or renal artery thrombosis.[22,23]

RESUSCITATION PHASE

The early detection of genitourinary trauma is important to optimal outcome in terms of organ salvage and patient survival. However, GU trauma does not take precedence over more life-threatening injuries to the head, chest, and abdomen. Genitourinary trauma may not present initially as a life-threatening situation, but delay in diagnosis and treatment can produce significant tissue loss from prolonged ischemia or blood and urine extravasation.

Assessment of GU trauma is based on multiple strategies. No one strategy is sufficient to diagnose genitourinary trauma specifically. An accurate diagnosis is obtained through the interpretation of diagnostic clues obtained from the history, physical examination, and radiologic and laboratory testing. However, a high index of suspicion, based on knowledge of the mechanism of injury, is key in the detection of GU trauma. Genitourinary trauma should be suspected in the following types of injuries:

- Fall or deceleration injury
- Motor vehicle collision
- Crushing incident
- Abdominal, flank, lower chest, back, or pelvis injury
- Powered personal watercraft events

- Straddle injury
- Sexual assault
- Penetrating abdominal trauma[2,3,5,6,11,14,19,20,24-29]

HEALTH HISTORY

A health history always begins with the circumstances causing the person to seek treatment within the health care system. The initial step of the assessment is to obtain an accurate history of the events leading to injury.[29] Details about the mechanism of injury provide valuable clues to the occurrence, nature, and extent of the genitourinary trauma.

For MVCs the estimated speed of the vehicle when it crashed, the type of vehicle, the use of seat belts, and the position of the victim within the vehicle should be determined. If a fall has occurred, the height of the fall, objects struck during the fall, the patient's body position on landing, and the type of landing surface should be noted. After penetrating trauma, information must be obtained regarding the type of weapon used (e.g., gun, knife, impaled object), the type and length of the knife if used, and the occurrence of other events following the penetrating trauma (e.g., a fall).

Various details about the condition of the patient at the scene of the trauma affect clinical management decisions. Was the patient pinned in the vehicle; what was the extrication time? Was there evidence of the use of drugs or alcohol? What care was provided in the field? Was there evidence of airway compromise or hemodynamic instability? Details such as these can be obtained from prehospital providers, witnesses, family, or police officers at the scene.[29]

In addition to the circumstances of injury, essential past medical history information includes allergies, medications, previous diseases or surgical procedures, last meal eaten and when, and the events before the trauma. Previous injuries, known anatomic abnormalities, and preexisting genitourinary conditions should be determined. The congenitally abnormal kidney is especially vulnerable to severe injury from minor trauma.[3,10] Anatomic abnormalities or preexisting pathologic conditions of concern include GU tumors, congenital hydronephrosis with cysts, renal calculi, polycystic disease, and horseshoe or pelvic kidney.

Previous genitourinary surgery may have contributed to the development of adhesions, strictures, or a predisposition to calculi formation or chronic GU infection, all of which can influence treatment modalities after trauma. Prior nephrectomy or preexisting genitourinary disorders such as chronic renal failure, renal artery stenosis, or one of the glomerulonephropathies may govern both the initial treatment and long-term management of the trauma patient with GU injury.

Part of the subjective data obtained should include the patient's feeling of an inability to void. Inability to void may indicate upper urinary tract injury, obstruction caused by blood clots, or bladder or urethra rupture.[29]

A quick way to remember the components of the essential health history is the AMPLE acronym, which stands for allergies, medications, past history of medical or surgical illnesses, last meal, and events preceding the injury.[29]

PHYSICAL EXAMINATION

During the resuscitation phase the assessment of life-threatening injuries to the cardiovascular, respiratory, and neurologic systems takes priority. Until the patient is stabilized and the genitourinary system can be assessed, a high index of suspicion should be maintained for GU trauma.

INSPECTION. The first phase of the physical examination is inspection. Abdominal and flank symmetry should be assessed; evidence of torso or pelvic trauma may extend to evidence of GU trauma.[11,29] The presence of a complex or open pelvic fracture, the number and position of wounds caused by penetrating trauma, and the position of impaled objects must be noted. Impaled objects should not be removed until the patient is in the operating room. Grey Turner's sign (ecchymosis over the posterior aspect of the eleventh or twelfth rib or the flank) may indicate renal trauma or a retroperitoneal bleed.[29] Frequently, renal injury is the result of a direct blow to the flank.[29] Absence of ecchymosis does not rule out renal trauma as a significant proportion of patients with renal trauma do not have Grey Turner's sign. Fractures of the eleventh or twelfth rib or the lumbar transverse process may contribute to renal or ureteral injury.[9]

Assessment of the perineum is integral to patient management. The urinary meatus must be inspected for signs of bleeding, a strong indicator of urethral injury.[28,29] The assessment of the urinary meatus is essential before placing a urinary catheter.[29] The perineal area should be assessed for evidence of trauma, including lacerations, hematomas, swelling, and ecchymosis.

The scrotum may be edematous or contused because of extravasation of urine or blood in patients with urethral injury, pelvic fracture, or retroperitoneal hematoma.[29] Diffuse perineal bruising is a later sign of fracture of the symphysis pubis or pelvic rami. Perineal swelling, vaginal bleeding, vulvar hematoma, and rectal tenderness are all indications of potential genitourinary injury in females from straddle injury, fall, MVC, or assault.[28] For women with an altered level of consciousness, a brief pelvic examination should be performed to ascertain any injury and to determine the presence of a tampon, diaphragm, or intrauterine device.

In blunt trauma patients with vaginal bleeding or pelvic fractures, the possibility of vaginal laceration should be considered. Evaluation for such injury is done under direct vision using a speculum or retractors. In the patient with a severe pelvic fracture, the examination usually must be done under anesthesia in an operating suite. Separation of the legs for examination of a patient with a severe pelvic fracture can result in hemorrhage from pelvic bleeding. This should be avoided at all costs. After the pelvis is stabilized, vaginal examination can occur in the operating suite.

In patients with blunt and penetrating trauma with suspected or confirmed vaginal lacerations or penetrating lower abdominal injury in both males and females, rectal injury must be assumed until proven otherwise. Such patients require a proctoscopic examination.

AUSCULTATION. The presence and quality of bowel sounds can be assessed. Although the absence of bowel sounds is not specific to genitourinary or gastrointestinal injury, the mechanism and identified injuries should guide assessment.

Auscultation around the renal arteries is essential. A bruit in these areas may reflect turbulence at an intimal tear in the artery.

PERCUSSION. Percussion of the abdomen and flank allows assessment of abnormal areas of fluid or air collection.[30] Excessive dullness in the lower abdomen or flank may indicate the extravasation of blood or urine or the presence of a retroperitoneal hematoma. Percussion over the kidneys determines their location in the retroperitoneum.

PALPATION. The flank, abdomen, lumbar vertebrae, and lower rib cage are palpated for evidence of pain, mass, or crepitus—all potential indicators of GU trauma.[29,31] Renal colic or costovertebral angle pain may indicate renal trauma.[29] Renal colic may be the result of clots obstructing the renal collecting system.[29] Severe costovertebral angle pain may be caused by ischemia from a renal artery thrombosis. Additional signs beyond abdominal tenderness, with or without distention, include a flank mass or a pelvic fracture.[29]

The pelvic area is palpated for evidence of tenderness or movable bony fragments, which may indicate pelvic fracture.[28] Palpation of the suprapubic area may reveal a distended bladder. Severe tenderness in the hypogastrium may signify bladder rupture.[4]

A rectal examination should also be performed before urinary catheterization, especially in men. The presence of a boggy or displaced prostate may suggest urethral injury.[29]

LABORATORY STUDIES

In addition to the history and physical examination, results from diagnostic and laboratory testing are essential to the assessment of the patient who has sustained trauma to the genitourinary tract.

On admission, blood work is drawn to establish baseline profiles. Hematologic studies may indicate hemorrhage, but other sources must be ruled out before making the assumption that the cause lies in the GU tract. From a genitourinary perspective, the primary laboratory study is urinalysis. Gross hematuria correlates with significant lower urologic injury.[4,11,31] Microscopic hematuria may indicate minor injury to the GU tract and requires follow-up.[4] Microscopic hematuria alone does not require further diagnostic studies.[31]

Because urine obtained by catheterization usually contains 5 to 10 red blood cells per microscopic field, it is optimal if the patient can be encouraged to void the initial specimen. This allows the differentiation between hematuria caused by catheterization and hematuria caused by genitourinary injury. The absence of hematuria, however, should not lead the trauma team to falsely assume that there is no GU injury. Laceration of a major renal vessel may or may not be associated with hematuria. In a study by Udekwu, Gurkin, and Oller, both the urine dipstick and urinalysis were poor predictors of urologic injury.[32]

In the case of penetrating trauma, neither gross nor microscopic hematuria is a reliable sign of ureteric injury and is usually present in only 45% of patients with ureteral injury caused by gunshot wounds to the abdomen.[14]

RADIOLOGIC STUDIES

Radiographic assessment of the patient with genitourinary trauma is the cornerstone of the diagnostic process. The primary study of value is computed tomography (CT), yet other studies can provide valuable information about the organs that they assess.

KIDNEY-URETER-BLADDER RADIOGRAPHY.

The kidney-ureter-bladder (KUB), a radiograph of these three structures, is usually performed after the patient is stabilized. The purposes of the test are to visualize the position and size of the kidneys; identify lower rib, pelvic, vertebral body, or transverse process fractures; identify the likely position of foreign bodies; and evaluate diaphragmatic displacement.

The psoas muscles may be obliterated or bulging, possibly the result of retroperitoneal hemorrhage or hematoma. The KUB itself is not specific for genitourinary trauma, so the lack of pathologic findings on this examination does not rule out renal trauma. It does, however, heighten the examiner's awareness of other possible associated injuries.

INTRAVENOUS PYELOGRAM.

The intravenous pyelogram (IVP), also known as the excretory urogram, is one of the fundamental diagnostic procedures in the assessment of patients with renal trauma. The IVP evaluates both structural integrity and excretory function of the renal system. It also allows visualization of renal parenchyma, calices, and pelvis; assessment of perfusion to the injured kidney; evaluation of the status of both the injured and noninjured kidney; and assessment of the continuity of the collecting system.[1,15,29]

With the patient in the supine position, an iodine-based dye is injected intravenously.[29] Before the injection the patient should be screened for allergy to the contrast medium. Patients who have experienced allergic reactions to shellfish or previous injections of contrast material should be given an initial test dose of the contrast dye and observed closely for hypotension with tachycardia or bradycardia, nausea, vomiting, or urticaria.

Two minutes after the dye injection, a radiograph is done, which allows visualization of the renal parenchyma. Additional films at 5-, 15-, and 30-minute intervals[10] allow visualization of the pelvicaliceal system, ureters, and bladder. In trauma patients a one-shot IVP is usually performed

to save time; this is used purely to confirm the presence of two functional kidneys or massive disruption of the kidneys before surgery.[15,29,33-35] In addition to urologic trauma, abnormalities such as polycystic kidneys, absent kidneys, renal calculi, hydronephrosis, and pyelonephritis may be identified. Presently use of the one-shot IVP is under question because CT is more valuable in genitourinary assessment.[29] One-shot IVP may be valuable during surgery to evaluate pedicle injury and contralateral kidney excretion.[1,34] The study is not accurate if osmotic diuresis is induced or when hypotension is present, resulting in decreased excretion of urine.[31] Patel and Walker found that 80% of one-shot IVPs were normal even though renal injury was detected during surgery.[33] In addition, 20% of patients with abnormal findings on IVP had no renal injury present on surgical exploration.

RETROGRADE URETHROGRAM.

The retrograde urethrogram (RUG) is the diagnostic procedure conducted before catheterization of a patient suspected of having an injury to the urethra.[11,25,29,36-38] To perform this test, an 8 French Foley catheter is attached to an irrigating syringe filled with contrast material. The catheter is gently inserted into the urinary meatus until the catheter balloon is 2 to 3 cm proximal to the meatus.[29] The balloon is inflated 1.5 to 2 ml, then 15 to 20 ml of contrast is gently injected into the urethra.[29]

Extravasation of the contrast material detects urethral injury. Partial urethral injury is identified through extravasation with bladder filling, whereas a complete tear of the urethra involves extravasation with loss of continuity.[27] If a catheter is already in place, a pericatheter RUG can still be performed to identify urethral injury.[11]

CYSTOGRAM.

The cystogram is used to detect intraperitoneal or extraperitoneal bladder rupture.[11,29,36] A urethral catheter is passed (after urethral injury is ruled out) and at least 300 to 500 ml of water-soluble contrast medium is instilled by gravity.[29,36] Anteroposterior and oblique radiographic films are obtained. The bladder is then emptied and an anteroposterior postdrainage radiograph is taken. The cystogram should be performed before the IVP.[29] Bladder contusions appear normal on a cystogram.[37] A false-negative study occurs if there is incomplete distention of the bladder or if no drainage radiograph is done.[39] CT cystograms have been found to be 85% to 100% accurate.[37]

RADIONUCLIDE IMAGING.

Renal radionuclide scanning provides information regarding renal injury. This test is especially useful for patients who are allergic to contrast dyes. Abnormal results of this test may indicate renal hypoperfusion, fractures, urinary extravasation, and delayed excretion. Renal blood flow can be assessed accurately, but parenchymal and collecting system injuries cannot be identified as accurately as with IVP or CT. Urine from patients receiving radionuclide injections should be handled with gloves after the procedure to avoid care provider exposure to the radioactive isotope.

ULTRASOUND.   Renal ultrasound is capable of detecting renal abnormalities with the use of high-frequency sound waves. The sound waves produce echoes, which are amplified and converted via a transducer into electric impulses that are seen on an oscilloscope screen as anatomic pictures. This test is seldom used for early identification of injury because it is imprecise in differentiating injuries. Ultrasonography is most useful for the identification and serial evaluation of perinephric hematomas and urinomas. In the acute resuscitative period, ultrasound is ineffective in GU evaluation.[4]

RENAL ANGIOGRAPHY.   Renal angiography is indicated when there is incomplete or absent visualization of one or both kidneys on IVP, prolonged bleeding without another source, suspicion of renal pedicle trauma, or questionable renal viability. Angiography provides information concerning the preservation of blood supply to the damaged renal parenchyma. Devitalized areas must be identified because necrosis or abscess formation may follow. These injuries may be diagnosed after initial damage control surgery of the abdomen.

Nonvisualization of the kidney on IVP is a potentially serious finding and may be caused by renal artery spasm, contusion, or intimal tear with thrombosis. Timely diagnosis of insufficient kidney perfusion can decrease the possibility of nephrectomy necessitated by ischemia.

Renal arteriography involves cannulation of the femoral artery. After the procedure, the site is monitored closely for bleeding and pulses distal to the site are evaluated for presence and quality.

COMPUTED TOMOGRAPHY.   CT provides the most precise delineation of genitourinary trauma. The test is particularly sensitive in staging renal lacerations (the extent of injury), and in identifying intrarenal and subcapsular hematomas, renal infarct, contrast extravasation, the size and extent of a retroperitoneal hematoma, renal perfusion, and associated injuries to abdominal organs.[1,3,16,35] Using contrast medium, arterial injury and lack of perfusion can also be demonstrated. CT is also used to monitor progress in nonoperative management of renal injury.[1] CT has essentially replaced IVP as the gold standard for renal evaluation.[40]

After administration of oral (PO) and intravenous (IV) contrast, a spiral CT scan with excretory delayed films is performed to diagnose upper urinary tract injury.[31] CT scan has also been used to identify bladder injuries. CT identified only 50% of bladder injuries in one study.[32] In contrast, Sivit, Cutting, and Eichelberger demonstrated that CT scanning done with a 5-minute delay after IV contrast administration while the bladder catheter was occluded was accurate in identifying intraperitoneal versus extraperitoneal bladder rupture in children.[40]

SPECIFIC ORGAN INJURY

Specific genitourinary injuries vary widely in severity, the need for immediate operative management, and sequelae. In the following section, specific injuries, diagnoses, and treatments are discussed.

TRAUMA TO THE PERINEUM

Trauma to the genital organs, although often not life threatening, can produce overwhelming loss and crisis for the patient and significant others. Genital trauma may be associated with injury to the perineum, bony pelvis, thighs, bladder, vagina, and rectum. Blunt trauma, direct blows, burns, penetrating trauma, and industrial events all may produce genital trauma. Fortunately trauma to the genitals is not frequent, and surgical intervention can produce good results in both function and appearance. Hemorrhage of the external genitalia is usually controlled by compression dressings, clamps, or ligation.[34] These wounds are further managed by wound irrigation and debridement to preserve tissue viability.

MALE GENITALIA

Testes.   The testes are usually spared from injury by their mobility, contraction of the cremaster muscle, and a tough capsular covering. However, injury can be produced by a direct blow that impinges the testes against the symphysis pubis, producing contusion or rupture. The tunica vaginalis sac may fill with blood (hematocele), and the patient may present with a large, tender, swollen scrotal mass.

Management.   Immediate surgical intervention is the treatment of choice, with every attempt made to salvage the testis. Blood clots are evacuated from the tunica vaginalis, and testicular rupture is repaired. Delayed treatment may increase the risk of infection of the hematocele or testis or testicular atrophy from the pressure of the tense hematocele. Orchiectomy is the least desired outcome of severe injury or complications of testicular trauma.

Scrotum.   Trauma to the scrotum may produce avulsion injuries, resulting in significant tissue loss. The mechanisms of injury are the same as for the testes.

Management.   When possible, the avulsed scrotum is reconstructed around the testes and usually regains normal size within a few months. If scrotal reconstruction is not possible, the testicles may be implanted into upper thigh pockets, where the temperature is similar to that of the scrotum.

Penetrating injury to the scrotum can result in injury to the spermatic cord and testes. Salvage rate for the testes is approximately 35%.[41] Early debridement and primary repair are essential. Associated injuries may be present, affecting the thighs, femoral vessels, small bowel, or colon.[41]

Penis. Trauma to the penis may be a result of blunt trauma, strangulation injury, mishaps during sexual intercourse, amputation, or penetrating injury (Figure 25-3).[41-43] Blunt trauma usually produces a penile fracture with rupture of the tunica albuginea, hemorrhage, and hematoma formation.[42] Of these injuries, 10% to 30% result in urethral injury as well.[42,43] The patient presents with pain, swelling, discoloration, and deviation. If the injury occurs from striking against a hard object, a direct blow, or abnormal bending, a snap or crackle may have been heard at the time of injury.[42]

Penetrating injuries to the penis involves the urethra in 22% of cases.[41] Indications that the urethra is involved are discussed later in this chapter. One study noted that 38% of the patients seen with penetrating penile trauma tested positive for hepatitis B, C, or both and that more than 60% of the incidents involved the use of alcohol.[41]

Management. Injuries to the penis comprise 0.25% of emergent urologic admissions.[42] Injury to the penis can be treated either conservatively or with immediate surgical repair.[2] Conservative treatment includes urethral catheterization or suprapubic cystostomy, application of ice, elevation, administration of antiinflammatory drugs, compression dressings, analgesics, and medication to temporarily suppress erections.[43] Complications of conservative treatment include penile abscess, urinary extravasation, pain, inadequate erection, and permanent deformity.[42,43] Patients with penile injury experience a 28% to 30% complication rate.[43]

Surgical intervention is advocated as the treatment of choice to decrease the incidence of complications and promote rapid recovery.[43] Early surgical repair reduces fibrosis and curvature.[42]

Strangulation injuries may be produced by foreign objects or human hair constricting the penis. The patient presents with pain and swelling distal to the constricting object. Urethral fistula formation and partial amputation may result from prolonged constriction. Immediate surgical intervention is necessary.

Traumatic amputation of the penis may produce severe physical and psychologic disability. Successful outcome requires the cooperation of a urologist, plastic surgeon, and psychiatrist. Surgical reattachment of the distal segment may be possible if ischemia time is 18 hours or less (this time may be longer if the segment is preserved in iced saline). Microvascular repair may be advisable. Immediate repair and local reshaping may be performed, with plastic surgery and cosmetic repair done at a later time.

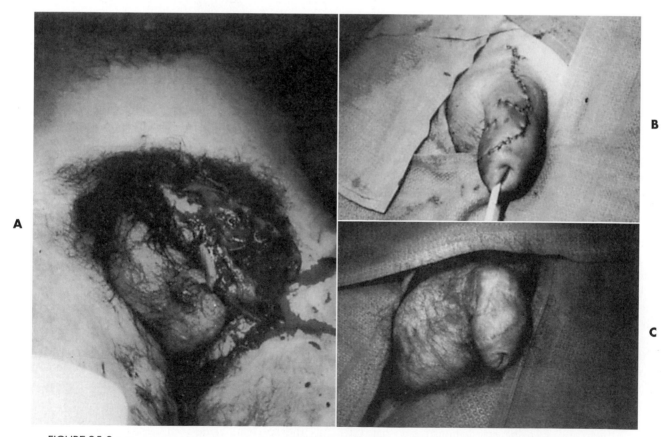

FIGURE 25-3 A, Power saw injury to the penis resulted in complete midline hemisection from symphysis through the glans penis, including the urethra. **B,** Appearance at the completion of reconstruction. A urethral stenting catheter was left in place. All tissue survived without additional debridement required. **C,** Genital appearance 6 months after injury. The patient had complete return of sensation, sexual function, and urethral voiding. (From McAninch JW, Kahn RI, Jeffrey RB et al: Major traumatic and septic genital injuries, *J Trauma* 24:291-298, 1984.)

FEMALE GENITALIA. Trauma to the female genitalia is caused by straddle falls, motor vehicle collisions, sexual assault, and powered personal watercraft (Jet Ski) incidents.[19,20,24,28] Pelvic fractures account for the majority of female external genital trauma and most often injure the vagina and perineum. Penetrating trauma also may injure the uterus and ovaries, which may require surgical repair, hysterectomy, or oophorectomy.

Perineum. External perineal injury may present as vulvar hematoma after a straddle event or sexual assault. Assault further involves tears of the introitus.[28] The most common injuries in young girls involve the vulva (63%) and vagina (53%).[28] Concomitant anorectal lacerations may be noted. Sexual assault may also result in lacerations to the urethra, especially in young girls or women with an imperforate hymen.[44] Use of a colposcope, a freestanding microscope used outside the speculum, has significantly increased the documentation of injuries sustained from sexual assault.[24] The colposcope allows increased visualization through magnification. Table 25-1 lists the genitalia injuries sustained in order of frequency by age group.[24]

Vagina. Vaginal tears occur during sexual assault and frequently during Jet Ski events. The pressurized water from the Jet Ski enters through the swimsuit or pushes the suit out of the way, causing vaginal laceration with or without intraabdominal extension, perianal abrasion, and perineal laceration. In addition, a high-speed fall onto water carries sufficient force that the water behaves as a solid object, resulting in vaginal and perineal laceration.[20] Injuries are considered severe when the cervix is involved or when profusely bleeding vaginal lacerations, which can result in hypovolemic shock, are present.[19] These injuries can be prevented by use of a wet suit.

The most common clinical sign of vaginal trauma is vaginal bleeding, which may be masked by spasm of the vagina. Consequently a speculum examination is essential in women who have sustained pelvic fracture after pelvic hemorrhage is under control. Evidence collection for sexual assault must be undertaken carefully, preferably by a sexual assault nurse examiner (SANE). Evidence of sperm and seminal plasma still can be obtained up to 48 hours after assault.[44] Swabs should be taken of the introitus and rectal cavity.

TABLE 25-1	**Female Genitalia Injury After Sexual Assault**
Age Group	**Injury in Order of Most to Least Frequent**
0-12	Hymen, labia minora, posterior fourchette, rectum into hymen, rectum
13-17	Hymen, posterior fourchette, labia minora, cervix/vagina into hymen, cervix
Adult	Hymen, cervix, posterior fourchette, vagina into labia minora, cervix, periurethral area

Management. Examination under general anesthesia provides a more complete assessment.[28] More than 75% of upper vaginal lacerations require surgical repair.[19] In the Jet Ski injury group, 80% of women with vaginal tears presented with bleeding, 10% with pain, 3% to 15% with shock, and only 1% with injuries that extended into the peritoneum.[19] During surgical repair, hypogastric artery ligation may be necessary to control reproductive hemorrhage. Interventional angiography for embolization can avoid retroperitoneal exploration. Packing is an alternative to control hemorrhage until other organ injuries are ruled out.[19]

Complications of vaginal tears include pelvic abscesses and sepsis. Lacerations from Jet Ski events require antibiotics for potential infection from lake, river, or ocean water exposure. Wounds are often left open to avoid retroperitoneal abscess formation.[19]

TRAUMA TO THE URETHRA

Injury to the female urethra is rarely seen because the urethra is shorter and more mobile than in males.[45] When injury is present, however, it is usually associated with significant pelvic fracture or disruption and injury to the bladder neck and vagina.[45]

High-risk events likely to result in urethral injury are straddle events and Malgaigne pelvis fractures. Straddle injuries can crush the urethra without pelvic fracture. These straddle scenarios are more common in children than adults.[26] Complete rupture of the urethra is also more common in children because the thin, delicate membrane of the urethra is less elastic than in an adult.[26] In children the most likely sites of urethral injury are the prostatic urethra and bladder neck.[26]

In male patients pelvic fractures shear the prostate from the urogenital diaphragm, rupturing the ligaments holding the urethra in place and disrupting the urethra.[11,37] Posterior urethral injury in males has an 80% association with lateral compression pelvic fractures.[8] Anterior pelvic ring disruption with pubic rami fracture results in bladder and urethra injury in either sex.[11] Unilateral pubic ramus fracture is associated with urologic injury in 15% of cases, which increases to 40% if bilateral pubic rami are involved.[11] The likelihood of urethral injury increases with open book and vertical shear types of pelvic fractures.

Penetrating trauma to the anterior urethra may be produced by gunshot wounds, stab wounds, or self-inflicted instrumentation of the urethra with foreign bodies.[41] Power takeoff (machinery) injury is another form of penetrating trauma and is sometimes seen in farm and industrial events. In these cases the clothing becomes caught in the power belt of a machine. The patient may sustain trauma involving the skin of the penis, the scrotum, and the urethra.

ASSESSMENT. Findings characteristic of urethral injury include identification of blood at the urinary meatus, an inability to void, gross hematuria, pelvic or perineal ecchymosis, perineal or scrotal edema, or a high-riding prostate.[24,29,45] A male patient with straddle injury may present

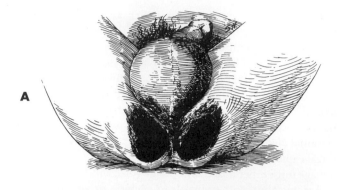

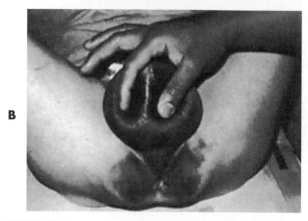

FIGURE 25-4 **A,** Diagram of a butterfly hematoma. **B,** Appearance of a patient with perineal butterfly hematoma. (From Peters P, Sagalowsky A: Genitourinary trauma. In Walsh P, Gittes R, Perlmutter A et al, editors: *Campbell's urology,* ed 5, vol 1, Philadelphia, 1986, WB Saunders.)

TABLE 25-2	**Urethral Injury Classification**
Grade	**Injuries**
I	Posterior urethra stretch
II	Partial/complete posterior injury with tear of membranous urethra above the urogenital diaphragm
III	Partial/complete combination anteroposterior injury with disruption of the urogenital diaphragm
IV	Bladder neck injury with extension into the urethra
IV A	Base of the bladder injury with periurethral extravasation simulating a grade IV injury
V	Partial/complete anterior urethra injury

Modified from Goldman SM, Sandler CM, Corriere JN et al: Blunt urethral trauma: a unified anatomical mechanical classification, *J Urol* 157, 1997.

with a characteristic butterfly-shaped ecchymotic area beneath the scrotum (Figure 25-4). Urethral injury is without any signs or symptoms in 5% to 12% of all patients.[11,25] It should be assumed that both male and female patients with pelvic fractures have urethral injury until proven otherwise.

In male patients urethral injuries are classified according to location. Table 25-2 lists the classification of urethral injury by Goldman, Sandler, Corriere, et al.[46] In general, urethral injuries below the urogenital diaphragm, involving the bulbous and penile urethrae, are classified as anterior urethral trauma. Those above the urogenital diaphragm, toward the bladder neck and involving the prostatic and membranous urethrae, are classified as posterior urethral trauma.

Posterior urethral injury should be suspected in any patient with a pelvic fracture or separation of the symphysis pubis and in patients in whom a displaced prostate or soft boggy mass is found on rectal examination. Injury to the membranous urethra is the most common and may extend into the bulbous urethra with disruption of the urogenital diaphragm.[25,37] Stretching usually precedes rupture at the bulbomembranous junction.[26] Complete tears occur 65% of the time in the posterior urethra.[26]

Any patient with an anticipated urethral tear must have an RUG before urethral catheterization.[11,25,27,34,37,38,47] Tears at the urogenital diaphragm demonstrate extravasation into the peritoneum. These are significant tears because cellulitis and sepsis can occur. Stricture is inevitable with these tears.[25]

MANAGEMENT. Catheterization by anyone other than the urologist should not be performed if any indication or potential for urethral injury is present. Catheterization can convert an incomplete tear of the urethra to a complete tear, increase the risk of infection, and infect a sterile hematoma.[37] Catheter placement should be avoided if a posterior tear is identified on RUG.[26] If the patient can void spontaneously, catheterization is ill advised because any tear is likely partial.[38] Complete disruption on RUG does not preclude only a partial tear of the urethra. A single attempt at catheterization should be made, and if this is not successful, a suprapubic tube should be placed.[11] When placing a Foley catheter in a male patient, it is imperative to remember that the first urine encountered is from passage through the membranous urethra. The catheter must be advanced another 3.5 cm before the bladder is reached.[25]

Management of urethral injury generally involves the placement of a suprapubic cystostomy (SPT) to divert urine from the area of injury if a catheter cannot be placed successfully or if the patient is critically ill.[8,27,34,38,47-49] To avoid infection the hematoma is usually not evacuated. Treatment varies and is still somewhat controversial with regard to outcomes and complications. The goals of treatment are to maintain patency of the urethra, continence, and potency.[49] Treatment options include direct repair, realignment, and nonoperative management with SPT placement.[38] A large-diameter catheter is essential with pelvic fractures to divert urine and allow fixation of the pelvis.[11] During pelvic repair the urologist may chose to perform primary realignment of the urethra.[11]

The most common management of prostatomembranous urethra injury involves SPT placement with delayed urethroplasty.[8,34,47] The incidence of incontinence and impotence is decreased with delayed repair although the occurrence of stricture is guaranteed.[27,49] Use of SPT avoids entry into the pelvic hematoma, thereby decreasing the risk of infection and blood loss and avoiding mobilization of the prostate.[49] If rectal injuries are present, immediate operation is required. During this time, evacuation of the hematoma with primary urethral realignment over a Foley catheter can be performed. Preservation of the bladder neck is essential to maintain continence.[27,48]

Acute realignment of injury to the urethra is becoming more common. The procedure increases the incidence of erectile dysfunction and incontinence but decreases the occurrence of stricture.[8,34,47,49] Early realignment reestablishes continuity and eliminates the need for delayed urethroplasty and long-term SPT placement.[47] Primary realignment is performed either by endoscopy or fluoroscopy.

Anterior urethral injuries are managed with a transurethral catheter or SPT for approximately 3 weeks.[8,27,34] Strictures are likely to occur and require urethroplasty after 3 months.[27] RUG is required before Foley or SPT removal to ensure urethral continuity.

Penetrating injuries generally require surgical intervention. Debridement and cleansing are done along with reconstruction of the injury. Management after debridement is the same as mentioned previously.

Missed urethral injuries in the female patient result in severe complications, which include sepsis and necrotizing infection.[11] A delayed diagnosis in the female patient results in incontinence, ureterovaginal fistulae, urethral diverticula, dyspareunia, hematuria, abscess, recurrent urethritis, or cystitis.[11]

TRAUMA TO THE BLADDER

The bladder of an adult rests within the pelvic region of the lower abdomen, well protected by the pelvis. Injury to the bladder occurs during a significant transfer of kinetic energy to the pelvis. Another mechanism of injury to the bladder occurs when the bladder is full and, as a result of its larger size, it is less protected by the bony pelvis. Although injury to the bladder is usually caused by blunt trauma, gunshot wounds to the bladder result in intraperitoneal rupture and urine leak.[17] Patients who present with bladder rupture after minor trauma should be suspected of having a preexisting bladder condition, such as cancer or an infiltrative disease (e.g., tuberculosis or amyloidosis), or having undergone previous radiation treatments.

When the pelvis is fractured or the bladder distended, the normal protective mechanisms are lost and the bladder is at higher risk for injury. As the number of pubic rami fractures increases, the risk of bladder rupture increases.[39,50] The bladder is relatively mobile except for the bladder neck. The dome is its weakest point and is vulnerable to rupture.[36]

The incidence of intraperitoneal bladder rupture is 15% to 45% and occurs primarily in children.[36] In children under 6 years the risk for bladder injury is high because the bladder is an abdominal organ.[36] Intraperitoneal ruptures usually result from a blow to the lower abdomen or a seat belt deceleration injury.[5,11,36,37,39] Increased intravesicular pressure results in a tear in the dome of a full bladder (Figure 25-5).

The incidence of extraperitoneal bladder injury is 50% to 85% among patients with pelvic fractures.[36] Fracture of the

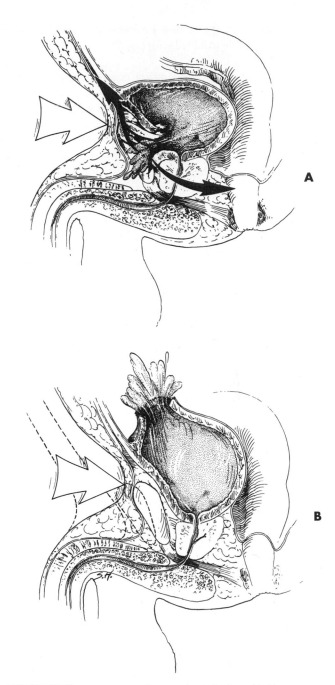

FIGURE 25-5 **A,** Mechanism of extraperitoneal urinary bladder rupture. The pubic rami are fractured, and the bladder is perforated by a bony fragment. **B,** Mechanism of intraperitoneal vesical rupture. A sharp blow is delivered to the lower abdomen of a patient with a distended urinary bladder. The distensive force is exerted on all surfaces of the bladder, and it ruptures at its weakest point, usually the dome. (From Peters P, Sagalowsky A: Genitourinary trauma. In Walsh P, Gittes R, Perlmutter A et al, editors: *Campbell's urology*, ed 5, vol 1, Philadelphia, 1986, WB Saunders.)

anterior pelvic arch is the most frequently associated injury.[5] In the case of pelvic fracture a bony spicule punctures the bladder.[5,8,37,39] Only 35% of extraperitoneal bladder ruptures occur on the same side as the pelvic fracture.[36] In addition to direct injury, the pelvic fracture may disrupt the bladder ligaments of attachment, resulting in injury.[39]

Combination intraperitoneal and extraperitoneal bladder injuries have a 5% to 12% incidence.[36,37]

ASSESSMENT. Bladder rupture is associated with gross hematuria (87%-98%), tachycardia, hypotension, and decreased hematocrit.[5,39] The patient with a ruptured bladder may present with pain in the shoulder area, a sign of urine in the peritoneal cavity. The patient may also be unable to void. A urine specimen reveals gross or microscopic hematuria.[5,39] Microscopic hematuria is indicative of a bladder contusion and should resolve over a few days.[5] The most common bladder injury is contusion.[11]

The patient may be in shock and have multiple associated injuries. The most common coexisting injuries include bowel lacerations and laceration of major vessels, including the vena cava, mesentery, and renal or iliac arteries or veins.

Definitive diagnosis of bladder rupture is made by cystogram.[11,36] Urethral injury must be ruled out before placement of a catheter for the procedure. On cystogram intraperitoneal bladder rupture is demonstrated by contrast material outlining bowel loops, filling the cul de sac, and extending into the paracolic gutters. Urine and blood may collect in the peritoneal space. Extraperitoneal bladder rupture demonstrates feathery flames of contrast on cystogram. Occasionally the cystogram may reveal a bladder that is teardrop shaped. This change in shape is due to the presence of large pelvic hematomas or urine extravasation.[27] The pressure of these hematomas on the bladder creates the teardrop configuration.

MANAGEMENT OF EXTRAPERITONEAL BLADDER RUPTURE.
Management of extraperitoneal bladder rupture consists of drainage via a large transurethral catheter or SPT.[36] Antibiotics may be administered to decrease urine colonization and resultant urinary tract infection.[36] Nonoperative management results in minimal morbidity. Drainage is necessary for approximately 10 days or until extravasation no longer occurs.[8,36,50] Cystogram is used to identify closure of the rupture.[8]

Spontaneous repair of bladder rupture occurs in 74% of patients within 10 to 14 days.[50] If severe bleeding with clots, sepsis, or persistent extravasation occurs, exploration is necessary. Extraperitoneal bladder injury results in a 26% delayed healing rate with vesicocutaneous fistula development, sepsis, bladder calculi, and death.[50] The mortality, though, is primarily associated with nonurologic causes.

Bacterial colonization of the bladder occurs within a few days as a result of catheterization despite adequate urine drainage.[50] Multiple catheterizations and bladder irrigation increase the colonization risk. Hence adequate bladder drainage is essential. In addition, antibiotic coverage for both gram-positive and gram-negative bacteria may be considered to decrease the risk of infection.[50] Inadequate bladder drainage results in retrograde infection and colonization of the pelvic hematoma.

Maintaining catheter patency within the first 24 to 48 hours is integral to successful nonoperative management. If patency cannot be maintained, exploration and closure of the bladder injury are necessary.[34,50] Ureteral stents may be used to ensure bladder drainage.[34]

MANAGEMENT OF INTRAPERITONEAL BLADDER RUPTURE.
An intraperitoneal bladder rupture must be surgically repaired, the pelvic hematoma left undisturbed, and extravasated urine and blood evacuated.[8,34,36] Nonviable bladder tissue is removed, the tear is sutured, and a suprapubic catheter tube is placed for urine drainage.

Unrecognized intraperitoneal bladder rupture can result in hyperkalemia, hypernatremia, uremia, and acidosis as a result of resorption of the extravasated urine.[11] Continued extravasation of urine may result in peritonitis, abscess, fistula, or uroascites with respiratory compromise.[36] Infected urine may contribute to septic complications. Delay in diagnosis may produce symptoms similar to an acute condition in the abdomen.

Mokoena and Naidu documented cases of isolated bladder rupture that presented as metabolic derangement and peritonitis.[51] The resorption of urea and creatinine through the peritoneum is a form of dialysis that results in increased serum blood urea nitrogen (BUN) and creatinine. Patients with delayed presentation were predominantly young males with minor trauma sustained while intoxicated, with a mean presentation of 5.4 days after injury.

TRAUMA TO THE URETER
The ureter is a muscular tube with an adventitial sheath that acts as a conduit for urine from the kidney to the bladder. The ureter is mobile with fixed points at the bladder and where the ureter crosses the pelvic brim.

Ureteral injuries are typically the result of iatrogenic injury during surgery or penetrating trauma.[6,9] Gunshot and stab wounds are common causes of penetrating ureteral injury and may produce partial or complete transection.[6]

Ureteral injury is rarely produced by blunt trauma but, when present, is usually in the form of disruption at the ureteropelvic junction.[9,31] Blunt ureteral injury may be caused by the excessive force produced by a fall or ejection from a motor vehicle or a major hyperextension of the lower thoracic or upper lumbar area.[9,31] UPJ and ureter injuries occur mostly in children.[6,9,31]

Ureteral trauma can be described as a silent injury, often with no presenting symptoms. Ureteral trauma is suspected when hematuria is present with a normal IVP or CT. The direction of penetrating trauma and hyperextension of the spine during blunt injury indicate that there is potential for ureteral injury.

ASSESSMENT. The patient may complain of pain only when the ureter is obstructed. Unilateral ureteral obstruction may produce a slight, transient increase in serum creatinine or BUN levels, but urine output typically does not change. A patient may lose complete kidney function secondary to unilateral ureteral injury yet remain asymptomatic if the contralateral kidney is able to maintain renal function. In patients with a solitary kidney, loss of function as a result of misdiagnosed ureteral injury can be life threatening. Bilateral ureteral injury is rare but may be induced iatrogenically.

Ureter injury is frequently diagnosed by IVP or intravenous urethrogram. Especially after penetrating injury, dye can be injected into the ureter and extravasation determined during the operative procedure for abdominal injury. CT is not a better method of identifying the injury.[6] Retrograde pyelogram is not usually feasible in the critically injured.[6]

Delayed diagnosis of ureteral injury is not uncommon because of the lack of signs and symptoms and the inaccessibility of the upper ureters.[6,14] Delayed diagnosis, however, carries a significant morbidity because of the loss of renal function.[14]

MANAGEMENT.   The goal of ureter repair is to preserve renal function and restore continuity of the collecting system.[6] Laceration of the ureter can be repaired surgically or stented to divert urine and prevent urinoma formation.[31] Definitive reconstruction occurs after the patient is stabilized and acidosis, hypothermia, and coagulopathies are reversed.[15] Gross bleeding must be controlled, but the time required for stenting or nephrostomy is not available. Primary ureter repair is the option during damage control surgery. The risk of bleeding as a result of delayed repair of the ureter is minimal.[34] Spontaneous drainage of urine into the abdomen must be avoided.[34] Drainage via stent or

ligation with nephrostomy is necessary. Significant delay in repair may result in loss of a kidney, especially when UPJ injury is involved.[9] Nephrectomy is avoided through rapid percutaneous ureterostomy,[15] although in the pediatric trauma patient with UPJ injury nephrectomy is common.[6]

Trauma to the lower third of the ureter may be repaired by reimplantation into the bladder or by ureteroureterostomy (the anastomosis of ureteral ends) (Figure 25-6). Injury to the upper and middle thirds of the ureter may be best managed by ureteroureterostomy.[9] Internal silicone stenting catheters are placed to maintain alignment, ensure patency, prevent urinary extravasation, and provide support. These stents remain in place for several weeks or months and are removed by cystoscopy. Complications of ureteroureterostomy increase when colon injury, multiple abdominal injury, intraoperative bleeding, or shock is present.[15]

Loss of extensive segments of ureter may necessitate a transureteroureterostomy, the anastomosis of the injured ureter into the contralateral ureter (Figure 25-7). If this procedure is not possible, the injured ureter may be replaced with ileum in an attempt to prevent loss of renal function.

Penetrating ureter injuries require irrigation and debridement followed by primary repair.[15] Vascular reconstruction in the face of urinary leak requires primary repair or stenting to decrease the leak.[6]

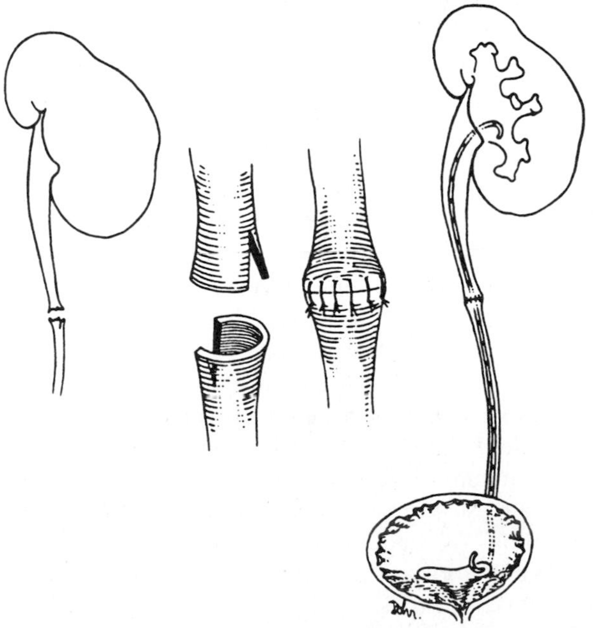

FIGURE 25-6 **Spatulation of Ureteral Ends Before Ureteroureterostomy Over an Internal Ureteral Stent.** Watertight closure is accomplished. (From McAninch J: Injuries to the urinary system. In Blaisdell WF, Trunkey D, editors: *Trauma management,* vol 1, *Abdominal trauma,* New York, 1982, Thieme Stratton.)

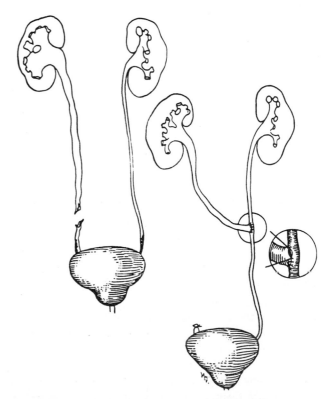

FIGURE 25-7 **Technique of Transureteroureterostomy.** (From McAninch J: Injuries to the urinary system. In Blaisdell WF, Trunkey D, editors: *Trauma management,* vol 1, *Abdominal trauma,* New York, 1982, Thieme Stratton.)

TABLE 25-3	Renal Injury Classifications				
	I	II	III	IV	V
Federle M, 1990	Contusion	Laceration into collecting system, extravasation	Shattered kidney, pedicle injury	UPJ avulsion	—
Moore, Shackford, Pachter et al, 1989	Contusion	Minor laceration without collecting system involvement	Major laceration into the medulla, extravasation	Vascular injury	Vascular and parenchymal injury
Thall et al, 1996	Contusion	Solitary laceration without collecting system involvement	Deep laceration with or without extravasation	Renal vascular-pedicle injury	—

Sources: Federle M: Evaluation of renal trauma. In Pollack HM, editor: *Clinical urography*, Philadelphia, 1990, WB Saunders, 1472-1494; Moore EE, Shackford SR, Pachter HL et al: Organ injury scanning: spleen, liver and kidney, *J Trauma* 29:1664-1666,1989; and Thall EH, Stone NN, Cheny DL et al: Conservative management of penetrating and blunt Type III renal injuries, *Br J Urol* 77:512-517, 1996.

After ureteral repair the patient must be observed for potential complications, which include obstruction, pseudocyst, obstructive hydronephrosis, fistula, and urinoma.[6,31] Fistulas may develop as a result of stricture or obstruction. Persistent leakage of urine may follow. If the ureteral injury is missed, fistula development may cause inflammation that may prevent repair.

Stricture formation leading to hydronephrosis is another complication of ureteral injury.[31] This problem may develop slowly and may not be evident for months. An IVP is recommended at 6 weeks and again at 3 months after stent removal to monitor the healing process and monitor for the development of stricture formation.

Retroperitoneal urinoma is a complication related to delay in diagnosis or prolonged extravasation at the repair site. Patients with penetrating ureteral trauma who have a low-grade fever, prolonged ileus, or flank pain may have developed a urinoma.[6] Drains are placed until urine leak ceases. These drains should be well protected from contamination and enclosed in a sterile bag. Urinomas can ultimately result in obstruction and local inflammation, both signs of late recognition.[6]

Infection is a threat to the patient who has experienced ureteral trauma. Infection of the urine during the perioperative period may produce retroperitoneal scarring, abscess formation, or pyelonephritis. Urine cultures are monitored carefully, and antibiotics are administered as required.

TRAUMA TO THE KIDNEY

The kidneys lie behind the liver and colon and are in close proximity to the spleen, stomach, jejunum, and pancreas. Injury to these viscera is often associated with renal injury.

The kidney is mobile and is attached by a pedicle consisting of the renal artery, renal vein, and ureter. Its mobility can be detrimental in an acceleration-deceleration injury, whereby the organ is put into motion, is contused by the ribs and abdominal viscera, and rotates on the pedicle.

Renal trauma is often classified according to mechanism of injury. Blunt renal trauma is caused primarily by motor vehicle collisions, pedestrian versus car events, assault, and sports injuries. Penetrating renal trauma is caused by knife

or gunshot wounds or impalement injuries. The majority of renal injuries are contusions, whether the cause is blunt or penetrating trauma.[2,4,15] In children the incidence of renal injury is second only to head injury and higher than that of all abdominal injuries.[4]

STAGING OF RENAL INJURIES. Renal injury is staged by severity as identified on CT scan. Table 25-3 lists the staging of renal injuries.[1,31] Staging guides treatment, thus influencing outcomes. Inadequate staging or underrepresentation of the severity of injury results in increased morbidity and mortality.[2] There is no universally accepted classification system for staging renal injuries. An example of a classification system for renal injury is seen in Figure 25-8.

ASSESSMENT. Patients with minor renal trauma usually present with costovertebral angle pain on palpation. A flank mass may indicate a tamponaded perirenal hematoma. Bruising may be evident over the eleventh and twelfth ribs. IVP is normal or shows a slight delay in function in patients with minor renal injury. Microscopic or gross hematuria may be present. Patients with microscopic hematuria can be discharged home with hydration and follow-up care to monitor clearance of the hematuria.[4]

MANAGEMENT. The management priority for renal trauma is salvage of renal function. Clinically unstable patients require surgery to repair or remove the injured kidney.[31] Nonoperative management of major renal lacerations may be safe in the patient that remains hemodynamically stable.[52] Timely percutaneous or endoscopic drainage of urine minimizes loss of renal tissue.[2] Grades I and II injuries are usually managed successfully without operative intervention.[1,4,16] Nonoperative management of renal injury requires monitoring of renal function through urine output and serum chemistries.

Hemodynamic stability is key to successful nonoperative management.[16,35] Decreasing hemoglobin and hematocrit requiring transfusion indicate changes in a previously stable patient with perinephric hematoma. Renal lacerations are surrounded by a perinephric hematoma, which provides a tamponade effect on bleeding. A perinephric hematoma

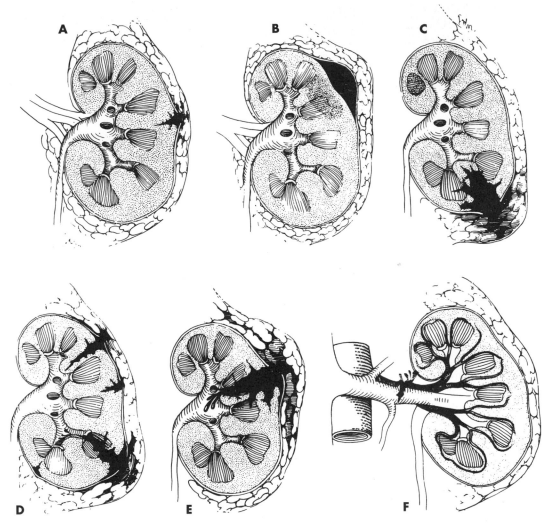

FIGURE 25-8 **Classification of Renal Injuries. A,** Minor parenchymal lacerations involving only the renal cortex. **B,** Contusion has evidence of injury without parenchymal laceration. **C,** Major parenchymal lacerations extend through cortex and into the renal medulla **(D)** and include lacerations of collecting system **(E). F,** Vascular injuries include injuries to the main renal artery or vein or their segmental branches. (From McAninch JW, Carroll PR, Loosterman PA et al: Renal reconstruction after injury, *J Urol* 145(5):993, 1991.)

with hemodynamic stability is an indication for nonoperative management. Operative procedures to repair the kidney have not demonstrated a decrease in complication rate.[35] Gentle palpation of any flank mass by the same examiner over time allows assessment of expansion in size of the perinephric hematoma. CT or angiography may be indicated to identify a source of the bleeding if hemodynamic instability occurs. Repeated CT scanning may be performed to monitor extravasation of blood and urine or expansion of a retroperitoneal hematoma. Indications for surgery include the development of sepsis, falling hemoglobin and hematocrit levels despite blood replacement, an expanding perirenal mass, or the inability to maintain hemodynamic stability despite supportive care.[35]

Patients with major renal trauma may present with a palpable flank mass, gross hematuria, shock, or microscopic hematuria. Ecchymosis may be evident over the flank and lower ribs. These patients may complain of abdominal and flank tenderness. The eleventh and twelfth ribs may be

fractured. Life-threatening hemorrhage may occur from renal arterial or venous bleeding.

Grade III injuries are also staged through the use of CT. An IVP is inadequate to accurately stage the injury. Grade III injuries in hemodynamically stable patients can be managed nonoperatively.[1,16] Reassessment and restaging of the injury are essential to nonoperative management because accumulation of free urine and blood in the collecting ducts and in the area surrounding the kidney may cause further renal damage and infection.[31]

Percutaneous drainage of the urinoma, often associated with a grade III injury, is necessary to prevent a delayed nephrectomy.[2,34] Fifty percent of grade III injuries with extravasation spontaneously resolve within 4 or 5 days.[4] Potential complications of nonoperative management of grade III lacerations with extravasation include abscess, hypertension, ureteral obstruction, renal cysts, and dystrophic calcification.[4] Nonoperative management of grade III and IV injuries is associated with a risk of delayed bleeding.[16]

Grade IV injuries involve pedicle or vascular injuries. All authors cited recommend immediate operation for Grade IV injuries.[1,2,4,16] Arteriography is indicated when vascular injury is suspected because a thrombosis at the site can partially or completely occlude the artery. Surgery is frequently necessary to treat not only the renal injury but also the associated injuries. Urinary extravasation is drained, and expanding retroperitoneal hematomas are explored. An expanding, pulsatile hematoma or spontaneous bleeding outside the fascia requires exploration.[34] Immediate exploration, although required as a life-saving procedure, results in a 20% to 43% incidence of nephrectomy.[1]

If the patient is hemodynamically stable, arterial reconstruction can be undertaken.[34] Early vascular control preserves renal function before reconstruction.[4] In the unstable patient selective renal artery embolization may be necessary.[34] Delays in definitive repair of vascular injuries result in renal tissue loss as a result of ischemia.[34]

Despite appropriate intervention, large parts of the injured parenchyma may be lost or may have sustained significant injury resulting in devitalized tissue before intervention. Devitalized segments can result in delayed hemorrhage; determination of the degree of devitalized tissue by CT is essential to management.[16] Devitalized renal tissue leads to an 85% risk of complications, which include urinoma and abscess of the pancreas and small bowel.[52] The presence of devitalized tissue of the kidneys requires surgery to improve patient outcome.

Extensive damage to the upper or lower pole of the kidney may necessitate partial or total nephrectomy. Damage to the midportion of the kidney may necessitate a renorrhaphy, in which the devitalized midportion of the renal parenchyma is removed and the parenchymal edges are approximated.

Before a nephrectomy it is essential to evaluate the uninjured kidney for function. An arteriogram should be considered before or during surgery if the noninjured kidney cannot be visualized by IVP and the patient is hemodynamically stable.

COMPLICATIONS.   Complications less than 4 weeks after renal injury include hemorrhage, abscess, infected urinoma, arteriovenous fistula, and prolonged extravasation.[2,31,52] Complications of nonoperative management of renal injury include ischemic renal atrophy, hypertension, and hydronephrotic nephrolithiasis.[4] Hypertension, cystitis, infection, arteriovenous fistula, infected hematoma, hydronephrosis, atrophy, and dystrophic calcification are considered late complications and occur more than 4 weeks after injury.[2,31]

Persistent extravasation of urine is a significant complication of renal injury, resulting in inflammation and sepsis.[34] Extensive extravasation along with devitalized segments and coexisting bowel and pancreas injury are relative indications for surgical renal exploration.[52] Delayed renal repair may be necessary if extravasation worsens.[1] In 87% of cases extravasation resolves spontaneously with the use of stents or percutaneous drains.[52] In this situation broad-spectrum antibiotics may be used to prevent infection by skin and fecal flora.[34] Closed system urine drainage also prevents colonization and resultant infection.[34]

Hypertension.   Another complication of renal trauma is hypertension. The incidence ranges from 1% to 40% and can develop from 2 weeks to 10 years after injury.[2,53] The duration is unknown.[53] Hypertension is associated with renal pedicle injury. Renal pedicle injury must be treated quickly and urinoma resolved.[4,53] Early onset hypertension is associated with laceration of the renal artery or its branches. Nephrectomy or revascularization relieves hypertension.[53] The etiology of hypertension is renal infarct, scarring, hydronephrosis, chronic infection, vascular injury, and Page kidney.[4] Page kidney is compression of the renal parenchyma resulting in ischemia and hence excess renin production.[4,53] Page kidney has a low incidence and usually resolves on its own.[31]

Renal injury-induced hypertension should be suspected when essential hypertension occurs in patients under age 40 or when new-onset hypertension occurs in the elderly.[53] Untreated hypertension in people under age 35 reduces life expectancy by 16.5 years.[53] Long-term follow-up of patients after renal injury is necessary to promptly identify and manage hypertension early.[2,4,53]

The majority of cases of hypertension are low grade and resolve spontaneously or with a short course of medication.[53] Operative intervention to relieve compression of the kidney is required if hypertension worsens, organ deterioration occurs, the side effects of the medications are intolerable, or the patient does not take the medications prescribed.

Hypertension may also be related to a renal arteriovenous fistula that causes ischemia distal to the fistula, stimulating excess renin production.[53] Renal arteriography with renal vein renin assays is necessary. A comparison is made between the renin production of the two kidneys. Increased renin production is diagnosed when the affected kidney to contralateral kidney ratio of renin is 1.5:1 to 2:1.[53] Arteriography and renal vein renin assay studies predict lesions amenable to surgery in more than 90% of cases.[53] Renal arteriovenous fistula repair eliminates hypertension by removal of the cause.

CRITICAL CARE PHASE

The critical care phase in the management of genitourinary trauma focuses the caregiver's attention on hemodynamic changes and potential complications. Many genitourinary complications are not associated with direct GU trauma but with the management or effects of associated injuries.

HEMORRHAGE

The potential for bleeding and hemorrhage is present after almost all genitourinary trauma as described previously for specific organ injuries. Care is directed toward correcting and maintaining adequate oxygen delivery to all organs. Hemodynamic and ventilation-perfusion parameters must be assessed at frequent intervals. Positive inotropic infusions are used only after adequate blood volume is ensured. Awareness of the effects of inadequate circulating volumes and vasoactive drugs on renal function is essential, especially if renal injury has occurred.

Serial hemoglobin, hematocrit, and coagulation studies are monitored. The patient must be observed closely for bleeding from surgical sites or drains, for evidence of hematuria or myoglobinuria formation, and for expansion of an abdominal or flank mass. A pulmonary artery catheter may be used to allow the evaluation of circulating volume and for the prevention of fluid overload.

Prevention of hypotension and hypothermia is essential because both may contribute to oliguria, anuria, and loss of renal function. Urinary output must be maintained. A rise in blood pressure during the critical care phase may indicate constriction of the renal parenchyma, vascular injury, or potential deterioration in renal function. Safeguarding the function of the renal parenchyma is essential to the patient after unilateral nephrectomy.

GENITOURINARY INFECTION

After surgery the critically ill patient with genitourinary injury will have a multitude of invasive monitoring and drainage devices. Consequently this patient is at high risk for infection. Strict aseptic technique must be maintained when caring for any drain, surgical site, or urinary drainage system. The urinary or suprapubic catheter must be secured to prevent accidental dislodgment. In female patients the urinary catheter is secured to the inner thigh by either adhesive tape or a Velcro strap. In male patients the urinary drainage catheter is secured to the abdomen. In this patient population a dislodged urinary drainage catheter should not be replaced until a careful evaluation has been made by the urologist. The urinary drainage system (urinary and ureterostomy catheters) must be kept closed to prevent the entrance of organisms.

A kinked or obstructed urinary catheter may allow the stagnation of urine and promote the growth of pathogens. An obstructed drain may produce pooling of extravasated blood or urine, leading to abscess formation and sepsis.[31]

The patient is observed for signs and symptoms of infection, including dysuria, frequency, low back pain, suprapubic pain, and foul, cloudy urine. Infectious processes include perinephric abscess, renal abscess, urinoma infection, and sepsis. Trends in temperature and white blood cell counts should be monitored. Urine must be sent for culture and sensitivity, and appropriate antibiotics are administered as ordered.

Perineal wounds should be monitored for signs of infection, including necrosis and soft, foul-smelling drainage, which may indicate a necrotizing infection. A colostomy is usually present to divert the fecal stream from the perineal wound.

PAIN MANAGEMENT

The patient with genitourinary trauma may experience severe pain caused by edema from hemorrhage, tissue damage, and associated injuries. Ice packs placed on the scrotal area and penis may be of benefit in reducing pain. Commercially available products may be used, or crushed ice may be placed in a surgical glove. When ice packs are used, extreme care is required to avoid cold burns because the skin over these organs is thin and fragile. For severe scrotal swelling a scrotal support may reduce pain aggravated by the additional weight of swollen tissue. Use of commercially available scrotal supports or providing support with a towel functioning as a sling are effective.

RHABDOMYOLYSIS AND MYOGLOBINURIA

Rhabdomyolysis is a syndrome of ischemia followed by reperfusion, resulting in the release of inflammatory mediators and further injury to the myocytes.[54,55] Injured muscle tissue releases myoglobin, which enters the circulation and results in acute renal failure if untreated.

Partial tissue perfusion has greater systemic effects than complete occlusion because of the effects of reperfusion injury. Tissue inflammatory mediators such as cytokines and eicosanoids cause endothelial disruption and cellular damage.[54] Lipid peroxidation from oxygen-derived free radicals causes increased cellular permeability and rupture.[54] The cellular damage results in the release of myoglobin, creatine kinase (CK), potassium, and phosphorous.

The causes of rhabdomyolysis include direct or indirect muscle injury.[56] Causes of muscle injury include crush injury, compartment syndrome, quail consumption, application of military antishock trousers (MAST), burns, lightning strikes, poisonous insect or reptile bites, and compression of one or more limbs caused by a prolonged period in one position.[54,55,57,58] Periods of ischemia to muscle of less than 1.5 hours usually allow full recovery. More than 4 hours of ischemia leads to irreversible injury, and more than 6 hours results in necrosis.[54]

Myoglobinuria is an accurate marker of rhabdomyolysis.[57] Myoglobin is an oxygen-binding protein with a higher affinity for oxygen than hemoglobin.[54] Thus oxygen is tightly bound to myoglobin, reducing oxygen delivery. Oxygen is released from myoglobin only when a hypoxic state exists. Myoglobinuria presents as dark, tea-colored urine that tests positive for blood with a urine dipstick but is without red blood cells on urinalysis.[58]

Myoglobinuria has a renal tubulotoxic effect because of the myoglobin degradation product ferrihematine. This byproduct results in tubular obstruction, altered renal blood flow, and ultimately reversible oliguria.[57] Mortality associated with rhabdomyolysis and myoglobinuria is 8%. The mortality rate is significantly lower than that associated with renal tubular destruction from aminoglycosides (25%-30%) and sepsis (70%-80%).[57]

ASSESSMENT. Rhabdomyolysis presents as a significantly increased serum CK (normal CK is 45-260 IU/L) with myoglobinuria. The serum CK is released from the injured muscle tissue.[54] Less specific indicators of rhabdomyolysis are elevated lactate dehydrogenase (LDH), aspartate aminotransferase, uric acid, and phosphorous levels and decreased serum calcium levels.[57] Calcium is decreased as it is deposited into the injured muscle tissue. Later, serum calcium levels rise as a result of the resolution of soft tissue calcification and increased parathyroid hormone excretion.[57]

MANAGEMENT. Treatment goals for patients with rhabdomyolysis/myoglobinuria are prevention or attenuation of acute renal failure (ARF) through intravenous fluid administration, diuresis, and alkalinization of urine.[57] Intravenous fluids maintain circulating blood volume and renal perfusion. The objective is to flush the myoglobin from the kidneys with a urine output of 100 to 200 ml/hr.[57] Diuresis with mannitol also protects the kidneys because mannitol acts as a scavenger of the oxygen metabolite hydroxyl radical.[58] Another free radical scavenger that may have potential for use in myoglobinuria is pentoxifylline, which decreases neutrophil adhesion and cytokine release.[58] Other antioxidants such as vitamins E and C, zinc, manganese, selenium, and glutathione have not been studied.

Alkalinization of urine prevents the breakdown of myoglobin into the ferrihematine byproduct, increases myoglobin solubility, and decreases cast formation.[57,58] The treatment goal is to raise urine pH to more than 6. Iron chelation therapy with mannitol may prevent hydroxyl radical release after muscle ischemia.

Inadequate management of rhabdomyolysis/myoglobinuria results in acute renal failure. Impending ARF may be signaled by a urine specific gravity greater than 1.025 and decreased urine output.[58] Venous bicarbonate is the most accurate predictor of ARF after rhabdomyolysis has occurred.[58] ARF associated with rhabdomyolysis is usually oliguric with increased creatinine, BUN, and potassium.[57] Temporary dialysis resolves the ARF.[57] These patients have an excellent potential for recovery if identified and treated rapidly.[56]

ACUTE RENAL FAILURE

Acute renal failure is a syndrome characterized by an acute deterioration in renal function. ARF results in the inadequate excretion of various end products of cellular metabolism and an impaired ability to regulate fluid, electrolyte, and pH balance.[59] Figure 25-9 provides a review of normal renal functional anatomy.

Renal failure is a serious complication of trauma and occasionally of renal injury. It is important to distinguish between renal failure and pseudorenal failure. Pseudorenal failure can occur when urine extravasates into the abdominal cavity.[60] The urine then dialyses across the peritoneum.

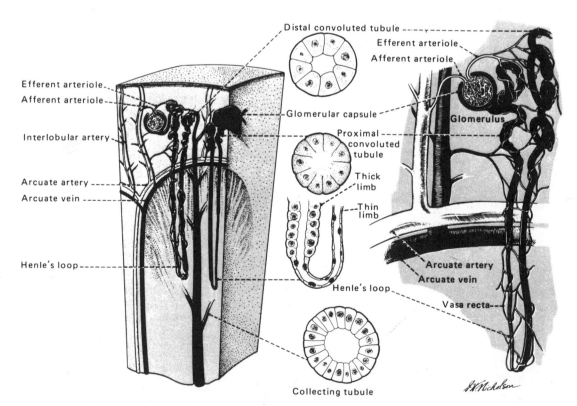

FIGURE 25-9 The Nephron and its Blood Supply are Shown at the Sides of this Figure. Sections of different portions of the tubule are shown in the center. (From Langley LL, Telford I, Christianson J: *Dynamic anatomy and physiology,* New York, 1980, McGraw-Hill.)

It is usually a delayed presentation after injury to a full bladder resulting in intraperitoneal bladder rupture. The patient demonstrates hyponatremia, dehydration, and apparent renal failure. Pseudorenal failure rapidly resolves when urine is drained away from the abdomen.[60]

Renal failure may result from direct renal injury or secondary injury as a result of hypovolemia and rhabdomyolysis/myoglobinuria. A cause of secondary renal failure is increased intraabdominal pressure or abdominal compartment syndrome. One of the earliest signs of abdominal compartment syndrome is decreased urine output.[61] As pressure in the abdomen increases, the renal artery is compressed. Renal perfusion is impaired, and renal failure ensues. Sugrue et al demonstrated that increased intraabdominal pressure in and of itself is significant enough to result in ARF.[62] Decompression of the abdomen through a laparotomy incision provides rapid treatment of abdominal compartment syndrome and the resultant ARF.[61]

Acute renal failure is a potentially life-threatening complication of trauma with or without primary genitourinary or renal injury. Acute renal failure results in a loss of normal function and is subclassified by its etiology. Prerenal failure is a result of inadequate perfusion of the kidney without actual renal tissue damage. Intrarenal failure results from direct insult to the renal parenchyma by prolonged ischemia, injury to the nephron, or infectious or immunologic processes. Postrenal failure occurs as a result of an obstruction in the drainage system.[63]

Causes of renal failure include hypotension, transfusion reaction, contract media, rhabdomyolysis, aminoglycoside administration, sepsis, systemic inflammatory response syndrome, and vasopressor administration.[58] Mortality from renal failure is greater than 50%, with a chronic medical history of renal dysfunction and nephrotoxic medications as contributing factors.[58] Less than one third of all cases of acute renal failure are the result of inadequate resuscitation.[58]

PRERENAL FAILURE.   Trauma patients are at great risk for developing prerenal failure. Hypotension caused by hemorrhage, hypovolemia, and cardiac failure cause decreased renal blood flow. Renal blood flow can remain relatively stable despite significant variance in the mean arterial pressure (MAP).[63] When the MAP falls below 50 mm Hg for any reason, autoregulatory mechanisms fail and urine output falls. Creatinine is not a good predictor of prerenal failure because there may not be a rise until 50% to 90% of glomerular filtration is lost.[58]

Mannitol administration and contrast media injection may result in diuresis but do not reflect true renal function.[58] Thus the renal function of trauma patients in the resuscitative phase and those with head injuries is more difficult to evaluate. Prerenal oliguria returns to normal if perfusion to the kidneys is reestablished.

INTRARENAL FAILURE.   The type of intrarenal failure is determined by the section of the kidney that is injured. The outer layer, or cortex, is the vascular portion containing the glomeruli and distal convoluted tubules. Damage occurs by vascular, infectious, or inflammatory processes that result in swelling at the capillary bed (Table 25-4).

The second type of intrarenal failure is caused by damage to the middle layer, or medulla. The medullary tissue is composed of the collecting tubules, ducts, and the long loops of Henle (Table 25-5). Nephrotoxic agents, particularly antibiotics or contrast media, release crystals that lodge in the tubules and obstruct the flow of filtrate. A source of ischemic injury frequently seen in trauma patients is rhabdomyolysis (see previous discussion). The myoglobin released from muscle injury is too large to pass through the tubules and may become lodged in the tubule system, resulting in acute tubular necrosis (ATN).

POSTRENAL FAILURE.   Primary injury to any part of the urinary collection system, such as a ruptured bladder, interruption in ureteral or urethral integrity, or pressure from hematomas, may lead to postrenal failure. Other potential causes arise from sources of urinary retention such as neurogenic bladder or a urinary tract infection (UTI).

TABLE 25-4	**Intrarenal Failure: Common Sources of Cortical Damage**
Infectious	
Acute glomerulonephritis	
Acute pyelonephritis	
Immunologic	
Goodpasture's syndrome	
Systemic lupus erythematosus (SLE)	
Severe hypercalcemia	
Malignant hypertension	

TABLE 25-5	**Intrarenal Failure: Common Sources of Medullary Damage**
Nephrotoxic Sources	
Antibiotics	
Aminoglycosides	
Cephalosporins	
Tetracyclines	
X-ray contrast media	
Heavy metals	
Arsenic	
Lead	
Pesticides and fungicides	
Ischemic Sources	
Burns	
Crush injuries	
Massive hemorrhage	
Prolonged hypotension	
Sepsis	
Transfusion reactions	

CLINICAL PRESENTATION. Acute tubular necrosis, an intrarenal failure, is the classic model for the clinical presentation of ARF. It consists of five stages: onset, oliguric phase, nonoliguric phase, diuresis, and recovery.[59]

The onset or actual event (prerenal, intrarenal, or postrenal) initiates the sequelae of renal failure. Initially the kidney is able to successfully compensate for changes in the renal blood flow or filtration pressures. The oliguric phase is characterized by a urine output of less than 25 to 30 ml/hr with the presence of serum and urine electrolyte abnormalities. This phase generally lasts 10 to 20 days.

In the case of a less severe insult to the tubules, nonoliguric or high-output renal failure may develop. Electrolyte abnormalities occur, and the urine is poorly concentrated. Urine output is abnormally high, as much as 1 L/hr; however, creatinine clearance remains low. The duration of this phase is usually 5 to 8 days.

By comparison, the urine output in the diuretic phase is also elevated, to 125 to 150 ml/hr. However, as the kidneys begin to regain their function, the urine is more concentrated and the electrolyte imbalances are corrected. The diuresis occurs because of an excess fluid volume and a hyperosmolar state created by the elevated urea level.

The final phase of renal failure is recovery, which can last between 3 and 12 months. It is characterized by gradual restoration of renal function. The degree of recovery is determined largely by the severity of the damage and by early recognition and treatment.

Table 25-6 outlines the general signs and symptoms that are commonly seen within the various phases of renal failure.

ASSESSMENT. The hallmark of acute renal failure is low urine output. The decrease in output reflects abnormalities in the glomerular filtration rate (GFR) and regulatory mechanisms. Laboratory analysis offers the clinician useful data for diagnosing and monitoring the progress of ARF. Pertinent values and their norms are summarized in Table 25-7.

Creatinine clearance is the gold standard for monitoring glomerular filtration.[58] Creatinine, a normal byproduct of tissue metabolism, is excreted via glomerular filtration into the urine. Because the rate of tissue metabolism is usually constant and clearance occurs solely at the nephron, renal function may be readily assessed by collecting urine over a fixed amount of time and measuring concurrent urine and serum creatinine levels. A 2-hour creatinine clearance accurately reflects the glomerular filtration.[58] The creatinine clearance calculation is as follows[58]:

$$\frac{\text{Urine creatinine}}{\text{Serum creatinine}} \times \text{Urine volume (ml/min)} \times \frac{1.73}{\text{BSA (m}^2\text{)}}$$

The urine to plasma creatinine concentration ratio is usually greater than 40. In ATN the ratio drops below 20. As the glomerular filtration rate decreases in renal failure, the amount of creatinine cleared by the kidney also is reduced, resulting in an elevation of serum creatinine levels. The best and most accurate measure of acute renal failure is the fractional excretion of sodium (FENa).[58] A FENa of less than 1% suggests prerenal failure, whereas FENa greater than 2% indicates acute renal failure. FENa (%) is calculated as follows[58]:

$$\frac{\text{Urine Na}^+/\text{Serum Na}^+}{\text{Urine creatinine/Serum creatinine}} \times 100$$

TABLE 25-6	**Phases of Renal Failure**		
	Symptoms		
System Involved	**Oliguric Phase**	**Diuretic Phase**	**Recovery**
Neurologic	Decreased level of consciousness, muscular twitches, fatigue, apathy, seizures, coma	Decreased level of consciousness, lessened potential for seizure activity, potential for fatigue, apathy, restlessness	Normal
Cardiovascular	Elevated blood pressure, heart rate, cardiac output; potential cardiac pump failure; anemia; cardiac arrhythmias; pitting edema	Low blood pressure, elevated heart rate, elevated temperature, atrial or ventricular cardiac arrhythmias	Normal; may have residual blood pressure or cardiac arrhythmia problems
Pulmonary	Pulmonary edema, rales, Kussmaul's respiration	Tachypnea, Kussmaul's respiration	Normal
Metabolic	Hyperkalemia, hypermagnesemia, acidosis, hypernatremia	Hypokalemia, acidosis, hyponatremia	Normal
Gastrointestinal	Gastrointestinal bleeding, negative nitrogen balance, anorexia, nausea	Gastrointestinal bleeding, negative nitrogen balance, anorexia, nausea, thirst	Anorexia, nausea, thirst
Genitourinary	Decreased urine output	Increased urine output	Normal urine output, potential chronic renal failure, potential for impotence

With the increase in the serum creatinine, BUN levels also rise. However, because the BUN level is affected by many other factors, such as hypovolemia, hypercatabolism, and gastrointestinal bleeding, it is an unreliable measure of the GFR when viewed in isolation from other values. A simultaneous rise in the BUN and serum creatinine levels in a ratio greater than 10:1 is a better indicator of renal failure. A creatinine level of more than 2 mg/dl and increase in creatinine of 0.5 over the baseline with an associated increase in BUN is predictive of ARF.[54]

Other serum and urine electrolyte values are affected as the ability of the nephron to regulate their movement becomes progressively more impaired. As the tubules reabsorb increasing amounts of sodium and free water, serum sodium levels rise and urine values fall. The failure of the collecting tubules to excrete potassium is responsible for elevated serum potassium levels. Hemoglobin and hematocrit levels may be normal initially, but as the kidneys fail to produce erythropoietin, chronic anemia may ensue.

Urinalysis, specific gravities, and microbiology tests are also useful in monitoring the progression of renal failure. Significant urinalysis findings are summarized in Table 25-8 for each of the categories of renal failure.

PREVENTION. Prevention of ARF after trauma involves maintaining intravascular volume and renal perfusion, avoiding nephrotoxic agents or ensuring adequate intravascular volume loading before administration, and treating myoglobinuria to prevent hematin deposition.[58,63] Awareness of the potential for acute tubular necrosis and prerenal failure after injury is imperative in the critical care phase.

MANAGEMENT. Treatment goals and nursing interventions for patients with ARF focus on reversing or compensating for the deterioration in renal function. This is particularly challenging when dealing with severely injured patients. Fluid, electrolyte, and pH abnormalities may be exacerbated by underresuscitation, postresuscitation fluid overload, osmotic diuresis, hypothermia, hypoxia, nephrotoxic medications, or fluid restrictions.

TABLE 25-7 Normal Laboratory Values

Serum Analysis		Urine Analysis	
		Appearance: pale yellow, clear	
		Odor: mild ammonia	
Chloride	96-109 mEq/L	Chloride	110-250 mEq
CO_2	24-30 mEq/L	Specific gravity	1.005-1.030
BUN	12-25 mg/dl	Osmolality	300-1200 mOsm
Creatinine	0.4-1.5 mg/dl	—	—
pH	7.35-7.45	pH	4.5-8.0
Glucose	70-115 mg/dl	Glucose	0
Magnesium	1.5-2.0 mEq/L	Magnesium	100 mg
Potassium	3.5-5.0 mEq/L	Potassium	25-120 mEq
Sodium	135-145 mEq/l	Sodium	40-220 mEq
Calcium	9.0-10.5 mg/dl	Calcium	50-150 mg
Phosphorus	3.0-4.5 mg/dl	Ketones	0
Total protein	6.0-8.5 g/dl	Protein	<150 mg/24 hr
Albumin	3.2-5.3 g/dl	Crystals	0
Hemoglobin	13.9-16.3 g/dl	Casts	0
RBC	4.84 m/mm^3	RBC	<3/HPF
WBC	4500-11000/mm^3	WBC	<4/HPF
MCV	41%-53%	Creatinine clearance	125 ml/min
Platelets	150,000-350,000/mm^3		

BUN, Blood urea nitrogen; *HPF,* high-power field; *MCV,* mean corpuscular volume; *RBC,* red blood cells; *WBC,* white blood cells.

TABLE 25-8 Urinalysis in Renal Failure

	Prerenal Etiology	Intrarenal Etiology	Postrenal Etiology
Specific gravity	≥1.020	1.010	Normal
Myoglobin	May be positive	May be positive	Usually negative
Urine sodium	Low	High (>30 mEq/L)	Normal (<20 mEq/L)
Sediment	Normal	Renal tubular cells and cell casts; pigmented granular casts	Normal
Protein	<1 g/24 hr	<1 g/24 hr	<1 g/24 hr
Red blood cells	Microscopic	Microscopic	Microscopic
White blood cells	Few	Few	Few

Adequate nutrition, which assists in maintaining electrolyte balances, poses a special problem because of the high protein requirements of trauma patients. Protein, vital for tissue healing, produces urea as a metabolic byproduct. In the patient with ARF the kidney is unable to remove the nitrogen byproducts of protein metabolism. Elevations in BUN occur and contribute to the risk of developing significant azotemia. Thus early continuous renal replacement therapy (CRRT) assists the patient in removing this increased protein load.[54]

Hemodynamic stability and adequate oxygen delivery are necessary for meeting the oxygen requirements of all tissues, including the kidneys. Prolonged hypotension or underresuscitation may exacerbate existing renal failure, which in turn diminishes the amount of renal function recovered. Hypertension is a common result of renal failure. As the kidneys perceive a decrease in the renal blood flow, the renin-angiotensin cascade is activated at the juxtaglomerular apparatus. Production of renal prostaglandins is also elevated. The resulting vasoconstriction, increases in the circulating plasma volume as a result of aldosterone production, and electrolyte imbalances contribute to systemic hypertension.

In some cases, such as prerenal pathology, patients with acute renal failure recover after treatment of the underlying cause with careful management of fluids. Patients who experience actual damage to the nephrons usually require some form of temporary dialysis until renal function returns.

Initial management includes administration of a fluid challenge to identify or rule out prerenal causes of ARF. If the pulmonary artery wedge pressure rises by 3 to 5 mmHg and the increase is sustained for more than 5 to 10 minutes, the patient most likely has an adequate circulating volume.[58] The patient who does not respond to diuretics such as mannitol or furosemide is likely in ARF. If not already ruled out, renal artery thrombosis, myoglobinuria (tea-colored urine), and increased abdominal pressure should be considered as causes of acute renal failure.[58] Treatment of the cause will attenuate the ARF.

Dialysis is the next line of management and should be initiated early in the process of ARF. All forms of dialysis strive to replicate normal kidney function, that is, to regulate excess fluid and electrolytes and to remove metabolic wastes.[62] This is accomplished through the use of a porous membrane that, like the glomerular capillary bed, is only permeable to water and small molecules. The dialysis filter membrane essentially creates two compartments, one containing blood and the other a hypertonic solution called dialysate (Figure 25-10).

The function of the system is governed by four principles. Hydrostatic pressure is the force that pushes the fluid through the system. In the kidney this is created by the systemic blood pressure. Osmosis is the movement of fluid across the semipermeable membrane from an area of greater concentration to an area of lesser concentration. Diffusion is the movement of small molecules across the semipermeable membrane from an area of higher concentration to an area of lower concentration. Both processes continue until

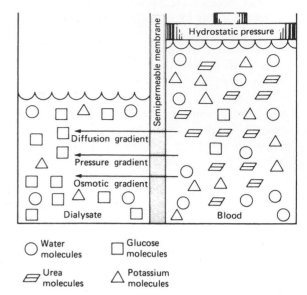

FIGURE 25-10 Osmosis, Diffusion, and Filtration in Dialysis Therapy. (From Baer CL: Dialysis therapy. In Kinney M, Dear CB, Packa DR et al, editors: *AACN's clinical reference for critical care nursing,* New York, 1981, McGraw-Hill.)

equilibrium is reached. Filtration is the movement of fluid from an area of greater pressure to one of lower pressure. Application of these principles is evident in all forms of dialysis.

Peritoneal Dialysis. Clinical use of peritoneal dialysis (PD) was reported as early as 1932.[54] Dialysis is accomplished using the mesenteric capillary bed as the semipermeable membrane. A hypertonic glucose solution is instilled into the abdominal cavity and left to dwell for 30 to 45 minutes. Water and solutes are pulled from the capillary bed to the dialysate (osmosis and diffusion). The greater the concentration of glucose, the more water and solutes are removed.[63]

Peritoneal dialysis has the advantage of being relatively simple and inexpensive to perform. No special preparation of the patient is required for bedside insertion of the abdominal trocar catheter. The procedure can be managed without use of costly equipment. Unfortunately, peritoneal dialysis is usually inadequate for the clearance of both solutes and nitrogenous waste in the acutely critically ill trauma patient.[54] The peritoneum must be intact as well. In trauma patients this is often not the case. The use of PD in the presence of abdominal trauma, vascular anastomosis, or hematoma is at best controversial.

Peritonitis is a major complication of peritoneal dialysis because of the use of the hypertonic glucose solution. Another disadvantage is the effects of the increased intraabdominal pressure during dwell times. Abdominal distention restricts diaphragmatic motion and may impair the patient's ventilatory status and increase abdominal compartment pressure, a cause of acute renal failure. Peritoneal dialysis is

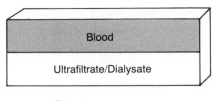

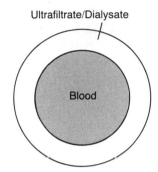

FIGURE 25-11 **Schematic Representation of Two Common Hemofilters.**

an effective treatment for acute fluid overload and stable renal failure; however, these disadvantages limit its use in the multitrauma population.

Hemodialysis. Hemodialysis involves the extracorporeal circulation of blood through a hemofilter, which uses a synthetic semipermeable membrane between the blood and the dialysate.[63] Figure 25-11 is a schematic representation of two commonly used filters. Blood is forced through the extracorporeal circuit by a mechanical pump. Because management of the system requires specially trained personnel, the bedside nurse's primary function is monitoring the patient during the treatment.

Hemodialysis has two distinct advantages over other forms of dialysis: (1) Treatments are brief, usually between 4 and 6 hours; and (2) the process is highly efficient in the removal of fluid, wastes, and electrolytes. These advantages are crucial to the survival of patients with life-threatening poisonings and those in uremic crisis.

However, the resulting rapid shift of fluid and electrolytes can lead to a disequilibrium syndrome.[54] This may be manifested by a decreased level of consciousness, dizziness, weakness, diaphoresis, vomiting, seizures, and hypotension. The neurologic symptoms reflect the entry of water into the cerebrospinal fluid (CSF). This occurs because of a transient concentration gradient in which urea cannot be diffused rapidly enough from the CSF into the blood because of the blood-brain barrier. The cardiovascular effects are related to the rapid shifts of intravascular volume, sodium, and potassium. These symptoms are most often evident when abnormal blood chemistries are corrected too rapidly. In addition, hemodialysis is intermittent, resulting in periods of normal levels of electrolytes and

wastes alternating with gradual increases until the next treatment.

Hemodialysis requires anticoagulation; therefore another significant disadvantage is the risk of hemorrhage.[54] Many trauma patients are already coagulopathic as a result of hepatic injuries, disseminated intravascular coagulopathy (DIC), thrombocytopenia, or multiple transfusions of banked blood. In addition, anticoagulation is contraindicated in head-injured patients and those with abdominal injuries who are being managed nonoperatively.

Continuous Renal Replacement Therapies. Continuous renal replacement therapies are effective in managing acute renal failure, especially in the critically injured patient. CRRT includes continuous arteriovenous hemofiltration with dialysis (CAVHD) and continuous venovenous hemofiltration/dialysis (CVVHD). Schematics of the various forms are presented in Figure 25-12. CRRT can maintain acid-base balance and fluid balance and enable administration of high-protein nutrition without need for systemic anticoagulation and with minimal effect on hemodynamic and pulmonary status.[54]

Continous arteriovenous hemofiltration (CAVH) was introduced in 1977. In this arrangement blood enters an extracorporeal circuit from an arterial access, passes through a hemofilter with a semipermeable membrane, and returns to the patient through a venous access. The hydrostatic pressure created by the patient's mean arterial pressure forces plasma water and some small molecules across the membrane and into a collection system. Structurally the hemofilter is similar to that used for hemodialysis.

In 1983 the addition of a countercurrent dialysate infusion allowed even greater removal of fluids and solutes because of the wider convective and diffusive gradients.[62] This new arrangement, continuous arteriovenous hemofiltration with dialysis, is similar to traditional hemodialysis in treating acute renal failure. This fact, coupled with the absence of capital investment for equipment, elimination of anticoagulation, and avoidance of rapid fluid shifts, has caused it to gain great popularity among critical care clinicians.[55,62]

Both CAVH and CAVHD filter arrangements rely on the arteriovenous (AV) pressure gradient being greater than or equal to 50 mm Hg to create the hydrostatic pressure in the filter.[54] The AV gradient (MAP CVP) is a more reliable indicator than MAP alone because it incorporates the resistance the blood must overcome in returning to the systemic circulation.

Disadvantages. Many trauma patients do not have a sufficient AV gradient to move the blood through the dialysis filter to support CAVH or CAVHD. Inadequate MAP may be related to hypovolemia or septic shock. Significantly elevated central venous pressure, such as that which occurs with the high airway pressures, may actually obstruct the blood in the filter from returning through the venous access. When the AV pressure gradient narrows, blood flow through

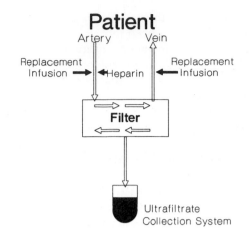

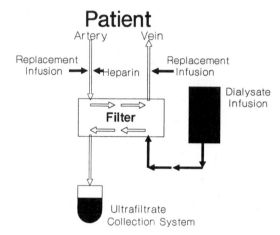

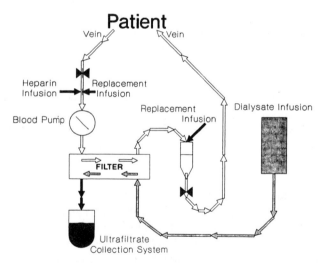

FIGURE 25-12 Schematic Representations of Various Forms of Continuous Acute Renal Replacement Therapies.

the filter slows and the blood clots. In these situations a mechanical blood pump may be used between the arterial and venous access to facilitate movement of blood through the CAVHD filter. In this case a slower blood flow rate is maintained than that used in hemodialysis.

Arterial access for CAVHD may be undesirable or contradicted in some patients. In these patients venous access sites can be used with a roller blood pump. This system, continuous venovenous hemofiltration with dialysis, has several advantages over CAVHD. Venous access can be established with one double lumen catheter, minimizing the need for repeated central venous cannulation. Use of the pump enables clinicians to dialyze patients who are hypotensive or have a narrow AV gradient and cannot support CAVH or CAVHD.

Heparinization is usually needed for CRRT. However, unlike hemodialysis, the goal is to localize the anticoagulation to the filter. This is accomplished using a low-dose heparin infusion located on the arterial side of the filter. Ideally the heparin is cleared by the filter before returning to the patient. However, sufficient clearance is not always achieved, and an alternative anticoagulant such as sodium citrate may be needed. Coagulation status is monitored via serial coagulation studies such as partial thromboplastin time (PTT) or activated clotting time (ACT).

Advantages. Because CRRT slowly removes nitrogenous wastes, therapy should be initiated early in the management of ARF.[54] In addition, it is believed that CRRT may also remove circulating inflammatory mediators such as myocardial depressant substances released with the systemic inflammatory response syndrome.[54,64] Clearance of inflammatory mediators remains controversial, as noted in a study by Rogiers et al (1999) in which significant removal of tumor necrosis factor could not be identified.[64] Another advantage of CRRT includes decreased blood loss by continuous return of circuit blood to the patient. To prevent complications during CRRT, a patent circuit is maintained, fiber rupture identified, and signs of excess anticoagulation recognized.[63] CRRT also allows warming of the replacement fluid to prevent or treat hypothermia.[63]

Critical care nurses have an active role in maintaining the patient on CRRT. Continuous assessment and monitoring focus on the prevention of fluid and electrolyte imbalance, blood and heat loss, infection, and poor ultrafiltrate production.[63] Blood flow through the CRRT circuit is maintained between 100 and 200 ml/min depending on the hemodynamic status of the patient.[63] Blood flow rates through the filter and IV replacement fluids are maintained to achieve the desired fluid balance. Net fluid loss may be desirable if the patient is in fluid overload, or no fluid loss (IV replacement) may be desired if the goal is only solute removal. Laboratory tests are monitored closely during this therapy.

During CRRT setup or during filter change, the filter is primed so that there are no air bubbles within the filter because they increase clotting and obstruct blood flow.[63] The filter integrity is monitored because clotting can occur even with anticoagulation. Signs of clotting include poor filtrate outflow and darkening of the filter fibers.

Regardless of the dialysis therapy selected to treat the patient with ARF, optimal renal function may not return for up to 12 months.[59] Monitoring renal function is required at regular intervals. This includes serial laboratory tests in addition to detailed physical assessment. Management of these patients is directed toward salvage and preservation of the kidney unless treatment compromises other vital organs such as the brain, heart, and lungs. Failure to do so condemns the surviving patient to a life restricted by chronic dialysis or transplantation.

INTERMEDIATE/REHABILITATION PHASES

Once the patient has progressed to the intermediate phase of care, the focus becomes rehabilitative in nature. The potential for complications remains with the genitourinary trauma patient through rehabilitation and after discharge. The long-term effects of GU trauma include both physical disability and emotional stressors.

DELAYED HEMORRHAGE

During the intermediate or rehabilitation phase the nurse continues to monitor the patient for signs of delayed or occult bleeding from genitourinary structures. The patient receiving nonoperative renal injury management is usually placed on bedrest. Trends in vital signs and serial hemoglobin and hematocrit results must be monitored for evidence of hemorrhage.

Any flank or abdominal mass must be evaluated for increase in size. Gentle palpation allows more direct assessment of size but risks the rupture of a tamponaded bleed. Observing for changes in abdominal girth may allow more indirect but safer evaluation of the mass.

URETHRAL STRICTURE, INCONTINENCE, AND IMPOTENCE

The family and patient require education about the care of any remaining drains or urethral or suprapubic catheters. Instruction includes information about potential delayed complications of genitourinary trauma, including infection, sexual difficulties, incontinence, stricture formation, calculus formation, hypertension, hydronephritis, pyelonephritis, and chronic renal failure.

Impotence, stricture, and incontinence were originally believed to be complications caused by treatment.[8,25,27,49] Studies have shown that, although management may have an impact, these are primarily caused by the original injury.[11,47,49] Stricture occurs with complete injuries and is frequently seen after nonoperative management. Treatment of stricture requires delayed urethroplasty. Primary realignment decreases the incidence of stricture but increases the incidence of impotence.

Before the availability of magnetic resonance imaging (MRI) it was believed that impotence was the result of injury to the neurovascular bundles during repair.[47] MRI has demonstrated that significant injury occurs to the corporeal bodies, which results in impotence. Hence in 80% of cases the cause is vasculogenic as a result of the original injury and not repair.[47] Avulsion of the corpus cavernosum from the ischium, separation of the corporeal bodies, corporeal body fracture, and displacement of the prostate are predictive of impotence.[47]

Bladder neck injury is usually associated with incontinence.[45] Every effort must be made to protect the sphincter and repair the bladder neck. A key component of rehabilitation after genitourinary injury is bladder retraining and management of incontinence at home.

CYSTITIS/BLADDER SPASM

Postoperative pain is not as likely to be present once the patient reaches the rehabilitation phase. However, bladder spasms may occur intermittently after bladder repair. Antispasmodic medications are often effective in relieving bladder spasm, and additional analgesia may be required for effective pain relief. If cystitis does occur postoperatively, pain medication may be needed in conjunction with medications, such as phenazopyridine hydrochloride (Pyridium), that produce an analgesic effect on the mucosa of the urinary tract and relieve burning, urgency, and frequency.

INFECTION

The prevention of infection remains a priority throughout the rehabilitation phase. Management of the drainage systems to prevent infection is the same as in the critical care phase.

PHYSICAL DISFIGUREMENT AND SEXUALITY

Patients sustaining genitourinary injury may have residual problems that can alter sexual functioning or bladder control. Patients whose injuries are not likely to produce such sequelae should be reassured as soon as they are stable enough to comprehend such information.

Patients whose injury will cause altered levels of normal body functions not only need intense psychologic support but also may require professional counseling that addresses sexual function. A referral for counseling should be obtained by the nurse. The usual phases of grief and loss related to sexual dysfunction or physical disfigurement can be expected (see Chapter 18).

Female patients who required a hysterectomy or oophorectomy also may experience significant psychologic adjustment. Depending on the woman's age and childbearing status, a hysterectomy may cause severe emotional impact. The surgery may have profound effects on how she perceives herself with respect to her reproductive role, sexuality, vitality, youth, and attractiveness. Each individual values these qualities differently. Depression and mood swings can often occur as a result of these altered body image perceptions and hormonal changes.

Sexual concerns should not be ignored or postponed until the patient is in a rehabilitation unit. Patients may have concerns about sex even during the acute phase after injury. Such concerns are significant, should be addressed, and warrant attention by the nurse.[65-67]

A first step toward initiating a conversation regarding sexual concerns of the patient is to recognize that patients may communicate their concerns about sexuality in a variety of ways, both verbally and nonverbally. Some patients may give no outward indication that they have concerns about sexuality. The nurse should verbally "allow" the patient to initiate a discussion by using a nonjudgmental yet interested approach. By taking time to listen to patients, the nurse creates an atmosphere wherein the patients feel free to talk about their injury and the meaning it has. The nurse should respond to these concerns with a balance of gentle reassurance and realism about the difficult adjustments that undoubtedly lie ahead.[65-67]

Offering the patient information about sexual function is an important intervention. Often in the acute postinjury phase patients simply need reassurance that their sexual function is not totally lost. Allowing patients to have private time with their spouse or significant others is an important nursing measure.

Another intervention that may be helpful is to arrange for the newly disabled person to talk with someone who has made a successful adjustment to a similar disability. The opportunity to explore issues with someone in a similar circumstance may be a good outlet for the patient's concerns.

The measures described previously are also appropriate for use with the patient's spouse or significant other. They too can have tremendous concerns about their future sexual relationship with the disabled individual.

One final consideration of utmost importance in any discussion of patients' sexual concerns is the nurse's own comfort level regarding both sexuality and disability. Attitude is a critical determinant of the nurse's effectiveness in this area. The intense issues surrounding sexuality and disability may be highly sensitive for the nurse for many reasons. It is crucial for nurses to take time for self-analysis regarding these issues because nothing is communicated more surely to the patient than one's own attitudes.

SUMMARY

Rapid identification and management of genitourinary injury can result in satisfactory outcomes. GU injuries are far from insignificant even though they are frequently not life threatening. Urethral injury must be identified early and managed with drainage to prevent complications and allow monitoring of urine output. Renal injuries can be life threatening if hemorrhage occurs. Acute renal failure, although involving the genitourinary system, is often the result of nonrenal causes. Prevention of acute renal failure in all multisystem-injured patients is critical to survival and a positive functional outcome. Long-term complications and disability involve the personal and emotional issues of sexual dysfunction and physical disfigurement, which can be devastating. Trauma nurses from resuscitation through rehabilitation play a vital role in the identification of genitourinary injuries and the prevention and management of short-term and long-term complications.

REFERENCES

1. Thall EH, Stone NN, Cheny DL et al: Conservative management of penetrating and blunt Type III renal injuries, *Br J Urol* 77:512-517, 1996.
2. Mansi MK, Aldkhudair WK: Conservative management with percutaneous intervention of major blunt renal injury, *Am J Emerg Med* 15:633-637, 1997.
3. Brown SL, Elder JS, Spirnak JP: Are pediatric patients more susceptible to major renal injury from blunt trauma? A comparative study, *J Urol* 160:138-140, 1998.
4. Elshihabi I, Elshihabi S, Arar M: An overview of renal trauma, *Curr Opin Pediatr* 10:162-166, 1998.
5. Wright DG, Taitsman L, Laughlin RT: Pelvic and bladder trauma: a case report and subject review, *J Orthop Trauma* 10:351-354, 1996.
6. Ghali AMA, El Malik EMA, Ibrahim AIA et al: Ureteric injuries: diagnosis, management, and outcome, *J Trauma* 46:150-158, 1999.
7. Sommers MS: Blunt renal trauma, *Crit Care Nurse* 10(3): 38-48, 1990.
8. Routt ML, Simonian PT, Defalco AJ et al: Internal fixation in pelvic fracture and primary repairs of associated GU disruptions: a team approach, *J Trauma* 40:784-790, 1996.
9. De La Taille A, Houdelette P, Houlgatte A et al: Ureteropelvic junction avulsion due to nonpenetrating abdominal trauma treated with caliceal ureterostomy, *J Urol* 157:1840, 1997.
10. Schmidlin FR, Schmid P, Kurtyka T et al: Force transmission and stress distribution in a computer-simulated model of the kidney: an analysis of the injury mechanism in renal trauma, *J Trauma* 40:791-796, 1996.
11. Taffett R: Management of pelvic fracture with concomitant urologic injuries, *Ortho Clin North Am* 28:389-396, 1997.
12. Smith DP, Klein FA: Renal injury in a child with airbag deployment, *J Trauma* 42:341-342, 1997.
13. Insurance Institute for Highway Safety: Congress mandates advanced airbags, extends unbelted test, *Status Rep* 33:7, 1998.
14. Medina D, Lavery R, Ross SE et al: Ureteral trauma: preoperative studies neither predict nor prevent missed injuries, *J Am Coll Surg* 186:641-644, 1998.
15. Azimuddin K, Ivatury R, Porter J et al: Damage control in a trauma patient with ureteric injury, *J Trauma* 43:977-979, 1997.
16. Wessells H, McAninch JW, Meyer A et al: Criteria for non-operative treatment of significant penetrating renal lacerations, *J Urol* 157:24-27, 1997.
17. Velmahos GC, Degiannis E: The management of urinary tract injuries after GSW of the anterior and posterior abdomen, *Injury* 28:535-538, 1997.
18. Swinburn EE: Serious injuries in jet skiers, *Med J Aust* 165:606-609, 1996.
19. Haefner HK, Andersen HF, Johnson MP: Vaginal laceration following a jet-ski accident, *Obstet Gynecol* 78:986-988, 1991.
20. Morrison DM, Pasquale MD, Scagliotti CJ: Hydrostatic rectal injury of a jet ski passenger: a case report and discussion, *J Trauma* 45:816-818, 1998.

21. Hamman BL, Miller FB, Fallat ME et al: Injuries resulting from motorized PWC, *J Pediatr Surg* 28:920-922, 1993.
22. Jeffrey RS, Caiach S: Waterbike injury, *Br J Sports Med* 25:232-234, 1991.
23. Shatz DV et al: Personal watercraft crash injuries: an emerging problem, *J Trauma* 44:198-201, 1998.
24. O'Brien C: Improved forensic documentation of genital injury with colposcopy, *J Emerg Nurs* 23:460-462, 1997.
25. Harrahill M, Eastes L: Traumatic urethral disruption: a protocol for diagnosis, *J Emerg Nurs* 24:615-616, 1998.
26. Koraitim MM, Marzouk ME, Atta MA et al: Risk factors and mechanisms of urethral injury in pelvic fracture, *Brit J Urol* 77:876-880, 1996.
27. Boon TA, Van der Werkern C: Urethral injuries revisited, *Injury* 27:533-538, 1996.
28. Okur H, Kucukaydin M, Kazez A, et al: GU tract injuries in girls, *Br J Urol* 78:446-449, 1996.
29. American College of Surgeons: Abdominal trauma. In American College of Surgeons' Committee on Trauma: *Advanced trauma life support*, ed 6, Chicago, 1997, American College of Surgeons, 193-218.
30. Jarvis C: Abdomen. In Jarvis C: *Pocket companion for physical examination and health assessment*, ed 2, Philadelphia, 1996, WB Saunders, 181-195.
31. Goldman SM, Sandler CM: Upper urinary tract trauma—current concepts, *World J Urol* 16:62-68, 1998.
32. Udekwu PO, Gurkin B, Oller DW: The use of computerized tomography in blunt abdominal injury, *Am Surg* 62:56-59, 1996.
33. Patel VG, Walker ML: The role of "one-shot" intravenous pyelogram in evaluation of penetrating abdominal trauma, *Am Surg* 63:350-353, 1997.
34. Coburn M: Damage control for urologic injuries, *Surg Clin North Am* 77:821-834, 1997.
35. Valmahos GC et al: Selective management of renal GSW, *Br J Surg* 85:1121-1124, 1998.
36. Bodner DR, Selzman AA, Spirnak JP: Evaluation and treatment of bladder rupture, *Semin Urol* 13:62-65, 1995.
37. Sandler CM, Goldman SM, Kawashima A: Lower urinary tract trauma, *World J Urol* 16:69-75, 1998.
38. Maharaji D, Naraynsingh V: Fracture of the penis with urethral rupture, *Injury* 29:483, 1998.
39. Hochberg E, Stone NN: Bladder rupture associated with pelvic fracture due to blunt trauma, *Urology* 41:531-533, 1993.
40. Sivit CJ, Cutting JR, Eichelberger MR: CT diagnosis and localization of rupture of the bladder in children with blunt abdominal trauma: significance of contract material extravasation in the pelvis, *Am J Roentgenol* 164:1243-1246, 1995.
41. Cline KJ, Mata JA, Venable DD et al: Penetrating trauma to the male external genitalia, *J Trauma* 44:492-494, 1998.
42. Morris SB, Miller MA, Anson K: Management of penile fracture, *J Royal Soc Med* 91:427-428, 1998.
43. Cortellini P, Ferretti S, Larosa M et al: Traumatic injury of the penis: surgical management, *Scand J Urol Nephrol* 30:517-519, 1996.
44. Pierce JT: A 14 y.o. victim of sexual assault with an imperforate hymen and urethral meatus tear, *J Emerg Nurs* 25:153-154, 1999.
45. Ahmed S, Neel KF: Urethral injury in girls with fractured pelvis following blunt abdominal trauma, *Brit J Urol* 78: 450-453, 1996.
46. Goldman SM, Sandler CM, Corriere JN et al: Blunt urethral trauma: a unified, anatomical mechanical classification, *J Urol* 157:85-89, 1997.
47. Kotkin L, Koch MO: Impotence and incontinence after immediate realignment of posterior urethral trauma: result of injury or management? *J Urol* 155:1600-1603, 1996.
48. Podesta ML, Medel R, Castera R et al: Immediate management of posterior urethral disruptions due to pelvic fracture: therapeutic alternatives, *J Urol* 157:1444-1448, 1997.
49. Koraitim MM: Pelvic fracture urethral injuries: evaluation of various methods of management, *J Urol* 156:1288-1291, 1996.
50. Kotkin L, Koch MO: Morbidity associated with nonoperative management of extraperitoneal bladder injury, *J Trauma* 38:895-898, 1995.
51. Mokoena T, Naidu AG: Diagnostic difficulties in patients with a ruptured bladder, *Br J Surg* 82:69-70, 1995.
52. Matthews LA, Smith EM, Spirnak JP: Nonoperative treatment of major blunt renal lacerations with urinary extravasation, *J Urol* 157:2056-2058, 1997.
53. Montgomery RC, Richardson JD, Harty JI: Posttraumatic renovascular hypertension after occult renal injury, *J Trauma* 45:106-110, 1998.
54. Slater MS, Mullins RJ: Rhabdomyolysis and myoglobinuric renal failure in trauma and surgical patients: a review, *J Am Coll Surg* 186:693-716, 1998.
55. Carriere SR, Elsworth T: Found down: compartment syndrome, rhabdomyolysis, and renal failure, *J Emerg Nurs* 24:214-217, 1998.
56. Naqui R et al: Acute renal failure due to traumatic rhabdomyolysis, *Ren Fail* 18:677-679, 996.
57. Szewczyk D, Ovadia P, Abdullah F et al: Pressure-induced rhabdomyolysis and acute renal failure, *J Trauma* 44:384-388, 1998.
58. Belzberg H, Cornwell EE, Berne TV: The critical care of the severely injured patient. II. Pulmonary and renal support, *Surg Clin North Am* 76:971-983, 1996.
59. Whittaker A: Patients in acute renal failure. In Clochesy JM, Breu C, Cardin S et al, editors: *Critical care nursing*, ed 2, Philadelphia, 1996, WB Saunders, 926-948.
60. Jerwood DC, Mason NP: Pseudo-renal failure after traumatic bladder rupture—the common features, *Brit J Urol* 76: 406-407, 1995.
61. Nayduch DA, Sullivan K, Reed RL: Abdominal compartment syndrome, *J Trauma Nurs* 4:5-11, 1997.
62. Sugrue M, Jones F, Deane SA: Intra-abdominal hypertension is an independent cause of postoperative renal impairment, *Arch Surg* 134:1082-1085, 1999. 1999.
63. Baldwin IC, Elderkin TD: Continuous hemofiltration: nursing perspectives in critical care, *New Horiz* 3:738-747, 1995.
64. Rogiers P, Zhang H, Smail N et al: Continuous venovenous hemofiltration improves cardiac performance by mechanisms other than tumor necrosis factor-attenuation during endotoxic shock, *Crit Care Med* 27:1848-1855, 1999.
65. Gamlin R: Sexuality: a challenge for nursing practice, *Nurs Times* 95:48-50, 1999.
66. Aylott J: Sense and sexuality, *Nurs Times* 94:34-35, 1998.
67. LeMone P, Jones D: Nursing assessment of altered sexuality: a review of salient factors and objective measures, *Nurs Diagn* 8:120-128, 1997.

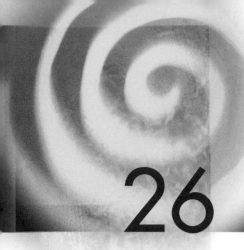

MUSCULOSKELETAL
INJURIES

Colleen R. Walsh

26

Management of traumatic musculoskeletal injuries rarely takes precedent during the initial phases of trauma care. The basic principles of trauma care stress resuscitation and therapeutic interventions for those life-threatening injuries most commonly associated with trauma. Musculoskeletal injuries are considered part of the secondary trauma survey unless those injuries result in significant hemodynamic instability, such as traumatic amputations and massive pelvic injuries. Musculoskeletal injuries require prompt recognition and appropriate management after stabilization of the cardiopulmonary and neurologic systems to maximize the patient's full recovery.

Musculoskeletal injuries, although not usually life threatening, take much longer to heal than most other injuries and often result in lifelong disability and lifestyle changes. This chapter addresses the major musculoskeletal injuries seen in trauma and the complications that require early diagnosis and emergency management.

ANATOMY AND PHYSIOLOGY

An understanding of the anatomy and physiology of the musculoskeletal system is necessary to enable nurses caring for trauma patients to plan interventions and care aimed at prevention of the complications that frequently occur in this population. Although this discussion is not meant to be inclusive, a basic review of the structures and functions of the musculoskeletal system assists the reader to identify at-risk patients based on their injuries.

FUNCTIONS

The musculoskeletal system is composed of two systems: the skeletal system and the skeletal muscles. The skeletal system is composed of bones and joints, and its main functions are to provide support, protection, storage of mineral salts and fats, and hematopoiesis (red blood cell production). The skeletal system also provides the leverage needed by skeletal muscles to produce movement through contraction of skeletal muscles and bending and rotation at joints.[1] Any injury to the musculoskeletal system can cause an alteration in or even cessation of any of these functions,

which then produces far-reaching detrimental effects on the patient.

STRUCTURES

Figure 26-1 illustrates normal bone architecture, including articular cartilage, spongy bone, epiphysis, epiphyseal plate, compact bone, medullary cavity, diaphysis, endosteum, yellow marrow, and periosteum. There are two types of bone tissue: compact bone (cortical bone) and spongy bone (cancellous). Compact bone is organized, strong, and solid and contains the main structural units, called the haversian system. The haversian system contains bone cells called osteocytes and carries out the major metabolic processes of compact bone, transporting nutrients to and removing wastes from the osteocytes.[1] Spongy bone is less organized and does not contain haversian systems. Spongy bone is characterized by trabeculae, or plates, that branch out to form an irregular meshwork. Stresses placed on the bone form the pattern of trabeculae, and the spaces between the trabeculae are filled with red bone marrow.[1]

The diaphysis, or shaft, is composed of a thick layer of compact bone that offers a tremendous degree of support and protection. This slender part of the bone is slightly curved in long bones to provide added strength and to enable the bone to withstand and absorb stress. The bone shaft can withstand shearing and compression forces but is at risk for injury from tension-producing mechanisms. For example, diaphyseal fractures most often occur as a result of tension failure produced by a bending, twisting, or pulling mechanism. Bone is strongest at the point where maximal forces or stressors are applied. This concept is discussed later in the chapter.

The epiphysis, or bone end, is made up primarily of cancellous or spongy tissue that houses red marrow in the large pores of the trabeculae. This segment of bone is at greater risk of injury from crushing mechanisms that cause compression or impaction of bone ends. The sequelae of an injury to this area of the bone increases in severity in prepubescent children because longitudinal bone growth occurs at the epiphyseal plate. Thus an injury there can permanently alter bone growth in children.

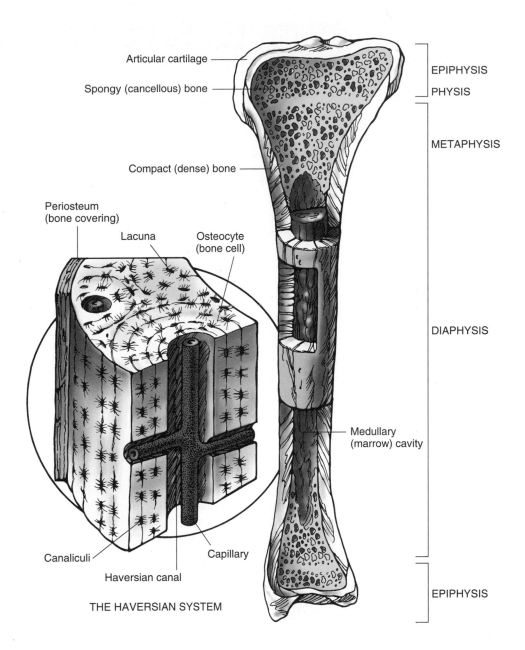

EPIPHYSIS

PHYSIS

METAPHYSIS

Articular cartilage

Spongy (cancellous) bone

Compact (dense) bone

Periosteum
(bone covering)

Lacuna

Osteocyte
(bone cell)

DIAPHYSIS

Medullary
(marrow) cavity

Canaliculi

Capillary

Haversian canal

THE HAVERSIAN SYSTEM

EPIPHYSIS

FIGURE 26-1 Diagram of Longitudinal Section of a Long Bone and Haversian System. (From Ignatavicus DD, Bayne MV: *Medical-surgical nursing: a nursing process approach,* Philadelphia, 1991, WB Saunders, 719.)

The periosteum is a fibrous membrane sleeve that covers the entire bone except the cartilaginous ends. The inner osteogenic layer consists of elastic fibers, vessels, and osteoblasts, which are responsible for new bone formation. The outer fibrous layer is made up of connective tissue and houses blood and lymphatic vessels and nerves. Bone growth, repair, and nutrition rely on an intact and healthy periosteum. This closely adherent covering is thickest where muscles surround the bone, such as at the diaphysis of the femur. Because it is a thin and tightly bound membrane in adults, it usually tears at fracture sites rather than separating from the bone. When a fracture occurs, one side of the periosteum remains intact (the periosteal hinge). The remaining portion of intact membrane aids fracture reduc-

tion and maintenance and serves as an osteogenic covering that promotes healing. The degree to which the periosteum is damaged during a fracture event often determines the course of healing of the fracture.

Injuries to the soft tissue, including muscle, nerves, vessels, subcutaneous fat, and skin, occur to some degree in conjunction with all fractures. The soft tissue injury may be more serious and have more significant ramifications than the fracture itself. Neglect or underestimation of soft tissue involvement may lead to serious fracture complications.

BONE CELLS

Bone contains three types of cells: osteoblasts, osteocytes, and osteoclasts. Each type of cell plays a major role in the formation, repair, and cyclic remodeling of bone. Osteoblasts are bone-forming cells whose major function is to lay down new bone. Once this is accomplished, they become osteocytes. Osteocytes are osteoblasts that have become trapped in the bone matrix.[1] Their major function is not well defined, but it is postulated that they function to maintain the bone matrix.[1] Osteoclasts are the major resorptive cells of bone and function primarily during periods of growth and repair.[1] Any process that interferes with the function of these bone cells can adversely affect the dynamic state of skeletal tissue. Approximately 18% of bone is removed and replaced every year in premenopausal women; after menopause this balance changes to an increase in bone resorption and a decrease in bone production, leading to the development of osteoporosis.

EPIDEMIOLOGY

Approximately 33 million musculoskeletal injuries occur annually, including 20 million fractures, dislocations, and sprains, with approximately 8000 deaths.[2] Musculoskeletal injuries found in the trauma patient result from a variety of causes. The major causes of significant musculoskeletal injuries are vehicular crashes; falls; industrial, home, and farming incidents; and assaults. Musculoskeletal injuries are often associated with serious injuries to other body systems.

RESUSCITATION PHASE

ASSESSMENT

PREHOSPITAL DATABASE.   A variety of energy forces can traumatize the musculoskeletal system. Each type of impact exerts a different amount of force on the body. The degree, direction, and duration of that force, along with the patient's age and health history, determine the severity of the injury and its resulting morbidity.

Knowing the type of incident and the mechanism of injury can greatly increase the clinician's index of suspicion during the assessment of the musculoskeletal system. A victim of a fall and a driver of a car striking another car head on may absorb similar amounts of energy from the impact, but the direction of the forces applied to the body, the body surface area involved, and the rate of deceleration that occurs are different, thus producing different injuries.

Information concerning the mechanism of injury should be obtained from the patient if possible and from the prehospital providers. Important information to obtain is summarized in Table 26-1. Similar injuries can occur in different environments, and the sequelae of an open fracture can be very different if the injury occurred in a farming incident versus a fall at home. Pathogenic organisms found in soil can cause serious, even fatal, infections. Early identification of environmental factors can decrease complications if appropriate interventions are started early in the treatment phase.

Each musculoskeletal injury is the result of absorbed and transferred energy. The fall victim who lands on his or her

TABLE 26-1   **Prehospital Database**
How did the incident happen?
Where did the incident happen?
Was it a high-energy incident or a low-energy incident?
What position was the patient in when the incident happened?
What position was the patient found in?
When did incident happen? How long ago?
In what environment did the incident happen?

feet may have obvious ankle injuries, but other injuries often associated with this type of mechanism, such as pelvic and lumbar spine fractures, may be occult (Figure 26-2). Other patterns of energy absorption and transfer are demonstrated in Figure 26-3. This patient was an unrestrained front seat occupant in a head-on collision in which he struck his knee against the dashboard. A minor abrasion of the knee was sustained without underlying fracture, but the energy transferred to the pelvis resulted in major pelvic ring disruption. Information concerning events of extrication, immobilization, and stabilization that occurred at the site of the incident is important and should be obtained from the prehospital providers. Knowing the degree of angulation of a fracture, attitude of a joint, neurovascular status of the extremity at the scene, amount of exposed bone, and estimated blood loss heightens suspicion and helps determine the type of treatment necessary. Review Chapter 11 for further discussion of mechanism of injury.

MUSCULOSKELETAL PHYSICAL ASSESSMENT.   The initial assessment of the patient with musculoskeletal injuries begins with the primary survey, which consists of the standard evaluation of airway, breathing, circulation, and neurologic status. Initiation of appropriate interventions to establish or maintain normal cardiopulmonary and neurologic function takes precedence regardless of obvious or suspected musculoskeletal injuries.

Attention is directed toward the musculoskeletal system during the secondary survey. Any suspected or obvious musculoskeletal injuries require baseline assessment of neurovascular and motor status, proper immobilization of affected extremities, and application of sterile dressings to open wounds. Additionally, an unstable pelvic ring disruption (as identified on initial radiographs) with possible vascular injury may require application of a C-clamp to prevent exsanguination.[3] Other interventions are not initiated until the total patient evaluation is completed and the patient is hemodynamically stable. Throughout the resuscitation process all personnel should be aware of potential or actual fracture sites to minimize further manipulation or injury. Severe pain from soft tissue or bony injuries may mask symptoms of other more significant injuries; thus a thorough total system evaluation is essential. Conversely, restlessness and agitation caused by other pathologic conditions may further disrupt bone fragments and increase the patient's pain.

Areas of suspected injury should remain immobilized

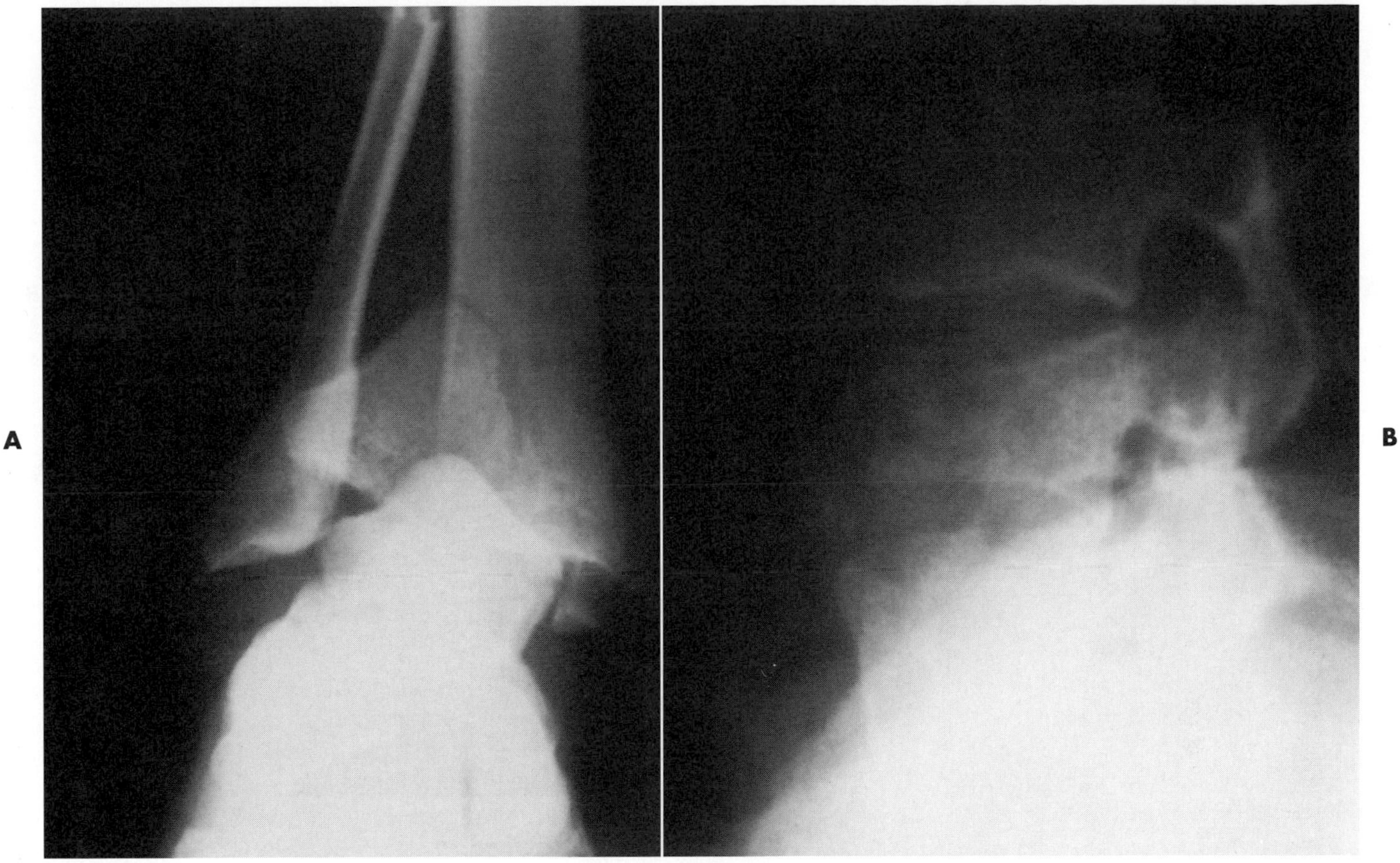

FIGURE 26-2 **Radiographs of a Fall Victim Who Landed on his Feet. A,** Fractured ankle. **B,** Associated compression fracture of the lumbar spine.

and their movement kept to a minimum. Whenever the patient requires turning or moving, one person assumes responsibility for the affected limb to maintain alignment and immobilization. This is critically important when caring for patients with suspected spinal column injuries because any motion at the fracture site may result in partial or total paralysis below the level of injury.

Continuous monitoring is an important concept for emergency personnel. After primary and lifesaving measures are instituted, it is essential that providers reassess the patient's status, especially the neurovascular function of extremities with obvious or suspected fractures. Physiologic events, such as muscle spasms, or environmental events, such as transports, can further displace fracture fragments and lead to serious neurovascular compromise of the affected extremity. If undetected, neurovascular compromise can cause permanent disability, loss of limb, or even death.

Inspection and Palpation. Assessment of the musculoskeletal system in a systematic fashion decreases the chance of missing an injury. Assessment involves inspection and palpation. The position of the patient and the extremities should be observed. Note is made of any deformities such as angulation, shortening, or rotation; open wounds; obviously protruding bone ends; abrasions, and road burns. Estima-

tion of external blood loss, including the blood on the patient's clothes and the ambulance stretcher and the amount of blood at the scene, is important to provide information about the patient's hemodynamic status.

The patient is inspected for additional findings that may indicate musculoskeletal injury:

- Ecchymosis: caused by vascular disruption with blood dispersing through soft tissue
- Muscle spasm: continuous muscle contraction over an injured part; considered a protective mechanism of the muscle to splint the injured part
- Swelling: caused by injury to the soft tissue and interruption of the venous and lymphatic return system
- Extremity color: pale color indicates inadequate arterial blood supply; dusky, bluish color indicates venous congestion

Each bone is palpated and any interruptions in the natural integrity are noted. Interruption in bone integrity may be difficult to identify; crepitus, pain, or muscle spasm may be the only indication that an injury exists. Palpation is used to assess the following:

- Capillary refill time: A filling time longer than 2 seconds is considered abnormal, but factors such as

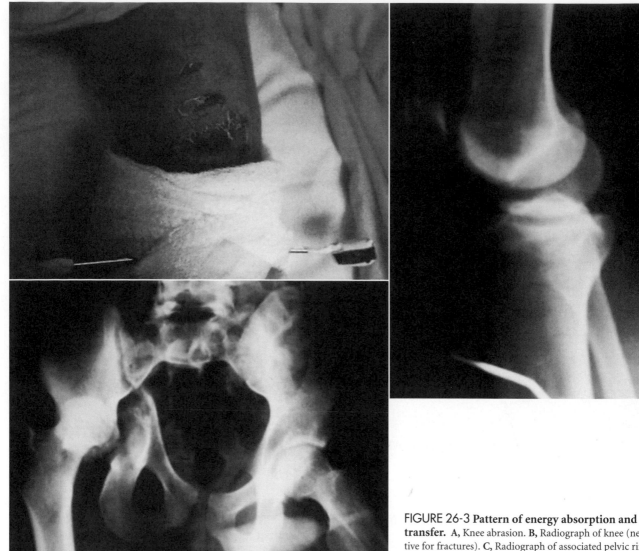

FIGURE 26-3 **Pattern of energy absorption and transfer.** **A,** Knee abrasion. **B,** Radiograph of knee (negative for fractures). **C,** Radiograph of associated pelvic ring disruption.

ambient air temperature, patient's core body temperature, and environmental exposure may affect the capillary refill time.

- Pulses: Quality and equality are evaluated over the entire length of an extremity, not just distal to an obvious injury; results are compared with pulses in the nonaffected extremity.
- Crepitus: A grating sound is heard and felt when fractured bone ends move.
- Muscle spasm: As noted above. Lack of spasms over an obvious fracture may indicate a neurologic lesion above the fracture, preventing contraction of the muscle.
- Movement: Range of motion, both passive and active, is assessed. Deviation from normal range or limitation of motion or muscle strength is noted. Obviously injured extremities should not be tested for range of motion because of the risk of increasing the damage to surrounding neurovascular structures.

- Sensation: Alterations in sensation in response to sharp and dull stimuli and proprioception are assessed.
- Pain: Bones are essentially insensitive. Pain is usually caused by injury to the periosteum (which has sensory innervation), muscle spasm, soft tissue injury, and swelling within fascial compartments.

Zone of Injury. The zone of injury is the area affected by traumatic forces, as seen in Figure 26-4. Injuries to the skeletal system are always accompanied by some degree of soft tissue injury. Damage to the soft tissue structures is greater than what is discovered on clinical assessment and radiologic examination. The exact zone of injury is often not fully appreciated until the operative or critical care phase; therefore continued physical assessment with a high index of suspicion includes areas both distal and proximal to any obvious or suspected injury.

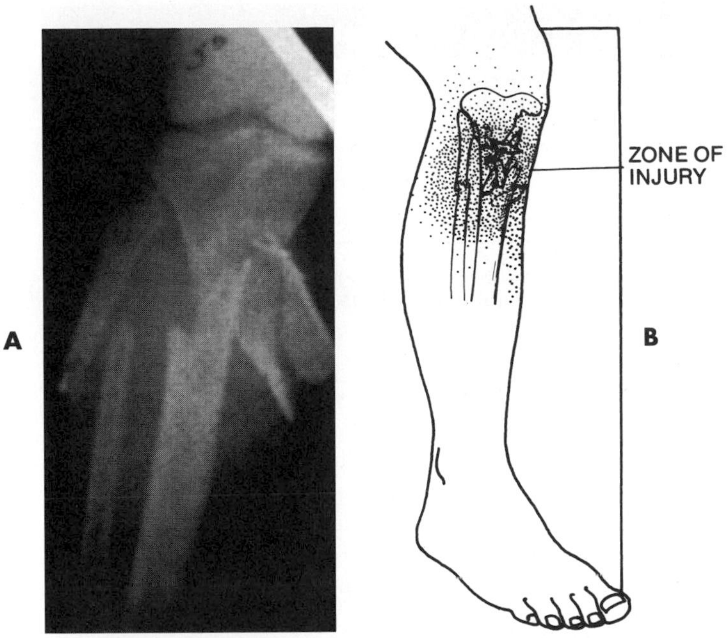

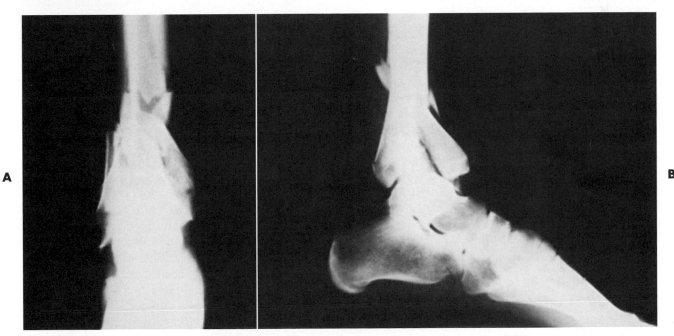

FIGURE 26-4 **The Mechanism of Injury Predicts the Zone of Soft Tissue Injury. A,** Radiograph of a grade III tibia fracture that resulted from a car bumper crush injury. **B,** The zone of injury *(stippled)* of the leg. The fracture pattern and the mechanism of injury predict the size of this zone. (From Manson PN, Yaremchuk MJ, Hoopes JE: Soft tissue injuries of the extremities. In Zuidema GD, Rutherford RB, Ballinger WF, editors: *The management of trauma,* Philadelphia, 1985, WB Saunders.)

FIGURE 26-5 **Radiographs of a Fracture of the Distal Tibia/Fibula and Ankle Showing the Degree of Angulation and Displacement. A,** Anteroposterior view. **B,** Lateral view.

Diagnostic Studies. Various radiographic studies are used to confirm musculoskeletal injuries. For plain radiographic films, at least two views are required to determine the degree of angulation and displacement (Figure 26-5). Surrounding anatomic structures and the structure of the bone or joint in question may reduce the effectiveness of plain films in diagnosing skeletal injuries and necessitate use of other techniques such as computed tomography (CT) scans, angiography, CT myelograms, and magnetic resonance imaging (MRI). CT scans aid in confirmation of hidden or minimally displaced fractures in areas such as the

pelvic ring, the ankle, and the knee. Angiography is usually necessary for severe fractures or dislocations near the knee joint, in pelvic injuries with persistent hemorrhage, and when distal circulation is compromised. Angiography also can provide added information concerning the true zone of injury. Myelography is useful as a delayed diagnostic procedure (at least 2 weeks after the injury) when nerve root avulsion is suspected. If conducted earlier, the study may yield a false-negative result because blood clots can obstruct the meningoceles, which are diagnostic of nerve root avulsion. MRI studies are often performed to aid in the diagnosis of suspected soft tissue injuries such as herniated intervertebral disks or ligamentous disruption. Inlet and outlet views of the pelvis, taken from a superior and inferior angle, can be done in the resuscitation room to quickly identify significant pelvic injuries and aid clinicians in early treatment of these injuries.

During the diagnostic process the nurse is responsible for the following:

1. Assisting with explanation of the procedure to the patient and obtaining consent when necessary
2. Assisting with safe patient positioning during and after the procedure to prevent further injury- or procedure-related complications. For example, after an angiogram in which the femoral artery was cannulated, hip flexion is restricted for 6 to 8 hours to prevent further bleeding at the insertion site.
3. Protecting the patient from unnecessary radiation exposure by shielding with a lead-lined apron whenever possible
4. Constantly monitoring the patient's overall status, including potential reaction to contrast media
5. Documenting the procedure, patient response, and follow-up evaluation

Patient Health History.   Eliciting a specific patient health history is an important part of the patient assessment. Information concerning health history can be obtained from the patient or, when necessary, from family members or friends. The nurse should determine whether the patient has ever had an allergic reaction to any medication or contrast material and the type of reaction that occurred. Previous reactions to pharmacologic agents can alter the choice of diagnostic studies, such as angiograms, or the choice of medications used for treatment. Current or recent use of medication, and the reason, dose, and frequency are ascertained if possible. Learning whether the patient has taken any anticoagulants, aspirin, nonsteroidal antiinflammatory drugs (NSAIDs), or similar medication is essential. The patient's tetanus immunization history is also important. Other helpful information includes previous hospitalizations and surgeries, anesthesia-associated problems, and any specific health problems. Previous fractures, ligamentous or soft tissue injuries, thromboembolic disease, neurologic disorders, and problems with infection or delayed healing potentially affect the patient's treatment and recovery. The importance of obtaining an AMPLE history during the initial assessment cannot be overemphasized because this history guides the clinician's assessment and treatment of the trauma patient (Table 26-2).

CLASSIFICATION OF INJURIES.   Extremity injuries include fractures, fracture-dislocations, amputations, and trauma to the soft tissue, nerves, vessels, and tendons. Soft tissue injuries involve skin, muscles, tendons, ligaments, and cartilage.

TABLE 26-2 "AMPLE" History	
A	Allergies (penicillin, latex, etc.)
M	Medications (steroids, cardiac)—including herbals and over the counter
P	Past medical illnesses—past medical history
L	Last meal—vomiting and aspiration
E	Events of incident—mechanisms of injury

From American College of Surgeons' Committee on Trauma: *Advanced trauma life support*, ed 6, Chicago, IL, 1977, American College of Surgeons.

Extremity Fractures.   The classification of a fracture is based on several factors: (1) type of fracture line (spiral, transverse, oblique); (2) whether the fracture is linear or comminuted; (3) anatomic location (distal, middle, proximal third of the shaft, intraarticular); (4) type of displacement (angulation, translation, impaction, distraction); and (5) position of the displacement in relation to other fragments[4] (Figure 26-6).

A fracture with associated interruption in skin integrity is an open fracture. An open fracture is further classified according to the degree of soft tissue involvement and the amount of disruption in skin integrity. A grade I open fracture wound is small with minimal soft tissue damage. A grade II open fracture wound is larger with a moderate amount of soft tissue injury. A grade III open fracture is associated with significant avulsion, soft tissue damage, muscle devitalization, or wound flaps, such as fractures caused by gunshot wounds or bumper mechanisms or fractures associated with open segments and neurologic or vascular involvement. Grade III fractures are further subclassified as III A, B, or C depending on the degree of skin, muscle, or bone loss or vascular injury[4] (Table 26-3).

The soft tissue injury in a grade I fracture may appear benign or occur away from the fracture site. This is attributed to the overriding of fractured bone ends at the time of injury. One end penetrates the skin some distance from the fracture site and then withdraws back through the soft tissue into relatively normal anatomic alignment.

Certain mechanisms of injury automatically classify an open fracture as grade III, such as a shotgun injury, a high-velocity gunshot wound, an open fracture occurring in a farm environment, and a crushing injury from a fast-moving vehicle. The time elapsed from open injury to definite irrigation and debridement of open fractures also influences fracture classification. Any open fracture left untreated for more than 8 hours has an increased incidence of significant infection of the fracture or surrounding tissue (Figure 26-7).

Traumatic Amputation.   Traumatic amputations are classified according to the degree of soft tissue, nerve, and vascular injury. A cut or guillotine amputation has well-defined wound edges and localized damage to soft tissue, nerves, and vessels. A crush amputation wound has more soft tissue damage, especially to the arterial intima.

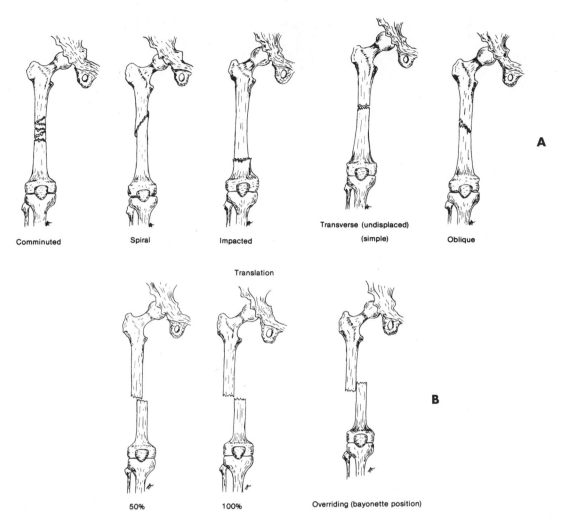

Comminuted   Spiral   Impacted   Transverse (undisplaced) (simple)   Oblique

Translation

50%   100%   Overriding (bayonette position)

FIGURE 26-6 A, Types of fractures. B, Translation. (From Stearns HC: Principles of lower extremity fracture management. In Hilt N, editor: *Assessment and fracture management of the lower extremities [monograph]*, Pitman, NJ, 1984, National Association of Orthopedic Nurses.)

TABLE 26-3 Classification of Open Fractures

Type	Description
I	Wound less than 1 cm
	Moderately clean, minimal contamination
	Fracture—simple transverse or oblique with skin pierced by bone spike
	Minimal soft tissue damage
II	Wound greater than 1 cm
	Moderate contamination
	Fracture—moderate comminution/crush injury
	Moderate soft tissue damage (flaps or avulsions)
III	High degree of contamination
	Fracture—severe comminution and instability
	Extensive soft tissue damage involving muscle, skin, and neurovascular structures
	Traumatic amputation
III A	Soft tissue coverage of fracture is adequate
	Fracture—segmental or severely comminuted
III B	Extensive injury to or loss of soft tissue, periosteal stripping, and exposure of bone
	Massive contamination
	Fracture—severe comminution
III C	Any open fracture associated with arterial injury that must be repaired regardless of degree of soft tissue injury

Modified from Snyder P: Fractures. In Maher AB, Salmond SW, Pellino, TA, editors: *Orthopaedic nursing*, Philadelphia, 1998, WB Saunders.

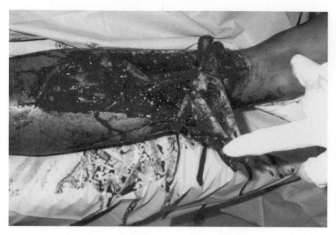

FIGURE 26-7 Grade III B open fracture of the tibial shaft with extensive soft tissue loss.

Injury to the soft tissue may be localized or extended some distance from the wound edge. An avulsion amputation wound is caused by forceful stretching and tearing away of the tissue. Neural and vascular structures are torn away at levels different from the actual site of the bone fracture.

The advent of newer and more sophisticated microsurgical techniques used for reattachment of severed limbs has made it imperative that all prehospital and hospital personnel correctly care for the limb until a determination can be made regarding the feasibility of surgical reattachment. The limb is placed in a plastic bag and then placed in another bag containing ice water and transported with the patient. Direct contact with iced solutions can cause freezing and crystallization with subsequent rupture of tissue cells, thus making successful reattachment unlikely. Dry ice should never be used as the cooling agent because it increases crystal formation. Amputations caused by crush or avulsion injuries have a low reattachment success rate; therefore the procedure is usually not attempted.

Dislocation. A dislocation occurs when articulating surfaces are no longer in contact because of joint disruption. Movement can be limited or impossible. The dislocation is described in terms of the distal component relative to the proximal component. For example, a dislocation of the elbow involving the radius alone can be anterior, posterior, or lateral. Hip dislocations may be classified as anterior, posterior, or central (Figure 26-8). The incidence of neurovascular injuries associated with major joint dislocations is high; thus careful assessment of neurovascular function is necessary. The ligamentous structures surrounding the dislocated joint are usually severely stretched or completely disrupted, leaving the joint unstable. Immobilization is essential to prevent or limit the neurovascular compromise often found with these injuries.

Subluxation. A subluxation is a partial dislocation in which a portion of the articular surface is not in contact. The subluxation is often accompanied by varying degrees of neurovascular compromise, and again immobilization is essential. Many subluxations spontaneously reduce during extrication or other procedures, but care must be taken to assess the affected joint for ligamentous instability.

Pelvic Ring Disruption. The pelvis is composed of three bones held together and stabilized by a ligamentous network. Anteriorly the symphysis pubis, a strong ligamentous structure, acts as a strut to prevent anterior pelvic collapse; it has little to do with weight bearing. The major stabilizing force in the pelvis is the posterior tension band that includes the following ligaments: iliolumbar, posterior sacroiliac, sacrospinous, and sacrotuberous (Figure 26-9). Pelvic ring disruptions are the third most often seen injury in fatal motor vehicle crashes.[2] Pelvic ring disruptions are clinically described as stable or unstable. Two thirds of pelvic ring disruptions are stable.[2] Although fewer in incidence, the unstable injury is potentially more life threatening because it is often accompanied by many complications. These include massive to exsanguinating blood loss, genitourinary trauma, sepsis, chronic pain, and long-term disability. The injury to the pelvic ring may be closed or open, as with an associated laceration or puncture of the skin, rectum, or vagina. The mortality rate associated with open pelvic fractures is 6% to 70 %.[5]

Various systems exist for classification of pelvic injuries, such as those described by Trunkey et al,[6] Pennal et al,[7] and Young and Burgess.[8] The current and most practical classification system, described by Tile,[9] categorizes pelvic ring disruptions by their mechanism of injury and their degree of stability. The four major types of injury are anteroposterior compression, lateral compression, vertical shear, and complex. Subdivisions exist within all categories; however, this chapter addresses only the four major categories. Refer to the text by Tile[9] for an excellent discussion of this subject.

An anteroposterior compression injury (Figure 26-10), or external rotation injury, may occur when a crushing force on the posterior superior iliac spine causes the symphysis pubis to spring open anteriorly. Continued external rotation causes rupture of the anterior sacroiliac and sacrospinous ligaments. This disruption is referred to as an "open book" injury. Conversely, direct pressure on the anterior superior iliac spines can disrupt the symphysis pubis and lead to sacrospinous and anterior sacroiliac ligament injury if the compression continues.

Lateral compression (Figure 26-11), or internal rotation, the most common type of pelvic injury, is a result of high-energy forces. Direct pressure to an iliac crest causes an internal rotation injury that crushes the anterior sacrum and displaces the anterior pubic rami. Pressure on the greater trochanter causes the femoral head to disrupt the pubic rami, which can extend into the anterior acetabulum. The ipsilateral sacroiliac complex is also injured by this force. This injury causes bone impaction and may not involve the posterior ligamentous complex.

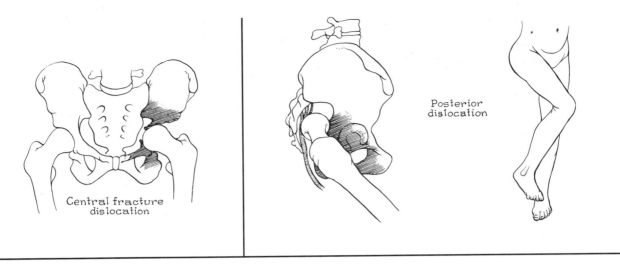

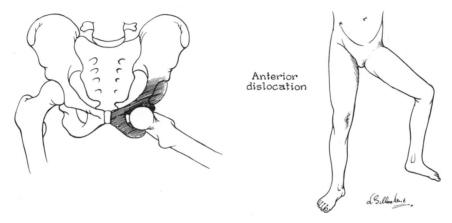

FIGURE 26-8 Basic Types of Hip Dislocation. (From Thomas C: Fractures of the pelvis and hip. In Zuidema GD, Rutherford RB, Ballinger WF, editors: *The management of trauma*, Philadelphia, 1985, WB Saunders.)

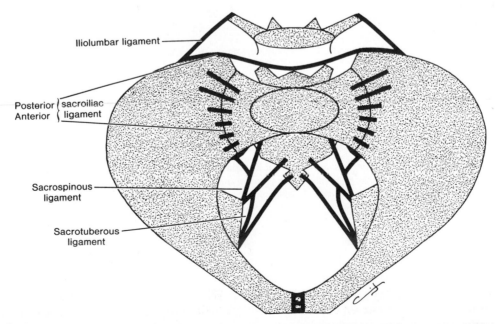

FIGURE 26-9 Diagrammatic representation of the major ligaments of the pelvis: the strong symphysis pubis anteriorly and the posterior tension band of the pelvis, including the iliolumbar, posterior sacroiliac, sacrospinous, and sacrotuberous ligaments. (From Tile M: *Fractures of the pelvis and acetabulum*, Baltimore, 1984, Williams & Wilkins.)

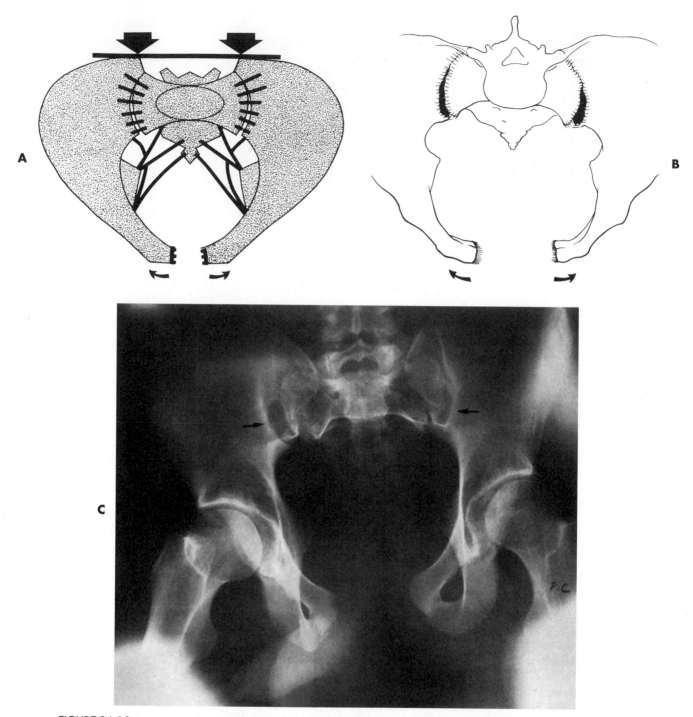

FIGURE 26-10 **Anteroposterior Compression (External Rotation).** **A,** A direct blow to the posterior superior iliac spines causes the symphysis pubis to spring open. **B,** A typical anteroposterior compression (open book) injury, showing a disruption of the symphysis pubis and the anterior sacroiliac ligaments. **C,** Anteroposterior pelvic radiograph of such a patient with markedly widened sacroiliac joints anteriorly. (From Tile M: *Fractures of the pelvis and acetabulum,* Baltimore, 1984, Williams & Wilkins.)

Most anteroposterior and lateral compression injuries are considered stable disruptions because the posterior sacroiliac complex remains intact or because the bone is impacted, thus preventing further disruption. However, the magnitude of the injuring force may be great enough to cause extensive soft tissue injury, leading to instability. Because these injuries are generally stable, they are associated with fewer long-term problems and have low morbidity and mortality rates.

Vertical shear, or Malgaigne fracture (Figure 26-12), is an unstable injury associated with bone and soft tissue disruption. Great force, such as that from falls and crush mechanisms, is in the vertical plane and is usually shearing in nature. Fractures may be unilateral or bilateral, the latter

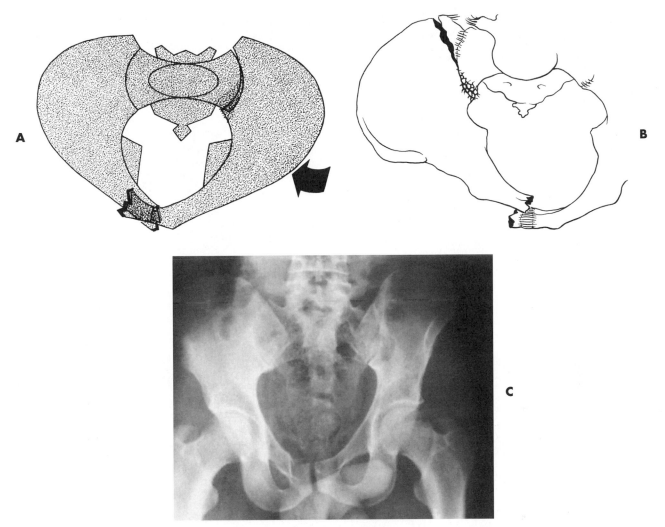

FIGURE 26-11 **Lateral Compression (Internal Rotation). A,** A lateral compressive force directed against the iliac crest causes the hemipelvis to rotate internally, crushing the anterior sacrum and displacing the anterior pubic rami. **B,** A typical ipsilateral type of lateral compression injury, showing a posterior injury and an anterior disruption of the pubic rami with internal rotation of the hemipelvis. **C,** Anteroposterior radiograph of such a patient. (From Tile M: *Fractures of the pelvis and acetabulum,* Baltimore, 1984, Williams & Wilkins.)

representing the most destructive type of unstable disruption. Anterior and posterior ring disruptions and injuries to the sacrotuberous and sacrospinous ligaments are present. Anterior injuries may involve disruption of the symphysis pubis and two to four pubic rami injuries. Posterior lesions involve the sacrum, sacroiliac joints, and the ilium. Skin and subcutaneous tissue may be torn as well. Vertical shear disruptions impose the greatest risk for associated injuries to the gastrointestinal, genitourinary, vascular, and neurologic systems and therefore have the highest morbidity and mortality rates.[2]

Complex pelvic ring disruptions, which result from very powerful forces, cause bizarre fracture-dislocation patterns that do not fit neatly into one of the previously mentioned classifications. These injuries generally represent combinations of applied forces and ligamentous injuries and are usually extremely unstable.

Pelvic ring disruptions such as vertical shear and complex fractures should alert the admitting team to the severity of injury sustained and the need for a comprehensive team approach to resuscitation. Hemodynamic status must be continually monitored because the incidence of severe vascular injury is high with these types of fractures.

Interruption in bone or joint continuity can cause severe muscle spasms that result in pain, angulation, and overriding of bone ends. These complications lead rapidly to decreased venous and lymphatic return, increased soft tissue injury, and swelling. Additionally, persistent bony disruption precipitates further risk for neurovascular injury and fat embolism syndrome.

BONE AND JOINT CONTINUITY MANAGEMENT PRINCIPLES

Early immobilization represents the first step in rehabilitation. Immobilization helps to preserve what function currently exists and prevents further injury. By minimizing

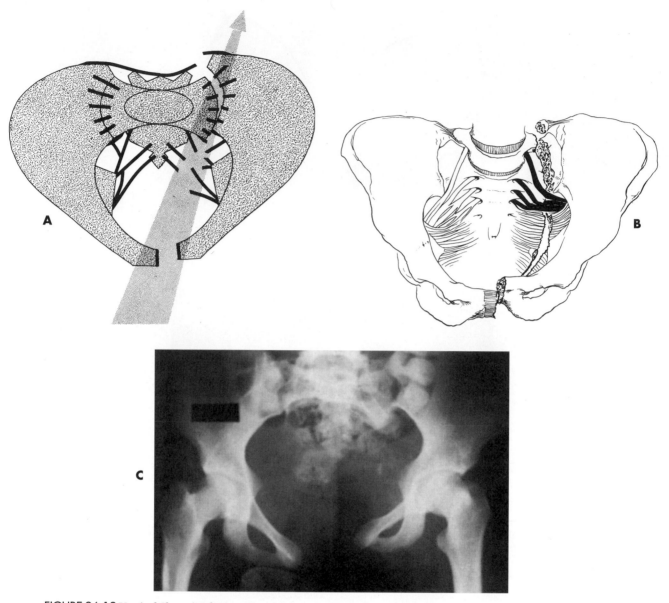

FIGURE 26-12 Vertical Shear (Malgaigne Fracture). A, A shearing force causes marked displacement of bone and gross disruption of soft tissues, resulting in major pelvic instability. **B,** Unilateral unstable (vertical shear [Malgaigne]) fracture causing massive disruption of the pelvic ring. **C,** Inlet view of pelvis shows severe posterior displacement and total disruption of the soft tissues on the left side, indicated by the avulsion of the ischial spine. (From Tile M: *Fractures of the pelvis and acetabulum,* Baltimore, 1984, Williams & Wilkins.)

muscle spasms, proper immobilization also decreases the risk of angulation and overriding of bone ends, helping to prevent closed fractures from becoming open fractures. Application of traction in the field in conjunction with immobilization may help align bone ends in a near-normal anatomic position, which often restores neurovascular and lymphatic function, reduces further soft tissue edema, and decreases pain.

Immobilization techniques and devices applied before admission should remain in place until appropriate radiographic studies are done. Frequent monitoring of neurovascular and motor status is required despite the presence of an immobilization or traction device. Compartment syndrome of the foot has been reported with use of splint-balanced

immobilization devices.[10] Monitoring the immobilization device is necessary to ensure proper placement and effectiveness. After radiologic evaluation, definitive immobilization modalities are initiated.

DISLOCATIONS. Dislocations are immobilized in the position in which they are found. Attempting to straighten a dislocated joint usually results in increased pain and may cause further neurovascular damage. Definitive management of dislocations is discussed later in this chapter.

ANGULATED FRACTURES. Realignment of a severely displaced fracture by a nonphysician depends not only on the presence or absence of vascular compromise and the

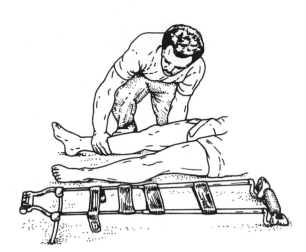

FIGURE 26-13 **Hare Traction Splint.** (From The Maryland Way: *EMT—a skills manual*, Baltimore, 1985, MIEMSS.)

amount of pain associated with realignment but, more importantly, on the established local emergency medical services (EMS) policies governing treatment of such an injury. When realignment is not possible, the injured area is immobilized in the position in which it is found. The neurovascular status of the affected limb should be closely monitored until the limb is properly aligned and immobilized.

EXTREMITY FRACTURES. Proper immobilization of a fracture includes the joints both above and below the site of injury. Manufactured devices such as the Thomas ring splint, the Hare traction splint (Figure 26-13), or the Sager emergency traction device are useful for fractures of the lower extremity that occur approximately 2 inches proximal to the ankle or above. These devices allow application of traction and immobilization of the affected area. Positioning of these devices usually requires two people, and established policies outline the specific procedure to follow to ensure safe, rapid application. The affected extremity must be monitored for swelling, especially with traction, preformed splints, and metal devices. These splints may require loosening of straps and padding to prevent further injury, such as compartment syndrome, which can occur when edematous tissue meets the resistance of such devices. Air splints or premolded rigid splints are useful for feet, ankles, and upper extremities. They decrease edema by applying pressure over the injured area and simultaneously provide tamponade of open, bleeding wounds.

Tissue ischemia can develop if the splint remains in place for an extended time, acting as a tourniquet. The length of time required to cause ischemia varies with each patient and is dependent on multiple variables. Distal pulses cannot be palpated with certain types of immobilization devices in place; therefore visual assessments are essential. The inflatable splint should be replaced with another device as soon as possible. Pressure area changes are common when a splint that has been applied outdoors in a cold environment warms with indoor temperatures. Neurovascular status may deteri-

orate, and warm air causes the splint to tighten. Direct pressure on an inflatable splint should result in some degree of depression, indicating that the splint is not overinflated.

Immobilization should never be prevented or delayed because of a lack of manufactured splints. Any rigid object padded with soft material can be used for effective immobilization. For example, a fractured lower extremity can be splinted against the opposite extremity with padding in between, or injured upper extremities can be immobilized against the torso. Ski boots or other heavy protective boots left in place act as splints and may effectively tamponade underlying vascular injuries.

PELVIC RING DISRUPTION. Initial evaluation of the trauma patient may not reveal obvious clinical evidence of a pelvic injury, such as extremity rotation, shortening, or abnormal movement on downward or inward compression of the iliac wings. However, any signs or symptoms indicative of pelvic ring disruption require patient immobilization before transport to minimize the risk of further neurovascular injury. Suspected pelvic injuries may be effectively immobilized with a pneumatic antishock garment (PASG). This garment provides a tamponade effect and bony immobilization. The use of the PASG is contraindicated in patients with head injuries because it can cause critical elevations in intracranial pressure (ICP). It also is contraindicated in patients who are pregnant and those with pulmonary edema, congestive heart failure, penetrating abdominal trauma, tension pneumothorax, and cardiac tamponade.[11] Obvious pelvic injuries with associated hip dislocations or blow-out injuries to the acetabulum often require creative techniques to achieve initial immobilization and stabilization. Injuries that cause shortening, rotation, or frog-leg positioning require support and stabilization of the patient's lower extremities in the position in which they are found. A long wooden backboard with pillows, rolled sheets, or blankets secured and taped under the patient's knees supports extremity position and ensures immobilization during transport. The patient with an unstable pelvic ring disruption may require formal stabilization (external fixator application) during the early phase of resuscitation to prevent exsanguination and restore hemodynamic stability (Figure 26-14). Use of a C-clamp in the resuscitation room can quickly stabilize the posterior sacroiliac joint if significant bleeding is present or suspected.[3] Caution is essential whenever moving a patient with a pelvic injury because disruption of the retroperitoneal tamponade can rapidly progress to hemorrhagic shock.

GENERAL MANAGEMENT PRINCIPLES AND COMPLICATIONS

The potential for serious, even fatal, complications from musculoskeletal trauma exists in all patients who sustain a musculoskeletal injury. It is mandatory that all persons providing care to injured persons be alert to the signs and symptoms of potential complications. These complications can occur during any phase of the trauma cycle.

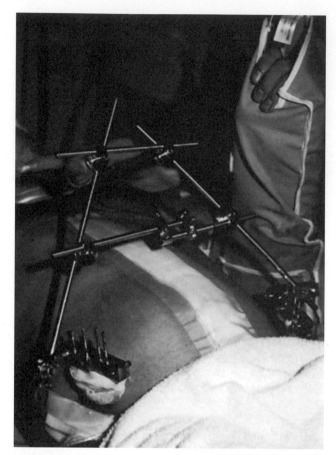

FIGURE 26-14 **Clinical Immobilization for Pelvic Ring Disruption.**

TABLE 26-4   Blood Loss Caused By Fractures*

Fracture	Blood Loss (ml)
Humerus	500-1500
Elbow	250-750
Radius/ulna	250-500
Pelvis	750-6000
Femur	500-3000
Tibia/fibula	250-2000
Ankle	250-1000

*Data from DeDoer AS, Mintjes-deGroot AJ, Severignem AJ et al: Risk assessment for surgical site infections in orthopaedic patients, *Infect Control Hosp Epidemiol* 20(6):402-409, 1999.
Note: One unit of whole blood equals approximately 500 ml.

HYPOVOLEMIA. Any musculoskeletal injury results in blood loss. The degree of hemorrhage and its effect on the patient's overall hemodynamic status depend on the type, location, and number of injuries. Generally, musculoskeletal injuries receive attention after stabilization of the cardiopulmonary and neurologic systems. However, there are times when musculoskeletal injuries become priorities and necessitate early, aggressive intervention. Two injuries associated with excessive blood loss, traumatic amputations and massive pelvic injuries, require priority care with a coordinated team approach to facilitate restoration and maintenance of cardiovascular stability. Other bony and soft tissue injuries can usually wait for definitive care, but the patient still requires adequate volume replacement to prevent hypovolemia related to blood loss.[12] It is difficult to estimate accurately the actual amount of blood lost, especially in patients with multiple extremity or pelvic fractures and soft tissue injuries. Hypovolemia should be anticipated in patients with these injuries, and measures to restore and maintain hemodynamics must be instituted. Table 26-4 approximates possible blood loss with open and closed fractures.

Any patient with actual or potential intravascular volume deficits requires vigilant observation and frequent reevaluation for the clinical indicators of shock. Patients with major musculoskeletal injuries such as traumatic amputations, multiple fractures, and unstable pelvic ring disruptions require close vigilance and should only be transported out of the resuscitation area if accompanied by qualified personnel. These patients can and do rapidly and unexpectedly deteriorate into a hemorrhagic shock state from massive blood loss. Thus constant monitoring, especially during transport, is essential. For example, the retroperitoneal hematoma associated with a massive or unstable pelvic ring disruption can break loose during transfer of the patient to the radiography table. The sudden release of the tamponade precipitates rapid cardiovascular deterioration to shock.

Adequate fluid replacement with colloids or crystalloids, blood, or component therapy is an integral component of successful fluid resuscitation. Early and substantial blood transfusions help prevent deterioration and the sequelae of late shock as a result of massive blood loss (see Chapters 12 and 13). The blood bank should be notified early and updated regarding needs. The amount of blood and blood products required for a patient with massive pelvic injuries can severely strain blood bank supplies. The team may need to consider transferring the patient to a major trauma center for this reason alone.

Obvious sources of external hemorrhage require immediate application of direct pressure and pressure dressings to obtain control. Options include a figure-eight bandage or a bandage wrapped in a spiral fashion, starting at a point distal to the wound and wrapped proximally. Pressure dressings minimize damage to soft tissue and neurovascular structures while achieving hemostasis. Properly applied pressure dressings almost always provide adequate control of hemorrhage, even for traumatic amputations. A tourniquet is not appropriate, except as a last resort for massive, uncontrollable hemorrhage, because it increases the extent of the injury on amputated parts by causing ischemic damage to nerves and vessels.

The benefits from the use of pneumatic antishock garments remain controversial, specifically concerning translocation of blood.[13-16] Their widely recognized values include immobilization and compression effects. PASGs extend the amount of time for resuscitation procedures and provide excellent external tamponade for major hemorrhage, as seen with pelvic injuries and open extremity fractures.

Significant blood loss, as indicated in Table 26-4, can occur within an extremity despite the fact that a specific fracture has been classified as closed. The areas surrounding and distal to the fracture site become swollen, and the skin tightens from the accumulation of blood within the soft tissue.

An open fracture can cause blood loss of at least 1 to 3 or more units, in addition to the amounts listed in Table 26-4. Not only does blood loss become apparent externally, but it also continues internally within the soft tissue.

Massive blood loss and hypovolemic shock can occur from traumatic amputations. This devastating injury requires priority intervention to restore cardiovascular stability. Direct pressure and pressure dressings must be initiated immediately at the scene of the injury and maintained during the initial evaluation and resuscitation phases.

Exsanguination represents the primary cause of early mortality after an unstable pelvic fracture.[12] As previously mentioned, the pelvis receives a rich blood supply through the arteries and venous plexus of the iliac system (Figure 26-15). This vascular network can easily sustain injury or disruption because of its close approximation to the bony structures. The retroperitoneal space can hold large volumes of blood before spontaneous tamponade occurs, making it difficult to determine actual blood loss. The patient with a pelvic injury is also at increased risk for hemorrhage from common associated injury sites, such as intraabdominal viscera, bladder, and urethra, which compounds the blood loss from bony and vascular injuries.[17,18] Hypovolemic shock must be anticipated in patients with massive pelvic injuries, and early interventions to restore hemodynamic status are required. Refer to Chapter 13 for further discussion.

INFECTION.   All open orthopedic injuries are considered contaminated and place the patient at risk for tetanus, gas gangrene, osteomyelitis, and other infections.[4,11] These wounds are contaminated by the prehospital environment and then may be exposed to resistant hospital organisms. Wound and bone infections are potentially disastrous and disabling complications associated with increased morbidity. These infections can lead to delayed union, nonunion, or acute or chronic osteomyelitis, prolonging hospitalization, increasing the patient's financial burden, and possibly resulting in loss of the affected extremity.[19,20] Therefore measures aimed at eliminating further wound contamination and preventing microbial growth are essential and take precedence early during resuscitation.[20-23]

During resuscitation, gross contaminants are removed from the wound and exposed soft tissue and bone are covered with a wet, sterile saline dressing. Prevention of reentry of a dirty bone end or soft tissue into the wound is important. Should reentry occur, it is imperative that the orthopedic specialist be notified. Saline-soaked dressings are recommended rather than those saturated with iodine-based solutions.[11] Soft tissue absorbs some of the solution, and iodine has been found to cause local tissue irritation, decreasing the tissue's resistance to infection. Additionally, iodine can create cellular toxicity.[11] Saline has replaced iodine solutions during surgery and in postoperative wound management as well. Frequent dressing manipulations are avoided because the risk of additional pathogens entering the wound increases with each examination. Sterile procedure must be observed by all personnel when handling open wounds and dressings (e.g., wearing a mask, hat, and sterile gloves).

Ideally the patient should proceed rapidly to the operating suite for irrigation, debridement, and definitive care. If a delay prevents this from occurring, early, aggressive wound irrigation in the emergency care area is necessary. The optimal method of irrigation includes use of large volumes of saline and pulse lavage systems.[23]

Tetanus is a preventable yet highly lethal complication caused by anaerobic bacterial growth in necrotic tissue. To reduce the risk of tetanus, all devitalized tissue must be surgically excised and the patient must be adequately immunized. The patient's recent tetanus immunization history is determined and a booster administered as indicated (see Chapter 14).

Wound contamination may occur from contaminants that enter at the time of injury, bacteria introduced in the hospital environment, and the products of necrosis. The trauma patient with multisystem and musculoskeletal injuries, especially open fractures and traumatic amputations, is at high risk for infection and therefore should receive antibiotics during the resuscitative phase.[19] Wound cultures done before initiating antibiotics can identify infecting organisms and allow for a more precise determination of appropriate therapy, but this may delay treatment. Environmental factors surrounding the incident are essential considerations when initiating antibiotic therapy. Broad-spectrum antibiotic therapy is typically started immediately, with organism-specific antibiotics added depending on environmental factors.

Prevention of microbial growth requires adequate concentrations of the antibiotic at the site of the bone or soft tissue injury or operative site. From the time the antibiotic is administered intravenously, it requires approximately 20 to 30 minutes to achieve saturation in the interstitial fluid of a healthy bone matrix.[19] Antibiotics are most beneficial when they are administered at the peak of bacterial wound contamination, when they satisfactorily invade the bony injury or wound, and when they are chosen specifically for the potential contaminating organisms.[19] For these reasons, administration of intravenous antibiotics begins in the resuscitative phase (or approximately 30 minutes before an elective operative orthopedic procedure) to achieve maximal antimicrobial effects.[19]

The use of prophylactic antibiotics in patients undergoing open reduction of closed fractures is controversial. A specific bacterial organism identified later during the critical

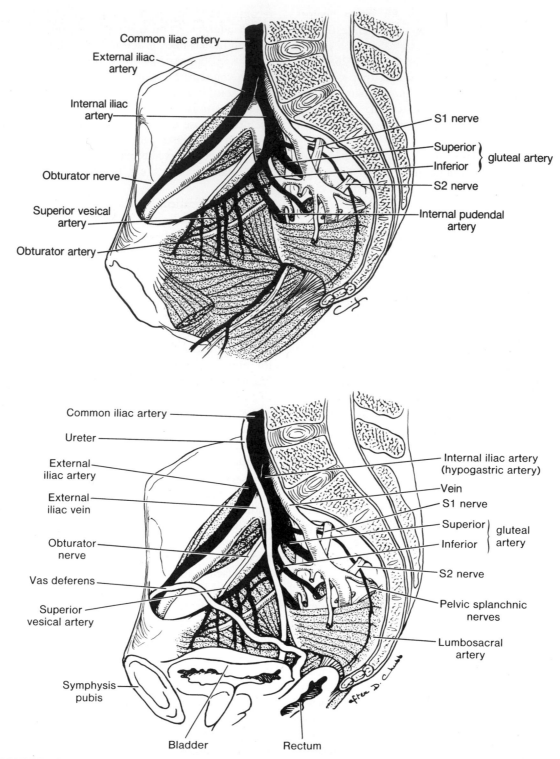

FIGURE 26-15 The Internal Iliac System of Arteries and Veins Showing the Position of the Pelvic Viscera. (From Tile M: *Fractures of the pelvis and acetabulum*, Baltimore, 1984, Williams & Wilkins.)

care or intermediate phase is easier to treat if the organism has not developed a resistance through the administration of prophylactic antibiotics. Many studies related to prophylactic antibiotic use predominately focus on elective orthopedic surgery patients. In the multiple trauma patient the risk of infection increases as the number of systems involved rises.[20] Studies also have shown that operative procedures

lasting longer than 90 minutes have a higher incidence of infection.[20]

NEUROLOGIC AND VASCULAR COMPROMISE. During the resuscitative phase, early recognition of patients at risk for neurologic and vascular compromise as a result of musculoskeletal injury is imperative. The following mechanisms and injuries are precipitants of neurologic and vascular complications:

- Compression or crushing mechanism
- Open or closed fracture
- Soft tissue injury
- Arterial involvement or injury
- Dislocation
- Prolonged use of PASG
- Hypovolemia or shock

Any musculoskeletal injury that involves bone or soft tissue can potentiate neurologic or vascular compromise. Muscle and nerve tissues are easily damaged because of their close proximity to the bony structures and extreme sensitivity to impaired circulation and compression. Regardless of the actual cause of the compromise, the same pathologic condition results: Disrupted vasculature decreases tissue perfusion causing ischemia. If the ischemic process continues, muscle tissue becomes edematous as a result of increased capillary permeability. Edema further increases pressure on the capillaries and eventually causes their collapse. The progression from ischemia to muscle necrosis occurs rapidly. Within 6 to 8 hours the nerves, muscles, and vascular structures may sustain irreversible damage both locally and distally.[24] Understanding the mechanism of injury and the specific types of injuries that carry the highest incidence of neurovascular compromise is the first step in preventing this common yet serious complication.

Injuries to the brachial plexus and lumbosacral plexus also may cause altered sensation and mobility. Neither of these injuries necessitates immediate intervention during the resuscitation and stabilization of the patient with multisystem injuries. However, the peripheral nerve involvement associated with both injuries may create an insensate and paralyzed extremity that renders the patient completely disabled in that limb.

Dislocations. Dislocations are often easily recognized clinically without the aid of diagnostic studies. However, a dislocation may occur at the time of impact and then either reduce spontaneously or during application of an immobilization device at the scene of the incident. For this reason it is important to obtain a history from either the patient or the prehospital care providers concerning any "popping" or "snapping" of a joint that may have been felt or heard.

Dislocations create orthopedic emergencies when bone impinges on nearby vessels or nerves. For example, dislocations of the elbow or the knee require immediate intervention by an orthopedist because of the extremely high incidence of associated neurovascular disruption. The nerve injury secondary to a dislocation may be actual, as in laceration by a bone fragment, or physiologic, as from compression, blast effect, or traction or stretching mechanisms. Clinical findings indicative of a physiologic nerve injury may resolve spontaneously after the bones have been reduced and properly aligned. Symptoms may, however, be of a more permanent nature, depending on the severity of

TABLE 26-5	Neurovascular Structures at Risk for Involvement in Joint Dislocation
Joint	**Nerve/Vessel**
Shoulder	Brachial plexus, axillary artery
Elbow	Ulnar nerve, brachial artery
Wrist	Median nerve
Hip	Sciatic nerve
Knee	Tibial/peroneal nerve, popliteal artery/vein
Ankle	Tibial artery

the injury and the length of time that elapsed before treatment. Vascular involvement may result from laceration, compression, crushing, and traction or stretching mechanisms. The potential resolution of vascular complications depends on the specific injury, the ischemic time, and the ability of collateral circulation to restore and maintain blood flow. Table 26-5 correlates joint dislocations with the potential neurovascular branches involved.

Fractures. Neurovascular compromise associated with fractures results from causes similar to dislocations. Injury to the neurovascular supply of the extremities may result from actual laceration or tearing, compression from bone ends or edematous soft tissue, and stretching by disrupted bone fragments.

Pelvic Injuries. The pelvis enjoys a rich vascular supply, as seen in Figure 26-15. Oxygenated blood enters the pelvis via the internal iliac artery. A venous plexus, consisting of valveless, thin-walled veins that allow bidirectional blood flow, drains the pelvic basin. Collateral networks exist on both the arterial and venous sides. The sciatic nerve arising from the lumbosacral plexus innervates the pelvis and the lower extremities. Any disruption of the bones or ligaments of the pelvis or hips can potentially cause severe neurovascular complications. Massive pelvic ring disruptions are considered lethal injuries because of the major vascular complications with which they are associated.

Brachial Plexus Injury. The brachial plexus, which incorporates the roots of the fifth cervical vertebra to the first thoracic vertebra, subdivides to form the axillary, musculocutaneous, median, ulnar, and radial nerves (Figure 26-16). These nerves are responsible for deltoid, biceps, and triceps function and innervation of the extensors and flexors of the forearm, wrist, and hand.

Traumatic injury to the brachial plexus may occur from blunt or penetrating mechanisms. Blunt injuries usually result from excessive forces that initially injure the muscle and its fascia and then cause extreme stretching of the nervous network, usually the nerve roots.[25] Associated injuries that often accompany brachial plexus injuries include closed head injuries and shoulder dislocations. Most frequently the blunt mechanisms that result in a plexus injury involve the patient's ejection from a car or off a

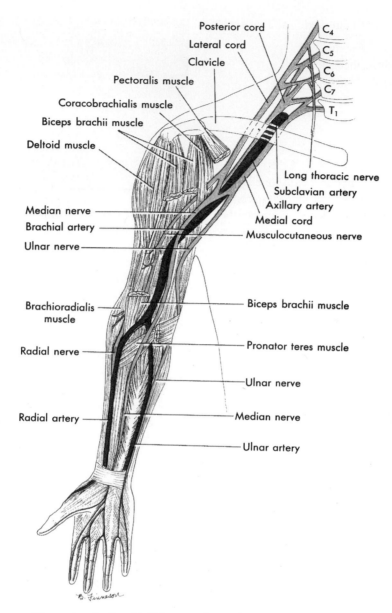

FIGURE 26-16 **Diagram Illustrating the Brachial Plexus and Distribution of Nerves.** Note their relation to arteries and to muscles (right arm). (From Kimber DC, Gray CE, Stackpole CE: *Kimber-Gray-Stackpole's anatomy and physiology,* New York, 1977, Macmillan.)

motorcycle with a landing such that the head is distracted from the affected shoulder and upper extremity.

Blunt brachial plexus injuries are subdivided into upper root and lower root classifications.[26] The upper roots, C5 to C7, may sustain injury when the head experiences significant lateral bending away from the shoulder and when the shoulder itself is forcefully depressed downward. Upper root injury usually does not affect motor function in the wrist and hand but leaves the patient with a motionless shoulder and elbow. The sensory deficit usually affects the deltoid muscle, arm, and forearm. A lower root injury involving C8 to T1 may occur when the arm is forcefully extended over the head. The shoulder and elbow maintain intact motor function, but the forearm and hand lose sensation and motor function. Any closed or blunt injury to the brachial

plexus may be complete or incomplete. Incomplete injuries often present confusing clinical pictures because the patient has inconsistent or unusual patterns of sensory or motor dysfunction. A complete lesion within the brachial plexus results in paralysis and complete sensory loss in the arm and hand.

Penetrating mechanisms, such as in missile or blast injuries or stabbings, that cause open wounds near the shoulder or clavicle may result in injury to the brachial plexus. Associated injuries to surrounding soft tissue and the subclavian vein or artery may precipitate upper extremity ischemia, which further clouds the clinical picture. Motor and sensory deficits can occur from either the ischemic process or the plexus injury, and conclusive differentiation may be difficult.

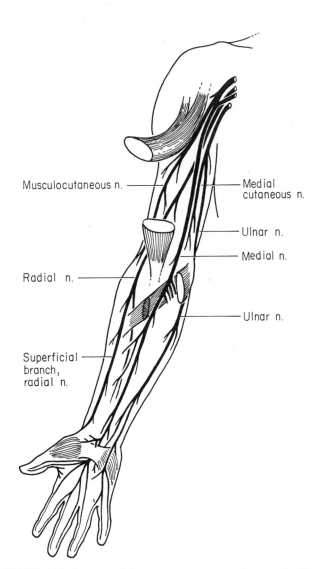

FIGURE 26-17 Nerves of the Arm and Forearm. (From Mubarak SJ: Anatomy of the extremity compartments. In Mubarak SJ, Hargens AR, Akeson WH, editors: *Compartment syndromes and Volkmann's contracture,* Philadelphia, 1981, WB Saunders.)

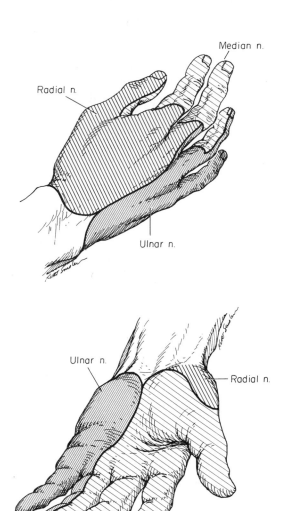

FIGURE 26-18 Distribution of the Cutaneous Nerves to the Hand. (From Mubarak SJ: Anatomy of the extremity compartments. In Mubarak SJ, Hargens AR, Akeson WH, editors: *Compartment syndromes and Volkmann's contracture,* Philadelphia, 1981, WB Saunders.)

Accurate and complete evaluation of the functional status of the brachial plexus in the critically injured multisystem trauma patient is a challenge. Often alterations in the patient's level of consciousness and sensory responses make assessment difficult if not impossible. Differentiation of this injury from a cervical spinal cord injury and from the flaccidity seen with devastating head injuries is essential. The patient should be assessed for Horner's syndrome, or Horner's pupil, which occurs with a preganglionic interruption of the T1 dermatome, causing loss of sympathetic innervation to and constriction of the ipsilateral pupil. The affected pupil remains reactive to light and is usually accompanied by ptosis of the eyelid and possibly loss of facial sweating on the same side. If the patient cannot abduct the affected arm over the head or

extend the elbow against resistance, a brachial plexus injury may have occurred. More specific neuromotor checks to evaluate the nerves in question include the following and are shown in Figures 26-17 and 26-18:

1. The musculocutaneous nerve is tested by evaluating the patient's biceps function and sensation over the lateral portion of the forearm.
2. The radial nerve primarily serves a motor function. Radial nerve injuries usually result in an inability to extend the wrist.
3. An intact median nerve allows apposition of the thumb to the little finger on the affected extremity. Sensory function is evaluated by stimulating the volar surface of the index finger.

4. The motor function of the ulnar nerve is assessed by requesting the patient to abduct and adduct the fingers on the extremity. Intact sensation on the distal volar surface of the little finger represents sensory function.

Early care of brachial plexus injuries is generally supportive, including protection of the affected extremity and proper immobilization, as previously discussed; these measures must continue during critical care. Early rehabilitation to prevent muscle wasting and joint contractures is essential. Prompt recognition of complications such as causalgia and prevention of secondary disabilities such as skin breakdown (see the immobility discussion in the critical care section on page 682) are of paramount importance for the patient with a brachial plexus injury. Early surgical exploration may be indicated in open injuries; at this time the nerves are tagged for later identification. Retrospective studies have demonstrated better functional outcomes if nerve repair, nerve transfers, or nerve grafts are done within 4 months of injury.[26] Unfortunately, despite the advances in microsurgical techniques, outcomes of patients with upper plexus injuries remain poor.[26,27]

Reflex Sympathetic Dystrophy (Causalgia). Brachial plexus injuries that tear sensory nerves at their central attachment may produce reflex sympathetic dystrophy (RSD).[5] This altered pain processing is most commonly associated with ulnar and median nerve involvement. RSD generally develops within the first month after injury. Changes in the affected extremity reflective of autonomic dysfunction may include alterations in skin color (e.g., discoloration, flushing, bluish coloring) and temperature (e.g., hot/flushed or cold/clammy, dry, or increased local perspiration). The most severely disabling problem is extreme, constant, burning pain in the extremity that may be impossible to alleviate. The intractable pain, often leading to behavioral and emotional changes, can interfere with the patient's cooperation and participation and intensify rehabilitation needs. Early administration of narcotics or sympathetic blocks (with a local anesthetic) may provide pain relief. Dorsal column stimulators that block pain transmissions may be effective. Severe, unrelenting pain may require sympathectomy. The emotional and behavioral changes generally improve or dissipate after satisfactory pain management. (Refer to Chapter 17 for further discussion.) This phenomenon also has the potential to occur with any musculoskeletal injury, including fractures, ligamentous or cartilaginous tears, and other soft tissue injuries.

Lumbosacral Plexus Injury. The lumbosacral plexus, incorporating the five lumbar spinal nerves and first four sacral spinal nerves, supplies the sensory and motor function to the lower extremities. The three major nerves arising from the lumbosacral network are the obturator, the femoral, and the sciatic, which divide into the posterior tibial and common peroneal nerves (Figure 26-19).
Injury to the lumbosacral plexus itself occurs much less

frequently than injury to the brachial plexus and must be differentiated from spinal injuries and associated root injuries. Lumbosacral plexus injury occurs rarely from blunt forces and more commonly from penetrating mechanisms such as gunshot wounds.[25] Three types of injuries to the lumbosacral plexus are (1) intradural nerve root avulsion or stretching injury, (2) individual nerve root transection or crushing injury, and (3) disruption or palsy of the plexus. The obturator nerve, protected by its position within the pelvis, rarely sustains injury, yet it may be affected by penetrating trauma to the perineum. Any penetrating or blunt forces to the anterior thigh, especially near the inguinal ligament, may injure the femoral nerve.

The major trunk of the sciatic nerve lies within the pelvis and therefore remains protected from most external trauma. It is at high risk for injury, however, when pelvic disruption or hip fracture or dislocation occurs. The gluteal folds represent the point of superficial appearance of the sciatic nerve, and any wounds in the area of the buttock or thigh may involve the nerve as well. After the division of the sciatic nerve, the most common site of injury to the peroneal branch is at the head of the fibula, where the nerve is afforded little protection from any type of applied force. Blunt or penetrating mechanisms of force may affect the tibial nerve in the popliteal space or in the calf. Elevated pressure within the compartments in the lower leg poses an increased risk for tibial nerve damage.

Evaluation of the integrity of the nerves that arise from the lumbosacral plexus may present a formidable clinical challenge in the multiple trauma patient. It is essential to perform initial and subsequent assessments in the patient suspected of having, or at risk for developing, peripheral nerve involvement. Figure 26-20 shows the peripheral nerves of the lower leg and foot, and Figure 26-21 shows their cutaneous distribution in the foot. (Review the sensory and motor dermatomal patterns found in an anatomy and physiology text.)[1]

1. The motor function of the obturator nerve can be assessed by having the patient adduct the thigh. This examination includes evaluation of the sensory status over the medial aspect of the thigh.
2. The femoral nerve supplies sensation to the anterior thigh and motor function to the quadriceps. Inability to extend the knee and altered sensation in the anterior thigh indicate injury to the femoral nerve.
3. Injury to the common peroneal nerve results in footdrop, the inability to dorsiflex and evert the foot and ankle. Sensory changes in the web space between the first and second toes or over the lateral aspect of the calf indicate peroneal nerve injury.
4. Tibial nerve dysfunction should be suspected if the patient is unable to plantarflex or invert the foot and ankle and experiences sensory changes on the plantar surface of the foot and heel.

Often nerve function can be restored with early reduction (closed or open) of a fracture or dislocation if the angulation

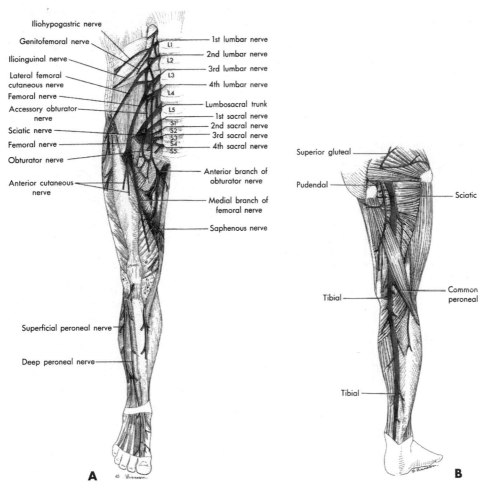

FIGURE 26-19 A, Diagram illustrating the lumbosacral plexus and distribution of nerves. Note their relation to muscles of the leg *(right)*. **B,** Nerve supply to right lower extremity, posterior view. (From Kimber DC, Gray CE, Stackpole CE: *Kimber-Gray-Stackpole's anatomy and physiology,* New York, 1977, Macmillan.)

or dislocation represents the probable cause of the dysfunction (as with posterior hip dislocation). Actual detection and diagnosis of a lumbosacral plexus injury may not occur until later in the acute care or recovery phases, as the patient becomes more alert and is permitted more spontaneous movement. Newer microsurgical techniques have the potential to offer patients more function, but the results are variable. As previously stated, surgical reduction of a posterior hip dislocation (with associated sciatic nerve involvement) may promote nerve recovery.

Compartment Syndrome. Compartment syndrome may affect any body compartment, including extremity compartments throughout the body. Most commonly affected are the lower leg and the forearm, which have two and four muscle compartments, respectively. Of the body's 46 compartments, 36 are found in the extremities.[24] Compartments are defined as closed spaces containing muscles, nerves, and vascular structures that are enclosed within tissue such as bone or fascia.[24] Sheaths of fascia tightly bind these closed muscle systems, which house neurovascular bundles. Compartment syndrome may result when either internal contents or external sources increase compartment pressure (Table 26-6). Internal causes of increased compartment pressures include increased volume and increased capillary filtration, which represent increased intracompartment content. External causes of increased compartment pressure decrease the size of the compartment. Both internal and external causes elevate pressures within the compartments, which compress the microvascular system, leading to ischemia of the muscle tissue (Figure 26-22). If elevated compartment pressures are not reduced, irreversible damage to the muscle and nerve tissue, including necrosis and scarring, results within 6 to 8 hours.

A common misconception is that open fractures are safe from compartment syndrome because they are open. Although an open wound may violate a fascial compartment, other compartments remain intact and are at risk for this syndrome. Additionally, traumatic wounds usually occur horizontally and are not large enough to decompress the compartment.[28]

After an injury to an extremity, an immediate inflammatory response results in decreased blood flow distal to the injury and tissue hypoxia.[24] Inflammatory mediators are released and cause the capillary wall to lose integrity and colloid proteins to leach into the soft tissue, drawing more

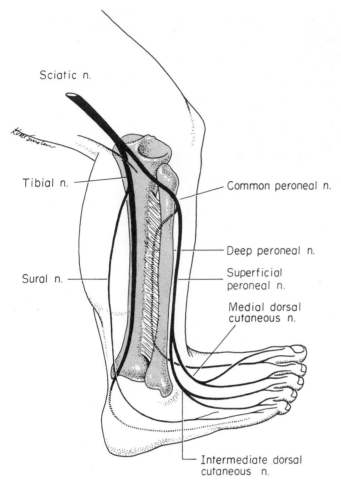

FIGURE 26-20 **Peripheral Nerves of the Leg.** (From Mubarak SJ: Anatomy of the extremity compartments. In Mubarak SJ, Hargens AR, Akeson WH, editors: *Compartment syndromes and Volkmann's contracture,* Philadelphia, 1981, WB Saunders.)

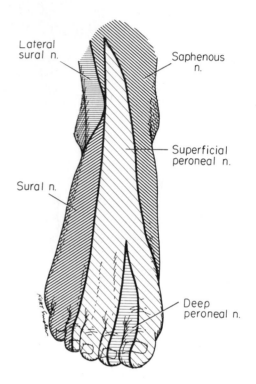

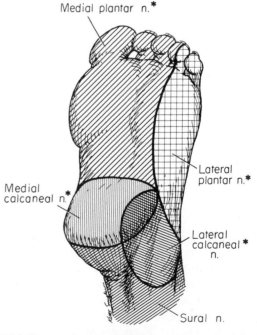

TABLE 26-6	**Causes of Compartment Syndrome**
Internal	**External**
Trauma compressing or crushing mechanisms, open/closed fractures	Prolonged or excessive use of pneumatic antishock garments, splints, traction devices, circumferential dressings
Soft tissue or vascular injuries	Prolonged pressure over compartment: lying or positioning, intraoperative
Burns: thermal, electrical, frostbite	Excessive skeletal traction
Venomous bites: spiders, snakes	Eschar from burns
Prolonged shock states: tissue ischemia, venous pooling	
Contusions	
Bleeding disorders or anticoagulation	
Infiltrated intravenous sites	

FIGURE 26-21 **Distribution of the Cutaneous Nerves to the Foot.** (From Mubarak SJ: Anatomy of the extremity compartments. In Mubarak SJ, Hargens AR, Akeson WH, editors: *Compartment syndromes and Volkmann's contracture,* Philadelphia, 1981, WB Saunders.)
*Branches of the tibial nerve.

SECTION OF MUSCLE COMPARTMENTS

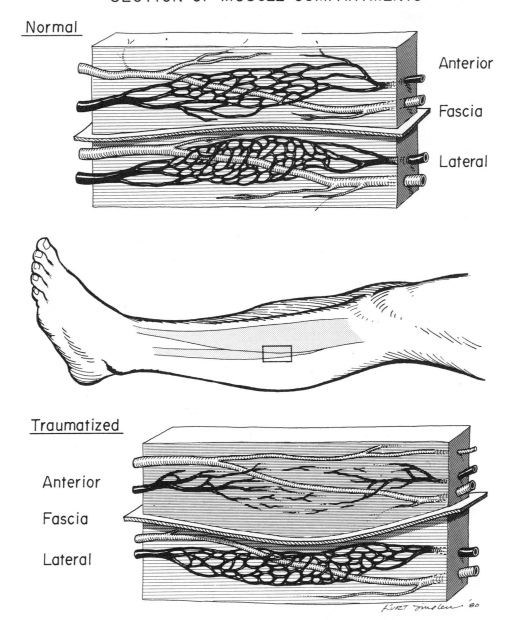

FIGURE 26-22 Unifying Principles of Compartment Syndrome. In the enlarged figure above the leg, normal microcirculation is viewed during rest in the anterior and lateral muscle compartments. These two compartments are separated by fascia. During rest, intracompartmental pressure in the anterior and lateral compartments is near zero, and blood flow in all capillaries *(network of black vessels)* and large arteries *(shaded vessels entering figure from the right)* is normal. If pressure in the anterior compartment reaches a threshold level near 30 mm Hg *(enlarged figure below leg)*, capillary perfusion is inadequate to maintain tissue viability. It is noteworthy that distal pulses are usually present in the foot primarily because intracompartmental pressure rarely rises above central artery diastolic pressure. (From Hargens AR, Mubarak SJ: Definition and terminology. In Mubarak SJ, Hargens AR, Akeson WH, editors: *Compartment syndromes and Volkmann's contracture,* Philadelphia, 1981, WB Saunders.)

fluid into the soft tissue.[24] This fluid shift causes increased edema, and the cycle is perpetuated. As the edema within the compartment increases, there is a change in the pressure relationships within the compartment.[24] The imbalance in the pressures between inflow of arterial blood and outflow of venous blood eventually cumulates in total cessation of blood flow into the affected extremity.[24] Intracompartmental pressures in excess of 30 to 40 mm Hg can cause muscle ischemia, and pressures greater than 55 to 65 mm Hg cause

irreversible muscle death.[24] Recent studies have implicated neutrophils and thromboxane A_2 in the microvascular dysfunction and blood flow distribution abnormalities found in the ischemia-reperfusion injury of acute compartment syndrome.[29,30] The use of cyclooxygenase inhibitors have demonstrated decreased thromboxane levels and intracompartmental pressures and may play a role in limiting tissue ischemia[29] (Figure 26-23).

Patients who are athletes or have sustained a prior injury

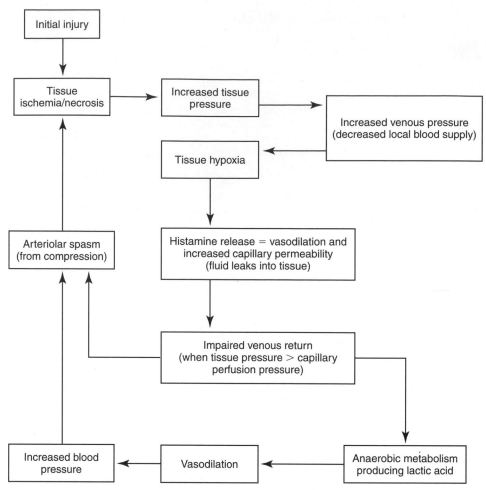

FIGURE 26-23 **Pathophysiology of Acute Compartment Syndrome.** (From Ross D, Evans R: A patient with acute compartment syndrome. In *Clinical simulations in medical-surgical nursing III: Medi-Sim computer assisted instruction,* Baltimore, 1994, Williams and Wilkins.)

with scar formation are at higher risk for development of compartment syndrome. The larger muscle mass associated with athletes, especially distance runners, decreases the available space within a compartment. Scar formation also limits the fascia's ability to expand to accommodate edema.[31,32]

Clinical signs of compartment syndrome include throbbing pain that is localized to the affected compartment; firmness of the entire compartment; and paresthesia, a later symptom, in the distal distribution of the nerve involved. When these symptoms—pain, firmness, and paresthesia—are found simultaneously, they signal impending extremity morbidity unless appropriate interventions begin immediately.

The pain associated with neurovascular compromise, often described as burning or searing, results from the ischemic process occurring at the site of injury and in surrounding and distal soft tissue structures. Bleeding and edema within the surrounding soft tissues, in addition to the specific injury, result in the pain associated with fractures and dislocations. Any type of movement of the extremity increases pain at the site of injury. Reported compartment syndrome pain usually seems out of proportion to the actual injury. Use of narcotics often cannot relieve the pain associated with this syndrome. The pain increases on passive stretching of the muscles. For example, flexion of the ankle and foot or the toes causes increased pain in the lower leg. It is therefore important to monitor and record trends in the patient's pain patterns and effects of the medication administered.

Edema becomes clinically evident soon after the initial injury as a normal response to trauma. Compartment pressure increases, however, as bleeding, interstitial edema, and muscle fiber swelling increase within the compartment space. As compartment pressures rise higher than 30 mm Hg, the affected compartment becomes extremely taut and feels hard. Pain and firmness of the compartment are the key symptoms of compartment syndrome.

Paresthesia, pulselessness, and paralysis are late signs of compartment syndrome. Waiting for all these symptoms to appear not only places the patient at risk for losing the limb but also may create a potentially life-threatening situation. It is important to note that in the early stages of compartment syndrome the extremity may be very warm to touch, with rubor, and pulses may be bounding. This is the body's

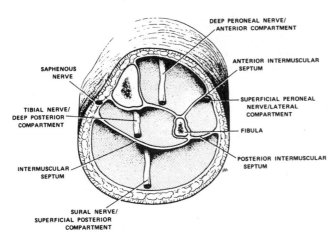

FIGURE 26-24 Cross-Section at the Junction of the Middle and Distal Thirds of the Leg, Illustrating the Four Compartments and Their Respective Nerves. (From Mubarak SJ, Owen CA: Double incision fasciotomy of the leg for decompression in compartment syndromes, *J Bone Joint Surg* 59A:184, 1977.)

compensatory attempt to increase local blood flow, but it eventually fails, and the extremity then demonstrates pallor, pulselessness, and eventually "polar" or ice-cold characteristics. This signifies death of tissue.

Altered sensation indicates probable pressure on nerves housed within muscle compartments. Described symptoms may include numbness, tingling, and "sticking" feelings. For example, paresthesia or dysesthesia over the medial aspect of the leg to the knee, such as that seen in posterior thigh compartment syndrome, indicates obturator nerve involvement. Deltoid compartment syndrome may present as paresthesia over the lateral shoulder and skin covering the deltoid muscle from compression of the upper lateral brachial cutaneous nerve, the sensory branch of the axillary nerve. Involvement of the superficial peroneal nerve, housed in the lateral compartment of the lower leg (Figure 26-24), results in altered sensation in the dorsum of the foot.

Decreased voluntary limb movement may occur initially as a result of extreme pain. However, actual paralysis is a later sign, signifying that the muscles have begun to necrose (e.g., the patient with compartment syndrome of the anterior compartment of the lower leg cannot dorsiflex the great toe). Alterations in distal pulse quality and capillary refill time are most commonly seen in compartment syndrome of the hand and foot and not in other compartments.

Prompt recognition and early institution of therapeutic measures must occur long before the late signs of compartment syndrome. The injured extremity should always be compared with the nonaffected extremity during this evaluation. This assessment must be performed at least every 1 to 2 hours or more frequently, depending on the patient's status and the examiner's clinical observations and judgment. Established protocols or nursing standards provide further guidelines. Early recognition and treatment decrease the risk of limb morbidity and minimize the risk of life-threatening complications.

Clinical signs of compartment syndrome indicate the need to measure the pressures within the muscle compartments. Pressure measurements may be performed prophylactically in the unconscious patient who has signs of increasing pressure. Controversy exists surrounding the upper pressure limits that mandate a fasciotomy, the treatment of choice for elevated pressures; the aggressive recommendation for fasciotomy uses 30 mm Hg[33] as the determining level, whereas the conservative recommendation uses 60 mm Hg.[34] Most authorities agree on a gray zone in which the pressure limits may be borderline. If the patient is conscious, can give reliable information, and has the ability to describe pain and other symptoms consistently, close clinical observation should continue, with possible follow-up pressure measurements as indicated. However, if the patient is unconscious and has borderline pressure measurements, fasciotomy is usually recommended.[34] Continuous monitoring is occasionally used in the patient with multisystem injuries to obtain a reliable trend in intracompartment pressures.[34] Recently it was reported that mannitol treatment was used to decrease intracompartmental pressures by promoting osmotic diuresis.[35]

There are several methods of measuring intracompartmental pressures.[34] The systems that are currently being used, the slit and wick catheters, consist of a fluid-filled catheter attached to an extracorporeal transducer that is placed into the muscle compartment.[34] The accuracy of these measurements depends on accurate calibrations and is affected by the position of the limb and the height of the pressure transducer above the tip of the catheter. These type of systems measure the intracompartmental pressures in relation to capillary pressures.[34] Recently an electronic transducer-tipped catheter, originally designed to measure intracranial pressures, has been used to measure intracompartmental pressures and does not rely on fluid-filled systems.[34] This new system is ideal for use in continuous monitoring of intracompartmental pressures because it does not require frequent saline flushes to maintain the patency of the catheter.[34]

Monitoring and Management. Potential or actual peripheral nerve or vascular compromise requires continuous, ongoing monitoring. Clinical findings commonly seen with dislocations, fractures, or plexus injuries include alteration in pulse quality, edema, change in skin color (e.g., pallor, arterial inadequacy, cyanosis, venous congestion), and altered sensory and motor function. Ongoing motor and sensory assessments are essential even after institution of traction devices to promote early detection of neurologic impairment. Devices such as Buck's skin traction, used preoperatively for hip fractures, can cause peroneal branch nerve compression if improperly applied or maintained.[36] Compression of the peroneal nerve as it passes over the fibular head leads to footdrop, a complication that can extend the patient's hospital stay and increase rehabilitation needs.

As discussed previously in this chapter, proper immobilization and alignment are essential elements in preventing further injury to the soft tissues, especially the vessels and nerves. The risk for further injury, such as laceration, continued hemorrhage, and additional impingement or compression, increases if proper immobilization techniques are not employed soon after injury. For example, splinting the entire upper extremity in the position of function is essential for the patient with a brachial plexus injury because further stretching of the deltoid muscle may result in humeral head dislocation. Proper positioning, realignment of fractures, or reduction of dislocations often must take precedence during resuscitation in an effort to reduce extremity morbidity.

Elevation. Maintaining an injured limb in a nondependent position, but not above the level of the patient's heart, may reduce further edema formation and improve venous return. Elevation above the level of the patient's heart may actually impede circulation because the local arterial pressure decreases 0.8 mm Hg for each centimeter of elevation.[37] Certain situations may call for elevation of an extremity above the level of the heart, but these are handled on an individual basis.

Cooling of the injured extremity should begin concurrently with elevation. Prepackaged coolant bags and plastic bags and gloves filled with ice-cooled water all work effectively. Use of frozen products or pure ice bags should be avoided because ice causes vasoconstriction, with a resultant decrease in local circulation and venous return, and may lead to thermal injuries in areas with decreased sensation.

Any extremity with neurologic impairment should be monitored closely for position and environmental factors. A paralyzed, insensate limb is at increased risk for accidental or secondary injury. Prolonged pressure on bony prominence can quickly lead to skin breakdown and ulceration, which are preventable and costly complications for the patient.[24] Measures that improve circulation and promote venous return, such as positioning and elevation, should be instituted.

PAIN MANAGEMENT. Injury to the musculoskeletal system produces pain of varying intensity depending on the type and location of the injury. Muscle spasms are the major cause of pain associated with fractures. The pain results from fractured bone ends moving, overriding, and passing through soft tissue. Lessening or elimination of muscle spasms by immobilization and stabilization or by reduction of the fracture often eliminates much of the pain. Placement of cool packs over the site of injury and administration of analgesics are required.

Pain associated with dislocation is often severe and continuous until the dislocation has been reduced. Additional pain is often caused by intentional or unintentional movement of the joint. Immobilization of the joint in the position in which it is found helps prevent or minimize movement and thereby minimize pain. Muscle relaxants and narcotics relieve some of the muscle spasms and pain, but complete elimination of the pain associated with dislocations usually can only be accomplished through reduction of the dislocated joint. Because of the time that elapses from injury to attempted reduction (usually more than 2 hours), increased muscle spasms and pain make muscle relaxants and narcotics necessary to attempt reduction. In severe cases general anesthesia is required to effect complete muscle relaxation.

Compartment syndrome pain is often described as deep, poorly localized, and continuous and is difficult to control with the usual analgesics required for musculoskeletal pain management. Compartment syndrome is often associated with crush injuries and severe fractures. It is easy to discount the pain as being caused by the original injury and not by compartment syndrome, a complication of the injury. Pain associated with compartment syndrome can only be relieved by eliminating the high fascial compartment pressures, such as by removal of constrictive bandages, elevation of the affected extremity (but not higher than the level of the patient's heart), application of cool packs to reduce swelling, and fasciotomy.

The therapeutic plan for acute pain management is often developed and initiated during the resuscitation or preoperative phases of care. For example, recognizing the pain associated with a complex acetabular fracture and realizing surgical intervention will be delayed for at least several days, the team may elect to insert an epidural catheter before transferring the patient to the intensive care unit after resuscitation. Early continuous analgesia given through this type of catheter provides pain relief, thus enabling the patient to cooperate with the prescribed physical therapy regimen to prevent muscle wasting. This catheter also may be inserted during the preoperative phase for both intraoperative and postoperative use. Continuous analgesia via an epidural catheter enables early patient mobility and nursing interventions to prevent or minimize complications such as pulmonary problems.[38]

Pain management, as with all aspects of trauma patient care, requires a comprehensive, team approach for effective, safe results. Management of acute and chronic pain, defined as pain lasting longer than 6 months,[39] is discussed in Chapter 17.

FAT EMBOLISM SYNDROME
Etiology. Fat embolism syndrome (FES) is an ambiguous and controversial process that has been studied and debated since the 1860s when it was first described in the literature. Controversy continues surrounding the etiology and appropriate therapy for FES. FES has been described in association with a variety of injuries and disease processes. The course of the syndrome and the developing symptomatology are often similar, with the end result being a form of acute respiratory distress syndrome (ARDS). FES may develop from hours to days after the injury, but usually occurs within 72 hours after injury.[40] Close monitoring of patients at high risk for FES should begin on admission and must continue throughout the early phase of critical care.

Although FES is usually discussed in association with musculoskeletal injuries, it also has been described in patients with burns, massive soft tissue injuries, severe infections, and nontraumatic medical problems such as diabetes and pancreatitis.[41] Long bone fracture, multiple rib fractures, pelvic injury, or a combination of multiple fractures, however, places the patient in the classic high-risk category. Recent studies have demonstrated that patients with multiple fractures usually have a higher Injury Severity Score (ISS) and therefore a higher incidence of other injuries, with resultant increases in the incidence of fat embolism syndrome.[42]

It is important to distinguish fat embolus from fat embolism syndrome. Fat embolus indicates the presence of fat globules in the lung tissue and peripheral circulation and may or may not cause systemic symptoms.[43] Fat embolism syndrome is a manifestation of fat emboli that results in clinical evidence of alterations in function of the respiratory, neurologic, and dermatologic systems.[43]

Two theories have emerged regarding the etiology of FES: active mobilization of fat globules and altered fat metabolism. The mobilization, or mechanical, theory focuses on the actual impact (e.g., the time a bone is stressed and sustains a fracture). The damaged bone and the injured veins, which lie close to the bone itself, allow the release of marrow components, including fat globules, into the circulation. Sauter and Klopper report that increased pressure and longer duration of the externally applied forces result in increased release of fat emboli.[44] The second theory, altered fat metabolism, has been referred to as the "physiochemical theory." The biochemical disturbances that occur after stress or trauma affect the stability and metabolism of fat and other circulating products. Increased catecholamine levels activated by the inflammatory response cause an increased release of free fatty acids and neutral fats into the circulation. The free fatty acids affect the pneumocytes, altering gas exchange.[24,43] The problem worsens as fibrinolysis, red blood cell aggregation, and platelet adhesiveness increase from the disrupted fat metabolism. The fat globules grow in size as they become coated with platelets.[43,45] It is felt that these two processes are not mutually exclusive and that synergism plays an important role in the development of the FES[43] (Figure 26-25).

The subsequent pathologic conditions that occur during the syndrome are the same regardless of the etiologic theories. The large fat globules are filtered out in the pulmonary vascular system and obstruct the blood flow in capillaries. This obstruction, in combination with the release of serotonin and other inflammatory mediators, increases capillary permeability, leading to fluid leaks into the interstitial space, hemorrhage, and ARDS, with alveolar collapse, impaired tissue perfusion, and tissue hypoxia.[24,46,47]

A latent period between the injury and appearance of clinical symptoms of FES, has been described and also disputed. Peltier noted that not giving this asymptomatic phase the attention that it warrants causes the early signs to be overlooked.[45] In actuality, acute signs and symptoms of FES have been reported as soon as 1 hour or less after the injury and as long as 96 hours after injury; the average time appears to be between 12 and 48 hours.[43] Mild cases of FES or the early signs of the syndrome may be overlooked if high-risk patients are not closely monitored and the syndrome is not anticipated.

The clinical manifestations of FES involve the pulmonary, neurologic, and cutaneous systems.[40,43] Tachypnea, dyspnea, cyanosis, tachycardia, and fever are common clinical findings.[24,40,43] Hypoxemia is the hallmark of FES, and use of continuous pulse oximetry may detect early changes in oxygen saturation.[40,43] Neurologic findings include subtle changes ranging from irritability to coma.[43] Petechiae are thought to be the result of occlusion of dermal capillaries by fat and increased capillary fragility and are

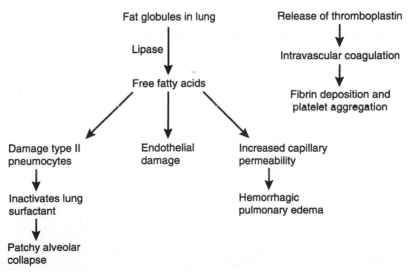

FIGURE 26-25 **Pathophysiology of Fat Embolism Syndrome.** (From Maher AB, Salmond SW, Pellino TA: *Orthopaedic nursing,* Philadelphia, 1998, WB Saunders.)

usually distributed over the chest, base of the neck, conjunctiva, mucous membranes, and axillae.[24,43] Treatment of FES is usually supportive and is aimed at correction of fluid volume deficits, improvement of oxygenation, and management of associated injuries.[24,40,43] Respiratory support is essential to correct hypoxemia and includes supplemental oxygen and mechanical ventilation with positive end-expiratory pressure (PEEP).[40,43]

Throughout the resuscitation and postresuscitation phases, high-risk patients require close monitoring. Acute awareness of the potential for FES and actively observation for suspicious signs facilitate prompt recognition of this syndrome.

Signs and Symptoms.   Efforts to restore normovolemia and sustain hemodynamic stability must continue throughout the early phases of trauma care. Insertion of a pulmonary artery catheter may become necessary to evaluate the patient's hemodynamic status in an effort to avoid fluid overload. The patient with FES usually develops tachycardia, hypotension, and decreased cardiac output in response to increased pulmonary resistance. The patient may complain of chest pain and exhibit signs of right ventricular heart dysfunction, as evidenced on serial electrocardiograms and elevated central venous pressure (CVP) or right atrial pressure (RAP). Arrhythmias, right bundle branch block, inverted T waves, prominent S waves in lead I, prominent Q waves in lead III, and depressed RST segments may all be seen with cardiac strain from FES.[45]

Analysis of serial arterial blood gases aids in early detection of hypoxemia. With the onset and progression of FES, the patient experiences tachypnea and dyspnea and may develop a productive cough. Auscultation of bilateral lung fields may reveal moist crackles. Cyanosis, bloody sputum, pulmonary edema, and findings of bilateral fluffy infiltrates on the chest radiograph are indicative of ARDS. Pulmonary support is the most important component of care for patients with FES. The patient may require therapy similar to that for ARDS: intubation, mechanical ventilation, and varying levels of PEEP for adequate alveolar aeration.[42] Some patients respond to oxygen and do not require intensive therapies.

Generally the first neurologic sign of deterioration is an abrupt change in behavior or mentation. A previously awake, alert, cooperative patient without an associated head injury becomes restless, agitated, uncooperative, and even disoriented in the presence of FES. Cerebral embolization may result in localized areas of anoxia because of specific vessel occlusion; generalized anoxia may occur from pulmonary dysfunction-induced hypoxemia.[43] The patient with cerebral involvement may rapidly deteriorate to a state of unresponsiveness, necessitating close neurologic monitoring.

In FES, oliguria or anuria commonly indicates inadequate circulating volume and reduced renal perfusion. Lipuria, fat in the urine, is believed to indicate a clinically

significant manifestation of FES.[45] Hematuria also may be present.

Analysis of arterial blood gases typically reveals low Pao_2 (less than 60 mmHg) and elevated $Paco_2$, indicative of hypoxemia and carbon dioxide retention. Thrombocytopenia with platelet counts as low as 50,000/mm³ develops as a normal process of the clotting mechanism after injury and also as a result of platelet aggregation around the fat globules. Platelet levels usually return to normal within 5 to 7 days. Decreases in hemoglobin of 3 to 5 g/dl reflect the sequestration of red blood cells to the fat globules.

The petechial rash seen with FES may develop 12 to 96 hours after injury. Flat red spots usually appear and disappear in waves, often going unnoticed by the unsuspecting observer, and generally cease within 48 hours of onset. Petechiae are not seen in all patients; therefore the absence of petechiae is not diagnostic.

A classic sign of FES is a rapid temperature spike to 38° C to 40° C (101.4° F-104° F) without other precipitating causes. Altered temperature regulation from cerebral emboli may be responsible for the fever.[40]

DEEP VEIN THROMBOSIS.   Deep vein thrombosis (DVT) is a significant hazard to the trauma patient with musculoskeletal involvement and may result in pulmonary thromboembolism (PTE). Approximately 630,000 patients in the United States develop pulmonary embolism each year, resulting in 200,000 deaths.[48] General data on all general surgery patients over the age of 40 indicate that DVT occurs in 16% to 30%, significant PTE episodes occur in 1.6%, and fatal PTE occurs in 1% of this patient population. Trauma-related DVT/PTE data are sparse because injuries are commonly multisystem, and tissue trauma can cause false-positive results in some diagnostic studies used for DVT/PTE. Generally, however, 20% of young adult trauma patients develop DVT.[49] More than 40% of elderly trauma patients with hip fractures experience DVT, and 14% have a fatal PTE episode.[49] Data on head- and spinal cord-injured patients reveal a DVT incidence of greater than 40% and fatal PTE of 5%.[49] Prevention of DVT/PTE is emphasized as better than any treatment modality.[49] The American College of Chest Physicians (ACCP) Consensus Committee on Pulmonary Embolism reviewed 8 clinically relevant issues and made recommendations regarding diagnosis and treatment (the reader is encouraged to review this consensus statement).[50] Currently there are multiple studies that address the issue of detection and diagnosis of pulmonary embolism.[51-54] A majority recommend combination prophylaxis with low-dose heparin, low-molecular-weight heparin, elastic stockings, and intermittent pneumatic compression.[49]

The major etiologic factors that predispose patients to DVT and subsequently PTE are called Virchow's triad: (1) venous stasis from decreased blood flow, decreased muscular activity, and external pressure on the deep veins; (2) vascular damage or concomitant pathologic state; and

(3) hypercoagulability. Predisposing factors within these three categories include the following:

- History of vascular disease
- Previous DVT or PTE episode
- Prolonged bed rest or immobility
- Lengthy surgical procedures
- Shock states
- Sepsis
- Spinal cord injuries
- Long bone, hip, or pelvic fractures
- Soft tissue injuries
- Vessel trauma
- Multiple venous punctures
- Intravenous infusion of irritating fluids or drugs
- Immobilization devices
- Prolonged use of pneumatic antishock garments
- Obesity
- Age greater than 40 years
- History of heart failure, acute myocardial infarction, stroke, or malignancy
- History of estrogen or anticoagulation therapy

Early identification of patients who are prone to DVT/PTE and initiation of measures that optimize venous return are integral components of care. Patients identified as high risk who require extensive surgery on admission, such as operative stabilization of cervical or thoracolumbar spine injuries or reconstructive plastic surgery, may benefit from preoperative application of graduated elastic stockings or an alternating pneumatic compression device. Low-molecular-weight or low-dose heparin is started in most trauma patients within a few hours of admission.[49]

Assessment and Diagnosis. Ongoing patient evaluation aids in early detection of signs of DVT. Patients should be regularly assessed for physical signs and symptoms although these are not specific or reliable, and such findings should be reported immediately:

- Calf pain on forced dorsiflexion of the foot (Homans' sign)
- Subtle to obvious swelling of the involved area
- Tachycardia
- Fever
- Distal skin color and temperature changes

An acute pulmonary thromboembolism episode may be the first indication of the presence of DVT. Any signs or symptoms of DVT should arouse suspicions in all trauma patients. Accurate assessment and patient history is important. Many trauma patients are women, and hormone therapy, either oral contraceptives or hormone replacement therapy (HRT) in postmenopausal women, is a major contributing factor in the development of DVT/PE.[55,56]

A number studies are available to diagnose DVT:

- Venography—rarely used because of serious complications
- Doppler flow studies
- Venous pressure measurement
- Impedance plethysmography (IPG)
- Plasma D-dimer studies
- Magnetic resonance imaging
- Computed tomography

Controversy remains regarding the benefits of serial screening for DVT in asymptomatic patients. Further research is needed to weigh the cost/benefit ratio.[49]

Prevention. Patient and family teaching should include the causes of DVT, common signs and symptoms, and self-preventive measures. Ongoing teaching and reinforcement promote patients' understanding and ideally their participation and compliance with the preventive regimen.

Mobilization should occur as soon as possible and as much as permitted within the limitations of the patient's injury because lower extremity muscle activity optimizes circulation and venous return. Early mobilization is a primary DVT preventive measure. If ambulation is impossible because of injuries or a critical patient condition, an exercise program should be initiated soon after resuscitation. Isometric exercises stimulate muscle contraction, which increases venous return. Ambulatory patients should be encouraged to remain as mobile as possible by ambulating for at least 20 minutes three to four times a day. Patients who are allowed out of bed in a chair should be assisted in getting out of bed several times a day even if for short periods, rather than one time a day for a lengthy period. While out of bed, patients should not be permitted to keep their legs in a dependent position for an extended time; rather, legs should be outstretched and elevated to promote venous return. Periodic lowering of the legs during sitting can reduce compression of the femoral vein. Pressure areas on the calves or under the knees should be avoided while positioning the patient in the chair. The patient should continue to perform isometric exercises and active dorsiflexion and plantar flexion while in the chair.

Awake patients confined to bed rest require frequent change in positions, active range-of-motion exercises, and isometric exercises within the limitations imposed by their injuries. Specific injuries or alterations in level of consciousness that preclude the patient's participation in an exercise regimen require a team approach to restore and maintain muscle activity and enhance venous return. A coordinated, planned exercise program includes active involvement of the physical therapy department, but primary responsibility rests with the bedside nurse.

Attention to extremity placement, positioning, and padding is important. For example, the lateral recumbent position without adequate padding between the legs increases external pressure on the veins in the lower extremities and increases the risk of intimal damage. Pressure or prolonged flexion of the knees impedes circulation and venous return. Elevation of the knees and upper torso above hips should be avoided.

Early recognition of patients who may require prolonged bed rest leads to early institution of DVT prophylaxis such as graded elastic stockings or plantar plexus pulsation intermittent pneumatic compression devices. Elastic bandages wrapped from the toes to the thighs or fitted elastic stockings can be applied soon after resuscitation.

Pneumatic compression devices (Figure 26-26) are indicated in trauma patients in whom anticoagulation is contraindicated or who are unable to actively perform exercises. Pneumatic compression devices have a tubular section for each leg, which is usually positioned between the ankle and knee. They continuously inflate to a predetermined pressure and deflate after a preset length of time. Such devices cause no positioning restrictions and should be initiated soon after resuscitation, for example, intraoperatively on patients requiring lengthy operative procedures on admission. Their effectiveness in preventing DVT is related to promotion of venous flow through vein compression and activation of fibrinolytic activity.[49]

High-risk trauma patients may require early prophylactic anticoagulation to aid in prevention of DVT.[49] Low-molecular-weight heparin is the current drug of choice.[49] Used in conjunction with other preventive modalities, subcutaneous injections every 12 hours or continuous intravenous infusion may be prescribed. Anticoagulation, performed cautiously in the trauma patient, can be started after achieving hemostasis and cardiovascular stability. Initially the clotting studies, partial thromboplastin time (PTT) and prothrombin time (PT), should be drawn daily until ideal therapeutic levels are obtained. Target range elevation of the PTT levels are usually approximately 60 seconds for patients receiving subcutaneous injections of heparin and 80 to 100 seconds for those receiving continuous infusions. Patients must be monitored for any significant bleeding episodes. Thrombocytopenia is a complica-

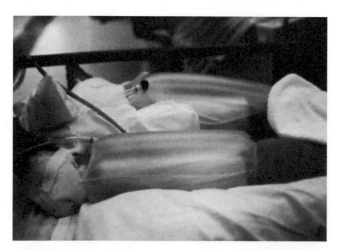

FIGURE 26-26 **Pneumatic Compression Device Applied to the Lower Legs.**

tion of anticoagulation that must be recognized promptly. Prophylactic therapy is generally discontinued after the patient is ambulatory.

Management. After the diagnosis of DVT is confirmed, therapeutic efforts focus on preventing propagation of existing clots and minimizing the risk of new clot formation. Therapeutic measures include the following:

- Bed rest: lowers the risk of clot dislodgment
- Anticoagulation: prevents clot propagation and new clot formation
- Thrombolysis: promotes lysis of thrombus formation
- Surgery: may become necessary to prevent pulmonary embolus[49]

The primary concern for the patient with DVT is the prevention of a fatal pulmonary thromboembolism.

PULMONARY THROMBOEMBOLISM. Pulmonary thromboembolism is a dangerous complication of musculoskeletal trauma. Injuries and factors that increase the patient's risk are cited earlier in this section. PTE occurs when a clot dislodges from a deep peripheral vein, usually in the lower extremity or pelvis.[51] The embolus circulates through the body to the heart and eventually lodges in a pulmonary artery or the smaller branches and obstructs blood flow. Both pulmonary and cardiovascular complications may ensue.[51]

The clot release may be spontaneous or precipitated by sudden movement, such as rapidly assuming a standing position or engaging in Valsalva's maneuver, that abruptly increases pressure and blood flow. The precipitating factors mentioned must be kept in mind when the patient begins to get out of bed, whether in the intensive care unit or later in less acute patient care areas.

Assessment and Diagnosis. Sudden-onset dyspnea is the classic signal of pulmonary thromboembolism. Symptoms of PTE vary according to the size and number of clots, the size of the pulmonary vessels affected, and the presence of lung infarction. Symptomatology is often vague or nonspecific; therefore a high index of suspicion is essential in high-risk patients.[51]

Signs and symptoms of PTE include the following:

- Substernal chest pain
- Hypovolemic relative shock
- Rapid, shallow respirations
- Shortness of breath
- Pale, dusky, or cyanotic skin coloring
- Bronchial breath sounds, rales, pleural friction rub
- Anxiety, feeling of impending doom
- Altered or decreased levels of consciousness
- Low-grade fever

Signs of a pulmonary infarction, a rare complication of PTE, can include cough and hemoptysis, pleuritic pain, and high fever.

Diagnosis can be difficult and usually cannot be confirmed by clinical findings alone. Studies that aid in confirmation of pulmonary thromboembolism are identified in Table 26-7.

Management. The objective of PTE management is to improve pulmonary gas exchange and maintain hemodynamic stability. Cardiopulmonary support, pain control, anticoagulation, and operative intervention may be necessary. The patient experiencing pulmonary thromboembolism requires support of both cardiovascular and pulmonary systems. The obstructive thromboembolus causes release of vasoactive substances that increase pulmonary vascular resistance and lead to right ventricular dysfunction. PTE may cause a relative hypovolemic shock state. Simultaneously the embolus causes a ventilation-perfusion mismatch (ventilation continues, but pulmonary perfusion is impaired), which impairs alveolar gas exchange. Hypoxemia, hypercarbia, ischemia, and pain are results of impaired pulmonary circulation.

TABLE 26-7 Diagnostic Studies for Pulmonary Thromboembolism

Laboratory Data

Arterial blood gases:
  May be normal initially or show relative hypoxemia
  Pao_2 less than 60 mm Hg
  Hypocarbia
  Decreased arterial saturation
  Respiratory alkalosis
Complete blood count:
  Elevated leukocytes (with pulmonary infarct)
Enzymes:
  Elevated LDH, CPK, SGOT
Echocardiogram:
  May only show tachycardia (if mild episode of PTE)
  Changes with massive PTE reflect right ventricular strain, failure, ischemia; may see new-onset atrial fibrillation
  Peaked T waves
  Widened QRS
  ST and T changes
  Right QRS axial shift

Chest Radiograph

Initial radiograph usually normal
Later films may reveal atelectasis or infarction pattern

Lung Scan (Ventilation-Perfusion)

Not an exclusive diagnostic study for PTE
Normal ventilation—air still enters and expands lungs
Perfusion defect—clot obstructs pulmonary circulation distal to clot, causing underperfused or nonperfused areas

Pulmonary Angiogram

Most definitive diagnostic study for significant PTE[75]
Reveals clots in the pulmonary vasculature
Identifies areas of impaired perfusion (caused by filling defects)

LDH, Lactate dehydrogenase; *CPK,* creatine phosphokinase; *SGOT,* serum glutamic-oxaloacetic transaminase; *PTE,* pulmonary thromboembolism.

Atelectasis commonly results after PTE because of the associated alveolar constriction and dead space and the loss of surfactant.[57] Frequent suctioning, and breathing and coughing exercises all promote alveolar gas exchange and improve arterial oxygen concentrations by clearing and removing secretions, thus preventing or minimizing atelectatic areas. Administration of supplemental oxygen provides more oxygen for exchange. Endotracheal intubation and mechanical ventilation may be necessary (see Chapter 23).

Pain and increased airway resistance can hinder the patient's breathing efforts. Placing the PTE patient in semi- or high Fowler's position, unless contraindicated, reduces the work of breathing. Analgesic agents can be used to reduce the patient's pain and associated anxiety. Pain control promotes patient compliance and participation in breathing exercises and pulmonary hygiene, which maximizes breathing efforts and oxygenation. Morphine sulfate is the choice for analgesia because it relaxes the smooth muscle of the bronchiole, thus easing breathing.[58] Narcotic analgesics must be used with caution because their use decreases respiratory drive and tidal volumes.[58]

Cardiovascular collapse from release of vasoactive substances or right ventricular failure necessitates hemodynamic support. Administration of positive inotropic agents and volume expansion may be required to optimize cardiac output. Analysis of vital sign and hemodynamic trends, including pulmonary artery pressure measurements, aids in evaluation of the effectiveness of resuscitative efforts.

Anticoagulation is typically indicated after confirmed PTE. Continuous intravenous heparin infusion is recommended because it reduces the overall amount of heparin needed each day, eliminates the "peaks and valleys" associated with intermittent injections, and minimizes the risk of bleeding.[59] Routine monitoring of coagulation profiles is essential to evaluate dose adequacy. Platelet counts, PT, and PTT are monitored because thrombocytopenia is a complication associated with anticoagulant therapy. Heparin therapy usually continues for 1 week, after which an oral anticoagulant regimen is begun, but newer approaches including starting warfarin at the same time the heparin infusion is initiated.[57]

Plasminogen activators such as streptokinase and urokinase, although rarely appropriate in trauma patients, are occasionally used to lyse fresh thrombi and may also inhibit future thrombus formation.[60] These agents, similar to anticoagulants, should be used judiciously in the trauma patient. Thrombolytic therapy is contraindicated in patients at risk for intracranial bleed (e.g., brain contusion, subdural hematoma) or massive hemorrhage (e.g., liver or spleen laceration).

Pulmonary embolectomy is indicated in patients with severe obstructive PTE or in whom other therapies are ineffective or contraindicated. Insertion of a caval filter or umbrella or vena caval ligation to prevent PTE may be necessary for patients in high-risk categories, which include head injury with spinal cord injury, head injury with long bone fracture, and multiple long bone fractures.[61] Although

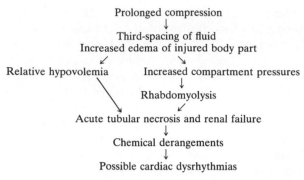

Prolonged compression
↓
Third-spacing of fluid
Increased edema of injured body part
↓   ↓
Relative hypovolemia   Increased compartment pressures
↓
Rhabdomyolysis
↓
Acute tubular necrosis and renal failure
↓
Chemical derangements
↓
Possible cardiac dysrhythmias

FIGURE 26-27 Events Associated With Crush Syndrome. (From Peck SA: Crush syndrome: pathophysiology and management, *Orthop Nurs* 9(3):33-40, 1990.)

there are currently no large, prospective randomized studies to support the prophylactic insertion of an inferior vena cava filter, a number of smaller trials support the use of caval filters in trauma patients.[62-68]

CRUSH SYNDROME. Crush syndrome results from prolonged entrapment or a crushing injury, which may occur with a structural collapse, cave-in, wringer-type industrial or farm incident, motor vehicle crash (as either a vehicle occupant or pedestrian), or other traumatic mechanisms that cause compression. This is a potentially life-threatening syndrome, in large part as a result of the number and severity of associated complications.

A predictable series of sequelae develops after a crush injury (Figure 26-27). Prolonged compression of the involved body part causes ischemia and anoxia of muscle tissue. Tissue ischemia leads to a cycle of events resulting in third-spacing of fluids, edema, increased compartment pressures, and impaired tissue perfusion precipitating further tissue ischemia.

Rhabdomyolysis, a result of muscle destruction and dissolution from the primary injury and from subsequent ischemia/edema damage, causes a release of myoglobin and potassium. Hypoperfusion from the initial traumatic insult and blood loss and from the relative hypovolemia caused by third space fluids combines with the myoglobinuria to cause renal dysfunction in the form of acute tubular necrosis and renal failure.[69] Impaired renal function, in the presence of a metabolic imbalance that already exists from the rhabdomyolysis, causes further chemical derangements that may precipitate cardiac arrhythmias. Liberation of potassium from cellular necrosis can dramatically raise serum potassium levels and lead to sudden cardiac arrest.

Additional complications inherent to crush syndrome include neurovascular compromise from compartment syndrome and infection from the original injury and subsequent ischemic changes.

OPERATIVE PHASE

The responsibilities of the perioperative nurse include completing a preoperative patient assessment, which in-

cludes a complete systems assessment and gathering information about confirmed and suspected injuries, potential complications, and therapies instituted. A systematic report from the prior caregiver provides continuity of care, an essential factor in preventing fragmented therapy. During the preoperative phase the nurse explains the activities that the awake patient will experience in the operating room and expected postoperative care. The perioperative nurse has the vital role of coordinator, especially for the multisystem-injured patient with musculoskeletal injuries. These patients may well undergo multiple simultaneous surgical procedures during their operative visit. General responsibilities, therefore, also include anticipating the length of stay in the operative suite, patient positioning, and use of different operating tables; confirming the sequence of the various planned procedures and the equipment needed for each; and ensuring patient safety and monitoring throughout the entire case. During the often lengthy orthopedic operative procedures, the perioperative nurse communicates with the patient's family to provide updates and progress reports as requested. After surgery a report of all prior procedures, resuscitation efforts, and operative procedures is given to the receiving nurse either in the postanesthesia room or in another patient care area. Again the systematic exchange of a complete report between primary care nurses promotes continuous and consistent patient management.

GENERAL MANAGEMENT PRINCIPLES

PREVENTION OF INFECTION. Early and aggressive wound irrigation and debridement are two of the most important treatments to prevent infection in an open fracture or traumatic amputation.[70] The most effective irrigation is done with copious amounts of normal saline. A minimum of 10 L of saline is typically used in open fractures.[23] Debridement of necrotic fascia, devitalized muscle tissue, and bone fragments is necessary to decrease the potential for infection and to promote wound healing.

The risk of infection associated with open fractures depends on the grade and location of the fracture.[20] The existence of other factors such as age, nosocomial infections, and wound contamination class also affect postinjury infection rates.[20] Wound care is important to remove devitalized tissue, and debridement is continued until the wound is clean.

Closure of an open wound is contraindicated during the initial operative phase. Allowing the wound to remain open promotes drainage of microscopic debris not removed during the initial irrigation. Closure of the wound at this time would impede this drainage, providing the perfect environment for bacterial growth and infection. Delayed primary or secondary closure is performed when the wound appears free of infection.[20]

REESTABLISHMENT OF BONE INTEGRITY. Restoring the fractured bone to normal alignment and length is necessary to initiate the healing process. Reduction of the dead space between fractured bone ends decreases the size of hematoma

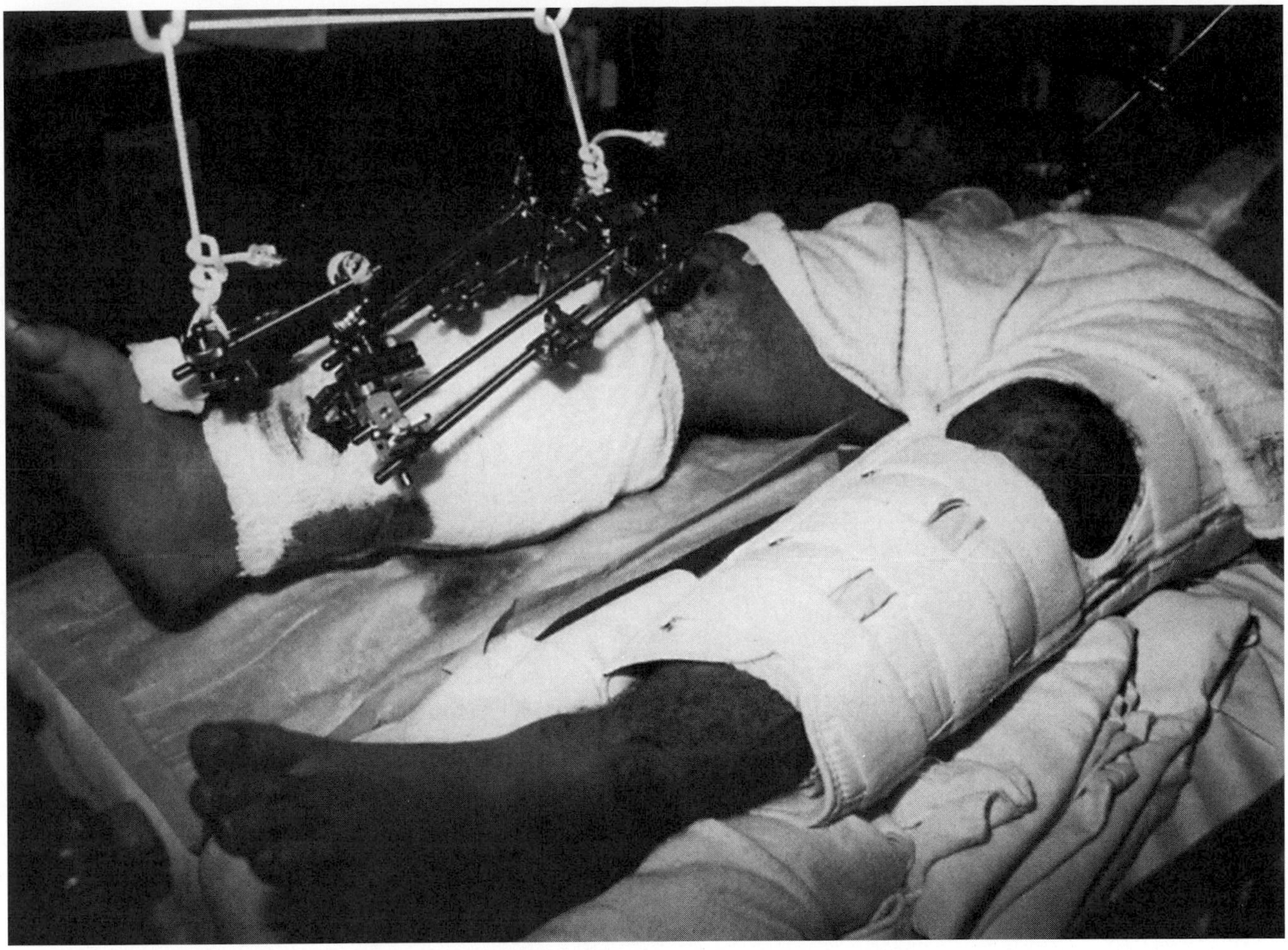

FIGURE 26-28 External Fixator Applied to the Right Leg (Tibia/Fibula Fracture).

formation, which in open fractures can become a site for infection. Restoring the bone to normal alignment improves venous and lymphatic return, which decreases soft tissue swelling and reduces the release of marrow components into the circulation. Early and aggressive operative intervention reduces the overall morbidity and mortality of the multisystem-injured patient.[71] In addition to the total clinical picture presented by the patient, including age, number and severity of injuries, and overall hemodynamic status, members of the trauma team need to consider other situational factors when making operative decisions. These factors include (1) effectiveness of closed reduction, (2) fractured or displaced articulating surfaces, (3) presence of arterial injury, (4) presence of multiple injuries, (5) contaminated wound, (6) length of time since the injury occurred, (7) contraindication of long-term immobility, and (8) cost of long-term immobility caused by closed reduction.

FRACTURE STABILIZATION. The method of stabilization used for an extremity fracture depends on the grade, type, and location of the fracture. The current philosophy of long bone stabilization supports the use of intramedullary devices.[23]

Reaming of the intramedullary canal consists of passing a device directly into the canal and "smoothing" the canal in preparation for passage of a rod for fracture fixation. The use of reamed nails in open fractures, once controversial because of evidence that they interrupt vascular supply to the fracture site, has again found a role in tibial fixation.[23] Recent clinical experience has shown that use of unreamed intramedullary nails has expanded the indications for nailing to now include grades I and II open fractures. Grade III open long bone fractures also may be treated with unreamed intramedullary nails if debridement was performed within 6 hours of the injury. Modern designs of first- and second-generation unreamed intramedullary nails now permit even very complex fracture patterns (e.g., combined femoral shaft and neck fractures) to be treated with a single device.[23] Recent studies have demonstrated that in reamed intramedullary nail placement, intramedullary pressures rise significantly and can increase the incidence of fat embolism syndrome.[72-74]

External fixation (Figure 26-28) continues to play a major role in acute fracture management and limb reconstruction procedures. Although an external fixator may be the definitive treatment option for a given fracture, it also can be used as a temporary stabilization device on a critically ill patient who cannot safely undergo a lengthy operative procedure on admission.

External fixation also plays an important role in management of a patient with a severely crushed lower leg with significant soft tissue and bone loss. The use of external fixators allows free access for wound care, soft tissue coverage (free tissue transfer), and bone transport or transplantation to fill the bony defect.

In unstable pelvic ring disruptions, external fixation provides provisional pelvic fixation and at times may be lifesaving. It does not, however, stabilize the posterior bony structures adequately, and therefore internal pelvic ring fixation must be performed as soon as the patient's condition permits. The preferred fixation method for pure sacroiliac joint dislocations is now anterior plating via the retroperitoneal approach rather than posterior screw fixation, which was frequently associated with wound complications.[75] Although early open reduction and internal fixation (ORIF) is the preferred method of pelvic fracture fixation, there may be isolated cases where skeletal traction is indicated.[76]

MANAGEMENT OF NEUROLOGIC AND VASCULAR COMPROMISE

Fasciotomies allow for the decompression of fascial compartments that have high pressures caused by swelling of tissues, as previously described. The fascial compartment is opened to allow the increased compartment volume caused by swelling to expand without increasing pressure on the microcirculation. The technique used to open the fascial sheath depends on the compartment requiring decompression. The forearm compartments can be opened with two incisions—one volar, one dorsal—placed 180 degrees to each other. Because the lower leg has four compartments, the lower leg fasciotomy technique involves an anterolateral incision between the fibular shaft and the tibial crest to relieve pressure in the anterior and lateral compartments. The deep posterior and superficial posterior compartments are approached through a posteromedial incision. The type of incision required for other compartments, such as those of the hip, thigh, shoulder, pelvis, upper arm, hand, or foot, is determined by the structure and number of fascial compartments involved.

The wounds created by the large incisions are left open and covered with wet saline dressings to prevent desiccation. (Wound care and dressing changes are discussed further in the critical care section.) Delayed primary closure or delayed secondary closure by skin grafting is then done when swelling has subsided.

PREVENTION OF COMPLICATIONS CAUSED BY IMMOBILITY

One of the fundamentals of perioperative nursing is prevention of immobility-related injuries, most commonly neurologic and vascular impairment. The length of the surgical procedure combined with the positions required during surgical interventions for musculoskeletal injuries increase the risk of iatrogenic injury if proper protection and padding are not provided to prevent compression of neurovascular structures. Coordinated preoperative planning between nurses, anesthesiologists, and surgeons regarding patient positioning on various types of operative tables, such as fracture frame or turning frame, facilitates optimal patient protection.

The potential for a brachial plexus injury as a result of improper positioning and alignment demands strict perioperative attention from the trauma operating room nurse. Postoperative brachial plexus palsy may result from hyperextension or hyperabduction of the upper extremity during surgery.[26] This complication usually represents a temporary alteration in regional or generalized motor and sensory function. Healing and full recovery commonly occur within hours to days after the insult.[26,27]

Pressure sores are another risk for the immobilized patient during surgery. Providing adequate padding over bony prominences and any body area that comes in contact with a rigid surface and keeping such areas dry minimize the risk of these pressure sores developing. Prevention is the primary intervention for these complications.

CRITICAL CARE PHASE

Principles of patient care regarding immobilization, skin breakdown, and potential complications that were discussed in the resuscitation section also apply during the critical care phase. One of the responsibilities of the critical care nurse is to review and update patient assessment data, including operative procedures, anesthesia time, and fluid volume replacement requirements.

PREVENTION OF INFECTION

During the critical care phase the patient with musculoskeletal injury continues to be at risk for infection. Injuries that require delayed primary or secondary skin closure, surgical incisions, and pin sites require close observation and meticulous care. Predisposing factors that influence whether an infection develops during the critical care phase include devitalized muscle tissue, dead space, hematomas, and foreign bodies. Other factors include impairment of the immune system as a result of traumatic injury, the patient's age, nutritional status, hemodynamic stability, pulmonary gas exchange, and the presence of any underlying disease.[77]

Early recognition of the signs and symptoms of infection is important in preventing or minimizing major infection, sepsis, and delayed healing. Trends in vital signs, including temperature, complete blood count with white blood cell differentiation, and electrolytes, must be monitored, documented, and evaluated. Wound incision and pin site appearance and drainage (i.e., amount, consistency, color, and odor) should be monitored and documented.

Because primary wound closure is not always performed

during the initial resuscitative or operative phases of patient care, wounds associated with open fractures, amputations, and fasciotomies require wet-to-wet or wet-to-dry sterile dressing changes. Wet-to-dry dressing changes provide some debridement of the wound. Wounds with exposed bone, veins, tendons, and fat are treated with wet-to-wet sterile dressing changes to prevent desiccation. For open fractures, crushing injuries, or traumatic amputations, continued operative irrigation and debridement are necessary every 24 to 48 hours until tissue granulation becomes apparent and the wound is free of infection and necrotic tissue.

Hematomas are avascular and are thus an excellent environment for bacterial growth. Closed-system evacuation drains, such as the Jackson Pratt or the Hemovac, inserted intraoperatively reduce hematoma formation in surgical wounds. These drains require close monitoring to maintain patency and proper function. Specific nursing care includes emptying and reactivating the suction every 4 to 8 hours (or more frequently with large amounts of drainage); measuring and documenting the amount and characteristics of the drainage (e.g., color, consistency, odor); performing dressing changes using aseptic technique every 8 hours (or as ordered); documenting the status of the skin and tissue surrounding the drain site; and preventing accidental drain removal. Drains are generally removed within 3 to 5 days after insertion or earlier if drainage has stopped.

There is no consensus concerning the proper method for carrying out pin site care.[78] The controversy is whether to remove dried exudate from nondraining pin sites or to leave it in place. One school contends that the dried exudate is part of the normal healing process, provides a tight pin-skin interface, and prevents skin flora from entering the bone via the pin tract. The opposing school believes that removing the dried exudate allows the pin holes to drain freely, reducing the bacterial concentration and decreasing the risk of pin tract infection. Generally pin sites (of simple percutaneous pins for skeletal traction or more complex pins from an external fixator) ooze after insertion. A gently wrapped, loose-fitting 4 × 4 opened gauze dressing (Figure 26-29) allows free drainage while containing the drainage. Frequent dressing changes and pin site care are necessary for the first 1 to 2 days after insertion. Pin care given every 8 or 12 hours is satisfactory after active drainage has stopped. Cleaning the exterior part of the pins helps prevent retrograde contamination of the pin tract, which can lead rapidly to osteomyelitis (see Chapter 14).

Short-term antibiotic therapy initiated during resuscitation typically continues during the critical care phase for any patient with an open fracture, crush injury, or traumatic amputation. The choice of antibiotic depends on the environment in which the injury occurred or on formal wound culture and sensitivity reports. The usual drug of choice is a second-generation cephalosporin such as cefazolin.[23] An aminoglycoside may be added if significant wound contamination is present.

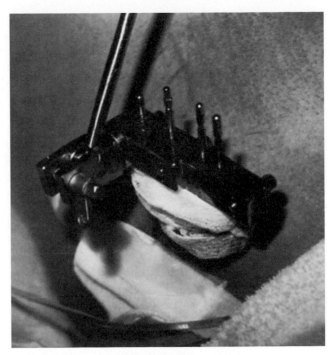

FIGURE 26-29 Insertion Site of a Percutaneous Pin, With Loose-Fitting Gauze Dressing Around the Pin Site.

NEUROVASCULAR COMPROMISE RELATED TO COMPARTMENT SYNDROME

As previously discussed, compartment syndrome may develop soon after the injury, during resuscitation, as a result of excessive bleeding or swelling into the compartments or the soft tissue. During the critical care phase, compartment syndrome remains a potential problem for the patient with musculoskeletal injuries. Despite definitive intraoperative care, soft tissue edema can persist because of sluggish venous return or persistent oozing of smaller injured vessels, which can increase muscle compartment volume, resulting in neurovascular compromise. Additional factors that can lead to compartment syndrome or less acute forms of neurologic or vascular impairment include tight-fitting casts, occlusive circular dressings, traction devices, and improper positioning of patients when on their side.

Close monitoring of the neurovascular status of the affected extremity remains the single most important intervention and preventive measure. Evaluation of the compartments includes comparisons of the injured limb with the noninjured limb. This assessment should be performed and the findings documented at least every 1 to 2 hours or more frequently as warranted by the patient's condition. Assessment criteria include presence or absence of peripheral pulses; location, strength, and quality of the pulses; capillary refill times; temperature and color of the extremity; and motion and sensation of the extremity.

Evaluation of immobilization and stabilization devices ensures maintenance of proper alignment and early identification of signs of local or generalized compression. If clinical findings suggest that a tight-fitting cast, for example, may be the causative factor of deterioration in the neurovascular status of the distal extremity, the cast should be bivalved and the top half removed. The posterior portion continues to serve as a stabilizing device while attention is given to the extremity.

The interventions described during resuscitation remain essential during critical care. The affected extremity should remain elevated and cooled for the first 24 to 48 hours after injury to promote venous return and minimize further edema. Elevation and extremity cooling are continued when the patient is positioned on one side or is out of bed in a chair. An injury managed by external fixation can be elevated easily with traction apparatus. More conventional methods of elevation include pillows, folded sheets, and preformed foam elevation blocks. Clinical signs of increased compartmental pressures necessitate compartment pressure measurements, as discussed previously.

FAT EMBOLISM SYNDROME

As extensively reviewed earlier in this chapter, the potential for severe respiratory compromise resulting from FES exists for approximately 96 hours after injury. The critical care nurse must be alert to the signs and symptoms of FES, and early interventions should be implemented to manage the syndrome.

IMMOBILITY-RELATED COMPLICATIONS

The degree of physical immobility for the patient with musculoskeletal injuries depends on the type of injury, the pain associated with the injury, the method of treatment chosen, and the presence of other system injuries. The goal of management is promotion of mobility as soon as feasible after injury.

Immobility, the usual common denominator in trauma patients with concomitant musculoskeletal injuries, stresses the body, mind, and spirit in a variety of ways. Not only does it cause altered feelings of self-esteem and a sense of powerlessness, but it also slows anabolic processes and accelerates catabolic activities.[79] Results of immobility often include tissue atrophy, protein catabolism, alteration in intracellular and extracellular exchanges, and fluid and electrolyte imbalances. More specifically, immobility increases the trauma patient's risk for secondary disabilities from pulmonary complications, vascular stasis with thromboemboli formation, skin breakdown, fecal impaction, renal calculi, muscle wasting, and contractures.[79] Appropriate nursing interventions can prevent or minimize the risk of these complications. Immobility remains one of the most frightening and psychologically significant components of musculoskeletal trauma, and patients often require emotional support from psychiatric liaison services or clinical nurse specialists.[79]

Different treatment modalities available for musculoskeletal injuries afford varying degrees of postoperative mobility. State-of-the-art orthopedic management, however, promotes early mobility after surgery.

Atelectasis and pneumonia are preventable sequelae of immobilization. Immobilized patients require chest physiotherapy, including turning with postural drainage and percussion every 2 to 4 hours, to aid clearance of secretions from the lung parenchyma. The patient should be placed in the lateral and prone positions and coached to cough frequently to clear secretions from the tracheobronchial tree. Instructions also include proper deep breathing techniques and use of an incentive spirometer.[79]

Skin breakdown in the immobilized or insensate patient is a costly complication that can be prevented. Each ulceration can potentially add thousands of dollars to a patient's health care bill in hospital cost, surgical skin repair, and control of infection.[80] Skin breakdown results from decreased arterial circulation to the localized area. Other factors that directly or indirectly predispose the patient to skin breakdown include friction from bed linen or from cast and traction devices; anemia, malnutrition, infection, and fever; decreased sensation or paralysis; use of anticoagulants, sedatives, or neuromuscular blocking agents; and age of more than 65 years.[79] Potential breakdown sites need to be monitored for redness, burning pain, and itching. Turning and repositioning the patient as frequently as allowed minimizes the length of time that pressure is exerted on any skin area.[79]

Immobilization reduces intestinal mobility, which is further compounded by the administration of medications such as narcotics. Thus bowel sounds and frequency of bowel movements in the immobilized patient are important to evaluate. If permitted, the patient's diet should include juices and roughage to help maintain normal bowel movement. Mild laxatives, stool softeners, or enemas may be required to maintain normal intestinal mobility. Often, as a result of intraabdominal injuries, long-term total parenteral nutrition (TPN) is required. Bowel movements are not frequent and are usually loose. A nutrition consultation may be necessary to assist with appropriate nutritional needs.[79]

Calcium or other crystalline salts can become concentrated in the urine beyond the point of solubility in the immobilized patient as a result of bone demineralization and inadequate fluid intake.[1] High concentrations can result in renal calculi formation. Adequate fluid intake helps to prevent urine concentration and calculi formation. Weight bearing reduces bone loss associated with bed rest. Early fracture fixation also prevents prolonged lying in the dorsal recumbent position, which increases pooling of urine in the renal pelvis.[79]

Immobility, especially of the antigravity muscle groups, precludes normal muscle stresses and leads to decreased muscle fiber size. Muscle atrophy, or a decrease in muscle mass, begins within 24 hours after the onset of immobility.[81] Approximately 3% of original muscle strength is lost each day a muscle remains immobile.[81] Connective tissue fibrosis around immobile joints also begins soon after immobilization, progressing to joint contractures and limiting range of motion. Muscle wasting, atrophy, and contractures can be prevented or minimized by range-of-motion exercises that are planned appropriately for the patient's degree of dependence or independence. Passive or active assisted range-of-motion movements are required during every shift for patients who are unable to carry out independent exercise. This exercise regimen should include noninjured joints required later for ambulation and affected joints within restrictions.

Range-of-motion maneuvers include moving all possible joints through their ranges of abduction, adduction, internal and external rotation, pronation, supination, eversion, and inversion and repeating each motion five times successively.[81] Complete range-of-motion exercises help prevent contractures, improve joint function, and promote circulation. These maneuvers, used in conjunction with isometric exercises, also increase the patient's tolerance and endurance. Optimal muscle strength, full joint movement, and endurance are all essential components of later mobility and ambulation.[81]

During range-of-motion exercises it is important to monitor and document the degree of each joint's range; any sign of inflammation, spasm, edema, or stiffness; and the patient's complaints of pain. A joint should not be forced to move beyond free range. Force and persistent range-of-motion movements when the patient describes an unusual amount of pain may precipitate joint or muscle strain or injury, which prolongs rehabilitation.

Neurologic injuries to an extremity that result in loss of motion require functional splinting of the extremity. The inability to dorsiflex the wrist or ankle can lead to permanent flexion contractures of the brachioradialis tendon and the Achilles tendon, making recovery of function difficult if not impossible. Premolded fiberglass or soft splints are used in the early phases of trauma to prevent these contractures.

Some patients, such as those with brachial plexus injuries, require splints during prolonged periods of immobility to maintain position of function and reduce the risk of contractures. Properly fitting splints and close monitoring of underlying skin integrity prevent or minimize skin breakdown. Physical and occupational therapy consultations are required during the critical care phase to evaluate and plan care. These therapists are an integral part of the critical care team. Occupational therapists fabricate custom-made splints and determine optimal wearing schedules. Physical therapists evaluate patients and customize physical therapy modalities that promote early range of motion and maintain and build strength.

INTERMEDIATE CARE AND REHABILITATION PHASES

OVERVIEW OF REHABILITATION

Trauma rehabilitation is the process of restoring the patient to physical, emotional, and economic usefulness. Not all trauma patients with musculoskeletal injuries can return to the level of functioning they enjoyed before their injury or illness. New, realistic levels must be defined and the patient assisted, through education and therapy, to attain these new goals.

Rehabilitation for the patient with musculoskeletal injuries begins at the time of injury. Prehospital care personnel initiate the first stage of rehabilitation by providing the proper care for injuries and preventing further injury. During the resuscitative and operative phases, injuries are diagnosed and definitive treatment is initiated. Prevention of secondary disabilities related to immobility during the critical care phase plays an equally important role. Pulmonary hygiene, skin care, and active and passive range-of-motion exercises help maintain the patient's existing capabilities and prevent delays in starting the more active rehabilitation process.

The intermediate and rehabilitative phases involve the most active efforts in educating and training the patient to adapt to new limitations. Family involvement is greater during these phases than at any other time since the patient's injury occurred. Both the patient and the family are reeducated and trained so that the individual may reach the highest possible functioning capability (see Chapter 10).

COMPLICATIONS DURING RECOVERY

DELAYED HEALING. Infection, causing delayed healing of fractures and soft tissue wounds, can postpone the initiation of the active rehabilitative process. Proper nursing care and patient and family education can help prevent or minimize the risk of infection in the patient with musculoskeletal injuries.

Osteomyelitis is a bacterial invasion of the bone that results from either a primary or secondary cause. Primary osteomyelitis is caused by direct introduction of microorganisms into the bone with the initial injury, such as open fractures or penetrating injuries, or during surgery. Secondary osteomyelitis results from microorganisms seeded into the bone from soft tissue infections or systemic infection.[82] Commonly isolated organisms include *Staphylococcus, Escherichia coli, Klebsiella,* and *Pseudomonas aeruginosa.* Acute osteomyelitis that becomes resistant to therapy can develop into chronic osteomyelitis.

Signs and symptoms of osteomyelitis include local pain with movement, edema, erythema, elevated temperature, chills, diaphoresis, muscle spasms, limited joint movement, weakness, and a direct wound tract with purulent drainage. Diagnosis of osteomyelitis is based on blood, wound drainage, or bone marrow cultures. Laboratory blood tests show an elevated white blood cell count and erythrocyte sedimentation rate. Approximately 10 to 14 days after onset of the infection in adults, radiographic examination shows elevated periosteum, areas of radiolucency secondary to bone lysis, and areas of density secondary to bone necrosis. Deep bone destruction is evident on CT scans, and radionuclide scans demonstrate areas of occult infection.

Treatments for osteomyelitis include antibiotic therapy, surgical debridement, and irrigation to eliminate the causative organism; immobilization to reduce the associated pain and the risk of pathologic fractures; nutritional support to optimize healing; and institution of a pain management regimen. Patients with chronic osteomyelitis may require bone grafting to increase the stability of the bone after extensive bone damage.[82]

Movement of the affected area should be minimized; immobilization is maintained by bed rest, casting, splinting, or traction. If movement of the area is required, full and gentle support must be provided. Analgesia is administered as required and before dressing changes, with the effectiveness closely monitored. Wound drainage monitoring includes a description of its amount, color, odor, and consistency.

Soft tissue injuries with significant tissue loss require tissue grafting to promote healing, provide soft tissue coverage of the bone, and prevent osteitis. Closing the wound and increasing the vascular supply through grafting can shorten the fracture healing time and decrease the risk of infection.[20] Soft tissue grafting is done when the wound is free of devitalized tissue, which may occur 4 to 7 days after injury. The presence of any wound infection will delay grafting. Dressing changes for soft tissue wounds are done every 4 to 6 hours from the time of injury until the wound is ready for grafting.[20]

Healing times for fractures depend on the location and type of fracture, associated traumatic injuries, and systemic complications. Bone healing has five distinct stages, each dependent on the successful completion of the stage before (Table 26-8). If healing does not occur within the expected time for the type of fracture present, delayed union is present. The diagnosis of nonunion is made when, after serial patient examinations, motion and pain at the fracture site persist and there are no progressive radiologic changes suggestive of healing 4 to 6 months after the injury.[4]

Many factors can lead to delayed union or nonunion of fractures: severity of fracture, amount of bone or soft tissue loss, loss of periosteum, excessive motion at the fracture site, poor nutritional status, smoking, improper weight bearing, and decreased vascular supply. Trauma nurses need to recognize the variables that affect fracture healing and institute measures to increase its likelihood.

Bone grafting enhances bone formation at the site of nonunion fractures. It is also used for fractures in which healing is expected to be delayed because of the severity of the fracture, bone loss, or extensive soft tissue injury. Many fractures with segmental bone loss, significant loss of the cortical diameter, or gross comminution with separation of fracture fragments require bone grafting to aid in bone healing.[4] The grafting may be done in the initial stages of treatment or several weeks after the injury, depending on the condition of the soft tissue surrounding the area of injury. Bone grafting during the initial repair or during the first several weeks after injury can significantly decrease the time required for healing.

MECHANICAL FAILURE OF FIXATORS. External fixators are frequently used to stabilize fractures and the length of time a fixator remains in place depends on the type of injury. The risk of complications increases with the length of time the fixator is in place. Components of the frame, including the transfixion pins, pin clamps, and couplings, can loosen, causing loss of bone alignment. At least weekly checks of the frame components are necessary to identify loosened parts. An increase in pain around the pin tract is often associated with pin loosening and may be the first sign that the pin-to-bone contact is decreased. Loose pins also can increase the risk of pin tract infection and need to be removed. The patient and family must be taught before discharge how to properly care for the fixator. This includes being able to check for frame tightness and recognizing early signs of pin loosening.

Metal fatigue from cyclic loading is a problem associated with internal fixators. There is competition between the process of bone healing and implant failure. Healing of uncomplicated fractures, however, usually occurs long before the implant fails.[4] With improved operative techniques and metallurgy and increased knowledge of the biomechanics involved in fractures and healing, the incidence of implant failure has been reduced. Although implants are usually removed after healing has occurred, removal may be delayed or abandoned if the risk associated with a second surgical procedure outweighs the benefits of hardware removal. Patients who undergo implant removal from weight-bearing bones must be taught to use protected weight-bearing techniques to prevent refracture.

Protected weight bearing is necessary for a minimum of 6 weeks after implant removal to allow the bone to regain its normal strength and allow for mineralization of the multiple pin tracks in the bone. Occasionally, soft splints may be used to protect the fracture site during final healing.

A fracture is considered completely healed when its strength is equal to that of normal bone and it tolerates

TABLE 26-8 **The Five Stages of Fracture Healing**	
Stage	**Activity**
First: hematoma formation	A hematoma forms at the fracture site.
Second: granulation	Within a few days after the injury, fibroblasts and capillaries invade the hematoma and form granulation tissue.
Third: callus formation	Within 6 to 10 days, plasma and white blood cells enter the granulation tissue and form a thick, sticky substance known as the callus. This material helps keep the bone fragments together.
Fourth: consolidation	Connective tissue and osteoblasts proliferate, bringing the bone ends closer together.
Fifth: remodeling	In this final phase of healing, bone fragments are united, excess cells have been absorbed, the bone is remodeled, and healing is complete.

normal stresses without refracture. Radiographic examination of a healed fracture shows dense and continuous bone cortices.[4]

IMPAIRED MOBILITY.   The effects of immobility caused by fracture, dislocation, plexus injury, or amputation can be psychologically and physically devastating. The nurse must anticipate potential problems and collaborate with the physical and occupational therapists to initiate actions to prevent the complications previously discussed.

Amputations.   Amputees require special attention to the residual limb. Active range-of-motion exercises prevent contractures of the joint immediately proximal to the incision. The patient should be taught isometric exercises of the targeted muscle groups if active range of motion is impossible or limited. Some activities promote contracture formation of the proximal joint and need be avoided or limited. For example, a patient with a below-the-knee amputation should not be in a sitting position without extension of the knee joint, and those with above-the-knee amputations must avoid long periods of sitting and must spend time in the prone position to promote extension of the hip joint. The positioning of the intact extremities and the muscles of the trunk also must be considered to avoid dysfunction of these muscle groups. The patient is taught the importance of promoting mobility by performing active exercises. Mobilizing as soon as possible the patient who has lost a weight-bearing limb enhances overall recovery and rehabilitation. It is necessary for the patient with a lower extremity amputation to develop a new sense of balance as new methods of mobility are learned.

Extremity Fractures.   Methods of ambulating the patient with a fracture of the lower extremity vary according to the type and location of the fracture and whether the bone affected is weight bearing. Crutch walking for the patient with a single lower extremity fracture and wheelchair transfer for the patient with bilateral lower extremity fractures facilitates mobility and reduces the complications of immobility. Active exercises of the upper extremities and trunk are necessary to increase the patient's physical strength and tolerance for these different types of activities.

External fixators have greatly increased the mobility of patients with fractures, who at one time were confined to prolonged bed rest with traction. Despite the advantages provided by the external fixator, it can still be intimidating to the patient, resulting in slow acceptance of the device and hesitation to become fully mobilized. Education and emotional support can help the patient understand the function of the external fixator, accept the change in body image, and reduce any fear associated with ambulation with the external fixator.

Patients with tibial plateau, supracondylar, patellar, or acetabular fractures are at risk of formation of joint adhesions and contractures. Limited passive range-of-motion exercises of the joint can help reduce these risks. Use of a continuous passive motion machine (CPM) has been shown to effectively restore or increase joint extension and flexion, reducing discomfort and decreasing the formation of degenerative bone changes.[81] Lubrication of the articular joint surface is optimized by the production of synovial fluid, which is stimulated by the motion. The CPM is most effective when applied within the first week after surgery. The nurse must be thoroughly familiar with the operation of the CPM and any potential complications that it can cause. Proper alignment of the CPM is necessary to reduce contact between skin surface areas and the CPM. Padding is necessary to prevent irritation or breakdown of those skin areas that come in contact with the machine. The nurse should be alert for any signs and symptoms of infection around incision sites and for any increased bleeding from surgical drains as a result of motion at the drain sites. Neurovascular checks and skin care should continue while the machine is operating. If the patient needs to get out of bed or requires turning for chest physiotherapy, the CPM can be removed.

Pelvic Fractures.   The degree of mobility permitted after a pelvic fracture depends on the type of fracture, the amount of pain associated with the fracture, and the method of treatment. Extended bed rest may be necessary, with the hip fixed in flexion, extension, adduction, or abduction. Progressive ambulation without weight bearing may be allowed according to the patient's pain tolerance. Internal or external fixation of pelvic fractures can decrease the amount of time required for bed rest. Myositis ossificans is the formation of heterotrophic bone and occurs anywhere in the body, but the hip and pelvic regions are especially susceptible. Heterotrophic bone is the rapid multiplication of osteoblasts in tissues that surround joints and can eventually lead to complete fusion of the joint.[81] Multiple modalities have been used to prevent the formation of heterotrophic bone, including use of low-dose radiation and indomethacin. Care must be taken with patients receiving indomethacin because of risk of gastric ulcerations, prolongation of bleeding times, and other hematologic abnormalities.

Plexis Injuries.   Functional recovery of a plexus injury depends on several variables, including the type of injury, the specific nerve and level injured, and the patient's age.[26] For example, a patient who sustained nerve impairment after an isolated anterior shoulder dislocation may recover fully within a few days to weeks, whereas a more violent injury, such as from a motorcycle crash with more than one nerve root injured, implies a worse prognosis for recovery. Despite months of intense rehabilitation, the patient with this type of injury may only recover minimal function, if any, of the affected extremity.[27]

Rehabilitation must begin soon after any type of plexus injury. If or when nerve regeneration occurs, optimal physical condition in the affected limb affords more rapid restoration of function and use of the extremity.

Closed plexus injuries generally require extensive rehabilitation for many months before any significant progress in function is seen, and both closed and open brachial plexus injuries may require early surgical intervention for associated soft tissue, vascular, or bony injuries.[26] Primary nerve repair is usually performed several weeks after injury, when soft tissue wounds are healed and the risk of infection is minimal. Primary repair of more peripheral nerve injuries may be appropriate and indicated for clean injuries in the distal aspects of the extremity. Surgical exploration may also be indicated for the patient who shows little functional improvement after an injury that has a good prognosis for recovery.[27]

CHRONIC PAIN.   Chronic pain is a potentially serious complication of musculoskeletal trauma that can delay and intensify rehabilitation. The therapies used for acute pain management are often different from those used in, and sometimes even are contraindicated in, the management of chronic pain. A planned, team approach affords the most effective and comprehensive pain management therapy (see Chapter 17).

The patient with a musculoskeletal injury may experience any one or a combination of the following types of pain:

1. Nociception: tissue damage-induced stimulus to the brain from the periphery, as with degenerative joint diseases
2. Central pain: abnormal activity along afferent pathways that have been severed from the peripheral connections, as in traumatic amputations
3. Psychologic pain: feelings of anxiety or depression mislabeled as pain sensations
4. Behavioral pain: for reasons such as attention, sympathy, compensated time off from work, and financial aid, patients continue to behave as though they still have pain

Because chronic pain can actually be a combination of these pain states, patients should undergo physical, psychologic, and social evaluation. Chronic pain may become the focal point of a patient's life and negatively affect all aspects of his or her being.[83] Therefore these patients require behavioral and psychologic therapy in conjunction with analgesic therapy. For example, patients with chronic pain often experience depression and may benefit greatly from a combined drug regimen that includes analgesics and antidepressants in addition to psychologic therapy. Because pain is often a combination of physical and psychologic components, when the pain is relieved, the emotional changes subside, and vice versa. When a serious psychologic issue is resolved, the pain described by the patient often ceases.

PATIENT AND FAMILY EDUCATION

The nurse can detect early signs of infection and promptly initiate therapy by frequent assessment of wounds, pin sites, and surgical incisions. In preparation for discharge, patient and family education related to aseptic technique, pin care, and dressing changes for wounds and incisions is necessary. The nurse should ensure that the patient and family can demonstrate their ability to perform these procedures accurately and that they can correctly identify the signs and symptoms of pin tract and wound infections. The education process is started early to allow time for the patient and family to become comfortable and competent with this responsibility.

Weight-bearing restrictions and use of assistive devices are key elements of patient and family teaching. Many patients require adaptive equipment after discharge, and the trauma team members can contribute to the discharge process by early identification of such needs and by assisting with the procurement of durable medical equipment (DME) to ease patients' transition to home. Continued medical therapies are often required, and referral to home health care agencies provides for expert continuity of care. Follow-up contact with the patient and family via telephone or clinic visits gives the trauma nurse the opportunity to evaluate the effectiveness of the teaching and discharge plan and is an important component of quality improvement functions.

SUMMARY

Musculoskeletal trauma promises to provide a continuing challenge to the entire health care team. Four major areas that demand further research and development are trauma reduction and prevention, prehospital trauma care, nursing and medical therapies, and trauma rehabilitation. Despite the many advances in all areas of health, trauma remains the major threat to the health of our citizens.[84] The reduction and prevention of musculoskeletal injuries require in-depth research, public education, and, in some cases, state and federal legislation. Safety for automobile occupants has become a major area of research not only for medical and trauma personnel but also for automotive engineers.[85] Siegel and associates demonstrated that lower extremity injury occurs more frequently in frontal crashes, whereas pelvic injuries occur more often in lateral crashes.[86]

Newer areas of research are focusing on the impact of air bags on trauma. The National Transportation Safety Administration estimated that air bags saved approximately 2700 lives in 1997.[85] Although this is an extremely important advance in trauma care, Burgess et al (1995) found that although air bags did decrease mortality, the incidence and severity of lower extremity injuries increased.[87] Other injuries associated with air bags include upper extremity fractures, abrasions, and ocular damage.[85]

Public education remains an important aspect in any injury prevention program. There are multiple community-based organizations and programs that address safety issues: Safe Kids (child safety seat use), Mothers Against Drunk Drivers (MADD), Students Against Drunk Drivers (SADD), and many others.

Improvements in prehospital stabilization techniques and the development of improved immobilization-traction devices for musculoskeletal injuries are essential. Advances need to occur in emergency care of traumatic amputations and partial amputations to optimize reattachment efforts.

Research must continue to develop improved assessment techniques and definitive care options. Potential nursing research topics may include acute and chronic pain assessment and management techniques; prevention of secondary injuries and complications, especially those related to immobility; early rehabilitation techniques; patient and family teaching and participation in care; and improved crisis management for families, patients, and staff. Medical issues that require further research and development in the realm of musculoskeletal injury include the stimulation and control of the fracture and soft tissue healing process, management of nonunion, improved microsurgical techniques to optimize reattachments, modalities to enable earlier mobility, and development of improved prosthetic and implant devices.

Rehabilitation of both physical and psychosocial injuries must be addressed concomitantly for the patient with musculoskeletal trauma. Improved chronic pain management, care of the amputee, and management of patients with osteomyelitis, nonunion, and paralysis are all worthy areas of research.

Advances in orthopedic surgery have changed the way in which many therapies and treatments are administered.[3] The development of new low-contact titanium plates used in fracture stabilization has decreased the incidence of osteoporosis found under fixation plates, and newer stainless steel low-contact plates, which are less expensive, are on the horizon.[3]

Outcome of care is a major topic in all areas of health care delivery. The outcomes movement in orthopedic surgery is relatively young, but concerted efforts are underway to identify outcome measurements, collect data, and improve patient outcomes.[88] This will be a major step in improving outcomes in trauma patients.

The future of musculoskeletal trauma patient care will demand a highly collaborative approach by health care providers during all cycles of trauma care. Continued research, with an increased emphasis on education and clinical application, is essential to the multidisciplinary search for excellence in patient care outcomes.

REFERENCES

1. Mourad LA: Structure and function of the musculoskeletal system. In McCance KA, Huether SE, editors: *Pathophysiology: the biological basis of disease in adults and children*, ed 3, St. Louis, 1998, Mosby.
2. James C: Orthopedic and neurovascular trauma. In Newberry L, editor: *Sheehy's emergency nursing: principles and practice*, ed 4, St. Louis, 1998, Mosby.
3. Browner BD: What's new in orthopaedic surgery? *J Am Coll Surg* 184:169-173, 1997.
4. Snyder P: Fractures. In Maher AB, Salmond SW, Pellino TA, editors: *Orthopaedic nursing*, ed 2, Philadelphia, 1998, WB Saunders.
5. Woods RK, O'Keefe G, Rhee P et al: Open pelvic fractures and fecal diversion, *Arch Surg* 133(3):281-287, 1998.
6. Trunkey DD, Chapman MW, Lim RC et al: Management of pelvic fractures in blunt trauma injury, *J Trauma* 14:912-923, 1974.
7. Pennal GF, Tile M, Wendall JP et al: Pelvic disruption: assessment and classification, *Clin Orthop* 151:12-21, 1980.
8. Young JWR, Burgess AR: *Radiological management of pelvic ring fractures: systemic radiographic diagnosis*, Baltimore, 1987, Urban and Schwarzenberg.
9. Tile M: *Fractures of the pelvis and acetabulum*, Baltimore, Williams & Wilkins, 1984.
10. Watson AD, Kelikian AS: Thomas splint, calcaneus fracture, and compartment syndrome of the foot: a case report, *J Trauma* 44(1):205-208, 1998.
11. Hefti D: Complications of trauma: the nurse's role in prevention, *Ortho Nurs* 14(6):9-16, 1995.
12. Bassam D, Cephas GA, Ferguson KA et al: A protocol for the initial management of unstable pelvic fractures, *Am Surg* 64(9):862-867, 1998.
13. Oxer H: No requiem for the MAST, *Prehosp Disaster Med* 6(2):231, 1991.
14. Jameel A, Vanderby B, Purcell C: The effects of pneumatic antishock garment (PASG) on hemodynamics, hemorrhage, and survival in penetrating thoracic aortic injury, *J Trauma* 31(6):849-851, 1991.
15. Schneider PE, Mitchell JM, Allison EJ: The use of military antishock trousers in trauma—a reevaluation, *J Emerg Med* 7(5):497-500, 1989.
16. Mattox KL, Bickell W, Pepe PE et al: Prospective MAST study in 911 patients, *J Trauma* 29(8):1104-1112, 1989.
17. Agnew SC: Hemodynamically unstable pelvic fractures, *Orthop Clin North Am* 25(4):715-721, 1994.
18. Burgess AR: Pelvic ring injuries, *Top Emerg Med* (15)1:78-90, 1993.
19. Woods RK, Dellinger EP: Current guidelines for antibiotic prophylaxis of surgical wounds, *Am Fam Physician* 57(11): 2731-2740, 1998.
20. DeDoer AS, Mintjes-deGroot AJ, Severignem AJ et al: Risk assessment for surgical site infections in orthopaedic patients, *Infect Control Hosp Epidemiol* 20(6):402-409, 1999.
21. Salmond SW: Infections of the musculoskeletal system. In Maher AB, Salmond SW, Pellino TA, editors: *Orthopaedic nursing*, Philadelphia, 1998, WB Saunders.
22. Walsh CR: Antimicrobial prophylaxis in surgery, *Med Lett Drugs Ther* 39(1012):97-101, 1997.
23. Keating JF, O'Brien PJ, Blachut PA et al: Locking intramedullary nailing with and without reaming for open fractures of the tibial shaft, *J Bone Joint Surg* 79(3):334-340, 1998.
24. Pellino TA, Polacek LA, Preston, MAS et al: Complications of orthopaedic disorders and orthopaedic surgery. In Maher AB, Salmond SW, Pellino TA, editors: *Orthopaedic nursing*, Philadelphia, 1998, WB Saunders.
25. Clark WK: Trauma to the nervous system. In Shires GT, editor: *Care of the trauma patient*, New York, 1979, McGraw-Hill.
26. Bentolila V, Nizard R, Bizot P et al: Complete traumatic brachial plexus palsy: treatment and outcome after repair, *J Bone Joint Surg* 81(1):20-30, 1999.
27. Barbier O, Malghem J, Delaire O et al: Injury to the brachial plexus by a fragment of bone after fracture of the clavicle, *J Bone Joint Surg* 79(4):534-535, 1997.

28. Blick SS, Brumback RJ, Polka A et al: Compartment syndrome in open tibial fractures, *J Bone Joint Surg* 68A(9):1348-1352, 1986.

29. Dabby D, Greif F, Yaniv M et al: Thromboxane A$_2$ in post ischemic acute compartment syndrome, *Arch Surg* 133: 953-956, 1998.

30. Sadasivam KK, Carden DL, Moore MB et al: Neutrophil mediated microvascular injury in acute, experimental compartment syndrome, *Clin Orthop Rel Res* 339:206-215, 1997.

31. Breit GA, Gross JH, Watenpaugh DE et al: Near-infrared spectroscopy for monitoring of tissue oxygenation of exercising skeletal muscle in a chronic compartment syndrome model, *J Bone Joint Surg* 79A(6):838-843, 1997.

32. Mittal R, Gupta V: Compartment syndrome of the thigh and the role of skin scars: case report and review of the literature, *J Trauma* 45(2):395-396, 1998.

33. Kalb RL: Preventing the sequelae of compartment syndrome, *Hosp Pract* 34(1):105-107, 1999.

34. Willy C, Gerngross H, Sterk J: Measurement of intracompartmental pressure with use of a new electronic transducer-tipped catheter system, *J Bone Joint Surg* 81(2):158-168, 1999.

35. James MD, Bregis RM: Mannitol treatment for acute compartment syndrome, *Nephron* 79(4):492, 1998.

36. Bryant GP: Modalities for immobilization. In Maher AB, Salmond SW, Pellino TA, editors: *Orthopaedic Nursing*, Philadelphia, 1998, WB Saunders.

37. Slye DA: Orthopedic complications, *Nurs Clin North Am* 26(1):113-132, 1991.

38. Gordon DB: Assessment and management of pain. In Maher AB, Salmond SW, Pellino TA, editors: *Orthopaedic nursing*, Philadelphia, 1998, WB Saunders.

39. Lamb S, Barbaro NM: Neurosurgical approaches to the management of chronic pain syndromes, *Orthop Nurs* 6:23-29, 1987.

40. Bulger EM, Smith DG, Maier RV et al: Fat embolus syndrome: a 10 year review, *Arch Surg* 132:435-439, 1997.

41. Lehman EP, Moore RM: Fat embolism: including experimental production without trauma, *Am Surg* 14:621-662, 1927.

42. Muller C, Rahn B, Pfister U et al: The incidence, pathogenesis, diagnosis, and treatment of fat embolism, *Orth Rev* 23: 107-117, 1994.

43. Varon AJ: Fat embolism: the trauma victim's bad break. Ryder Trauma: www.trauma.org/anaesthesia/fatembolism.html, 1999.

44. Sauter AJM, Klopper PJ: Fat embolism after static and dynamic loads: an experimental investigation, *Acta Orthop Scand* 54: 94-100, 1983.

45. Peltier LF: The diagnosis of fat embolism, *Surg Gynecol Obstet* 121:371-379, 1965.

46. Defrainge JO, Pincemail J: Local and systemic consequences of severe ischemia and reperfusion of the skeletal muscle: pathophysiology and prevention, *Acta Chir Belg* 98(4):176-186, 1998.

47. Tollens T, Janzing H, Broos P: The pathophysiology of acute compartment syndrome, *Acta Chir Belg* 98(4):171-175, 1998.

48. Layish DT, Tapson VF: Pharmacologic hemodynamic support in massive pulmonary embolism, *Chest* 111:218-224, 1997.

49. Clagett PC, Anderson FA, Geerts W et al: Prevention of venous thromboembolism, *Chest* 114(5):531S-560S, 1998.

50. ACCP Consensus Committee on Pulmonary Embolism: Opinions regarding the diagnosis and management of venous thromboembolic disease, *Chest* 113:499-504, 1998.

51. Goldwater SO: Pulmonary embolism, *N Engl J Med* 339(2): 93-104, 1998.

52. Keaton C, Ginsberg JS, Harsh J: The role of venous ultrasonography in the diagnosis of suspected deep venous thrombosis and pulmonary embolism, *Ann Intern Med* 129:1044-1049, 1998.

53. Rau J, Olson AJ, Palace PA: Clinical recognition of pulmonary embolism: problems of unrecognized and asymptomatic cases, *Mayo Cain Proc* 73:873-879, 1998.

54. Perrier A: Noninvasive diagnosis of pulmonary embolism, *Hosp Pract* 15:47-55, 1998.

55. Grady D, Sawaya G: Postmenopausal hormone therapy increases risk of deep vein thrombosis and pulmonary embolism, *Am J Med* 105:41-43, 1998.

56. Lewis MA: The epidemiology of oral contraceptive use: a critical review of the studies on oral contraceptives and the health of young women, *Am J Obstet Gynecol* 179:1086-1097, 1998.

57. Stauffer JL: Lung. In LM Tierney, SJ McPhee, MA Papadakis, editors: *Current medical diagnosis and treatment*, Norwalk, Conn, 1999, Appleton & Lange.

58. Wilson BA, Shannon MT, Stang CL: *Nurses drug guide*, Norwalk, Conn, Appleton & Lange, 1996.

59. Sue DY: Pulmonary disease. In Bongard FS, Sue DY, editors: *Current critical care diagnosis and treatment*, Norwalk, Conn, Appleton & Lange, 1994.

60. Dalen JE, Alpert JS, Harsh J: Thrombolytic therapy for pulmonary embolism: is it effective? Is it safe? When is it indicated? *Arch Intern Med* 157:2550-2556, 1997.

61. Winchell RJ, Hoyt DB, Walsh JC et al: Risk factors associated with pulmonary embolism despite routine prophylaxis: implications for improved protection, *J Trauma* 37:600-606, 1994.

62. Cipolle M, Marcinczyk M, Pasquale M et al: Prophylactic vena caval filters reduce pulmonary embolism in trauma patients [Abstract], *Crit Care Med* 23:A93, 1995.

63. Greenfield LJ, Proctor MC, Rodrigues JL et al: Post trauma thromboembolism prophylaxis, *J Trauma* 42:100-103, 1997.

64. Rodriguez JL, Lopez JM, Proctor MC et al: Early placement of prophylactic vena caval filters in injured patients at high risk for pulmonary embolism, *J Trauma* 40:797-804, 1996.

65. Rogers FB, Shackford SR, Ricci MA et al: Routine prophylactic vena cava filter insertion in severely injured trauma patients decreases the incidence of pulmonary embolism, *J Am Coll Surg* 180:641-627, 1995.

66. Rosenthal D, McKinsey JF, Levy AM et al: Use of the Greenfield filter in patients with major trauma, *Cardiovasc Surg* 2:52-55, 1994.

67. Willson JT, Rogers FB, Wald SL et al: Prophylactic vena cava filter insertion in patients with traumatic spinal cord injury, *Neurosurgery* 35:234-239, 1994.

68. Zolfaghari D, Johnson B, Weireter LJ et al: Expanded use of inferior vena cava filters in the trauma population, *Surg Ann* 27: 99-105, 1995.

69. Sparger G, Shea SS, Selfridge J: Patients with trauma. In Clochesy JM, Breu C, Cardin S et al, editors: *Critical care nursing*, Philadelphia, 1998, WB Saunders.

70. Chapman MW: Open fractures of the shaft of the tibia, *West J Med* 168(2):122-123, 1998.

71. Sangwan SS, Sharma V, Siwach RC: Role of pin traction in wound closure, *Orthopaedics* 22(4):419-422, 1999.

72. Aoki N, Soma K, Shindo M et al: Evaluation of potential fat emboli during placement of intramedullary nails after orthopedic fractures, *Chest* 113:178-181, 1998.

73. Kropfl A, Berger U, Neureiter H et al: Intramedullary pressure and bone marrow fat intravasation in unreamed femoral nailing, *J Trauma* 42(5):946-954, 1997.

74. Richards RR: Fat embolus syndrome, *Can J Surg* 40(5):334-338, 1997.

75. Smith JM: Pelvic fractures, *West J Med* 168(2):124-125, 1998.

76. Walsh CR, McBryde AM: Cost effectiveness of the orthopaedic advanced practice nurse: a joint protocol for home skeletal traction, *Orthop Nurs* 16(3):28-33, 1997.

77. Porter JM, Ivatury RR, Azimuddin K et al: Antioxidant therapy in the prevention of organ dysfunction and infectious complications after trauma: early results of a prospective randomized study, *Am Surg* 5(65):478-483, 1999.

78. Jones-Walton P: Clinical standards in skeletal traction pin site care, *Orthop Nurs* 10(2):12-15, 1991.

79. Szaflarski NL: Immobility phenomenon in critically ill adults. In Clochesy JM, Breu C, Cardin S, Rudy EB, Whittaker AA, editors: *Critical care nursing*, Philadelphia, 1998, WB Saunders.

80. O'Keefe GE, Maier RV, Diehr P et al: The complications of trauma and their associated costs in a level 1 trauma center, *Arch Surg* 132(8):920-926, 1997.

81. Jagmin MG: Assessment and management of immobility. In Maher AB, Salmond SW, Pellino TA, editors: *Orthopaedic nursing*, Philadelphia, 1998, WB Saunders.

82. Salmond SW: Infections of the musculoskeletal system. In Maher AB, Salmond SW, Pellino TA, editors: *Orthopaedic nursing*, Philadelphia, 1998, WB Saunders.

83. Gordon DB: Assessment and management of pain. In Maher AB, Salmond SW, Pellino TA, editors: *Orthopaedic nursing*, Philadelphia, 1998, WB Saunders.

84. D'Ambrosia RD: Orthopaedics in the new millennium: a new patient-physician partnership, *J Bone Joint Surg* 81(4):447-453, 1999.

85. Jordan KS: Air bags: a major advancement in injury control, *Orthop Nurs* 18(1):37-41, 1999.

86. Siegel J, Mason-Gonzales S, Cushing BM et al: A prospective study of injury patterns, outcome and cost of high speed frontal versus lateral motor vehicle crashes. In *Proceedings of the 34th Conference of the Association for the Advancement of Automotive Medicine*, Scottsdale, Ariz, 1990, 289-313.

87. Burgess A, Dischinger P, O'Quinn T: Lower extremity injuries in drivers of air bag equipped automobiles: Clinical and crash reconstruction correlations, *J Trauma* 38(4):509-516, 1995.

88. Swintowski M: The outcomes movement in orthopaedic surgery: where we are and where we should go, *J Bone Joint Surg* 81(5):731-741, 1999.

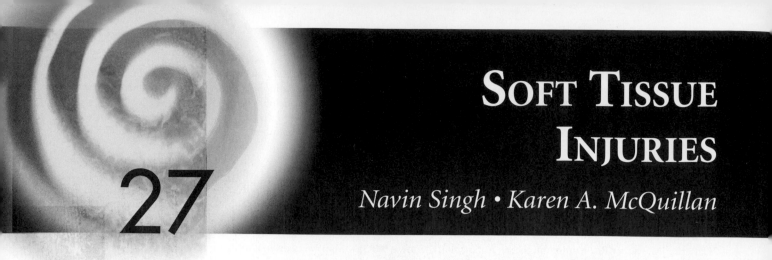

SOFT TISSUE INJURIES

Navin Singh • Karen A. McQuillan

Because the skin is the enveloping external organ of the human organism, it is the first line of defense in any injury and thus is nearly always injured when trauma occurs. Although a soft tissue injury may not be the critical illness from which a trauma victim suffers, it can contribute to the challenges of clinical management. Injury to skin and soft tissues predisposes the individual to secondary complications such as (1) localized and systemic infection, (2) hypoproteinemia, (3) hypothermia, and (4) sequelae related to tissue necrosis. Soft tissue injury and subsequent complications incur a high financial cost—not only from direct health care costs, but also from workdays lost for the patient and decreased quality of life secondary to having to live with scars or deformity.

Minimizing the risk of secondary complications and maximizing wound healing foster achievement of optimal outcomes for the patient with soft tissue injury. This chapter describes soft tissue injuries and their optimal assessment and management by the multidisciplinary health care team throughout the trauma cycle.

Skin is an organ with great variety: It is thin and mobile in some parts, such as the eyelids, and thick and immobile in others, such as the back and soles of the feet. It overlies other soft tissues in some areas and various bony protuberances in others (e.g., the mandible, zygoma, and malleoli). Therefore the pattern and degree of injury vary. Injurious modalities may impart low, medium, or high amounts of energy to the soft tissue envelope, depending on the particular mechanism of injury (e.g., motor vehicle crash, animal or human bites, blunt assault, or ballistic penetrating trauma). The skin may be abraded, avulsed, amputated, lacerated, contused, punctured, crushed, or bitten. When the patient is seen at the hospital, the soft tissue envelope may have already developed complications such as necrotizing infection if a prolonged period elapsed from injury to rescue and hospitalization.

SOFT TISSUE ANATOMY

SKIN

Skin is the largest organ in the body, having the largest surface area of all the organs and accounting for 16% of body weight. Intact skin provides many functions that are essential to survival. It serves as a barrier to invasion by microorganisms and chemicals. Skin also prevents loss of proteins and assists with regulation of electrolytes and fluid. Intact skin retains body heat, yet cutaneous vasodilation and activation of sweat glands help cool the body. Finally, skin provides sensory feedback about pressure, thermoperception, proprioception, touch, and pain.

Skin is a composite of several elementary tissues, including (1) connective tissue (collagen, elastin); (2) epithelium, including secondary skin appendages such as sweat glands and hair follicles; (3) nerves, including sensory structures such as Meissner's and pacinian corpuscles; and (4) blood vessels (Figure 27-1). The skin consists of two layers, the epidermis and dermis. The epidermis, the external surface of the skin, is composed of keratinized squamous epithelial cells. These cells produce a protein keratin, which is the same protein in hair and nails. Thickness of the epidermis varies depending on the functional forces to which it is subjected. For instance, it is thickest on the soles of the feet and on the palms.

The epidermis consists of five layers of cells (Figure 27-2). First is the stratum basale, which is the germinative layer of the epidermis. It is from this layer that cells divide by mitosis and undergo maturational changes to go on to produce keratin. Next is the stratum spinosum layer, which contains cells in the process of growth and early keratin synthesis. Stratum granulosum, a granular layer 1 to 4 cells thick,[1] is next followed by the stratum lucidum, which is present only in thick skin such as on the palms or soles of the feet. Most superficial is the stratum corneum layer, which consists of nonviable flattened fused cells composed mainly of the fibrous protein keratin. This superficial layer constantly

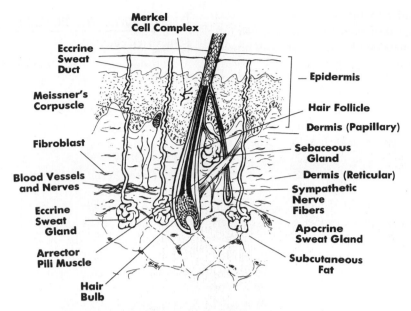

FIGURE 27-1 Schematic Vertical Cross-Section of Skin. (From Johnson TM, Nelson BR: Anatomy of the skin. In Baker SR, Swanson NA, editors: *Local flaps in facial reconstruction,* Chicago, 1995, Mosby, 4.)

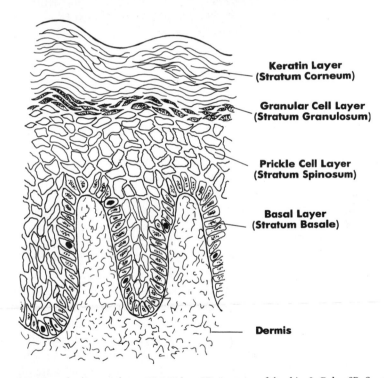

FIGURE 27-2 Layers of Epidermis. (From Johnson TM, Nelson BR: Anatomy of the skin. In Baker SR, Swanson NA, editors: *Local flaps in facial reconstruction,* Chicago, 1995, Mosby, 7.)

sheds. Melanin is also present in the epidermis and is elaborated by melanocytes, which migrate through and are scattered in the basal layers of the epidermis.

Immediately subjacent to the epidermis is the dermis, a highly vascular layer that contains many sensory receptors. The basement membrane zone connects the epidermis and dermis. This zone blocks passage of certain substances (e.g., chemicals) and provides mechanical support to the epidermis.[1,2] At the interface of the dermis and epidermis there are rete ridges. These are interdigitations of the epidermis and dermis, which prevent the epidermis from sheering off. The most superficial layer of the dermis is the papillary dermis, which is highly vascular with fine interlaced collagen fibers. The main bulk of the dermis is in the reticular layer, which contains most of the collagen. The cells of the dermis are largely fibroblasts, which produce collagen, elastin, and ground substance.

Skin appendages such as hair follicles, sebaceous glands,

and sweat glands extend into the deep dermis. Hair is a highly modified keratinized structure produced by hair follicles. Associated with them is a bundle of smooth muscle cells called the arrector pili, which are responsible for raising hair and producing goose pimples. Sebaceous glands secrete an oily substance called sebum onto the hair surface to provide waterproofing and moisturizing. Sweat glands are coiled tubular glands that secrete a watery fluid onto the skin surface to cool the body by evaporative heat loss. Beneath the dermis lies subcutaneous tissue, a variable thick layer of fat.

MUSCLE

Another soft tissue is muscle, which directly underlies skin everywhere except at the bony protuberances. In this chapter the discussion is limited to the skeletal musculature. From a functional viewpoint, muscles accomplish motion—acting on bones across joints or acting directly on skin, as with the muscles of facial expression. Muscle has a high metabolic demand and is relatively intolerant of ischemia. Vascularity to muscle is immense, serving its higher metabolic demand. Although muscles provide important functions, some are expendable because of either redundancy in the system, whereby many muscles accomplish the same motion (e.g., gracilis and adductor magnus, which both adduct the thigh, or extensor digitorum communis and extensor indicus proprius, which both extend the index finger), or the vestigial nature of some muscles (e.g., palmaris longus or plantaris longus, which perform no function whatsoever in humans but are used by lower primates to cup the palm or sole).

NERVES

Nerves in the soft tissue serve two functions. The first is an afferent function, the retrieval of sensory information from the periphery to the central nervous system. These sensory nerves relay information on temperature, pain, pressure, position, and vibration from the joints and skin. The second function is efferent, signaling nerves leaving the central nervous system to execute action in the periphery. These motor nerves are directed to muscles or autonomic nerves that regulate involuntary functions such as sweating or vessel dilation.

Nerve injuries can be classified according to the Sunderland system (Table 27-1), which prognosticates the time and degree of functional recovery.[3] Extent of nerve damage is often unclear at the initial evaluation and can be surmised only by neurometric tests and serial examinations to evaluate functional progress.

TYPES OF SOFT TISSUE INJURIES

CONTUSION

A contusion or bruise arises from rupture of subcutaneous blood vessels and extravasation of erythrocytes (Table 27-2). There is no break in the skin, but discoloration or ecchymosis, swelling, and pain are present at the site of contusion. A hematoma may accumulate at the site of ecchymosis.

HEMATOMA

A hematoma, resulting from rupture of a deeper and larger vein or artery, will expand in soft tissues until pressure in the area of hemorrhage exceeds the pressure within the disrupted artery or vein (see Table 27-2). Thus arterial hematomas, elaborated by arteries under greater pressure (mean arterial pressure is approximately 80-100 mm Hg) accumulate at a more rapid rate and to a larger size than hematomas of venous origin. The size of the hematoma is also related to the capacitance of the tissues in which it forms. For instance, in the hand, where the tissues are not so distensible, the pressure will rise quickly as the skin starts to distend and tamponade the extravasation. However, in a region such as the thigh, several liters of blood may extravasate because the soft tissue envelope is more accommodating.

If a hematoma is present, fluid fluctuance or a doughy ballotable mass is appreciated on palpation. Postinjury edema makes distinguishing between hematoma and profound edema challenging. Focal ecchymosis overlying an area of swelling should signify a hematoma as well.

ABRASION

Abrasions suggest a friction mechanism of injury such as dragging (see Table 27-2). These injuries may be superficial (i.e., involving only the epidermis or partial thickness of the dermis) or they may be deep (i.e., violating the full thickness of the dermis). A partial-thickness abrasion demonstrates erythema and punctate bleeding and is painful. It is not unlike a partial-thickness burn. A full-thickness abrasion is white, does not bleed, and is painless because of injury to the sensory nerves as well. A partial-thickness abrasion may progress to a full-thickness loss of skin if it is not treated appropriately or, if systemic resuscitation is suboptimal, from infection, ischemia, or hypoxia.

Traumatic abrasions are often contaminated with debris implanted into the skin, resulting in traumatic tattooing.[4] Gravel or road debris may become imbedded, for instance, in a patient ejected during a motor vehicle crash. This

TABLE 27-1   The Sunderland Classification System for Nerve Injuries

Grade	Structures Injured	Name	Prognosis
I	Loss of myelin sheath	Neurapraxia	Complete recovery in days to months
II	Neural death but intact sheath	Axonotmesis	Complete return in months
III	Neural and endoneurial injury		Mild/moderate reduction in function
IV and V	Disruption of all nerve structures	Neurotmesis	Marked reduction in function

TABLE 27-2 Summary of Traumatic Wounds

Type	Description	Mechanism of Injury	Assessment	Therapeutics	Complications
Contusion/ hematoma	An injury that does not involve the breaking of the skin. Characterized by swelling, pain, and discoloration. The rupture of small blood vessels causes extravasation of blood into the tissues, forming a hematoma.	Caused by blunt trauma.	Test for sensation and movement. Assess vascular involvement by measuring changes in the surface area of the bruise. Check for any underlying fractures.	Elevate the injured part and apply cold packs. Administer mild analgesics as required. May require up to 2-3 weeks for the hematoma to be reabsorbed.	Development of compartment syndrome, in which blood collects and increases pressure within the fascial compartment, compromising in the circulation and function of the affected area.
Crush injury	A composite injury involving two or more tissue types and graded severity of injury.	Incident involving high energy exchange such as a fall of significant distance or a motor vehicle crash in which a part of the body is run over and crushed.	Assess for size and anatomic location of crushed area. Check neurologic status and test for loss of function. Assess for tissue and blood loss and effect on underlying structures. Use invasive or noninvasive transcutaneous monitoring to detect increased compartment pressure (pressure exceeds diastolic arterial pressure).	Apply a pressure dressing, elevate, and cool. Treat open portions as described above. Surgical intervention may be required for serial debridement, fasciotomy, and fracture stabilization. Measure urine myoglobin when extensive muscle damage is present.	Complications include those of abrasions, avulsions, amputations, lacerations, and contusions. High risk of compartment syndrome. Amputation of crushed extremity may result.
Abrasion	A scraping or rubbing away of a layer or layers of the skin caused by friction with a hard object or surface. Abrasions vary in depth but are never deeper than the dermis.	Often caused by motorcycle crash or any incident in which the patient is dragged or slides across a rough surface.	Assess for size, depth, location, and degree of contamination. An abrasion covering a large amount of the body surface should raise concern for lost body fluids. Depth and number of exposed nerve endings affect the amount of pain experienced. Location affects limitation of movement, especially if the abrasion occurs over a joint. Dirt and debris are commonly embedded.	Local infiltration or topical application of anesthetic. Parenteral sedation for extensive abrasions. Meticulous cleansing by scrubbing with a saline- or surfactant cleanser-soaked sponge or surgical brush and copious irrigation. Do not use detergents because they produce additional pain. A needle, No. 11 surgical blade, or forceps may be required to remove embedded particles. Coat with antibiotic ointment and leave open or cover with nonadherent or occlusive dressing. Healing time varies with depth, location, and degree of contamination.	Direct sunlight may cause changes in skin pigmentation. "Traumatic tattooing," or the retention of foreign debris such as gunpowder, asphalt, and sand in the wound after healing, is characterized by a blue hue and a rough appearance.

Continued

TABLE 27-2 Summary of Traumatic Wounds—cont'd

Type	Description	Mechanism of Injury	Assessment	Therapeutics	Complications
Avulsion	A tearing away of tissue, resulting in full-thickness loss. Wound edges cannot be approximated. Degloving injuries, which result from shearing types of force, are one type of avulsion.	Caused when an extremity is cut by a meat slicer or saw or when an individual is thrown through the window in a motor vehicle crash.	Assess for amount of lost tissue, location, loss of function, and damage to underlying structures. The amount of tissue lost determines the course of treatment (e.g., grafting vs. revision and use of a flap). A large avulsion may result in fluid loss. Disability and disfigurement particularly occur when the avulsion involves the hand or face.	Thorough cleansing as described above. Control bleeding by direct pressure. Thorough irrigation with saline and early debridement of damaged tissue. Split-thickness grafting for closure when required. Complex avulsions may require use of a free flap placed with microvascular surgical techniques.	Disfigurement and loss of function of the affected limb may result in changes in patient's body image and may affect vocation and avocations.
Amputation	An avulsion in which the affected limb is completely separated from the body	Caused when a digit or extremity is caught in a piece of equipment and is sheared off. Guillotine type of injury is caused when a digit or extremity is cleanly cut off by a power saw or similar tool.	As with avulsion, assess for amount of lost tissue, location, loss of function, and damage to underlying structures. In addition, the separated part must be assessed for its viability after transport.	Thorough cleansing as described above. Wrap amputated part in a dry, sterile dressing and place in a sterile plastic bag or container. Place wrapped part in an insulated cooler with ice. Do not freeze the amputated part. Properly managed, the part may be maintained for 6-12 hours before replantation.	Infection and hypertropic scarring are the most frequent complications of amputations. Loss of viability or inability to replant the amputated part is related to mechanism of injury and warm ischemic time. Muscle in the amputated part is sensitive to ischemia and a large amount of muscle may have an adverse effect on the part's viability.
Laceration/incision	An open wound resulting from tearing or cutting of the skin. It is termed *superficial* if it involves only the dermis and epidermis and *deep* when it extends into the underlying tissues or structures.	Caused by rupture of the skin when struck by a blunt force, producing a torn, jagged wound; or a sharp object such as a shard of glass can cut the soft tissue.	Assess for damage to underlying structures and degree of contamination. Perform neurovascular checks to determine any sensory or motor deficits. Assess age of injury for degree of contamination and desiccation.	Thorough cleansing and irrigation, with hemostasis by pressure and elevation. Necrotic wound edges should be excised and edges approximated and closed with suture or skin tape. Use antibiotic ointment and nonadherent or occlusive dressing. Dressing should provide some pressure to reduce swelling and hematoma formation. Splints or casts are used when immobilization is required.	Sutures too tight or left in too long cause unsightly cross-hatching; sutures too loose cause wide scars. Improper approximation of the wound edges causes raised scars or tunnels that permit infection and hematoma formation. A loose dressing permits the wound to bleed and gapping to occur; a dressing applied too tight causes wound ischemia.

	Description	Cause	Assessment	Treatment	Complications
Puncture wound	A wound in which there is a small external opening in the skin but deep penetration of the underlying tissue.	Caused by the penetration of the skin by a sharp or pointed object. A high-pressure spray gun or similar equipment produces numerous punctures.	Assess for depth of penetration, degree of contamination, and any retained or injected foreign material. Appearance of surface injury may be benign. Assess for underlying tissue damage.	Soak the wound and examine the tract of the penetrating object. Remove any foreign bodies and irrigate the wound. Filling the wound space may be required for adequate healing.	Complications most frequently involve infection related to retained foreign material.
Mammalian bites	An animal or human bite causing puncture and a crushing wound by the teeth and jaws of the mammal and resulting in a grossly contaminated injury.	Caused by animal or human teeth and pressure from jaw force.	Determine the source of the bite and potential for infection. Assess wound's age, depth, and size and damage to underlying tissue.	Scrub and irrigate with povidone-iodine solution and apply cold pack. Bites more than 12 hours old should not have primary closure except in the face. Hand bites should be covered with a large bulky dressing. Plastic surgery may be required for facial bites. Antibiotic treatment is required in human and some animal bites. Tetanus and rabies prophylaxis may be needed.	Infection from microorganisms in the saliva. Human bites produce both gram-negative and gram-positive infections.

mechanism of injury is suggested by linear streaking within the abrasion.

AVULSION

Avulsions result from stretching or tearing away of the soft tissues, creating a full-thickness loss (see Table 27-2). Unfortunately, the magnitude of an avulsion injury is often underestimated. Tissues that appear viable and salvageable today are simply not so 24 hours later. This scenario is often repeated every 24 hours, with progressive loss of tissue. The tissue that remains behind is thus significantly compromised and declares itself viable or not over 48 to 96 hours.

LACERATION

Lacerations, compared with other soft tissue injuries, can appear to be a more elementary problem (see Table 27-2). Lacerations may be caused by sharp trauma such as glass or a knife wound. The adjacent area of crush and devitalization in these mechanisms may be small, approaching surgical incisions. These linear lacerations approximate well and have an optimal chance to heal. Facial lacerations that arise from blunt trauma generally occur along relaxed skin tension lines (normal skin creases), which are in areas of "skin fault lines," where skin is attenuated and susceptible to tearing[5] (Figure 27-3). This laceration pattern represents cleavage of the skin overlying the skeleton. If the laceration occurs at a right angle to the relaxed skin tension lines, healing generally takes longer and scarring is wider than if the laceration occurs within these lines.[6,7] Lacerations from

a blunt mechanism of injury are associated with larger margins of contused and compromised tissues. Often visible around the laceration is a halo of erythema or ecchymosis, indicating that the absolute zone of injury is larger than that of a laceration caused by a sharp object (e.g., a knife), and the relative zone of injury is quite large. Repair of this type of laceration is more challenging.

Lacerations that disrupt muscular tissues gap widely because of muscle contraction. Thus lacerations that divide muscles (e.g., across the full-thickness lip or eyelid) often give the appearance that tissue has been avulsed and is absent. By meticulously examining the functional elements, it can be ascertained that the tissues are present and can be reapproximated.

PUNCTURE WOUND

Puncture wounds carry a heightened risk of infection (see Table 27-2). Although they do not cause vast soft tissue destruction or lacerations, puncture wounds can set up an aggressive infection because they deliver bacteria or foreign inoculum deep into the body. Puncture wounds should not be closed, so that any infections that may develop can exit. Animal bites are notorious causes of puncture wounds. A bite from a dog with large teeth often causes lacerations that have a lower likelihood of getting infected because the bacteria can work their way out. However, in contrast, because of their fine, needlelike teeth, cats can cause a deeper bacteria inoculum that seals over. Bacteria then flourishes and cannot egress, leading to a virulent infection.[8,9]

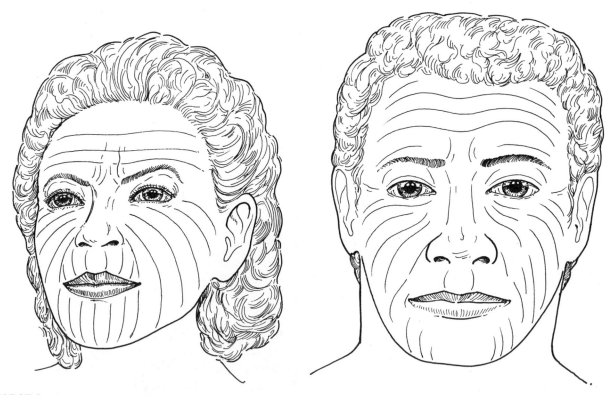

FIGURE 27-3 **Relaxed Skin Tension lines.** (From Cook TA, Brownlee RE: Rotation flaps. In Baker SR, Swanson NA, editors: *Local flaps in facial reconstruction,* Chicago, 1995, Mosby, 76.)

ASSESSMENT OF SOFT TISSUE INJURY

On encountering the patient, the organ we cannot help but examine is the skin. Immediately, from seeing the tone of skin, the examiner can ascertain whether the patient is flushed and well oxygenated, blue and dusky from hypoxia, or pale and mottled from anemia or tissue hypoperfusion. From the turgor, indirect cues about the hydration and volume status of the patient can be ascertained. Wrinkles convey information regarding the age of the patient. From the temperature, as hands are laid on the patient, hypothermia, physiologic warmth, and febrile response are assessed.

INJURY DATABASE

Information should be obtained from the prehospital care providers about the mechanism and environment of injury and treatment provided at the injury scene. Although external evidence of soft tissue injury may be present and obvious to the trauma team, information about the mechanism of injury may direct the practitioner to explore other less suspicious areas for soft tissue disruption. Any sustained pressure application over soft tissue and periods of hypoxia or hypotension in the prehospital phase should be noted because these factors can threaten the viability of soft tissues.

The health care team should also appreciate the time elapsed from the injury until hospital admission and definitive treatment of the wound. As this time interval increases, so does the likelihood of wound infection.[9,10] Decisions about wound closure and antibiotic prophylaxis may be based in part on this factor.[8,9]

In addition to the vectors of force directed and amount of kinetic energy delivered to the patient, the environment in which the injury occurred must be considered. Injuries sustained in environments with exposed soil (e.g., farms, construction sites) are likely to be highly contaminated with numerous pathogens, including gram-positive anaerobic bacteria (e.g., *Clostridia*). Wounds contaminated with certain species of *Clostridia* (e.g., *Clostridia perfringens*) can develop clostridial myonecrosis (gas gangrene) if provided an area of decreased oxidation-reduction potential (e.g., necrotic tissue, tissue lacking perfusion, hematoma, foreign body). Gas gangrene has a rapid and fulminating clinical course that can lead to tissue destruction, limb loss (sometimes within 24 to 48 hours), toxemia, and death.[11] Therefore, wounds acquired in a dirty or farm environment require aggressive, serial debridement at regular intervals.

Aquatic injuries are often contaminated with gram-negative bacteria. Brackish water in intertidal zones such as bays and estuaries is conducive to the proliferation of these organisms. Virulent bacteria from marine environments include *Vibrio*, *Aeromonas*, and *Mycobacterium* species. Wounds infected with these organisms require coverage with third-generation cephalosporins, quinolones, or other broad-spectrum antibiotics.

Industrial injuries, which deliver large loads or high pressure, can pose unique challenges. Chemical caustic agents used in industrial settings can penetrate skin. Material data sheets from the site of the injury are important to obtain in order to evaluate the cytotoxic effects of these chemicals. High-pressure injection of these agents into subcutaneous tissues can lead to unsuspected wide dissemination of caustic agents underneath the skin. These wounds require aggressive debridement. In blunt trauma suffered in industrial settings, large loads, such as those typically manipulated by cranes or forklifts, are brought to bear on small areas such as the lower or upper extremities. This leads to large amounts of soft tissue devitalization and crush injuries. The patient often requires multimodality stabilization, including possible placement of an external fixator for fracture stabilization, control of hemorrhage with interventional radiologic or operative techniques, and surgical debridement of nonvital tissues.

INITIAL ASSESSMENT PRIORITIES

Initial assessment and management priorities for trauma patients are to ensure a patent airway, adequate breathing, and sufficient circulation. Skin characteristics may provide clues about insufficient oxygenation, poor tissue perfusion, location of life-threatening injuries, and sources of hemorrhage, which are considered during the primary survey. However, a detailed soft tissue assessment is typically delayed until the ABCDE (airway, breathing, circulation, neurologic disability, exposure/environmental control) priorities of the trauma resuscitation protocol have been assessed and managed and the patient has been stabilized.[12]

SOFT TISSUE ASSESSMENT

INSPECTION AND PALPATION.   Starting in the head and neck region and proceeding downward, the soft tissue is evaluated carefully for injury. The patient should be disrobed completely to expose the entire skin surface. Care is taken to evaluate between all skin folds and beneath hair. The patient should be log-rolled to the side as soon as possible to permit thorough evaluation of the posterior aspect.

Location, size, and appearance of any wound or area of skin discoloration should be well documented in the medical record. It is important to note the amount, character, and odor of any wound exudate. Tissue swelling may be noted at or near the site of soft tissue injury, and the nurse should monitor the patient closely for any edema that impairs tissue perfusion or obstructs the airway. Extremity girth may be measured serially to detect increased soft tissue swelling. Any change in the appearance of a wound or wound drainage should be reported to the physician.

Soft tissue perfusion is evaluated by assessing capillary refill time, pulses, skin color, and temperature. Sluggish capillary refill time; absent or weak pulses; and pale, mottled, or bluish skin color are all symptoms of impaired tissue perfusion. When the skin is cool to touch, it signals the presence of systemic hypothermia or tissue hypoperfusion. Skin very warm to touch may provide evidence of underlying inflammation or systemic fever.

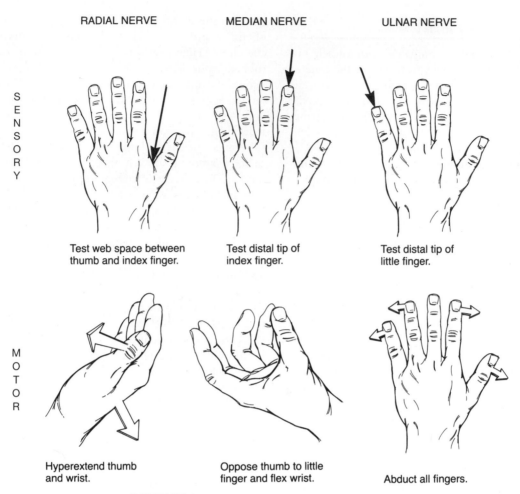

RADIAL NERVE   MEDIAN NERVE   ULNAR NERVE

S
E
N
S
O
R
Y

Test web space between   Test distal tip of   Test distal tip of
thumb and index finger.   index finger.   little finger.

M
O
T
O
R

Hyperextend thumb   Oppose thumb to little
and wrist.   finger and flex wrist.   Abduct all fingers.

FIGURE 27-4 **Upper Extremity Sensory-Motor Assessment.**

When evaluating a wound, in addition to inspecting for erythema, purulence, and tenderness, the patient must be assessed for crepitus. Crepitus is produced by subcutaneous air or gas. Subcutaneous emphysema develops when air is trapped benignly along soft tissue planes or is being produced by an anaerobic organism (e.g., *C. perfringens*, coliforms, anaerobic streptococci, bacteroides).[11]

NEUROMUSCULAR FUNCTION. A neuromuscular examination is performed to discern the presence of muscle or nerve damage. In the alert and cooperative patient, a detailed motor and sensory examination, including assessment of the cranial nerves (see Chapter 19) and peripheral nerves distributed to the extremities, is performed (Figures 27-4 and 27-5). Sensation in other areas of the body should also be evaluated by determining if the patient can distinguish sharp versus dull stimulus in other sensory dermatomes. (Refer to Chapter 22 for an explanation of sensory assessment.)

Injuries to various regions of the body may prohibit certain components of the assessment from being carried out fully. For example, lower extremity fractures preclude obtaining a full motor function examination of the leg. Patients with an altered level of consciousness are usually unable to reliably perform tests of motor function or sensation and require modifications to the neuromuscular examination. Examination of specific involuntary reflexes (e.g., pupillary light reflex, corneal reflex, gag reflex) evaluates some cranial nerve functions. (Refer to Chapter 19 for a thorough explanation of cranial nerve assessment.) In the comatose patient, motor function assessment is performed by examining the type and strength of patient movement in response to noxious stimuli. The only means of evaluating peripheral sensation is to observe responsiveness to noxious stimuli applied to the extremities.

Motor or sensory deficits should raise a signal of alarm not only for direct injury to the nerve but also for the possibility of limb-threatening compartment syndrome. After soft tissue injury, compartment syndrome occurs if bleeding and edema within a fascial compartment elevates the intracompartment pressure, resulting in compromised blood flow to the muscles and nerves of the compartment. (Refer to Chapter 26 for more information on compartment syndrome.) Diminution of sensation is the most reliable early diagnostic symptom of compartment syndrome.[11] Patient complaint of pain out of proportion to the injury and motor weakness may also be noted. Pulselessness is a

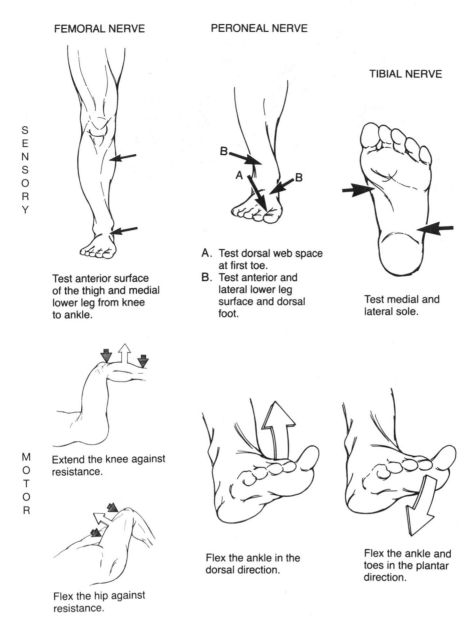

FEMORAL NERVE

PERONEAL NERVE

TIBIAL NERVE

S
E
N
S
O
R
Y

Test anterior surface of the thigh and medial lower leg from knee to ankle.

A. Test dorsal web space at first toe.
B. Test anterior and lateral lower leg surface and dorsal foot.

Test medial and lateral sole.

M
O
T
O
R

Extend the knee against resistance.

Flex the hip against resistance.

Flex the ankle in the dorsal direction.

Flex the ankle and toes in the plantar direction.

FIGURE 27-5 **Lower Extremity Sensory-Motor Assessment.**

very late finding, by which time tissue necrosis may have begun.[11,13]

LABORATORY STUDIES. A number of abnormal laboratory values may provide clues about underlying problems that require timely intervention. Low hemoglobin and hematocrit levels accompany substantial blood loss from soft tissue injury and may necessitate blood transfusion. Abnormal coagulation parameters require prompt correction to prevent excessive blood loss from soft tissue disruption. Persistent elevations of the white blood cell concentration may provide evidence of soft tissue infection. Elevation in the serum creatine phosphokinase (CPK) level or the presence of myoglobinuria implies muscle necrosis, which may result from development of compartment syndrome.[14]

OTHER DIAGNOSTIC STUDIES. Soft tissue damage often overlies other injuries such as fractures. For instance, periorbital ecchymosis ("black eyes" or "raccoon's eyes") is virtually pathognomonic for orbital, nasal, or basilar skull fractures. Findings of soft tissue disruption often trigger additional diagnostic studies to rule out or determine the extent of underlying injury.

Concern about the presence of an embedded foreign body may prompt additional diagnostic tests to confirm the presence, size and location of the object. Radiographs can usually detect foreign objects that are radiopaque (e.g., metal, gravel, glass) if they are large enough to be visualized.[15,16] A computed tomography (CT) scan may also be useful in locating a foreign body and determining what disruption the object caused to surrounding tissues.

RESUSCITATION

INITIAL PRIORITIES

First and foremost, the multidisciplinary trauma team focuses on ensuring a patent airway, adequate breathing, and sufficient circulation.[12] Soft tissue injury of the neck or maxillofacial region may precipitate airway obstruction, requiring immediate attention. (For specific information on injury to the maxillofacial region, see Chapter 20.) Hemorrhage from soft tissue disruption may also cause significant depletion of intravascular volume, leading to impaired circulation.

CIRCULATION

Hemorrhage from soft tissue injury is cause for immediate concern. Hemorrhage from injured soft tissue can cause exsanguination, especially if large blood vessels are involved. Bleeding into the soft tissues or body cavities although less obvious than external hemorrhage, may also lead to hypovolemia and shock.

External hemorrhage is treated initially by application of direct pressure on the bleeding site.[13] A pressure bandage applied around the circumference of a bleeding area may effectively tamponade the hemorrhage until more definite treatment can be rendered. Care must be taken when applying a circumferential dressing to ensure that compression does not completely obstruct flow for a prolonged period, thereby causing ischemia to the distal portion of the affected body part. When compression fails to control soft tissue hemorrhage, the wound requires surgical exploration to clamp and ligate the bleeding vessel. The nurse should continuously monitor wound dressings and drainage, and the physician should be kept informed of the estimated blood loss.

Soft tissue injury also causes fluid loss via a number of other mechanisms. Disruption of the skin integrity, especially over large body surface areas, increases the volume of insensible fluid loss. Tissue injury can cause vascular damage and inflammation at and around the affected site, allowing fluid to extravasate out of the intravascular space and into the interstitium. Both these mechanisms contribute to depletion of the intravascular volume, which can lead to inadequate tissue perfusion.

Crystalloids, colloids, and, when appropriate, blood products are administered intravenously to restore adequate intravascular volume. The patient's hemodynamic parameters (e.g., heart rate, systemic blood pressure, central venous pressure) and indicators of tissue perfusion sufficiency (e.g., mentation, capillary refill time, urine output, acid-base balance, lactate levels) should be used to guide the appropriate volume of fluid therapy. If concern about persistent hemorrhage exists, serial evaluation of hemoglobin, hematocrit, and coagulation parameters may be prescribed.

NORMOTHERMIA

Disruption of skin integrity allows loss of body heat through the skin opening. When a large area of the skin covering is affected, body temperature may drop. Systemic hypothermia in turn causes vasoconstriction in an attempt to conserve the body's heat, which reduces peripheral circulation and impedes oxygen delivery to the tissues.[17,18] Vasoconstriction-induced tissue hypoxia reduces collagen deposition, which is necessary to provide tensile strength to healing wounds.[18] Low body temperatures also slow down all chemical reactions, including those needed to lay down collagen and heal wounds. Hypothermia also impairs immune function, which, together with decreased tissue oxygenation caused by vasoconstriction, increases the risk of wound infection.[17-19] Other deleterious consequences of hypothermia can include coagulopathy; diminished cardiac output; slowed cardiac conduction; arrhythmias; decreased level of consciousness; loss of motor and reflex function; hemoconcentration; respiratory depression; and reduced hepatic, renal, and adrenal function.[20] Body temperature should be monitored closely, and measures to warm the patient (e.g., use of warming blankets, heated ventilator circuits, warmed intravenous fluids) should be employed as necessary to normalize body temperature.[12,20] Refer to Chapter 13 on Initial Management of Traumatic Shock for more information on hypothermia and its management.

WOUND CARE

Cleansing and repair of simple or minor soft tissue injury can typically be performed in the resuscitation area, whereas repair of more complex wounds requires surgical intervention in the operating room. Depth and direction of the wound should be assessed to predict deep structure involvement and detect contamination. Wounds should be cleansed of all nonviable tissue and foreign material, which, if not removed, predispose the wound to infection, causing a delay in healing.[21-23] Wounds are cleansed by scrubbing, pulsed irrigation, and minimal but judicious sharp debridement of contused wound edges.[22] Inadequate cleansing of the wound may result in traumatic tattooing, wherein road debris (e.g., gravel) is embedded into the dermis, making later excision impossible. Conservative debridement is indicated in those areas with little local tissue laxity, such as the distal nose, ears, eyelids, and vermilion of the lips. Superlative results are obtained when nonvital and compromised tissues are excised and the wound is closed primarily. Thus meticulous attention must be paid to closure and debridement at the time of repair; reliance should not be placed on later scar revision. The goal of complete excision of contused tissues is not always accomplishable because there may not be enough local tissue laxity to close the wound primarily if generous debridement is undertaken. In those situations, secondary scar revision is usually necessary. A layered repair then achieves an optimal result. Nurses should clarify with the physician specific care desired for wounds after closure or while awaiting closure.

Attention must be given to the soft tissue in contact with stabilization and immobilization devices applied in the field (i.e., backboard, cervical collar, traction, and splinting devices). These devices typically lack sufficient padding and pose a substantial risk for skin breakdown if left on for an excessive time. The nurse should collaborate with the rest of the health care team to pursue removal of these devices in a timely fashion.

PREVENTION OF INFECTION

Controversy surrounds the use of prophylactic antibiotics for traumatic wounds. Sufficient levels of antibiotics need to be present in the tissues at the time of injury to optimize their effectiveness, which is impossible in the case of unanticipated trauma. When given after injury, antibiotic effectiveness is significantly diminished.[8,17] Needless antibiotic use for minor decontaminated wounds is discouraged to decrease the risk of creating antibiotic-resistant infections. Administration of antibiotics may be considered when a clean wound cannot be created by debridement. Antibiotics may also be considered if there is major soft tissue disruption, an associated open injury to a joint or bone, or the patient has a premorbid history of immunosuppression or cardiac valvular disease.[8] Prophylactic antibiotics must be present in high concentrations before and during wound closure or surgical manipulation of the wound to be effective.[8,17] Consideration of the environment where the injury occurred is important when selecting an antibiotic so that the drug selected covers likely pathogens. Prophylactic antibiotics are not a substitute for thorough wound debridement, meticulous wound care, and adequate tissue perfusion and oxygenation to prevent infection.[8,17,19,24]

When the patient is admitted with an established infection of the soft tissue caused by delay in hospitalization after injury or demonstrates onset of infection during the resuscitation phase, the infection should be treated with thorough wound debridement and irrigation and appropriate antibiotics. Early onset of a rapidly progressing wound infection should trigger an investigation to rule out clostridial or group A streptococcal infection, which can develop within hours of injury.[25] Cultures of the wound bed and exudate provide essential information about the causative organism and which antibiotic would be most appropriate.

Adult patients who have not had a tetanus shot within the past 10 years should receive a tetanus toxoid booster. In severely contaminated wounds that are tetanus prone and for patients who have an inadequate immunization history, tetanus immune globulin should also be administered for passive immunization. The tetanus immune globulin should be administered at a different site than the tetanus toxoid so that the antibody and antigen do not neutralize each other in the same injection site.[8]

PAIN MANAGEMENT

Soft tissue injury may cause a significant amount of patient discomfort. Pain can have an adverse effect on wound healing because it stimulates catecholamine release, causing vasoconstriction and reduced peripheral tissue perfusion and oxygen delivery.[17,26] The nurse should carefully assess and document the location and severity of the patient's pain. Once a baseline neurologic assessment is performed, pre-

scribed pain medication should be administered and the patient's pain relief should be evaluated. Increasing pain should not be dismissed or simply medicated with increasing doses of analgesics; instead the cause of the increasing pain should be investigated. Refer to Chapter 17 for more extensive information on pain management.

OPERATIVE PHASE

SOFT TISSUE RECONSTRUCTION

The "reconstruction ladder" is an important concept used to plan the repair of soft tissue deficits[27] (Figure 27-6). This construct includes all the interventions that may be used to achieve stable closure of a wound, from the most elementary technique at the bottom of the ladder to the most complicated at the top. The simplest technique that achieves the optimal functional and most cosmetically acceptable outcome with the least risk to the patient is selected.[8,27,28]

PRIMARY VERSUS SECONDARY WOUND CLOSURE.   Primary closure of a wound, when wound edges can be approximated and closed with sutures, staples, or tape, is the first option considered for wound closure. When that is not possible because of tissue loss or not advisable because of wound infection or marginal tissue, secondary intention healing is recommended if it will not cause a functional or cosmetic deformity. Secondary intention healing occurs when an open wound is allowed to granulate and eventually close on its own. Small wounds in cosmetically unimportant areas such as the abdomen, trunk, or legs can be treated with wet-to-dry saline dressings and allowed to granulate. Open management of wounds in the head and neck region is not advocated because of the unique vascularity, ability to heal, and social significance of this region.[8] Primary closure of facial wounds is preferred, with serial debridements and closures staged at 24 and 48 hours.

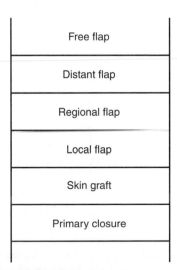

FIGURE 27-6 **The Reconstructive Ladder.** The simplest wound closure technique that achieves the most desirable outcome with the least risk to the patient is selected. Simplest techniques start at the bottom of the ladder.

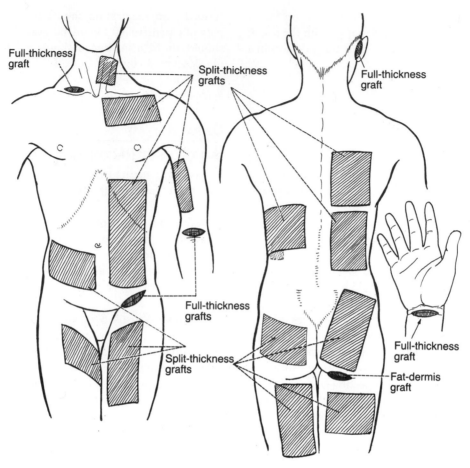

FIGURE 27-7 **Available Donor Sites for Skin Grafts.** (From Rudolph R, Ballantyne DL. Skin grafts. In McCarthy JG, editor: *Plastic surgery,* vol 1, *General principles,* Philadelphia, 1990, WB Saunders, 227.)

As neovascularization (formation of new blood vessels) occurs, a healthy wound bed will take on a beefy red appearance. The wound bed reepithelializes from the edges because the epithelial cells lose their contact inhibition and start to proliferate, creeping into the wound. If a wound bed has full-thickness skin loss and the skin is allowed to granulate, the new skin will lack a dermis and will have only a friable epidermis layer. Over the ensuing months, as greater collagen deposition occurs, the wound will regain up to 80% of its original strength.[28] This is cosmetically inferior and does not provide durable coverage. Secondary closure is recommended only for small wounds because a large wound may take months, even up to 1 year, to fully reepithelialize. This time to full healing may be further prolonged in the nutritionally compromised patient.[17,26]

The Sure-Closure device (Life Medical Sciences, Princeton, NJ) may be used to stretch and increase the surface area of skin to enable wound closure. This skin-stretching device recruits the viscoelastic properties of skin, namely "creep" and "stress relaxation," using incremental traction. Wound edges initially not coapted can be stretched together within minutes to days with this device simply by turning a screw.[29,30] Application of elastics is another method used to dynamically recruit the viscoelastic properties of skin to achieve wound closure.

SPLIT-THICKNESS SKIN GRAFTS. Wounds that have a healthy, viable bed with sufficient blood supply and that are too large to granulate over can be managed with skin grafts. Skin grafts can be split thickness or full thickness. Split-thickness skin grafts contain less tissue requiring revascularization and have greater capillary exposure, making them more likely to tolerate a recipient site with some vascular compromise. In contrast, full-thickness skin grafts require a recipient site that has a rich vascular supply.[31]

A split-thickness skin graft is harvested, when possible, from relatively hidden areas, using a dermatome device (Figures 27-7 and 27-8). Skin is harvested through the mid-dermis so that the split-thickness skin graft includes partial-thickness dermis and all of the epidermis (Figure 27-9). Typical thickness for a harvested split-thickness skin graft is .0012 of an inch to .0015 of an inch. When the skin graft is applied to an appropriately healthy wound bed, it should "take" to the bed. The skin graft may be meshed (meaning cut into a lattice format) to allow the skin graft to expand (Figure 27-10). Meshing is done to achieve closure of a large wound when donor sites are at a premium, for instance in a severely burned patient with only a few donor sites available. Mesh ratios typically used for skin grafts are 1.5:1 or 3:1, which respectively provide 150% or 300% coverage. An additional reason for meshing is to allow fluid collections beneath the graft to escape through the mesh

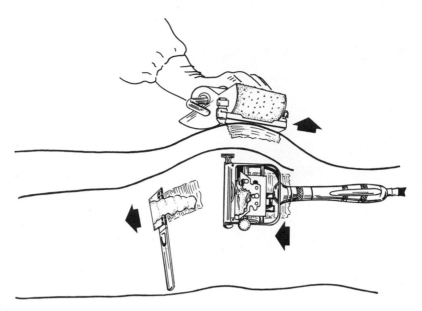

FIGURE 27-8 Split-thickness skin grafts should be harvested from relatively hidden areas such as the thighs and buttocks whenever possible. Drum dermatomes are generally used across a convex surface whereas power dermatomes and hand-held knives are best used longitudinally on an extremity. (From Rudolph R, Ballantyne DL. Skin grafts. In McCarthy JG, editor: *Plastic surgery,* vol 1, *General principles,* Philadelphia, 1990, WB Saunders, 227.)

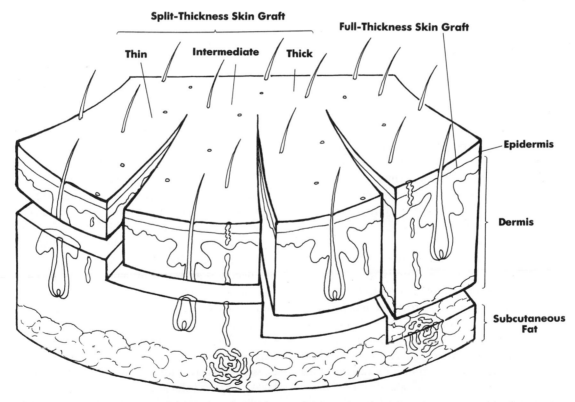

FIGURE 27-9 Relationship of Skin Graft Type to Thickness of Skin. (From Glogan RG, Haas AF: Skin grafts. In Baker SR, Swanson NA, editors: *Local flaps in facial reconstruction,* Chicago, 1995, Mosby, 249.)

openings. Whereas meshed skin grafts can give greater coverage and are more resistant to the development of a seroma (localized collection of serous fluid within tissue), hematoma, or even infection beneath the graft, they give a cosmetically inferior result because the mesh pattern is retained.

Skin graft "take" is a process that lasts several days. For the first 36 hours or so, a skin graft lives off imbibition. Imbibition, from the Latin for drinking, is essentially osmosis, whereby nutrients diffuse from a healthy wound bed to the skin graft and cellular waste products diffuse from the skin graft into the wound bed, where they are taken away

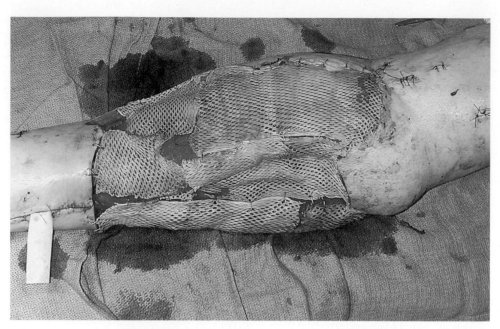

FIGURE 27-10 Meshed Skin Graft Applied to the Leg.

by the circulation. Because the success of diffusion is determined by close approximation of the skin graft to the wound, it is important that no fluid collections, such as seroma or hematoma, arise between the skin graft and the wound bed, because this will impair diffusion and lead to graft loss.[27,31] After the first 36 to 48 hours of dependence on imbibition, the skin graft starts to undergo revascularization by anastomoses of the host and graft vasculatures (inosculation) and ingrowth of the recipient site vessels into the capillary architecture of the skin graft dermis.[32]

Because a split-thickness graft contains only a partial amount of the dermis, it undergoes contracture after healing. Fibroblasts and myofibroblasts in the wound bed pull the edges of the wound together. This may provide a cosmetically inferior result if a split-thickness graft is used in an area such as the face.[31] More importantly, it may provide a functionally inferior result, leading to a contracture across a joint, when applied in an area such as the elbow, wrist, dorsum of the hand, axilla, knee, or ankle. If there are concerns about cosmesis or delayed development of a contracture, the patient can be managed with secondary scar revision using a full-thickness skin graft, or a full-thickness skin graft can be chosen as the initial mode of treatment.

Meanwhile, the donor site for a split-thickness skin graft harvest heals spontaneously because only a partial thickness of the dermis has been harvested. Skin appendages such as sweat glands and hair follicles contain epithelial nests, which start to bud and volcano out of their roots in the deep dermis. These epithelial nests spread across the injured surface until they meet the epithelial cells from the adjacent accessory skin appendage. A harvest site reepithelializes within 7 to 10 days.

FULL-THICKNESS SKIN GRAFTS. A full-thickness skin graft is harvested by designing an ellipse matched to the dimensions of the skin needed. This ellipse may be taken from a convenient inconspicuous area such as a groin crease. Then a full-thickness skin graft is excised from this ellipse, defatted down to the dermis, and applied to the wound bed. The donor site can usually be closed primarily as a straight line if there is sufficient soft tissue laxity in the chosen site. For skin grafting in the head and neck region, the color match is superior if the skin graft donor site is chosen from above the shoulders (e.g., the postauricular, preauricular, or supraclavicular region).[31] These donor sites can also be closed primarily with a linear closure.

Full-thickness skin grafts also may be harvested from an expanded area. A tissue expander is placed in the subcutaneous region of an area from which a full-thickness skin graft will be harvested later[33] (Figure 27-11). This implant is inflated serially to allow the overlying skin and soft tissue to stretch out. Once enough new skin has been created and recruited, the tissue expander is removed, the excess skin is harvested for a full-thickness skin graft, and the wound is closed primarily. This technique is useful for patients who need a large full-thickness skin graft and would otherwise be unable to undergo primary closure of the donor site if so much skin was excised. Alternatively, a full-thickness skin graft can be excised from a donor area that can then be closed itself with a split-thickness skin graft from yet another area.

OTHER TYPES OF SKIN REPLACEMENT. Additional biologic, synthetic, and biosynthetic skin replacement products are available. A number of grafts are available for temporar-

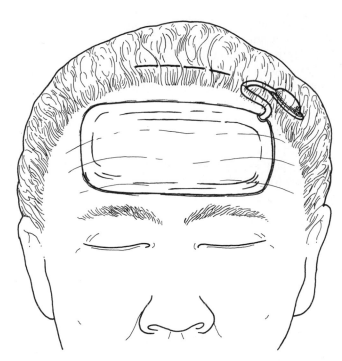

FIGURE 27-11. Large Rectangular Tissue Expander is Placed Beneath Frontalis Muscle Through Small Incision Above Hairline. (From Argenta LC: Controlled tissue expansion in facial reconstruction. In Baker SR, Swanson NA, editors: *Local flaps in facial reconstruction*, Chicago, 1995, Mosby, 528.)

ily covering a wound to prevent infection, excessive discomfort, body fluid evaporation, and heat loss.[27] Xenografts, harvested from pigs, and allografts, from human cadavers, are temporary grafts used primarily for burns.[27,34,35] Several synthetic dermal coverings have also been developed (e.g., Integra, Alloderm).[34,36] Epithelial cells have been cultured and grafted onto wounds with limited success. Cultured cells have also been used to develop epidermal grafts, dermal replacements, and composite grafts, containing dermal and epidermal components.[34,37] Although most of these skin replacement products have been used and tested primarily with burns, they may have a role in healing selected traumatic soft tissue injuries. New developments in skin replacement offer tremendous hope for other more effective alternatives to manage soft tissue injury.

FLAPS. Wounds that are not suitable for primary closure, secondary intention healing, or closure with skin grafts may require a flap for closure. Flaps are required when vital structures such as nerves, blood vessels, tendons, or bones without any overlying vascular tissue are exposed. Because these vital structures need more padding than can be provided by a skin graft or they are no longer vascularized to support a skin graft (e.g., tendon without paratenon or bone without periosteum), they must be covered with tissue that brings its own vascularity—namely, a flap.

Flaps may be composed of various tissues. Skin and subcutaneous tissue flaps are called fasciocutaneous flaps. Flaps may also incorporate muscle, in which case they are termed musculocutaneous flaps. Complex composite tissues including bone, muscle, skin, and fat may also be moved as a flap. These are termed osseomusculocutaneous or osseofasciocutaneous free flaps. Examples of these include the free fibula, in which a vascularized piece of the fibular bone from the lower extremity is transferred, using microsurgical techniques, to reconstruct other bony losses such as the humerus, radius, or mandible. This technique of free tissue transfer with complex composite tissue flaps represents the dawning of a new era of plastic surgery reconstruction. With advances in tissue engineering, a flap can essentially be designed and engineered in a remote location to replace detailed areas such as half of a face or portions of an arm. Once mature, the flap can be transported by microsurgical techniques to the desired location.

The type of flap used is based in part on patient habitus. In a slightly obese patient for whom bulk is needed to fill the wound bed, a fasciocutaneous flap may be well suited. However, when a pliable surface is required, such as on the face or the back of the hand, a thinner flap composed solely of fasciocutaneous tissues and underlying fat may be harvested from the back or abdomen of an appropriately thin patient.

Abundant vascularity is tremendously beneficial when muscles are used as flaps to provide soft tissue coverage and to ablate dead space in traumatic wounds. Because of augmented vascularity, a muscle flap that has been rotated to cover an exposed critical area can deliver polymorphonucleocytes, mononuclear lineage cells, and lymphocytes in the inflammatory phase of wound healing to enhance removal of debris and combat infection. Animal studies show that muscle flaps demonstrate greater resistance to infection than fasciocutaneous (skin) flaps when subjected to the same bacterial inoculum.[38-40] Enhanced vascularity provides greater traffic of erythrocytes and increases the oxygen tension in a wound, which expedites wound healing. Muscle flaps, compared with skin flaps, are more pliable and conform to complex surfaces and curves in three-dimensional space to ablate dead space and enhance final contour.

Flaps may be obtained from local or remote tissue. A flap from local tissue involves leaving the blood supply intact and rotating, transposing, or tunneling locally available tissue into the wound.[41] For example, the rectus abdominis muscle can be harvested and flipped from the abdomen to cover an exposed femoral artery and vein in the groin. Another example is a nasal labial flap, whereby vascularized tissue from the nasolabial crease is raised with its intact blood supply from the angular artery and vein and tunneled to cover defects on the sides of the nose.

When local tissues are not available, such as in the distal third of the leg where there is a paucity of soft tissue covering, remote tissues must be used for closure. An example of remote tissue use includes an across-leg flap, where tissue from one leg is bridged to the opposite injured leg. After 2 to 3 weeks, when the injured leg has adopted tissue from the healthy leg, the soft tissue is divided between the two legs. Remote tissue is also used when a hand stripped of a soft tissue covering is "tucked in" to the abdomen for 2 to 3 weeks until it has revascularized and incorporated soft tissue from the abdomen.

Over the past 20 to 30 years the microsurgical technique for placement of free flaps has largely supplanted other techniques using remote tissue. A free flap does not initially retain its own vascularity. Using microsurgical techniques, the flap is harvested from its donor site (e.g., the rectus abdominis muscle is harvested from the abdomen or the latissimus dorsi muscle is harvested from the back) with its artery and vein intact. Then, under an operating microscope, the artery and vein are anastomosed with extremely fine suture (8.0 or 9.0 nylon) to suitable blood vessels in the region. This muscle flap now is revascularized because it is connected to a regional blood vessel. Large studies show that microsurgical techniques have a 95% to 98% success rate.[42,43]

Appropriate flap selection requires attention not only to the needs of the recipient site but also to minimizing undesirable alterations at the donor site. When possible, donor sites are located in inconspicuous areas and leave little scarring to minimize undesirable appearance of the site. Preservation of function at the donor site is probably a more important consideration when selecting tissues (i.e., muscle, nerves, and blood vessels) for transfer. Preferably tissues selected for transfer should be expendable or cause minimal functional loss at the donor site.[44]

ADDITIONAL SOFT TISSUE REPAIR CONSIDERATIONS. Consideration always needs to be given to involvement of underlying structures when establishing a plan for soft tissue repair. For example, injury of the lacrimal apparatus may accompany inner eyelid lacerations, or parotid duct injury may be present beneath trauma to the cheek. These underlying structures may require surgical repair in addition to the surface laceration.

Thorough description of repairs and reconstruction done to remedy motor deficits remains beyond the scope of this chapter but is mentioned to increase awareness. Motor defects may be corrected by repairing, grafting, or transplanting nerves, tendons, and muscles. For example, cranial nerve VII (the facial nerve), which innervates all the muscles of facial expression, can be reconstructed by (1) nerve grafts from the contralateral uninjured facial nerve to the intact muscles or (2) transplanting muscles and nerves from the back (latissimus dorsi and thoracodorsal nerve) or thigh (gracilis muscle and obturator nerve branch). Motor defects in the upper extremity, where precision is of the utmost concern, can similarly be reconstructed by (1) nerve grafts (e.g., using the sural nerve, which supplies sensation to the lateral foot); (2) tendon transfers, whereby expendable muscles are rerouted and reconnected so that they assume functions of the critical muscles that have been irretrievably traumatized; or (3) muscle transplantation (free flaps) using muscle such as the gracilis.

Neural deficits may be corrected immediately if the wound is not contaminated and is not associated with a broad zone of injury. If the zone of injury is not clear, then watchful waiting to determine if injured tissues remain viable or not is the modus operandi. Once the extent of the neural deficit is determined, reconstruction can be performed with primary nerve repair or, if the gap is too large, by interpositional nerve grafts harvested from expendable nerves such as the antebrachial cutaneous nerve, which supplies sensation to the proximal forearm, or the sural nerve.

Especially in upper extremity reconstruction, but applicable elsewhere, it is important to make good use of "spare parts." In the case of an amputation, for example, bone, nerves, or blood vessels may be harvested from the nonsalvageable part to facilitate replant of another amputated part.

HEMATOMA MANAGEMENT
Whereas small hematomas should absorb spontaneously, large ones should be aspirated or incised and drained. The risks of reaccumulation are minimized with use of a soft compressive dressing. An organizing hematoma is not amenable to large-bore needle aspiration. Early reports indicate that a liposuction cannula can be used to successfully remove a hematoma.[45] Large hematomas left in situ have a risk of getting infected or causing pressure necrosis of surrounding tissues.

CRITICAL CARE PHASE
Management during the critical care phase focuses on promoting graft and flap survival; optimizing wound healing; and preventing, recognizing, and appropriately treating potential complications. Maintenance of airway patency, breathing, and circulation, which still may be threatened in this phase, continues to be critical not only for the survival of the patient but also to ensure sufficient supply of oxygen-rich blood to damaged soft tissues. Adequate perfusion and oxygen supply to wounded tissue is extremely important for healing and resistance to infection.[17,26] In addition to adequate tissue perfusion and oxygenation, sufficient nutrition, balance of fluid and electrolytes, and avoidance of infection are also important for wound healing.[17,22,26] Meticulous wound assessment and care are essential to achieve optimal outcomes from soft tissue injury.

TISSUE PERFUSION
Adequate tissue perfusion depends in large part on ample intravascular volume and sufficient blood pressure to drive blood into the tissues. Hypovolemia eventually causes hypotension, but initially the body compensates for decreased intravascular volume by shunting blood from the periphery to more vital organs to sustain adequate blood pressure. Therefore it is essential that adequate intravascular fluid volume be maintained to promote tissue perfusion.[26] The nurse should closely monitor the patient's hemodynamic parameters (e.g., heart rate, blood pressure, central venous pressure, pulmonary artery pressures) and tissue perfusion indicators (e.g., capillary refill time, urine output, mentation, lactate levels, acid-base balance, gastric intramu-

cosal pH) for evidence of hypovolemia or compromised tissue perfusion. Abnormal findings should be reported promptly to the physician so that appropriate therapy can be rendered to replete intravascular volume and improve blood flow to the tissues. Once adequate intravascular fluid volume is provided, vasoactive or inotropic agents may be considered to support the patient's blood pressure and improve oxygen delivery. Normal blood pressure in the setting of vasopressor use (e.g., epinephrine, norepinephrine) can also lead to peripheral vasoconstriction and reduced perfusion so that blood is shunted to the vital organs.[17] Patients with a flaps or skin grafts, where perfusion is dependent on the peripheral vasculature, are particularly intolerant of hypotension, hypovolemia, and vasopressor use because circulation to the flap or graft may be compromised. The plastic surgeon of record must be informed immediately if vasopressors are being used in a patient with flaps. Caution must also be taken when administering sedation, analgesics, diuretics, or other agents that may reduce blood pressure, which could be deleterious to flap survival and wound outcome.

Maintaining systemic normothermia and pain control remain important during the critical care phase to avoid vasoconstrive-induced tissue hypoxia.[17,26] Body temperature should be monitored frequently, and warming interventions should be employed if hypothermia becomes evident. Likewise, the presence of pain should be regularly evaluated and treated with prescribed analgesics to achieve patient comfort.

Anticoagulants are typically used to keep the vascular anastomosis patent in a free flap. Agents commonly prescribed by microsurgeons include aspirin, heparin, warfarin, or dextran. Because the microvascular anastomosis usually reendothelializes within 5 days, anticoagulants are used for 3 to 5 days to prevent occlusion. During this time the nurse should closely monitor coagulation studies to ensure appropriate levels, employ bleeding precautions, and frequently assess the flap site for evidence of inadequate perfusion.

TISSUE OXYGENATION

Maintaining peripheral perfusion with well-oxygenated blood optimizes oxygen delivery to the healing tissues. The patient's oxygenation status must be monitored closely with a device such as a pulse oximeter so that hypoxia can be readily detected and remedied. Supplemental oxygen is administered to increase the partial pressure of dissolved oxygen in the blood and thus deliver more oxygen to a healing wound. Data suggest that oxygen supplementation, even in a patient with normal arterial oxygen saturation at room air, is beneficial.[46] Adequate tissue oxygenation reduces wound infection, hastens collagen synthesis, and accelerates the rate of healing.[17,19,24,26,46]

If the pectoralis major muscle from the chest wall or the rectus abdominis from the abdomen is used for a flap, splinting during respiration as a result of pain on the side of the flap donor site may cause atelectasis. This complication can cause or exacerbate problems with the oxygenation status of the patient. It is essential that pain be controlled so

that the patient can fully participate in deep breathing exercises to prevent or resolve the atelectasis.

Regardless of the modality used for wound closure, hyperbaric oxygen may have a role in fostering healing of soft tissue injury. Hyperbaric oxygen may accelerate the clinical course of wound healing by increasing oxygen tension in wound beds, which prevents certain adverse inflammatory reactions, reduces tissue ischemia, protects from reperfusion injury, promotes neoangiogenesis and collagen production, and acts against infection.[47-51] Hyperbaric oxygenation acts against bacteria by inhibiting toxin formation of certain anaerobes, directly killing the anaerobic organisms and enhancing the activity of polymorphonuclear leukocytes to expedite bacterial clearance.[48,51,52]

WOUND CARE

Astute assessment of wounds at regularly scheduled intervals is essential to evaluate progression of healing and to detect onset of potential complications (e.g., infection, tissue necrosis). Size and depth of the wound should be measured and recorded at least daily. Wound appearance, including color, odor, approximation of closed wound edges, and drainage characteristics, are also noted. Specific assessment parameters evaluated with grafts and flaps must also be monitored meticulously (as described later in this chapter).

Abrasions, incision lines, and wounds should be cleaned as prescribed to remove exudate and nonviable tissue. Occasionally a thin layer of antibiotic ointment (e.g., bacitracin) is prescribed for application after wound or incision cleansing to help prevent infection.[53] Because most antibiotic ointments are irritative to the eyes, ophthalmic antibiotic ointments are generally ordered for patients with head and neck wounds so that if they enter into the eye, no harm is done. After cleansing, an incision may be left open to air or a prescribed wound dressing is applied. Numerous wound-dressing products are now available, and the wound characteristics should determine the best dressing for optimal wound healing.[54] An effective dressing should protect the wound and create an environment that promotes wound healing. It is desirable to have a dressing that maintains a moist but not macerated wound surface and allows surrounding tissues to remain dry.[8,54,55] Pain at the wound site is likely to increase during dressing changes and irrigations, necessitating administration of analgesics or sedatives before the procedure.

Factors that may compromise a skin graft include hematoma or seroma formation beneath the graft, shear factors, desiccation, and infection.[27,31] If a hematoma or seroma develops, it can raise the skin graft off the wound bed, thus cutting off its nutrient supply, which the skin graft obtains initially by diffusion. Nurses should remain vigilant for evidence of a fluid collection beneath the graft and, if present, should notify the physician immediately. A hematoma or seroma must be evacuated to allow the skin graft to "take." Shear forces can also disrupt the skin graft and prevent its initial adherence to the wound bed. Thus the patient's skin graft site must be immobilized appropriately and protected with a dressing or splint. It is important not to rub the graft site while repositioning or providing other care to the patient. It is also important to keep the grafted area elevated when possible to minimize edema at the site.[27] Because skin grafts may dry out, a dressing is applied with mineral oil, saline, or oxychlorosene sodium (Clorpactin). Many surgeons, particularly in burn units, recommend wet downs of the skin grafts. This involves pouring 30 ml of oxychlorosene onto the dressings placed over a skin graft. Oxychlorosene is a potent antimicrobial that protects the skin graft from bacterial degradation, in addition to preventing graft desiccation in the early phase. Early after placement, when a skin graft has not yet revascularized, it is susceptible to infection because it is essentially dead tissue and consequently a great medium for bacteria. Care must be taken to avoid contamination of the graft site and to monitor closely for evidence of infection during this period.

After 5 days, when the skin graft has "taken," it changes from pale to pink as capillary buds from the wound bed reach and join the dermal vascular architecture. Seven to ten days after grafting, the patient begins application of a topical antimicrobial lubricant, such as bacitracin, to the skin-grafted area to help prevent infection as the site continues to reepithelize through its small raw surfaces. Two weeks after grafting, the patient starts to apply regular skin emollients such as vitamin E oil or cocoa butter to keep the skin graft lubricated because it contains no functional sebaceous glands.[31]

Skin grafts require frequent assessment of color, which should be pink once the graft has taken[27,31] (Table 27-3). Next in order of importance during assessment, turgor of the site is evaluated. Evidence of excessive edema or bulging may indicate the presence of fluid collection beneath the graft. The graft should be warm to touch, and drainage from the site should appear unremarkable. Grafts should adhere to the wound. If a skin graft appears to be falling off the wound or if any other abnormal findings are evident, the physician should be notified immediately.

Condition of the skin graft donor site should also be assessed regularly to determine if healing is occurring or if

TABLE 27-3	**Plastic Surgery Skin Grafts and Flaps**		
	Skin Grafts	**Local Flaps/Rotational Flaps**	**Free Flaps**
Description	Transfer of full- or partial-thickness skin for wound coverage; requires an intact vascular bed	Transfer of local skin or muscle tissue, maintaining the native blood supply	Transfer of distant skin, muscle, or bone tissue with microscopic reconnection of the blood supply
Most Important Issues	Type of dressing to avoid graft displacement from wound bed and bacterial overgrowth	Checking flap viability via color, edema, turgor, and temperature	Checking flap viability via color, edema, turgor, and temperature
		Checking native blood supply via Doppler not usually required	Assessing Doppler arterial and venous signals (critical)
		Nothing compressing graft; dressing should be loose and moist	Nothing compressing graft; dressing should be loose and moist
Mobility with Leg Grafts*	POD 1-4: OOB to chair/wheelchair with leg up unless otherwise specified	POD 3-4: OOB to chair/wheelchair with leg up unless otherwise specified	POD 6: OOB to chair/wheelchair with leg up unless otherwise specified
	POD 5 (if interstices are epithelized): Dangle 5 minutes BID	POD 5-6 (if interstices are epithelized): Dangle 5 minutes BID	POD 6-7 (with interstices epithelized): Dangle 5 minutes BID
	POD 6 (if tolerated POD 5 dangling): Dangle once for 10 minutes	POD 6-7 (if tolerated 5 minute BID dangle): Dangle once for 10 minutes	Stop if there is excessive pain
			POD 7-8 (if tolerated 5 minute BID dangle): Dangle once for 10 minutes
	Continue to dangle leg once/day increasing dangle time 5 minutes/session as tolerated	Continue to dangle leg once/day increasing dangle time 5 minutes/session as tolerated	Continue to dangle leg once/day increasing dangle time 5 minutes/session as tolerated
Diet and Medication		No caffeine, nicotine, or vasoconstrictive drugs	No caffeine, nicotine, or vasoconstrictive drugs
		If dopamine, epinephrine, norepinephrine, or other vasoactive drugs are required, notify plastic surgeon	If dopamine, epinephrine, norepinephrine, or other vasoactive drugs are required, notify plastic surgeon

Modified from an unpublished table developed by Gena Stanek and Bradley Robertson.
POD, Postoperative day; *OOB,* Out of bed; *BID,* Twice a day.
*This is a sample protocol. Preferences for when and how to get the patient OOB or dangle the extremity with a graft or flap vary between institutions and among surgeons and should consider the individual patient needs.

Continued

any complications (e.g., infection) are present. Petroleum jelly gauze dressings applied to the split-thickness skin graft harvest site intraoperatively should be allowed to dry and spontaneously fall off the site. Another way to manage the donor site for a split-thickness skin graft is using a closed technique, whereby a semipermeable occlusive dressing (e.g., Opsite) is placed over the site. This technique decreases pain and provides a moist environment that shortens healing time.[31]

Flaps require greater and closer monitoring than skin grafts because they are vascularized viable tissues that bring their own blood supply. Local or rotational flaps should be

TABLE 27-3 **Plastic Surgery Skin Grafts and Flaps—cont'd**			
	Skin Grafts	**Local Flaps/Rotational Flaps**	**Free Flaps**
Room Temperature	To the patient's comfort	Avoid cold temperature	Avoid cold temperature
Standard Assessment Parameters	In order of importance: color (pink) edema/flap turgor temperature drainage	In order of importance: color (pink) edema/flap turgor temperature drainage flap "sweat" (open muscle should look moist) Doppler (not usually required)	In order of importance: color (pink) edema/flap turgor temperature drainage flap "sweat" (open muscle should look moist) Doppler—listen to both arterial and venous signals (nurse must know exact location to check signal)
Frequency of Checks (as Designated by Physician)	Every 8 to 12 hours.	Every 4 hour checks of above parameters	Every 30 minutes for first 4 hours Every hour from 4-24 hours Every 2-4 hours for next 24 hours
When to Call Physician with a Concern	Graft discoloration Fluid collection noted beneath graft Appearance of graft falling off the wound Any other abnormal change from baseline graft condition	Acute changes in vital signs, especially hypotension Any change from baseline flap condition Infection/sepsis	Acute changes in vital signs, especially hypotension Any change from baseline flap condition Infection/sepsis Difficulty obtaining Doppler signal Venous problems (swelling, purple color; classic reason for losing flap is the result of venous outflow problems at site of anastomosis) Arterial problems (graft shrinkage, pale color) (Flaps can be salvaged 40% of the time within the first 72 hours postop if insult identified and surgical intervention obtained within 2 hours)
Communication on Patient Transfer	RN to RN transfer should include status of skin graft and any special care	On patient transfer, attending/ fellow should review necessary monitoring parameters with RN and write specific orders addressing required parameters and frequency of monitoring RN to RN transfer should include the same specifics related to appropriate graft care	On patient transfer, attending/ fellow should review necessary monitoring parameters with RN and write specific orders addressing required parameters and frequency of monitoring RN to RN transfer should include the same specifics related to appropriate graft care

assessed every 4 hours to evaluate the flap color, pulse, edema, turgor, temperature, drainage, and moisture (see Table 27-3). The flap should appear pink and moist (flap sweat) and should have a palpable or audible pulse. Flap sweat is cellular exudate, which is absent in the presence of flap necrosis. There should be no excessive edema or atrophy of the flap, and drainage from the site should be unremarkable. Skin graft adherence to the flap is also noted because early nonadherence is a sensitive indicator of poor flap condition. Local flaps may become ischemic from arterial insufficiency or congested from venous insufficiency caused by postoperative edema or kinking of blood vessels that perfuse the flap. Hematoma formation beneath the flap may also compromise flap perfusion by compressing the vascular pedicle. The patency of the lower pressure venous circuit is particularly threatened. Any evidence of flap ischemia must be reported immediately to the physician. If such a complication develops, the patient may have to return to the operating room to evacuate any hematoma or to reposition the flap so that the vascular pedicle is unkinked or no longer under tension.

Free flaps require extremely close monitoring, particularly for onset of vascular thrombosis, the most common cause of flap failure (see Table 27-3). Early recognition and communication to the surgeon of symptoms pathognomonic of vascular thrombosis is important so that corrective interventions (e.g., operative flap revision) can be initiated to attempt salvage of the compromised flap.[42] If the reconstructed artery supplying perfusion to the flap clots off, the flap becomes pale, looses its turgor, and fails to make flap sweat. In addition to these symptoms, the flap becomes cool to the touch compared with normal body temperature. It takes on a limp appearance, and the overlying skin graft is no longer adherent. If the venous anastomosis clots off, venous blood backs up into the flap, creating venous congestion; the flap becomes swollen and takes on a deep blue hue. The exact locations to evaluate venous and arterial Doppler signals should be marked clearly or well communicated between care providers. Doppler signal monitoring has only a limited role in flap assessment. Loss of an arterial Doppler signal signifies arterial occlusion; however, the presence of a Doppler signal does not pacify the surgeon when the clinical appearance of the flap is not satisfactory.

Other techniques for monitoring the condition of free flaps are available and are regularly used in some institutions. Implantable Doppler probes and probes to monitor tissue oxygenation are available. Transcutaneous oxygen tension ($P_{TC}O_2$) monitoring can alert the nurse if perfusion is inadequate ($P_{TC}O_2$ below 20 mm Hg). A rapid decline in $P_{TC}O_2$ below 20 mm Hg that is unresponsive to increased supplemental oxygen suggests occlusion of the artery supplying the flap.[27] Measures of tissue pH also provide a reliable index of flap perfusion. A sustained decline in tissue pH signals vascular occlusion. An arterial occlusion causes a more rapid drop in tissue pH than venous occlusion.[27] Because ischemic muscle looses its contractility, evaluation of muscle contraction in response to applied electrical stimulation also provides information about muscle flap perfusion. Photophethsmography uses an infrared light to measure pulsatile changes in blood flow of the free flap. Pulse oximetry can effectively monitor oxygen saturation in digital free flaps. A decline in oxygen saturation below 85% suggests venous occlusion, and a loss of pulsatile flow indicates arterial obstruction.[27] Although these monitoring techniques may prove to be helpful adjuncts in evaluating flaps, there is agreement that physical assessment of the flap remains the best method for determining flap condition. Adverse clinical findings should never be ignored, even if adjunctive monitoring parameters are normal.

Manipulation and external compression of any flap must be avoided to prevent impairment of perfusion or injury to the tissue. When caring for a patient with a flap in the head and neck region, the nurse must ensure that tracheostomy ties are not secured too tight and that no face mask elastic band is placed around the neck. These bands can occlude the artery or vein that is perfusing the flap. Other intravenous lines, tubings, monitoring wires, cables, and bed linens also should be kept away from the flap site to prevent external compression. The patient needs to be reminded not to touch the flap. If the patient is uncooperative, restraints may be needed. Dressings should be kept moist and applied loosely to the flap site. Any drains placed around the flap should be emptied regularly to prevent excessive pressure beneath the flap.

Positioning a patient with a flap should be carried out with the intention of minimizing postoperative edema, promoting venous outflow, and avoiding interference with arterial supply. The extremity with a flap should be elevated to promote venous return as long as arterial flow is not impaired.[27] Patients with a flap in the head or neck region should have the head of the bed elevated to expedite venous drainage from the flap. The surgeon typically indicates how to position the flapped area (e.g., whether the patient's head is to be kept neutral, to the left side, or to the right side). It is important to position the patient as prescribed to avoid putting the vascular pedicle or anastomosed vessels under tension or kinking them. Splints may be used to help immobilize an area with a flap. When positioning the patient, care must be taken to prevent compression of the flap. Positioning restrictions should be posted clearly so that all health care providers caring for the patient can readily visualize them.

Early intervention with medicinal leeches may effectively reduce postoperative venous congestion that can impair flap perfusion and threaten flap survival.[56,57] Leeches applied directly to the flap consume blood until full and then detach spontaneously. Because leech saliva has anticoagulant properties, the bite wound continues to ooze blood even after the leech has detached, further reducing flap engorgement.[56,57]

In addition to preventing systemic hypothermia that might threaten flap perfusion, the flap itself should be protected from exposure to cold. The room should be kept warm, and cool air from an air-conditioning vent should not be directed onto the wound. Sometimes the surgeon prescribes an air-warming device to be placed loosely around the flap to encourage blood flow to the area.

PREVENTION OF INFECTION

Prevention of infection is paramount for successful wound healing and graft or flap survival.[21,22,40] Measures to prevent wound contamination, such as frequent hand washing and sterile dressing changes, must be used regularly by health care team members. Close assessment for evidence of local wound infection, as evidenced by erythema, purulent drainage, or malodor at the site, should be performed with each dressing change. Wound infection can also cause systemic symptoms, such as fever and increased white blood cell count, and should always be considered when performing a fever workup.

Antibiotics to treat contaminated wounds or identified wound infections should be administered as prescribed. Debridement of necrotic tissue remains important because antibiotics cannot perfuse nonviable tissue to effectively reduce or eliminate pathogens harbored there.[17,22] Abrasions may be treated with topical antimicrobials. Just as in burn management, bacitracin provides some antimicrobial coverage but not deep penetration into an eschar. Silver sulfadiazine (Silvadene) provides broader coverage and is more effective in managing a larger partial-thickness abrasive injury. Leukopenia is a potential side effect of silver sulfadiazine use, so blood counts should be monitored in patients receiving this drug. Mafenide acetate cream (Sulfamylon) provides even broader coverage and is particularly useful over cartilaginous injuries such as abrasions of the ear or nose.[58]

NUTRITION

Adequate nutrition is imperative for optimal healing of soft tissue injuries. Intake of adequate protein, carbohydrates, fats, vitamins, and minerals is essential.[17,26,59] Referred to Chapter 16 for a more in-depth review of metabolic and nutritional management. A registered dietitian can be consulted to determine the patient's individualized nutritional needs.

INTERMEDIATE AND REHABILITATION PHASES

Hospitalization may be prolonged for the patient with soft tissue injury because of associated injuries, onset of complications, or need for repeated surgical intervention to repair the injured site. During the intermediate and rehabilitation phases of trauma care, the focus continues to be on optimizing conditions for wound healing and prevention of complications that may impair the healing process. More intense focus on increasing the patient's independence and preparation for discharge occurs. In addition to the physical healing of the wound, the psychologic impact of the injury also requires care.

CONTINUED WOUND CARE

Wound healing may require a lengthy period of time, depending on the severity of the wound, the condition of the patient, and the presence or absence of factors that promote wound healing. Wound care should continue to be provided as prescribed. Measures that foster perfusion and oxygen delivery to the wound site and prevent infection remain imperative as healing continues.

Subatmospheric pressure, applied with a specialized sponge dressing that attaches to a vacuum-assisted closure (VAC) device (Kinetic Concepts Inc., San Antonio, Texas), may be used on open wounds to assist with wound healing and closure. This device removes interstitial fluid from the wound, which improves localized blood flow and decreases local inflammatory mediators that may inhibit granulation tissue formation. These improvements in the local wound environment increase the rate of granulation tissue formation and accelerate wound healing.[60-63] Exposure to negative pressure also encourages wound contracture.[61] Nurses working with this device need to ensure that the wound dressing remains occlusive to retain the vacuum effect and should know how to troubleshoot the system.

Caffeine, a vasoconstrictive agent, must be avoided in the diet of a patient with a flap. Smoking is forbidden outright because of its deleterious effect on wound healing and also because of the explosive hazards it presents if oxygen is in use. Even a nicotine patch, which is often applied to patients who smoke to prevent cravings, can be deleterious because it delivers nicotine, a powerful vasoconstrictive agent that compromises peripheral tissue perfusion.[17,27]

INCREASED MOBILITY AND SELF-CARE

Once the skin graft or flap of the lower extremity has taken, the leg needs to be dangled by a physical therapist (sample dangling protocol in Table 27-3). Procedures for how and when to mobilize the leg with a graft or flap can vary according to the physician or institution preference or patient-specific requirements. The surgeon specifies when the patient can get out of bed to a chair with the leg elevated. On the postoperative day prescribed the extremity can be dangled cautiously using the following procedure: A compressive dressing is applied to the lower extremity over the graft or flap, and the lower extremity is allowed to dangle off the side of the bed for 5 minutes. At 5 minutes the leg is elevated, the dressing is taken down, and the graft or flap is evaluated. The graft or flap site may take on a bluish hue as it develops venous congestion when dependent because its venous drainage system has not matured completely. Once the patient is returned to the recumbent position and the leg is elevated, the bluish hue resolves and the pinkish vascular color returns. Dangling an extremity with a graft or flap acclimates the graft to its new position and to its relative venous insufficiency. A graft or flap that becomes venous congested from dangling for too long may necrose, just as a venous stasis ulcer necroses in patients with insufficiency in their native tissue. Once the graft or flap is able to tolerate longer periods of dependent positioning, the length of time the leg can dangle can be increased as prescribed by the plastic surgeon.

Wounds, grafts, and flaps may restrict movement during the healing phase. A physical therapist should be consulted to assist the patient in movement after activity is permitted by the plastic surgeon. Prescribed range-of-motion exercises as tolerated by the patient can be initiated. Range-of-motion exercises are particularly beneficial when a wound, graft, or flap extends over a joint. The condition of the wound should be monitored closely as movement is increased to detect any adverse effects on the healing process. An occupational therapist can help to establish alternative means of accomplishing activities of daily living while the soft tissue is healing and grafts and flaps are immobilized.

ALTERED BODY IMAGE

After a soft tissue injury has healed, patients literally carry battle scars. In the past a scar was worn proudly as a symbol of chivalry, heraldry, or bravery. In modern society an obvious scar may be perceived as a symbol of a criminal or violent past. This can lead to stereotyping, resulting in fewer employment opportunities, and social outcasting. Although patients' reactions to soft tissue injury vary, soft tissue wounds can significantly affect self-esteem, role performance, and interpersonal relationships. Individuals often respond to such alterations in body image by grieving, and some experience depression.[64]

Nurses need to be sensitive to the patient's psychologic responses to injury and should implement strategies that assist patients in dealing with their altered body image. Patients should be encouraged to ask questions and ventilate feelings about their injury. They should be allowed to visualize their wound as desired.[27] Nurses should demonstrate an accepting and positive attitude when caring for the wound, taking care not to send negative nonverbal messages.[64] Choices about personal care (e.g., when to get out of bed or bathe) should be offered when possible to increase the patient's sense of control. Reinforcing the patient's positive attributes and accomplishments can help foster self-worth. Consultation with a crisis counselor or psychiatric liaison may assist the patient and family in coping with the injury and altered body image. Refer to Chapter 18 for more in-depth content on the psychologic aspects of trauma care.

Sudden changes in body image can cause anxiety, which may trigger use of defense mechanisms such as denial, withdrawal, repression, suppression, avoidance, and regression.[64] Desire for isolation from others and refusal of treatment for the wound may become evident. Discussion about feelings that foster these behaviors should be encouraged. Prescribed analgesics and anxiolytics should be provided as needed during dressing changes. Only desired visitors should be allowed to see the patient, and no one should force the patient into unwanted social interactions. A supportive significant other may prove helpful in reducing anxiety and apprehension about the wound and socialization.

REINTEGRATION INTO THE COMMUNITY

Ultimately the goal is to reintegrate the traumatized patient back into society. Wound healing usually continues for some time after the patient's hospital discharge, necessitating continued care of the wound and of the psychologic aspects of the injury while at home. Clear, comprehensive patient and family education and assurance of adequate home health resources foster successful reintegration back into society after soft tissue injury.

PATIENT AND FAMILY EDUCATION

Patients and their families should be kept apprised by the surgeon of the anticipated course for wound healing and likely outcomes. This information can be reiterated and reinforced by the nursing staff. The patient should be encouraged to ask questions and solicit information. The Internet is a new medium for gaining information and also misinformation. Patients and families should be directed to a reputable site for information on wound care, such as the American Society of Plastic Surgeons web site (www.plasticsurgery.org). This learning process is also important for concerned family members who must make decisions in proxy for a disabled patient. Gaining knowledge and information can be empowering and helps decrease fears of uncertainty.

Care of the wound should be demonstrated for the patient and family. Then the individual who will be performing the wound care after discharge should demonstrate the procedure to validate accurate learning. Patients and family members should be instructed to wash their hands frequently and avoid touching the wound. For several months after reepithelialization the skin graft harvest site requires twice-daily external lubrication with emollients such as vitamin E oil or cocoa butter because the sebaceous glands have been transected and fail to provide normal lubrication to the skin. In some patients, because of the depth of harvest, sebaceous glands may never regain function.

Patients should also be instructed to avoid exposure of wounds, incisions, grafts, and flaps to direct sunlight and ultraviolet rays. The wound may develop hyperpigmentation if exposed to the sun.[31] If sunlight exposure is anticipated, the wound should be covered or strong sunscreen should be applied.

Measures for fostering graft and flap survival that were initiated in the hospital setting must be taught to the patient and family so that they are continued after hospital discharge. The interventions include avoiding caffeine in the diet, not smoking, preventing compression or manipulation of the graft or flap site, restricting movement or positioning as prescribed, elevating the affected area, and avoiding extreme cold. The patient should practice the range-of-motion exercises prescribed by the surgeon with the physical therapy staff before discharge. The importance of maintaining a healthy diet to foster wound healing should also be emphasized.

Patients and families also require education on potential wound healing complications and their symptoms, such as wound infection or impaired wound healing. Symptoms of graft or flap failure must also be well described to patients. Other long-term wound healing complications, described later in this chapter, should also be discussed with the patient and their family. The patient and family need to have a clear understanding of what actions should be taken if complications become evident.

Adaptation and psychologic adjustment to soft tissue injury and its subsequent scarring may take several weeks to months. Patients and families should be informed that depression, altered mood, increased anxiety, and nightmares or flashbacks about the injury event are common reactions to traumatic injury.[64] Referral to a counselor or therapy group may be suggested if these symptoms become evident or problematic.

HOME HEALTH CARE RESOURCES

Home health care resources may be necessary if extensive dressing changes are required, intravenous antibiotics are continued, or the condition of a graft or flap requires follow-up evaluation. The home health nurse can assist with the dressing changes or at least confirm that the patient or family member is performing them correctly. The nurse should ensure that sufficient supplies and necessary home health resources are available before discharge from the hospital.

POTENTIAL FOR LONG-TERM WOUND HEALING COMPLICATIONS

SCARS AND KELOIDS. Not all wounds heal optimally. There are many factors that can interfere with one or more of the three wound healing phases, resulting in excessive scarring[6] (Table 27-4). For example, wounds that have been abraded or healed with minor degrees of infection in the patient with a propensity toward abnormal wound healing may develop hypertrophic scars or keloids. A hypertrophic scar is excessive or exuberant and appears indurated and raised from the wound edges but remains within the boundaries of the original injury. It represents an abnormal amount of collagen deposition.[17] Keloids, on the other hand, exceed the bounds of the original injury.[65,66] Risk of keloid formation is higher in African-Americans and Asians and lowest among Caucasians. Individuals who develop keloids are believed to have genetically abnormal wound healing.[6] Microscopically keloids also have an abnormal amount of disorganized collagen.[6,66] Pathologically there is

little difference between the two entities, and only a clinical distinction is made.

Hypertrophic and keloid scars are managed similarly. Initial early management includes the application of compression stockings. Silicone gel contact sheeting is also recommended.[6,65-67] Silicone gel sheeting reduces scar formation by an unclear mechanism. It has been hypothesized that gel sheeting may exert a beneficial effect by increasing skin temperature, moisturizing the scar, occluding the involved area, increasing pressure, or creating a small electrical current by friction contact across the immature scar.[6,66,68] At approximately 3 months, if evidence of hypertrophic scarring or keloid is present, steroid injections, typically of triamcinolone acetonide (Kenalog), may be administered. Steroid injections are not without complications. They may cause hypopigmentation of the surrounding wound and even of the normal skin, the development of telangiectasis, and weakening of the wound.[66] Scars that remain unsuitable at 1 year may be considered for surgical revision. However, before undertaking revision of a scar, it must be determined what is to be done differently this time as opposed to the initial repair. If the cause of the initial dissatisfactory scar is related to contusion or contamination, for example, then a new surgical wound may achieve the desired results. If the dissatisfactory scar is felt to arise as a result of the patient's biology, then scar revision will not achieve a satisfactory result and recurrence of excessive scarring is likely.[6] When surgery is combined with other therapies, such as intradermal corticosteroids, compression treatment, or radiation, results may be improved and the likelihood of recurrence is reduced.[6,69]

Certain lasers (e.g., Er:YAG or CO_2) have been shown beneficial for resurfacing posttraumatic scars.[65,70] The mechanism of action for laser surfacing is to produce a photothermal injury to the dermis, which enhances new collagen production, remodeling, and reepithelization.

Contractures occur when scars shrink and restrict mobility or cause cosmetic deformity. Initially pressure dressings, range-of-motion exercises, braces, and serial casting or splinting are used to prevent and treat contractures.[17,66] Established contractures that resist stretching or that recur may require surgical intervention.[17] Z-plasty may be entertained to release a linear contracture (Figure 27-12). Simi-

TABLE 27-4 Factors That Predispose to Excessive Scarring in Each Phase of Wound Healing

Inflammatory Phase	Transitional Repair Phase	Remodeling Phase
• Hematoma or foreign body	• Physical or chemical irritants	• Mechanical tension
• Infection or allergic reactions	• Infection or allergic reactions	• Anatomic location
• Repetitive trauma (e.g., scratching)	• Genetic factors	
• Edema	• Adolescence	
• Chronic open wound	• Pregnancy	
• Poorly aligned wound edges	• Endocrine disorders	
• Deep partial-thickness burn wound	• Neurofibromatosis	
• Crush injury		

Modified from Su CW, Alizadeh K, Boddie A et al: The problem scar, *Clin Plast Surg* 25:453, 1998.

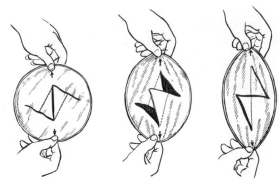

FIGURE 27-12. Z-plasty. (From McCarthy JG: Introduction to plastic surgery. In McCarthy JG editor: *Plastic surgery,* vol 1, *General principles,* Philadelphia, 1990, WB Saunders, 56.)

larly a double opposing z-plasty,[71] running z-plasty, or w-plasty may be required across linear contractures.[65] Larger contractures may require full-thickness skin grafting.

Trauma patients often require multiple procedures to achieve satisfactory scar revision. What may be satisfactory at one point in the patient's life may become dissatisfactory later on. Camouflage and makeup techniques can make wounds essentially imperceptible and scars entirely acceptable. For larger defects, such as an ear or nose defect, a bioprosthesis may be indicated.

TRAUMATIC TATTOOING.   Traumatic tattooing from foreign debris (e.g., gravel, metallic substances) embedded into the skin can also present an aesthetic challenge. Because pigments are buried in the deep dermis, they are visible and typically not amenable to dermabrasion (skin sanding). Tattooing can be minimized by meticulous debridement of the wound at initial presentation. However, absent that, these deformities may be managed with laser resurfacing.[4,72] Lasers with various frequencies, each suitable to a particular pigment, are available. For example, yellow-light lasers may be employed for red-pigmented tattoos. Some caution must be exercised when using lasers because red tattoos containing iron may be turned black by oxidation and thereby worsened. Similarly, titanium-containing tattoos turn from white to black by laser oxidation. Results of laser therapy to repair traumatic tattooing remain somewhat unpredictable.

SUMMARY

Optimizing outcomes from soft tissue injuries provides numerous opportunities for research. Further investigation into which interventions and techniques optimize wound healing and prevent infectious and long-term healing complications is necessary. How to best deal with the psychologic aspect of these injuries also requires further study. Additional research exploring the efficacy of alternative skin replacements and determining the usefulness of emerging technologies such as lasers and microdermabrasion is also under way.

Nurses work in collaboration with other health care team members to create and implement a plan of care that allows optimal outcomes to be achieved. Nurses caring for trauma patients must be knowledgeable about soft tissue trauma and the techniques used to repair and reconstruct these injuries. Astute nursing assessment and meticulous care of soft tissue injuries can have a tremendous impact on the outcome of graft or flap survival and wound healing.

REFERENCES

1. Johnson TM, Nelson BR: Anatomy of the skin. In Baker SR, Swanson NA, editors: *Local flaps in facial reconstruction,* St. Louis, 1995, Mosby, 3-14.
2. Stotts NA: Integumentary clinical physiology. In Kinney MR, Dunbar SB, Brooks-Brunn JA et al, editors: *AACN's clinical reference for critical care nursing,* ed 4, St. Louis, 1998, Mosby, 1055-1059.
3. Sunderland S: The anatomy and physiology of nerve injury, *Muscle Nerve* 13:771-784, 1990.
4. Troilius AM: Effective treatment of traumatic tattoos with a Q-switched Nd: YAG laser, *Lasers Surg Med* 22:103-108, 1998.
5. Lee RH, Gamble WB, Mayer MH et al: Patterns of facial laceration from blunt trauma, *Plast Reconstr Surg* 99: 1544-1554, 1997.
6. Su CW, Alizadeh K, Boddie A et al: The problem scar, *Clin Plast Surg* 25:451-465, 1998.
7. Cook TA, Brownlee RE: Rotation flaps. In Baker SR, Swanson NA, editors: *Local flaps in facial reconstruction,* St. Louis, 1995, Mosby, 75-90.
8. Stewart RM, Page CP: Wounds, bites, and stings. In Mattox KL, Feliciano DV, Moore EE, editors: *Trauma,* New York, 2000, McGraw-Hill, 1115-1135.
9. Wolff K-D: Management of animal bite injuries of the face: experience with 94 patients, *J Oral Maxillofac Surg* 56:838-843, 1998.
10. Robson MC, Duke WF, Krizek TJ: Rapid bacterial screening in the treatment of civilian wounds, *J Surg Res* 14:426-430, 1973.
11. Hoover TJ, Siefert JA: Soft tissue complications of orthopedic emergencies, *Emerg Med Clin North Am* 18:115-139, 2000.
12. American College of Surgeons' Committee on Trauma: *Advanced trauma life support for doctors student course manual,* ed 6, Chicago, 1997, American College of Surgeons.
13. Modrall JG, Weaver FA, Yellin AE: Diagnosis and management of penetrating vascular trauma and the injured extremity, *Emerg Med Clin North Am* 16:129-144, 1998.
14. Swain R, Ross D: Lower extremity compartment syndrome: when to suspect acute or chronic pressure buildup, *Postgrad Med* 105:159-168, 1999.
15. Chisholm CD, Wood CO, Chua G et al: Radiographic detection of gravel in soft tissue, *Ann Emerg Med* 29:725-730, 1997.
16. Manthey DE, Storrow AB, Milbourn JM et al: Ultrasound versus radiography in the detection of soft-tissue foreign bodies, *Ann Emerg Med* 28:7-9, 1996.
17. Hunt TK, Hopf HW: Wound healing and wound infection: what surgeons and anesthesiologists can do, *Surg Clin North Am* 77:587-606, 1997.
18. Kurz A, Sessler DI, Lenhardt R: Perioperative normothermia to reduce the incidence of surgical-wound infection and shorten hospitalization, *N Engl J Med* 334:1209-1215, 1996.
19. Hopf HW, Hunt TK, West JM et al: Wound tissue oxygen tension predicts the risk of wound infection in surgical patients, *Arch Surg* 132:997-1004, 1997.

20. Kirkpatrick AW, Chun R, Brown R et al: Hypothermia and the trauma patient, *Can J Surg* 42:333-343, 1999.

21. Ramasastry SS: Chronic problem wounds, *Clin Plast Surg* 25:367-396, 1998.

22. Robson MC: Wound infection: a failure of wound healing caused by an imbalance of bacteria, *Surg Clin North Am* 77:637-650, 1997.

23. Masem M, Greenberg BM, Hoffman C et al: Comparative bacterial clearances of muscle and skin/subcutaneous tissues with and without dead bone: a laboratory study, *Plast Reconstr Surg* 85:773-781, 1990.

24. Knighton DR, Halliday B, Hunt TK: Oxygen as an antibiotic: a comparison of the effects of inspired oxygen concentration and antibiotic administration on in vivo clearance, *Arch Surg* 121:191-195, 1986.

25. Rabinowitz RP, Caplan ES: Management of infections in the trauma patient, *Surg Clin North Am* 79:1373-1383, 1999.

26. Whitney JD, Heitkemper MM: Modifying perfusion, nutrition, and stress to promote wound healing in patients with acute wounds, *Heart Lung* 28:123-133, 1999.

27. Black JM: Surgical options in wound healing, *Crit Care Nurs Clin North Am* 8:169-182, 1996.

28. Stotts NA: Promoting wound healing. In Kinney MR, Dunbar SB, Brooks-Brunn JA et al, editors: *AACN's clinical reference for critical care nursing*, ed 4, St. Louis, 1998, Mosby, 237-245.

29. Caruso DM, King TJ, Tsujimura RB et al: Primary closure of fasciotomy incisions with a skin-stretching device in patients with burn and trauma, *J Burn Care Rehabil* 18:125-132, 1997.

30. Hirshowitz B, Lindenbaum E, Har-Shai Y: A skin-stretching device for the harnessing of the viscoelastic properties of skin, *Plast Reconstr Surg* 92:260-270, 1993.

31. Ratner D: Skin grafting: from here to there, *Dermatol Clin* 16:75-90, 1998.

32. Converse JM, Smahel J, Ballantyne DL et al: Inosculation of vessels of skin graft and host bed: a fortuitous encounter, *Br J Plast Surg* 28:274-282, 1975.

33. Argenta LC: Controlled tissue expansion in facial reconstruction. In Baker SR, Swanson NA, editors: *Local flaps in facial reconstruction*, St. Louis, 1995, Mosby, 517-544.

34. Hansbrough JF, Franco ES: Skin replacements, *Clin Plast Surg* 25:407-423, 1998.

35. Spence RJ, Wong L: The enhancement of wound healing with human skin allograft, *Surg Clin North Am* 77:731-745, 1997.

36. Winfrey ME, Cochran M, Hegarty MT: A new technology in burn therapy: Integra artificial skin, *Dimens Crit Care Nurs* 18:14-20, 1999.

37. Choucair MM, Phillips T: What is new in clinical research in wound healing, *Dermatol Clin* 15:45-58, 1997.

38. Gosain A, Chang N, Mathes S et al: A study of the relationship between blood flow and bacterial inoculation in musculocutaneous and fasciocutaneous flaps, *Plast Reconstr Surg* 86:1152-1162, 1990.

39. Calderon W, Chang N, Mathes SJ: Comparison of the effect of bacterial inoculation in musculocutaneous and fasciocutaneous flaps, *Plast Reconstr Surg* 77:785-794, 1986.

40. Murphy RC, Robson MC, Heggers JP et al: The effect of microbial contamination on musculocutaneous and random flaps, *J Surg Res* 41:75-80, 1986.

41. Heniford BW, Bailin PL, Marsico RE: Field guide to local flaps, *Dermatol Clin* 16:65-74, 1998.

42. Khouri RK, Cooley BC, Kunselman AR et al: A prospective study of microvascular free-flap surgery and outcome, *Plast Reconstr Surg* 102:711-721, 1998.

43. O'Brien CJ, Lee KK, Stern HS et al: Evaluation of 250 free-flap reconstructions after resection of tumors of the head and neck, *Aust N Z J Surg* 68:698-701, 1998.

44. Hallock GG: "Microleaps" in the progression of flaps and grafts, *Clin Plast Surg* 23:117-138, 1996.

45. Ascari-Raccagni A, Baldari U: Liposuction surgery for the treatment of large hematomas on the leg, *Dermatol Surg* 26:263-264, 2000.

46. Grief R, Akca O, Horn E-P et al: Supplemental oxygen to reduce the incidence of surgical-wound infection, *N Engl J Med* 342:161-167, 2000.

47. Fulton JE: The use of hyperbaric oxygen (HBO) to accelerate wound healing, *Dermatol Surg* 26:1170-1172, 2000.

48. Clark LA, Moon RE: Hyperbaric oxygen in the treatment of life-threatening soft-tissue infections, *Respir Care Clin N Am* 5:203-219, 1999.

49. Zhang F, Cheng C, Gerlach T et al: Effect of hyperbaric oxygen on survival of the composite ear graft in rats, *Ann Plast Surg* 41:530-534, 1998.

50. Niezgoda JA, Cianci P, Folden BW et al: The effect of hyperbaric oxygen therapy on a burn wound model in human volunteers, *Plast Reconstr Surg* 99:1620-1625, 1997.

51. Bouachour G, Cronier P, Gouello JP et al: Hyperbaric oxygen therapy in the management of crush injuries: a randomized double-blind placebo-controlled clinical trial, *J Trauma* 41:333-339, 1996.

52. Jain KK: *Textbook of hyberbaric medicine*, ed 3, Seattle, 1999, Hogrefe & Huber, 189-210.

53. Kaye ET: Topical antibacterial agents, *Infect Dis Clin North Am* 14:321-339, 2000.

54. Ladin DA: Understanding dressings, *Clin Plast Surg* 25:433-441, 1998.

55. Winter GD: Formation of the scab and the rate of epithelization of superficial wounds in the skin of the young domestic pig, *Nature* 193:293-294, 1962.

56. Mortenson BW, Dawson KH, Murakami C: Medicinal leeches used to salvage a traumatic nasal flap, *Br J Oral Maxillofac Surg* 36:462-464, 1998.

57. Utley DS, Koch RJ, Goode RL: The failing flap in facial plastic and reconstructive surgery: Role of the medicinal leech, *Laryngoscope* 108:1129-1135, 1998.

58. Greenfield E: Integumentary disorders. In Kinney MR, Dunbar SB, Brooks-Brunn JA et al, editors: *AACN's clinical reference for critical care nursing*, ed 4, St. Louis, 1998, Mosby, 1065-1087.

59. Flanigan KH: Nutritional aspects of wound healing, *Adv Wound Care* 10:48-52, 1997.

60. Fabian TS, Kaufman HJ, Lett ED et al: The evaluation of subatmospheric pressure and hyperbaric oxygen in ischemic full-thickness wound healing, *Am Surg* 66:1136-1143, 2000.

61. Mooney JF, Argenta LC, Marks MW et al: Treatment of soft tissue defects in pediatric patients using the V.A.C.™ system, *Clin Orthop Rel Res* 376:26-31, 2000.

62. Argenta LC, Morykwas MJ: Vacuum-assisted closure: a new method for wound control and treatment: clinical experience, *Ann Plast Surg* 38:563-576, 1997.

63. Morykwas MJ, Argenta LC, Shelton-Brown EI et al: Vacuum-assisted closure: a new method for wound control and treatment: animal studies and basic foundation, *Ann Plast Surg* 38:553-562, 1997.

64. Magnan MA: Psychological considerations for patients with acute wounds, *Crit Care Nurs Clin North Am* 8:183-193, 1996.

65. McGillis ST, Lucas AR: Scar revision: the cellular and molecular basis for therapy, *Dermatol Clin* 16:165-180, 1998.

66. Tredget EE, Nedelec B, Scott PG et al: Hypertrophic scars, keloids, and contractures The cellular and molecular basis for therapy, *Surg Clin North Am* 77:701-729, 1997.

67. Berman B, Flores F: Comparison of a silicone gel-filled cushion and silicon gel sheeting for the treatment of hypertrophic or keloid scars, *Dermatol Surg* 25:484-486, 1999.

68. Hirshowitz B, Lindenbaum E, Har-shai Y et al: Static-electric field induction by a silicone cushion for the treatment of hypertrophic and keloid scars, *Plast Reconstr Surg* 101:1173-1183, 1998.

69. Berman B, Bieley HC: Adjunct therapies to surgical management of keloids, *Dermatol Surg* 22:126-130, 1996.

70. Jacobson D, Bass LS, VanderKam V et al: Carbon dioxide and ER:YAG laser resurfacing, *Clin Plast Surg* 27:241-250, 2000.

71. Gahhos FN, Cuono CB: Double-Z rhombic technique for reconstruction of facial wounds, *Plast Reconstr Surg* 85:869-873, 1990.

72. Chang S-E, Choi J-H, Moon K-C et al: Successful removal of traumatic tattoos in Asian skin with a Q-switched Alexandrite laser, *Dermatol Surg* 24:1308-1311, 1998.

UNIQUE PATIENT POPULATIONS

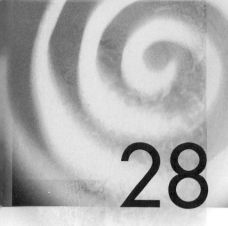

THE PREGNANT TRAUMA PATIENT

Lynn Gerber Smith

The pregnant trauma patient presents a double challenge: two lives must be treated concurrently. When the trauma patient is pregnant, response to shock is different and unique injuries, life-threatening to both the mother and the fetus, can occur. While caring for the pregnant trauma patient from resuscitation through rehabilitation, the nurse must assess the patient, interpret the assessment findings, and make decisions pertinent to the patient's care. The nurse is the integral link between the many specialists consulting with the pregnant trauma patient. Therefore, it is essential for the nurse to develop a firm knowledge base and proficient assessment skills regarding the needs of this unique patient population so that sound decisions can be made to enhance the care of both mother and child.

EPIDEMIOLOGY

The national birth rate increased from 1985 to 1993 and remained stable during the last half of the 1990s.[1] Considering the large number of pregnant women in our society, it has been estimated that 7% of active pregnant women will suffer some type of unintentional injury during their pregnancy.[2] The most common causes of traumatic injuries for the pregnant population include motor vehicle crashes, battering or spouse abuse, falls, firearm injuries, and burns.[3] National statistics on the specific incidence of trauma during pregnancy are not known.[4] Early studies identified the number of pregnant patients treated at specific trauma centers and emergency departments and their mechanisms of injury. At one major trauma center, 79 injured patients admitted over a 9-year period were pregnant. This total represents less than 1% of total acute admissions, 1.7% of all female admissions, and 2.6% of women of childbearing age (14 to 45 years) admitted.[5] In this study, blunt mechanisms of injury had been incurred by 96% of the study population and penetrating mechanisms had injured 4%.

Timberlake and McSwain report that, over a 10-year period at Charity Hospital of Louisiana at New Orleans, 28 patients were diagnosed as pregnant and incurred a traumatic injury.[6] Of the 25 patients studied, 68% were found to have a blunt mechanism of injury and 32% a penetrating mechanism of injury.[6]

During a 5-year period in another center, 318 pregnant women were identified as suffering traumatic injury. Twenty-five of these patients had injuries that warranted admission to the trauma service, and they represented 0.3% of the general trauma admissions.[7] Within the subset of 25 pregnant women, 16 (64%) sustained blunt trauma secondary to a motor vehicle crash, 4 (16%) sustained burns, and 2 (8%) had been assaulted. One had an abdominal stab wound, one sustained a gunshot wound, and one had fallen.

Finally, in a multicenter study with a combined trauma registry base of 30,000 patients, 73 pregnant women were admitted to four level I trauma centers in Pennsylvania. The most common mechanism of injury was blunt trauma (76.7%), followed by falls (15.1%), penetrating trauma (6.8%), and burns (1.4%).[8]

More recent studies have attempted to characterize patterns of injury and risk factors to predict fetal mortality. A 1992 study of 114 injured pregnant patients found that motor vehicle crashes accounted for 70% of the injuries (46% had not used seat belts or helmets) and violence accounted for 12%.[8] Violent assault was the second most common injury mechanism. Fetal loss was higher in patients with higher Injury Severity Score (ISS), evidence of shock state, and abdominal injuries.[9]

A 5-year Canadian study also looked at factors identified with high fetal mortality in patients with an ISS of more than 12. The most common mechanism of injury was motor vehicle crash. Fetal death was correlated with maternal ISS, maternal hemoglobin level, and number of blood transfusions plus presence of disseminated intravascular coagulation (DIC).[10]

Motor vehicle crashes are the leading cause of death for women ages 14 to 44, which are generally considered the childbearing years.[11] There are nearly 10 times more fatalities from motor vehicle crashes than from any other mechanism of injury during the reproductive years.[12] This is clearly supported in numerous multicenter studies that reviewed trauma during pregnancy and found that motor vehicle crashes continue to be the most significant mechanism.[4-9] In years past, pregnant women secluded themselves, traveling less often, but pregnant women of today continue to drive and ride in vehicles until the time of delivery, and many of them do not use protective restraints properly or at all.

Physical abuse, or interpersonal violence, is a common source of blunt trauma during pregnancy. Parker et al found that 20.6% of pregnant teenagers and 14.2% of pregnant adults were physically abused during pregnancy.[13] Gazma-rarian et al reviewed 13 studies on violence against pregnant women in an attempt to summarize the findings. Their review indicates that the reported prevalence of violence during pregnancy ranges from 0.9% to 20.1%.[14] Physical abuse during pregnancy has been associated with low fetal birth weights, low maternal weight gain, maternal infections, anemia, and maternal alcohol and drug abuse. Women who claim to have fallen but whose injuries do not seem to match the described event may have been victims of assault. They must be interviewed in private, with assurances of nondisclosure, to investigate the possibility of abuse.

For anatomic and physiologic reasons, falls are more common during pregnancy. During the first trimester the woman is more easily fatigued and prone to fainting. As the pregnancy progresses, the uterus extends beyond the pelvic confines and may alter the mother's gait and balance, thus increasing the potential for falls. Relaxation of the pelvic girdle ligaments causes pelvic tilt and increases lordosis, and a change in balance occurs. Falls can occur while going down stairs, when walking on ice, and when performing even simple tasks such as putting on boots. During late pregnancy the woman may desire to redecorate for the new baby (nesting syndrome) and is likely to climb on a ladder or a chair, further placing herself at risk.

Penetrating injuries secondary to ballistic trauma and stab wounds also occur during pregnancy. Historically firearms have been second only to motor vehicle crashes as a cause of fatal injury. A study from the Cook County Medical Examiner found that of the 44 maternal deaths resulting from trauma between 1986 and 1989, 22% were from gunshot wounds and 13.6% were from stab wounds.[3] It has been suggested that penetrating trauma is more common in the urban environment; however, it is a problem faced in every emergency department.[15] The pregnant abdomen may be the target of penetrating trauma when angry behaviors are displayed or when attempts to abort the fetus are made. Domestic violence does occur in an estimated 20% of pregnancies; the pregnancy may actually be the precipitating factor for such action.[13]

Pregnant women also can receive burn and inhalation injuries although these types of injuries occur less frequently than those previously mentioned. Traumatic injuries that result from the aforementioned etiologies account for the leading nonobstetric causes of death in pregnant women.

NURSING DATABASE

All female trauma patients of childbearing age should be considered pregnant until proven otherwise. Sherer and Schenker[16] suggest that it is difficult to determine the actual incidence of trauma during pregnancy because of lack of questioning and documentation. They cite two clinical examples in which this information may not be recorded: the mild traumatic event that is poorly documented in the medical record and the life-threatening situation in which pregnancy may not be considered. Therefore, it is of utmost importance that an accurate database and patient health history be obtained as soon as possible. This information not only helps to establish a pregnant condition but can often provide information that aids in both the diagnosis and management of traumatic injuries during pregnancy. Therefore, an obstetric history, starting with questions about pregnancy, should be initiated immediately. If the patient is unconscious and the family is not available to answer questions, a pregnancy test should be performed. A description of the events preceding an injury and, whenever possible, of the actual event itself is important to obtain, particularly when the trauma patient is pregnant. When a pregnant woman sustains a traumatic injury, obstetric complications such as eclampsia must be ruled out as a precipitator. If loss of consciousness, headache, back pain, or abdominal pain precedes an incident, an underlying obstetric problem that precipitated the event should be suspected. Information concerning the actual event can help the nurse to relate the mechanism of injury to possible injuries and must be included as part of the nursing database.

MECHANISM OF INJURY

MOTOR VEHICLE CRASH.   The information important to obtain following a pregnant woman's involvement in a motor vehicle crash includes whether she was a driver or passenger in the vehicle, whether she was wearing a seat belt and shoulder harness, and whether the air bag deployed. The dynamics of the crash are significant (see Chapter 11) and should be considered in anticipating maternal and fetal injuries. If the woman was the driver of the vehicle, then the protuberant abdomen may have been injured by the steering column, particularly if safety restraints were not used. Proper use of seat belts may decrease the severity of maternal injuries and increase maternal survival[17] (Figure 28-1). Seat belts prevent ejection from the vehicle, decrease the likelihood of severe head injury, and in general lower mortality. Because the overall leading cause of fetal death is maternal death after motor vehicle crashes, seat belts also increase the chance of fetal survival.[18]

When prehospital care providers have information about the events that precipitated a crash or its severity, this information should be conveyed to the health care providers at the receiving facility. One study examined the relationship between type of collision and resultant maternal injuries in 441 pregnant women who were involved in motor vehicle crashes.[19] When there was minor damage to the vehicle, less than 1% of the women were injured. When the damage to the vehicle was severe, more serious injuries were found, as expected. Seven percent of those who were involved in severe crashes died and 12.9% suffered injury. More recent studies have focused on maternal factors as predic-

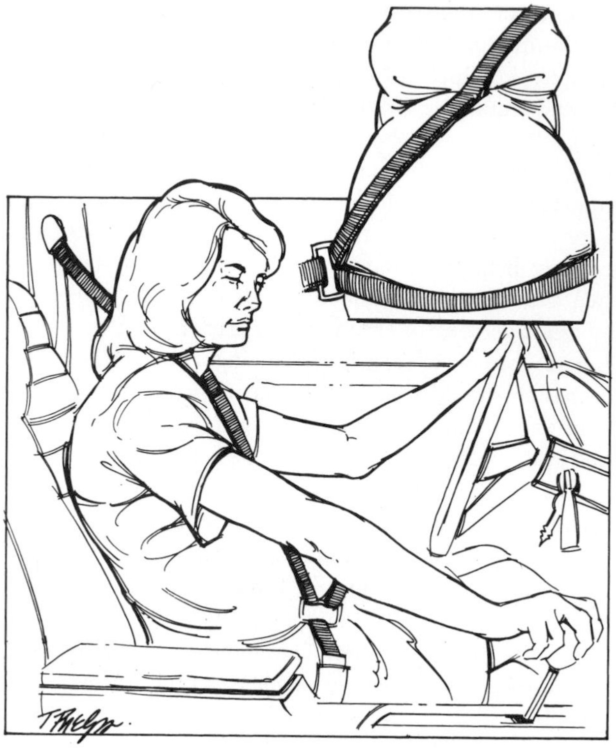

FIGURE 28-1 **Proper Use of a Seat Belt During Pregnancy.**

tors of fetal outcome more than vehicle damage and seat belt use.[9,10]

FALLS.   The enlarging uterus, loosened pelvic joints, and possible pain and neuromuscular dysfunction from pelvic pressure predispose pregnant women to falls. An accurate history of the events preceding the fall and of the fall itself is helpful in determining an underlying pathologic process that may have precipitated the fall and resultant injuries.

If possible, details of the actual fall event should be described because the type and severity of injuries, which are related to the dissipation of mechanical energy, may be predicted. The height a person falls in part determines velocity and may reflect injury severity. If a person is able to break the fall by grasping on to something, the velocity can be decreased. Impact forces also can affect injury severity. The energy-absorbing qualities of the structure on which the woman fell is another important factor to consider.

As previously noted, if the pattern of injuries does not match the fall event, abuse should be considered. A private, confidential interview might elicit this information.

When a pregnant woman falls, she generally lands on her buttock or side, not her abdomen. Injuries are therefore more likely to be sustained by the mother than by the fetus. Head and spinal cord injuries and fractures of the pelvis and lower extremities are common; however, caregivers must still be wary of obstetric injuries such as abruptio placentae.

FIREARMS AND OTHER WEAPONS.   Gunshot wounds are the most common type of penetrating trauma during pregnancy. Other sources of penetrating trauma include stabbings with knives or other sharp objects. When the woman is pregnant, the enlarged abdomen is the most likely body part to be targeted, causing possible damage to the underlying uterus.

Events surrounding a shooting are often vague, and witnesses or even the woman herself may claim that the incident was unintentional. However, such violent crime may represent an attempt to damage or abort the fetus, and that motive must be suspected. The nurse must make every attempt to elicit this information from the patient, family members, or significant others. Information about the type of firearm involved and the distance between the individual and the weapon can aid in determining the severity of underlying injuries. Gunshot wounds usually require early surgical exploration and repair.

Stab wounds require that a description of the weapon be given to the emergency care personnel if the weapon does not accompany the patient. This information may need to be elicited from the victim or witnesses. The length and width of the object and how far it penetrated the abdomen or other body part are clues to possible underlying injury. Stab wounds may be explored locally to determine the extent of injury and the possible need for further surgical intervention.

ABUSE.   Abuse, battery, and intentional physical violence constitute a major problem affecting the health and welfare of women today. An estimated 1.8 million women are severely assaulted by male partners or cohabitants in the United States annually.[20,21] As many as one in three women has been battered by her male partner. Abuse during pregnancy is common; depending on the survey and how the data were collected, studies show that as many as 20% of pregnant women suffer from abuse during their pregnancy.[13]

The complications of pregnancy are significantly higher in women who are abused. These patients tend to have less weight gain and a higher incidence of anemia, infections, and first and second trimester bleeding.[22] Additionally, abuse during pregnancy is associated with significantly higher maternal rates of depression; suicide; and tobacco, alcohol, and drug use.[23,24]

When the patient presents with a pattern of injuries that does not match the reported mechanism, the nurse should suspect abuse and administer an abuse assessment screening to the patient in a private area separate from the mate. If abuse is suspected, the patient must receive follow-up care. Currently there is a focus on teaching the pregnant woman safety behaviors to prevent future abuse. Safety behaviors include hiding money, having extra keys, having a family code, and removing weapons.[25] All women should be aware that the National Domestic Violence Hot Line is available to them by calling 1-800-799-SAFE.

In view of this strong epidemiologic basis for violence during pregnancy and the potential obstetric complications, nurses must maintain a high index of suspicion and probe to

1. Have you ever been emotionally or physically abused by your partner or someone important to you?

YES ☐   NO ☐

2. Within the last year, have you been hit, slapped, kicked or otherwise physically hurt by someone?

YES ☐   NO ☐

If YES, by whom_____

Number of times_____

3. Since you've been pregnant, have you been hit, slapped, kicked, or otherwise physically hurt by someone?

YES ☐   NO ☐

If YES, by whom_____

Number of times_____

Mark the area of injury on body map.

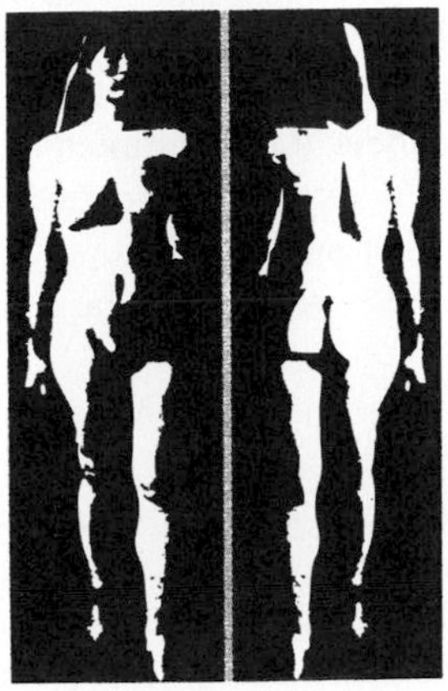

4. Within the last year, has anyone forced you to have sexual activities?

If YES, who_____

Number of times_____

5. Are you afraid of your partner or anyone you listed above?

YES ☐   NO ☐

Developed by the Nursing Research Consortium on Violence and Abuse of which both authors are members. 1989. Readers are encouraged to reproduce and use this assessment tool.

FIGURE 28-2 **Abuse Assessment Screening Tool.** (From Parker B, McFarlane J: Identifying and helping battered pregnant women, *Am J Matern Child Nurs* 16:161-164, 1991.)

ascertain information detailing the events leading to injury. Parker and McFarlane suggest that routine prenatal assessment provides an excellent opportunity to conduct an abuse assessment screening.[21] Hospitalization for an unexplained traumatic event is also a time to conduct such an assessment. As stated by Parker and McFarlane, a nonjudgmental, gentle approach is essential, but the questions must be direct. An abuse assessment screening tool developed by the Nursing Research Consortium on Violence and Abuse is presented in Figure 28-2.

BURNS AND INHALATION INJURIES. Thermal injuries during pregnancy usually occur at home or in the work environment and are caused mainly by flame or hot liquids. The incidence of thermal injuries to pregnant women is low in the Western world, but it is higher in developing countries.[26] Burns are detrimental to fetal survival. Survival is related primarily to gestational age and maternal survival. A prospective study of 27 pregnant burn patients found a correlation between fetal death and total body surface area (TBSA) burned. A fetal loss rate of 56% with no maternal loss was recorded in patients with 15% to 25% TBSA burns. Maternal and fetal morbidity increased to 65% when the burns covered 25% to 50% of the TBSA.[27] Initial management strategies include calculation of the extent of the burn (% TBSA) and rapid resuscitation efforts that focus on the provision of adequate oxygenation and restoration of circulating fluid volume[28] (see Chapter 31).

It has been suggested that early burn wound excision and skin grafting can improve maternal and fetal survival.[29] Urgent delivery has been suggested when the baby is of viable age and the maternal TBSA is greater than 50%.[30]

If the pregnant patient suffers a suspected inhalation injury, carbon monoxide (CO) intoxication should always be suspected and carboxyhemoglobin (COHb) levels measured. Carbon monoxide intoxication is a leading cause of all poisoning deaths, including fetal poisoning deaths, in the United States.[31] Fires, automobile exhaust, and faulty heating systems are major causes of CO poisoning.

The fetal effects of CO poisoning are more severe than maternal effects because the concentration of carboxyhemoglobin is 10% to 15% higher in the fetus as a result of the higher affinity of fetal hemoglobin for CO.[32]

Fetal effects include teratogenicity, neurologic dysfunction, decreased birth weight, and increased fetal death because the fetal partial arterial oxygen concentration (Pa_{O_2}) decreases in direct proportion to the increase in carboxyhemoglobin. Carbon monoxide poisoning impairs the release of oxygen from the mother to the fetus and from fetal hemoglobin to fetal tissue. Prompt diagnosis and appropriate management of inhalation injuries are therefore essential.

Extensive research by Long and Hill in 1977 demonstrated that fetal COHb concentration rises slower than the maternal level but surpasses maternal levels after 5 hours.[33] Maternal CO will reach a steady state in 7 to 8 hours, but fetal concentrations continue to rise for 36 to 48 hours.[33] The CO half-life in the fetus is twice as long as the maternal half-life. Therefore the fetus is more susceptible to CO poisoning.

The treatment for acute carbon monoxide poisoning is administration of oxygen. There had been some uncertainty regarding the use of hyperbaric oxygen (HBO) in the pregnant patient because of possible adverse fetal effects from oxygen at high partial pressures. However, because of the disastrous consequences to the fetus, HBO at 2.8 atmospheres absolute (ATA) should be used more liberally for the treatment of women to prevent fetal hypoxia.[31,34]

Based on Hill's model, it is recommended that a pregnant woman receive 100% oxygen up to five times as long as necessary to reduce her own COHb level to normal. If HBO is not available, 100% oxygen can be administered via a tightly fitting mask.

OBSTETRIC HISTORY

When pregnancy is suspected, an obstetric history should be considered an important component of the patient's health history. The gestational age of the fetus and status of the pregnancy must be established, and a complete obstetric history should be obtained as soon as possible. Suspicion of pregnancy increases if more than 4 weeks have lapsed since the last menstrual period (LMP) or if the LMP was unusual in any way.

To determine gestational age, a reliable historian can be most helpful. The LMP is the most accurate factor in determining the gestational age of the fetus and the expected date of confinement, or due date.[35]

A more thorough obstetric history includes parity (Table 28-1), which indicates any previous abortions or premature deliveries. Delivery history, including the number of hours of labor and types of birth (vaginal or cesarean), also should be obtained along with the maternal Rh factor. This information can alert medical personnel to potential problems, including premature labor and delivery and other fetal and maternal injuries. A spouse, family member, or significant other should be interviewed to obtain this information when possible. Information should also be obtained concerning what, if any, form of contraception was used and how assiduously it was used.

RESUSCITATION PHASE

Early recognition that the trauma patient is pregnant can lead the nurse through the dual ongoing assessment of mother and fetus. Early signs of pregnancy may be easily overlooked. Therefore the astute nurse is alert to even the most subtle changes that can occur during pregnancy (Table 28-2).

The general principles on which trauma management is based must not be ignored when caring for a pregnant trauma patient. The implementation of a rapid primary survey followed by a secondary assessment is imperative, with the ABCs (airway, breathing, circulation) being acknowledged as first priorities.[29] Early recognition of pregnancy should trigger the nurse to be suspicious of unique injuries and to be alert for the pregnancy-related changes that may alter assessment findings and mask signs of shock.

CLINICAL MANAGEMENT/TEAM APPROACH

The key to successful management of the pregnant trauma patient is a team approach. Both emergency/trauma personnel and obstetric personnel should be involved in the patient's care. Although obstetric management is imperative, the ABCs of trauma resuscitation remain the first priority because the best guarantee of fetal survival is prompt maternal care after traumatic injury.

TABLE 28-1   **Parity**

In many institutions, obstetric history is summarized by digits and dashes (e.g., 3-1-0-4).

First digit:	Number of term infants (38 weeks)
Second digit:	Number of premature infants (20-37 weeks)
Third digit:	Number of abortions (any loss before 20 weeks, including ectopics and induced abations)
Fourth digit:	Number of children currently alive

In the example above (3-1-0-4), the woman had 3 term births and 1 premature infant and has 4 children alive. (Many recall this with the mnemonic Florida Power And Light, which stands for Full term, Preterm, Abortions, and Living.)

Data from Pritchard J, MacDonald P, Gant NF: *Williams' obstetrics*, ed 17, Norwalk, Conn, 1990, Appleton-Century-Crofts, 246.

TABLE 28-2   **Presumptive, Probable, and Positive Signs of Pregnancy**

Presumptive Signs
Amenorrhea
Breast changes
Fatigue
Frequent micturition
Nausea and vomiting
Quickening
Skin changes
Cervical changes

Probable Signs
Uterine contractions
Fetal outline
Laboratory pregnancy tests
Uterine changes

Positive Signs
Fetal heart movement recorded by sonogram
Fetal heart sounds
Fetal movement felt by examiner

Data from Pilliteri A: *Maternal-newborn nursing care of the growing family*, ed 3, Boston, 1985, Little Brown, 320.

In 1974 Crosby[36] identified complications associated with the management of injured pregnant women:

Among physicians who man emergency rooms, there is a lack of familiarity with the state of pregnancy and the physiological changes that accompany it. . . . Thus a state of therapeutic paralysis is often seen when the trauma victim is recognized as being pregnant. Attention is all too often directed away from the pregnancy, which may be unfamiliar, but potentially of major importance. . . . Lacerations are sutured, fractures are set, x-ray [films] taken and abrasions cleaned while the fetus may die; a retroplacental clot may grow with shock-inducing speed during the time spent dealing with lesser problems.

The situation as Crosby describes it may not be as common in the trauma setting today, but the concept of therapeutic paralysis does persist. The development of an Advanced Life Support in Obstetrics course for improved obstetric emergency management suggests that concerns continue about the management of obstetric emergencies.[37] The fact that aggressive maternal care is essential for the best fetal outcome must be emphasized.[2,38,39]

MATERNAL ASSESSMENT

To render prompt and aggressive care to the pregnant trauma patient during the resuscitation phase, the nurse must have knowledge not only about initial trauma management interventions but also about the normal anatomic and physiologic changes that occur during pregnancy and the significance of the changes[40] (Table 28-3). This knowledge must be applied during the initial assessment process and as resuscitation efforts continue. Care of the pregnant trauma patient becomes more complex when obstetric complications are encountered in addition to traumatic injuries. These assessment considerations are not limited, however, to the resuscitation phase of care; they must be considered throughout all phases of care.

NEUROLOGIC CONSIDERATIONS. Neurologically a pregnant woman has an increased risk of fainting and is more easily fatigued as a result of the unpredictable physiologic changes that occur during pregnancy.[2] The pregnant woman also may experience changes in gait and balance, primarily during the third trimester. Changes in vision, history of headaches, and seizure activity are abnormal and, when present, suggest obstetric complications such as preeclampsia and eclampsia (Table 28-4). Prompt identification of an obstetric complication can guide care and prevent both maternal and fetal compromise.

RESPIRATORY CONSIDERATIONS. The respiratory system is also altered during pregnancy. The upper respiratory passages become engorged by capillaries, making the pregnant patient more prone to nasopharyngeal bleeding and subsequent upper airway obstruction.

TABLE 28-3 **Normal Anatomic and Physiologic Changes During Pregnancy**		
Body System	**Alteration**	**Significance of Change**
Neurologic	Increased risk of fainting	More prone to fall
	Easily fatigued	Increased risk of trauma
Cardiovascular	Hypervolemic (increased volume of as much as 50% above prepregnancy levels)	Signs of blood loss subtle to develop
	Supine hypotension	Increased fluid needs for resuscitation
	Physiologic anemia	Vital signs, lab tests must be assessed against normal
	Increased heart rate	pregnancy values (see Tables 25-5 and 25-6)
	Hypercoagulability	
Respiratory	Engorged upper respiratory passages	Decrease in blood buffering capacity
	Increased tidal volume	Altered response to inhalation anesthetics
	Increased vital capacity	Early use of oxygen therapy essential secondary to
	Increased respiratory rate	functional residual capacity
	Elevated diaphragm	Potential for nasopharyngeal bleeding
	Decreased functional residual capacity	Gentle oral intubation with smaller well-lubricated tube
Gastrointestinal	Physiologic ileus	Increased risk of aspiration
	Increased gastric acidity	Altered internal injury patterns
	Compartmentalization of abdominal contents	
Genitourinary	Increased urinary frequency	Altered appearance in intravenous urogram
	Increased glomerular filtration rate	Bladder susceptible to abdominal trauma
	Dilation of renal calyces, renal pelvis, and ureter	
	Bladder pulled into abdomen	
Musculoskeletal	Alterations in gait and balance	Increased risk of fall
	Widened symphysis pubis	Possible increased risk of spinal subluxation
	Lordosis	

TABLE 28-4	**Signs and Symptoms of Preeclampsia**
Mild Preeclampsia:	**Severe Preeclampsia:** When any of the following exists:

• Systolic blood pressure of at least 140 mm Hg or a diastolic blood pressure of at least 90 mm Hg
• Associated with either
  1. Proteinuria
     OR
  2. Edema
	• Blood pressure >160 mm Hg systolic, >110 mm Hg diastolic
	• Proteinuria >5 g/24 hr
	• Oliguria defined as <500 ml/ 24 hr
	• Cerebral or visual disturbances
	• Pulmonary edema
	• Epigastric or right upper quadrant pain
	• Impaired liver function
	• Thrombocytopenia
	• Fetal intrauterine growth retardation or oligohydramnios
	• Elevated serum creatinine
	• HELLP Syndrome (an acronym that stand for hemolysis, elevated liver enzymes, and low platelets)

Seizures = Eclampsia

From American College of Obstetricians and Gynecologists: *Hypertension in pregnancy,* ACOG Tech Bull 219, 1996.

During pregnancy there may be as much as a 40% increase in tidal volume and a rise of 100 to 200 ml in vital capacity. There also may be an increase in respiratory rate by 15%,[41] or it may remain unchanged. The combined effects of these respiratory changes place the pregnant woman in a chronic state of hyperventilation that results in arterial blood gas alterations. $Paco_2$ levels drop to approximately 30 mm Hg, and Pao_2 increases to 101 to 104 mm Hg. A normal pH is maintained by the excretion of bicarbonate via the kidneys (Table 28-5).

As pregnancy progresses, the diaphragm becomes elevated, decreasing functional residual capacity by 20% at times. This decreases the pregnant woman's oxygen reserve, predisposing her to hypoxia. Therefore the airway and breathing of a pregnant trauma patient must be monitored carefully and supported as necessary to prevent maternal and subsequent fetal hypoxia.

Supplemental oxygen should be given to all pregnant trauma patients, and pulse oximetry should be used. If the patient is intubated, capnography is useful; $Paco_2$ is normally 30 mm Hg during pregnancy.

CARDIOVASCULAR CONSIDERATIONS. Cardiovascular changes are perhaps the most profound physiologic alterations that occur during pregnancy and the most critical to interpret when assessing the pregnant trauma patient. The pregnant woman is normally hypervolemic. Blood volume during pregnancy begins to increase by the tenth week of gestation; by the thirty-fourth week of gestation, a pregnant woman's circulatory volume can increase by as much as 50%. This increase can mask a 30% gradual loss of maternal blood volume or a 10% to 15% acute blood loss. When this occurs, although the maternal vital signs may remain unchanged, the fetus can be at risk because of a decrease in uterine perfusion; the woman's risk is also increased because these stable vital signs may change precipitously. Because the uterus cannot autoregulate, its flow is directly related to the pressure it receives from maternal circulation.

The electrocardiogram can be altered during pregnancy as well. As the uterus enlarges and elevates the diaphragm, the heart is pushed upward and rotated, causing a shift of the electrical axis by 15 degrees. This may precipitate changes such as T-wave flattening or inversion in lead III, Q waves in lead III, and augmented V lead (aVF), which are considered normal in pregnancy.[42]

HEMATOLOGIC CONSIDERATIONS. Although erythrocyte production increases during pregnancy, adequate levels cannot be maintained as plasma volume increases; therefore the pregnant woman is physiologically anemic. A normal prepregnancy hematocrit of 40% to 41% may drop to 31% to 34% in late pregnancy.[41]

The coagulation profile of the pregnant woman is also altered because fibrinogen and concentrations of factors VII, VIII, and IX are increased during pregnancy. Bleeding time, clotting time, and prothrombin time should remain unchanged during pregnancy. The increase in fibrinogen and other factors, coupled with a decrease in circulating plasminogen activator, can actually benefit the pregnant patient if hemorrhage occurs. These same changes, however, pose a problem. The risk of venous thromboembolism is five times higher in a pregnant woman than in a nonpregnant woman of similar age. Immobility after a traumatic event puts the pregnant patient at even greater risk.[43]

The leukocyte count is normally elevated in pregnancy to approximately 5000 to 15,000/mm^3 and becomes even further elevated during labor and delivery. Except for an increase in phagocytes and a decrease in lymphocytes during pregnancy, the differential remains unchanged. Other laboratory study adjustments for pregnant women are listed in Table 28-5.

HEMODYNAMIC CONSIDERATIONS. The most dramatic hemodynamic change that occurs during pregnancy is supine hypotension, also known as vena cava syndrome. In the supine position, after 16 to 20 weeks' gestation, the enlarging uterus compresses the vena cava and aorta, impeding venous return and decreasing blood pressure and cardiac output. Therefore the pregnant trauma patient should never be placed in the supine position. Traditionally the pregnant woman is placed in the left lateral position, which displaces the uterus and decreases compression of the major abdominal vessels (Figure 28-3). During prehospital transport and until spinal injuries are ruled out, the supine position can be avoided by tipping the backboard 30

TABLE 28-5 Laboratory Value Adjustments During Pregnancy

	Nonpregnant	Pregnant
Electrolytes and Acid-Base Values		
Sodium (mEq/L)	135-145	132-140
Potassium (mEq/L)	3.5-5.0	3.5-4.5
Chloride (mEq/L)	100-106	90-105
Bicarbonate (mEq/L)	24-30	17-22
P_{CO_2} (mm Hg)	35-50	25-30
P_{O_2} (mm Hg)	98-100	101-104
Base excess (mEq/L)	0.7	3-4
Arterial pH	7.38-7.44	7.40-7.45
BUN (mg/dl)	10-18	4-12
Creatinine (mg/dl)	0.6-1.2	0.4-0.9
Creatinine clearance (ml/min)	3.5-5.0	2.0-3.7
Osmolality (mOsm/kg)	275-295	275-285
Lipids and Liver Function Tests		
Total bilirubin (mg/dl)	1.0	1.0
Direct bilirubin (mg/dl)	0.4	0.4
Alkaline phosphatase (IU/ml)	13-35	25-80
SGOT (IU/ml)	10-40	10-40
Total protein (g/dl)	6.0-8.4	5.5-7.5
Albumin (g/dl)	3.5-5.0	3.0-4.5
Globulin (g/dl)	2.3-3.5	3.0-4.0
Total lipids (mg/dl)	460-1000	1040
Total cholesterol (mg/dl)	120-220	250
Triglycerides (mg/dl)	45-150	230
Free fatty acid (g/L)	770	1226
Phospholipids (mg/dl)	256	350
Hematologic Laboratory Values		
Complete blood count:		
Hematocrit (%)	37-48	32-42
Hemoglobin (g/dl)	12-16	10-14
Leukocytes (count/mm^3)	4300-10,800	5000-15,000
Polymorphonuclear cells (%)	54-62	60-85
Lymphocytes (%)	38-46	15-40
Fibrinogen	250-400	600
Platelets	150,000-350,000	Normal or slightly decreased
Serum iron (g)	75-150	65-120
Iron-binding capacity (g)	250-410	300-500
Iron saturation (%)	30-40	15-30
Ferritin (ng/ml)	35	10-12
Erythrocyte sedimentation (mm/hr)	<20	30-90

Modified from Elrad H, Gleicher N: Physiologic changes in normal pregnancy. In Gleicher N, editor: *Principles of medical therapy in pregnancy*, New York, 1985, Plenum, 51-52.
BUN, Blood urea nitrogen; *SGOT,* serum glutamic-pyruvic transaminase (aspartate aminotransferase).

degrees, simulating the left lateral position[44] (Figure 28-4). The right-sided tilt can be equally effective if left-sided injuries make that position difficult.

Hypotension therefore can occur normally in a pregnant woman in a supine position. When this occurs, the patient becomes uncomfortable or nauseated until she is repositioned and blood pressure increases. Hypertension is never normal during pregnancy and suggests an obstetric complication. During pregnancy the heart rate increases approximately 10 to 20 beats/min above prepregnancy levels. Data on pregnant patients' central venous pressure and pulmo-nary artery wedge pressure were collected by Clark et al in 1989. They assessed the central hemodynamic status of 10 normal pregnant patients who were screened carefully both in their third trimester and postpartum. In late pregnancy the patients had a 43% increase in cardiac output (4.3 to 6.2 L/min). Other significant findings included a 21% decline in systemic vascular resistance, a 34% decline in pulmonary vascular resistance, and a 28% decline in the colloid oncotic pressure-pulmonary capillary wedge pressure gradient.[45] There was no significant difference in mean arterial pressure, central venous pressure, or pulmonary capillary wedge

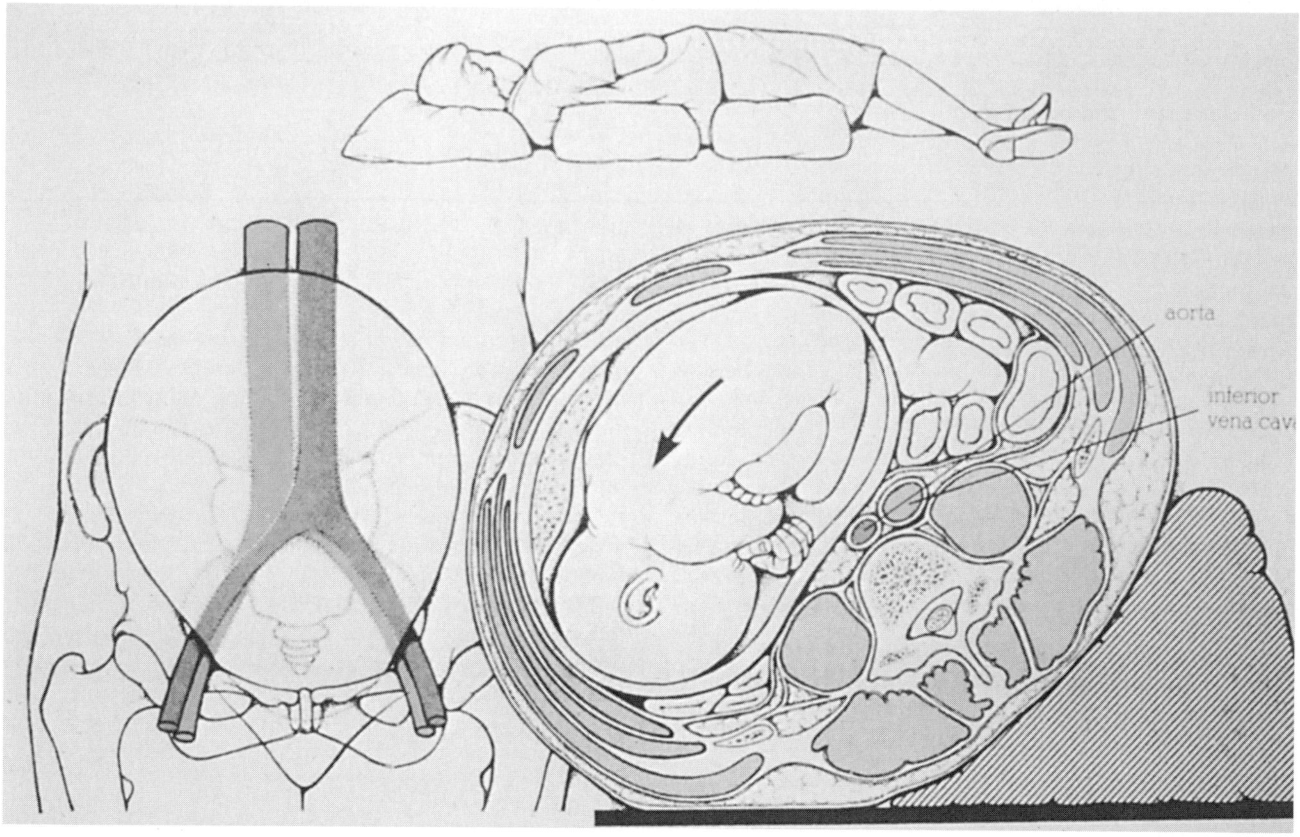

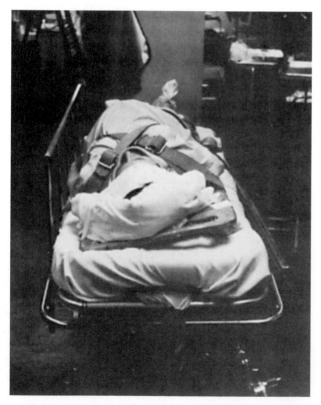

FIGURE 28-3 Left lateral positioning displaces the uterus and decreases compression of major abdominal vessels.

FIGURE 28-4 Placing a small roll under the right side of the backboard and tipping the backboard 30 degrees displaces the uterus to the left side.

pressure during late pregnancy compared with the nonpregnant state (Table 28-6).

The hemodynamic changes that occur normally during pregnancy cause confusion as the resuscitation team assesses the patient's condition. Tachycardia and hypotension that occur when the pregnant trauma patient is in a supine position may not be indicative of a shock state but may instead represent normal changes. Caution must be exercised, however, because the pregnant trauma patient, as previously stated, can mask a 15% to 30% blood loss without evidence of shock while uterine perfusion decreases, risking fetal anoxia and dire maternal consequences. Changes in laboratory values, including hematocrit and leukocyte count, further confuse the clinical picture.

GASTROINTESTINAL CONSIDERATIONS. A physiologic ileus, or diminished emptying time of the bowel, normally occurs during pregnancy. In addition, the placental production of gastrin and progesterone increases the acidity of the stomach contents. On auscultation, bowel sounds may be absent, making interpretation difficult. It should always be assumed that the pregnant trauma patient has a full stomach and is at risk for vomiting, aspiration, and pulmonary complications.

GENITOURINARY CONSIDERATIONS. Genitourinary changes include an increase in urination frequency through-

TABLE 28-6 **Central Hemodynamic Changes**		
	Nonpregnant	**Pregnant**
Cardiac output (L/min)	4.3 ± 0.9	6.2 ± 1.0
Heart rate (beats/min)	71 ± 10.0	83 ± 10.0
Systemic vascular resistance (dyne cm sec^{-5})	1530 ± 520	1210 ± 266
Pulmonary vascular resistance (dyne cm sec^{-5})	119 ± 47.0	78 ± 22
Colloid oncotic pressure (mm Hg)	20.8 ± 1.0	18.0 ± 1.5
Colloid oncotic pressure-pulmonary capillary wedge pressure (mm Hg)	14.5 ± 2.5	10.5 ± 2.7
Mean arterial pressure (mm Hg)	86.4 ± 7.5	90.3 ± 5.8
Pulmonary capillary wedge pressure (mm Hg)	6.3 ± 2.1	7.5 ± 1.8
Central venous pressure (mm Hg)	3.7 ± 2.6	3.6 ± 2.5
Left ventricular stroke work index (g-m/m^{-2})	41 ± 8	48 ± 6

From Clark S, Cotton O, Lee W et al: Central hemodynamic assessment of normal term pregnancy, *Am J Obstet Gynecol* 161:1439-1442, 1989.

out pregnancy. The increase in frequency during the first trimester is the result of a rise in the glomerular filtration rate (GFR) by approximately 30.5% of prepregnancy values. During the third trimester the further increased frequency is a result of compression of the bladder by the enlarging uterus, in addition to an increased GFR.

After blunt trauma to the abdomen during late pregnancy, the bladder is more likely to empty spontaneously or rupture because the bladder may be elevated and out of the protection of the pelvic ring. Assessment of the pregnant woman should include gentle palpation of the bladder above the symphysis pubis. If a stable condition allows, the patient should be encouraged to void. If she is unable to void spontaneously and bladder trauma is plausible given the mechanism of injury, the patient should be catheterized using strict aseptic technique. Glucosuria revealed by urine testing is common during pregnancy, but the presence of frank or microscopic blood suggests genitourinary trauma. Diagnostic tests may be performed, including cystography, intravenous (IV) pyelography, and cystoscopy. Physiologic dilation of renal calyces, renal pelves, and ureter (particularly on the right side) may be evident. These conditions are present from approximately the tenth week of pregnancy until after delivery and are believed to be caused by ureteral obstruction from the ovarian vein plexuses, dextrotorsion of the uterus, and increased progesterone concentrations.

METABOLIC CONSIDERATIONS.   As a normal change of pregnancy, the pituitary gland nearly doubles in weight. Shock or hypoxia in the pregnant patient can precipitate a sudden drop in pituitary blood flow, leading to necrosis[46] (known as Sheehan's syndrome). Calcium, phosphate, mag-

nesium, creatinine, and blood urea nitrogen (BUN) levels fall during pregnancy. There is also an increased risk of glucose intolerance during pregnancy.

OBSTETRIC AND FETAL CONSIDERATIONS

When the trauma patient is pregnant, primary and secondary assessment must also focus on the fetus and the possible obstetric complications that can result after traumatic injury. The fetus may be compromised while the mother appears stable. As an initial response to shock, uterine perfusion decreases, causing stress to the fetus. Unique injuries to the uterus must be detected and treated immediately or the lives of both fetus and mother are threatened.

OBSTETRIC ASSESSMENT.   The obstetric assessment must determine the viability of the fetus, establish the potential for impending delivery, and identify unique injuries.

Gestational Age.   Accurate assessment of gestational age or the estimated date of delivery is important during the initial resuscitation to determine if the fetus is viable. As previously mentioned, the date of the LMP is the most accurate indication of gestational age if the patient is a reliable historian. However, in the emergency setting it may not be possible to obtain this information.

For a rapid assessment (including prehospital assessment), fundal height can be measured quickly. Fundal height is the distance from the symphysis pubis to the top of the fundus. From 16 to 32 weeks this measurement approximates the weeks of gestation (Figure 28-5).

Ultrasound has become a routine assessment tool for obstetricians, trauma surgeons, and emergency physicians.[47] An ultrasound examination can be used to estimate gestational age; it is most accurate when performed before 13 weeks of gestation.[48] Ultrasound is considered consistent with menstrual dates if there is agreement on gestational age within 1 week at 6 to 11 weeks or within 10 days at 12 to 20 weeks.[48]

Determination of the gestational age of the fetus is also helpful in identifying possible injuries to both the mother and fetus. During the first 12 to 14 weeks (early pregnancy), the uterus is well protected in the pelvic confines. Cases of uterine and fetal injury in this stage have been documented, but they are rare. After the first trimester (12 to 14 weeks), the uterus becomes an abdominal organ and is no longer protected by the pelvis. The uterus and fetus may therefore absorb the impact of traumatic forces and consequently sustain unique injuries.

Premature Rupture of Membranes (PROM).   After the estimation of gestational age and establishment of fetal well-being, the patient's amniotic membrane status (intact or ruptured) must be assessed. Indications of labor, if any, also must be noted. A history of a sudden gush of fluid after abdominal impact suggests premature rupture of amniotic membranes but must be differentiated from a spontaneous bladder void. If a pool of vaginal fluid is present, it should be

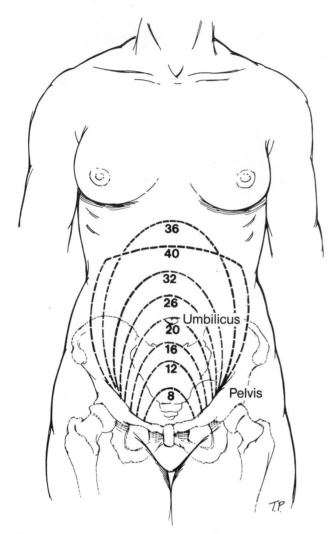

FIGURE 28-5 **Uterine Size and Location, Reflecting Gestational Age.**

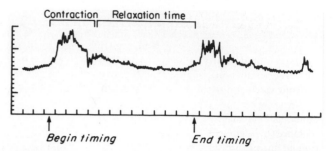

FIGURE 28-6 **A Uterine Contraction Consists of Two Periods: Contraction Time and Relaxation Time.** The frequency of contractions is the interval of time from the beginning of one contraction period to the beginning of the next contraction period.

TABLE 28-7	Signs and Symptoms of Uterine Damage

Mild uterine injuries (e.g., lacerations and contusions):
   Varied and mild symptoms
Uterine rupture:
   Sudden onset of abdominal pain with increased uterine
     irritability
   Maternal hypovolemic shock
   Loss of fetal heart tones or evidence of fetal distress
   Uterine tenderness to palpation and increased tone
   Palpation of two abdominal masses (uterus and fetus)
   Vaginal bleeding (variable)

Source: Pearlman M, Tintinalli J: *Emergency care of the woman,* New York, 1998, McGraw-Hill, 69-76.

tested for pH. The normal pH of amniotic fluid is 7 to 7.5; that of urine is 4.8 to 6. The fluid also should be checked microscopically (place a drop on a slide and allow to dry) for the appearance of ferning, which is a more reliable sign of the presence of amniotic fluid. It is unlikely that membranes have ruptured if ultrasound reveals normal amniotic fluid volume.[47]

Premature Labor. Determining if the patient is in labor is also a component of the obstetric assessment. Labor consists of three stages: dilation of the cervix, expulsion of the baby via the birth canal, and the separation and expulsion of the placenta. Labor is defined as cervical change in response to uterine contractions. Identification of the onset of labor is particularly important if the woman is not at term. Signs and symptoms of the onset of labor include bloody show, ruptured membranes, and contractions. Contractions can be difficult for the nonobstetric staff to assess; therefore, obstetric team expertise is most valuable. Contractions causing dilation of the cervix indicate that the patient is in labor. The duration and frequency of contractions must be assessed. The frequency of contractions is determined by noting the time from the beginning of one contraction to the beginning of the next (Figure 28-6). Premature labor after trauma may indicate the presence of fetal or uterine injury. As measures are taken to inhibit the progression of labor, additional obstetric assessment should be obtained to rule out fetal or uterine injury.

Uterine Damage. As pregnancy progresses, the uterus becomes an abdominal organ and can be damaged after blunt or penetrating trauma. Uterine damage can consist of laceration, a tear, or a partial or complete rupture. If the uterus has ruptured, it is usually, but not always, tender on palpation. The abdomen may be distended, and vaginal bleeding may occur (Table 28-7). When uterine rupture is severe, two distinct masses may be palpable in the abdomen: the uterus and the fetus. Milder forms of uterine damage are more common although clinically less distinct. The most reliable indicator of uterine rupture is fetal distress.

Abruptio Placentae. Placental abruption, the premature separation of the placenta from the uterine wall, also can occur after trauma. It is second only to maternal death among the causes of fetal death.[49] Abruption in mild forms can be difficult to diagnose. An abnormal fetal heart rate

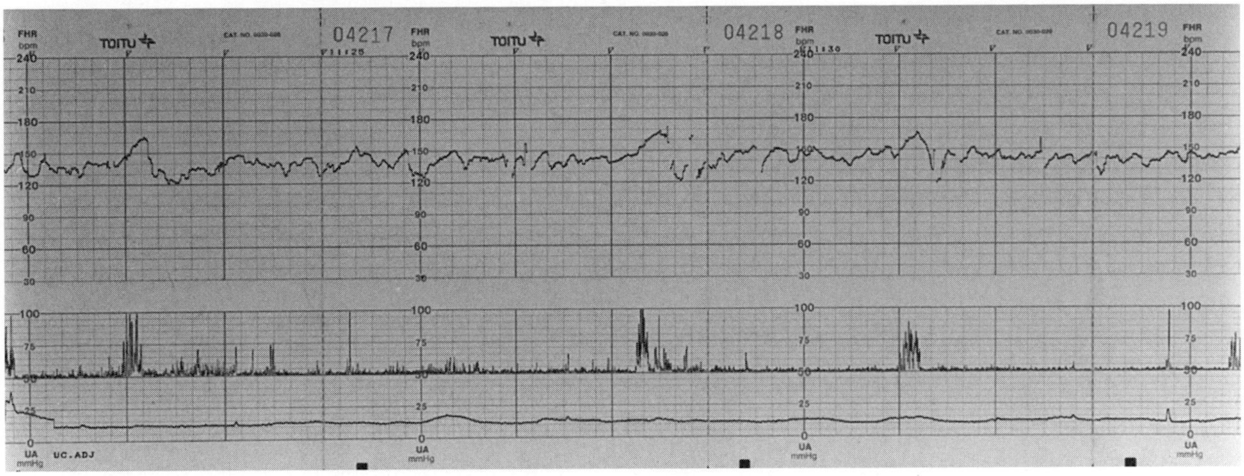

FIGURE 28-7 Monitor strip segment showing a normal fetal heart tracing *(upper tracing)* with significant variability, acceleration of heart rate associated with fetal movement *(middle tracing)*, and no decelerations below the baseline. Uterine irritability detectable as small irregular contractions *(bottom tracing)* indicates potential for problems such as placental separation (abruptio), other bleeding, and preterm labor. Monitoring should be continued until the uterus is quiescent.

TABLE 28-8 **Signs and Symptoms of Abruptio Placentae**

The symptoms of an abruptio placentae can be variable depending on the degree of the placentae separation. They include:

- Vaginal bleeding (may not be always present)
- Premature labor
- Sudden onset of abdominal or back pain
- Uterine tenderness to palpation
- Uterine tetany or rigidity (uterine tone may be increased with small, frequent contractions superimposed)
- Expanding or rising fundal height
- Maternal hemodynamic instability and coagulopathy
- Fetal distress or absence of fetal heart tones, no fetal cardiac

Source: Pilliteri A: *Maternal and child health nursing,* ed 3, New York, 1999, JB Lippincott, 384-386.

pattern (identified by obstetric staff with expertise in this area) can be helpful in identifying a placental abruption in women at more than 20 weeks' gestation.[49,50] (Figure 28-7) Fetal heart rate pattern irregularity is the most reliable indicator of placental abruption. The grave sign of decreased or absent fetal heart tones may indicate too late that the placenta was injured. Other signs and symptoms are listed in Table 28-8. Placental abruption can occur more than 48 hours after the initial traumatic incident, though rarely.[51] The incidence of abruptio placentae after severe trauma ranges from 6.6% to 66%.

The mechanism causing the abruption is directly related to the trauma. Higgins and Garite describe the placenta in the uterus as a potato chip inside a tennis ball.[51] The uterus is elastic; the placenta is seemingly less so. On impact the placenta cannot reshape as rapidly as the uterus; instead it separates or pulls away from the uterine wall, causing

disruption of the maternal-fetal circulation and hemorrhage. Early detection of an abruption and appropriate action increase the chances of fetal survival.

Coagulation changes are rare after a mild abruption, but if the abruption is severe enough to cause fetal demise, as with any situation involving significant hemorrhage, the mother can develop a severe coagulopathy.

Fetomaternal Hemorrhage.   Fetomaternal hemorrhage is the transplacental bleeding of fetal blood into the maternal circulation.[52] Its incidence among pregnant injured women is four to five times higher than among noninjured pregnant women.[49] To detect fetomaternal hemorrhage, the Kleihauer-Betke acid-elution assay can be performed on maternal blood. This test also can estimate fetal blood loss. Positive results are especially important for Rh-negative mothers with Rh-positive infants; in this scenario an appropriate amount of Rh immune globulin can be administered to prevent isoimmunization. The authors of a study involving the results of 523 Kleihauer-Betke tests concluded that the assay should be reserved for patients with severe trauma or evidence of fetal compromise.[53]

FETAL ASSESSMENT.   Ongoing fetal assessment is essential because the mother can mask signs of shock and the fetus can be the first to show evidence of compromise.

Fetal condition is easiest to evaluate by assessing the fetal heart rate. Normal fetal heart rate is 120 to 160 beats/min and can be detected by an ultrasound device (Doppler) by 10 to 12 weeks of gestation. If the fetus is viable, its heart rate should be monitored continuously with an electronic fetal monitor (EFM) once the mother's condition has been stabilized. The variability of the fetal heart tones and the rate should be evaluated by a clinician experienced in fetal monitoring (see Figure 28-7). Fetuses older than 23 weeks are considered viable if neonatal resources are available;

infants born at 21 to 22 weeks have survived. If an EFM is not available, only a Doppler designed for obstetric evaluation should be used because its frequency is adjusted to assess fetal heart tones. An adult Doppler of higher frequency such as those used for vascular studies may not have sufficient range, so that nothing is heard even though the fetus is viable, thereby confusing the clinical picture. Fetal tachycardia followed by the more grave sign of fetal bradycardia suggests fetal anoxia, and if the mother's condition permits, immediate action should be taken so that the fetus can survive.

When the pregnant trauma patient is conscious, she is a resource for detecting an alteration in fetal activity, which is also an indicator of fetal well-being. Quickening, or the maternal perception of fetal movement, usually occurs in approximately the sixteenth week of gestation in a second pregnancy and in the twentieth week of a first. Although the fetus is not in constant motion, a prolonged period during which fetal movement is lacking can suggest fetal demise.

Additional diagnostic procedures that can aid in assessing the condition of the fetus include ultrasound and amniocentesis. Real-time ultrasound can identify fetal cardiac movement and detect fetal heart tones and fetal death. Fetal biophysical assessment by ultrasound is a method used to determine if a fetus is being asphyxiated. Fetal biophysical profile scoring is based on five biophysical variables, four of which are monitored simultaneously by dynamic ultrasound imaging. The variables are fetal breathing movement, gross body movement, fetal tone, reactive fetal heart rate, and qualitative amniotic fluid volume.[54] Each is coded as normal or abnormal according to set criteria and given a rating of 2 (normal) or 0 (abnormal).

Based on the biophysical profile score, a management protocol is recommended. The biophysical profile looks for an alteration in the fetal central nervous system as an indication of fetal asphyxia. In the emergency setting, biophysical profile scoring may be helpful, but the test requires up to a 30-minute ultrasound observation period, which may not be appropriate during initial trauma resuscitation. The scoring and observation can be done after resuscitation while the patient undergoes acute monitoring.

Amniocentesis can test for fetal maturity. Maturity of the fetal lungs is determined by the lecithin/sphingomyelin ratio and the presence of phosphatidyl glycerol. It is difficult to imagine, however, how this information would be obtained and used in an acute care setting. If it is important to consider an early delivery, gestational age assessment, as outlined above, provides sufficient knowledge about the risks of prematurity and associated morbidity.

SPECIAL MANAGEMENT CONSIDERATIONS

Other factors must be considered when caring for the pregnant trauma patient during intubation, radiographic examinations, medication administration, medical or pneumatic antishock garment (PASG) use, and invasive abdominal assessment procedures. The cardiac arrest situation is also unique for this patient population.

INTUBATION. Use of nasal airways or nasotracheal tubes should be avoided to prevent nasal bleeding. When intubation is required, a smaller (≤7 mm), well-lubricated endotracheal tube should be gently inserted by an experienced clinician.[55] This is to prevent posterior pharyngeal bleeding from engorgement of the area, which occurs during pregnancy.

RADIOGRAPHIC EXAMINATIONS. Radiographic examinations considered essential for diagnosing injuries after trauma should never be omitted during pregnancy. Care must be taken, however, to protect the patient from unnecessary exposure. When possible, the uterus should be shielded with a lead apron during radiographic examination (Figure 28-8). Duplication of radiographs should be avoided, and the purpose of each exposure should be validated regarding its clinical implications. The patient should be assured that essential tests must be done to diagnose her injuries properly.

Assessment of fetal radiation risk is a complex process. Qualitative radiation risks are categorized as low, intermediate, and high based on the quantity of radiation the patient has been exposed to in milligrays (mGy) (Table 28-9).[56,57] If questions arise after resuscitation, early consultation with a perinatologist is appropriate.

MEDICATIONS. All medications are, as a rule, relatively contraindicated during pregnancy. Decisions concerning medication use during pregnancy must weigh the benefits to the mother against the risks to the fetus. The highest risk period for the fetus is during organogenesis (days 10 to 56 after conception).[58] It is during this time that medications are most likely to have a teratogenic effect.

Tetanus prophylaxis with toxoid, commonly administered after trauma, should be given if the pregnant patient has not been immunized in the past 5 years because there is no risk to the fetus.

The pregnant trauma patient who is immobile after her injury is at risk for venous thromboembolism (VTE). There is strong evidence that a pregnant patient is more at risk than a nonpregnant patient. The agents currently available for the prevention for VTE are heparin, heparinlike compounds (unfractionated heparin, low-molecular-weight heparin [LMWH], and heparinoids), and coumarin derivatives.[59] The two potential fetal complications of anticoagulant therapy are teratogenicity and bleeding. Heparin does not cross the placenta and cannot cause either fetal bleeding or teratogenicity; therefore it is thought to be safe for the fetus. There is also evidence that LMWH and heparinoids do not cross the placenta. However, coumarin derivatives cross the placenta and have the potential to cause both fetal bleeding and teratogenicity; thus they are seldom used, with the exception of the rare patient with a mechanical heart valve.

PNEUMATIC ANTISHOCK GARMENT. PASGs are no longer commonly used in trauma resuscitation to augment circulatory support. Should they be used on a pregnant

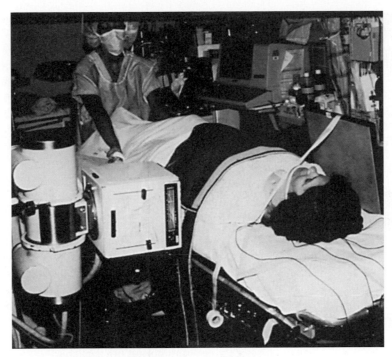

FIGURE 28-8 The pregnant patient's abdomen should be shielded by a lead apron from above the fundus to below the pelvic area.

TABLE 28-9	**Radiation Risk Categories**
Risk Category	**Dose Range (mGy)**
Low	<10
Intermediate	10-250
High	>250

From Mann FA, Nathens A, Langer SG et al: Communicating with the family: the risks of medical radiation to concept uses in victims of major blunt-force torso trauma, *J Trauma* 48(2):354-357, 2000.

trauma patient, it is suggested that only the leg compartments be inflated. The effects of inflating the abdominal portion over a pregnant uterus are not known; therefore this procedure is not recommended.

Numerous clinical case reports have documented the use of PASGs during obstetric emergencies. These include abortion complications, ectopic pregnancies, hydatidiform mole bleeding, hypocoagulation states, postoperative hemorrhage, and uterine atony.[60,61] In these cases the uterus has been emptied and the abdominal portions were used to tamponade hemorrhage.

ABDOMINAL ASSESSMENT (ULTRASOUND, COMPUTED TOMOGRAPHY, AND DIAGNOSTIC PERITONEAL LAVAGE).
Abdominal assessment of the pregnant trauma patient is somewhat unique because of the stretching of the abdominal wall and the enlarging uterus. It is important to determine the presence of abdominal injury in the resuscitation phase. Ultrasound, computed tomography (CT), and diagnostic peritoneal lavage (DPL) are all useful for this patient population. The hemodynamic stability of the

patient and the risk assessment for injury should guide clinical decision making. (See Chapter 24 for additional abdominal test information.)

Ultrasound is commonly used in the evaluation of abdominal trauma in the United States.[47] In the gravid trauma patient, ultrasound may have particular merit because it is noninvasive and does not expose the fetus to radiation. Ultrasound can be used to assess fetal well-being, gestational age, and placental and uterine injuries. A skilled radiologist also can employ ultrasound to evaluate abdominal viscera and pelvic fluid.

CT is also a popular modality for assessment of abdominal trauma. It has the advantages of being noninvasive and providing information on the retroperitoneum and genitourinary tract. Uterine injuries can be identified and defined with an abdominal CT scan and fetal injuries noted in a sleeping, sedated, or dead fetus (Figure 28-9). The amount of radiographic exposure to the fetus during abdominal CT depends on a number of factors, including patient age, type of machine, shielding of fetus, and fetal position.

DPL is considered both safe and appropriate in pregnant trauma patients.[62] The stomach and bladder should be emptied before the procedure, and the uterus should be well defined. During pregnancy, DPL may be more safely accomplished using a minilaparotomy instead of a catheter inserted with a needle. If clinical inspection after penetrating trauma suggests penetration of the abdominal wall, the lavage may be omitted in lieu of emergency laparotomy. This modality is less commonly used today because of the availability and utility of imaging.

Another diagnostic test that has been employed during

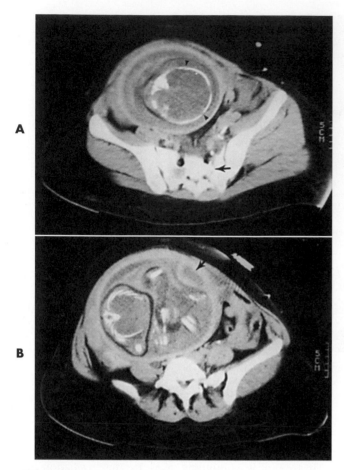

FIGURE 28-9 CT Scan of Trauma to the Gravid Uterus and Fetus. A, Axial CT image through the level of the fetal head, obtained after blunt trauma to the maternal abdomen and pelvis at 7 months' gestation, shows two fetal skull fractures *(arrowheads).* A maternal left sacral fracture is present *(arrow).* **B,** CT image through the fetal torso reveals placental abruption with elevation of a portion of the placenta from the uterine wall *(arrow).* Fetal demise was confirmed by sonography before performing abdominal CT to assess extent of injury. (Courtesy Stuart E. Mirvis, M.D., Department of Diagnostic Radiology, University of Maryland Medical Center, Baltimore.)

pregnancy is culdocentesis. In selected patients, culdocentesis has been of clinical value,[17] but most traumatologists do not use this procedure because of the possibility of causing fetal damage.

CARDIAC ARREST. When the pregnant trauma patient is in cardiac arrest, the principles of resuscitation are the same as those for nonpregnant patients. Standard cardiopulmonary resuscitation (CPR) procedures should be performed and advanced cardiac life support (ACLS) measures instituted to ensure survival of both the mother and fetus. A team member should be assigned to manually displace the uterus to improve venous return. Defibrillation should be performed if necessary.[63] Drugs commonly administered during the cardiac arrest activities should be used during pregnancy as well.[64] If the resuscitation is not going well, consideration may be given to emptying the uterus because this may improve venous return and expose an other-

wise unsuspected intraabdominal (retrouterine) source of blood loss.

POSTMORTEM CESAREAN SECTION. When the patient is in irreversible cardiac arrest on admission, the decision to perform a postmortem cesarean section must be made. Obstetric and neonatal personnel must be notified immediately. More than 150 cases of successful postmortem cesarean section have been documented.[65] The cesarean section should be performed while CPR is in progress and as soon after maternal death as possible. Two key factors that must be considered when making the decision to perform a postmortem cesarean section are gestational age of the fetus and the amount of time the patient has been in arrest. Neonatal resuscitation almost always is necessary after delivery of the infant and should be managed by neonatal personnel, who must have emergency equipment immediately accessible (Table 28-10). Postmortem cesarean section should never be performed if the fundus of the uterus is below the umbilicus, if the mother died of subacute or chronic asphyxia, or if someone capable of resuscitating the newborn is not available.

MATERNAL AND FETAL INJURIES UNIQUE TO PREGNANCY AFTER BLUNT TRAUMA

MATERNAL HEMORRHAGIC SHOCK. Although hemorrhagic shock is not unique to the pregnant trauma patient, this patient does present a confusing clinical picture during resuscitation. Hypotension can occur normally in a supine position during pregnancy and may be subtle. Turning the pregnant patient to the left lateral position can markedly increase cardiac output and should always be done as a resuscitative measure (see Figure 28-3). Care must be taken to stabilize the neck and maintain the spine in proper alignment when repositioning. When the patient is immobilized on a backboard, the board can be slightly elevated toward the left lateral position (see Figure 28-4). If the patient's injuries or resuscitation procedures prohibit this positional change, the uterus can be displaced manually. The vital signs should be monitored closely for indications of shock throughout the resuscitation phase so that aggressive volume replacement can be initiated as necessary. Laboratory value trends must be monitored closely as well and compared with normal pregnancy values (see Table 28-5).

As the initial assessment of the pregnant trauma patient progresses systematically, knowledge of the anatomic and physiologic changes that occur during pregnancy must be integrated into the scenario. Injuries to the liver and spleen commonly cause shock during pregnancy. The patient's abdomen should be assessed carefully for pain, guarding, and rebound tenderness. Additional minutes should be spent in auscultating bowel sounds because the diminished emptying time of the bowel can mimic a silent abdomen. An orogastric tube should be inserted early during the resuscitation phase of care.

The patient should be prepared for abdominal tests. She may perceive the procedure as harmful to her baby and

TABLE 28-10 Neonatal Resuscitation Supplies and Equipment

Suction Equipment
Bulb syringe
Mechanical suction and tubing
Suction catheters, 5F or 6F, 8F, 10F or 12F
8F feeding tube and 20-mL syringe
Meconium aspirator

Bag-and-Mask Equipment
Neonatal resuscitation bag with a pressure-release valve or pressure manometer (the bag must be capable of delivering 90% to 100% oxygen)
Face masks, newborn and premature sizes (cushioned-rim masks preferred)
Oxygen source with flowmeter (flow rate up to 10 L/min) and tubing

Intubation Equipment
Laryngoscope with straight blades, No. 0 (preterm) and No. 1 (term)
Extra bulbs and batteries for laryngoscope
Endotracheal tubes, 2.5-, 3.0-, 3.5-, 4.0-mm internal diameter (ID)
Stylet (optional)
Scissors
Tape or securing device for endotracheal tube
Alcohol sponges
CO_2 detector (optional)
Laryngeal mask airway (optional)

Medications
Epinephrine 1:10,000 (0.1 mg/mL)—3-mL or 10-mL ampules
Isotonic crystalloid (normal saline or Ringer's lactate) for volume expansion—100 or 250 mL
Sodium bicarbonate 4.2% (5 mEq/10 mL—10-mL ampules
Naloxone hydrochloride 0.4 mg/mL—1-mL ampules, or 1.0 mg/mL—2-mL ampules
Dextrose 10%, 250 mL
Normal saline for flushes
Feeding tube, 5F (optional)
Umbilical vessel catheterization supplies
   Sterile gloves
   Scalpel or scissors
   Povidone-iodine solution
   Umbilical tape
   Umbilical catheters, 3.5F, 5F
   Three-way stopcock
Syringes, 1, 3, 5, 10, 20, 50 mL
Needles, 25, 21, 18 gauge, or puncture device for needleless system

Miscellaneous
Gloves and appropriate personal protection
Radiant warmer or other heat source
Firm, padded resuscitation surface
Clock (timer optional)
Warmed linens
Stethoscope (neonatal head preferred)
Tape, ½ or ¾ inch
Cardiac monitor and electrodes or pulse oximeter and probe (optional for delivery room)
Oropharyngeal airways (0, 00, and 000 sizes or 30-, 40-, and 50-mm lengths)

From American Academy of Pediatrics: *Textbook for neonatal resuscitation,* ed 4, Elk Grove Village, Ill, 2000, American Academy of Pediatrics.

should be encouraged to verbalize her fears. Reinforcing the value of the procedure as a diagnostic tool that is not harmful to the baby may ease some of the mother's fears.[66] Preparation for surgical intervention is indicated if abdominal exploration is deemed necessary.

FETAL ANOXIA. Once the mother has achieved a degree of stability, continuous fetal monitoring is ideal because any change in maternal condition can be compared with fetal well-being (see Figure 28-7). If continuous monitoring is not available and something comparable is desired, the fetal

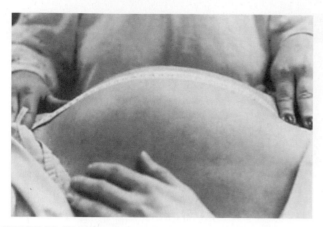

FIGURE 28-10 Measuring Fundal Height. The fundus is measured in centimeters from the symphysis pubis to the top of the fundus.

heart rate should be checked every 10 to 15 minutes or with each assessment of maternal vital signs. Because uterine perfusion is sensitive to maternal blood volume and vascular tone, the fetus may be the first to evidence shock. The only action that can be taken if the fetus is anoxic and not of viable age is to continue resuscitating the mother. A sudden change in fetal heart rate in a nonviable fetus rarely prompts a change in maternal care and at the same time is emotionally traumatic for the staff and the mother, who feel helpless in facing the probability of fetal demise. Thus continuous fetal monitoring is appropriate only once the mother is stable and if the information will be used in her care.

UTERINE INJURIES. When uterine damage is suspected, the patient's abdomen must be reassessed frequently (every 15 to 30 minutes) (see Table 28-7). Fundal height should be measured and marked on the patient's abdomen with tape or indelible marker on admission and every 30 minutes thereafter until the concern has passed (see Figure 28-10). A rise in fundal height may indicate intrauterine hemorrhage.

If a uterine laceration or tear is suspected, surgical intervention to repair the uterus is probable; disruption of the pregnancy depends on the severity of the uterine injury and on fetal assessment.

PLACENTAL ABRUPTION. As stated previously, the most common cause of fetal death after maternal death is abruptio placentae. As many as 40% to 50% of pregnant women who suffer major trauma may have an abruption.[66]

A complete abruption results in maternal shock and fetal distress. The presentation of partial or delayed abruption is not as obvious, so the patient must be observed for indications of this condition during resuscitation. The inclusion of obstetric personnel during the resuscitation is ideal because their expertise in assessing the subtle signs or symptoms of an abruption are helpful (see Table 28-8). Although there is a reported case of delayed abruption after

injury, more recent studies indicate that virtually all abruptions become evident within 6 hours.[50] A plan of care for the patient who is experiencing placental abruption is presented in Table 28-11.

The patient must be monitored for symptoms of DIC (Table 28-12). Coagulation studies should be obtained routinely, and arrangements for possible blood component therapy must be made, depending on the circumstances of the trauma.

PREMATURE RUPTURE OF MEMBRANES (PROM). The rupture of amniotic membranes may occur secondary to trauma and should be ruled out with a pelvic examination. The sterile speculum exam should be done gently. Fluid should be checked for pH and ferning. Membrane rupture can be associated with ascending infections, chorioamnionitis, preterm labor, and umbilical cord prolapse.[67] The potential for these injuries makes collaboration with obstetric personnel imperative. In addition, ultrasound procedures are indicated to determine gestational age, amniotic fluid level, and fetal status.

If the membranes rupture, the perineum and vagina should be inspected for visualization of the umbilical cord. If the umbilical cord is present, immediate interventions are indicated, depending on gestational age (Table 28-13). Rupture of membranes at or after 34 weeks is usually managed by inducing labor.

Core body temperature must be monitored closely in a patient who has PROM. If signs of amnionitis develop (fetal tachycardia, maternal tachycardia, tender uterus, or temperature higher than 38° C), consideration should be given to labor induction.

PREMATURE LABOR. Preterm labor is diagnosed by cervical change. The frequency and duration of contractions can be determined, and the patient must be assessed continually for signs of uterine and fetal distress because premature labor may indicate fetal and uterine injuries. Strict bed rest (lateral position) is essential.

Because dehydration can precipitate premature labor, the patient must be kept well hydrated. Accurate intake and output records must be maintained. After maternal hydration has been ensured and uterine and fetal injuries ruled out, preterm labor should be inhibited. The medications that inhibit labor have consequences in the trauma setting. Magnesium sulfate can decrease deep tendon reflexes and alter spinal cord assessment. Terbutaline and other β-agonists cause cardiac stimulation, including tachycardia, increased oxygen consumption, and possible hypotension. With an already confusing maternal clinical picture, these drugs make identification of maternal shock more difficult.[68] Calcium channel blockers and nonsteroidal antiinflammatory agents are often preferred for tocolysis in this setting. The patient's labor activity and cardiovascular status should continue to be monitored. If measures to inhibit labor appear unsuccessful, the obstetric and neonatal personnel should prepare for impending delivery.

TABLE 28-11 Abruptio Placentae Plan of Care

Interventions	Rationale
1. Monitor maternal vital signs every 15 minutes and fetal heart rate continuously as appropriate. Note any trends or changes.	Abruption and subsequent hemorrhage can occur after the traumatic event. Maternal hypervolemia can mask signs of shock. Fetal distress may be the first indication of maternal hemorrhage.
2. Ensure placement of two large-bore intravenous catheters and maintain aggressive fluid resuscitation as ordered.	Maternal hypervolemia can mask a 15% to 30% blood loss. Early aggressive fluid resuscitation is recommended to prevent maternal hypovolemia. Large volumes of fluid are necessary to maintain maternal hypervolemia.
3. Obtain and compare maternal laboratory values based on normal pregnancy values (include coagulation profile).	Laboratory values change acutely in pregnancy; an early, accurate baseline is essential for clinical observation. Coagulation profile is necessary because DIC is a possible complication.
4. Measure and mark fundal height on admission and every 30 minutes.	A rising fundal height may indicate intrauterine hemorrhage from abruptio placentae.
5. Monitor patient for clinical signs of abruptio placentae for 6 to 24 hours or longer. Vaginal bleeding Abdominal pain Uterine tenderness Uterine tetany or rigidity Rising fundal height Maternal shock/fetal distress	Symptoms can often be vague, and all do not necessarily occur. Abruption can occur 24 hours or more after injury.
6. Maintain continuous electronic fetal monitoring in patients beyond 20 weeks' gestation until risk of fetal distress is minimal.	Early, continuous monitoring identifies signs of abruption. Continuous monitoring can show fetal distress such as late decelerations and decreased beat-to-beat variability. Uterine contraction patterns should be noted because uterine irritability and preterm labor can indicate uterine hemorrhage.

From Smith LG: Assessment and resuscitation of the pregnant trauma patient. In Hoyt KS, Andrews J, editors: *Contemporary perspectives in trauma nursing*, Berryville, Va, 1991, Forum Medicum.

TABLE 28-12 Disseminated Intravascular Coagulation

Clinical Assessment
Uncontrolled bleeding at IV sites, from mucous membranes, and from traumatic wounds
Petechia, ecchymosis, and development of hematomas
Thrombosis of extremities evidenced by cyanosis and mottling
Organ dysfunction, including decreased urine production and impaired oxygenation

Laboratory Coagulation Value Alteration
Decreased platelet count
Prolonged prothrombin time (PT)
Prolonged partial thromboplastin time (PTT)
Decreased fibrinogen level
Prolonged clotting time

Goal of Therapeutics
Identify and eliminate cause
Restore circulating blood volume
Provide adequate amount of red blood cells for oxygen transport
Replace hemostatic components

Nursing Therapeutics
Assist in identification and resolution of underlying cause
Continued assessment of bleeding sites for changes and blood estimation
On-going assessment of organ function, including oxygenation and urine production
Administration of blood products, including whole blood or packed red blood cells, fresh frozen plasma, and platelets per physician orders
Administration of fibrinogen and cryoprecipitate per physician orders

From Eberst ME: Evaluation of the bleeding patient. In Tintinalli JE, Ruiz E, Krome RL, editors: *Emergency medical*, ed 4, New York, 1996, McGraw-Hill, 973-976.

TABLE 28-13   Immediate Treatment for Prolapsed Cord

Goal: Relieve cord compression and ensure safe urgent fetal delivery.

Nursing Intervention	Rationale
1. *Gently* insert a gloved hand into the patient's vagina, don't touch the cord if possible, and elevate the fetal presenting part. Do not remove the examining hand until the fetus is delivered.	1. If the cord is being compressed by the presenting part, this maneuver will help relieve the compression.
2. *Extreme gentle* handling of the cord is essential; avoid manipulation, compression, additional exposure of the cord to air.	2. Manipulation of the cord and its exposure to air can cause cord spasm, further compromising the fetus.
3. Position the mother in the knee-chest position and place the stretcher in Trendelenburg. (The Sims' lateral position may also be utilized.)	3. Positioning of the mother is aimed at helping to elevate the presenting part. If a long period of time passes before delivery of the fetus, the Sims' lateral position may be less tiring for the mother.
4. Prepare the patient for emergency cesarean section.	4. Sometimes these patients may have a vaginal delivery, but a cesarean section is often clinically indicated and must be done in an emergent manner.
5. Monitor the fetal heart tones with an electronic monitor.	5. Determine fetal heart rate and note effectiveness of the emergency treatment.
6. Provide emotional support to mother and family during the procedures.	6. Answering patient and family questions and explaining the procedures may help decrease anxiety.

Make sure that the emergency department has a clinical plan in place for such obstetric emergencies.
If obstetric and neonatal personnel are available, they should be notified immediately to respond to the emergency department.

From Smith LG: Assessment and resuscitation of the pregnant trauma patient. In Hoyt KS, Andrews J, editors: *Contemporary perspectives in trauma nursing*, Berryville, Va, 1991, Forum Medicum.

DIRECT FETAL INJURY. Fetal injuries such as skull and clavicular fractures and fetomaternal hemorrhage must be suspected after a pregnant woman experiences blunt abdominal trauma. The fetal fractures are caused by disruption of the maternal pelvic ring (see Figure 28-9). A pelvic fracture in a pregnant woman is more serious because of the increased vascularity of the pelvis during pregnancy and the increased risk of bleeding. Fetomaternal hemorrhage is thought to occur in as many as 25% of cases of blunt trauma.[69]

A woman who has been subjected to blunt abdominal trauma should be prepared for ultrasound and CT scan to determine the existence of fetal injuries and to approximate gestational age. The fetal heart rate should be assessed with each determination of maternal vital signs. If the fetus is of viable age and is distressed, preparation should begin for an emergency cesarean section if in utero resuscitation is unsuccessful. If fetal death has occurred, the fetus may be removed by cesarean section or allowed to remain in utero for a vaginal delivery. A dead fetus in a critically injured patient needs to be removed via a cesarean section if DIC is present and felt to be caused by abruption or if a retroplacental clot is expanding; if the clot is stable, induction is indicated.

MATERNAL AND FAMILY ANXIETY. The traumatic event and sudden hospitalization certainly cause maternal and family anxiety. The patient must be reassured that prompt, aggressive care offers the fetus the best chance for survival, and she should be kept informed of impending diagnostic tests and results. Allowing the patient to listen to

the fetal heart beat and observe ultrasound images may lessen anxious feelings. The family needs to be kept informed of the status of the mother and baby. The family members should be permitted to be with the patient. In addition to fears concerning the baby, the patient and family may experience guilt feelings about the events leading to the incident. They should be encouraged to express their feelings, and nonjudgmental support should be offered.

CASE STUDY

A 34-year-old woman was admitted to a trauma center after a motorcycle crash. She was a passenger on the vehicle and was not wearing a helmet.

On initial nursing assessment the patient had a compromised airway with blood in her nasopharynx and labored breathing with diminished breath sounds on the left. The patient was tachycardic (133 beats/min), hypotensive (88 systolic/56 diastolic), and decerebrate bilaterally.

Care focused on the ABCs of resuscitation. The patient was intubated orally, and two large-bore IVs and a left-sided chest tube were inserted. Vital signs were assessed every 5 minutes. Continued tachycardia and hypotension were noted.

Further assessment identified a rigid abdomen, an open femur fracture, and left tibia fracture. With the airway maintained by intubation and fluid resuscitation with crystalloids and blood products, the patient was taken for a CT scan and then prepared for repair of a liver laceration and fractured spleen. Patient history obtained from family at this time revealed that the patient had been pregnant approximately 14 weeks.

The patient and fetus survived through the resuscitation and months of intensive care and rehabilitative care. A healthy full-term male, small for gestational age, was delivered via cesarean section near term.

COMMENT

During resuscitation of the pregnant trauma patient, the ABCs must remain the priority. The best guarantee of fetal survival is aggressive maternal care. At 14 weeks' gestation, the fetus is not viable; therefore, continuous monitoring of the fetal heart at this time is not appropriate. Early knowledge or identification that the patient is pregnant is useful in assessing for possible uterine injuries although they are uncommon at this early gestation. Because all women of childbearing age should be considered pregnant until proven otherwise, the abdomen should be shielded during radiographic procedures and left lateral positioning should be used. Once the patient is identified as pregnant, medication use may be altered.

PENETRATING TRAUMA IN PREGNANCY: MATERNAL HEMORRHAGE, SHOCK, AND FETAL INJURY.

As pregnancy progresses, the enlarging uterus displaces the bowel and becomes the most dominant abdominal organ; thus it is more likely to be damaged in a penetrating traumatic event. After a gunshot wound or stab wound to the abdominal area, the pregnant patient should be monitored for signs and symptoms of uterine damage (see Table 28-7). In viable pregnancies, fetal heart rate must be monitored continuously and fetal activity should be assessed in conjunction with maternal assessment. Local wound exploration may be necessary, and the patient should be prepared for emergency laparotomy if the wound extends into the abdominal cavity. Operating room personnel must be informed of the patient's pregnant condition (see Intraoperative Phase).

Obstetric and neonatal personnel should be available for consultation during the surgery. The decision to empty the uterus intraoperatively is based on gestational age, fetal distress, and control of hemorrhage around the uterus.

INTRAOPERATIVE PHASE

When a pregnant trauma patient is admitted to a trauma center or emergency department, operating room personnel should be notified of the possibility of an emergency cesarean section. A general surgery pack can be opened and additional surgical equipment added (Table 28-14), or an obstetric cesarean section pack can be opened. Other useful instruments are a small French suction catheter (8 Fr) and several end clamps. Neonatal or pediatric personnel need to be in the operating suite to manage the initial resuscitation and stabilization of the newborn.

ANESTHESIA

Anesthetic management of the pregnant trauma patient requires the expertise of anesthesia personnel familiar with

TABLE 28-14	**Surgical Tools to be Added to General Surgery Pack for Cesarean Section**

Bladder blade
Obstetric forceps
Sponge sticks
De Lee suction trap and bulb syringe
Suture for uterine closure

both trauma and obstetric anesthesia. If the pregnant trauma patient requires anesthesia, the care should be planned, recognizing that these patients are unique.[70] First, they have an increased metabolic demand secondary to pregnancy. Second, there are changes in hormonal activity. And finally, there are mechanical changes caused by the enlarging uterus and breasts. The decision whether to administer regional or general anesthesia is one of many to be made before and during surgery.

When the pregnant trauma patient has multiple injuries or needs immediate surgery, general anesthesia may be the best choice. The pregnant trauma patient given general anesthesia does have an increased risk of vomiting and aspiration, which is best controlled by first emptying the stomach with a gastric tube and administering 30 ml of a nonparticulate antacid (0.3 ml sodium citrate), which increases gastric pH.[70] Cimetidine or ranitidine can be given to decrease acid production. Intubation using a cuffed endotracheal tube after rapid sequence induction with cricoid pressure and 5 minutes of preoxygenation should protect the airway and provide adequate oxygenation.

Local or spinal anesthesia may be given during pregnancy. The location of injuries; length of procedure; cardiovascular, neurologic, and psychologic status of the patient; and risk of fetal distress are all determinants of the appropriateness of local or spinal anesthesia. For example, local anesthesia is appropriate for repair of a facial laceration, whereas repair of extensive facial trauma requires general anesthesia. Lower extremity injuries resulting from trauma can be repaired with spinal or epidural anesthesia or another regional block, but general anesthesia may be more appropriate for other injuries. There is no difference in morbidity or mortality in pregnancy between regional or general anesthesia.[71] The circulating nurse must ensure that specialty drugs such as oxytocin (Pitocin) and methylergonovine maleate (Methergine) are available in the operating room suite for the anesthesia and obstetric providers.

SURGICAL PROCEDURES

OBSTETRIC PROCEDURES.

Exploratory laparotomy may be indicated to identify the type and severity of uterine injuries. Uterine lacerations, contusions, and tears are common after abdominal trauma and may need repair. Cesarean section for removal of the fetus is appropriate only if the fetus is in distress and of viable age (>24 weeks' gestation) or, if necessary, to effect adequate uterine repair.

If the fetus has died secondary to trauma and the patient is stable, a cesarean section is considered inappropriate in most instances because it burdens the mother with the probability of cesarean section as the method of delivery for future pregnancies. A critically injured patient who is hemorrhaging can develop DIC, and in this instance a cesarean section may be necessary (although the fetus is dead) to prevent additional complications (e.g., DIC, sepsis). Cesarean section for an immature infant is also considered inappropriate; here too a vaginal delivery is preferable.

When uterine rupture is identified in emergency surgery, the first task is to stop sources of hemorrhage. The removal of the fetus is left to the discretion of the physician. The fetus should be removed via a low transverse incision unless the tear is nearly large enough to remove the fetus. The fetus should be handed immediately to the neonatal personnel. When possible, the uterus is then repaired to preserve future childbearing capabilities. If there is uncontrollable hemorrhage, a hysterectomy, uterine artery embolization, or bilateral hypogastric ligation may need to be performed.[2]

NONOBSTETRIC PROCEDURES.

Abdominal laparotomy, multiple orthopedic procedures, and neurosurgery may be more common than obstetric surgery during pregnancy.

When the fetus is of viable age, the fetal heart rate may be monitored continuously during the surgical procedures to detect early signs of fetal distress if recommended by the obstetrician.

To diminish surgical time and the anesthesia risk to the fetus, multiple surgical procedures may be done simultaneously, which may require that several scrub nurses assist with the operative procedures. The perioperative nurse preparing for this contingency must notify the charge nurse of the need for additional personnel. The procedures also can be done consecutively, which requires planning by the circulating nurse. When managing lower extremity orthopedic trauma during pregnancy, several factors must be considered. Although internal fixation of fractures exposes the patient to general anesthesia, it markedly reduces the pregnant patient's length of immobility. A woman who must remain immobile during pregnancy faces the risk of developing venous thromboembolic disease; therefore, early fixation is desirable to reduce prolonged immobility.

PERIOPERATIVE NURSING CARE

PATIENT AND FAMILY FEAR AND ANXIETY.

The nurse in the operating room is in a unique position to coordinate procedures and provide a therapeutic environment for the pregnant patient. A calm preinduction environment must be maintained for the patient in the operating room, with discussions kept to a minimum. As time permits, the patient should be allowed to voice concerns and fears. The family should be kept informed of the surgical progress and fetal outcome.

IMPORTANCE OF POSITIONING.

The proper positioning or padding of a surgical patient is the primary responsibility of the operative team, including the surgeon, anesthesiologist, and perioperative nurse.[72] When a pregnant patient is in the operating room, it is a challenge to prevent the enlarging uterus from causing decreased cardiac output as a result of vena cava compression. Patient positioning in the left lateral position is ideal but probably unrealistic during surgical intervention. An alternative is to displace the uterus using a towel roll or wedge under the hip and small of the back. A second alternative is to tilt the operating table laterally. If maternal injuries prohibit both these positions, manual displacement of the uterus by a team member or with a displacer is required.

When a pregnant patient with a fetus of viable age is having surgery after trauma, the surgical table should be prepared for possible cesarean section with the addition of several surgical instruments (see Table 28-14). Neonatal personnel must be alerted, and space must be provided in the surgical suite or adjoining area for neonatal resuscitation at the time of delivery.

The circulating nurse must coordinate the intraoperative plan of care to include several disciplines (e.g., surgeons, labor and delivery nurses, neonatologists, and neonatal nurses). All these services must be ready within the operating room suite when the skin incision is made if fetal delivery is believed to be a possible outcome.

The time of birth and other birth-related details must be noted as part of routine documentation procedures. The placenta must be obtained and prepared as a specimen for pathology test procedures.

As the patient's and fetus's conditions allow, attempts should be made to provide an environment that facilitates maternal-infant bonding. If the patient is awake and the infant is alive and in no distress, the mother should be permitted to see and hold her baby.

If the infant is premature or in distress, the mother must be kept informed of the infant's progress and permitted to see the infant, even for a brief moment, if possible. If the mother is under anesthesia, she should be told about the birth as soon as she is through the postanesthesia recovery stage. The family or significant others should be permitted to see the baby when possible and kept informed of the baby's progress. Many intensive care nurseries (and labor/delivery suites) use an instant camera to take a snapshot of the infant; the photograph provides the mother with what may be her only glimpse of the child for days.

CASE STUDY

A 32-year-old woman at 38 weeks' gestation was admitted to a trauma center after being struck by an automobile. The patient was admitted directly to the operating room on a backboard with cervical collar in place for immediate intervention. The obstetric and neonatal staff were on hand in the operating room when the patient arrived.

Immediate care included insertion of large-bore intrave-

nous lines, infusion of fluids, and anteroposterior and lateral cervical spine films. Obstetric and abdominal assessment was difficult. The patient's tachycardia made it impossible to differentiate fetal heart tones. The patient's abdomen was contused, bruised, and tender to palpation. While the patient was tipped in the left lateral position, an emergency cesarean section was performed by the obstetricians and a female infant was delivered. The infant had 0/2 Apgar scores and was aggressively resuscitated and stabilized by the neonatal staff. After completion of the cesarean section by the obstetric staff, the trauma surgical team performed a laparotomy, repairing liver lacerations, splenic hematoma, and mesenteric tears.

The patient was placed in a pelvic Hoffman device, and her open fractures were irrigated and debrided. She was then moved to the critical care unit.

CRITICAL CARE PHASE

After initial resuscitation the pregnant trauma patient should be transferred to an appropriate care unit. The team approach, involving both the obstetric and the trauma staff, affords the patient the most comprehensive care. The bedside trauma nurse is the most likely person to detect subtle changes in the patient's status. It is therefore essential for the nurse to have a sound knowledge base in regard to the care of the pregnant trauma patient. The nurse assumes an important role in coordinating and integrating the care provided by the various services.

The general goal of care for the pregnant trauma patient after resuscitation is to provide aggressive maternal care while minimizing fetal stress. The patient should be kept well hydrated and provided with immediate nutritional support. Care should be focused on the immediate treatment of traumatic injuries and problems while recognizing that the patient is pregnant.

The potential for delayed obstetric complications, such as abruptio placentae and premature labor, should be considered. The critical care staff should be aware of the signs and symptoms of obstetric emergencies and of the immediate action that must be taken, and obstetric personnel must be notified (see Tables 28-7, 28-8, and 28-11). An emergency delivery plan and a neonatal resuscitation plan should be established. Maintaining active communication with both the obstetric and neonatal teams improves the quality of care.

Assessment for signs and symptoms of these obstetric complications may be difficult in the critically injured patient for a number of reasons. Sedation or an unconscious state imposes limitations on the ability to communicate with the patient. Communicating with an intubated patient may be difficult as well. After spinal cord injury, although the patient may be able to communicate, sensations that would otherwise indicate the onset of labor or signify the development of other problems may be lacking.

A communication link with the obstetric staff should be prearranged. If an obstetric complication is suspected or delivery appears imminent, the obstetric staff should be notified immediately. If the patient cannot be moved from the critical care unit, obstetric personnel should administer the appropriate treatment in the unit. Necessary emergency delivery equipment should be kept at the bedside. The potential need for neonatal personnel and emergency neonatal resuscitation equipment also should be addressed.

Collaboration with the obstetric staff is essential. As the patient's hospitalization course continues, the obstetric staff, as part of the critical care team, should monitor the status of the pregnancy and provide useful information for the staff caring for the patient. The frequency with which the obstetric personnel have direct contact with the patient depends in part on the patient's unique needs and clinical condition.

ANTEPARTUM CONCERNS

INCREASED METABOLIC DEMANDS. Good nutrition is essential during pregnancy because of the metabolic demands of the fetus, placenta, and uterus, in addition to the metabolic demands secondary to the normal physiologic changes of pregnancy. When the pregnant patient is in critical condition after traumatic injury, meeting the metabolic demands of both the pregnancy and maternal healing becomes a challenge.

Dietary consultation should be initiated on admission to the critical care unit so that the patient's nutritional requirements can be determined. Tube feeding, parenteral nutrition, or a combination of the two may be necessary to meet metabolic demands. The goal is to prevent maternal protein-calorie malnutrition. In some cases, total parenteral nutrition (TPN) may be necessary. TPN has been used successfully in selective pregnant cases.

For patients who are able to tolerate oral feedings, food preferences should be acknowledged when possible. Smaller, more frequent meals are recommended for the pregnant patient to avoid unnecessary discomfort resulting from a full stomach. The nutritional status should be assessed continually so that adjustments can be made accordingly (see Chapter 16).

MATERNAL POSITIONING. Positioning is an important aspect of nursing care and is especially important for the pregnant trauma patient. Although the patient should be turned to the left or right side to prevent compression of the vena cava and aorta by the enlarging uterus and thus improve cardiac output, a single position cannot be maintained for long periods without increasing risk of atelectasis. A turning schedule should be developed and followed to prevent the pregnant patient from remaining on her back for any length of time. The turning schedule should emphasize side-to-side turning with little, if any, time spent in the supine position. The patient's injuries may dictate the need to devise unique positioning strategies (i.e., musculoskeletal stabilization devices). Such requirements should be detailed in the patient's plan of care or pathway.

VENOUS STASIS AND POSSIBLE PULMONARY EMBOLI. The normal physiologic changes that occur during pregnancy place the pregnant woman at a greater risk for venous stasis and phlebitis. Although the true risk of venous thromboembolic disease is not known, it is thought to be increased.[59] Immobility during the critical care phase places the patient at further risk. It is therefore important for the pregnant patient to be mobilized as soon as possible to prevent such complications. Intermittent pneumatic compression of the calves is a safe and effective treatment modality that can be initiated. Low-molecular-weight heparin therapy is indicated in this patient population if there are no other contraindications for its use. Heparin does not cross the placenta and does not cause fetal bleeding or have teratogenic effects.[59]

A thorough respiratory assessment must be completed on every shift and as often as indicated. Vital signs, including pulse oximetry, must be monitored continually and arterial blood gas trends must be examined routinely during the initial postresuscitation phase.

PAIN CONTROL.   Pain control is an important aspect of every patient's care, but the pregnant patient presents a challenging situation. Pain, if not managed effectively, can cause stress to the mother and fetus and increase metabolic demands. The team approach of critical care, obstetrics, and pain specialists can determine appropriate pain management options that have minimal fetal effects.

POSTPARTUM CONCERNS

The trauma patient who has aborted or delivered during the resuscitation phase presents different concerns during the critical care phase; therefore, appropriate priorities must be established. Immediately postpartum the patient must be monitored closely for hemorrhage and shock. The potential for infection also must be considered.

Telling the patient and family of a fetal loss, although a difficult task, also must be accomplished as soon as possible, and comfort measures should be provided as needed. Most obstetric and neonatal units have a grief management team. A group such as this can be invaluable not only to the patient and her family but also to the trauma team during what, even for them, can be a very difficult time.

POSTPARTUM HEMORRHAGE.   After a normal delivery a woman commonly loses up to 300 ml of blood. This blood loss is compensated by the relative hypervolemia of pregnancy. If the bleeding exceeds 500 ml, it is considered a primary postpartum hemorrhage.[73] (It is not uncommon for clinicians to underestimate blood loss.) Uterine atony is the most common cause of postpartum hemorrhage. Therefore the critical case nurse must include postpartum care in his or her plan.

The fundus should be assessed and massaged every 15 minutes for the first hour postpartum and then every hour for at least 4 hours thereafter. A rise in fundal height, increased lochia, or a "boggy" uterus should be reported to the obstetric staff. The amount of vaginal bleeding should be monitored closely. Pad counts are often helpful in assessing the extent of bleeding. An excessive amount of bleeding should be reported to the obstetrician immediately. If hemorrhage is occurring, the fundus should be massaged vigorously while the patient is given 10 to 30 U of oxytocin in 1 L of intravenous fluid. Oxytocin should never be given as an intravenous bolus because that practice often causes hypotension. If the uterus does not become firm, the patient may be given methylergonovine, 0.2 mg intramuscularly, but this drug must be used cautiously in hypertensive patients. Continued hemorrhage may indicate a hidden vaginal or cervical problem, and the critical care nurse should prepare the patient for possible damage control surgery and, more importantly, manage the patient's hypovolemic shock state.[74]

POSTPARTUM INFECTION.   The patient's temperature should be monitored routinely. A slight elevation can be expected after delivery; however, persistent elevation should be reported. The quantity and quality of vaginal drainage (lochia) should be monitored routinely for several days. The obstetric team should be notified if a foul-smelling discharge is noted.

The perineum should be inspected routinely as well. Swelling is normal immediately after delivery but should decrease after several days. Ice should be applied directly to the perineal area to reduce swelling and alleviate local pain.

BREAST ENGORGEMENT.   If necessary, a breast binder should be obtained and applied for the patient who is planning to bottle feed or who has experienced a loss, provided that it does not restrict respiratory movement or interfere with necessary treatment activities. A snugly fitted bra can suffice.

MATERNAL GRIEVING.   When the fetus is lost during resuscitation, the decision of when to tell the mother is difficult. The father and other appropriate family members should be immediately notified. The multidisciplinary team members should collaborate in making this decision. The mother's level of consciousness and clinical condition are strong determining factors; once the mother can listen and comprehend, telling her should not be delayed. Input from family members is often helpful in determining the patient's ability to cope with such devastating news. Requests from family members should be respected and incorporated into the management plan if possible. Family members should be present when the patient is told of the loss.

During the grieving process the mother may request detailed information such as the time of birth, the baby's weight, or the color of the baby's hair. If possible, the fetus should be held in the area if it is anticipated that the mother might be able to see and hold her infant. Pictures of the baby are often helpful. The grieving process extends beyond the critical care phase. A consistent approach allows continued nursing support through all phases of care as grieving continues (see Chapter 18). Even though the mother may not request them at the time, it is appropriate to collect a lock of hair, a photograph, hand and foot prints, and baby's first cap and blanket and archive them, letting the mother know that the materials are hers whenever she wants them. Many mothers request these keepsakes after their loss.

MATERNAL-INFANT BONDING. The patient who has delivered a healthy or premature infant during the resuscitation phase of care presents an equal challenge to the critical care nurse. Every effort must be made to provide as much contact as possible between the mother and baby. The family should be encouraged to take frequent photographs of the baby to share with the mother. The mother needs to be assured that the baby is being cared for properly in the neonatal unit or at home. It might be suggested that the family keep a log of the baby's progress, which can be helpful to the mother as she becomes more stable. If the mother is not interested in the infant, however, her feelings should be accepted by the staff. The patient's injuries may be the focus of her attention during the critical care phase. During family visits, time also should be spent concentrating on the mother's injuries and concerns. Conversations should not always focus on the baby. Continued disinterest in the infant may signal excessive guilt or denial. These feelings should be explored further with the patient.

FAMILY STRESS. After the delivery process the disruption of the family unit inevitably alters role functions. Family members should be encouraged to express their needs, concerns, and problems. Appropriate referrals should be made to social service personnel as necessary. The family needs assistance in developing a plan for maternal and infant care upon discharge from the hospital.

INTERMEDIATE CARE AND REHABILITATION PHASE

The pregnant trauma patient in the intermediate care and rehabilitation phases presents a challenging nursing situation. The patient and family have had to adapt to a sudden hospitalization and perhaps months of continuous care in the critical care setting. Depending on the patient's injuries and critical care course, the adaptation process may be more profound as the patient prepares for discharge.

Team members caring for the patient during this phase may include not only obstetric personnel and trauma specialists but also physical, occupational, and speech therapists.

During the critical phase of care the primary goal was to provide aggressive maternal care with minimal fetal stress. As the pregnancy progresses and the patient's clinical condition shows continued improvement, the focus must be placed on the impending delivery. The family may begin to express fears about the fetal outcome. Changes in birthing plans must be made, and discharge planning should include delivery and home care requirements.

Concerns that existed during the critical care phase of care may carry over to the intermediate care/rehabilitation

phases. The patient's nutritional status should continue to be a primary concern. Altered mobility and pain management concerns, although less intense, may continue to require consistent nursing intervention. However, the patient's involvement in managing each of these concerns becomes more active.

If the fetus was lost during the resuscitative or critical care phase, the patient and family must now deal with that loss and the effects of the trauma on the mother. The mother may feel guilt over the loss of the baby. Depending on the events leading to the injury, other family members may feel guilt about the incident. The adjustment process may be slow and tedious, and the family needs constant support. Pictures and a description of the baby may be appropriate to share with the mother for the first time. A Christian mother may need assurance that her baby was baptized.

An assessment of how the mother and family are coping with the loss of the baby must be performed on a continual basis. Although the fetal death may have occurred weeks earlier, the rehabilitation phase may be the time when the family has the energy to focus on their grief and possible guilt. As the patient stabilizes, an obstetric staff member should meet with the patient and family to review the fetal loss and discuss future pregnancies. In the grave event that the patient's injuries required a hysterectomy to be performed, the grieving process may be prolonged as the loss of future pregnancies is mourned. Many women equate loss of the uterus with a loss of femininity and desirability, a myth shared by some men as well. Therefore the patient and family need continued counseling. Appropriate referrals should be made as needed.

LABOR AND DELIVERY PLANS

As the patient enters the third trimester, decisions should be made and plans established for the impending delivery. Initially it must be decided where labor and delivery will take place. The decision should be a collaborative one, with both the obstetric and rehabilitation staffs involved. Where the patient will receive optimal obstetric care should be a strong consideration. Transfer from the rehabilitation setting to an acute care facility may be necessary. Transportation should be arranged for either an interunit or interhospital transfer at the time a decision is made concerning delivery plans. The transportation means should be available 24 hours a day and be clearly stated in the patient's plan of care or pathway.

Signs and symptoms of labor should be assessed routinely. An organized plan of action should be included as part of the patient's pathway so that appropriate staff members are notified. All efforts should be made to ensure a smooth transfer when labor occurs.

The obstetric staff should be educated by the rehabilitation advanced practice nurse concerning the patient's current limitations. This may be accomplished during a meeting with the obstetric staff, when a patient profile may be presented. The patient's neurologic deficits and orthopedic limitations should be emphasized. If the patient has suffered a closed head injury and requires cognitive retraining, detailed information about her current level of functioning should be presented to the obstetric staff.

Orthopedic injuries that require special nursing interventions or that limit a patient's movement also should be explained. The obstetric staff may not be familiar with musculoskeletal stabilization devices such as a Hoffman apparatus and need detailed instructions.

Plans also should be made regarding alternative positions for vaginal delivery. The patient's bedside nurse and the advanced practice nurse may be able to help the obstetric staff plan alternative positions. The obstetric staff may need to be reminded of the advisability of the lateral Sims position. A birthing bed allows flexibility in patient positioning and patient accessibility during delivery.

Childbirth classes should not be neglected and need to be individualized according to the patient's special needs. The obstetric educator may need to give bedside education to the pregnant patient and father or other support person. This allows the obstetric team to become familiar with the patient's special care needs while concurrently providing the opportunity for the patient and the father to ask questions and express concerns about the upcoming labor and delivery process. If the patient has suffered a head injury, she may have difficulty understanding instructions; therefore, alternative plans may need to be made.

The importance of planning ahead for the upcoming delivery must be emphasized. The establishment of a strong, supportive relationship between the trauma and obstetric staffs fosters effective communication patterns and facilitates a smooth delivery process.

POSTPARTUM CARE

Many trauma patients, as a result of their injuries, are limited in their ability to care for themselves after delivery. This may be difficult for the postpartum nursing staff, who are not accustomed to caring for trauma patients and therefore are unfamiliar with their special care needs. Postpartum staff members should be educated by either the rehabilitative advanced practice nurse or the patient's nurse concerning the patient's ability to meet her own needs and those of the baby. Thorough attention will likely be focused on rehabilitation plans for discharge, but there must be some consideration of family planning/contraception. The patient may have become sexually active during rehabilitation, and now in the postpartum period family planning should be discussed. The obstetric staff should remind the team of this important aspect of postpartum care.

FAMILY NEEDS.   The situation is far from ideal when the newborn baby is in the nursery, the mother is in intermediate care or rehabilitation, and the family members are home. The nursing plan of care should include provisions to minimize family disruptions.

When possible, the patient should be allowed to care for her infant. At times it may be necessary for the nursing staff to offer alternative solutions if limitations imposed by the patient's injuries impede her caregiving abilities. For example, the patient may not be able to both hold and feed the baby, in which case the postpartum staff may assist the patient by holding the baby while allowing the patient to feed him or her. Early and frequent maternal-infant interaction is an important component of the bonding process; there should be open visitation rights. The attachment or bonding that occurs between a mother and a newborn is a complex, unique emotional relationship.[75] Efforts should be made to allow the mother to hold the infant or to have the infant lie by her side. Physical communication between the newborn and mother allows the newborn to utilize sensual abilities (Table 28-15) and therefore is imperative.

When the patient's needs as a trauma patient are extensive, she may be transferred back to the rehabilitation or intermediate care unit after the immediate postpartum period (first 24 hours). This may be the most practical alternative for the patient's care but produces maternal-infant separation. In this situation, every attempt should be made to arrange for regular and frequent maternal-infant interactions.

It is also necessary for the family to identify who will provide infant care in the home after the baby's discharge. If infant care cannot be provided by family members or friends on a 24-hour basis, other alternatives must be explored. Reliable and competent contractual care providers may be identified by contacting an appropriate community agency.

BREASTFEEDING.   If at all possible, the mother's desire to breastfeed should be respected and accommodated. However, because the metabolic and emotional demands on the nursing mother are intensified, the status of the patient's clinical condition should be considered carefully by the rehabilitation team before a final decision regarding breastfeeding is made. An important aspect of this decision-making process is any medications required by the mother. Virtually all maternal medications appear in breast milk, and the amount of the medication, how it is bound with breast milk, and how much the fetus absorbs are not clearly known for all medications.[58] The American Academy of Pediatrics publishes lists of drugs safe for use during pregnancy. Also the time between the mother taking

TABLE 28-15	**Parental-Infant Bonding: Newborn Sensual Responses or Abilities Used in Bonding**
Touch	Voice
Eye-to-eye contact	Entertainment
Odor	Biorhythmicity
Body warmth	

Data from Lowdermilk DL: Family dynamics after childbirth. In Bobak IM, Jensen MO, editors: *Essentials of maternity nursing*, ed 3, St. Louis, 1991, Mosby, 560-577.

the medication and the infant nursing is important. The risk/benefit ratio should be evaluated.[58] If it is determined that breastfeeding is a viable option, the mother may need assistance while nursing the baby during visits.

It is necessary for milk to be extracted from the breasts between visits; therefore a breast pump must be made available to the patient, and instruction and assistance for use should be provided as needed. Plans for milk storage and a routine for delivery to the baby must be arranged in conjunction with the family.

FETAL DEATH

When a newborn dies or a pregnancy is lost, parents should be expected and encouraged to grieve. The death of an infant or a fetus is experienced as a deep loss to the mother, father, and other family members, and a variety of reactions and responses are displayed by those who have invested emotional energy in the growth and development of the new life. A supportive and accepting attitude by the nurse caring for the patient and family are valuable as they address their feelings of grief (see Chapter 18). Consultation should be obtained from the perinatal grief management service.

COMMUNITY REINTEGRATION PHASE

Preparation of the antepartum or postpartum trauma patient for discharge begins the day the patient is admitted. After weeks or possibly months of hospitalization, the patient must be prepared to return to home and to the community. The patient's obstetric status is an important consideration when planning care during this phase. If delivery occurred during the patient's hospitalization and the baby was discharged weeks before the mother, the priorities should be focused on maternal-infant interactions. For the patient who is pregnant during the discharge planning process, special attention must be placed on prenatal care and delivery plans, with careful consideration of injuries and restrictions imposed.

PERINATAL REFERRALS

The antepartum trauma patient being discharged to home must continue to receive prenatal care. Referral should be made to the patient's private obstetrician or to a high-risk maternity center if deemed necessary. The referral should include information about the patient's injuries and clinical course, current medications and treatment interventions, limitations that may affect the delivery process, and potential postpartum home care needs.

HOME HEALTH CARE

The standard of care is to plan for the patient's early discharge and to provide for continuation of care through home health services in order to decrease medical costs. Early discharge is a possible alternative for the antepartum or postpartum trauma patient, but it requires special planning and the educational preparation of home health providers.

Weeks before the patient is discharged, contacts should be made to the agency that will provide care to the pregnant or postpartum trauma patient on her release from the hospital. Discharge planning conferences should be scheduled as needed and should include the patient, family, nurse, physician team members, social service team members, and members of the home health care team. This structured approach provides a forum for the patient's special care needs to be addressed and for the patient's and family's concerns to be expressed. These meetings also provide the opportunity for the patient and family members to begin to develop a trusting relationship with the home health care providers, thus fostering a smoother transition from hospital to home.

Family counseling sessions may be necessary. Physical or cognitive changes may alter the mother's ability to assume various role responsibilities. For example, the patient who returns home during the postpartum period with some cognitive dysfunction cannot assume full responsibility for the newborn baby. Another family member or a contractual infant care provider may be needed to assist with the care of the baby while allowing the patient short and frequent interactions with the baby to encourage maternal-infant bonding.

FUTURE TRENDS AND PREVENTION

Pregnant women in modern society usually remain active well into their third trimester of pregnancy. They continue to work outside the home and travel until the time of delivery. Driving or riding in automobiles is a reality for today's pregnant women, placing them at risk for traumatic injury. Trauma is often preventable, and public education that focuses on the proper use of safety belts during pregnancy may significantly decrease the number and severity of injuries resulting from vehicular crashes during pregnancy.

Safety belts should be worn during pregnancy because they prevent ejection from the vehicle and impact against the steering wheel and dashboard. The seat belt should be worn low or under the fundus, across the pelvis.[76,77] The shoulder harness should be worn in the normal position, not against the neck but between the breasts and off the shoulder (see Figure 28-1). Padding the seat belt for comfort is discouraged because the belt can shift upward on impact, causing injury to the thinner portion of the fundus.

Women are more likely to wear their seat belts than are men, but fewer women wear their seat belts when pregnant.[78] The major myth concerning seat belt use during pregnancy is that the belt will hurt the unborn child. Lack of safety belt use by anyone increases the chances of ejection from the vehicle, which increases chances of death twenty-fold.[78] This, in turn, dramatically increases the risk of fetal death.[79,80] Mandatory seat belt legislation and, more important, public education and enforcement may serve as major catalysts in increasing seat belt use during pregnancy and thus preventing injuries.

In addition to road traffic crashes, the number of injuries during pregnancy can be decreased by preventive measures. Pregnant women should be educated concerning the normal changes that occur during pregnancy, which may place them at risk for injuries. A pregnant woman should be encouraged to take short breaks from work or exercise. For example, if a teacher is pregnant, she should be encouraged to sit down and prop her feet up between classes. This may decrease her fatigue in early pregnancy. In late pregnancy a pregnant woman's altered gait and balance should be of concern. Safety measures should be taken by pregnant women, including care in climbing on ladders and avoiding climbing on chairs (Table 28-16).

Legislative changes may affect the incidence of penetrating injuries. Stricter weapon control measures may decrease the number of penetrating injuries sustained by the American public, including those experienced by pregnant women.

Violence and abuse are serious health problems in the United States. In the past decade, great advances have been made in research regarding this problem in the pregnant population.[13] Interventions that can protect pregnant women are being defined. We must encourage such research because it can bring about improvements in outcomes.

TABLE 28-16	**Safety Precautions During Pregnancy**
Area	**Precaution**
Home	Do not stand on stools or stepladders because it is difficult to maintain balance on a narrow base.
	Avoid throw rugs without a nonskid backing.
	Keep small items such as toys out of pathways because it is difficult for a pregnant woman to see her feet.
	Use caution when stepping in and out of a bathtub because the surface is slippery.
	Do not overload electrical circuits because it is difficult for a pregnant woman to escape a fire as a result of poor mobility.
	Do not smoke (many fires are started by a person's falling asleep with a cigarette).
	Do not take medicine in the dark (an error may be made because of limited vision).
Work	Avoid handling toxic substances.
	Avoid working to a point of fatigue, which lowers judgment.
	Avoid long periods of standing, which can lead to orthostatic hypotension and fainting.
Automobile	Use a seat belt at all times.
	Refuse to ride with anyone who has been drinking alcohol or whose judgment might be impaired.

Adapted from Pilliteri A: *Maternal and child health nursing*, ed 3, New York, 1999, JB Lippincott, 356.

NURSING RESEARCH AND EDUCATION

The first step in research on the topic of trauma during pregnancy is clarification of the scope of the problem. It is estimated that 7% of pregnant women suffer trauma or injury during pregnancy.[2] It is unclear how this figure was derived and whether it includes mild falls (which may not be recorded in hospital records) and severe trauma. Establishing a database of pregnant trauma patients—their injuries and outcomes (both fetal and maternal)—would yield a wealth of information. The National Trauma Registry lists pregnancy as a preexisting medical condition and not a specific question, which makes it hard to gather national data. There has been a great increase in studies addressing two clinical issues: predicting fetal outcome and determining how long to monitor a pregnant patient after a traumatic event.[10,49,79,80]

The results concerning how to predict fetal outcomes are not surprising. After motor vehicle crashes, unbelted women have lower birth weight infants and are more likely to give birth within 48 hours.[81] This supports the general idea that seat belts prevent injuries. It is not surprising that women with higher Injury Severity Scores have poorer fetal outcomes.[9,10] Maternal shock, as evidenced by decreased hemoglobin and increased lactate levels, is predictive.[9,10] Maternal vital signs, which can mask or mimic shock, are not always reliable indicators.

The length of time a pregnant patient requires electronic fetal monitoring has been debated. There have been documented cases of delayed abruption up to 48 hours after injury, and a second study found a high incidence of fetal death after mild maternal injury. These observations suggest that pregnant women with mild injuries should be monitored for 24 to 48 hours.[79,80] Larger, more recent studies suggest that within 4 to 6 hours of minor trauma, if there is no labor or fetal distress, monitoring can be safely discontinued.[79] It is fairly clear that in patients who do not have contractions and who have good variability in fetal heart tones the need for additional monitoring is slight. Patients who contract clearly require additional monitoring. Once the decision has been made to continue obstetric monitoring, the collaborative team of trauma and obstetric professionals must identify the appropriate nursing unit in which the patient will receive care and diligent fetal monitoring. More studies of pregnant patients who have contractions after trauma may help identify additional predictive factors for fetal complications. Investigation of the adaptation of the antepartum or postpartum trauma patient after discharge home could affect future trends in discharge planning. Because current literature is limited on this topic, it should be targeted in future nursing research endeavors.

A final area of research is how to increase seat belt use during pregnancy. Antepartum prevention strategies that increase women's seat belt use would be helpful in preventing injuries.

REFERENCES

1. National Center for Health Statistics: *Natl Vital Stat Rep* 47(18):1-30, 1999.
2. Lavery JP, Staten-McCormick M: Management of moderate to severe trauma in pregnancy, *Obstet Gynecol Clin North Am* 22:69-90, 1995.
3. Fildes J, Ried L, Jones N et al: Trauma, the leading cause of maternal death, *J Trauma* 32:643-645, 1992.
4. Stiffman L: The impact of injuries on the medical system. In Frey C, editor: *Initial management of the trauma patient,* Philadelphia, 1976, Lea & Febiger, 3-8.
5. Esposito T, Gens R, Smith LG et al: Trauma during pregnancy: a review of 79 cases, *Arch Surg* 126:1073-1078, 1991.
6. Timberlake G, McSwain N: Trauma in pregnancy: a 10-year perspective, *Am Surg* 55:151-153, 1989.
7. Drost TF, Rosemurgy AS, Sherman HF et al: Major trauma in pregnant women: maternal/fetal outcome, *J Trauma* 30:574-578, 1990.
8. Hoff WS, Amelio LF, Tinkoff GH et al: Maternal predictors of fetal demise in trauma during pregnancy, *Surg Gynecol Obstet* 172:175-180, 1991.
9. Shah K, Simons R, Holbrook T et al: Trauma in pregnancy: maternal and fetal outcomes, *J Trauma* 45(1):83-86, 1998.
10. Ali J, Yeo A, Gana TJ et al: Predictors of fetal mortality in pregnant trauma patients, *J Trauma* 42(5):782-785, 1997.
11. Jackson F: Accidental injury; the problem and the initiatives. In Buschbaum HJ, editor: *Trauma in pregnancy,* Philadelphia, 1979, WB Saunders, 1-21.
12. National Safety Council: *Injury facts,* Chicago, 1999.
13. Parker B, McFarlane J, Soeken K: Abuse during pregnancy: effects on maternal complications and birth weight in adult and teenage women, *Obstet Gynecol* 84(3):323-328, 1994.
14. Gazmararian JA, Lazorick S, Spitz AM et al: Prevalence of violence against pregnant women, *JAMA* 275:1915-1920, 1996.
15. Mauro LH, Cockrane SO, Cockrane P: Trauma and pregnancy in the urban environment, *Trauma Q* 6:69-82, 1990.
16. Sherer DM, Schenker JG: Accidental injury during pregnancy, *Obstet Gynecol Surv* 44:330-338, 1989.
17. Pepperill R, Rubinstein E, MacIsaac I: Motor car accidents during pregnancy, *Med J Aust* 1:203-205, 1977.
18. Crosby WM, King AI, Stout LC: Fetal survival following impact: improvement with shoulder harness restraint, *Am J Obstet Gynecol* 112:1101-1106, 1972.
19. Crosby WM, Costiloe JP: Safety of lap-belt restraint for pregnant victims of automobile collisions, *N Engl J Med* 284(12):632-636, 1971.
20. Straus M, Gelles R: *Physical violence in American families: risk factors and adaptations in violence in 8,145 families,* New Brunswick, NJ, 1990, Transaction.
21. Parker B, McFarlane J: Identifying and helping battered pregnant women, *Am J Matern Child Nurs* 16:161-164, 1991.
22. Parker B, McFarlane J, Soeken K: Abuse during pregnancy: effects on maternal complications and infant birth weight in adult and teenage women, *Obstet Gynecol* 84:323-328, 1994.
23. Martin SL, English KT, Clark KA et al: Violence and substance use among North Carolina pregnant women, *Am J Public Health* 86:991-998, 1996.
24. McFarlane J, Parker B, Soeken K: Abuse during pregnancy: associations with maternal health and infant birth weight, *Nurs Res* 45:37-42, 1996.
25. McFarlane J, Parker B: Safety behaviors of abused women after an intervention during pregnancy, *J Obstet Gynecol Neonatal Nurs* 27(1):64-69, 1998.
26. Akhtar MA, Mulawkar PM, Kulkarni HR: Burns in pregnancy: effect on maternal and fetal outcomes, *Burns* 20:351-355, 1994.
27. Makrouk AR, El-Feky AE: Burns during pregnancy: a gloomy outcome, *Burns* 23(7-8):596-600, 1997.
28. Esposito T: Pitfalls in resuscitation and early management of the pregnant trauma patient, *Trauma Q* 5:1-22, 1988.
29. Prasana M, Singh K: Early burn wound excision in "major" burns with "pregnancy": a preliminary report, *Burns* 22(7):234-237, 1996.
30. Ullmann Y, Blumnfeld Z, Hakim M et al: Urgent delivery, the treatment of choice in the pregnant woman with extended burn injury, *Burns* 23(2):157-159, 1997.
31. Van Hoesen KB, Camporesi EM, Moon RE et al: Should hyperbaric oxygen be used to treat the pregnant patient for acute carbon monoxide poisoning? A case report and literature review, *JAMA* 261(7):1039-1043, 1989.
32. Longo LD: The biological effects of carbon monoxide on the pregnant woman, fetus, and newborn infant, *Am J Obstet Gynecol* 129(1):69-103, 1977.
33. Longo LD, Hill EP: Carbon monoxide uptake and elimination in fetal and maternal sleep, *Am J Physiol* 232:H324-H330, 1977.
34. Silverman RK, Mortano J: Hyperbaric oxygen treatment during pregnancy in acute carbon monoxide poisoning: a case report, *J Reprod Med* 42(5):309-311, 1997.
35. Anderson H, Johnson T, Barclay M et al: Gestational age assessment, *Am J Obstet Gynecol* 139:173-177, 1981.
36. Crosby W: Trauma during pregnancy: maternal and fetal injuries, *Obstet Gynecol Surv* 29:683-697, 1974.
37. Bealsey J, Damos J, Roberts R et al: The advanced life support in obstetrics course, *Arch Fam Med* 3:1037-1042, 1994.
38. American College of Surgeons: *Advanced trauma life support for doctors,* Chicago, 1997, The College.
39. Pearlman MD: Motor vehicle crashes, pregnancy loss and preterm labor, *Int J Gynaecol Obstet* 57:127-132, 1997.
40. Valzey C, Jacobson M, Cross F: Trauma in pregnancy, *Br J Surg* 81:1406-1415, 1994.
41. Knudson M, Rozycki GS, Strear C: Reproductive system trauma. In Mattox KL, Feliciano D, Moore EE, editors: *Trauma,* New York, 2000, McGraw-Hill, 879-906.
42. Vander Veer J: Trauma during pregnancy, *Topics in emergency medicine: special aspects of trauma care* 6(1):72-77, 1984.
43. National Institutes of Health Consensus Development Conference: Prevention of venous thrombosis and pulmonary embolism, *JAMA* 256:744-749, 1986.
44. Kuhlmann RS, Cruikshank OP: Maternal trauma during pregnancy, *Clin Obstet Gynecol* 37:274-293, 1994.
45. Clark S, Cotton O, Lee W et al: Central hemodynamic assessment of normal term pregnancy, *Am J Obstet Gynecol* 161:1439-1442, 1989.
46. Jacobs H: Hypothalamus and pituitary gland. In Hytten F, Chamberlain G, editors: *Clinical physiology in obstetrics,* Oxford, 1980, Blackwell, 383-399.
47. Ma OJ, Mateer JR, DeBehnke DJ: Use of ultrasound for the evaluation of pregnant trauma patients, *J Trauma* 40(4):665-668, 1996.
48. Hauth J, Merinstein G: *Guidelines for perinatal care,* ed 4, Elk Grove Village, Ill, 1997, American Academy of Pediatrics and American College of Obstetrics and Gynecologists.

49. Pearlman MD, Tintinalli JE, Lorenz RP: A prospective controlled study of outcome after trauma during pregnancy, *Am J Obstet Gynecol* 162:1502-1510, 1990.

50. Goodwin TM, Brun MT: Pregnancy outcome and fetomaternal hemorrhage after noncatastrophic trauma, *Am J Obstet Gynecol* 162:665-671, 1990.

51. Higgins S, Garite T: Late abruptio placenta in trauma patients: implications for monitoring, *Obstet Gynecol* 63:105-109, 1984.

52. Pearlman MD, Tintinalli JE, Lorenz RF: Blunt trauma during pregnancy, *N Engl J Med* 323:1609-1613, 1990.

53. Emery CL, Moreway LF, Chung-Park M et al: The Kleihauer-Betke test: clinical utility, indication, and correlation in patients with placental abruption and cocaine use, *Arch Pathol Lab Med* 119:1032-1037, 1995.

54. Manning FA: Fetal biophysical assessment by ultrasound. In Creasy RK, Resnick R, editors: *Maternal-fetal medicine: principles and practice,* ed 2, Philadelphia, 1989, WB Saunders.

55. Shnider S, Levinson G: Obstetric anesthesia. In Miller R, editor: *Anesthesia,* New York, 1986, Churchill Livingstone.

56. Wagner LK, Leslie RG, Saldona LR: *Exposure of the pregnant patient to diagnostic radiations,* Philadelphia, 1985, JB Lippincott, 1-34.

57. Mann FA, Nathens A, Langer SG et al: Communicating with the family: the risks of medical radiation to concept uses in victims of major blunt-force torso trauma, *J Trauma* 48(2):354-357, 2000.

58. Briggs GG, Freeman RF, Yaffe S: Drugs in pregnancy and lactation, ed 4, Baltimore, 1994, Williams & Wilkins, xi-xvii.

59. Gensburg J, Hush J: Use of antithrombotic agents during pregnancy, *Chest* 114:5245-5305, 1998.

60. Pearse CS, Magrina JF, Finley BE: Use of MAST suit in obstetrics and gynecology, *Obstet Gynecol Surv* 37:416-422, 1984.

61. Gunning J: For controlling intractable hemorrhage, the gravity suit, *Contemp Obstet Gynecol* 22:23-32, 1983.

62. Esposito TJ, Gens DR, Gerber-Smith L et al: Evaluation of blunt abdominal trauma occurring during pregnancy, *J Trauma* 29:1628-1632, 1989.

63. Curry J, Quintana J: Myocardial infarction with ventricular fibrillation during pregnancy treated by direct current defibrillation with fetal survival, *Chest* 58:82-84, 1970.

64. Songster G, Clark S: Cardiac arrest in pregnancy: what to do, *Contemp Obstet Gynecol* 26:141-155, 1985.

65. DePace NL, Betesh JS, Kotler MN: Postmortem cesarean section with recovery of both mother and offspring, *JAMA* 248:971-973, 1982.

66. Hill D, Lense J: Abdominal trauma in the pregnant patient, *Am Fam Phys* 53(3):1269-1274, 1996.

67. Towery R, English P, Wisner D: Evaluation of pregnant women after blunt injury, *J Trauma* 35(5):731-735, 1993.

68. Henderson S, Mallon W: Trauma in pregnancy, *Contemp Issues Trauma* 16(1):209-228, 1998.

69. Rose PG, Strohm PL, Zuspan FP: Fetomaternal hemorrhage following trauma, *Am J Obstet Gynecol* 153:844-847, 1985.

70. Mokriski BLK, Malinov AM: Anesthesia for the pregnant trauma patient, *Probl Anesth* 4(3):530-540, 1990.

71. Sendak M: Anesthesia in pregnancy, *Emerg Med* 18:111-131, 1986.

72. Association of Operating Room Nurses: *Standards, recommended practices, and guidelines,* Denver, 1998, The Association, 265-266.

73. Chamberlain G, Steer P: Obstetrical emergencies, *Br Med J* 318(7194):1342-1345, 1999.

74. Moice K, Belfont M: Damage control of the obstetric patient, *Surg Clin North Am* 77(4):834-852, 1997.

75. Bobak I, Jensen M: *Essentials of maternity nursing,* St. Louis, 1991, Mosby, 560-577.

76. American College of Obstetricians and Gynecologists: Automobile passenger restraints for children and pregnant women, *ACOG Tech Bull* 16(15), 1991.

77. Tringa G: Medical aspects of seatbelt usage, *J Traffic Med* 8:32-35, 1980.

78. Agran P, Dunkle D, Winn D et al: Fetal death in motor vehicle accidents, *Ann Emerg Med* 16:1355-1358, 1987.

79. Dahmus MA, Sibai BM: Blunt abdominal trauma: Are there any predictive factors for abruptio placentae or maternal-fetal distress? *Am J Obstet Gynecol* 169(4):1054-1059, 1993.

80. Wolf M, Alexander B, Rivara F et al: A retrospection cohort study of seat belt use and pregnancy outcome after a motor vehicle crash, *J Trauma* 34(1):116-119, 1993.

81. Biester EM, Tomich PG, Esposito TJ et al: Trauma in pregnancy: normal Revised Trauma Score in relation to other markers of maternofetal status: a preliminary study, *Am J Obstet Gynecol* 176(6):1206-1212, 1997.

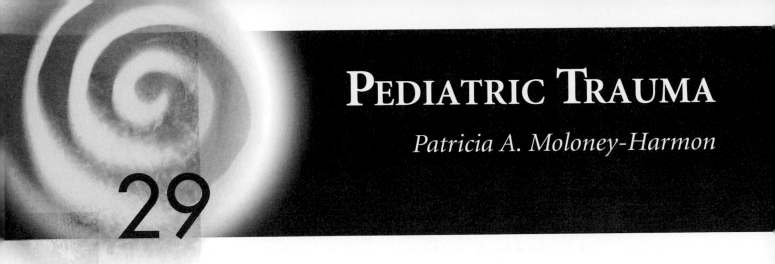

PEDIATRIC TRAUMA

Patricia A. Moloney-Harmon

29

Trauma is the leading cause of death in children from 1 to 14 years of age. In addition, each year another 100,000 children suffer permanent disability from injury.[1] But the impact of pediatric trauma extends far beyond statistics and is often seen in the tragedy that the family and society must endure. Therefore nurses must be able to recognize the patterns of pediatric injury and the appropriate treatment.

The purpose of this chapter is to explain the similarities and differences between critically ill children and adults and to bring the nurse up to date on the practical management of the pediatric trauma patient. The pathophysiologic mechanism of traumatic injuries is basically the same for children and adults. In many respects, however, the management of trauma in children differs from that in adults. This chapter describes in detail appropriate assessment and management strategies in caring for a critically injured pediatric patient through the resuscitation, critical care, and intermediate care/rehabilitation phases of care. Special emphasis is placed on nursing management considerations as they pertain to the child rather than on specific injury types. Refer to other sections of the book for injury-specific information.

Nurses often have the primary responsibility for recognizing and interpreting changes in the child's condition. The nurse must therefore understand how the child's normal circulating blood volume, cardiac output, thermoregulation, fluid and electrolyte requirements, and renal function are different from the adult's. Small variations may cause significant changes in the child's condition. These changes must be immediately recognized and acted on by the nurse. The intent of this chapter is to provide a systematic framework that allows nurses to relate to the pediatric trauma patient on the basis of the unique physiologic and psychologic dynamics inherent in this age group.

EPIDEMIOLOGY/INCIDENCE

In the United States, children between the ages of 1 and 19 years are more at risk of dying from injury than from all other diseases combined. Injury in this population is also the leading cause of disability.[1] The single largest cause of all trauma-related deaths is motor vehicle incidents. Other causes of traumatic injury in children include burns, drownings, poisonings, firearms, falls, and abuse.

Two of three childhood traumatic incidents occur in males. The peak unintentional injury age range is between 4 and 12 years, with the highest incidence at 8 years. The reason is because children in this age group are starting school, and parents generally are allowing them to experience some independence. Unintentional injury is not the leading cause of death in children under 1 year of age; however, a recent study demonstrated 32.1 injury deaths per 100,000 infant years.[2]

PATTERNS OF INJURY

The most common injuries seen in children are blunt as opposed to penetrating injuries. At least 80% of life-threatening injuries in children occur from blunt trauma.[3] Blunt injuries are associated with rapid deceleration, which can occur in automobile incidents or with direct blows resulting from child abuse or contact sports activities. Blunt injuries can complicate the management of the child because they are commonly associated with multiple injuries, including head injuries.[1] Few signs of injury may be visibly apparent after blunt trauma, but life-threatening internal damage may result. Nurses need to exercise a high index of suspicion when caring for these children.

Penetrating injuries represent approximately 20% of pediatric trauma. These are not as difficult as blunt injuries to evaluate and manage in children because the injury is obvious and therefore appropriate interventions may be determined and initiated earlier. After the child has been totally evaluated and has relatively stable vital signs, preparation for surgical exploration usually begins.

The anatomy of children renders them especially vulnerable to traumatic injury. The head of the child is proportionately larger in relation to body mass as compared with these proportions in an adult; therefore the child's head is especially vulnerable to injury. Head injury is the most common cause of traumatic death in children.[4]

In pedestrian trauma, injuries to the left side of the patient are predominant, perhaps because vehicles are driven on the right side of the road in the United States. Skeletal injuries usually involve long bones, especially of the lower limbs.[5] Chest injuries generally occur as a result of blunt trauma. Because of differences in the child's compliant chest wall, rib fractures and flail chest are less common than in adults, but pulmonary contusions are more frequent.[5] Injuries to the liver and spleen are the most common blunt abdominal injuries seen in children; other injury sites include the bowel and pancreas. Because the kidneys in children are less protected and more mobile than in an adult, genitourinary system injuries often involve the kidneys, and less frequently, the bladder and urethra.[5]

TRAUMA AND CHILD ABUSE

Child abuse and neglect are the causes of approximately 4000 deaths a year in the United States. It is estimated that an overwhelming 2.9 million children in our population experience some form of child abuse and neglect.[6] Child abuse and neglect are broadly defined as the maltreatment of children and adolescents by their parents, guardians, or other caretakers. The nurse has two main responsibilities in such cases: detecting and reporting. The laws on child abuse reporting are clear. In all states it is mandatory for nurses to report suspected cases of child abuse and neglect to the local protective service agency. The law protects health professionals from liability suits if suspicion proves to be wrong. Reluctance to report such information can lead to a recurrence of abuse and injury. The opportunity to help these children lies in the ability of the emergency department staff not only to appropriately treat the child but also to recognize the recurring nature of the underlying problem.

An important facet of the evaluation of pediatric trauma should be a careful examination of the child for other signs that might suggest the possibility of intentional or inflicted injury. Inconsistencies between the trauma history and the injuries sustained should alert the nurse to potential child abuse.[7] Diagnostic signs of child abuse include orbital ecchymosis in the absence of a clear causative factor. This is a serious concern because of the high incidence of subdural hematoma formation associated with vigorous shaking or jarring of an infant's head. Skull fractures, particularly if out of magnitude with the history, should always alert one to the possibility of inflicted injury. The general appearance and nutritional state of the child also may suggest intentional injury. Other diagnostic signs may include cigarette burns; unusual bruising, especially over the back or soft tissue areas of the body; and any situation in which the circumstances are not clearly defined as causative of the injury. Old fracture sites revealed on radiographic examination also should raise suspicion. Careful examination of the genitalia and anal areas always need to be part of the evaluation of the injured child. Any injury in these areas should raise suspicion of sexual abuse.

In addition to detecting and reporting, the nurse's role is to give the child the necessary emergency treatment and protection while at the same time helping to alleviate the parents' distress. Informing the parents of the need for the child's treatment and protection and verbalizing an interest in helping the parents through the crisis are important roles for the nurse. This is a difficult task for nurses who are experiencing feelings of anger toward the parents; therefore, it is imperative for nurses to explore and come to terms with their own feelings regarding child abuse before therapeutic intervention can be expected. A helping relationship needs to be established early with the family to lay the groundwork for future intervention. If intentional injury is raised as a legitimate consideration in the causation of the child's injury, the child protection team must be alerted so that they can help clarify the circumstances surrounding the injury.

PREVENTION STRATEGIES

With the recognition that nonintentional injury and death are major public health problems, nurses play a major role in injury prevention. Based on clinical experiences and the identification of patterns and trends related to pediatric trauma, nurses' contributions are paramount in all multidisciplinary efforts to determine sound trauma prevention strategies.[5]

Most children who are killed or injured in automobile-related mishaps are passengers. These casualties occur when an automobile collides with another vehicle or a fixed object. The use of restraints decreases fatalities from motor vehicle crush injuries by 13% to 46%.[8] By communicating these facts, health professionals involved in the care of pediatric patients have been instrumental in promoting the passage of safety restraint laws in all states. Because nurses are frequently in teaching roles, they are instrumental in bringing the legislation to the user level by instructing parents in how to protect their children and how to use restraint devices correctly.

Bicycle injuries are now the most common cause of injuries requiring treatment in an emergency department. Epidemiologic studies indicate that 76% of deaths resulting from bicycle crashes involving either motorized or nonmotorized vehicles were the result of severe head injuries. The single most effective way to make bicycle riding safer is to insist that riders wear helmets. Improved bicycle design also contributes to the reduction of injury and injury severity.

Drowning, the fourth leading cause of death in children, is most common in children under 4 years of age and in adolescent males 15 to 19 years of age.[9] Prevention strategies to decrease the incidence of drowning include teaching parents never to leave an infant or young child alone during a bath, providing supervised swimming instruction for children, and installing safety fences around pools. Cardiopulmonary resuscitation (CPR) helps to decrease the number of deaths if initiated early and executed effectively; therefore, CPR education is paramount. Adult supervision, however, is by far the most effective defense strategy, although difficult to teach and impossible to legislate.

Fire-related deaths among children can be reduced in several ways. Because many fires are started by ignited cigarettes, the incidence of fires could be decreased by manufacturing cigarettes that self-extinguish. Parents also should be taught never to leave small children home alone, even for brief periods, and matches and lighters need to be kept out of the reach of children. Smoke detectors in the home can provide early warning of fires and are therefore considered valuable devices in preventing asphyxiation and burns. Nurses are instrumental in preventing fire-related injuries by teaching parents the necessity of having smoke detectors in the home and the importance of checking the battery routinely. Home fire drills involving all family members are important to establish and reinforce safe practices.

Falls by children are not uncommon, and even though many are minor, they account for a large number of injuries and deaths each year. Deaths are often caused by falls from second-story windows by wandering toddlers. Nurses need to educate parents about the importance of constant adult supervision in and around the home, the installation of safety gates at the tops and bottoms of stairwells, and diligent use of window locks.

Playground safety is also an area that requires community education and awareness. Playground design should be in accordance with available safety standards. Standards include using wood chips instead of concrete on the ground, reducing the height of equipment, and replacing metal pieces with plastic or wood.

RESUSCITATION PHASE

The priorities of management for the pediatric trauma patient during the resuscitation phase are affected by a broad spectrum of factors. Immediate interventions depend on the severity of injuries and the critical nature of the patient's responses. The primary and secondary surveys provide a structured and systematic approach to the physical assessment of the patient. Other factors that must be considered are the growth and development patterns of the child. In addition, the child's family must be cared for as they face the traumatic experience with their child.

ASSESSMENT CONSIDERATIONS

PEDIATRIC TRAUMA HISTORY. A thorough history is obtained during the early evaluation of a child who has sustained multiple injury and is included as part of the nursing database. The purpose of the history is to determine and record the nature, location, and time of injury. The history of the injury is crucial to the child's treatment and begins at the scene of the incident. The history includes events leading to the incident, mechanism and time of injury, clinical course after the injury, contamination of wound sites, previous history of chronic illness or injury, allergies, medications, and time of the last meal eaten before injury. The American College of Surgeons recommends taking an AMPLE history[10]:

A = allergies
M = medications
P = past medical history
L = last meal
E = events leading to the accident

An allergy history is obtained in children, as with all patients. The parents are asked if the child is allergic to any medicine, adhesive tape, latex, or environmental substances.

The nurse establishes if the parents have given the child any medications recently. In addition, the nurse determines if the child takes medication routinely for diabetes, seizures, lung disease, cardiac disorders, or other disease entities.

In gathering the medical history, the nurse establishes if the child is under medical care for reasons other than routine well-child health care. Important questions include: Does the child have any chronic illness, such as diabetes, seizures, lung disease, or heart disease? Has the child been hospitalized previously? If so, for what reason? Are the child's immunizations up-to-date?

Determination of when the child's last meal was eaten is important if the child needs to be intubated, sedated, or needs surgery.

Finally, whatever the presenting injuries, specific questions can give more insight into the extent of the injuries and sequelae or potentially overlooked injuries. What were the events leading to the injury? What were the mechanisms and time of injury?

Because of limitations in verbal and communication skills, neither the infant nor the very young child can give a complete history, but it is useful to obtain whatever information is possible from the child. Younger children are likely to remember recent events. Events somewhat further back in time may be better remembered by a parent or caretaker, even though their accuracy may be clouded by their emotional state after the injury. In general, once a child reaches school age, obtaining a history becomes considerably easier.

The nurse begins to establish a relationship with the family and the child during this information-gathering session. As the nurse gathers this information, serious consideration must be given to the fact that this crisis has disrupted the entire family unit and that fear and anxiety prevail. The family needs as much feedback from the medical and nursing professionals as possible on an ongoing basis. Establishing a supportive rapport with the family during this initial phase helps to foster a closer working relationship among the child, the parents, and the health care team members throughout the child's hospitalization. Early interactions with family members and the information presented should be documented in the nurse's notes. An assessment of the family's initial reactions, responses, concerns, and coping abilities serves as a baseline for other nurses who continue to care for the patient and family.

GROWTH AND DEVELOPMENT

Physical Development.   The initial encounter with the child includes an assessment of the child's growth and physical development, which helps to identify existing alterations that determine the approach used during the examination. This assessment is done quickly because of the critical nature of the child's injury. An accurate estimate of the size and weight (Table 29-1) is made as soon as possible so that therapy can be initiated. When time allows, however, an exact weight should be obtained because medical treatment that involves drug and fluid therapy, calculated on a per-kilogram basis, must be accurately determined.

Psychosocial Factors.   The multisystem injuries and hospitalization of a critically ill child are devastating for the child and the family. Nurses have the responsibility to do everything possible to minimize the psychologic trauma that accompanies this traumatic incident. Because stressful medical situations can become the focus of fears and the source of new symptoms for the child, pediatric emergency care must include not only physical management but also consideration of the child's psychologic reactions to the illness. By relying on basic age-appropriate developmental characteristics, nurses can be astute to the general psychologic responses expected of the child. Table 29-2 summarizes the essential issues in this assessment process based on the age of children; their state of language, motor, and social development; and related fears. Appropriate nursing implications are also outlined.

General Principles.   Several general principles are applicable when working with a pediatric patient regardless of the age or developmental level of the child. For most children, security in the world comes from their parents. Wanting their parents with them may be the children's first priority, even above that of relieving pain. When taking care of children, the nurse should observe the following guidelines:

- Let the child know someone will call the parents, and tell the child when they arrive.
- If the child brought a toy, let the child hold it.
- When speaking to the patient, get down to the child's eye level so that the child can see your face. Speak clearly and slowly so the child can hear you.
- Never assume the child has understood you. Find out by questioning the child.
- Do not let the child witness treatment given to a seriously ill adult. Take the time to segregate the child to avoid additional emotional trauma.

TABLE 29-1   Approximate Weights for Children

Age	Weight (kg)
Newborn	1
6 months	6
1 year	10
3 years	15
5 years	20
8 years	25
10 years	30
16 years	50

TABLE 29-2   Developmental Approach to Pediatric Emergency Care Patients

Age (yr)	Important Development Issues	Fears	Appropriate Interventions
Infancy (0-1)	Minimal language Feel an extension of parents Sensitive to physical environment	Stranger anxiety	Keep parents in sight Avoid hunger Use warm hands Keep room warm
Toddler (1-3)	Receptive language more advanced than expressive See themselves as individuals Assertive will	Brief separation Pain	Maintain verbal communication Examine in parent's lap when possible Allow some choices when possible
Preschool (3-5)	Excellent expressive skill for thoughts and feelings Rich fantasy life Magical thinking Strong concept of self	Long separation Pain Disfigurement	Allow expression Encourage fantasy and play Encourage participation in care
School age (5-10)	Fully developed language Understanding of body structure and function Able to reason and compromise Experience with self-control Incomplete understanding of death	Disfigurement Loss of function Death	Explain procedures Explain basic pathophysiology and treatment Project positive outcome Stress child's ability to master situation Respect physical modesty
Adolescence (10-19)	Self-determination Decision making Peer group important Realistic view of death	Loss of autonomy Loss of peer acceptance Death	Allow choices and control Stress acceptance by peers Respect autonomy

From Fleisher GR, Ludwig S: *Textbook of pediatric emergency medicine*, Baltimore, 1993, Williams & Wilkins.

- Never lie to the child. Be honest about the possibility of pain during the physical examination. If the child asks about being sick or hurt, tell the truth, but give reassurance by telling the child that you are there to help. It is important to smile at the child. If you appear calm and in control, it is more reassuring to the child.
- Touch the child and hold the child's hand. Acceptance of you by the child shows in the reaction to your touch. Talking with the child and smiling can provide comfort.
- Always explain to the child what you are going to do during the primary and secondary surveys.
- Do not try to explain the entire procedure at once. Explain one step, do the procedure, then explain the next step.
- Children of all ages should be respected for feelings of bashfulness and modesty. In particular, school-age children and adolescents are modest about exposing their bodies to strangers. Keep all children covered with a hospital gown, only allowing exposure of different body parts during the physical examination.

Children are a unique patient population because they are in a dynamic state of growth and development. By practicing these few general principles while considering appropriate developmental tendencies, the nurse can lessen the trauma that the child experiences. Some children, however, are not able to remain calm and cooperative for the physical examination and interventions. Sedation may be necessary, based on the needs of the child and the child's physiologic stability.

PHYSICAL EXAMINATION. Nurses caring for children must be familiar with the normal physiologic parameters for children at different ages. A small child responds differently to major injuries than an older child or adult. Special considerations that can compromise management in children include less respiratory reserve, development of abdominal distention, fluid/electrolyte and caloric imbalances, differences in blood volume, and heat loss.

Vital Signs. Pulses are obtained at the radial, brachial, carotid, or femoral arteries and are counted for a full minute because there are often irregularities in an anxious or injured child. A child under normal circumstances has a faster heart rate and respiratory rate and a lower blood pressure than an adult. Tachycardia is usually found in children with such conditions as fever and shock and during the initial response to stress. Bradycardia can result from increased intracranial pressure, spinal cord injury, hypoxia, hypothermia, and hypoglycemia. Table 29-3 provides normal heart rates for children.

The respiratory rate is also counted for a full minute because of irregular breathing patterns. Tachypnea is a normal initial response to stress in children. If a stressed child does not hyperventilate, head injury, spinal cord injury, or other reasons such as a distended abdomen are

considered and investigated. Table 26-4 provides normal respiratory rates for children.

Blood pressures should be obtained using a cuff size that is no less than half and no more than two thirds the length of the upper arm. If pediatric cuffs are not available, an adult cuff can be used on the child's thigh. In the field a palpable systolic blood pressure is adequate; precious time should not be wasted to obtain a diastolic reading. The normal systolic blood pressure for individuals from 1 to 20 years of age is 80 plus two times the age in years. The diastolic pressure should be approximately two thirds the normal systolic pressure. Table 29-5 provides the normal blood pressure ranges in children.

Fear and distress can increase the child's heart rate and respiratory rate. The nurse may have to differentiate between emotional stress and hypoxia or shock. In addition, referring back to the medical history is important to provide insight into abnormal vital signs. For example, a pediatric trauma patient may have a congenital heart defect and normally be tachypneic; if that child has a normal respiratory rate, ventilatory assistance may be required.

Respiratory Reserve. The infant has less respiratory reserve than the adult for several reasons: (1) the infant's

TABLE 29-3	**Normal Heart Rates in Children**
Age	Beats/Min
Infants	120-160
Toddlers	90-140
Preschoolers	80-110
School-age children	75-100
Adolescents	60-90

TABLE 29-4	**Normal Respiratory Rates in Children**
Age	Breaths/Min
Infants	30-60
Toddlers	24-40
Preschoolers	22-34
School-age children	18-30
Adolescents	12-16

TABLE 29-5	**Normal Pediatric Blood Pressure Ranges**	
Age	Systolic (mm Hg)	Diastolic (mm Hg)
Infants	74-100	50-70
Toddlers	80-112	50-80
Preschoolers	82-110	50-78
School-age children	84-120	54-80
Adolescents	94-140	62-88

TABLE 29-6	**Calculation of Maintenance Fluids (per 24 Hours) in Children**
Weight (kg)	**Kg Body Weight Formula**
0-10	100-120 ml/kg
11-20	1000 ml for the first 10 kg and 50 ml/kg for each kg over 10 kg
21-30	1500 ml for the first 20 kg and 25 ml/kg for each kg over 20 kg

vital capacity is smaller, (2) the chest wall is soft because the ribs and sternum are cartilage, and (3) the ribs are horizontal, with poorly developed intercostal muscles.

An infant whose lung capacity is decreased compensates by increasing the respiratory rate and using auxiliary respiratory muscles, as evidenced by retractions. Retractions are an early sign of respiratory difficulty and compromise the infant's tidal volume. Most of the child's normal respiratory activity is affected by abdominal movement until age 6 or 7 years, and there is very little intercostal motion. A child who develops a paralytic ileus after blunt abdominal trauma may develop respiratory distress because abdominal distention elevates the diaphragm and interferes with pulmonary function. As a result, children in respiratory distress who are spontaneously breathing should be treated in semi-Fowler position when spinal injury has been ruled out.

Fluid and Electrolyte Balance.   The daily fluid requirement of the child is larger per kilogram of body weight than that of an adult because the child has greater insensible water losses per unit of body weight. This is because of the fact that the child has a larger surface area and a higher metabolic rate than the adult. Even with these factors, the absolute amount of fluid required by a child is small. Nurses must be alert to the fluid volume administered to the child to avoid overhydration. The calculation of maintenance fluid requirements is shown in Table 29-6.

If the child's fluid intake is adequate, the urine volume should average 0.5 to 1 ml/kg/hr. The nurse keeps accurate records of all possible sources of fluid loss, including laboratory blood samples, blood loss from any source, gastric drainage, vomitus, and diarrhea.

The child's higher metabolic rate dictates a requirement of more calories per kilogram of body weight. The critically ill child, even if immobile, still requires most of the normal maintenance calories if not more. This is discussed in more detail in the critical care phase.

Some forms of electrolyte imbalance are more likely to occur in children than in adults. Serum glucose, calcium, and potassium are monitored closely in the child. Infants have high glucose needs because of high metabolic rates and low glycogen stores; therefore the infant can become hypoglycemic quickly during periods of stress. A $D_{25}W$ bolus (0.5-1.0 gm/kg) helps correct this. Changes in serum potassium concentration can occur with changes in acid-base status and diuretic administration. The critically ill child does not seem to be as sensitive to hypokalemia as the adult, so cardiac arrhythmias from hypokalemia are not often seen in pediatric patients until the serum potassium is less than 3 mEq/L.[11] Ventricular fibrillation is rarely seen in pediatric patients but may result from severe hypokalemia or hyperkalemia. There are also reports of ventricular fibrillation produced by sudden blunt force trauma to the chest.[12]

The administration of citrate phosphate dextran (CPD) blood produces precipitation of serum ionized calcium.[13] An infant who requires frequent transfusions is at risk for developing hypocalcemia, a condition that can interrupt normal cardiovascular function. The ionized calcium levels are monitored closely so that calcium supplements can be administered as needed.

The child's circulating blood volume (80 ml/kg) is larger per unit of body weight than the adult's. The loss of a small amount of blood in a child, however, is proportionately more significant than in an adult because of the child's miniature total blood volume and may potentially lead to hypovolemic shock. A closed fracture of the femur, for example, in a 10-year-old may result in a loss of 300 or 400 ml of blood. The same amount of blood loss in an adult may not cause a significant problem, whereas in the child this may represent 15% to 25% of the total circulatory blood volume. The child's total circulating blood volume is calculated on admission, and all blood lost as a result of hemorrhage or drawn for laboratory tests is accurately tabulated and recorded.

Body Temperature.   Major heat losses can occur in a young child who is unclothed for even a short time. Infants and young children have a large surface area and therefore lose more heat to the environment through radiation, conduction, convection, and evaporation. During resuscitation, children are often unclothed and exposed, losing much of their body heat and therefore experiencing a lowered core body temperature. Hypothermia hinders the resuscitation attempt by causing apnea, coagulopathies, progressive metabolic acidosis, decreased cardiac output, and ventricular arrhythmias. The nurse can minimize this stress by monitoring the child's temperature rectally, keeping the child covered as much as possible, using heat lamps and warming blankets, and warming all fluids before infusion.

ASSESSMENT IN HEAD TRAUMA.   Head injuries are common in children. Each year approximately 22,000 acutely brain-injured children in the United States die and another 29,000 are left with a permanent disability.[14] In children the brain tissues are thinner, softer, and more flexible; the head size is greater in proportion to the body surface area; and a relatively larger proportion of the total blood volume is in the child's head. Thus the child's response to head injury differs significantly from that of an adult. Mass lesions after head injuries are less common. Intracranial hypertension and cerebral hypoxia occur commonly in children, rendering them highly susceptible to secondary brain injury.

TABLE 29-7 **Glasgow Coma Scale**			
Response	**Adults and Children**	**Infants**	**Points**
Eye opening	No response	No response	1
	To pain	To pain	2
	To voice	To voice	3
	Spontaneous	Spontaneous	4
Verbal	No response	No response	1
	Incomprehensible	Moans to pain	2
	Inappropriate words	Cries to pain	3
	Disoriented conversation	Irritable	4
	Oriented and appropriate	Coos, babbles	5
Motor	No response	No response	1
	Decerebrate posturing	Decerebrate posturing	2
	Decorticate posturing	Decorticate posturing	3
	Withdraws to pain	Withdraws to pain	4
	Localizes pain	Withdraws to touch	5
	Obeys commands	Normal spontaneous movement	6
Total score			3-15

From Nichols D, Yaster M, Lappe D et al: *In golden hour: the handbook of advanced pediatric life support,* St. Louis, 1991, Mosby, 180.

Secondary brain injury is, in part, considered to be more treatable than primary brain injury. This contributes to a significantly better outcome in the pediatric patient. Mortality in children with severe head injuries is 6% to 10%, as opposed to 30% to 50% in the adult with severe head injuries.[15] Expandable fontanelles and opening sutures allow increased room for swelling, providing an advantage for the head-injured infant. The primary disadvantage in the evaluation of the head-injured child is the developmentally imposed limitation in verbal expression, which can complicate assessment endeavors.

Neurologic Assessment. A thorough neurologic assessment should be done as soon as possible after the primary survey is complete and initial stabilization interventions are underway. The neurologic examination consists of the determination of level of consciousness, pupillary response, and motor response.

Evaluation of the level of consciousness after a head injury is probably the single most important aspect of the neurologic assessment but often the most difficult to perform in an infant or young child. Because level of consciousness means different things to different people, a uniform system like AVPU or the Glasgow Coma Scale should be used. The AVPU method is described below:

A Patient is *alert*
V Patient responds to *vocal* stimuli (This unfortunately is of little value in a very young child.)
P Patient responds to *painful* stimuli
U Patient is *unresponsive*

The Glasgow Coma Scale (GCS) is used worldwide as a neurologic assessment tool. The scale consists of three sections, each of which measures a separate function of the person's level of consciousness: the patient's eye opening response, verbal response, and motor response. The total score ranges from 3 to 15, with the higher scores indicating more intact neurologic function. However, because it is difficult to use this tool to evaluate verbal response in infants and preverbal children, many clinicians use a modified GCS (Table 29-7).[16]

With children, as with adults, pupil reactivity, size, shape, and symmetry are responses used to assess brainstem function. When increased intracranial pressure develops, the oculomotor nerve is compressed by general expansion of the brain, an intracranial lesion, or herniation of the brain; the pupil dilates but does not constrict in response to light. Eye movements are also noted. Abnormal eye movements include deviation of one or both eyes from midline and back and forth movements.

Any difficulty in movement of the extremities is evaluated; the nature of the movement is described as spontaneous or in response to pain. The extremity in which the response is elicited is also recorded. The child with increased intracranial pressure has a decrease in motor function and abnormal posturing or reflexes. Babinski's reflex is positive when the toes fan out and the great toe moves dorsally. The reflex is assessed by scratching the sole of the foot with an object such as the blunt tip of a tongue depressor. A positive reflex is normal in a child under 18 months but abnormal in any child who is walking and may indicate the presence of increased intracranial pressure.

Continuous monitoring is essential. After the initial neurologic examination, serial neurologic checks are repeated as often as every 15 minutes in the acutely ill child. Any changes are reported to the physician immediately and documented in the nurse's notes or flow record.

Vital Signs. In addition to the importance of the vital signs in the assessment of the general status of the pediatric trauma patient, the vital signs may be an observable manifestation of activity inside the patient's cranial vault.

An increase in the child's core body temperature may cause increased cerebral blood flow, increased intracranial volume, and therefore increased intracranial pressure. Because children are sensitive to environmental temperatures and their body temperature can drop quickly, care should be taken to keep the child in a neutral thermal environment.

Bradycardia in the presence of increasing blood pressure (Cushing's phenomenon) may indicate increasing intracranial pressure. A rapid pulse rate is a grave and late sign in a head-injured patient unless it is the result of some other cause. In children, shock is associated with tachycardia even if intracranial pressure is increased. Cushing's phenomenon, often not seen in infants, is a late sign and should not be relied on as an early indication of deterioration.

Elevated blood pressure can also indicate a rise in intracranial pressure although hypertension in a child with multiple injuries should never be assumed to be the direct result of a head injury. Hypertension may be precipitated by anxiety or pain or may be present as a result of preexisting illness. Generally, increased intracranial pressure is accompanied by an increase in systolic arterial blood pressure, producing a widening of the pulse pressure. This compensatory mechanism occurs as the body attempts to maintain adequate cerebral perfusion pressure by initiating a rise in blood pressure.

The child with a head injury may have several types of abnormal respiratory patterns. When intracranial pressure rises and signs of Cushing's phenomenon are evident, the child typically develops apnea. Development of Cheyne-Stokes pattern of breathing (alternating hyperpnea and bradypnea) after the presence of a normal respiratory pattern should alert the nurse to suspect neurologic deterioration. Hyperventilation usually indicates injury to the brainstem at the level of the pons.[16]

Head and Neck Examination.   All pediatric trauma patients must be suspected of having a cervical spine injury, especially those who have sustained facial or head trauma or who complain of pain in the neck or back. Anteroposterior, lateral, and open-mouth radiographic views of the cervical spine are necessary diagnostic studies.[1] Although spinal cord injury occurs infrequently in children, any time the cervical spine radiographs appear normal but the child is symptomatic, it is imperative that a neurosurgical consultation is obtained. Children may have a spinal cord injury without radiographic abnormality (SCIWORA), which mandates ongoing assessment for neurologic symptoms if the child's mechanism of injury is associated with a potential spinal cord injury.

After the initial examinations for head and neck injury have been obtained (vital signs and cervical spine films), the child's head and neck are assessed rapidly to look for obvious injury, including depressed or open skull fractures, lacerations, and leakage of cerebrospinal fluid (CSF). The nurse looks in the child's ears for blood or otorrhea and behind the child's ears for obvious ecchymosis (Battle's sign), indicating the presence of a basilar skull fracture. CSF

drainage from the nose may indicate the presence of a fractured cribriform plate. Finally the face and oral cavity are examined closely for lacerations or possible fracture sites.

Further neurodiagnostic evaluation is indicated in children with head injuries to identify the type and extent of injury. The need for skull radiographs in the management of severely head-injured patients has been under debate in recent years. Skull radiographs do not aid to the diagnosis in patients who require a computed tomography (CT) scan for possible intracranial lesions. Skull radiographs, however, can complement CT scan results in diagnosing depressed fractures and identifying the location of foreign bodies. They are indicated in cases of suspected child abuse.[7]

In patients with a head injury less than 72 hours old, CT scanning remains the procedure of choice for several reasons, including the limited potential for magnetic resonance imaging (MRI) to diagnose acute subarachnoid hemorrhage or acute parenchymal hemorrhage; the ease of monitoring unstable patients during the CT scan procedure; and the short time frame required to complete the procedure.[17] MRI is a technique used for imaging intracranial structures and is superior in imaging the posterior fossa, spinal cord structure, small vascular lesions, and most brain tumors. Lengthy procedure time, difficulty in monitoring critically ill patients during the procedure, cost, and the inability to visualize bone directly are among the limitations of this diagnostic procedure.

Many children do not cooperate with the need to remain still during these diagnostic procedures. Sedation is required in these situations.

ASSESSMENT OF THORACIC TRAUMA.   Although chest trauma in children is not as common as it is in adults, it can cause a number of problems related to diagnosis and management. Because of advances in the transport and treatment of the injured child, the mortality rate associated with thoracic trauma has decreased. The absence of preexisting disease states in children also contributes to the low morbidity rate associated with thoracic trauma.

One of the unique features of the child who has sustained thoracic trauma is the amazingly compliant thorax resulting from the flexibility of the bony and cartilaginous structures. It is not unusual, therefore, for the child to have major internal injury from compression of the chest without fracture of the bony thorax. A child's mediastinum is freely mobile and capable of wide anatomic shifts. This creates the potential for life-threatening situations such as dislocation of the heart, angulation of the great vessels, compression of the lung, and angulation of the trachea. Children with any type of traumatic injury experience aerophagia (swallowing of air), which results in gastric dilation that limits diaphragmatic excursion and leads to reflex ileus. In a small child this also can compromise ventilation and gas exchange.

Cardiopulmonary Examination.   Many injuries to the thorax can cause severe cardiorespiratory dysfunction soon after injury with fatal results if prompt and accurate diagnosis and treatment are not initiated. Continual reassessment of the child's condition after the initiation of therapy is imperative.

Abnormalities in the child's breathing pattern, such as flaring nostrils, chest wall retractions, and prominent use of accessory muscles, suggest ventilatory impairment. If the child is inadequately oxygenated, cyanosis of the fingers, toes, and lips are observed. When the airway is obstructed, cyanosis becomes prominent on both the face and trunk.

A flail chest is usually apparent on visual inspection. The child moves air poorly, and movement of the thorax is asymmetric and uncoordinated. A child with tension pneumothorax and massive hemothorax exhibits poor respiratory exchange, unilateral chest wall movement, or decreased unilateral chest wall movement. The presence of a tension pneumothorax results in distended neck veins and a tracheal and mediastinal shift to the opposite side. A child with cardiac tamponade also presents with distended neck veins; however, with a massive hemothorax the neck veins are often flat as a result of blood loss and decreased cardiac output. Any penetrating wounds to the thorax are noted and treated immediately. When an entrance wound is found, an exit wound also is sought. In the traumatized child, all aspects of the thorax, neck, and upper abdomen are examined for abrasions, lacerations, and contusions.

Palpation is performed gently and in a nonthreatening manner using warm hands. The area of injury is palpated last during the examination. Talking softly may have a calming effect on the child and may lessen the pain experienced as injured portions of the chest are assessed.

The nurse palpates the neck, clavicles, sternum, and thorax. Any signs of tenderness, swelling, or crepitus are noted. Subcutaneous emphysema is a finding of significant concern. Subcutaneous air can be palpated near penetrating chest wounds. When found in the neck area, it suggests a proximal tear or avulsion of the tracheobronchial tree or an esophageal perforation.

During examination of the thorax, any instability is noted. Unilateral tenderness in the upper abdomen may indicate a chest injury such as a fractured rib.

The small size of the chest in infants and children makes it difficult to use auscultation and percussion to determine the exact location of injury. Despite this limitation, however, these procedures are considered to be valuable in assessing thoracic injury. The presence of a pneumothorax is partially diagnosed through auscultation of breath sounds; because the chest wall of the young child is so thin, breath sounds are easily transmitted from other areas of the lung. Decreased breath sounds may not be heard over the involved lung; however, the nurse may note a difference in the quality or pitch of the breath sounds between the right and left sides. The nurse also should assess for the presence of any specific sounds, such as inspiratory stridor or expiratory wheezes, that might result from bronchial injury. Auscultation also can be used to identify a shift in the heart sounds corresponding to a tracheal shift caused by a tension

pneumothorax on one side of the chest. Cardiac tamponade is associated with muffled heart tones. In massive hemothorax, dullness to percussion is present although the limited thoracic surface area in an infant makes this assessment technique difficult.

Radiographic and Laboratory Studies. Roentgenograms of the chest should include anteroposterior (AP) and lateral views done in an upright position after cervical spine injury has been ruled out. With an upright chest radiograph the clinician can better visualize the degree of mediastinal shift. It is easier to diagnose abnormalities in the lung, pleural cavity, and diaphragm with this view as well.

Standard blood studies for any pediatric trauma patient include an arterial blood gas determination. Other more involved studies, such as pulmonary function tests, tomograms, barium contrast studies, sonograms, and CT scans, may be indicated depending on other clinical findings.

ASSESSMENT OF ABDOMINAL TRAUMA. Serious abdominal injury tends to be quite subtle compared with injuries of the head, chest, or limbs. Isolated abdominal injuries are relatively easy to treat and manage; however, confusion in establishment of priorities is common when evaluating a child with multiple trauma and possible abdominal injury.

Physical Examination. The physical examination of an acute abdominal condition in children is similar to the procedure for adults, but objective findings are often masked or misinterpreted. This assessment may be difficult because the child, if conscious, is often apprehensive and may be unwilling to cooperate. In the unconscious child, many of the voluntary responses are gone; therefore, few clinical signs are available to facilitate diagnosis. The key to making an accurate diagnosis of serious abdominal injury is careful examination with constant reassessment and the initiation of several diagnostic studies.

The abdomen and lower chest are examined for contusions, abrasions, and lacerations that may indicate compression injury. It should be noted whether the abdomen is scaphoid or distended. If a conscious child is pulling up the lower extremities, it may be in an attempt to relieve tension on the abdominal wall, thereby reducing pain.[18]

Penetrating wounds must be checked for involvement of intraabdominal organs. The back is examined for signs of surface injury, bony instability, and pain.

Because children up to about 6 years of age breathe primarily with their diaphragms, peritoneal irritation from blood or intestinal contents may result in an alteration of the breathing pattern. This child may display shallow breathing with the chest muscles to avoid pain. A distended abdomen may indicate significant injury and be caused by the accumulation of gas or liquid, such as blood, bile, pancreatic juice, urine, or intestinal contents. To examine the abdomen adequately, a nasal or orogastric tube is inserted. The drainage from the nasogastric tube should be examined for blood, which might indicate upper abdominal injury.

The abdomen is auscultated although absence of bowel sounds may be normal or may indicate an ileus. An intraabdominal hemorrhage or bowel perforation may initially give hypoactive or hyperactive bowel sounds. A quiet abdomen can be suggestive of an acute intraperitoneal injury.

Palpation.   Frightened children are often uncooperative, making palpation of the abdomen a difficult part of the examination. The nurse must be gentle and creative in the approach to this portion of the assessment. Palpation involves separate evaluation of the anterior and posterior abdominal wall and intraabdominal contents. Gentle pressure may bring about a voluntary response or guarding by the child, which may be localized to the abdominal wall or intraabdominal organs. Any physical signs of trauma are compared with this response to help identify injuries. With deeper palpation, an involuntary response of muscle spasm may be present. In the pediatric trauma patient, this peritoneal irritation is usually a sign of intraabdominal bleeding. Rebound tenderness may be difficult to interpret because it causes pain, crying, and voluntary guarding. The best way to elicit rebound tenderness in a child is by gentle percussion, shaking the child, or asking the child to cough rather than by rapidly releasing manual pressure over portions of the abdomen. This part of the examination helps to determine the presence of peritoneal irritation.

Pelvic and Genitourinary Assessment.   The last part of the abdominal examination is evaluation of the pelvis and genitourinary system. A pelvic fracture is suspected if pain is present on compression of the wings of the ilium or symphysis pubis or with abduction of the legs. Rupture of the bladder frequently accompanies pelvic fractures although a full bladder may rupture without a pelvic fracture. This injury is suspected when the child has lower abdominal pain, hematuria, and an inability to void. Urethral injuries are suspected when the child presents with perineal swelling, blood at the meatus, a floating prostate, a distended bladder, and an inability to void. Use of a urethral catheter is contraindicated because it may change an incomplete urethral tear into a complete urethral disruption. A rectal examination is necessary to evaluate the tone of the anal sphincter, position of the prostate, and integrity of the bony pelvis and bowel wall. The presence of blood strongly indicates perforation of the colon or rectum.

Injury to the kidney is common in pediatric trauma patients. Parenchymal contusion is the most common injury seen and most often results from blunt trauma.[19] An indication of this injury may be hematuria, with flank pain and tenderness also present. Further radiologic studies may be indicated, including contrast-enhanced CT scan, intravenous pyelogram, and renal scan.

Diagnostic Studies.   CT scan is a definitive method of evaluation for the child with blunt abdominal trauma. The CT scan provides superior detail of anatomy and allows for clear imagery of multiple abdominal organs simultaneously. An enhanced scan allows for the assessment of organ perfusion and evaluation of intraperitoneal bleeding, clearly defining the nature and extent of the injury.[17] Some recent reports recommend the use of ultrasound as the means to evaluate blunt abdominal trauma.[20]

Penetrating abdominal trauma is rare in the child and is often the result of a rib fracture. Because of the unpredictable nature of penetrating injuries, surgical exploration is usually indicated.[19]

Peritoneal lavage is not performed as frequently in children as in adults because it interferes with serial abdominal examination and because an isolated posttraumatic intraabdominal bleed is not necessarily an indication for surgery in pediatric patients.[20] Peritoneal lavage irritates the peritoneum for 24 to 48 hours, so it is not performed early in the clinical setting. In children with isolated abdominal trauma, the main determinations for surgical intervention are physical findings, deteriorating vital signs, and falling hematocrit. In a child with multitrauma, especially a head injury, clinical findings may not be as accurate in reflecting intraabdominal bleeding. Peritoneal lavage may be an appropriate diagnostic tool in the following circumstances[19]:

1. Altered pain responses
   a. Head injury
   b. Alcohol or drug ingestion
   c. Fractures of ribs, pelvis, lumbar spine
   d. Chest wall injury
2. Equivocal abdominal findings
3. Hemodynamic instability
4. General anesthesia
5. Stab wound with no peritonitis

Initially the abdominal examination may be negative, but continual reassessment is needed to rule out the development of a significant problem. It may take 12 to 24 hours for intraabdominal findings to become obvious in a child with suspected abdominal injury.

After the physical examination, appropriate laboratory studies are obtained. These include a complete blood count, type and crossmatch, blood gas analysis, prothrombin time, partial thromboplastin time, platelet count, and serum amylase determination.

ASSESSMENT OF MUSCULOSKELETAL TRAUMA.   Injuries to the extremities are usually obvious or readily identified with radiographic examination. Except for cervical and displaced pelvic fractures, orthopedic trauma is rarely life threatening. However, the importance of extremity injuries should never be underestimated because mismanagement could result in serious sequelae, such as infection, growth disturbance, deformity, or paralysis.

The high incidence of fractures in children can be explained by the combination of their relatively slender bone structure and their high activity level. Some of these injuries, such as buckle and greenstick fractures, are not serious compared with intraarticular and epiphyseal plate fractures, which can impair normal bone growth if they are not treated properly.

Examination of the Extremities. During the secondary survey the nurse palpates all extremities to detect pain, swelling, bruising, lacerations, and deformities. The neurovascular status of each limb should be noted and documented. The presence of a distal extremity pulse does not exclude an associated proximal artery tear. Soft tissue injuries should be thoroughly inspected for the presence of foreign bodies or dead tissue.

Temperature of the extremities is noted, with special care being given to determine whether the temperature is equal on both sides. Differences in temperature are usually caused by neurologic or vascular abnormalities. Extremities may be cold and pale after sympathetic nervous system stimulation. This condition also can be a sign of venous or arterial thrombosis or embolism.

Radiologic studies are used to confirm the diagnosis. Roentgenograms include the joint above and below the fracture to avoid missing an associated dislocation. Taking roentgenograms in two projections (e.g., AP and lateral) helps to avoid overlooking a fracture with deformity in only one location. Fractures in children often do not present a clear-cut picture; diagnosis may require additional effort. It is possible to overlook a severe injury, such as an epiphyseal separation with only a small degree of displacement or a fracture involving unossified epiphyses. Radiologic examination of both limbs, allowing for comparison of the injured and uninjured extremities, assists in avoiding this error.

SHOCK IN CHILDREN. In essence, shock is a generalized failure of adequate tissue perfusion resulting in impaired cellular and subcellular respiration. The basic cellular responses and general pathophysiologic mechanisms of the disease appear to be identical among different age groups. However, because of the differences between children and adults previously mentioned (e.g., vital sign parameters, thermoregulation, and response to head injury), shock is quite different in pediatric patients than in the adult population. The pediatric trauma patient is in shock most often because of hypoxia and blood loss. Children rarely suffer from diseases that predispose them to the development of other kinds of shock. In addition, there is a small margin of error in the recognition and treatment of pediatric patients with multisystem injury.

In infants and younger children, 70% of the total body weight is water and 50% of the total body water is located in the child's extracellular space. Therefore, hypovolemia occurs more rapidly in the child than in the adult, whose extracellular space contains only 23% of total body water.

Children have the ability to vasoconstrict effectively and can compensate for up to a 25% blood loss. Therefore, when hypotension does occur in the pediatric patient, it usually indicates a significant degree of blood loss. A traumatized child who is tachycardic; has cold, mottled extremities; and is hypotensive should be considered to be in shock.

Clinical Presentation. In assessing the child in shock, several clinical signs become apparent. Tachycardia and tachypnea are present. Because of the peripheral vasoconstriction, the extremities are cold, clammy, and mottled and the pulses are weak or nonpalpable. The child's level of consciousness is altered because of decreased cerebral perfusion. Urinary output is decreased or absent. The decrease in the systolic blood pressure is a late indicator; a narrowing of pulse pressure is usually seen first. Table 29-8

TABLE 29-8	**Classes of Hemorrhage for Children**		
Class	**Blood Loss**	**Signs**	**Treatment**
Class I	15% or less 40-kg child = 500 ml blood	Pulse: slight ↑ BP: normal Respiration: normal Capillary refill: normal Tilt test*: normal	Crystalloids
Class II	20%-30% 40-kg child = 800 ml blood	Pulse: tachycardia > 150 BP: ↓ systolic; ↓ pulse pressure Respiration: tachypnea > 35-40 Capillary refill: delayed Tilt test: positive Urine output: normal (1 ml/kg/hr)	Crystalloids
Class III	30%-35% 40-kg child = 1200 ml blood	BP: decreased Narrow pulse pressure Urine output: decreased	Crystalloids Packed red cells
Class IV	40%-50% 40-kg child = 1600 ml blood	Pulse: nonpalpable BP: nonpalpable No response to verbal or painful stimuli	Crystalloids Packed red cells

BP, blood pressure.

*A tilt test is done by sitting the child upright. The test is normal if the child can stay up for more than 90 seconds and maintain blood pressure.

differentiates the four classes of hemorrhage and lists the clinical signs and treatment for each.

Infants in shock may present differently than children or adults in shock. They may develop erratic hemodynamic parameters, mottling, hyperventilation or hypoventilation, glucose intolerance, and metabolic instability. The process is often insidious and requires accurate assessment.

The key elements involved in the successful management of hemorrhagic shock in the pediatric population are early recognition of hemodynamic instability, replacement of circulating blood volume, and arrest of further bleeding. Nurses should be aware of the pathophysiologic processes of shock and the signs and symptoms that these processes produce. If inadequate tissue perfusion continues, a potentially correctable problem may well lead to a fatal outcome.[21]

CLINICAL MANAGEMENT

In order to provide efficient and effective care to pediatric trauma patients, it is imperative that appropriate equipment and supplies be readily available. A general emergency department where both adults and children are seen must have equipment specifically for children. The availability of a separate pediatric trauma cart and pediatric resuscitation drug dosages improves the potential for a successful resuscitation. Table 29-9 presents essential equipment for a pediatric resuscitation.

In managing the critically ill child who has sustained multiple injuries, a systematic approach is used. This approach is practiced frequently so that it becomes automatic and can be applied even in a disorganized setting.

Children are assessed and treatment priorities are established on the basis of existing and potential life-threatening problems and the stability of the child's vital signs. The primary survey involves assessing the airway (while protecting the cervical spine), breathing, and circulation, with attention given to the diagnosis and treatment of shock. When indicated, appropriate resuscitative measures must be instituted concurrently with the primary survey.

PRIMARY SURVEY

Airway and Breathing.   The first priority in the sequential evaluation and management of the traumatized child is assessment of the airway. Airway patency must be ensured. There exists a great variation in the anatomy of the upper airway depending on the age of the child. In infants the oral cavity is small and the tongue is relatively large. The infant's larynx is more cephalad than the adult's. The glottis is higher than in adults; it is located at the level of the third cervical vertebra at birth and descends about one to two vertebrae with maturity. The vocal cords slant upward and backward behind a narrow, U-shaped epiglottis. However, for all ages the best method for initial assessment of the airway is to apply the chin-lift or jaw-thrust maneuver.

As with an adult, in-line cervical traction should always be applied in the traumatized child to maintain stability of the neck until a cervical fracture has been ruled out. Although cervical injury is rare in children, they are treated as if such injury has occurred until it is ruled out by roentgenogram. In addition to positioning for airway patency, foreign matter is quickly removed with a finger or gentle suction. This is done carefully, especially if a facial injury or basilar skull fracture is suspected. Close, continuous observation is essential because the child's ineffective efforts to clear the airway may quickly result in an obstructed airway once again.

The Conscious Child.   In a conscious child who is breathing spontaneously but whose airway is obstructed despite the foregoing measures, a nasopharyngeal airway device is useful. The length of the nasopharyngeal airway is estimated by measuring the distance from the nares to the tragus of the ear. The tube is lubricated, advanced gently along the floor of the nasal cavity, and rotated if resistance is met. If unsuccessful, the procedure is repeated on the opposite side. Epistaxis, avulsion of adenoid tissue, or damage to conchae can occur if a gentle technique and

Age	0-6 mos.	6-12 mos.	1 yr.	18 mos.	3 yrs.	5 yrs.	6 yrs.	8 yrs.	10 yrs.	12 yrs.	14 yrs.
TABLE 29-9 Recommended Resuscitation Equipment for the Infant and Child											
Weight (kg)	3-5	7	10	12	15	20	20	25	30	40	50
Resuscitation Mask	0-1	1	1-2	2	3	3	3	3	3	4	4-5
Laryngoscope (Miller/Mac)	0	1	1	1	2	2	2	2	2	2	3
ETT	3.0	3.5	3.5	4.0	4.5	5.0	5.5	6.0	6.0	6.5	7.0
Suction Catheter (ETT/Tracheal)	6	6	8	8	10	10	10	10	10	14	14
Suction (OP/NP)	10	10	10	10	14	14	14	16	16	16	16
Chest Tube	10-12	10-12	16-20	16-20	16-20	20-28	20-28	20-28	28-32	28-32	32-42
NG/OG	8	8	8	8	10	10	10	10	12	12	14
Foley	5	5	8	8	10	10	10	10	12	12	12
Trach (pediatric)	00	1	1	1-2	2-3	3	3	4	4	5	6

ETT, Endotracheal tube; *OP,* Oropharyngeal; *NP,* Nasopharyngeal; *NG,* Nasogastric; *OG,* Orogastric.
Modified from Widner-Kolberg MR, 1989, Maryland Institutes for Emergency Medical Services Systems.
Reprinted from Moloney-Harmon P, and Rosenthal CH: Nursing care modifications for the child in the adult ICU in Stillwell S, editor: *Critical care nursing reference book,* 1992, St Louis: Mosby, 590.

lubrication are not used during insertion. This method is contraindicated if rhinorrhea is present.

The Unconscious Child. In an unconscious child an oropharyngeal airway can be used. The selection of an appropriately sized airway is of paramount importance and can be facilitated by placing the airway alongside the child's face so that the flange is at the level of the central incisors and the bite block portion is approximately at the angle of the mandible. An airway device too small or too large can obstruct the airway (Figure 29-1).

The airway is inserted by opening the child's mouth and lifting the tongue with a tongue depressor. The airway is slid into position with care to avoid pushing the tongue backward and thus obstructing the airway. The practice of inserting the airway in an inverted position and rotating it 180 degrees is not recommended in pediatric patients because trauma to the teeth or soft tissue may occur. In the conscious child, gagging may occur during insertion of an oral airway and it is generally tolerated poorly.

After a clear and stable airway has been established, the child is reassessed continually. The nurse looks, listens, and feels for evidence of air exchange. In infants, adequacy of ventilation is assessed by observing for expansion at the lower chest and upper abdomen. This differs from the reassessment of older children and adolescents, in whom adequate ventilation and expansion are checked at the upper chest. Air exchange is assessed through auscultation, listening first over the trachea to establish that air exchange is occurring through the central airway and then listening for breath sounds bilaterally to assess for peripheral air exchange. Observing for symmetrical lung expansion is also essential.

Once the airway has been established and the child is spontaneously breathing, supplemental oxygen (50% to 100%) is provided. Although children are quite resistant to the effects of hypercarbic and respiratory acidosis, they do not tolerate even short periods of oxygen deprivation.

Bag-mask ventilation with 100% oxygen is indicated in children who do not resume spontaneous breathing. When using a bag mask to ventilate, the fingers should be kept on the lower jaw to avoid compressing the soft tissue under the infant's chin. Placing the fingers on the soft tissue forces the tongue back into the posterior pharynx and then obstructs the airway (Figure 29-2).

Endotracheal intubation is indicated for children who cannot be ventilated adequately via the bag-mask method and who need prolonged control of the airway, including prevention of aspiration. The oral route for endotracheal intubation is preferred for the child in the emergent phase. A nasotracheal tube is generally more stable in the pediatric patient, but nasal intubation usually takes longer and is not recommended in patients who are not breathing or who have cranial, maxillary, or facial injuries. Children are also likely to have hypertrophied lymphoid tissue (adenoids and tonsils), which can cause problems with the passage of a nasotracheal tube. The higher location of the larynx in the pediatric patient creates a more acute angle from the nasopharynx, making successful nasal intubation less likely. When cervical injury is suspected, oral intubation must be done with in-line traction applied and without extension of the neck, as in the adult population.

Uncuffed tracheal tubes are used in pediatric patients up to 7 years of age to avoid subglottic edema and stenosis. The appropriate interior diameter (ID) of the tracheal tube for a

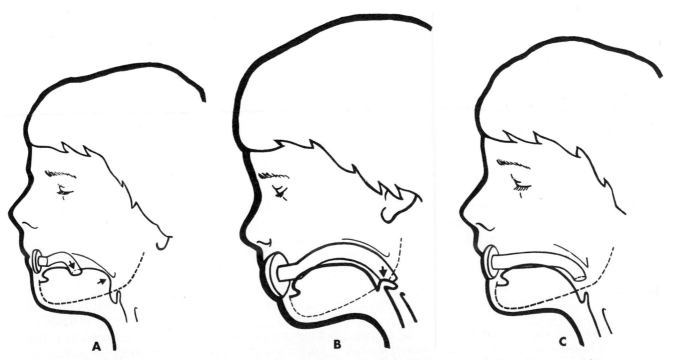

FIGURE 29-1 **Choosing the Appropriate Size Airway. A,** Airway too small. **B,** Airway too large. **C,** Airway correct size.

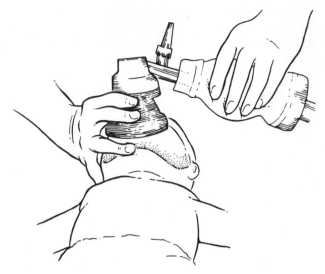

FIGURE 29-2 **Proper Placement of Hand and Fingers on Lower Jaw When Using a Bag Mask.** (From Eichelberger MR et al: *Brady's pediatric emergencies,* Englewood Cliffs, NJ, 1992, Prentice Hall, 49.)

particular child can be estimated by using the following formula:

$$16 + \text{age in years}/4 = \text{ID of tracheal tube}$$

For example, for a 2-year-old child, the following calculation applies:

$$16 + 2/4 = 4.5 \text{ mm}$$

This is an approximate rule, so it is recommended that tubes of the next higher and lower sizes also be readily available. Another approximate measure often used to determine tracheal tube diameter is the size of the internal naris. If the tube fits into one naris, it will probably fit comfortably down the trachea.

Rapid-sequence intubation is indicated in the child with a full stomach or in the child with a potential for increased intracranial pressure. All pediatric trauma patients are assumed to have a full stomach, and a rapid-sequence intubation minimizes the possibility of regurgitation.[19] This technique also blunts the response of increased intracranial pressure that can be stimulated by intubation. Intubation should always be preceded by ventilation with 100% oxygen. The medications commonly administered in a rapid-sequence intubation are atropine, a sedative, and a muscle relaxant.

The technique of cricoid pressure (Sellick maneuver) is used during a rapid-sequence intubation to prevent passive regurgitation of stomach contents into the pharynx. In this technique the upper esophagus is compressed against the cervical vertebral column by applying anteroposterior pressure on the cricoid cartilage. Cricoid pressure must be maintained until correct placement of the tracheal tube is confirmed.

If a tracheal tube cannot be placed within 30 seconds, ventilation is resumed for several minutes before a second attempt. After the tube has been placed, to ensure proper placement of the tube in the trachea, the nurse auscultates both lung fields and observes for symmetrical chest expansion. However, because clinical confirmation may be unreliable, confirmation of tracheal tube placement is achieved by exhaled CO_2 detection. As in adults, it is extremely easy for the tracheal tube to slide into the child's right mainstem bronchus, causing atelectasis and further decreasing ventilation. After the nurse's assessment by auscultation and observation of chest expansion and exhaled CO_2 detection, the tube is secured to the upper lip with tincture of benzoin and adhesive tape until proper tube position is verified by chest roentgenogram. Securing the tracheal tube carefully and restraining the child's hands are necessary interventions because dislodgment can occur easily because of the short length of the child's trachea.

Surgical Intervention. If the airway obstruction persists after implementation of the preceding methods, direct injury to the larynx or trachea or uncontrollable hemorrhage should be suspected. Although cricothyroid puncture may be a lifesaving procedure, it is virtually never the first choice for establishing an airway and adequate ventilation. Almost all children can be adequately ventilated and oxygenated without surgical intervention. When necessary, the preferred surgical method in children is needle cricothyroidotomy. Great care is taken to ensure that the catheter remains patent. Arterial blood gases are drawn to assess the adequacy of oxygenation and ventilation endeavors.

If inadequate ventilation is the result of chest injury, such as tension pneumothorax, open pneumothorax, or large flail segment, these alterations must be addressed immediately. A tension pneumothorax may be relieved by needle insertion or chest tube placement; an open pneumothorax must be covered with a sterile petrolatum gauze dressing; a flail segment must be supported and, if necessary, positive-pressure controlled ventilation should be instituted. Adequate ventilation does not ensure adequate tissue oxygenation; therefore the potential for impaired gas exchange remains a concern throughout the emergent and critical phases of care. An attempt should be made to maintain arterial Po_2 in the 80 to 100 mm Hg range.

Circulation. During the primary survey the adequacy of circulation is first assessed by noting the quality, rate, and regularity of central and peripheral pulses. Peripheral perfusion is also assessed initially by capillary refill. Capillary refill is easily tested by applying pressure to the nail beds and observing the time required for return of skin color. Under normal circumstances the color should return within 2 seconds. If the child has been in a cold environment, refill in the extremities may be prolonged, in which case it is assessed on mucous membranes.

Circulatory support is initiated as soon as it is deemed necessary. Active bleeding is controlled immediately with a direct pressure dressing. Intravenous access is critical in infants and children in severe shock or cardiac arrest. However, it is in this clinical situation that venous access may be most difficult and time-consuming because of the smaller vessel size in children and the fact that veins often collapse when children are in shock. Intravenous access is attempted via percutaneous catheter placement, intraosseous needle insertion, or central venous line placement.

Intraosseous Infusion. Intraosseous infusion is a technique used to establish venous access that was described more than 60 years ago. For intraosseous infusion, a bone marrow needle is inserted into the medial flat surface of the anterior tibia, approximately 2 finger breadths below the tibial tuberosity. The needle is inserted perpendicular to the bone or at a 45-degree angle away from the growth plate to avoid injury to this structure. This is considered an effective route for the administration of sodium bicarbonate, calcium, bretylium, and glucose, none of which can be given via the endotracheal route. In addition, infusions of crystalloids, colloid, blood, dopamine, epinephrine, and dobutamine can be given while attempts at intravenous cannulation are under way. The main advantages of intraosseous infusion are that it is a readily available route, requires little skill, and has a low rate of complications. The most common complications attributed to this procedure are the subcutaneous infiltration of fluid (although minimal) and leakage from the puncture site after the removal of the needle. Osteomyelitis and subcutaneous infections have been noted, but they occur only after the intraosseous infusion is maintained for extended periods of time or when hypertonic fluids are infused via this route.

Volume Replacement. Volume replacement with a crystalloid solution of lactated Ringer's solution (20 ml/kg) is given to raise blood pressure and improve circulation. If vital signs do not stabilize with the administration of one bolus, a second bolus of 20 ml/kg should be given as quickly as possible, keeping in mind that half the child's blood volume has been replaced. If blood pressure returns to normal, the intravenous infusion is set at a maintenance rate. If the child remains hypotensive, then blood replacement is needed. In children with exsanguinating hemorrhage, either type-specific or type O packed cells are immediately infused.

Fluid therapy is guided by special attention to preinfusion and postinfusion vital signs and indicators of systemic perfusion because these indicate whether a child has continued fluid losses. In the past, platelets and clotting factors were routinely administered when patients received large amounts of blood products. At present it is recommended that platelets and fresh frozen plasma be given only when the patient's clinical status and laboratory studies indicate that they are necessary.[21]

Resuscitation drug therapy may be indicated for the pediatric trauma patient. Table 29-10 lists the common resuscitation drugs and their dosages. For use in emergency situations, when the exact weight of the child is not known, completed emergency drug cards for various weights (e.g., 2 kg, 5 kg, 10 kg, 15 kg) assist in quickly determining the correct dosages. The approximate weight card can be pulled out and used during the emergency situation. (Approximate weights for children are discussed earlier in the chapter.) The key to successful resuscitation efforts is being prepared with predetermined charts for drug dosages before the arrest takes place. Nurses need to be knowledgeable about the actions, indications, and adverse effects of the standard drugs used in resuscitation.

Defibrillation. Because ventricular fibrillation is an infrequent occurrence in pediatric cardiopulmonary arrest, defibrillation is a relatively uncommon intervention. Before any attempt to defibrillate, the rhythm is confirmed; unmonitored defibrillation is not recommended. When fibrillation is monitored, defibrillation is attempted only after the child has been prepared. Coarse fibrillation may be more easily treated than fine fibrillation. Fine fibrillation may be converted to coarse fibrillation with the administration of epinephrine or calcium.

Pediatric paddles are smaller in diameter than those used for an adult and are available with most defibrillators. The electrodes are prepared with electrode paste or gel pads. The paste or pads are placed carefully. Electrical bridging results in ineffective defibrillation and burning of the skin surface. Both electrodes may be placed on the anterior chest wall, one at the right of the sternum below the clavicle and the other at the level of the xyphoid along the left midclavicular line. Anteroposterior placement of the electrodes on an infant or young child is also acceptable; however, this is sometimes difficult to achieve during resuscitation.

Current for the initial shock is 2 watt-sec/kg. If the first defibrillation effort is unsuccessful, cardiopulmonary resuscitation should be continued for 3 to 5 minutes before the current is doubled to 4 watt-sec/kg for a second attempt.

SECONDARY SURVEY. After the primary survey, initial stabilization of the cardiopulmonary system, and aggressive treatment of shock, each child should undergo a secondary survey. As in adults, this secondary survey consists of a timely, systematic, and directed evaluation of each body region to assess for injury. Specific injuries more common to the pediatric population are discussed earlier in the chapter.

While performing the systematic head-to-toe survey in children, several principles are used. First, any child with one injury is assumed to have additional injuries until proven otherwise. Second, isolated head injuries rarely cause shock; therefore, a child with a head injury who is in shock requires a thorough evaluation. Third, verbal reassurance is offered to the child who is conscious, and the treatment plan is explained in terms that are easily understandable. Finally, appropriate physiologic parameters and laboratory studies are obtained and recorded frequently, and the child is monitored closely and reassessed continually. Laboratory study trends are analyzed consistently as well.

TABLE 29-10   PALS Medications for Cardiac Arrest and Symptomatic Arrhythmias

Drug	Dosage (Pediatric)	Remarks
Adenosine	0.1 mg/kg Repeat dose: 0.2 mg/kg Maximum single dose: 12 mg	Rapid IV/IO bolus Rapid flush to central circulation Monitor EGG during dose.
Amiodarone for pulseless VF/VT	5 mg/kg IV/IO	Rapid IV bolus
Amiodarone for perfusing tachycardias	Loading dose: 5 mg/kg IV/IO Maximum dose: 15 mg/kg per day	IV over 20 to 60 minutes Routine use in combination with drugs prolonging QT interval is *not* recommended. Hypotension is most frequent side effect.
Atropine sulfate*	0.02 mg/kg Minimum dose: 0.1 mg Maximum single dose: 0.5 mg in child, 1.0 mg in adolescent. May repeat once.	May give IV, IO or ET. Tachycardia and pupil dilation may occur but *not* fixed dilated pupils.
Calcium chloride 10% = 100 mg/mL (= 27.2 mg/mL elemental Ca)	20 mg/kg (0.2 mL/kg) IV/IO	Give slow IV push for hypocalcemia, hypermagnesemia, calcium channel blocker toxicity, preferably via central vein. Monitor heart rate; bradycardia may occur.
Calcium gluconate 10% = 100 mg/mL (= 9 mg/mL elemental Ca)	60-100 mg/kg (0.6-1.0 mL/kg) IV/IO	Give slow IV push for hypocalcemia, hypermagnesemia, calcium channel blocker toxicity, preferably via central vein.
Epinephrine for symptomatic bradycardia*	IV/IO: 0.01 mg/kg (1:10,000, 0.1 mL/kg) ET: 0.1 mg/kg (1:1000, 0.1 mL/kg)	Tachyarrhythmias, hypertension may occur.

Epinephrine for pulseless arrest*	First dose:
	  IV/IO: 0.01 mg/kg (1:10,000, 0.1 mL/kg)
	  ET: 0.1 mg/kg (1:1000, 0.1 mL/kg)
	Subsequent doses: Repeat initial dose or may increase up to 10 times (0.1 mg/kg, 1:1000, 0.1 mL/kg)
	Administer epinephrine every 3 to 5 minutes.
	IV/IO/ET doses as high as 0.2 mg/kg of 1:1000 may be effective.	

Glucose (10% or 25% or 50%)	IV/IO: 0.5-1.0 g/kg 1-2 mL/kg 50% 2-4 mL/kg 25% 5-10 mL/kg 10%	For suspected hypoglycemia; avoid hyperglycemia.
Lidocaine*	IV/IO/ET: 1 mg/kg	Rapid bolus
Lidocaine infusion (start after a bolus)	IV/IO: 20-50 µg/kg per minute	1 to 2.5 mL/kg per hour of 120 mg/100 mL solution or use "Rule of 6" (see Table 3)
Magnesium sulfate (500 mg/mL)	IV/IO: 25-50 mg/kg, Maximum dose: 2 g per dose	Rapid IV infusion for torsades or suspected hypomagnesemia; 10- to 20-minute infusion for asthma that responds poorly to β-adrenergic agonists.
Naloxone*	≤5 years or ≤20 kg: 0.1 mg/kg >5 years or >20 kg: 2.0 mg	For total reversal of narcotic effect. Use small repeated doses (0.01 to 0.03 mg/kg) titrated to desired effect.
Procainamide for perfusing tachycardias (100 mg/mL and 500 mg/mL)	Loading dose: 15 mg/kg IV/IO	Infusion over 30 to 60 minutes; routine use in combination with drugs prolonging QT interval is *not* recommended.
Sodium bicarbonate (1 mEq/mL and 0.5 mEq/mL)	IV/IO: 1 mEq/kg per dose	Infuse slowly and only if ventilation is adequate.

From: American Heart Association: Guidelines 2000 for cardiovascular care, *Circulation 2000*, 102(suppl): 1308, 2000.
IV indicates intravenous; *IO*, intraosseous; and *ET*, endotracheal.
*For endotracheal administration use higher doses (2 to 10 times the IV dose); dilute medication with normal saline to a volume of 3 to 5 mL and follow with several positive-pressure ventilations.

THE FAMILY OF THE CHILD

An important aspect of the care of the pediatric trauma patient is care of the family. The family experiences the circumstances surrounding trauma as a crisis. Because trauma is unexpected, the parents do not have time to adjust to the possible death or disability of their child. Parents initially may experience shock and disbelief. Normal reactions include confusion, disorganized behavior, and an increase in tension and anxiety.[22] They may also have difficulty in accepting the situation as real. The normal coping mechanisms they have always used to deal with previous crises may no longer be effective. Decision-making abilities may be impaired.[22] The parents often experience feelings of guilt that may be indicated by anger at themselves, each other, the child, or the health care team. These feelings of anger may occur immediately or later as the family passes through the shock and disbelief phase to the developing awareness phase.[23]

These families require compassionate support throughout their adjustment to this crisis in their lives and need to be informed about what is happening to their child. Too often parents are whisked away to a waiting area and left to wonder about what is happening. Parents require information from the health care team as soon as possible because they are often imagining the worst; they wonder if the child is still alive. If parents are in a waiting area, an important priority is allowing them to see their child. As the child stabilizes, other concerns that the family members may have must be addressed.

An important consideration for the health care team is family presence during the resuscitation. Boie et al[23] determined that most parents whose children require resuscitation in the emergency department wish to be in attendance. Nurses take on the important responsibility of preparing families to stay with their child.

FAMILY ASSESSMENT.   The family network is assessed as soon as possible. Information is gathered about the family's knowledge of the situation. Does the family have any kind of support system, such as friends, relatives, or clergy? Where will they stay while their child is in the hospital? Does the family have other children? From this assessment, some inferences can be made about the family's perception of the situation and their ability to cope. Information about the family's medical insurance coverage is obtained as well. Many families express early concerns about hospitalization and health care costs and may require the services of a financial counselor. Referrals are made accordingly.

PROVIDING INFORMATION.   Information about their child is given to parents in a simple, straightforward manner because it is often difficult for them to process a great deal of information at this time. Any misconceptions that the family may have about the situation or their child's injuries and treatment plan are addressed. In preparing the family to see the child, they are told about the change in their child's appearance and about the equipment and personnel that are at the bedside. Parents are asked how the child appears to them, and explanations can then be based on their perceptions.

RESPONSE TO THE DEATH OF A CHILD.   Some children may not survive resuscitation efforts; after emergent efforts to save the child, care shifts to the family. These parents need support from the nursing staff when the news about the death of the child is shared. The immediate reactions of the family are shock, numbness, and disbelief—a period when parents often feel out of touch with reality. They are often immobilized and unable to make decisions.[24] Guilt also is a feeling that parents often experience when a child dies, especially if it is an unintentional death.

After the initial shock of a child's death, the phase of intense grief begins. This may begin immediately or may be delayed for weeks. During this phase, parents may experience loneliness and an intense yearning for their child. They may feel extremely helpless, which often leads to feelings of anger and despair. At this time they are also at risk for the development of physical symptoms, such as loss of appetite, and may experience sleep disturbances as well.[25]

The phase of reorganization follows. Parents report that they never recover completely from a child's death, but most are able to regain their previous level of functioning with support and care from others. This is evidenced by a return to normal daily activities, more happy memories of the child, and a decrease in feelings associated with intense grief.

Nursing Interventions.   For nurses working in an emergency department setting, telling the family of a child's death is an extremely difficult task. Initial interactions with the family usually occur as they experience the shock and numbness of their loss. At this time it is important to let parents know that all extraordinary measures were taken to save the child. The family is often comforted, too, to know that the child did not suffer. Further conversation should be guided by the family's expressed need for more information. Quiet time is often needed and appreciated. The nurse's physical presence while the family begins to experience their loss is often helpful. Many families are comforted to know of the health care team's care and concern, which often can be expressed more effectively in silence.

Some parents may feel a need to express their great pain and sorrow. Guilt feelings also may surface as the family begins to grieve. Such feelings should not be negated because they are a significant part of the process through which the family must progress in order to come to terms with their loss.

Anger and rage also may be experienced at this time and are often directed toward hospital personnel. Such feelings often pass once expressed, and the family members may become extremely confused by the various emotions that have overcome them. The most appropriate intervention at this time is for the nurse to listen, reinforce the positive aspects of their parenting role, and explain the normalcy of their feelings.

Parents may need assistance with problem solving as they face the many decisions that must be made during this time of great stress. Many families benefit from the support offered through social service programs. Appropriate referrals should be made at this time. Clergy members and social workers may assist the family by providing guidance in making funeral arrangements and by offering emotional and spiritual support.

It is also helpful if the nurse who cared for the child makes contact with the family shortly after the child's death. This conveys to the family that they have been remembered and provides them the opportunity to ask questions and express feelings that have surfaced since the child's death. Many parents need reassurance and continued support as they experience various aspects of their personal grief (see Chapter 18).

CRITICAL CARE PHASE

Once resuscitation and stabilization measures have been taken, the child is prepared for the definitive treatment regimen. Although not always the case, surgical intervention may be necessary at this time. The patient then progresses through a critical period that requires close observation and intensive interventions. Identified in this text as the critical care phase, it is during this phase of care that complications resulting from earlier resuscitation efforts may become evident. It is imperative that the pediatric critical care nurse develop and refine the necessary skills for detecting signs of impending danger. Early recognition of even the most subtle changes and rapid and efficient intervention may positively affect the outcome of care.

TOTAL SYSTEMS ASSESSMENT

As in the resuscitation phase of care, the pediatric trauma patient requires a systems assessment that helps to identify priorities for critical care management. The assessment during the critical care phase focuses more broadly on the integrated function of the child's body systems, psychologic status, and response to resuscitative and operative therapies. For example, the neurologic status requires close monitoring. The child's level of consciousness, pupillary response, movement, and reflexes are assessed continually. The child's movements are evaluated as spontaneous or in response to pain. The type of movement is documented as well. Does the child withdraw or posture? Is the child able to grasp? Grasp activity is evaluated for strength, equality, and the ability to release on command. The Glasgow Coma Scale (see Table 29-7) is a useful assessment tool used during the critical care phase and during the resuscitation phase of care (see Chapter 19).

The child's cardiovascular status, including heart rate and rhythm, blood pressure, quality of pulses, and perfusion, are assessed routinely. Clinical examination findings and hemodynamic parameters are part of the assessment data. The child continues to be assessed for the presence of shock, either septic or hypovolemic. Hypovolemic shock may be present if the child continues to bleed as a result of the traumatic injuries.

The potential for respiratory distress and failure necessitates a thorough respiratory assessment. Assessment parameters include respiratory rate, pattern and effectiveness of respirations, and quality of breath sounds. For infants an increase in respiratory rate is the mechanism of compensation for respiratory dysfunction because they cannot increase the tidal volume. If the child is intubated and mechanically ventilated, the presence or absence and quality of the child's own respirations are assessed. The ventilator is routinely checked and respiratory patterns monitored closely to ensure that the child's breathing is synchronized with the ventilator. Note the amount of oxygen being delivered, the positive end-expiratory pressure, and the peak inspiratory pressure. An increase in peak inspiratory pressures indicates difficulty in delivering tidal volume, which may be the result of progressive atelectasis or the development of a pneumothorax (see Chapter 23).

Serial arterial blood gases are obtained to determine the adequacy of oxygenation and ventilation. Pulse oximetry is useful for continuously monitoring oxygen saturation, and end-tidal CO_2 monitoring may be performed in patients with head injury or severe lung injury. Thoracic roentgenograms are monitored for the development of a pathologic respiratory process, such as atelectasis or pneumothorax. If the child has chest or mediastinal tubes in place, the color and amount of drainage are noted.

Abdominal assessment includes monitoring abdominal girth and the presence or absence and quality of bowel sounds. The amount and quality of nasogastric drainage are noted and recorded. The child is monitored for bleeding by noting hematocrit, abdominal girth and tension, and bleeding through the nasogastric tube. If the child has had surgical repair of the abdomen, a postoperative ileus is often present because of surgical manipulation and the body's response to trauma. There may be signs of hypovolemia and shock if the child has intraabdominal bleeding. The nasogastric fluid is tested for the presence of occult blood and obvious bleeding. Ranitidine is administered to prevent the development of a stress ulcer.

Renal assessment includes monitoring the amount and characteristics of urine output, the presence of hematuria, specific gravity, serum blood urea nitrogen and creatinine, urine electrolyte levels, and creatinine clearance. Hematuria may be associated with the trauma of inserting a urinary catheter or may be the result of genitourinary trauma related to the child's injury. Monitoring the renal parameters is important in assessing for the development of acute tubular necrosis. Acute tubular necrosis is a postresuscitation complication that may be seen in children who have experienced a profound decrease in circulating blood volume.[26] It also can result from hypoxia or sepsis. A significant decrease in circulating fluid volume leads to hypotension, causing a decrease in renal perfusion. This reduces the glomerular filtration rate and renal cortical blood flow, stimulating renin and aldosterone secretion and producing sodium and water retention and diminished urine output (see Chapter 25).

The condition of the child's skin is assessed, noting any lacerations or abrasions that may have been overlooked during the resuscitation phase. The condition of dressings, casts, traction, and pin sites are noted. Fracture reduction, necessitated as a result of musculoskeletal trauma, may be accomplished in a number of ways: closed reduction with immediate casting, continuous traction using Buck's or skeletal traction, external fixation devices such as a Hoffmann device, or open reduction and internal fixation. The child in any traction device is assessed for skin breakdown related to immobility or resulting from cast pressure sites. The child also is assessed for signs of infection at pin sites and under the cast. The potential for circulatory compromise in the injured extremity exists and is assessed by checking pulses, color, temperature, capillary refill, and sensation (see Chapter 26).

Body temperature remains an important parameter to monitor in the child. Hypothermia may produce arrhythmias during the critical care phase and during the resuscitation phase. A temperature of less than 30° C (86° F) can produce a life-threatening arrhythmia with a resultant decrease in cardiac output. Elevated temperatures may signal the development of an infection. Early detection and intervention may prevent the development of serious complications that increase the morbidity and mortality associated with the initial injury.

Infection is a risk in any posttrauma patient, including the pediatric patient. When the body's normal defense mechanisms are disrupted, septic shock may occur after exposure to infectious agents.[27] Because of their immature immune systems, infants are more prone to infection. Vital signs (including core body temperature), white blood cell (WBC) count, and the condition of all wounds, surgical sites, and vascular sites should be monitored closely.

Intravenous infusion sites are examined. Signs of infection such as redness, swelling, and purulent drainage are noted.

CLINICAL MANAGEMENT

The clinical management of the pediatric trauma patient in the critical care unit requires the same team approach that was necessary during the resuscitation phase. Coordination of disciplines is required to provide the best care for the child. The purpose of placing the child in the critical care unit is to provide continued monitoring and treatment.

The first step of clinical management is preparation. A report is given to the receiving unit from the emergency department/resuscitation area, operating room, or radiology department to facilitate continuity of care. The report includes the child's injuries and interventions, the level of consciousness, fluids received, estimated blood loss, airway and ventilatory support, intravenous lines and location, and any special equipment that is needed or that is accompanying the child. It is the nurse's responsibility to ensure that all

TABLE 29-11	Normal Pressure Values in Children
Central venous pressure	4-12 mm Hg
Systolic pulmonary artery pressure	20-30 mm Hg
Diastolic pulmonary artery pressure	<10 mm Hg
Mean pulmonary artery pressure	<20 mm Hg
Pulmonary artery wedge pressure	4-12 mm Hg

necessary pediatric equipment and supplies are in the receiving area and functioning properly.

MONITORING HEMODYNAMIC STABILITY. Ongoing management depends on the injuries and resultant problems. One of the main objectives of clinical management in the postresuscitation period is to restore hemodynamic stability and adequate perfusion to ensure viability of all organs and to prevent complications related to decreased perfusion, such as renal failure and hypoxic encephalopathy. This objective is accomplished by close, astute monitoring. Vital signs (including blood pressure, pulse, and respirations) are checked every 15 minutes until the child stabilizes.

Central venous lines, often inserted during the resuscitation phase of care, allow for trend analysis during the critical care phase. Pulmonary arterial pressure catheters may be inserted in the critical care unit for the following indications: (1) poor peripheral perfusion despite maximal fluid therapy, (2) pulmonary edema, or (3) a need for measurement of cardiac output or pulmonary venous oxygen levels. Central venous and pulmonary artery pressure trends provide information regarding fluid volume status and cardiac function, thus serving as a guide for fluid and pharmacologic therapy. Normal values are shown in Table 29-11. Decreased central venous pressure typically indicates fluid deficit; elevated pressure indicates fluid overload, congestive heart failure, or cardiac tamponade. The readings also may be elevated as a result of positive-pressure ventilation.

Intake and output should be monitored and recorded accurately. If possible, the child should be weighed daily so that appropriate fluid and nutritional calculations can be determined. Serum electrolytes should be measured daily or more often if appropriate. Depending on the goals of the treatment regimen, the child may be receiving maintenance or less than maintenance fluids.

RESPIRATORY SUPPORT. Ventilatory support may be provided via a tracheal tube and mechanical ventilation. Determination of ventilator settings is based on the child's ability to breathe spontaneously and on arterial blood gas trends, with consideration of the presence of pulmonary disorder. The child may need to be pharmacologically paralyzed and sedated. If the child has sustained a flail chest injury, mechanical ventilation with positive pressure are necessary for internal stabilization. The child is observed closely for the development of posttraumatic respiratory insufficiency. Early signs include increased respiratory rate, nasal flaring and retractions, and cyanosis on room air. Auscultation may reveal sparse rales. The nurse monitors the patient for hypoxemia that does not respond to increased levels of inspired oxygen, decreased lung compliance, and diffuse infiltrates that may progress to consolidation. If the child does develop posttraumatic respiratory insufficiency, massive respiratory and hemodynamic support are necessary (see Chapter 23).

Bronchial hygiene is provided for the intubated child to promote adequate ventilation and clearing of secretions. The frequency is individualized and depends on the respiratory disorder and the child's condition.

Extubation.　Once the child has passed through the critical phase and is able to oxygenate and ventilate adequately and clear secretions, extubation is the next step. Enteral feedings are discontinued 2 to 4 hours before, and sedation is stopped to ensure that the child has cough and gag refexes present.

MONITORING NEUROLOGIC STATUS.　The child with neurologic impairment as a result of head injury requires close monitoring and prompt intervention if evidence of increased intracranial pressure exists. The management of the pediatric patient with head injury is similar to that of an adult. A more detailed discussion of neurologic management is presented in Chapter 19.

Intracranial pressure monitoring devices are used in managing pediatric head trauma. If an intracranial pressure monitoring device is in place, the child's intracranial pressures should be monitored closely and recorded accurately. If it is necessary to remove excess CSF or to drain blood, a ventricular drain is inserted; physician orders should include the frequency and amount of fluid to be drained. Meticulous care of the catheter and insertion site is imperative to prevent infection. Specific instructions for intraventricular catheter site care and dressing changes are included in the child's plan of care. Methods of caring for these catheters are standardized in many institutions.

The child may be hyperventilated to reduce intracranial pressure. By lowering the $Paco_2$, cerebral blood flow is decreased, which reduces intracranial pressure. This therapy is controversial because the reduction in cerebral blood flow can result in ischemia. The current recommendation is that this therapy be used only for acute increases in intracranial pressure resulting in neurologic deterioration or that are refractory to other methods of reduction.[27] Mild hyperventilation ($Paco_2$ 30-34 mm Hg) is instituted to decrease cerebral blood flow but prevent cerebral ischemia associated with severe vasoconstriction.[28] The child's head is kept in a midline position and, if not contraindicated, may be slightly elevated (15-30 degrees) to facilitate venous drainage from the brain.

If the child is not in hypovolemic shock, fluids may be restricted to one half to two thirds of maintenance levels. Hypotonic fluids are avoided to prevent exacerbation of brain edema caused by free water. Hypertonic saline may be used for resuscitation of the severely head-injured child. A recent study demonstrated that hypertonic saline (3% NaCl) maintains blood pressure and cerebral oxygen delivery, decreases overall fluid requirements, and results in overall improved survival rates.[29] Simma et al[30] compared two groups of head-injured children who required resuscitation. One group received lactated Ringer's solution and the other group received hypertonic saline solution. The group who received hypertonic saline had lower intracranial pressures; higher cerebral perfusion pressures; required fewer interventions to maintain a lower intracranial pressure; had fewer complications, especially pulmonary complications; and had a shorter length of stay in the intensive care unit.

Osmotic diuretics such as mannitol (0.25 g/kg) may be given to children with increased intracranial pressure who are not responsive to other forms of therapy; however, these agents should be used with caution. After head trauma, children are at risk for the development of malignant brain edema. Malignant brain edema is a significant cerebral hyperemia. As many as 50% of head-injured children may develop this condition.[31] Because mannitol can increase cerebral blood flow dramatically as a result of the shift of fluid from the cellular to the vascular space, it is used with caution. When mannitol is used, boluses of 0.25 g/kg are recommended. Continuous administration of mannitol may lead to a reverse osmotic shift, resulting in increased brain osmolarity and increased intracranial pressure.[28] Serum osmolality is monitored every 6 hours and should not exceed 320 mOsm.

Posttraumatic seizures, which can occur in the child as a result of a severe head injury (GCS 3-8), diffuse cerebral edema, or an acute subdural hematoma, must be pharmacologically controlled.[32] Diazepam (0.1-0.3 mg/kg) or phenobarbital (20-30 mg/kg) may be given in an acute situation, with phenytoin (5 mg/kg/day) used for long-term control. Posttraumatic seizures may occur for 1 to 2 years after injury.

Steroids may be used because of their ability to reduce cerebral edema although their efficacy with cerebral edema related to head trauma has not been proven. Because of the absence of any positive effect of steroids in treating head-injured patients, administration of steroids is no longer recommended.[28]

If all measures to control increased intracranial pressure have failed, barbiturate coma may be initiated. High-dose barbiturates reduce cerebral blood flow and decrease cerebral metabolic demand. Pentobarbital is given in an initial dose of 5 to 10 mg/kg. This is followed by a continuous infusion of 1 to 5 mg/kg/hr (to maintain serum levels between 20 and 40 μg/ml).[33] High-dose barbiturates significantly reduce systemic vascular resistance and may produce profound hypotension requiring fluid therapy and vasopressors. Patients receiving high-dose barbiturates require close supervision with continuous blood pressure, cardiac output, and pulmonary artery wedge pressure monitoring.

Spinal cord injury is an infrequent occurrence in children, yet the implications for rehabilitation are far-reaching. Some of the complications that may develop in the spinal cord-injured patient are systemic hypotension, cutaneous vasomotor instability, constipation, neurogenic bladder, urinary tract infections, stress ulcers, pneumonia, pulmonary embolism, decubitus, and deformities such as scoliosis. Nursing interventions such as frequent turning, effective pulmonary toilet, range-of-motion exercises, monitoring of bowel movements, and initiation of a bladder training program may help to prevent complications (see Chapter 22).

Reorientation of the child to the surroundings is important as the child awakens. Family members, in conjunction with the nursing staff, can play an important role in stimulating the child's memory and assisting with mobility and activities of daily living.

COMPLICATIONS OF ABDOMINAL INJURIES. Many children who experience liver or splenic trauma are managed nonoperatively and therefore require close observation for the possible development of complications. Indications for intraoperative management include hemodynamic instability, signs of increasing peritoneal irritation, and the requirement of a transfusion of more than 30% to 50% of the child's total estimated blood volume (20-40 ml/kg).[5]

COMPLICATIONS OF IMMOBILITY. The child is at risk for developing complications, such as pneumonia and skin breakdown, resulting from immobility. As soon as the child's condition has stabilized, a referral is made to a physical or occupational therapist so that appropriate range-of-motion exercises can be incorporated into the plan of care. Splints are used as soon as possible to prevent contractures. Collaboration between the nurses caring for the child and the occupational or physical therapist enhances the benefits of the treatment regimen. When appropriate, the child and parents or significant others are included in the treatment plan as well.

Skin care must be meticulous. Placement of the child on a special mattress or bed, depending on the length of time of critical care intervention, may be necessary.

NUTRITIONAL SUPPORT. Adequate nutrition is essential for the pediatric trauma patient. Children are more at risk than adults for developing protein-calorie malnutrition in the critical care unit. They have increased energy requirements, small nutritional reserves, and greater obligate energy needs than adults. Protein-calorie malnutrition can develop in 5 to 7 days in critically ill children who were previously healthy. Nutritional support should be started as soon as possible after resuscitation is complete. Wound healing and immunocompetence depend on the provision of adequate nutrition.

Enteral feedings are preferable because they are more physiologically normal and more efficient. Individual caloric requirements and the child's general tolerance of a particular formula are among the factors that must be considered when choosing from a variety of available enteral formulas. Excess protein is not beneficial because it is not used efficiently by the body.[34] For children whose oral intake has been restricted for an extended period, a lactose-free formula is necessary because after a period of no gastrointestinal intake, the gut does not produce lactase, which is essential for the breakdown of lactose.

If the child is unable to tolerate enteral formulas, as evidenced by diarrhea or large residuals, total parenteral nutrition (TPN), including lipids, is initiated via a central venous catheter. The choice of TPN formulas greatly depends on the child's individual calorie needs. Once the child is receiving TPN, response to the therapy must be monitored. Metabolic complications may result from electrolyte, glucose, and fat imbalances. Therefore, serum levels should be monitored routinely. Weight gain and progressive wound healing indicate the child's positive response to nutritional support.

Close observation for complications resulting from TPN therapy is indicated as well. Infection is the most frequent complication and is most often the result of poor aseptic technique during catheter placement, during the solution preparation process, or while performing routine catheter care. Care also must be taken to avoid dislodgment of the catheter on insertion or during routine maintenance activities. Such mechanical complications may result in the development of a pneumothorax or air embolism. Close, continuous observation and meticulous catheter care serve as the best preventive methods.

PAIN MANAGEMENT. Pain is a part of every child's experience in the critical care unit. The nurse caring for the child must develop an individualized plan for helping the child cope with alterations in comfort levels. The child's developmental level is the most influential factor in the child's pain response. The ability to understand the reason for pain and to develop ways to cope with it is dependent on the child's level of psychologic maturity.[35]

Analgesics are useful for all age groups to decrease painful impulses and may enhance the effectiveness of other nursing interventions as well. Pain medication should never be withheld from the child if it seems to be the only effective means of pain relief. A combination of narcotics and benzodiazepines is often indicated to control pain and relieve anxiety.

Serving as adjuncts to analgesic therapy, nursing interventions that may assist the child to deal with pain include the use of touch therapy, relaxation or distraction techniques, and the provision of verbal explanations and support. The presence of parents and other family members often helps to lessen the burden of pain as well.

With infants, touching and holding—especially when movements are rhythmic—may be effective because they may stimulate some cutaneous receptor sites that decrease the perception of pain by inhibiting painful impulses.[36] Toddlers seek out parents for comfort and use self-regulating behaviors such as sucking and rocking.

Toddlers are often comforted by parents' talking to them because it serves as a distraction. Also used as a distraction technique, a discussion about siblings or family pets is a useful method to initiate conversation with preschool children. School-age children can be taught methods for relaxation such as deep-breathing exercises, which often work as a distraction technique and as a tension release modality. Touch therapy in the form of massage can also reduce a child's perception of pain.[37]

Before painful procedures, verbal explanations should be given in simple terms, geared specifically to the child's level of understanding. To help prepare for the procedure, the nurse can allow the child to think through how he or she might deal with the pain and to verbalize fears and concerns.

Adolescents may respond favorably to many of the same techniques as younger children, such as distraction and relaxation. They also use verbalization as a method of pain relief. Preparation via verbal explanations is as important for this age group as it is for the younger patient population.

The stimulating atmosphere and fast-paced routines of the critical care unit can contribute to the development of altered sleep patterns. The child's normal sleep patterns are accommodated if at all possible. Special efforts is made to reduce activity at the bedside and to create a quiet environment to promote quality sleep time.

INTERMEDIATE CARE AND REHABILITATION PHASES

Many of the clinical management strategies that were addressed in the critical care phase may be appropriate during the intermediate care and rehabilitation phases as well. To avoid unnecessary repetition, refer to the discussion of these issues in previous sections. The discussions in this section focus primarily on general rehabilitation issues as they pertain to the pediatric trauma patient.

Many children, resilient by nature, tend to recover quickly. They often progress rapidly from the critical care phase to the rehabilitation phase of care, breezing quickly through or skipping entirely a clearly identifiable intermediate care stage.

Rehabilitation issues are addressed at the time of admission. Even during the resuscitation phase, the nurse is astute to the measures that can be taken to lessen or prevent conditions that may otherwise result in short- or long-term disability. All efforts must be taken to assist the child and parent in adapting to the life changes that the trauma experience has elicited. Early recognition of available or lack of available support systems for the pediatric patient and family can facilitate the process of rehabilitation planning as assistance is offered from appropriate resource programs (e.g., social services and financial assistance services). Information elicited for further development of the nursing database should include details that greatly potentiate the creation of a comprehensive rehabilitation plan of care. (Refer to Chapter 10 for more detailed information.)

Trauma, in addition to being the leading cause of death in children, is also a major cause of long-term disability. An estimated 100,000 children or more suffer permanent disabilities resulting from injury every year.[38] The goal of rehabilitation is to provide a better quality of life for the child and to return the child to maximal potential within the family and social unit.

ASSESSMENT OF ADJUSTMENT AND ADAPTATION TO INJURY

It is important to first understand how children adjust to illness based on their individual cognitive/affective developmental level.[39] This affects how the child perceives the situation and what range of responses are available to the child (see Table 29-2).

TODDLER.   The first 2 years of life are a difficult time for the child because of a smaller repertoire of coping skills.[39] The child does not understand the reasons for the illness or treatments, and neither parents nor the health care team can explain them. The child's coping ability is greatly influenced by the parent's presence.

PRESCHOOL-AGE CHILD.   Preschoolers (3-6 years) have acquired some inner resources for coping with stress and thus have more coping abilities than the younger child.[39] The parents remain the major source of coping strength; however, children tolerate short periods of separation from their parents. The child at this age fears bodily intrusion and injury because of an inability to perceive long-term effects. Fantasy and guilt can distort the child's perception of the injury.

SCHOOL-AGE CHILD.   The school-age child (7-12 years) has made enough developmental progress to have enhanced coping abilities. This child has usually developed a peer group by this time and can tolerate longer periods of separation from the parents. Because of increasing cognitive abilities, the child is able to more fully understand cause-and-effect relationships and can think about the future.[40] However, the child still fears bodily injury and loss of control of bodily function.

ADOLESCENT.   The adolescent (13-18 years) has developed skills that enhance the ability to cope.[40] The adolescent is working to establish identity and does not rely as heavily on parents for coping strength. The adolescent is able to think abstractly and can apply general principles to specifics. Two of the biggest fears of the adolescent, however, are bodily disfigurement and loss of control. This becomes a critical issue with an adolescent trauma patient who has suffered an amputation, a spinal cord injury, or some other disfiguring injury. Part of the challenge of rehabilitation with this age group involves helping the adolescent adjust to an altered body image and a level of dependency during a developmental period when independence is being sought.[41]

CLINICAL MANAGEMENT

Interdisciplinary conferences that include the parents and, if appropriate, the patient are held on a regular basis. Mutual goal setting is imperative; goals that have been established by the health team without the involvement of the family and adolescent can actually hinder progress.

The child and family need much support during the rehabilitation phase. Families need to be involved in the child's care and long-range plans. They need honest, accurate information from the health care team. Many times these families are feeling guilt, frustration, and anger. These feelings need to be recognized and channeled appropriately. The nurses working with the families may help them assess their own support systems. It is helpful that families know that it is beneficial for them to maintain relationships with other family members and friends during this time. Other support systems, such as community and government agencies that provide assistance with financial problems or child care, should be discussed.

PLANNING FOR DISCHARGE.

As the child continues to improve, plans for discharge are discussed by the team, again including the parents. Some children may require total care and have little or no rehabilitation potential because of they are in a persistent vegetative state. Other children may make progress toward higher levels of consciousness and rehabilitation with proper stimulation. Children with spinal cord injury require an extended rehabilitation program to help them become as functional as possible relative to their injury. Because of the restorative and regenerative powers of the child and the potential for a long and productive life, every attempt should be made to locate a rehabilitation program that provides all that the child needs to become a functional member of the family and social unit.[42]

Some parents may choose to take their child home. For some families this is a viable alternative, but one that requires a tremendous amount of preparation. Families that are considering this option need to take into consideration the impact this child will have on the family unit. Does the child require special equipment, such as a ventilator and monitors? Will the child need home care nurses? How does the family feel about having a stranger in the home? How will bringing this child home affect the parents' relationships with each other and with their other children?

Once these considerations have been addressed and the decision is made to take the child home, preparations are begun. The family must be taught new skills, such as skin care, catheter care, tracheostomy care, or suctioning procedures, so that care of the child continues in the home environment. Education and instruction about bowel and bladder regimens and range-of-motion exercises also must be accomplished. Electrical safety in the home environment is an issue that must be addressed if special equipment will accompany the child. Family members also must learn to operate and maintain the equipment, such as ventilators and monitors. The tremendous advantage of home care is that children do benefit from the stimulation they receive from their home environment. These families should be encouraged to make contact with rehabilitation centers and appropriate community or government agencies as soon as possible for continued support, guidance, and direction as needed.

COMMUNITY REINTEGRATION.

As the child progresses through the rehabilitation phase, discharge planning continues. Discharge planning, although it can be exciting for the child and family, may also be extremely frightening. They are losing the protective environment of the health care facility.

A comprehensive discharge plan adequately prepares the family and child to go home and helps make the transition back into the community easier. The discharge plan is a component of the rehabilitation plan because the success or failure the family experiences after leaving the hospital depends on how the staff has assessed and worked with the family during the hospital stay. The family is involved from the very beginning of the discharge planning process.

The discharge planning process includes a thorough assessment of the family dynamics and their outside support systems and their ability to cope with stress. Assessment takes place by observing the family with the child in the hospital and by asking pointed questions. These details need to be incorporated into the discharge plan, and appropriate referrals to community agencies must be initiated.

It is often helpful for the child to go home for a day or weekend before the actual discharge date. A home visit gives the family an idea of unforeseen difficulties and helps them gain insight into living with their child again. It also helps the family gain a level of confidence as they realize that they can cope outside the hospital environment.

Another alternative is to have the family spend the weekend at the hospital caring for the child. This approach is especially useful for families of ventilator-dependent children who are going home. Children with spinal cord injuries are included in this population. These families can gain experience with special equipment such as ventilators and feeding pumps. Having a supervised period where they care for their child helps them attain a more realistic view of what it will be like to live with the child and gain a higher level of confidence while receiving the support of the nursing staff.

The development of the discharge plan requires a team effort, often coordinated by the primary nurse. The family should be included in the plan because they will be implementing the care measures at home.

Topics that need to be considered along with the discharge plan include finances, equipment, and supplies. Decisions must also be made about the child's caregivers. It is not uncommon for one or two family members to inadvertently be singled out by other family members as the primary caregivers. The burden of caregiving inevitably falls to one or two family members if a plan for shared responsibilities is not arranged and agreed on by all involved family members before the child's homecoming. The most effective plan is one that takes into consideration the needs of the caregivers and provides periodic relief. A good plan lessens the stress experienced by all involved.

Anyone who will be caring for the child at home also must master skills such as suctioning, tracheostomy care, and CPR, which are necessary to safely care for that child. Family members must be taught to problem-solving skills to deal with any emergencies that may arise, such as power outages and equipment failure. They also need to be made aware of the resources that are available in the hospital and in the community. The family should be encouraged to contact the local emergency response agency before the child's discharge to home to inform them of the situation. Notification helps to ensure that the response team arrives at the home with appropriate equipment and supplies and is adequately prepared to care for the child if called on for an emergency at a later date. It often helps for the family to be linked with a support group as well. Support groups provide the opportunity for families to be in touch with others who can relate to what they are experiencing and with whom they can exchange information.

Family involvement in the discharge plan and reintegration into the community is imperative. A comprehensive plan that prepares the child and family and takes into account all aspects of their physical, emotional, intellectual, and spiritual well-being has a favorable chance for success. Families can provide a strong motivation for the child to work toward recovery by being prepared to take the child home and support him or her through the reintegration process.

SUMMARY

Trauma is the primary killer of children between the ages of 1 and 14 years. One of every two children who die during these years does so because of an unexpected injury. Trauma is also a major cause of disabling injuries in children. This has serious implications for the expenditure of resources and personnel at a time when more constraints are occurring in the health care system. The resulting need for rehabilitation also has tremendous implications regarding the termination of work potential, the length of rehabilitation, and the adjustments affecting the growth and development of the child.

Further research endeavors should attempt to answer the following questions: Is the use of touch effective in reducing intracranial pressure in children? What is the relationship between the nutritional status of children and long-term outcomes? What are the long-term psychologic effects of head injury on children? What nursing interventions are most effective in supporting children in the adjustment to an altered body image? Many of the studies undertaken in the area of adult trauma should be redesigned to study the pediatric trauma population as well.

Efforts are needed to improve pediatric emergency medical systems. Such efforts must be focused on regional centers that can develop a systematic approach to the care of pediatric trauma patients. The health care team caring for the pediatric trauma patient must be well trained in the area of pediatric trauma. The facility also must be equipped to handle an injured child.

Legislators and other community leaders must be made aware of the devastating sequelae of traumatic injury. Pediatric trauma can be considered to be at epidemic proportions in our society today. Mandatory car seat and seat belt laws, when enforced, result in the saving of many young lives. Motorcycle and bicycle helmet laws can do the same. More attention needs to be focused on safety issues that affect the child. Nurses can do this by writing letters to senators, congressional representatives, and editors and by testifying at legislative hearings concerning pediatric trauma and safety issues.

Nurses, by virtue of their expert knowledge and skills, can provide educational leadership in a variety of ways. Nurses should expand their scope of practice by speaking to local agencies, parent groups, and children themselves about child safety issues and by teaching other colleagues about caring for the pediatric trauma patient. Legislators should be kept informed of all issues that currently affect the pediatric trauma population. Funding that supports extensive public awareness programs must be sought. Training and instruction must be provided by knowledgeable professionals, and more stringent safety laws must be pursued with diligence. The nurse's role in supporting all aspects of preventive care is paramount. Prevention remains the most effective treatment regimen for preserving the precious young lives in our society.

REFERENCES

1. Knapp JF: Practical issues in the care of pediatric trauma patients, *Curr Prob Pediatr* 20:309-320, 1998.
2. Scholer SJ, Hickson GB, Ray WA: Sociodemographic factors identify U.S. infants at high risk of injury mortality, *Pediatr* 103:1183-1188, 1999.
3. Hall JR, Reyes HR, Meller JL et al: The outcome for children with blunt trauma is best at a pediatric trauma center, *J Pediatr Surg* 31:72-77, 1996.
4. Zuckerman GB, Conway EE: Accidental head injury, *Pediatr Ann* 26:621-632, 1997.
5. Moloney-Harmon PA, Adams P: Trauma. In Curley MAQ, Moloney-Harmon PA, editors: *Critical care nursing of infants and children,* Philadelphia, 2001, WB Saunders, 947-980.
6. Widner-Kolberg MR: Child abuse, *Crit Care Nurs Clin North Am* 9:175-182, 1997.
7. Duhaime A, Christian CW, Rorke LB: Nonaccidental head injury in infants—the "shaken-baby syndrome," N Engl J Med 338:1822-1829, 1998.
8. Centers for Disease Control and Prevention: Motor-vehicle safety: a 20th century public health achievement, *MMWR* 48:369-375, 1999.
9. Swick D: Submersion injuries in children, *Int J Trauma Nurs* 3:59-64, 1997.
10. American College of Surgeons Committee on Trauma: *Advanced trauma life support manual,* ed 6, Chicago, 1997, American College of Surgeons.

11. Roberts KE: Fluid and electrolyte regulation. In Curley MAQ, Moloney-Harmon PA, editors: *Critical care nursing of infants and children*, Philadelphia, 2001, WB Saunders, 369-392.

12. Van Amerongen R, Rosen M, Winnick G et al: Ventricular fibrillation following blunt chest trauma from a baseball, *Pediatr Emerg Care* 13:107-110, 1997.

13. Brinker D, Moloney-Harmon PA: Hematologic critical care problems. In Curley MAQ, Moloney-Harmon PA, editors: *Critical care nursing of infants and children*, Philadelphia, 2001, WB Saunders, 821-850.

14. Fisher MD: Pediatric traumatic brain injury, *Crit Care Nurs Q* 20:36-51, 1997.

15. Mansfield RT: Head injuries in children and adults, *Crit Care Clin* 13:611-627, 1997.

16. Larsen GY, Vernon DD, Dean JM: Evaluation of the comatose child. In Rogers MC, editor: *Textbook of pediatric intensive care*, Philadelphia, 1996, WB Saunders, 735-746.

17. Grasso SN, Keller MS: Diagnostic imaging in pediatric trauma, *Curr Opin Pediatr* 10:299-302, 1998.

18. Martin S, Derengowski S: Gastrointestinal system. In Slota MC, editor: *Core curriculum for pediatric critical care nursing*, Philadelphia, 1998, WB Saunders, 424-460.

19. Tobias J, Rasmussen GE, Yaster M: Multiple trauma in the pediatric patient. In Rogers MC, editor: *Textbook of pediatric intensive care*, Philadelphia, 1996, WB Saunders, 1467-1504.

20. Partrick DA, Bensard DD, Moore EE et al: Ultrasound is an effective triage tool to evaluate blunt abdominal trauma in the pediatric population, *J Trauma* 45:57-63, 1998.

21. Morgan WM III, O'Neill JA Jr: Hemorrhagic and obstructive shock in pediatric patients, *New Horiz* 6:150-154, 1998.

22. Carnevale FA: Striving to recapture our previous life: the experience of families with critically ill children, *J Can Assoc Crit Care Nurs* 10:16-22, 1999.

23. Boie ET, Moore GP, Brummett C et al: Do parents want to be present during invasive procedures performed on their children in the emergency department? A survey of 400 parents, *Ann Emerg Med* 34:70-74, 1999.

24. Mangini L, Confessore MT, Girard P et al: Pediatric trauma support program: supporting children and families in emotional crisis, *Crit Care Nurs Clin* 7:557-567, 1995.

25. Pearson LJ: Separation, loss, bereavement. In Broome ME, Rollins JA, editors: *Core curriculum for the nursing care of children and their families*, Pitman, NJ, 1999, Jannetti, 77-92.

26. Grehn LS, Kline A, Weishaar J: Renal critical care problems. In Curley MAQ, Moloney-Harmon PA, editors: *Critical care nursing of infants and children*, Philadelphia, 2001, WB Saunders, 731-764.

27. Wichmann MW, Ayala A, Chaudry IH: Severe depression of host immune functions following closed-bone, soft-tissue trauma, and hemorrhagic shock, *Crit Care Med* 26:1372-1378, 1998.

28. Allen CH, Ward JD: An evidence-based approach to management of increased intracranial pressure, *Crit Care Clin* 14:485-495, 1998.

29. Shackford SR, Bourguignon PR, Wald SL et al: Hypertonic saline resuscitation of patients with head injury: a prospective, randomized clinical trial, *J Trauma* 44:50-58, 1998.

30. Simma B, Burger R, Falk M: A prospective, randomized, and controlled study of fluid management in children with severe head injury: lactated ringer's solution versus hypertonic saline, *Crit Care Med* 26:1265-1270, 1998.

31. Bruce DA, Alavi A, Bilaniuk L et al: Diffuse cerebral swelling following head injuries in children: the syndrome of "malignant brain edema," *J Neurosurg* 54:170-178, 1981.

32. Hahn YS, Fuchs S, Flannery AM et al: Factors influencing post-traumatic seizures in children, *Neurosurgery* 22:864-867, 1988.

33. Poss WB, Brockmeyer D, Clay B et al: Pathophysiology and management of the intracranial vault. In Rogers MC, editor: *Textbook of pediatric intensive care*, Philadelphia, 1996, WB Saunders, 645-666.

34. Verger JT, Schears G: Nutrition support. In Curley MAQ, Moloney-Harmon PA, editors: *Critical care nursing of infants and children*, Philadelphia, 2001, WB Saunders, 393-424.

35. Abu-Saad HH: Pain in children: a state of the art. In Tibboels D, van der Voort E, editors: *Intensive care in childhood: a challenge to the future*, Berlin, 1996, Springer-Verlag, 517-526.

36. Franck LS: The ethical imperative to treat pain in infants: are we doing the best we can? *Crit Care Nurs* 17:80-86, 1997.

37. Oakes LL: Caring practices: providing comfort. In Curley MAQ, Moloney-Harmon PA, editors: *Critical care nursing of infants and children*, Philadelphia, 2001, WB Saunders, 547-576.

38. Kirk JA: Pediatric trauma, *Clin Forum Nurse Anesth* 8:135-143, 1997.

39. Baroni MA: Cognitive and psychosocial development. In Broome ME, Rollins JA, editors: *Core curriculum for the nursing care of children and their families*, Pitman, NJ, 1999, Jannetti, 31-44.

40. Smith JB, Martin SA: Caring practices: providing developmentally appropriate care. In Curley MAQ, Moloney-Harmon PA, editors: *Critical care nursing of infants and children*, Philadelphia, 2001, WB Saunders, 17-46.

41. Bindler R: Health behavior. In Broome ME, Rollins JA, editors: *Core curriculum for the nursing care of children and their families*, Pitman, NJ, 1999, Jannetti, 63-76.

42. Holbrook TL, Anderson JA, Sieber WJ et al: Outcome after major trauma: 12-month and 18-month follow-up results from the trauma recovery project, *J Trauma* 46:765-773, 1999.

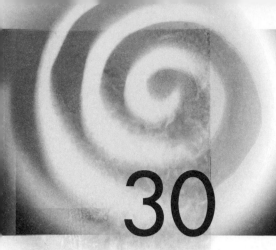

TRAUMA IN THE ELDERLY

Sharon L. Atwell

30

Projections by the U.S. Bureau of the Census[1] indicate that in 2030 20% of the population of the United States will be age 65 years or older. The elderly are the fastest growing segment of our population. The aging of our population represents a significant change in the national character, which has a major impact on the delivery of health care. Treatment costs are higher for elderly trauma victims than for the young, and outcomes for the elderly may be less satisfactory.[2] However, one recent study concluded that the actual per capita cost to a trauma center for elder care was less than for younger patients because 98% of the elderly were insured.[3]

Normal aging is a gradual process. From the moment of conception, a person undergoes progressive change: Youth and immaturity give way to adulthood and maturation. The summation of all the unique experiences of an individual is known as *aging.*

Research regarding the effects of aging on human function has provided greater understanding of the process but has also generated many new questions. To date no universal agreement exists as to when a person becomes "old." The chronologic age of 65 years is most often cited although some authors now differentiate between the young old (those between the ages of 65 and 74), the old (ages 75 through 84), and the oldest old (those over the age of 85).[4] Such designations, however, fail to adequately differentiate between the "healthy" old and the "infirm" old. It is clear that chronologic age alone is not adequate to explain the term *elderly.* At this time there is no omnibus process for assessing human biologic age.

Within the natural human life span, each person's experience is like no other. Illness and injury may contribute to shortened life expectancy, and the biologic clock that regulates function may begin to slow. Differences among individuals are expressed as differences in the capacity to function. Because of the wide variability among people, it becomes more and more difficult to estimate when an individual becomes "old." That is, any two 40-year-old persons are more alike than they are different; any two 70-year-old persons are more different than they are alike. Although chronologic age is clearly an inadequate measure,

in this chapter *elderly* is defined as an individual of chronologic age 65 years or more.

The ambiguity surrounding the definition of the elderly patient population creates difficulty for the nurse who is trying to anticipate potential problems related to trauma. It is unlikely that protocols developed for a younger population are as effective for older persons. However, currently available research does not provide sufficient information to indicate where changes should be made. The primary problem is that the available information does not adequately distinguish between elderly patients' responses to trauma apart from their altered responses as a result of chronic disease.

This intent of this chapter is to provide nurses with a brief summary of what is presently known about age-related physiologic changes in their patients, as well as the alterations in functional capacity that may result. It also explains the impact of these changes on elderly trauma patients and describes how nurses can optimize their care for this rapidly growing population.

EPIDEMIOLOGY

Injury is the seventh most frequent cause of death in persons age 65 years and over.[5] Injury deaths are preceded by mortality as a result of cancer, heart disease, chronic obstructive pulmonary disease, stroke, and pneumonia or influenza.[5] Although the elderly are injured less frequently than younger individuals, when they do sustain injuries, older patients are much more likely to die. In addition, injuries of relatively low severity in the elderly population have a significantly higher probability of resulting in death than they do in younger individuals.[5,6]

Between 1986 and 1996 the death rate from unintentional injuries decreased by more than 25% for all ages less than 25 years and by approximately 10% for people ages 25 through 74. Yet the unintentional injury death rate for people age 75 and older only decreased by half of 1% (Table 30-1). Also, the death rate from unintentional injuries is more than three times higher for those 75 years and older than for those who are 65 to 74.[5]

TABLE 30-1	Unintentional Injury Death Rates by Age in the United States		
Age Group	1986*	1996*	% Change
All Ages	39.7	35.2	−11
<5	21.4	15.0	−30
5-14	12.6	9.4	−25
15-24	50.5	37.8	−25
25-44	36.1	32.7	−9
45-64	33.0	30.2	−8
65-74	49.6	43.9	−11
≥75	141.5	140.9	−1

Data from National Safety Council: *Accident facts*, Chicago, 1997, National Safety Council.
*Per 100,000 population.

TABLE 30-2	Motor Vehicle Death Rates by Age in the United States		
Age Group	1986*	1996*	% Change
All Ages	19.9	16.3	−18
<5	6.6	5.2	−21
5-14	7.0	5.5	−21
15-24	38.5	29.3	−24
25-44	21.0	17.4	−17
45-64	15.2	13.8	−9
65-74	18.1	17.1	−6
≥75	28.3	29.0	+2

Data from National Safety Council: *Accident facts*, Chicago, 1997, National Safety Council.
*Per 100,000 population.

Comparative data from the National Safety Council[5] indicate that 68% of unintentional injury deaths in individuals 65 and older are due to three causes: motor vehicle crashes, falls, and thermal injuries. Motor vehicle crashes (including injuries to both vehicle occupants and pedestrians) account for 27% of the deaths. However, motor vehicle crashes are the most common cause of death from trauma through age 79, after which falls take the lead. Falls are the leading cause of death for both elderly men and women, accounting for approximately 38% of all trauma fatalities and almost 50% of the trauma-related deaths in persons more than 80 years of age. The literature suggests that an acute alteration in health status sometimes proceeds a fall. However, deficits in muscular strength and dexterity, often in combination with balance impairment, are more often the contributing factors. Prescription drugs and excessive alcohol intake may also contribute to falls in the elderly.[7]

Approximately 15% of licensed drivers in the United States are 65 years and older, totaling more than 25 million as of 1996.[5] These elderly drivers are involved in only 7% of the total motor vehicle crashes. However, on the basis of the lower number of miles they drive, individuals 75 years and older have a higher rate of involvement in fatal crashes than those in any other age group.[5] These statistics yield no information about the causes of the crashes but suggest that someone is more likely to die in a collision involving an elderly driver than in a collision involving a younger driver. That is not surprising when one considers the increased trauma mortality of the elderly driver alone.

A complicating factor is the nonlinear relationship between the total number of miles a person drives and the number of motor vehicle crashes that occur.[8] This may be at least partially explained by the fact that high-mileage drivers tend to travel more on major roadways, where the risk of collision is lower, than on the smaller roads (with respectively more intersections) that are negotiated by low-mileage drivers. From 1986 to 1996 the death rates for motor vehicle crashes decreased for all age groups by 18%. In contrast, the death rate for persons age 75 years and older increased.[5] Table 30-2 illustrates these death rates as a result of motor vehicle crashes according to age.

Death as a result of thermal injury accounts for approximately 4% of all accidental deaths in those 65 years of age and older.[5] Thermal injuries include flame burns and inhalation injury, direct and indirect contact with sources of heat, and electrical injury.[5] Scalds, flame burns, and contact with hot objects are the types of thermal injuries suffered most commonly by the elderly population.

PATTERNS OF INJURY

Falls are the most frequent cause of injury in the elderly population. Approximately 30% of individuals age 65 years and older fall each year.[9] Ninety-five percent of these elderly people live in the community.[7] Falls usually occur on level surfaces, and approximately 10% result in serious injury.[10,11] The majority of the injuries classified as serious are fractures of the hips, arms and hands, legs and feet, ribs, vertebrae, and pelvis, but head trauma and other nonfracture joint injuries occur as well.[11,12] The incidence of fractures is higher in elderly women than in men; however, the mortality rate is higher in men.[13]

Studies of the biomechanics of motor vehicle crashes indicate that crashes involving the elderly should be expected to result in injury patterns similar to those seen in younger patients. Comparisons between the young and the elderly are difficult because of variations in the manner of documenting injury in published reports and the fact that the elderly are seldom analyzed separately from the young.

The elderly are less likely than their younger counterparts to be involved in crashes after ingesting alcohol. They are more often involved in low-velocity crashes than younger adults. Although the incidence of injury to the abdominal and pelvic regions in the older age group is remarkably low, the mortality from abdominal injuries is significantly greater for the elderly.[14,15] The risk of rib cage fractures secondary to motor vehicle crashes is 10 times higher for elderly drivers than for younger drivers, with shoulder harness design implicated as a contributing factor.[5,6]

Thermal injuries in the elderly are associated with higher mortality compared with similar injuries in the young. When burn-related mortality is compared with age, it is usually expressed as the percentage of burn that leads to a 50% mortality.[16] The estimated 50% mortality for individuals between age 3 years and early adulthood is near 80% total body surface area (TBSA).[17] However, for patients older than 70 years old, there is an estimated 50% mortality for 20% to 30% TBSA.[18]

Members of the elderly population often have difficulty preventing burn injuries because of sensory deficits, increased reaction times, and limited dexterity. The same characteristics may contribute to increased burn severity, primarily because of longer contact time with the heat source. For example, impaired thermal perception predisposes older individuals to scalds that are often sustained from tap water in their own residences. The elderly are also more likely to sustain burns from ignited clothing and less able to escape from burning buildings.

INJURY THRESHOLD

INCREASED PERSONAL RISK

The aging process produces unique changes in an individual's functional status, which contribute to increased susceptibility to injury and increased mortality. These age-related physiologic changes vary immensely between individuals, and these changes, rather than the older age itself, contribute to the elderly patient's response to trauma.[15] Body systems most often cited as showing evidence of age-impaired function include the cardiovascular, respiratory, renal, musculoskeletal, and endocrine systems. Neurologic function is generally considered intact, with one notable exception: deterioration in special senses. The elderly also tend to accumulate the effects of chronic disease, which may add further limitations to those imposed by aging alone.

Age-related deterioration in function and chronic diseases have been implicated as causative factors in traumatic injury. Among community dwelling older individuals, falls are a strong predictor of placement in a skilled-nursing facility.[11] Mishaps such as tripping over furniture, steps, scatter rugs, and other obstacles are often cited as the immediate precursor to a fall. Other factors leading to falls are decreasing function of the special senses (such as loss of peripheral vision), syncope, postural instability, transient impairment of cerebrovascular perfusion, alcohol ingestion, and medication use.[7] The elderly also seem more susceptible to falls when exposed to a new environment.

Alterations in perception and delayed response to stressors also may contribute to injury. Diminished or impaired proprioception reduces awareness of an impending fall. The onset of corrective measures may then be too late to avoid falling. Loss of visual acuity limits the elderly person's ability to see traffic hazards and avoid them.

Preexisting diseases have been implicated as contributing factors in injuries sustained by the elderly. Chronic conditions that are associated with loss of consciousness, such as epilepsy, certain cardiac arrhythmias, and cerebrovascular disease, have been documented as leading to falls.[7] Preexist-

ing organ dysfunction (cardiovascular, hepatic, respiratory, renal, and endocrine) has been reported to have "a profound effect on patient outcome"[19] after injury, even after controlling for age and other factors. A 1997 retrospective study[20] reported that preexisting disease adversely affected the long-term survival of elderly patients. The same report stated, however, that the best overall predictor of adverse outcomes in trauma is the patient's age. Research results must be compared cautiously because of the many variations in study design. In addition, the diversity of the elderly population makes generalization of research findings extremely difficult.

Many older adults regularly use multiple medications. Although the use of specific medications by the elderly has not been clearly related to increased injury rates, it contributes at least in an indirect fashion.[21] Often an individual is under the care of more than one physician for more than one condition that requires medication. Drug interactions among prescribed medications (in addition to over-the-counter self-medication) are likely causes of impaired perception and response.[22] The number of adverse reactions to polypharmacy increases with the number of drugs taken and the consumption of alcohol.[7,21,23] Approximately 10% of elderly individuals are believed to be alcoholics.[24]

INCREASED SOCIETAL RISK

We live in a society that has been dominated by the fantasy of everlasting youth and health. Most communicable diseases have all but been eradicated, life spans have increased, and in many ways we are indeed enjoying healthier lives. However, as our society celebrates youth and long life, both the number of elderly citizens and the hazards to which they are regularly exposed are increasing rapidly. For example, the average traffic signal in the United States is designed for people who walk at four feet per second, a rate that is too fast for many persons more than 60 years of age.[25] A 1994 study[26] illustrated that more than 25% of older pedestrians were unable to cross all lanes of traffic at a busy intersection in the time allowed by the traffic signal.

Environmental hazards abound. Many road traffic areas were designed approximately 50 years ago, when the standard automobile was larger and heavier and the average age of drivers was younger. Increases in the number of distractions on modern streets and highways may overload the information processing capabilities of anyone, but especially those of elderly drivers and pedestrians. In the home, designs and furnishings favor the decorating tastes of younger persons. Scatter rugs, tables with sharp corners, open flames on stoves, cabinets located above eye level, stairs without railings, tap water heated to more than 130° F, and inadequate lighting increase the risk of accidental injury for the elderly.

As we look toward a future with greater numbers of elderly citizens, it becomes apparent that not enough is known about the special needs of our aging citizens. Health care providers must become aware of the many risks faced by the elderly. Nurses are well positioned to support the efforts of epidemiologists seeking to reduce environmental hazards. They can also have a positive effect on the attitudes and values of society at large.

RESUSCITATION PHASE

There are two major problems confronting health care providers responsible for the resuscitation of elderly trauma patients. First is the wide variability in prior function that exists in this patient population. Generalizations concerning injuries and responses to injury are possible with younger patients but are difficult, if not impossible, in the elderly. Second is the lack of adequate documentation concerning the initial response of older adults to injury. As a result, much is assumed about the elderly trauma patient but little is known. Widespread belief that all elderly individuals have significantly impaired cardiovascular function sometimes leads to inadequate fluid replacement and persistent hypovolemia. Conversely, the elderly are sometimes treated without due consideration of potential cardiovascular impairment, and fluid overload may result.

The inaccurate impression that all older individuals have significantly impaired function is easily acquired from the literature. Many reports primarily document disease and disability in the elderly, without regard for the resiliency of the healthy aged population. Many of our elderly citizens are healthy; therefore, generic patient management decisions based on chronologic age alone are unjustifiable.

ASSESSMENT. Resuscitation of the trauma patient is characterized by a need for speed and efficiency. To determine the magnitude of injury, the individual's response, and the potential for complications, the nurse relies on knowledge and experience to direct patient assessment. Experience is limited in resuscitation of elderly patients compared with that of younger populations. Rapid and thorough assessment is crucial in all emergencies; it is more difficult to perform in elderly patients because assumptions may not be valid. Assessment itself is especially complicated in cases when an older person presents with the accumulated effects of prior disease and injury. Table 30-3 lists normal physiologic changes that are part of aging.

An increase in the degree of monitoring is indicated because the elderly have higher mortality rates even when apparent injury is of low severity. In younger populations, increases in Injury Severity Score parallel increases in mortality. For the older population, however, death often results from injuries that would be survived by younger persons.[27] One study of long-term survival in older trauma patients illustrated that mortality related to their injuries is increased for as many as 5 years after the injury.[20] However, this increased mortality should not be allowed to eclipse the fact that significant numbers of elderly patients not only survive their acute injuries but eventually return to reasonable function and independent living.[28]

CARDIOVASCULAR CONSIDERATIONS. The general decline in cardiovascular function noted in the aged implies a diminished ability to respond to traumatic stresses. Age-related changes of the cardiovascular system include an increased amount of collagen, causing a stiffened left ventricle and increased rigidity of the cardiac valves.[29] Stress response and catecholamine release are not altered, but sensitivity to catecholamines is decreased, presenting as a decreased β-adrenergic response.[16,29] Elasticity of arterial walls declines with age, causing an increase in pulmonary and peripheral vascular resistance. These changes may be characterized by a delay in activation of responses, diminished magnitude of compensatory responses, a failure to sustain life after injuries usually survived by younger persons, or a combination of all these factors.

As is true for all trauma patients, initial measurements of blood pressure are likely to be misleading because of compensation or prior dysfunction. For example, the elderly have an increased incidence of hypertension.[30] Thus an initial normal blood pressure may mask true hypotension. Likewise, medications taken for chronic conditions, such as β-blockers, alter physiologic compensatory mechanisms and often obscure signs of shock.

Continuous monitoring should be instituted rapidly in elderly patients in order to assess trends and patterns of response. Early invasive monitoring (e.g., arterial lines, central venous pressure lines, and pulmonary artery catheters) should be considered despite some iatrogenic risk because it provides more reliable assessment of cardiovascular performance and guidance of fluid replacement therapy. Scalea et al[31,32] suggested that the elderly may appear hemodynamically stable while experiencing inadequate perfusion. Their data showed that delays in recognition and treatment of underperfusion were associated with increasing mortality. Although the sample was small, their study illustrated that invasive monitoring could assist in the identification of elderly patients with cardiovascular impairment, thereby reducing the risk of complications and death.

Arrhythmias in the elderly are essentially the same as those in younger populations; however, the incidence of atrial fibrillation, premature atrial and ventricular contractions, and heart block is considerably higher.[33] Nurses should evaluate cardiac arrhythmias for causes related to injury, such as hypoxemia or myocardial contusion, rather than assume they are due to cardiac disease. Myocardial infarction is often hypothesized as a cause of accidents, but there is little evidence to support this assumption. However, acute infarction may be found by the time the patient is admitted. Therefore, the patient should be assessed to rule out an acute process. A 12-lead electrocardiogram (ECG) should be obtained initially to provide baseline data. When clinical or electrocardiographic evidence supports a diagnosis of myocardial infarction, serial ECGs, serial cardiac enzymes, and troponin levels should be obtained. Elevation of the myocardial fraction of creatine kinase (CK-MB isoenzyme) with a normal creatine kinase (CK) level occurs

TABLE 30-3   Effects of Increasing Age on Organ Systems

Body System	Effects
Cardiovascular System	
Main pathologic disease	Hypertension, atherosclerosis
	Decreased ability to adapt to demands
	Decreased hypertrophic growth in response to stress
Increased risk for heart failure	Increased aortic impedance (increased diameter, stiffness)
	Increased left ventricular and papillary muscle thickness
	Decreased velocity of ventricular contraction and relaxation
	Decreased response to catecholamines (decreased β-adrenergic and muscarinic receptors)
	Decreased atrial contraction
	Increased myocardial fibrosis
	Increased risk for arrhythmias
Increased ischemic risks	Decreased vascularity
	Decreased vasodilator reserve
	Decreased capillary and arteriolar density
	Decreased autoregulation of coronary flow
	Decreased tolerance for ischemia
	Decreased cellular response to stress
Systemic changes	Increased fatigue
	Decreased ability to extract and utilize oxygen
	Decreased maximal oxygen consumption
	Decreased arterial-venous oxygen difference
Pulmonary System	
Generalized changes	Decreased vital capacity
	Decreased elasticity
	Decreased ciliary function
	Decreased respiratory muscle strength
	Increased work of breathing
Central Nervous System	
Cognitive changes	Decreased brain weight/mass
	Regional loss of neurons
	Increased neuronal death rate
	Decreased muscarinic receptors
	Increased intracranial and extracranial atherosclerosis
Increased CVA risk	Decreased cerebral perfusion
	Decreased blood flow
	Decreased cerebrovascular autoregulation
	Decreased sensory nerve and organ function (decreased vision, hearing, touch)
Peripheral nerve function changes	Increased sensitivity of peripheral nerves to injury
	Decreased muscle innervation
Skeletal Muscle System	
	Decreased ability to extract and utilize oxygen
	Decreased strength force
	Increased fatigue (increased need for recruitment to obtain strength)
	Decreased muscle mass (decreased cross-sectional diameter and decreased fibers)
Renal System	
Generalized changes	Decreased renal blood flow
	Decreased glomerular filtration rate
	Decreased sodium-conserving ability
	Decreased ability to tolerate ischemia, toxins
Decreased bladder muscular tone	Increased residual urine
Mucosal cell surface changes	Increased susceptibility to infection

Modified from Greenhalgh DG: Preexisting factors that effect care. In Carrougher GH, editor: *Burn care and therapy,* New York, 1998, Mosby, 383-385.

CVA, Cerebrovascular accident.

TABLE 30-3 Effects of Increasing Age on Organ Systems—cont'd

Body System	Effects
Gastrointestinal System	
Generalized gastrointestinal tract changes	Decreased gastric acid secretion
	Decreased intestinal motility
Generalized hepatobiliary changes	Decreased hepatic mass
	Decreased liver enzyme activity
	Decreased microsomal enzyme function
Hematopoiesis System	
Hematopoiesis	Decreased active bone marrow
	Decreased marrow fat
	Decreased hematopoiesis with demand
Decreased leukocyte function	Decreased killing
	Decreased chemotactic ability
	Decreased T-cell function
	Infection risk
Endocrine System	
Generalized changes	Increased basal and stimulated norepinephrine levels
	Mild changes in glucocorticoid regulation (decreased feedback control at pituitary and hypothalamus)
Glucose regulation dysfunction	Decreased insulin release
	Decreased glucose regulation
	Increased insulin resistance
Other Systems	
Generalized skin changes	Thinner skin
	Decreased hair follicles (impaired healing?)
	Decreased fat (more prone to pressure)
Weakened bone	Decreased bone mass
	Increased osteoporosis (increased fracture risk)
Decreased wound healing	Decreased inflammatory and proliferative responses
	Decreased angiogenesis
	Decreased fibroblast function (decreased collagen, decreased breaking strength)
	Decreased reepithelialization
	Decreased remodeling capabilities

twice as often in elderly patients with myocardial infarction than in younger patients.[34]

PULMONARY CONSIDERATIONS. Aging reduces lung mass and elasticity and calcification of the costal cartilage and osteoporosis limit the expansion of the rib cage, decreasing vital capacity. As a person ages, the trachea and bronchi tend to calcify, causing an increase in dead space ventilation. The pulmonary arteries thicken, decreasing vessel distensibility and increasing pulmonary vascular resistance. The lung parenchyma alveolar surface declines progressively with aging.[29] Alveolar ducts enlarge and alveoli become flatter and shallower, decreasing the amount of lung volume available for gas exchange. Respiratory muscle fibers atrophy, decreasing respiratory muscle strength and thus heightening the elderly patient's risk for respiratory fatigue in the face of traumatic injury. Cilia atrophy with age, increasing the risk for pulmonary infections. These age-related changes should not be mistaken for chronic lung disease. Common clinical findings in the elderly include a lowered arterial oxygen tension, a decrease in lung mechanics, and a marked tendency to develop pneumonia when hospitalized.[35,36] Arterial blood gas measurements typically show a moderately reduced oxygen tension (e.g., Pao_2 of 80 mmHg), whereas other values are within normal limits. Changes in values other than the Pao_2 should be interpreted in the context of the injury. Measurements across time remain essential for determining trends.

NEUROLOGIC CONSIDERATIONS. Initial neurologic assessment should include a brief examination of the patient for impairments of the special senses, especially vision and hearing, because alterations in these functions may cloud further assessment. Cognitive function can be tested superficially if the patient is capable of verbal response. Assessment of cognitive function may also be complicated by loss of short-term memory, the presence of senile dementia, or slow responses caused by an overload of sensory input.

Careful assessment should be made for evidence of intracerebral bleeding, particularly in trauma associated with falls and motor vehicle crashes. Younger trauma victims tend to sustain closed head injuries with cerebral edema, but older victims are more prone to bleeding incidents. Pupillary responses tend to be sluggish in the elderly, and assessment may be further complicated by eye disease or previous surgery.

MUSCULOSKELETAL CONSIDERATIONS.   Musculoskeletal assessment should be performed with consideration of age-related changes: limitations in mobility and joint flexibility, muscle atrophy, loss of subcutaneous fat, and preexisting deformity. Hip fractures are often associated with additional injuries, such as other fractures or head trauma. This suggests that the nurse should be alert to the potential for fractures of the wrists, humeri, ribs, and vertebrae, in addition to hip or femur fracture in patients admitted after falls.[11]

Large ecchymoses often result from minor injuries in the elderly because of their capillary fragility. Older individuals also have a tendency to develop large hematomas that migrate to dependent locations. Osteoarthritis is a common finding that results in deformity and limitation in joint mobility.[37] Especially when the cervical spine is involved, considerable difficulty may be encountered during initial assessment of the neck.[25]

Although conventional assessment techniques are presumed effective, some fractures may be missed if the patient has impaired perception of pain. The absence of pain should not be relied on to rule out the possibility of fracture. Where any question exists, radiologic confirmation is indicated.

RENAL CONSIDERATIONS.   The effects of age on renal function can be summarized as decreased renal blood flow (reduced glomerular filtration rate), impaired water reabsorption, decreased bladder capacity, decreased diluting ability, and delayed accommodation to stresses.[38] These changes may manifest through inappropriately high urinary output in the face of hypovolemia. Insertion of an indwelling urinary catheter carries a greater risk of infection in older persons but is justified for its monitoring value. Elevations in blood urea nitrogen (BUN) level (up to 69 mg/dl) and serum creatinine (1.9 mg/dl) are reflective of age.[39]

METABOLIC CONSIDERATIONS.   Little evidence exists that there is a decline in endocrine functions essential to the stress response, such as epinephrine or norepinephrine secretion. Adaptive responses in the elderly seem to be intact, but greater time is required for adaptation to occur. Some endocrine secretions, most notably estrogen, do diminish with age. The most frequent endocrine disorders found in the elderly are diabetes mellitus and hypothyroidism.[40]

PSYCHOSOCIAL CONSIDERATIONS.   The unique personal and health history of the individual should be obtained as soon as possible. If the patient is a reliable historian, immediate information concerning relevant medical history, including use of medications, should be obtained. If this is not possible, family members or friends often can provide valuable information. Contact with the patient's primary health care provider provides valuable insight into the prior health of the patient and should not be overlooked. Questions concerning the individual's daily activity and degree of independence prove helpful not only during initial assessment and treatment but later as well, when formulating long-term plans.

MANAGEMENT CONSIDERATIONS.   The same principles and concepts that underlie nursing management in young trauma patients apply to care of the elderly. Nursing care should emphasize communication with the patient through combined mediums, including vision, touch, and hearing. Although it is difficult to accomplish during resuscitation, the nurse should seek eye contact in the patient's direct line of vision and should speak slowly, clearly, and in low tones when talking to the patient. Questions should be phrased simply with limited use of medical terms. Verbal communication should be reinforced by purposeful touch that is gentle yet firm.

Elderly patients often experience tremendous fear in the midst of resuscitation procedures. Although physical and chemical restraints are sometimes used to facilitate resuscitation efforts, they can be justified only to protect the patient or staff from harm. Restraints should be considered a last resort after all attempts to communicate have failed and when it is clear that the patient lacks decision-making capacity. Also, restraints are appropriate to facilitate care only when the patient's condition is emergent.[41] Firm manual restraint is always preferable to tying the patient down. Restraint should be employed only for as long as necessary and should be accompanied by ongoing attempts to explain resuscitation procedures.[42,43] It is especially crucial that trauma nurses remember their role as patient advocate when caring for injured members of the elderly population.

Although the priorities of initial assessment and treatment of elderly patients do not differ from those of the young, specific procedures may have to be modified. In an elderly person requiring intubation, potential difficulty with positioning should be anticipated if the patient has cervical osteoarthritis. When required, intubation should be attempted under the best possible conditions in order to minimize incidental damage to the larynx or friable mucous membranes. Asepsis is essential because of the great risk of pulmonary infection in the elderly.

Mechanical ventilation should be instituted rapidly, if indicated, because the elderly have limited ventilatory reserve. Most elderly patients with blunt chest trauma who require mechanical ventilation sustain their injuries in motor vehicle crashes. Successful ventilatory management of these elderly patients is facilitated by the use of intercostal nerve blocks, intrapleural analgesia, and epidural blocks to augment other pain control measures.[32]

Fluid resuscitation must be monitored closely to ensure adequate, rapid replacement without excess administration of fluids. The general belief that rapid rates of administration tend to produce fluid overload in the elderly has not been substantiated through research. Conservative treatment based on this belief may prolong periods of hypovolemia and hypoperfusion, increasing morbidity and mortality.

In elderly trauma victims there is an increased possibility of prolonged periods of hypoperfusion, which may contribute to increased mortality.[31,32] Central venous pressure or pulmonary artery lines may provide clinical measurement for determining if fluid replacement therapy is adequate. Also, the greater incidence of preexisting cardiac disease among the elderly suggests that hemodynamic pressure monitoring should be considered early.[31,32] For the same reason, early consideration should be given to the use of inotropic support when the patient fails to respond adequately to fluid replacement.

Peripheral vascular changes and diminished thermoregulatory ability contribute to poor toleration of cold environments by the elderly.[44] This is a major problem during resuscitations. Injury responses and exposure to ambient temperatures produce significant heat loss, indicating a need for close monitoring of core body temperatures. It is difficult to keep the skin covered during resuscitation when access to the body is necessary for assessment and routine procedures, but it is essential to reduce heat loss. Overhead heat lamps are especially useful to augment heated blankets, and warmed intravenous fluids are essential.

Health care providers, like others in our society, are undergoing a revision of attitudes toward the elderly. However, there still exists a tendency to limit aggressive therapy at some point merely because of the individual's age. Age alone is not a justifiable criterion for limitation of resuscitation efforts.[27,28,45]

PERIOPERATIVE PHASE

Advancing age is associated with increased perioperative morbidity and mortality.[46] Although management of the elderly should adhere to the same general principles that are applied to the young, some age-related adaptation is necessary for many older individuals. In nonemergency situations, additional time should be allowed for obtaining operative consent. The elderly may have difficulty understanding the choices offered or arriving at a decision. Additional visits by the health care team may be indicated, and consultation with family or other support persons is often useful. Extreme care must be exercised to ensure that the patient understands the consequences of consent and of refusal to consent.

Because of the higher mortality associated with surgery in the elderly compared with the young,[46,47] every possible step should be taken to reduce the risk for these patients. Effective pain management, continuous nourishment, and maintenance of normothermia are essential strategies for reducing the stress response.[46,47] When time permits, underlying physiologic deficits should be corrected before operative intervention.

Potential problems with airway management should be anticipated. Vigorous manipulation of the head and neck must be avoided because of the risk of impairing vertebral circulation. Missing teeth can make mask ventilation difficult. Endotracheal intubation provides airway protection but may be difficult to accomplish because of deformity or rigidity of the cervical spine. Laryngeal mask airways may be a viable alternative.

Positioning in the operating room should be done with consideration for fragile skin and bones, suboptimal subcutaneous tissue depth, and stiff joints. Protective padding should be applied to all pressure-sensitive areas and bony prominences[47] because age-related changes contribute to the propensity to develop pressure sores. In addition, vigorous movement and positioning may cause musculoskeletal injuries, including iatrogenic fractures.

Prevention of heat loss is critical in elderly patients undergoing surgery.[46,47] Diminished function of the thermoregulatory mechanisms in the elderly makes them especially vulnerable to hypothermia. Core body temperature should be monitored continuously regardless of the length of the operative procedure. The skin at surgical sites should be prepared with warmed solutions. The nurse should also be alert to the need for warmed intravenous fluids, warming blankets, and possibly warmed inspired gases during the operative procedure.

All medications should be administered with caution to elderly patients because of age-related decreases in renal and hepatic function. Anesthesia has the potential to disrupt regulatory systems for perfusion, whether it is general or regional. General anesthesia is indicated for upper abdominal, thoracic, and intracranial procedures, as well as for patients in whom airway control is essential. Regional anesthesia is often used for lower extremity procedures and when preexisting respiratory disorders would be adversely affected by general anesthetics.

CRITICAL CARE PHASE

Two considerations, over and above those for trauma alone, govern nursing care planning for the elderly in critical care units. The first is to anticipate complications that are related to aging rather than to trauma. The second is modification and negotiation of rehabilitation goals.

ANTICIPATING COMPLICATIONS

As noted earlier, the cardiovascular, respiratory, and neurologic systems require scrupulous assessment and management during the resuscitation phase. They continue to play a major role during the critical care phase, along with the renal, endocrine, and integumentary systems.

The older person has a greater propensity for chronic diseases that may impair cardiac contractility or systemic perfusion. The individual may function quite adequately during usual activities but may decompensate under the stresses of trauma. The health care team must be diligent in assessing the actual impact of chronic health problems rather than assuming they play a major role.

ASSESSMENT

CARDIOVASCULAR CONSIDERATIONS.   Cardiac and vascular system changes do not necessarily increase the risk of death to the elderly unless there is significant underlying heart disease. In the past three decades, correction of underlying defects during the preoperative and postoperative phases of care has resulted in reduced surgical mortality.[48] Trauma, however, provides little opportunity for preoperative intervention, so much of the corrective therapy must be attempted in the critical care setting.

Continuous hemodynamic monitoring is indicated until the patient is stable. Inotropic support may be needed during the acute phase, along with close attention to fluid balance. Because of potential renal dysfunction, monitoring should include frequent electrolyte measurements, with attention given to the development of hypoosmolality and hyponatremia.[38] This finding could indicate potential fluid overload, even when intravascular pressures are within acceptable limits.

The prevalence of peripheral vascular stiffening that accompanies aging increases the likelihood that perfusion may be compromised at some time despite adequate volumes and contractility. Extremities should be inspected frequently for adequate pulses, sensation, temperature, and color changes. Keeping the patient warm is essential. Extra coverings for the hands and feet ward off some effects of vasoconstriction and often add to the patient's comfort. For those who are critically ill, monitoring of systemic vascular resistance helps detect indications for vasodilator therapy.

The incidence of cardiac arrhythmias, particularly atrial in origin, increases with age.[29,30,34] In some cases they are secondary to previous myocardial infarction. Each arrhythmia should be evaluated for its impact on perfusion before therapy is instituted. All rhythm changes should be examined for origin because they often provide clues to ventilatory problems, inadequate perfusion, and electrolyte imbalance. They may also reflect a preexisting diagnosis, but this should never be assumed. Continuous electrocardiographic monitoring is essential.

Every patient has the potential for pulmonary edema. Early fluid therapy should be monitored carefully, but rates of administration need not be slow just because of the person's age. Patient responses, including pulmonary artery pressures (PAP) and pulmonary vascular resistance (PVR), should provide individual guidelines. Fluid challenges can be administered to assess the impact of fluid volume and type, and ventricular function graphs are sometimes helpful.

RESPIRATORY CONSIDERATIONS.   The incidence of postoperative complications is higher for patients requiring emergency procedures than for those having elective surgery. Elderly surgical patients have up to a 40% incidence of respiratory complications, with specific operative sites contributing to varying risk. As with young patients, surgery involving the abdomen produces greater potential for respiratory compromise in the elderly. Preoperative oxygen tension deficits and abnormal pulmonary artery pressures are often present in elderly trauma patients. Older patients also have a propensity to develop respiratory infections.[35]

The pulmonary system is the leading site of posttraumatic complications. The elderly are predisposed to pulmonary complications in general, and impaired ventilatory effort is a prime contributor to increased mortality. Inadequate pain relief, a major cause of impaired ventilation in critically injured older patients, must be aggressively addressed by nurses.

Despite the risk of infection, the elderly frequently require airway and ventilatory support. They are less able to protect the airway because of decreased sensitivity of the gag reflex and diminished strength of the respiratory muscles. The early institution of mechanical ventilation may be followed by a long period of ventilatory support. Just as the older person may be slow to respond to stresses initially, the recovery of function takes longer. Weaning from ventilatory support may take as much as twice the time needed for a younger person with similar injuries. The mode of ventilatory weaning must allow for respiratory muscle strength to be regained. A tracheostomy may assist with the weaning process. Weaning should be monitored closely, and it should be initiated only after the patient has had sufficient time to recover from the injuries.

COGNITIVE CONSIDERATIONS.   Delirium develops in 14% to 56% of hospitalized elderly patients.[49,50] This is especially likely to occur postoperatively and in the critical care setting. Frequently mentioned precipitating factors include information and sensory overload, short-term memory losses, delays in information processing, decreased visual acuity, and hearing losses. However, other significant causes of confusion in the elderly are inadequate pain relief, medication reactions or intolerance, stress, metabolic imbalance, infection, alterations in thermoregulation, and brain disorders. Delirium is most likely to occur in frail elderly persons,[49-51] and it is associated with increased mortality. The need for comprehensive differential diagnosis is readily apparent.

PSYCHOSOCIAL CONSIDERATIONS.   Psychosocial factors also may contribute to deterioration in neurologic functions. The best outcomes noted for the hospitalized elderly occur in those persons who were relatively independent at the time of injury and who did not live alone. Family dynamics also appear to play a significant role, with increased chances of a good outcome when the older person feels needed and wanted. Conversely, factors such as social isolation, loneliness, residence in a nursing home, and infirmity seem to contribute to increased levels of dependence after injury.

RENAL CONSIDERATIONS.   Major derangements in renal function are evident from laboratory assessment. The number of nephrons, renal blood flow, and glomerular filtration rate decline with age, resulting in a decreased ability of the kidneys to concentrate and excrete waste products. Baseline laboratory values of the patient's BUN and creatinine are necessary to allow meaningful evaluation of renal function. The potential for fluid overload exists, as does a possible need to alter drug dosage. In some cases the kidneys may respond to trauma with development of acute renal failure. This condition most often presents as polyuric failure. Routine examination of renal function studies is indicated for each patient.

MUSCULOSKELETAL CONSIDERATIONS. Musculoskeletal system injury, particularly hip fracture, has been documented extensively in the literature. Hip fracture is often accompanied by other injury, and it is often associated with a poor outcome when return to preinjury state is used as a criterion.[52] Recovery from musculoskeletal injury seems to be related to age, gender, intellectual functioning, and multiple psychosocial factors.

Isolated hip fracture occurs most often in women, especially patients with evidence of osteoporosis. The incidence also increases with advancing age and where there is evidence of decreased intellectual capability. Beyond age 70, the incidence of hip fracture is similar for men and women. Those persons who are active before injury, independent in the activities of daily living, and relatively free of the need for social services appear to have the best opportunity for recovery of preinjury function.[52]

The major musculoskeletal complication to be anticipated is loss of mobility. Older bones and muscles tend to develop stiffness and loss of motion more quickly, and they also tend to recover function more slowly. Recovery may be complicated by arthritic changes. Nursing care should be directed toward the maintenance of mobility early in the critical care phase. Passive and active range-of-motion exercises are essential while bed rest is indicated. At the earliest opportunity, the patient should be out of bed and potentially walking. The benefits of early mobilization cannot be stressed enough. It helps reorient the older person, improves cardiac and pulmonary performance, maintains musculoskeletal integrity, minimizes damage to the integument, promotes gastrointestinal motility and wound healing, provides evidence of progress to the patient, and generates a sense of hope.

IMMUNE SYSTEM CONSIDERATIONS. Elderly trauma patients are at increased risk of wound infections and sepsis. However, research studies in this area have not adequately controlled for co-morbidity and malnutrition.[53] There is considerable evidence that aging is associated with immune system dysregulation, as opposed to the more often suggested immunodeficiency status.[53] The activity of helper and cytotoxic T cells declines with advanced age, resulting in decreased cell-mediated immunity and increased susceptibility to fungal, viral, and bacterial infections.[29] When combined with malnutrition, co-morbity, and the immunosuppressive effects of major trauma, this dysregulation is thought to account for much of the increased risk of sepsis.

Because the presentation patterns of infectious diseases and sepsis in the elderly are often atypical,[54,55] diagnostic delays may contribute to morbidity and mortality. Onset of infection may present as change in mental status, restlessness, slight or absent elevation in temperature, mild elevation in white blood cell count in the presence of immature white cells, and limited catecholamine response. Any deterioration in patient status dictates an immediate and thorough search for infection. Horan and Parker[53] recently asserted that rectal or core[29] temperature should always be measured before deciding that an elderly patient is afebrile.

CHRONIC DISEASE CONSIDERATIONS. Many researchers have attempted to correlate preexisting chronic disease with mortality. Using a history of recent physician care or medical diagnosis as evidence of chronic disease has been essentially unsuccessful. It is clear that prior diagnosis does not give sufficient information about the patient's physiologic reserve to draw conclusions or make predictions of mortality. Yet it seems both reasonable and logical that some chronic diseases could lessen the physiologic reserve to the point where survival is in jeopardy. A classic study by Finelli et al[14] provided support for this hypothesis through autopsy results of a sample of geriatric nonsurvivors. They found a high incidence of coronary artery and cerebrovascular disease, along with left ventricular hypertrophy and renal and hepatic pathologic conditions. These findings, along with those of Scalea et al,[31] imply that preexisting disease does make a difference in survival rate. What is lacking is an acceptable measure of the impact of such disease on the individual's ability to survive.

MANAGEMENT CONSIDERATIONS

In any discussion of management of trauma care in the elderly, it is important to recognize that age alone does not dictate changes in therapeutic approach. The elderly should not be treated more or less conservatively than younger patients merely because they are 65 years of age or older. What age does point out is the need for more intensive assessment and monitoring in order to determine which patients require modification of care plans for age-related changes.

Previous health status and the level of preinjury activity the individual enjoyed may be the best predictive parameters of functional recovery. Planning for long-term care must begin on hospital admission. The ultimate goal of treatment is return to the best possible functional state.

Assessment and treatment priorities should parallel those indicated by the nature and extent of the injuries. Cardiovascular and respiratory functions take priority. Intensive monitoring of both systems is indicated because aging does increase the probability that chronic disease are present and may negatively influence the outcome.

CARDIOVASCULAR AND RESPIRATORY CONSIDERATIONS. The need for pulmonary artery pressure measurements should be indicated by the patient's status. Placement of a pulmonary artery catheter increases the probability that dysfunction will be assessed more rapidly, and it may provide some protection against fluid excesses. It also offers the opportunity to measure cardiac output and to monitor trends in ventricular function curves. Because the elderly may be slow to respond to stress mediators, the use of vasoactive support of cardiovascular function should be considered early in the treatment course. Scalea et al[31] suggest that invasive monitoring is of greatest benefit in patients who have no obvious serious injury. They also suggest that optimizing oxygen delivery and oxygen consumption may lower mortality.

Respiratory support, in the form of tracheal intubation and mechanical ventilation, is not without risk. Once such devices are in place, they increase the risk of pulmonary infection in a population especially susceptible to pneumonia. Even under optimal circumstances, the elderly are at increased risk of aspiration, atelectasis, and pulmonary sepsis.

In elderly patients with blunt chest trauma, multiple fractured ribs are the most common injury after both falls and motor vehicle crashes. Adequate pain relief is essential to optimize pulmonary function. Inadequate pain relief may cause decreased respiratory effort, leading to atelectasis and decreased oxygen exchange, thus necessitating mechanical ventilation. The indicators leading to consideration of mechanical ventilation include a high Injury Severity Score (25 or more), flail chest, and preexisting pulmonary disease.

When the patient requires ventilatory support, the full range of nursing care measures should be instituted. Special attention should be placed on pulmonary asepsis. Measures to facilitate removal of secretions, such as turning and humidification of inspired gases, should be intensified in light of the elderly patient's diminished pulmonary clearance capability. Strategies should be formulated to maximize coughing effectiveness, such as planned cough exercises in the upright position. Weaning the elderly patient from ventilatory support should be achieved through a well-defined plan of alternating spontaneous and supported ventilatory modes. End goals for work of breathing, Pa_{CO_2}, and Pa_{O_2} should be communicated clearly to team members. Nursing interventions and activities of daily living need to consider the work of breathing and the weaning process to avoid unnecessary fatigue. Astute assessment is necessary during the weaning process to differentiate anxiety and confusion from alterations in adequate ventilation and oxygenation.

RENAL CONSIDERATIONS.   Close attention to renal function through laboratory measurements is indicated. Even brief periods of hypovolemia and hypotension may compromise the kidneys. Evidence of rising serum creatinine level or decreased creatinine clearance should trigger assessment of the patient's free-water clearance. Constant monitoring of fluid balance and serum electrolytes are necessary to avoid volume overload. Care providers must also assess for the need to modify drug dosages.

MUSCULOSKELETAL CONSIDERATIONS. Priorities for musculoskeletal system management include decisions about the timing and type of operative procedures. The full range of options should be explored, with the goals of achieving early mobilization and providing the best possible outcome for the individual. It is conceivable that some operative procedures may be delayed in order to correct underlying functional deficits. All possible interventions should be used to keep bed rest to a minimum.

COGNITIVE CONSIDERATIONS.   Several alternatives exist for the nurse to deal with confusion. Short-term memory loss indicates the need for frequent repetitions of the same information, such as orientation to time and place. The physical and personal environment should be maintained in a constant state. Alterations in levels of lighting help adjust for loss of visual acuity and reduce the incidence of day-night disorientation. The patient's family, significant others, and personal familiar objects are critical to improvement in and maintenance of orientation; they provide engagement in familiar relationships and a sense of comfort and security.

NURSING MANAGEMENT

Nursing management includes participating in the trauma team's goal formulation for the elderly patient. In addition, nurses have special responsibilities in the areas of monitoring, communication, nutrition, and protection from further injury. Monitoring needs have been outlined previously. During the critical care phase the cardiovascular, respiratory, and renal systems are most vulnerable to disruption.

Communication with older patients may be difficult. In addition to potential problems associated with artificial airways, the older person may have a communication impediment as a result of diminished hearing and vision. Sensory overload, loss of short-term memory, and delays in information processing may also contribute to the need for special communication strategies.

COMMUNICATION STRATEGIES.   Gaining the individual's attention is the first step in the communication process. Verbal communication begins with facing the individual. Words should be kept simple, spoken slowly in low tones, and repeated as often as necessary. If a hearing deficit is determined, speaking into the better ear is desirable. Speech should be enunciated clearly in a volume that is loud enough to be both audible and understandable. Beware of shouting because this tends to garble spoken words.

Nurses should identify themselves to the patient clearly and repeatedly if needed. They should verify that the patient heard what was spoken (hearing losses may cause words to sound garbled). Communication techniques should be included in the patient's plan of care to foster consistency in methods of approach and to provide a database to facilitate changes in communication strategies when indicated.

Touch is a useful form of communication, but the patient's preferences should first be ascertained. Touch reinforces verbal communication and can convey caring and worth, as well as comfort. Older persons are often deprived of this form of communication because their perception of touch may be decreased. There is also a tendency by some individuals to avoid touching the older person.

Visual communication occurs through written materials and facial expressions. Visual communication also includes pictures of pets and grandchildren, religious medallions, and other symbolic objects located within the patient's field of vision. These and similar items may lift the spirits of elderly trauma victims, providing hope while directing their thoughts toward the future.

NUTRITIONAL STRATEGIES.   Providing for the nutritional needs of critically ill trauma patients can be challenging at best. Castenada et al[56] demonstrated that the elderly respond to malnutrition with markedly decreased functional capacity. If age, infirmity, and poverty combine to produce prior undernutrition, significant modifications in medical therapy are indicated. Present nutritional needs must be met and prior deficits must be corrected. Initially, intravenous feedings are indicated if the gastrointestinal system recovers function slowly. Decreases in gastric secretions and intestinal motility are features of aging that predispose the individual to intolerance of enteral feedings. Postpyloric enteral feedings can be attempted early even in the absence of bowel sounds. Caution should be used to ensure the airway is protected. Elevation of the head of the bed is usually advised. Diminished sensitivity of the gag reflex increases the potential for aspiration, particularly if the level of consciousness is impaired.

INFECTION CONSIDERATIONS.   The elderly are especially susceptible to infection. Careful monitoring of vascular access sites and indwelling devices, such as urinary catheters, is indicated. Removal of such devices should be attempted at the earliest opportunity. Nursing interventions are aimed at protecting the patient's natural immunity barriers through universal precautions and pulmonary, renal, and skin integrity assessments for early signs of infectious compromise.

INTEGUMENTARY CONSIDERATIONS.   Early mobilization of the older patient helps reduce the potential for integumentary injury. Aging reduces the elasticity of the skin, decreases the subcutaneous fat layer, and may reduce perfusion. The skin becomes vulnerable to pressure and abrasion, but breakdown can be prevented in most cases. Normal care of the aged skin includes minimal bathing, avoidance of harsh soaps, use of lubricating lotions, and avoidance of abrasive and irritating materials, including tape. The patient's skin should be kept free from prolonged wetness and contact with irritating secretions. Frequent changes in position are necessary in order to minimize pressure areas. Complete reliance on devices (e.g., foam pads or rings) to minimize pressure is inappropriate. If the patient is not capable of moving independently,

nursing interventions must incorporate frequent position changes.

MODIFICATION OF GOALS

Advancing age is recognized as a time when individuals experience and adapt to multiple losses. It is also a time when attitudes, goals, and values may undergo significant revision. Critical care nurses must ensure that their own values and goals for patient outcome do not overshadow those of their elderly patients.

It is important for the patient and family to be directly involved in the process of planning care. Because the goals usually set for younger people may not be achievable in the aged, more effort must be placed on determining the goals of individual patients. After a hip fracture, for example, an older person may expect to walk with a cane and may (or may not) be satisfied with this achievement. On the other hand, the patient may know friends who have been placed in nursing homes after fractures and may perceive death as a better goal. Talking with the patient and family helps elucidate attitudes and values that must be considered when care is planned.

The foundation for rehabilitation of the patient is developed during the critical care phase. Assessment of the potential for return of function is shared with the patient and family in a realistic manner. Advising them of available health care support services allows them time to investigate and to begin necessary arrangements. For the patient and family, this is a time to concentrate on short-term goals; both may become discouraged when anticipating a long recovery period.

Primary attention should be placed on maintaining function as near to the preinjury state as possible. Emphasis on prevention of complications and early mobility is needed. When the stress of critical care is eased, more specific objectives can be defined.

Unfortunately, many of the elderly do not recover from injuries.[27] Nonsurvivors tend to die either during the resuscitative phase or in the critical care unit after a prolonged stay. When the prognosis and outlook are poor, the patient's attitudes and values toward death need to be determined. For some, "death with dignity" is paramount; for others, it is a need to feel that everything possible was done. When the patient cannot be consulted, the family is the main source of information. However, the family must be encouraged to consider the expressed wishes of the individual, as well as their own desires. Documentation of the patient's wishes through advance directives is helpful with health care and patient and family goal setting and decision making.

INTERMEDIATE CARE AND REHABILITATION PHASES

Once the patient is transferred from the critical care environment, plans for return to the community and rehabilitation become more specific. The patient's potential for return to the preinjury functional state should be assessed. Underlying problems secondary to chronic disease or nutritional deficits should be corrected and support services mobilized.

The functional assessment should determine the patient's degree of change from the preinjury state. The patient's attitude, participation in the activities of daily living, mobility, and social activities and the type of support systems available should be considered. Comparison of preinjury function with the limitations imposed by the type and nature of present injuries permits the formulation of initial rehabilitation goals. When formulating these goals, it is best to recall that some of the aged do not return to their prior functional state. This is especially true for those who have sustained fractures of the lower extremities.[52,57] Positive prognostic indicators for elderly individuals with hip fractures include activity level and independence of the person before injury; younger age; and the patient's outlook toward life, social support, and participation in a geriatric rehabilitation program.[57] The active aged have the best chance of returning to an independent functional state.

Nutritional evaluation should not be limited to the hospital course. Estimation of prior status provides clues to preexisting problems, whether of a financial or a social nature. Nutritional management must attempt to correct past and present deficits. Potential obstacles to adequate nutrition include physiologic changes, psychosocial factors, and sensory alterations. Inadequate nutrition may be related to limited income, social isolation, poor dental health, medication use, depression, and loneliness. Dietary patterns are also governed by social and cultural values that tend to be fixed in the older person.[58] If assessment reveals an underlying problem, this must be included in the nutritional plan for the individual. In general, baseline nutritional requirements should be age adjusted to the reduced needs of the older person. The increased nutritional requirements imposed by recovery from acute injury should then be added to this baseline.

Nursing Management

The patient's needs for communication become, if anything, more important at this time. It is likely that verbal methods will be used more often at this stage. Frequent repetition of instructions and communication that orients the patient are required because of short-term memory loss. Plans for moving the patient should be communicated early to allow the patient time to adjust. Constancy of the physical environment is more important as the patient becomes increasingly aware and mobile. Tables, chairs, and other items become part of the patient's personal space and contribute to orientation and a sense of security.

Once the dietary requirements are determined, attention to the particular likes and dislikes of the individual can help ensure adequate intake. Frequent small feedings may be better tolerated than traditional meals. Elderly patients often enjoy family contributions of foods prepared at home. Meals should provide a variety of tastes, textures, and colors but be limited in the amount of salt and sugar.

Meals should also be enjoyed in the company of others whenever possible.

Loneliness, fear, and depression often accompany hospitalization of the older person. The nurse should investigate the availability of the patient's support systems. These might include family, local church or civic groups, friends, neighbors, and beloved pets. Visitors can partially alleviate the sense of isolation the patient may feel.

Establishment and revision of and movement toward rehabilitation goals for the patient are continued through the intermediate phase of care. When restoration of "normal" function is not probable, the emphasis should be placed on achieving the maximal function possible. Advanced age is not an appropriate reason to deny patients the optimal benefits of rehabilitation.

The family and other support systems should be included in planning rehabilitation goals. Assessment of the family's ability to assist in care needed by the patient is crucial to discharge planning. Consider the following questions: Will the patient require support in mobility, such as a walking device? How will nutritional needs be met? Will there be assistance in complying with complicated medication regimens? The home environment is another consideration: Are modifications necessary? Can the elderly person manage such modifications financially?

Community Reintegration

The outlook for return of elderly people to the community can be good. The probable outcome for a given individual should be assessed early in the hospital course so plans can be developed for alternative care if that proves necessary. For some a return to independent living is likely. For others it may be possible to provide limited assistance in the form of home health care as an alternative to placement in a long-term care facility.

Support systems that have been identified previously can be mobilized just before discharge. Health care teaching needs for professionals and nonprofessionals alike should be implemented early enough to allow time for assessment of learning. Written reinforcement of teaching should accompany the patient on discharge.

Part of the health care teaching should include measures that can be taken to prevent future injury. Assessment of the home environment by interview or by home health visits can help identify and correct hazards. When financial considerations limit preventive strategies, social services may offer access to additional financial support.

Nursing Research Implications

There is a tremendous need for further research about optimal trauma care for the elderly. With the possible exception of hip fractures, too little is known about how the elderly respond to traumatic injury compared with younger victims of similar injury. As the number of elderly people increases, there is an even greater need for guidance in the care of these patients. Epidemiologists have described the problem in terms of incidence and expense, but they offer little clinical data. If trauma is today's neglected disease, then trauma to the elderly is yet to be recognized as a problem. The need for systematic research is widespread. The scope of research potential in this population can be best addressed by considering unanswered questions.

Still undefined in the realm of epidemiology are questions dealing with the mechanism of injury. Falls are the most common mechanism, but the circumstances surrounding them are less clear. How many falls (or other injuries) are related to age alone? Are injuries often or seldom preceded by transient losses of consciousness? What is the relationship between injury and psychosocial factors? Are falls causally related to nutritional status, thermoregulation, or osteoporosis? What environmental factors are associated with injury? How does preinjury functional status compare with that of those who are not injured? What role does chronic disease play with regard to injury severity? How should chronic disease be measured? Are there differences in injury severity or response to injury between those who fall and those injured in motor vehicle crashes? Are the disabled more prone to injury than the active? Do the elderly actually succumb to injuries of low severity, as it appears, and if so, why? What factors contribute to the inability to return to preinjury functional level? Is there a time in health care when the wisest action is no action at all? Should a goal of health care include attention to the quality of life to which the patient returns?

These questions and many more need to be answered simultaneously with evaluation of current nursing care strategies. The need for data is immense, especially related to elderly responses to nursing care in the intensive care setting. Previous data from this age group have been obtained almost exclusively from patients with significant medical problems, as opposed to those individuals who were essentially healthy before injury. As nurse researchers develop a better grasp on how elderly trauma patients respond differently from younger ones, research in alternative and complementary therapies may be pursued.

PREVENTION

Data available from studies of nonintentional injury show that the elderly have a high risk of death from three major causes: falls, motor vehicle crashes, and thermal injuries. Unintentional injury is the seventh leading cause of death in the elderly population. Because most "accidents" are not accidents at all, prevention of injury should be a priority for health care professionals.

Public health history indicates that individual change is the prevention strategy least likely to succeed. A more successful approach includes environmental modification and modification of support systems. Nurses can participate in public decisions through professional organizations and legislative action.

Despite the fact that modification of individual behavior has the least potential for success, there are situations when

this is the only available approach. The foundation of patient teaching rests on the professional's ability to persuade an individual to change. Health status, financial limitations, values, and attitudes that make change difficult to accomplish complicate education and training of the elderly individual.

PREVENTION OF FALLS

Factors that increase the probability of falls in the elderly include deterioration in health, physical changes associated with aging (e.g., loss of visual acuity), use of prosthetic devices (e.g., canes, walkers), and environmental hazards (e.g., slippery surfaces, stairs, poor lighting, unexpected objects in walkways).[7,9,11] Correcting underlying medical problems can sometimes reduce the chance of falls. For example, placement of a pacemaker can eliminate syncope resulting from some cardiac arrhythmias. Flexibility, strength, and gait-training exercises may be useful in reducing the frequency of falls.

Home and public environments are not designed with the elderly in mind. To lessen the chances of falls, floor surfaces should be covered with nonslip materials and handgrips provided on both sides of walkways. Handgrips are especially helpful in bathrooms. Floors and stairs can be covered with resilient materials that lessen the chance of injury if a fall occurs. Improved lighting in hallways and on stairs helps the elderly avoid tripping. Lighting should be concentrated on landings, where falls are most likely to occur. Levels of lighting should be as uniform as possible so that the elderly do not have to make rapid visual adjustments to variable light intensity.

PREVENTION OF MOTOR VEHICLE CRASHES

Many elderly pedestrian fatalities occur when the individual attempts to cross the roadway between intersections. In addition, the elderly account for almost half the pedestrian injuries in crosswalks. Education of elderly pedestrians, and drivers in general, can increase their awareness of the potential problems. The elderly should be alerted to driver behaviors, such as turning right on red without looking for pedestrians, that increase the risk of collisions. Pedestrians walking at night also should wear light-colored clothing or reflective material to increase their visibility to drivers.

Elderly drivers tend to voluntarily restrict their driving to familiar conditions and daytime hours. This behavior can be encouraged in the individual. Training in defensive driving skills also may be of benefit to the older driver. As important, perhaps, is education of younger drivers to the behaviors of elderly drivers.

PREVENTION OF BURNS

A frequent cause of burns in the elderly is hot liquid. Many of these injuries are caused by tap water at a temperature higher than 130° F. This temperature is enough to produce a full-thickness burn in 30 seconds.[59] The simple reduction in hot water heater temperatures to 120° F or less can reduce the frequency and severity of scalds. Hot liquids from cooking are another source of burn wounds. Use of special aprons and specially designed containers while cooking has been recommended as a prevention strategy.[59]

Causes of flame injuries include smoking, open flames (gas stoves), and house fires. The elderly are overrepresented in the burn fatalities from house fires, possibly because they are less able to escape once fire starts. Carbon monoxide and smoke detectors should be required in all elderly housing, along with use of flame-retardant materials in construction and furnishings. The elderly homeowner should be cautioned against household storage of flammable materials such as old newspapers and gasoline. Lastly, smoking in bed should be eliminated.

SUMMARY

In a health care environment in which initial care is based on rapid institution of protocols, the elderly trauma patient presents a unique challenge to the nurse. The protocols designed for younger trauma victims may not be appropriate for the elderly. In addition, the tremendous physiologic diversity of older adults may prevent any protocol from being appropriate for the entire age group. Elderly patients offer the nurse a true opportunity to individualize nursing care. They present with a great potential for altered responses to trauma. This may be the result of normal aging, or it may reflect the impact of chronic disease on their response to the stresses of injury. Because little guidance is available from protocols, nurses must maintain an intense degree of monitoring to discern deviations from expected norms. The nurse should be prepared to modify the plan of care based on the specific responses of each individual elderly patient.

REFERENCES

1. United States Bureau of the Census: *Current population reports: www.census.gov/population/projections/nation/nas, 1990.*
2. Sartorelli KH, Rogers FB, Osler TM et al: Financial aspects of providing trauma care at the extremes of life, *J Trauma* 46(3):483-487, 1999.
3. Young JS, Cephas GA, Blow O: Outcome and cost of trauma among the elderly: a real-life model of a single-payer reimbursement system, *J Trauma* 45(4):800-804, 1998.
4. Horan MA: The attributes of old age. In Horan MA, Little RA, editors: *Injury in the aging,* Cambridge, 1998, Cambridge University, 9-21.
5. National Safety Council: *Accident facts,* Chicago, 1997, National Safety Council.
6. Martinez R, Sharieff G, Hooper J: Three-point restraints as a risk factor for chest injury in the elderly, *J Trauma* 37(6): 980-984, 1994.
7. Downton JH: Who falls and why? In Horan MA, Little RA, editors: *Injury in the aging,* Cambridge, 1998, Cambridge University, 64-78.
8. Janke MK: Accidents, mileage and the exaggeration of risk, *Accid Anal Prev* 23:183-188, 1991.

9. Tinetti ME, Baker D, McAvay G et al: A multifactorial intervention to reduce the risk of falling among elderly people living in the community, *N Engl J Med* 331(13): 821-827, 1994.
10. Tinetti ME, Doucette J, Claus E et al: Risk factors for serious injury during falls by older persons in the community, *J Am Geriatr Soc* 43:1214-1221, 1995.
11. Tinetti ME, Williams CS: Falls, injuries due to falls, and the risk of admission to a nursing home, *N Engl J Med* 337(18): 1279-1284, 1997.
12. Schwab CW, Kauder DR: Trauma in the geriatric patient, *Arch Surg* 127(6):701-706, 1992.
13. Center JR, Nguyen TV, Schneider D et al: Mortality after all major types of osteoporotic fracture in men and women: an observational study, *Lancet* 353(9156):878-882, 1999.
14. Finelli FC, Jonsson J, Champion HR et al: A case control study for major trauma in geriatric patients, *J Trauma* 29(5): 541-548, 1989.
15. Evans JG: Epidemiology of trauma in the elderly. In Horan MA, Little RA, editors: *Injury in the aging,* Cambridge, 1998, Cambridge University, 22-50.
16. Greenhalgh DG: Preexisting factors that affect care. In Carrougher GJ, editor: *Burn care and therapy,* St. Louis, 1998, Mosby, 381-399.
17. Mueller MJ, Herndon D: The challenge of burns, *Lancet* 343:216-220, 1994.
18. Merrell SW, Saffle JR, Sullivan JJ et al: Increased survival after major thermal injury: a nine year review, *Am J Surg* 154: 623-627, 1987.
19. Sacco WJ, Copes WS, Bain LW et al: Effect of preinjury illness on trauma patient survival outcome, *J Trauma* 35(4):538-543, 1993.
20. Gubler KD, Davis R, Koepsell T et al: Long-term survival of elderly trauma patients, *Arch Surg* 132:1010-1014, 1997.
21. Ruppert SD: Alcohol abuse in older persons: implications for critical care, *Crit Care Nurs* Q 2(19):62-70, 1996.
22. Birnbaumer D: Geriatrics: unique concerns. In Rosen P, Barkin R, Danzl DF et al, editors: *Emergency medicine: concepts and clinical practice,* ed 4, St. Louis, 1998, Mosby, 162-167.
23. Pepper GA: Drug use and misuse. In Stone JT, Wyman JF, Salisbury SA, editors: *Clinical gerontological nursing: a guide to advanced practice,* ed 2, Philadelphia, 1999, WB Saunders, 589-621.
24. Gupta K: Alcoholism in the elderly, *Postgrad Med* 93(2): 203-206, 1993.
25. Mandavia D, Newton K: Geriatric trauma, *Emerg Med Clin North Am* 16(1):257-274, 1998.
26. Hoxie RE, Rubenstein, LZ: Are older pedestrians allowed enough time to cross intersections safely? *J Am Geriatr Soc* 42:241-244, 1994.
27. van der Sluis CD, Klasen HJ, Eisma WH, ten Duis HJ: Major trauma in young and old: what is the difference? *J Trauma* 40(1):78-82, 1996.
28. Perdue PW, Watts DD, Kaufmann CR et al: Differences in mortality between elderly and younger adult trauma patients: geriatric status increases risk of delayed death, *J Trauma* 45(4):805-810, 1998.
29. Stanley M: The aging cardiovascular system. In Stanley M, Beare PG, editors: *Gerontological nursing,* ed 2, Philadelphia, 1999, FA Davis, 130-138.

30. Lakatta EG: Circulatory function in younger and older humans in health. In Hazzard WR, Blass JP, Ettinger WH Jr et al, editors: *Principles of geriatric medicine and gerontology,* ed 4, New York, 1999, McGraw-Hill, 645-660.

31. Scalea TM, Simon HM, Duncan AO et al: Geriatric blunt multiple trauma: improved survival with early invasive monitoring, *J Trauma* 30:129-136, 1990.

32. Scalea TM, Kohl L: Geriatric trauma. In Feliciano DV, Moore EE, Mattox KL, editors: *Trauma,* ed 3, Stamford, Conn, 1996, Appleton and Lange, 899-915.

33. Crossley GH: Arrhythmias in the elderly. In Hazzard WR, Blass JP, Ettinger WH Jr et al, editors: *Principles of geriatric medicine and gerontology,* ed 4, New York, 1999, McGraw-Hill, 701-704.

34. Wei JY: Coronary heart disease. In Hazzard WR, Blass JP, Ettinger WH Jr et al, editors: *Principles of geriatric medicine and gerontology,* ed 4, New York, 1999, McGraw-Hill, 661-668.

35. Cantrell M, Norman D: Pneumonia. In Hazzard WR, Blass JP, Ettinger WH Jr et al, editors: *Principles of geriatric medicine and gerontology,* ed 4, New York, 1999, McGraw-Hill, 729-736.

36. Enright PL: Aging of the respiratory system. In Hazzard WR, Blass JP, Ettinger WH Jr et al, editors: *Principles of geriatric medicine and gerontology,* ed 4, New York, 1999, McGraw-Hill, 721-728.

37. Loeser RF, Osvaldo D: Aging and musculoskeletal system. In Hazzard WR, Blass JP, Ettinger WH Jr et al, editors: *Principles of geriatric medicine and gerontology,* ed 4, New York, 1999, McGraw-Hill, 1097-1112.

38. Beck LH: Aging changes in renal function. In Hazzard WR, Blass JP, Ettinger WH Jr et al, editors: *Principles of geriatric medicine and gerontology,* ed 4, New York, 1999, McGraw-Hill, 767-776.

39. Fletcher KR: Physical and laboratory assessment. In Stone JT, Wyman JF, Salisbury SA, editors: *Clinical gerontological nursing: a guide to advanced practice,* ed 2, Philadelphia, 1999, WB Saunders, 85-128.

40. Gruenewald DA, Matsumoto AM: Aging of the endocrine system. In Hazzard WR, Blass JP, Ettinger WH Jr et al, editors: *Principles of geriatric medicine and gerontology,* ed 4, New York, 1999, McGraw-Hill, 949-966.

41. Trandel-Korenchuk DM, Trandel-Korenchuk KM: *Nursing and the law,* ed 5, Gaithersberg, Md, 1997, Aspen, 161-192.

42. Wilson EB: Physical restraint of elderly patients in critical care, *Crit Care Nurs Clin North Am* 8(1):61-70, 1996.

43. Brungardt GS: Patient restraints: new guidelines for a less restrictive approach, *Geriatrics* 49:43-50, 1994.

44. Tappen RM, Andre SP: Inadvertent hypothermia in elderly surgical patients, *AORN J* 3(63):639-644, 1996.

45. Broos PLO, D'Hore A, Vanderschot P et al: Multiple trauma in elderly patients. Factors influencing outcome: importance of aggressive care, *Injury* 24(6):365-368, 1993.

46. Roy RC: Anesthesia for older patients. In Hazzard WR, Blass JP, Ettinger WH Jr et al, editors: *Principles of geriatric medicine and gerontology,* ed 4, New York, 1999, McGraw-Hill, 377-389.

47. Keough V, Letizia M: Elder care: perioperative care of elderly trauma patients, *AORN J* 63(5):932-937, 1996.

48. Bell R, Rosenthal RA: Surgery in the elderly. In Hazzard WR, Blass JP, Ettinger WH Jr et al, editors: *Principles of geriatric medicine and gerontology,* ed 4, New York, 1999, McGraw-Hill, 391-412.

49. Inouye SK: The dilemma of delirium: clinical and research controversies regarding diagnosis and evaluation of delirium in hospitalized elderly medical patients, *Am J Med* 97(3): 278-288, 1994.

50. Bross MH, Tatus NO: Delirium in the elderly patient, *Am Fam Physician* 50(6):1325-1332, 1994.

51. Juneau B: Special issues in critical care gerontology, *Crit Care Nurs Q* 19(2):71-75, 1996.

52. Cooney LM: Hip fractures. In Hazzard WR, Blass JP, Ettinger WH Jr et al, editors: *Principles of geriatric medicine and gerontology,* ed 4, 1999, New York, McGraw-Hill, 1547-1551.

53. Horan MA, Parker SG: Infections, aging and the host response. In Horan MA, Little RA, editors: *Injury in the aging,* Cambridge, 1998, Cambridge University, 126-146.

54. Chassagne P, Perol MB, Doucet J et al: Is presentation of bacteremia in the elderly the same as in younger patients? *Am J Med* 100(1):65-70, 1996.

55. Werner GS, Schultz R, Fuchs JB et al: Infective endocarditis in the elderly in the era of transesophageal echocardiography: clinical features and prognosis compared with younger patients, *Am J Med* 100(1):90-97, 1996.

56. Castenada C, Charnley JM, Evans WJ et al: Elderly women accommodate to a low-protein diet with losses of body cell mass, muscle function, and immune response, *Am J Clin Nutr* 62(1):30-39, 1995.

57. Anders RL, Ornellas EM: Acute management of patients with hip fracture: a research literature review, *Orthop Nurs* 2(16): 31-46, 1997.

58. Anding R: Nutrition support for the critically ill older patient, *Crit Care Nurs Q* 2(19):13-22, 1996.

59. Forjuoh SN: The mechanisms, intensity of treatment and outcomes of hospitalized burns: Issues for prevention, *J Burn Care and Rehabilitation* 19(5):456-460, 1998.

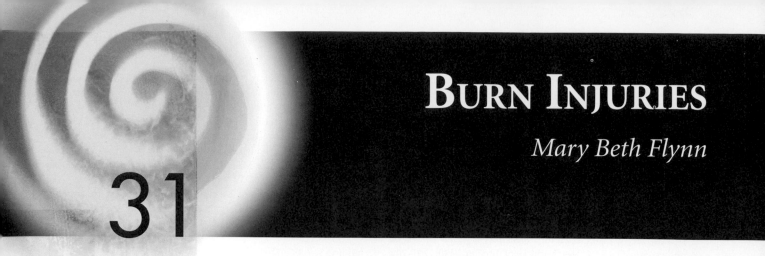

BURN INJURIES

Mary Beth Flynn

CARE OF THE BURN-INJURED PATIENT

More than 1.2 million people are burned in the United States every year. Burn injuries are the fourth leading cause of unintentional deaths, accounting for 3% of all deaths as a result of injury.[1] The majority of burn injuries are minor and are treated in outpatient settings. However, approximately 45,000[2] burns are moderate to severe and require hospitalization. The average size of a burn injury among people admitted to burn centers is about 14% of total body surface area (TBSA).[2] Burns of 10% TBSA or less account for 54% of burn center admissions, and burns of more than 60% TBSA account for 4% of burn center admissions.

Between 1971 and 1991 the number of deaths attributed to burns decreased by 40%, with a concomitant 12% decrease in deaths associated with inhalation injury.[3] Before the 1970s a patient with a 50% TBSA burn had a 40% chance of survival. Today a patient with a 75% TBSA burn has a 50% chance of survival.[4] Only about 6% of people admitted to burn centers do not survive, most of whom have suffered severe inhalation injury in fires.[2]

Advances in burn prevention strategies (e.g., increased public education, better fire retardant product design, and legislation)[5] and the medical treatment of burned patients have improved survival significantly. Reasons for the dramatic improvements in mortality after massive burns include advances in understanding of resuscitation, improvements in wound coverage, better support of the hypermetabolic response to injury, more appropriate infection control, and improved treatment of inhalation injuries.[4,6,7] Some patients require specialized burn units because of dedicated resources and the expertise of the various health care disciplines necessary to maximize outcomes of patients with large burn injuries. The American Burn Association has established guidelines to determine which patients should be transferred to a specialized burn center to maximize survival from the burn injury (Table 31-1).

PATHOPHYSIOLOGY OF BURN INJURY

TISSUE INJURY

Tissue injury is related to the coagulation of cellular protein caused by heat produced by thermal, chemical, electrical, or radiation energy. The coagulation associated with thermal injury is relative to the temperature of the wounding agent and the length of exposure to a given temperature (Figure 31-1).[8] The coagulation associated with chemical injuries is related to the type, strength, concentration, duration of contact, and mechanism of action. Chemical agents may be divided into several groups, depending on the mechanism by which they coagulate protein and cause tissue necrosis. Chemicals are categorized into broad groups of acidic or alkaline, and attempts to neutralize the agent can increase the thermal reaction and extent of injury.

Electrical injury is produced by the conversion of electrical energy into heat and from the direct physicochemical effects of electric current on tissue. The amount of current flowing in a circuit is directly proportional to voltage and inversely proportional to resistance. The quantity of heat produced by an electric current is related to the amount of voltage, the resistance of the conductor, and the duration of contact. Each type of tissue within the body absorbs the heat energy according to its own electrical resistance. Electrical current proceeds down the path of least resistance, which is via nerves, blood vessels, and muscles, thus sparing the skin, except at the entry and exit points of the current.[5] Thus most injuries caused by this mechanism consist of internal tissue damage.

Burn wounds can be conceptualized as having three zones (Figure 31-2)[9] representing damage to the tissues resulting from transfer of heat. The central zone of coagulation is an area of irreversible tissue necrosis, or full-thickness burn. Immediately surrounding the necrotic zone is the zone of stasis, characterized by a pronounced inflammatory reaction.[7] This zone may not show areas of coagulation initially but may proceed to tissue necrosis if adequate tissue perfusion is not restored to the area during the resuscitation

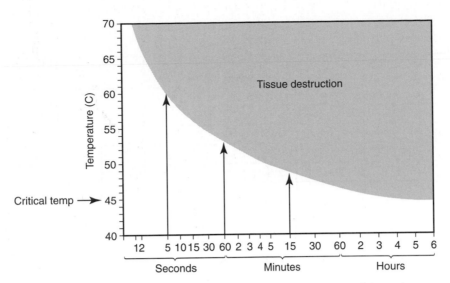

FIGURE 31-1 **Temperature Duration Curve.** Tissue destruction proceeds logarithmically, with increasing temperatures as a function of time exposure.

TABLE 31-1	American Burn Association Criteria for Burn Center Transfer and Referral

Patients meeting the following criteria should be transferred/ admitted to a burn unit:

Second-degree burns greater than 10% TBSA

Full-thickness burns greater than 5% TBSA

Any burn involving the face, hands, feet, eyes, ears, or perineum

Any burn that may result in cosmetic or functional disability

Circumferential burns of the chest or extremities

Inhalation injury and associated trauma

Chemical burns

Electrical burns, including lightning injury

Significant co-morbid conditions (diabetes mellitus, chronic obstructive pulmonary disease, cardiac disease)

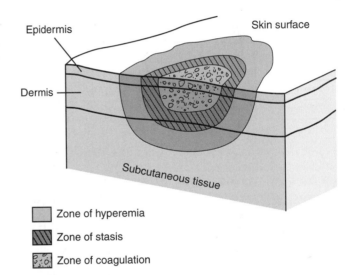

FIGURE 31-2 **Zones of Thermal Injury.** (From Pruitt BA, Goodwin CW, Cioffi WG: Thermal injuries. In Davis JH, Sheldon GF, editors: *Surgery: a problem solving approach,* ed 2, St. Louis, 1995, Mosby.)

period. The release of local mediators such as histamine, serotonin, kinins, arachidonic acid metabolites, xanthine oxidase products and complement cytokines, and catecholamines[4,6,7] results in arteriolar and venular dilation and increased microvascular permeability. Concurrently the co-agulation system is activated, causing platelet aggregation. Polymorphonuclear neutrophil leukocytes (PMNs) and macrophages are present and release multiple cytokines that are essential to wound healing. The summation of the activation of the intense inflammatory response is vascular stasis and rapid formation of tissue edema. Goals of initial burn therapy focus on providing adequate fluid resuscitation, maintaining normal tissue oxygenation, and attempting to block some of the inflammatory mediators in an effort to limit the conversion of the zone of stasis to coagulation necrosis. The outer zone of hyperemia has sustained minimal injury and therefore usually heals rapidly.

EXTENT AND DEPTH OF INJURY

Two important concepts in the clinical diagnosis and management of burn injuries are the extent and depth of burn injury. The *extent of burn* refers to the total surface area of injured tissue. This is usually calculated as percentage of TBSA using either the Berkow,[10] Lund-Browder,[11] or rule of nines formula. With any of the burn estimation tools, the clinician's goal is to estimate the amount of tissue damaged by the exchange of thermal energy. The Berkow and the Lund-Browder charts are more accurate assessment tools. They divide the body into multiple areas and take into consideration changes in the contribution of the head and lower extremities over the age range from infancy to adulthood (Figure 31-3).[12] The rule of nines is easy to

BURN ESTIMATE AND DIAGRAM
AGE vs. AREA

AREA	Birth 1 yr	1 – 4 yr	5 – 9 yr	10 – 14 yr	15 yr	Adult	2°	3°	Total	Donor Areas
Head	19	17	13	11	9	7				
Neck	2	2	2	2	2	2				
Ant. Trunk	13	13	13	13	13	13				
Post. Trunk	13	13	13	13	13	13				
R. Buttock	2¹/₂	2¹/₂	2¹/₂	2¹/₂	2¹/₂	2¹/₂				
L. Buttock	2¹/₂	2¹/₂	2¹/₂	2¹/₂	2¹/₂	2¹/₂				
Genitalia	1	1	1	1	1	1				
R.U. Arm	4	4	4	4	4	4				
L.U. Arm	4	4	4	4	4	4				
R.L. Arm	3	3	3	3	3	3				
L.L. Arm	3	3	3	3	3	3				
R. Hand	2¹/₂	2¹/₂	2¹/₂	2¹/₂	2¹/₂	2¹/₂				
L. Hand	2¹/₂	2¹/₂	2¹/₂	2¹/₂	2¹/₂	2¹/₂				
R. Thigh	5¹/₂	6¹/₂	8	8¹/₂	9	9¹/₂				
L. Thigh	5¹/₂	6¹/₂	8	8¹/₂	9	9¹/₂				
R. Leg	5	5	5¹/₂	6	6¹/₂	7				
L. Leg	5	5	5¹/₂	6	6¹/₂	7				
R. Foot	3¹/₂	3¹/₂	3¹/₂	3¹/₂	3¹/₂	3¹/₂				
L. Foot	3¹/₂	3¹/₂	3¹/₂	3¹/₂	3¹/₂	3¹/₂				
						TOTAL				

BURN DIAGRAM

AGE _____

SEX _____

WEIGHT _____

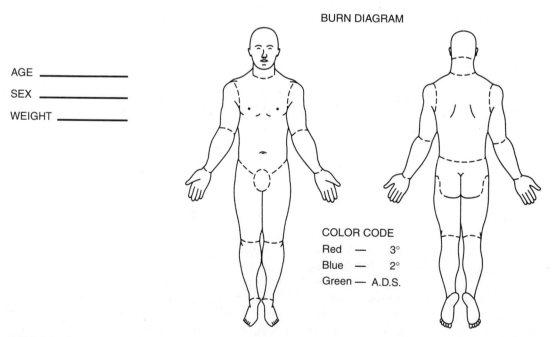

COLOR CODE
Red — 3°
Blue — 2°
Green — A.D.S.

FIGURE 31-3 **Burn Diagram and Table Based on the Lund-Browder Method of Calculating Burn Size.** Based on the Lund and Browder chart with Berkow's formula, it allows for more accurate assessment of the extent of burn injury based on age and depth of injury. *Ant.,* Anterior; *Post.,* Posterior; *L.,* Left; *R.,* Right; *R.U.,* Right upper; *R.L.,* Right lower; *L.U.,* Left upper; *L.L.,* Left lower; *A.D.S.,* Available donor site. (From LaBorde P, Willis J: Burns. In Sole ML, Lamborn ML, and Hartshorn JC, editors: *Introduction to critical care nursing,* ed 3, Philadelphia, 2000, WB Saunders, 612.)

remember and provides a rapid, gross estimate of the extent of burn. The body is divided into seven areas that represent 9% or multiples of 9% of the body surface area, with the remaining area, the genitalia, representing 1% of TBSA (Figure 31-4).[13] The last method of determining extent of TBSA injured uses the size of the patient's hand, assuming

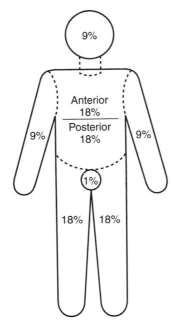

FIGURE 31-4 An estimate of the percentage of total body surface area (% TBSA) burned can be obtained using the rule of nines, whereby TBSA is divided into 9% segments of the total. Second- and third-degree burns are added and presented as a percentage of total skin. (From Greenfield E: Integumentary disorders. In Kinney MR, Dunbar SB, Brooks-Brunn JA et al: editors: *AACN's clinical reference for critical care nursing*, ed 4, St. Louis, 1998, Mosby, 1066.)

the palmar surface of the hand is roughly 1% of TBSA. Visualizing the patient's hand covering the burn wound approximates the amount of body surface area involved.[14]

Regardless of the method used to calculate TBSA, estimation of the burned area is somewhat subjective, with areas of clinical discrepancy. The primary goals in estimating the TBSA involved in the burn are to predict morbidity/survival, physiologic response in relation to fluid shifts and fluid resuscitation requirement, and metabolic and immunologic responses.

The concept of depth of burn injury is an important predictor of survival, overall morbidity, including surgical management, functional outcome, and cosmesis. Descriptions of the depth of burn are often confusing because a variety of nomenclature is used (Table 31-2). In general the *burn wound depth* describes tissue damage according to anatomic thickness of the skin involved, as determined by the clinician. As a general rule, the more superficial the burn wound, the more rapidly the wound heals.

TISSUE INJURY AND THE IMMUNOLOGIC RESPONSE

In the past decade, much knowledge has been amassed about the relationship of tissue injury and immunologic response to burn injury. Research into the histochemical response to tissue injury continues to elucidate the mechanisms of inflammation, infection, acute respiratory distress syndrome (ARDS), sepsis, systemic inflammatory response syndrome (SIRS), and multiple organ dysfunction syndrome (MODS).[7,15,16] The *tissue injury related to burns* refers not only to the local response of the coagulation produced by heat but also to the local and systemic responses that lead to inflammation, fluid shifts, and ultimately MODS if proper treatment is not provided. Ryan

TABLE 31-2	**Classification of Depth of Burn Injury**			
	First Degree	**Second Degree**		**Third Degree**
By skin thickness	Superficial	Superficial partial thickness	Deep partial thickness	Full thickness
By anatomic description	Epidermal	Epidermal and superficial dermal	Deep dermal	Full dermal tissue loss and possibly subdermal (fat, muscle, bone)
Appearance/ description of depth	Pink to red; no blisters; skin remains intact when rubbed gently; may appear slightly edematous	Red or mottled red to pink; blisters; skin easily rubbed off; moist, weeping, edematous; if pulled, hair remains intact; blanches with pressure	Pink to pale ivory; can see reticulated pattern; wound may appear somewhat dry; contains blisters and bullae; hair removes easily; does not blanch with pressure or return of color is slow	White, cherry red, brown, or black; may or may not contain blisters; may contain thrombosed vessels; appears dry, hard, leathery; may be depressed
Pain response	Uncomfortable/ painful to touch	Very painful	Pain response is variable, hyperalgesia and hypoalgesia	Insensate; pain is aching in nature
Time to heal	3-5 days	<3 weeks	>3 weeks	Requires grafting

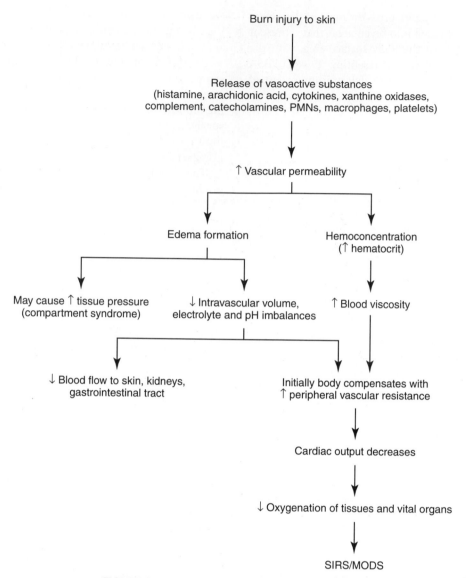

Burn injury to skin

↓

Release of vasoactive substances
(histamine, arachidonic acid, cytokines, xanthine oxidases,
complement, catecholamines, PMNs, macrophages, platelets)

↓

↑ Vascular permeability

Edema formation   Hemoconcentration
                         (↑ hematocrit)

May cause ↑ tissue pressure   ↓ Intravascular volume,   ↑ Blood viscosity
(compartment syndrome)   electrolyte and pH imbalances

↓ Blood flow to skin, kidneys,   Initially body compensates with
gastrointestinal tract   ↑ peripheral vascular resistance

Cardiac output decreases

↓ Oxygenation of tissues and vital organs

SIRS/MODS

FIGURE 31-5 **Physiologic Response to Burned Skin.**

et al[16] evaluated 1665 burn patients over 4 years and found that one third of them died of MODS. States of malperfusion, excessive edema, and negative effects of unbalanced inflammatory mediators remain the primary cause of MODS in burn victims. Research continues to enhance our understanding of and treatments for the local and system inflammatory processes that result in fluid shifts and altered tissue perfusion (burn shock) (Figure 31-5).

The pathophysiologic effects related to thermal injury (>20% TBSA)[17] and acute inflammatory processes are both local and systemic. The microcirculation is compromised to the worst extent 12 to 24 hours after a burn is sustained.[4,6,7,15] Goals of therapy are aimed at controlling the exaggerated inflammatory cytokine cascade[15] response and restoring the microcirculatory perfusion of tissues. Collectively the inflammatory mediators produce vasoconstriction, vasodilation, increased capillary permeability, activation of the coagulation cascade, and progressive and rapid edema formation with altered microcirculatory perfusion.

These complex interactions of inflammatory mediators are tightly interwoven in both physiologic and pathophysiologic states. With burn trauma, excessive Hageman factor (factor XII) is activated, initiating an interdependent activation of all the inflammatory cascade systems in an effort to reestablish homeostasis (Figure 31-6).[18] In the protective state this process is efficient and immune protective; however, in a poorly regulated situation, as seen with large burns and traumas, overwhelming inflammation, coagulation, and fibrinolysis can ensue and constantly be reactivated.[7,18] Mediators then leave the confines of the local tissue injury and move to the systemic circulation, causing alterations in organ function remote from the site of injury.[18] In large burn injuries, cytokine activities appear to be chaotic[15] and reactivated, creating a state of exaggerated or reactivated inflammation, causing distant organ involvement (i.e., ARDS, SIRS, and eventually MODS).[4,6,7,18]

Summation of the exaggerated activation of the inflammatory cascades produces microvasculature-induced car-

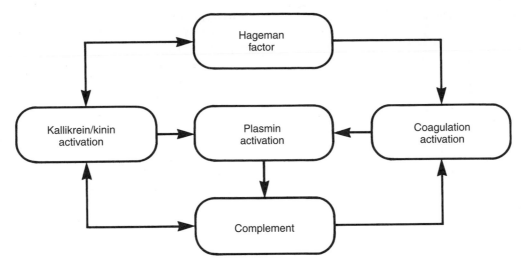

FIGURE 31-6 **Hageman Factor as the Link in the Interlocking Network of the Plasma Enzyme Cascades.** (From Secor Huddleston V: The systemic inflammatory response syndrome: role of inflammatory mediators in multiple organ dysfunction syndrome. In Secor Huddleston V, editor: *Multiple organ dysfunction and failure*, ed 2, St. Louis, 1996, Mosby, 56.)

diopulmonary changes marked by loss of plasma volume, increased peripheral vascular resistance, and subsequent decreased cardiac output.[4] Renal blood flow is altered, resulting in renal dysfunction. Activation of the stress response causes mild respiratory alkalosis and hypoxemia, which is complicated by increased pulmonary capillary permeability, resulting in decreased pulmonary compliance and function. Metabolic changes are highlighted by an early depression followed by marked and sustained increases in resting energy expenditure, lipolysis, proteolysis, and oxygen consumption.[4,6] Eventually, generalized impairment of host defenses, depression of immunoglobulins, and fatigued immune response make the burned patient prone to infections.

METABOLIC RESPONSE TO TISSUE INJURY

The metabolic response to burn injury has been studied extensively. As early as 1930, Cuthbertson[19] described the biphasic metabolic response to injury. He noted increased fluid shifts, urinary nitrogen losses, and losses of other intracellular substances such as potassium and phosphorus. In subsequent years the studies of the catabolic response to injury documented increased oxygen consumption, negative nitrogen balance, exaggerated hypermetabolism and catabolism, excessive muscle wasting, and weight loss in burned patients.

The intensity of the metabolic changes experienced by burn patients is directly related to the extent of injury.[6,20] The resting energy expenditure (REE) after a burn injury can be as much as 50% to 150% higher than that in the average trauma patient,[6,21] creating a hypermetabolic drive. Burn hypermetabolism is the result of multiple mechanisms associated with hormonal changes. After a burn injury, the inflammatory mediators stimulate the hypothalamus, increasing the body's central thermoregulatory set point and altering endocrine functions. Levels of catecholamines, cortisol, and glucagon are markedly elevated, initiating the

catabolic response seen in the burn patient. The presence of catecholamines increases the rates of glycogenolysis and hepatic gluconeogenesis and promotes lipolysis and peripheral insulin resistance.[6,21] The exaggerated metabolic response and excessive mobilization of glucose for energy requirements are necessary for wound healing. When adequate glucose cannot be supplied, the result is excessive protein catabolism.[6,20] Thus early nutritional interventions, with particular importance on meeting the REE, cannot be overemphasized in the treatment and survival of the burned patient.

Because the sympathetic response seems to be the major determinant of the metabolic response to burn injury and the sympathetic nervous system can be stimulated by a variety of responses, including lower than normal environmental temperatures, pain, psychologic responses, and the body's response to inflammatory mediators, it would seem that the use of nutritional replacement formulas based only on the size of the burn injury may not be accurate. Caution must be used in the application of standard nutritional replacement formulas; nutritional goals and endpoints should be reassessed and adjusted more frequently as the burn wound heals. Refer to Chapter 16 for a thorough discussion of nutritional assessment parameters and formulas.

Optimally, nutritional replacement therapy in the burn patient should be based on frequent measurements of oxygen consumption obtained with the use of a metabolic cart. (See Chapter 16 for a discussion of the advantages and disadvantages of metabolic carts.) Nutritional formulas[22] vary as much as resuscitation formulas, and there is little consensus as to which is most appropriate. In part this lack of consensus has to do with the great variability in nutritional needs from patient to patient and for the same patient over time. This is why actual measurement of oxygen consumption allows more accurate nutritional repletion.

MANAGEMENT OF THE PATIENT WITH BURN INJURY

PHYSIOLOGIC RESPONSE: CHANGES IN HEMODYNAMICS

The initial host-defense response leads to a shift in fluids from the vascular space into the interstitial and intracellular spaces. When the burn involves large areas of skin (e.g., >20% TBSA), this response may become an overall systemic response, with fluids shifting into interstitial spaces throughout the body. This massive fluid shift may lead to hypovolemic shock. To prevent shock, fluid resuscitation after burn injury is maintained for 24 to 48 hours after injury[6,23-25] while avoiding complications of inadequate or excessive therapy until signs of hypovolemia resolve. A number of formulas have been suggested for optimal replacement of this fluid. Some of the early formulas, such as the Evans formula and the original Brooke formula, recommended a mixture of sodium-containing fluids and colloid because both sodium-rich fluids and plasma proteins are lost as a result of this fluid shift. The Baxter (Parkland) formula supports that plasma given in the first 24 hours is no more effective than Ringer's lactate alone in maintaining normal plasma volume. Monafo and Warden formulas focus on the administration of hypertonic saline as a means of limiting edema and require a lower total amount of fluids than crystalloid and colloid formulas. The Demling formula incorporates the use of low-molecular-weight dextran in resuscitation formulas, with the goal of preventing edema in nonburned tissues. The consensus formula[26] combines concepts, using crystalloid and colloid administration at various times in the fluid resuscitation process. Table 31-3 outlines the available formulas for calculating the fluid resuscitation requirements for burned patients. No matter what formula is used, it must be viewed only as a guideline[15,25,27] and fluids should be titrated to physiologic endpoints.

The controversy over which resuscitation formula to use is similar to the controversy over what parameters to follow to assess the adequacy of resuscitation. Adequacy of organ perfusion is usually assessed by measurement of the normal function or output of the individual organ system. The function of the central nervous system is measured by noting the level of consciousness. The normal function of the gastrointestinal system is inferred by the return of normal bowel sounds and absence of ileus. The function of the kidneys is monitored by measurement of urine output, urine specific gravity, urine glucose level, and urine electrolyte content. Urine volume is a parameter cited frequently, yet the recommended hourly rate ranges from 0.5 to 1 ml/kg body weight.[4,6,27] In evaluating urine output as a parameter of adequate perfusion, the practitioner should keep in mind that diuresis can occur as a result of glucosuria in response to stress or as a response to hypertonic saline or dextran administration during resuscitation; therefore, other endpoint parameters should be used to ascertain the adequacy of the fluid resuscitation.[24,27,28]

Because of the early release of catecholamines, the blood pressure may be elevated artificially in relation to the degree of hypovolemia.[28] Thus trends obtained from the frequent monitoring of blood pressure may not reflect the status of resuscitation. Pulse pressure is easy to measure and correlates well with stroke volume. Narrowing or decreased pulse pressure is an earlier indicator of shock than systolic blood pressure.[29] Frequent monitoring of heart rate trends may be more useful in monitoring the cardiovascular response to resuscitation. In the well-resuscitated patient the heart rate should be in the upper limits of normal for age (<110 beats/min).[29] For the elderly patient or the patient with preexisting cardiac disease, the heart rate may not increase as the patient becomes hypovolemic; thus heart rate is a less reliable resuscitation parameter in these patients, and trends in increased heart rate need to be evaluated.

Other cardiovascular parameters that may be monitored include central venous pressure, pulmonary artery wedge pressure (PAWP), and cardiac output. Filling pressures are frequently very low for the first 24 hours after a burn, and any efforts to improve filling pressures during this period may result in overresuscitation. As long as other measurements of tissue perfusion are within normal ranges, the temptation to improve filling pressures should be resisted.[4,6,24,27] Likewise, cardiac outputs are often very low in the first 24 hours and then trend upward over the second and third 24 hours until they are 1.5 to 2 times normal. This is thought to be the result of the hypermetabolic response observed in patients with larger burns. Thus the use of invasive monitoring devices, such as pulmonary artery (PA) catheters for measurement of PAWP and cardiac output, adds little to the ability to monitor resuscitation and may increase long-term morbidity because of the increased risk of infectious complications. However, in the elderly patient, the cardiac patient, or the patient with severe inhalation injury, the use of a PA catheter to guide fluid resuscitation is advised.[4,6,27,30,31]

Controversy continues to surround the concept of hyperdynamic resuscitation as a predictor of improved survival of burned patients. Burn resuscitation guided by oxygen transport and consumption parameters is based on the premise that supranormal cardiac index (CI) is required to increase oxygen supply to cells and enhance cellular oxygen consumption.[27,30,32-34] Schiller et al[32] and Bernard et al[33] suggested the importance of using crystalloid and colloid resuscitation combined with PA catheter measurements and vasoactive agents to achieve maximal hyperdynamic variables without overresuscitation. The goals of effective resuscitation and hyperdynamic resuscitation are to maximize oxygen delivery to organs and prevent negative sequelae of MODS.

Acid-base balance is another indicator of the effectiveness of fluid resuscitation. A base deficit and elevated serum lactate levels are formed in hypoxic conditions. Base deficit manifests as metabolic acidosis and quickly corrects to normal with adequate resuscitation.[27,29] Jeng et al[35] discovered high base deficit and serum lactate levels were present

TABLE 31-3 Fluid Resuscitation Formulas

Crystalloid Formulas

Baxter (Parkland) formula	**First 24 Hours** Lactated Ringer's (4 ml/kg/% TBSA), half given over first 8 hours after injury; remaining half given over next 16 hours **Second 24 Hours** Dextrose in water, plus K+ Colloid-containing fluid at 20%-60% of calculated plasma volume (0.35-0.5 ml/kg/% TBSA)
Consensus formula	**First 24 Hours** Adults: Lactated Ringer's (2-4 ml/kg/% TBSA) Children: Lactated Ringer's (3-4 ml/kg/% TBSA), half given over first 8 hours; remaining half given over next 16 hours **Second 24 Hours** Adults: Colloid-containing fluid (0.3-0.5 ml/kg/% TBSA) and electrolyte-free fluid to maintain adequate urine output Children: Colloid-containing fluid (0.3-0.5 ml/kg/% TBSA) and half normal saline to maintain adequate urine output
Evans formula	**First 24 Hours** 0.9% normal saline (1 ml/kg/% TBSA) plus colloid solution (1 ml/kg/% TBSA), half given over first 8 hours; remaining half given over next 16 hours **Second 24 Hours** 0.9% normal saline (0.5 ml/kg/% TBSA) plus 5% dextrose in water (2000 ml)
Brooke formula	**First 24 Hours** Lactated Ringer's (1.5 ml/kg/% TBSA) plus colloid solution (0.5 ml/kg/% TBSA), half given over first 8 hours; remaining half given over next 16 hours **Second 24 Hours** Lactated Ringer's (0.5-0.75 ml/kg/% TBSA) plus 5% dextrose in water (2000 ml)
Modified Brooke formula	**First 24 Hours** Lactated Ringer's (2 ml/kg/% TBSA), half given over first 8 hours; remaining half given over next 16 hours **Second 24 Hours** Colloid solution (0.3-0.5 ml/kg/% TBSA) plus 5% dextrose in water to maintain adequate urine output
Monafo formula (hypertonic saline solution)	**First 24 Hours** Na+ 250 mEq/L, volume infused to maintain urine output at 0.5 ml/kg/hr (approximately 30 ml/hr) **Second 24 Hours** 33% isotonic salt solution (0.6% ml/kg/% TBSA) plus replacement of insensible losses
Modified Warden formula (hypertonic saline solution) for burns <40% TBSA	**First 8 Hours** 180 mEq/L Na+ (mix 50 mEq/L NaHCO^3 in Lactated Ringer's), 4 ml/kg/% TBSA; adjust to maintain urine output of 30-50 ml/hr **Second 8 Hours After Burn** Lactated Ringer's at rate to maintain urine output of 30-50 ml/hr
Dextran (Demling) formula	**First 8 Hours** Dextran 40 in saline (2 ml/kg/hr) Lactated Ringer's solution infused to maintain urine output at 30 ml/hr **Second 8 Hours After Burn** Fresh frozen plasma (0.5 ml/kg/hr) for 18 hours, plus additional crystalloid to maintain adequate urine output

in a group of patients believed to be adequately resuscitated based on blood pressure, heart rate, and urine output parameters. Shin et al[36] observed metabolic acidosis in the presence of normal blood pressure, heart rate, and urine output, suggesting base deficit to be a more sensitive indicator of hypoperfusion.

In summary, adequate fluid resuscitation is necessary for survival of a burn injury. For most burned patients, frequent monitoring of urine output, urine glucose level, heart rate, pulse pressure, sensorium, and base deficit allows assessment of the adequacy of resuscitation. These parameters, when monitored together, allow the evaluation of tissue perfusion.

NUTRITIONAL MANAGEMENT

The nutritional needs of most burn patients can be met with a mixture of glucose, essential amino acids, and fats. In addition to the major nutrients, vitamins and minerals are important in wound healing. As mentioned previously, multiple formulas exist for estimating the nutritional needs of the burned patient. Regardless of which formula is used, several principles need to be followed: (1) Nutritional assessment and reassessment must be frequent and ongoing throughout the course of the healing process. (2) Enteral tube feedings should begin within 24 hours after the burn to decrease the production of catabolic hormones, improve nitrogen balance, and maintain gut mucosal integrity.[6,31,37] (3) Increased protein consumption is critical to survival and rehabilitation of the burned patient.[38,39] (4) Anabolic hormone administration should be considered.[4,6,38-40]

As a part of nutritional management, electrolyte balances should be evaluated and imbalances corrected. Frequent measurement of serum sodium, potassium, chloride, phosphorus, calcium, and magnesium levels is necessary to prevent major electrolyte derangements. In addition, deficiencies in trace metals may occur in the burn patient; thus it is recommended that zinc, copper, manganese, and chromium levels be measured periodically and replaced if found deficient. Zinc is an important cofactor in wound healing and tends to be deficient after burn injury.

Nutritional support teams for the burned patient should be used. All efforts to maximize nutritional status of the burn patient are necessary for successful recovery, wound healing, and rehabilitation. See Chapter 16 for further discussions on nutritional interventions.

MANAGEMENT OF PULMONARY INJURY

Pulmonary injury may be the result of inhalation of the byproducts of smoke or the result of a systemic process related to SIRS or MODS. Inhalation injury may or may not injure lung tissue directly. One component of inhalation injury is carbon monoxide (CO) intoxication. Carbon monoxide does not affect the lining of the lung but produces its effect on the body by competing with oxygen for uptake by hemoglobin, thus acting as an asphyxiant. Because hemoglobin has 200 times more affinity for carbon monoxide than for oxygen, carbon monoxide replaces oxygen,

reducing the delivery of oxygen to tissues. This may lead to severe anoxia and related brain injury. In addition, carbon monoxide combines with myoglobin in muscle cells and the cytochrome oxidase system of the brain, producing muscle weakness and coma, respectively. The initial effects of muscle weakness and confusion from decreased oxygen uptake occur within approximately 5 minutes of exposure and may contribute to the inability of the person to escape from the fire. The long-term neurologic effects occasionally associated with smoke inhalation are most likely related to both prolonged anoxia and inhibition of the cytochrome oxidase system of the brain. A carboxyhemoglobin (COHb) level above 40% at the time of exposure is necessary to produce significant neurologic effects.[41] Carbon monoxide has a half-life of 4 hours if the patient breathes room air and 1 hour if the patient is breathing 100% oxygen. COHb levels measured in the emergency department must be interpreted in relation to the time after exposure and the concentration of oxygen administered to the patient since the exposure. Thus a person with a level of 25% COHb after breathing 100% oxygen for an hour probably had a level of approximately 50% COHb at the time of exposure. In addition, caution must be exercised with the use of pulse oximetry equipment as an evaluative tool for oxygen saturation. Pulse oximetry is inaccurate in the presence of elevated COHb.

Abdominal compartment syndrome, a clinical complication associated with the development of burn edema, presents as respiratory compromise. The increased, diffuse capillary leak seen in patients with large burns produces increased fluid translocation into the abdominal compartment, elevating intraabdominal pressures and peak airway pressures and causing oliguria.[42] Rapid detection of abdominal compartment syndrome and prompt corrective decompressive laparotomy may be required to support pulmonary function.

Other components of inhalation injury are upper airway injury and chemical injury to the lung parenchyma. Upper airway injury is the result of inhalation of superheated air, which may cause blisters and edema in the supraglottic area around the vocal cords. This may cause upper airway occlusion and is best treated by early endotracheal intubation. Tracheobronchial and parenchymal lung injuries are caused by the inhalation of a variety of chemicals (e.g., oxides of sulfur and nitrogen, aldehydes, and acrolein) that are byproducts of combustion. Although the exact mechanics of injury may differ, thermal and chemical insult to the major airways and lung parenchyma cause the ciliated epithelial cells to separate from the basement membrane and the systemic and bronchial circulation of the lung to dilate.[41] The loss of the mucociliary system results in ineffective bacterial clearing and predisposes the patient to pulmonary infections and sepsis.[6,43] Damage to type II pneumocytes[43,44] decreases surfactant production, causing the development of microatelectasis and ventilation-perfusion mismatches. Hemorrhagic tracheobronchitis, increased interstitial edema, and decreased macrophage function are additional sequelae seen with inhalation injury. Management efforts are focused on limiting the inflammatory response and fluid sequestration in an effort to avoid the complications of ARDS and pneumonia. As previously stated, 6% of all burned patients do not survive, most of whom have suffered an inhalation injury.

The treatment of inhalation injury primarily consists of supportive care. Of early primary concern is the need for increased volume of fluid resuscitation.[6,23,37] Although patients with inhalation injury require additional fluid resuscitation to maintain organ perfusion, excessive fluid resuscitation may lead to fluid overload and further compromise pulmonary function. For the patient with minimal injury, the administration of warm, humidified oxygen and incentive spirometry may allow adequate oxygenation. In patients with mild injury, maintenance of ventilatory and oxygenation support, pulmonary hygiene, and prevention of infection and atelectasis are of prime importance. For the patient with more severe disease, endotracheal intubation and mechanical ventilation are necessary. The preferred mode of ventilatory support remains undecided; suggested modes include interrupted-flow, high-frequency positive pressure ventilation; pressure control ventilation; permissive hypercapnia ventilation; and low versus high tidal volume ventilation.[4,37] Adjunctive oxygenation therapies and high positive-end expiratory pressure (PEEP) may prove to be beneficial in the management of the burn patient with severe inhalation injury. Prophylactic antibiotic therapy is typically contraindicated; however, when pneumonia is suspected, broad-spectrum antibiotic coverage is indicated.[43,44]

Diagnosis of inhalation injury is based on the patient's presentation (Table 31-4) and the findings on fiberoptic bronchoscopy or xenon 133 ventilation-perfusion scan. A chest radiograph is helpful in establishing baseline data but typically does not assist in the early diagnosis of inhalation injury. Ongoing evaluation of the response to therapy, decreased airway edema, adequate oxygenation and ventilation parameters, and absence of infection remain the management goals for the patient with inhalation injury.

MANAGEMENT AND PREVENTION OF INFECTION

The skin, the body's largest organ, acts in part as a natural mechanical barrier to microbial attachment, growth, and penetration.[45] After burn injury, the protective nature is lost, and the resultant avascular, denatured protein eschar provides an ideal medium for the growth of microorganisms. In addition, invasive devices (e.g., intravenous and Foley catheters, endotracheal tubes, nasogastric tubes) provide ports of entry for organisms. The overwhelmed inflammatory response tires, and the patient's ability to fight infection may decrease as the burn healing process progresses. Infections in the burned patient may involve the urinary tract, pulmonary system, bloodstream, or wound. Differentiation of active infection and colonization is an important element of medical management.[46]

In the not too distant past, the goal of wound care was to find an antimicrobial cream or solution that would prevent infection and allow the wound to heal or granulate so that a graft could be used to close the wound. During this time a number of the wound care products used today were developed (Table 31-5): mafenide acetate cream, silver sulfadiazine cream, and silver nitrate. More recently the emphasis in wound care has been on early removal of eschar (devitalized tissue) of deep dermal and full-thickness burns and use of a variety of biologic and synthetic dressings to cover the wound and promote healing and early wound closure. This change in focus has had a dramatic effect on burn care. The length of hospital stay has decreased, patients have fewer septic episodes, and wound cosmesis may be enhanced.[4,6,45]

In all areas of wound management the maintenance of a clean, well-nourished wound through meticulous nursing care is imperative. Initially, several careful cleansings of the wound with a nontoxic solution such as a mild soap or chlorhexidine gluconate solution may be necessary to remove wound debris associated with the traumatic event.[47,48] Healing wounds require adequate circulation, so care must be taken to apply a snug dressing that will remain on the wound but will not restrict blood flow. Maintaining a moist wound environment enhances wound healing and decreases the risk of infection. Similarly, the patient's position must be changed frequently to reduce pressure and maintain blood flow to dependent areas. Adequate nutrition is also imperative to prevent infection and maximize wound healing.

The use of systemic antibiotics in burn care has been reduced significantly except in those patients with positive cultures[49,50] and extensive injuries (>70 %).[46] Systemic antibiotics are used often in the perioperative period as prophylaxis against infection. In this case it is important to administer the antibiotic so that its peak period of effectiveness is during the surgical procedure.[47] When systemic antibiotics are used to treat bacteremias or sepsis, it is important to follow blood levels to ensure maximal effectiveness without toxicity and untoward effects. The burn patient handles a variety of drugs differently than other patients because of the hypermetabolic response. Drug pharmacokinetics must be considered when administering medications to a burn patient. Prevention of infection remains a priority goal.

TABLE 31-4 Signs and Symptoms Suggesting Inhalation Injury

- Burn injury occurred in a closed space
- Edema and redness of the oropharynx/nasopharynx
- Hoarse, brassy voice
- Shortness of breath
- Tachypnea, wheezing, stridor
- Carbonaceous sputum, singed nasal and facial hair
- Anxiety
- Disorientation progressing to obtundation and coma

TABLE 31-5 Wound Management Products

Wound Management Option	Clinical Considerations
Silver nitrate solution	Effective against most gram-positive and some gram-negative organisms
	Decreased penetration of eschar
	May produce hyponatremia, hypokalemia, and hypochloremia
Mafenide acetate cream	Effective against wide range of gram-positive and gram-negative organisms
	Rapidly diffuses through eschar (improved effectiveness in established infections)
	Painful application
	Hypersensitivity reactions may occur
	Acid-base derangements may occur
Silver sulfadiazine cream	Effective against wide range of gram-positive and gram-negative organisms
	Softens eschar and increases joint mobility
	Absorbed slowly; reduced chance of nephrotoxicity
	Hypersensitivity and leukopenia may occur
Enzymatic debridement agents	Provides nonsurgical debridement of denatured tissue
	May require concurrent antimicrobial coverage to prevent wound infection
	May be painful and cause bleeding in wound bed
Antibiotic-impregnated dressings	Provide continuous antimicrobial coverage over >24 hours
	Decreased frequency of dressing changes required although antimicrobial coverage is maintained
	Dressings must remain moist
	Hypersensitivity may develop
Biologic dressings	Provide immediate wound coverage and protection until autografting is possible
	Decrease bacterial proliferation
	Decrease evaporative water loss
	Prepare granulation tissue for autografting
	Hypersensitivity may develop
	Expense may be prohibitive
Cultured epithelial cells	No rejection
	Requires 3 weeks to grow skin
	Cultured skin has decreased tensile strength and may sheer easily after grafting
	Expense may be prohibitive

ASSOCIATED TRAUMA

Major burn injury in association with polytrauma poses an unusual and complex management problem.[51] In the military, up to 24%[51,52] of burn injuries are complicated by trauma; 7% of all burn admissions and 36% of those burn injury admissions with associated injuries are related to motor vehicle crashes.[51] Initial management of the burn trauma patient requires that the health care practitioner focus on the primary and secondary assessments, not on management of the burn wound. Priorities surrounding the burn injury are to stop the burning process with water; remove clothing, including metals and leather products; and cover the patient and burns with clean dry cotton materials, such as a sheet. Fluid volume resuscitation is initiated during the primary survey and may be adjusted after the secondary survey.[53] Attention to the "ABCDEs" of trauma survey are equally important in the burned and injured patient, especially in the event of suspected inhalation injury. Careful attention to the mechanism of injury is important. For example, the practitioner needs to determine if an altered neurologic response is due to a blow to the head or carbon monoxide toxicity. Concomitant fractures[54] may present an additional challenge to the management of the burn patient after hemodynamic stabilization. Although treatment strategies vary, goals in the management of burns and fractures revolve around early stabilization and mobilization of the fracture, with early coverage or closure of the burn wound.[54] As with any trauma, prevention of deep vein thrombosis should be part of the plan of care.

NURSING MANAGEMENT OF THE BURN PATIENT

Management of the burn patient can be divided into several phases. These phases lend themselves well to a discussion of nursing management. The initial phase, resuscitation, usually extends over the first 72 hours. The second phase, the reparative or acute cycle, spans the time from resuscitation until complete wound closure. The time varies depending on the depth and extent of burn, the method of wound management employed, and the variety of complications that may extend this phase, such as ARDS, sepsis, or MODS. The third phase, rehabilitation and reconstruction, may extend over years. The three phases associated with management of the burn patient are similar to those involved in the management of the trauma patient (resuscitation, critical care, intermediate care, rehabilitation). Nursing management during each of these phases depends on accurate assessment and development of evidence-based nursing care.

RESUSCITATIVE PHASE

Nursing management during this phase centers on maintenance of homeostasis and tissue perfusion, treatment of life-threatening complications, prevention of infection, management of pain, and management of anxiety and fear.

FLUID VOLUME RESUSCITATION.

The burned patient is prone to fluid and electrolyte disorders until the wound is healed or covered with a permanent or semipermanent cover. Initially fluid volume deficit is a major concern. As fluid shifts occur in relation to the initial injury, the circulating volume decreases rapidly. Without rapid infusion of fluids, the patient develops hypovolemia and shock. The importance of burn fluid resuscitation has been discussed previously. Monitoring the patient frequently to assess response to fluid therapy is a major nursing priority in the first 24 to 48 hours. The well-resuscitated patient should have adequate, glucose-free urine (at a flow of at least 0.5 ml/kg/hr), a pulse rate in the upper limits of the normal range for age, normal pulse pressure, clear sensorium, hematocrit less than 50%, no ileus, and normal acid-base balance.

Urine output can be a highly sensitive measure of adequate organ and tissue perfusion, but a variety of things should be considered when monitoring urine output. First, there is a normal variation in urine output from hour to hour; therefore, when using urine output as a monitor of resuscitation efforts, an average of 2 or 3 hours of urine flow should be assessed before changing intravenous fluid flow rates unless other signs of hypovolemia are present. Urine flow rates usually decrease over time in response to hypovolemia rather than drop abruptly. An abrupt decrease or absence of urine flow usually is related to a mechanical problem, such as a kink in the catheter or drainage system or a clot or plug in the catheter. Manipulation or irrigation of the catheter may correct this problem immediately. Glycosuria is a common response to stress and may cause the urine output to be falsely elevated. If the patient has other signs of hypovolemia and a high urine output, glycosuria is often the cause. The use of dextran or mannitol also may cause the urine output to increase in the face of hypovolemia. Thus although urine output can be a sensitive measure of organ perfusion, each of these issues should be considered when monitoring urine output.

In patients with electrical injuries the urine may contain hemochromogens, such as hemoglobin or myoglobin. The treatment for myoglobin in the urine is to flush the kidney to prevent permanent injury. In this case, fluids are given to increase hourly urine output to twice or three times normal (i.e., 1-1.5 ml/kg/hr).[4,55,56] In addition, osmotic diuretics are given to increase urine output. Thus normal parameters of urine output are no longer appropriate for monitoring.

Pulse rate also varies for a number of reasons. Age is a common cause of variation: infants and young children have significantly higher pulse rates, and elderly patients tend to have lower pulse rates and may not be able to significantly increase their rate in response to hypovolemia because of preexisting heart disease and medications (e.g., β-blocking agents). Young athletes often have a normal pulse rate of 50 to 60 beats/min. When stressed by hypovolemia, their rate may increase to low-normal values (80-90 beats/min) and seem a little low for the normal response to hypovolemia. Pain may cause an increased pulse rate and may be associated with agitation, both of which may mimic some of the signs of hypovolemia. Upward trends in pulse rate should be monitored and assessed as an indication of hypovolemia.

Unless the burned patient also has experienced head trauma, the sensorium should be clear; that is, the patient should be oriented to time, place, and person. Patients may appear to be somnolent and confused because they have been given narcotics or sedatives for pain management. For the most part, however, patients without associated head trauma are oriented to time, place, and person when aroused.

A hematocrit higher than 50% is usually a clear indication of hypovolemia and hemoconcentration (a normal hematocrit above 50% is rare). Ileus is another indication of decreased organ perfusion. This is common in the early hours of burn management, but once fluid replacement is well under way, it should no longer remain a problem. Lastly, evaluation of base deficit as a measure of adequate fluid resuscitation may be the most sensitive element in evaluating resuscitative interventions.

Again, each of these parameters has its limitations. It is only when all the parameters are considered in combination that a true picture of the patient's volume status can be assessed. When more than one of these parameters indicate that a fluid volume deficit has occurred, the volume of administered fluid should be adjusted. This may be done by administering boluses of fluid or increasing the flow rate for a specified time. It is important to monitor the patient's response to this fluid challenge continuously to note whether the monitored parameters return to normal. If the parameters continue to be abnormal, other causes of hypovolemia should be considered.

OTHER FLUID AND ELECTROLYTE IMBALANCES.

Although hypovolemia is the most common fluid and electrolyte problem in burn patients, one must be alert to a variety of other fluid and electrolyte issues. Fluid overload caused by overresuscitation may present problems during the resuscitative phase of burn management. Fluid overload is a rare problem except in infants, patients with preexisting cardiac conditions, patients with severe inhalation injury, patients with preexisting renal disease, and patients who have had delayed resuscitation intervention and have sustained a renal insult. Assessment parameters used to evaluate overresuscitation include elevated cardiac filling pressures and decreased cardiac performance (cardiac index and pulse rate), confusion, dyspnea, rales, inadequate oxygenation, normal or increased urine output, decreased urine specific gravity, normal or decreased heart rate, peripheral edema unrelated to burn site, decreased serum sodium level, and decreased serum and urine osmolality. Therapy may include more judicious administration of fluids, administration of diuretics, administration of oxygen if dyspnea is present, and evaluation and treatment of any underlying problems.

Hyponatremia, hypernatremia, hypokalemia, or hyperkalemia also may occur with some frequency during the resuscitation phase as fluids continue to shift between the extracellular and intracellular compartments. Frequent monitoring of electrolytes and adjustments in fluid replacement regimens may be necessary to prevent complications associated with electrolyte imbalances.

PULMONARY DYSFUNCTION.   Impaired gas exchange is a priority second only to hypoperfusion. Altered pulmonary function should be suspected when any signs indicate the presence of inhalation injury, fluid overload, abdominal compartment syndrome, or inadequate expansion of the chest wall related to full-thickness circumferential third-degree burns. Nursing goals prioritize assessment of the pulmonary system, including visual, auscultative, and laboratory data for evaluation of the adequacy of oxygenation and ventilation. If inhalation injury is suspected, establishment of an artificial airway (insertion of an endotracheal or nasotracheal tube) should be the highest priority for the nurse. Tissue edema is significant within the first 8 hours of injury,[25] so establishing an airway before the first 8 hours after burn may be the defining factor in a patient's survival.[51,53] The parameters to be monitored are rate and character of respiration, signs of increasing hoarseness, increased pulmonary secretions, decreased chest wall expansion, chest wall retractions in children, subjective complaints of dyspnea, changes in mentation, and increased facial edema. If an endotracheal tube is placed, it should be observed frequently for placement and the straps securing the tubes should be tightened or loosened accordingly to account for increases and decreases in edema formation over time. In addition, care should be taken when securing the nasally placed endotracheal tube not to put pressure on the nares or the burn-injured face, ears, or scalp. Pressure on the nares may lead to necrosis and loss of the normal contour of the nose. Pressure on injured tissue of the face, ears, and scalp may cause further loss of tissue and result in a poorer cosmetic result. Intubation may increase the burn patient's already altered sensory perception. Patients who have facial burns often have eyes that are swollen shut, so they cannot see. If they can no longer talk, they are likely to become even more agitated. This may make it more difficult for them to cooperate with mechanical ventilation. Frequent explanation, reassurance, and sedatives are necessary to ensure their cooperation.

Because these patients often have increased pulmonary secretions, diligent pulmonary toilet, including frequent suctioning, turning, and chest physiotherapy, are necessary to decrease the risk of pneumonia. Pneumonia is a major cause of morbidity and mortality in the intubated burn patient.

BURN WOUND MANAGEMENT.   The management of burn wounds is a collaborative process; the major goals of therapies have been discussed previously. The ongoing assessment of wound healing and adjustment of wound therapies frequently are nursing concerns. Initially the extent and depth of injury must be assessed accurately. Once the patient is hemodynamically stable, an accurate assessment of the extent of the wound should be made by an experienced burn health care professional. Again the Berkow or Lund-Browder formula provides more accurate assessments than the rule of nines formula. These formulas should be used to determine the extent of burn injury. Fluid resuscitation formulas should then be recalculated based on the more precise estimate of TBSA burned and adjustments made to avoid complications of underresuscitation or overresuscitation.

Assessment of the depth of injury requires even more judgment (see Table 31-2). The very superficial first-degree burn and the truly deep third-degree burn are fairly obvious. The difficulty comes in distinguishing the different depths of second-degree, or dermal, injuries. Again experience is helpful, but even the most experienced observer may be wrong as much as 50% of the time, especially during the first 24 hours.[14] The wound is dynamic, and its depth may change over time if edema, pressure, and low-flow states decrease circulation to the wound; extending a zone of stasis to a zone of coagulation. Careful documentation of wound appearance over time as the nurse provides wound care is useful in the assessment of depth and in the early recognition of wound infection. Increased erythema, tenderness, or pain around the wound; exudate that becomes more yellow or green; and discoloration within the wound (black or purple areas) are all signs of infection. Wound changes should be documented and followed carefully. An easy way to monitor increasing erythema is to use a marker to delineate the edges of the reddened area, noting the date and time. If the redness extends past these margins over the next few hours, this may indicate the need for a change in wound therapy or administration of systemic antibiotics to control infection. Many newer dressings are applied to the wound bed and remain intact for several hours to days. Assessment of the patient's response to the dressing and signs of infection are essential elements of the nursing plan of care.

Compartment syndrome may be an early complication as fluid shifts and maximal edema occur in the burn wound bed. Neurovascular assessment and direct compartment tissue pressures should be assessed in patients with circumferential extremity burns. Tissue compartment pressures greater than 20 mm Hg indicate compromised perfusion[4,6,51,54] and pressures greater than 40 mm Hg indicate significantly compromised perfusion. In these cases an escharotomy is necessary to release the pressure and expand the tissue compartment.[4,6,23,53] Patients with circumferential deep and full-thickness wounds are at the greatest risk of developing compartment syndrome.

MAINTAINING NONBURNED SKIN INTEGRITY. In the burn patient, alteration of skin integrity usually is considered in relation to the burn injury; the potential for other alterations in skin integrity also exist. The mobility of burn patients is usually restricted by invasive line placement, application of splints or skeletal traction, ventilatory management, neck immobilization, sedation and narcotic administration, or positioning necessary to prevent graft loss. Any or all of these may contribute to prolonged bed rest, decreased ability to move in bed, and development of pressure ulcers.[57] The severely burned and immobilized patient benefits from the use of low air loss or kinetic therapy mattresses. Although patients still require turning on a low air loss surface, pressure is reduced, decreasing some of the risks associated with the development of pressure ulcers. Nonburned skin should be assessed daily, and a valid pressure ulcer risk assessment tool (e.g., Braden Risk Assessment Tool) should be used to help identify patients at risk for skin breakdown (see Chapter 15). With each bath and dressing change, the dependent areas of the body should be inspected carefully for evidence of increased pressure and presence of skin breakdown. Common areas for the development of pressure ulcers in burn patients are the heels and the occiput. Burns involving these areas and edema often mask the beginning of pressure problems; thus ongoing assessment is extremely important in maintaining the tissue integrity of nonburned skin.

PREVENTION OF INFECTION. The burn patient is significantly immunocompromised by the loss of the protection normally provided by the skin; the loss of proteins, including immunoglobulins, during the acute resuscitative phase of injury; and exhaustion of the inflammatory mediators that orchestrate immune competence against invading microorganisms. Nursing management directed toward the prevention of infection focuses on four areas of concern: (1) vigilant monitoring for signs of impending wound infection, systemic sepsis, and pneumonia; (2) maintenance of the external and personal hygienic environment to reduce the reservoir of microorganisms; (3) use of aseptic technique for wound care and all invasive procedures; and (4) timely administration of antibiotics and appropriate use of topical antibacterial agents. Because the assessment of wounds for infection was discussed previously, this discussion is limited to signs of systemic infection.

The diagnosis of sepsis in the burn patient is complicated by the hypermetabolic response and by pain and anxiety, which may account for abnormalities in a variety of parameters monitored. The diagnosis of sepsis depends on the presence of abnormalities in several parameters: mental acuity; changes in body temperature, heart rate, respiratory rate, blood pressure, urine output, and gastrointestinal function; and changes in laboratory values such as urine glucose level, blood pH, white blood cell count, C-reactive protein, platelet count, and positive blood cultures.[58] Thus frequent, accurate monitoring of these parameters leads to timely diagnosis and treatment of systemic infections.

The second concern for prevention of infection is to provide an external environment that limits the access of microorganisms to the wounds of the burn patient. This includes the environment that is external to the patient (the patient's room; other areas of the hospital to which the patient is exposed [e.g., operating room, treatment rooms, hydrotherapy rooms]) and the staff who care for the patient. The most important aspect of providing a protective environment is to place a barrier between the patient and the environmental hazards. This may sound complicated but in fact can be quite simple. Inanimate objects in the environment, as long as they are cleansed with standard hospital disinfectants and dried, should present little, if any, risk to the patient. The major concern in the environment is porous materials that cannot be cleaned, such as chairs with cloth covers, mattresses without intact plastic covers, and similar hard to clean items. The biggest problem in maintaining a protective environment is personnel. Most transfers of microorganisms in the hospital environment occur via the hands of the hospital staff. Meticulous handwashing, wearing of gloves, and covering the clothing of the health care workers during direct patient care eliminate the major sources of microorganisms from the patient's immediate environment.[45,46] During wound care and invasive procedures, the use of surgical mask and hair covers may increase protection. These simple precautions can produce an acceptable external environment.

The other environment of concern is the patient's own body. Providing meticulous hygienic measures is important to reduce infection. Especially of concern is hygiene of hair-bearing areas, skin folds in the groin and axilla, and under nail beds. Oral care is also important, especially for the intubated patient.

Wound care should be managed aseptically. Careful attention to the removal of exudate and devitalized tissue reduces the bacterial load and maximizes the effectiveness of antibacterial creams or solutions to control bacterial proliferation. The choice of antibacterial agents should be based on knowledge of the usual bacterial flora prevalent within devitalized burn tissue; routine, periodic cultures of the patient's wounds may be appropriate to discern active infection versus colonization.[46] The type of infection and antibiotic sensitivity should be evaluated as an element in treatment to decrease the emergence of drug-resistant organisms typically seen in burn centers (e.g., methicillin-resistant *Staphylococcus aureus*[50] and vancomycin-resistant enterococci[49]).

Invasive procedures in burned patients carry increased risk for infection. Often, intravenous or arterial lines must be placed through burned areas, increasing the risk of infection. Meticulous care should be taken to keep the area around venous and arterial access lines as clean as possible. Usually the topical antibacterial agent used on the surrounding burn wound is also applied at the insertion site to decrease the risk of infection.[46] Suturing lines in place keeps them from being easily displaced or slipping within the vein, which increases the chance of infection. Intravenous catheters should be changed if infection is suspected or according to hospital policy. The advent of antibiotic-coated invasive catheters may also decrease the incidence of line sepsis in burn patients.

As mentioned previously, burn patients often exhibit altered pharmacokinetics in response to the administration of certain drugs. For this reason it is important to draw frequent peak and trough levels when administering antibiotics, so that the dose and frequency of administration can be adjusted to obtain appropriate drug levels necessary to combat the infection.

MANAGEMENT OF PAIN.   Altered tissue perfusion caused by extracellular and intracellular fluid shifts characteristic of the resuscitative phase encourage the use intravenous analgesia to provide adequate pain relief. Remember, the more superficial the burn wound, the greater the pain because of the associated exposed nerve fibers. When possible, a standardized pain assessment tool (e.g., WILDA[59]) should be used to ensure consistent evaluation of the patient's pain and treatment. Concurrent treatment of anxiety may also be beneficial. Additionally, care should be taken to differentiate and treat procedural pain (pain associated with burn wound care) and background pain (pain related to tissue injury and the inflammatory response, which may be exacerbated by movement, breathing, or pressure).[60,61] Procedural pain is brought on by manipulation of the wound, as in dressing changes, debridement, or intensive exercise to prevent skin contractures and improve mobility.

The mainstay of pain management in the acutely injured burn patient is opioids. Morphine or fentanyl may be used during the initial phase of care to manage both background and procedural pain. Usually small, frequent doses are administered intravenously or by intravenous drip. During the first 24 to 48 hours an adequate level of medication to relieve background pain can be established and background medication needs can be converted to oral opioid equivalents. When the patient's condition permits, a long-acting oral opioid can be used to manage background pain. Slow-release oral morphine preparations can be used for background pain control. The most important aspect of background pain control is to realize that this pain is always present to some degree and is best relieved by administering pain medication on a non-pain-contingent schedule. Background pain control in patients with high anxiety levels may be supplemented with an anxiolytic such as a benzodiazepine.[61] Patient-controlled analgesia (PCA) is another method that may be used to control background pain. This technique works especially well in young adults, who want and need to have some control over their care.

Procedural pain is intermittent and of high intensity. It is also best managed by opioids.[60] During the initial cycle of care, intravenous morphine or fentanyl may be used. An intravenous morphine bolus should be given 15 to 20 minutes before the procedure, and smaller boluses may be given during the procedure as necessary. Allowing the patient to deliver small doses every 5 minutes using a PCA

pump is often very effective during wound care. Fentanyl has a much shorter half-life than morphine and can be used when a short-acting drug is needed. Fentanyl is also useful for the patient with decreased cardiac reserve, exhibited by a labile blood pressure and periods of hypotension when given morphine. Once the patient's condition improves, oral opioids can be used for procedural pain. Immediate-release morphine, hydromorphone, oxycodone, and other opioids or synthetic opioids can be used. Unlike patients with cancer pain, with whom the objective is to begin with the weaker opioid and work up, the objective with burn patients is to begin with potent opioids for the severe pain associated with the fresh open wound and use opioids of decreasing strength as the wounds heal and the pain is less intense. Anxiety and fear, especially fear of the unknown, is a major component of procedural pain. Many patients report that the use of anxiolytics in conjunction with pain medication is helpful.[61] In this case the benzodiazepines are useful. When opioids and benzodiazepines are both administered for pain management, the time of peak effectiveness may be different and may necessitate giving them at different times before procedures to obtain maximal effectiveness.

Lastly, burn hypermetabolism and issues of pain tolerance may require that the pain treatment plan be reevaluated frequently, with medication regimens adjusted to meet the patient's pain relief needs.

NUTRITIONAL CONCERNS.   As discussed previously, hypermetabolism and nutritional needs must be addressed early in the treatment of burn patients. Goals to establish enteral nutrition are important in blunting translocation of gut microflora and negative sequelae of burn catabolism. Nursing care focuses on obtaining and maintaining enteral tube placements and aseptic management of central venous access used for infusion of total parenteral nutrition. Ongoing assessment of the patient's nutritional status guides the wound management plan because adequate protein intake is essential to wound healing.[4,6,38,39,62]

REPARATIVE PHASE

The second phase of care is the reparative phase. The major focus in this period is to support the body's natural healing properties and provide psychosocial support to allow both physical and psychologic repair. Nursing priorities focus on the provision of adequate nutritional support, wound and pain management, prevention of contracture formation, management of sensory and sleep disturbances, and psychologic interventions to help the patient cope with the injury and its consequences. Many of these nursing issues are common to all critically ill or injured trauma patients.

NUTRITIONAL SUPPORT.   Burn patients have greatly increased metabolic needs. The increased metabolic demands actually begin during the resuscitation cycle and continue for some time after wound closure, as evidenced by increased oxygen consumption for several months after complete wound closure.[39,40] The goal of the health care team is to continually assess the nutritional requirements and assist the patient in meeting these needs. The nutritional team is helpful in measuring and calculating the patient's nutritional needs. The nutritionist is also usually responsible for estimating the total calorie and protein requirements for the individual patient. To determine if the patient's nutritional needs are being met, measurement of weight, intake and output, serum proteins (albumin, prealbumin, transferrin), and nitrogen balance are usually considered. Accurate measurements are extremely important. Indications of inadequate nutrition include weight loss greater than 10% of preinjury weight; low serum albumin, prealbumin, and transferrin levels; and a negative nitrogen balance.

The delivery of appropriate nutrition is a major nursing consideration. Because most burn patients experience lack of appetite or may not be able to cooperate with attempts to get them to eat the large amounts of food required, alternative methods of alimentation may be necessary.

Enteral feeding is initiated early in the management of the burn patient and may be used for nighttime supplemental feedings. Concerns to be considered when tube feedings are administered include hyperosmolar diarrhea, hyperglycemia, ileus, aspiration, and fluid and electrolyte imbalance. Hyperosmolar diarrhea may occur if the osmolarity of the enteral feeding product is high or if the tube feeding is infused too rapidly. Careful monitoring of flow rates and feeding of progressively concentrated solutions usually eliminate this problem. Some patients experience hyperglycemia related to the high carbohydrate content of enteral tube feeding. This can be controlled by a change in the components of the feeding solution or administration of insulin. Symptoms of hyperglycemia include osmotic diuresis, glycosuria, and an increased serum glucose level. Ileus related to fluid and electrolyte imbalances and sepsis is a common problem in the burn patient and may complicate the administration of tube feedings. Often duodenal feedings are used to bypass the stomach and reduce the risk of aspiration associated with gastric feedings. The debate as to whether to use gastric or duodenal feeding routinely centers around two factors: (1) Duodenal feedings are less likely to be related to vomiting and aspiration but leave the lining of the stomach unprotected, which may lead to gastric ulceration. (2) Enteral feedings administered into the stomach protect the gastric mucosa but may leave patients more prone to aspiration. To prevent ulceration when duodenal feedings are used, antacids or histamine blockers are routinely prescribed. To reduce the risk of aspiration, it is also recommended that the head of the patient be maintained at 30 degrees of elevation. There is little evidence that elevation of the patient's head reduces the incidence or severity of aspiration, but it is generally believed that it may be beneficial.

Although tube feedings may be the primary means of nutritional support during the early phases of care, consideration should be given to beginning oral feedings. Offering small amounts of food that the patient likes or is craving may stimulate the patient's appetite and improve his or her overall morale. In some patients, to make the transition from enteral feedings to oral alimentation, it may be necessary to use enteral tube feedings at night to make up the calories not consumed during the day. All too often health care workers use the threat of enteral tube feeding to encourage the patient to eat. This rarely accomplishes an increase in oral intake and often leads to feelings of failure for the patient who just cannot eat enough. If it is apparent that the patient cannot eat enough, enteral tube feedings should be presented as an adjunct or alternative rather than as a threat. Additionally, anabolic hormones may prove beneficial in creating an environment of anabolism versus the catabolic, hypermetabolic state of burn injury, especially if the patient is struggling to consume adequate calories.

When oral feeding is the sole means of nutritional support, frequent, small feedings and high-calorie, high-protein supplements are useful in increasing calorie and protein intake. The intake of fluids low in calories and protein, such as coffee, tea, and diet sodas, should be discouraged or offered as positive reinforcers when adequate oral intake has been achieved.

MANAGEMENT OF PAIN. Pain is a major problem for the burn patient. Although its character and intensity may vary throughout all phases, it is no less a problem. Pain is related to tissue injury and the healing process and is complicated by fear, anxiety, depression, and the chronicity of the healing process. The goal of pain control throughout burn care should be to provide maximal comfort given the nature of the injury and the treatments required for recovery.

Establishing a partnership with the patient early in the course of care regarding how to manage pain relief may prevent problems and disappointments. One of the first goals in pain management is to establish an objective system by which the patient can measure and communicate the intensity of pain. Simple adjective scales may be used with patients from early school age to the elderly. In the event that the patient cannot communicate verbally or actively engage in the assessment of his or her pain, observation of some physiologic responses or behaviors may provide guidance. These include increased pulse rate, diaphoresis, increased agitation, grimacing, and rhythmic movements or lack of movement.

Assessment of pain is extremely important; however, the effectiveness of various pain relief measures is equally important. The absence of symptoms or pain behaviors or verbal reports of relief using adjective or numeric scales are necessary to tailor pain management therapies.

Once the wounds are essentially healed, the need for opioids should diminish. At this point most of the patient's pain can be managed with regularly scheduled doses of nonsteroidal antiinflammatory agents. During the later phases of care, antidepressants may be useful in some patients and may act as an adjunct to pain management.[61,63]

Nonpharmacologic therapies may be useful throughout the phases of burn care as adjuncts to other pain management regimens. The goal of this type of therapy is to help the patient relax and to control the perception of pain. The type of nonpharmacologic therapy depends on individual coping styles and the age of the patient. Techniques include distraction, imagery, breathing techniques, hypnosis, and biofeedback. A variety of distraction techniques may be used, such as music, television, or talking to the patient about hobbies. Imagery, breathing techniques, and hypnosis are similar and require that the patient actively concentrate on an activity (e.g., breathing) or a mental image that allows him or her to perceive something other than the pain and thus relax. Biofeedback, like imagery, breathing techniques, or hypnosis, requires the patient to concentrate on something other than the pain. In biofeedback, a body function, such as lowering the heart rate, is used to assist the patient with the intense concentration required and gives a specific measurement regarding when relaxation is maximized. Distraction techniques are external to patient control and require less energy and less cognitive effort on the part of the patient. Imagery, breathing techniques, hypnosis, and biofeedback all require intense patient participation and are energy consuming. When these techniques are used, the patient often complains of being tired and drained of energy and may have increased pain after the procedure. Administering less potent pain medications at the end of the procedure may prevent the letdown feeling and decrease pain complaints when nonpharmacologic therapies are used.

PREVENTION OF WOUND CONTRACTURES. Prevention of contractures begins immediately and continues until the scar has matured and the patient has completed the rehabilitation phase. Physical and occupational therapists play a major role in this aspect of care by providing a variety of splints and positioning devices and detailed exercise programs aimed at maximizing function and reducing contracture formation. The nurse must provide consistent and frequent monitoring of the patient's position, use of splints, and adherence to an exercise regimen. Understanding the importance of positioning the patient in an anticontracture position and integrating these positions into overall management maximizes functional outcome.[64,65] Understanding the importance of each aspect of care allows the nurse to work with the therapist to maximize care, reduce tissue breakdown, and prevent contractures at the same time. Likewise, elevation of the patient's head to prevent aspiration or improve respiratory effort may be contrary to the usual positioning techniques that reduce neck contractures; continued assessment and adjustment in patient positioning may allow all objectives to be accomplished over time. Another area that may pose problems is the need for intravenous access in extremities, which may limit the use or require alteration of the usual splints used to prevent contractures of the extremities. A thorough understanding of all treatment goals and priorities allows the nurse to optimize patient care.

WOUND MANAGEMENT. Wound management is a significant priority in the reparative phase of care. Therapeutic goals of burn wound management focus on rapid closure of the denuded tissue and provision of the optimal environment for wound healing. Techniques for optimal wound closure are diverse, and surgical preference dictates wound management techniques. Regardless of the technique, some principles cross all methods, as discussed below. Wound cleansing is required to keep the wound bed free of contaminants and decrease the risk of infection. Methods for cleansing include aseptic technique, use of a nontoxic agent such as a mild soap or chlorhexidine, and nonsubmersion hydrotherapy.[48] During wound cleansing processes the patient's body may be entirely exposed; therefore, precautions to prevent hypothermia and associated complications (e.g., increased metabolic response, sympathetic stimulation, and altered coagulopathy)[66] need to be avoided by prewarming the treatment room and limiting the amount of time the patient's body is exposed.

Topical antimicrobial agents (Table 31-5) may be used to prevent wound infections and maintain moisture on the tissue bed or eschar until effective wound debridement may be surgically completed. Topical antimicrobial agents have penetrating properties to prevent burn wound infections in deep dermal wounds,[48,67] but caution should be exercised when applying these agents on viable tissue. Antibiotic ointments may be more appropriate therapy as a means of decreasing microbial counts on wound beds with viable tissue.

Enzymatic debridement of necrotic tissue may be beneficial for a burn patient for whom surgical excision of denuded skin is not the optimal therapy. Klasen[68] reviewed the use of nonoperative removal of necrotic tissue, stating that enzymatic debridement should be individualized for each patient, debridement results may be variable within the wound bed, successful use of enzymatic agents requires maintenance of a moist wound bed, and concurrent antimicrobial treatment may be necessary to prevent wound infection. Despite the limitations cited by Klasen,[68] enzymatic debridement may be appropriate for the treatment of some burn wounds[48,69] and may enhance healing of partial-thickness burns by rapid debridement of necrotic tissue.

Anabolic hormones and growth factors have provided conflicting results in regard to their benefit in expediting wound healing.[70] Use of growth factors should be reserved for patients whose wounds are difficult to heal and those whose wounds involve significant TBSA. Anabolic hormones assist the wound-healing process through enhanced anabolic metabolism and tissue regeneration.[38]

Choice of dressing depends on factors such as the location and depth of burn wound, age of the patient, frequency of dressing change required, exudate management, and maintenance of a moist (not wet) wound environment. Traditional dressings consist of the application of an antimicrobial agent and fine gauze dressings reinforced with coarse gauze dressings to absorb exudates and provide protection. A variety of moist wound dressing therapies exist for the management of burn wounds,[71] but the characteristics of the dressing and wound bed must be evaluated when selecting a dressing that will provide an optimal outcome. (Refer to Chapter 15 for a discussion of the characteristics of dressing products.) Wound dressing choices may include hydrocolloid, nonadherent gauze, polyurethane (transparent) films, composite synthetic dressings, alginates, and hydrogel dressings.

A new category of antimicrobial wound dressings provides optimal healing conditions for partial-thickness burn wounds. Kerlix A.M.D. is a gauze dressing that contains polyhexamethylene biguanide, an antimicrobial agent used to fight bacterial colonization within and through the dressing.[72] Early research suggests that the dressing provides protection against gram-negative, gram-positive, and fungal microorganisms. Atomic silver and silver salts have been used as antiseptic agents for years.[73,74] As early as 1965, interest in the application of silver-based antimicrobial agents emerged in an effort to prevent microbial growth in burn wounds. Silver nitrate solutions, silver sulfadiazine, and mafenide acetate are all silver-based antimicrobial agents used in the treatment of deep partial-thickness and full-thickness burn wounds.[6,46,67,73,74] Silver-coated dressings (Acticoat and Silveron) are silver-impregnated dressings that provide a moist wound healing environment and antimicrobial action and do not require daily dressing changes.

Biologic and biosynthetic dressings are temporary skin substitutes that provide wound bed protection until skin grafting can be achieved. Biologic dressings provide a moist wound healing environment; however, the body may recognize the dressing as foreign, initiating an inflammatory response. The use and development of optimal biologic dressings has been an area of extensive research. Biologic dressings include allograft (cadaver skin), xenograft (porcine skin is most commonly used), Biobrane (a flexible nylon fabric impregnated with collagen), collagen derivatives, and artificial dermis (Integra and Apligraf).[71,75-79] Cultured epithelial autograft (CEA) has shown some promise as a means of providing an autograft skin covering, which is grown under sterile conditions from the replication of keratinocytes taken from a tissue biopsy of the patient. Concerns with cultured skin relate to the time required to grow the harvested tissue and the expense of the procedure.

Autografts remain the primary wound covering method used for deep burns. Autografts may be full-thickness or split-thickness grafts. Elements considered in the decision to use a full- or split-thickness skin graft include cosmetic concerns, necessity of graft durability, and area of denuded skin to be covered. Regardless of the type of graft used, principles of postoperative nursing care are as follows: (1) immobilization of the graft site to maximize graft adherence, (2) splinting of the immobilized grafted area in the position of greatest functionality, and (3) assessment of perfusion and gentle expression of accumulated drainage or blood.[80] Typically the grafted wound is protected with a thick, absorbent dressing that remains intact for several days. *Graft take down* refers to the removal of the protective dressing and assessment of the amount of autograft adherence ("take") to the wound bed. In addition to the autograft, the tissue donor site also requires wound care. The process of autografting creates a superficial partial-thickness donor wound that requires nursing management. A variety of dressings may be used to cover the donor site wound (e.g., nonadherent, hydrocolloid, polyurethane transparent, alginates).[81] Care focuses on the management of pain and daily assessment of the healing of the donor site.

Wound management and wound closure are significant nursing priorities during the reparative phase. Successful wound management encompasses nutritional support, management of pain, prevention of infection, and promotion of psychologic wellness.

PSYCHOLOGIC AND SLEEP DISTURBANCES. During the reparative phase the patient begins to struggle with the severity of the injury, injury-imposed lifestyle adjustments, and long-term consequences such as reconstructive surgeries. In addition, environmental noise and continued close monitoring of the patient results in frequent interruptions of sleep. Davis et al[61] advocate aggressive management of the patient's pain and anxiety as a means of providing psychosocial interventions and enhancing coping skills. Taal and Faber[82] evaluated posttraumatic stress and maladjustment among adult burn survivors. They concluded that although it remains difficult to identify patients at risk of developing psychologic morbidity after being burned, once psychologic difficulties are evident, interventions for successful coping need to be initiated. Nurses are in an optimal position to identify ineffective coping and sleep disturbance patterns. Involving the burn team in the management of the patient's psychologic wellness is an important aspect of burn nursing.

REHABILITATIVE AND RECONSTRUCTIVE PHASE

Goals of the rehabilitative and reconstructive phase focus on maximal rehabilitation and reconditioning of the burn patient, management of ongoing nutritional concerns, and psychologic adjustment to the burn injury, including interventions for depression.

ONGOING SKIN INTEGRITY CONCERNS AFTER HEALING. Burn wounds may break down after primary healing for a variety of reasons, such as thinner than normal epithelial cover, excessive dryness, sheering, trauma to scar tissue, exposure to sun or extremes of temperatures, and pressure from pressure garments and splinting devices. Burn wounds are especially prone to blistering and tissue breakdown for several months after healing. Without proper cleansing and application of therapies to encourage reepithelialization and prevent infection, these small wounds may become infected and cause additional tissue loss. If treated with gentle cleansing and small, nonadherent wound dressings, these wounds usually heal in 5 to 7 days. In addition, if the wounds are caused by excessive pressure or active exercise, then splints, pressure garments, and exercise routines should be adjusted immediately. It is imperative that discharge teaching review this type of preventative care so that infection and large open wounds can be minimized. A booklet of simple instructions about the aftercare of burns, splints, and pressure garments and the telephone number of a nurse or therapist who can answer questions should accompany discharge information.

ACTIVITY INTOLERANCE.   Activity intolerance is prevalent during all phases of burn care but becomes a special concern during this period, when the patient is striving to regain independence in the activities of daily living and return to work or school. The problem is related to the prolonged metabolic consequences of the burn injury and decreased range of motion caused by scar maturation and contraction. The goal is for the patient to increase activity tolerance gradually as the scars mature, range of motion improves, and physical stamina increases. Indications of activity intolerance include concern about not being able to complete desired activities; the need for frequent rest periods; and exercise intolerance as evidenced by shortness of breath, need for more sleep at night, and a general complaint of malaise. Often the diagnosis of activity intolerance is confused with depression, either or both of which may be prevalent. Usually, over time, if the problem is activity intolerance, a program of increasing activity with planned periods of rest results in improvement. This type of plan should be a part of discharge planning. If the patient and the patient's family recognize that this is a normal part of rehabilitation, they will be able to plan for it and cope with it. It is often helpful, as the patient prepares to return to work or school, for a member of the burn team to contact the supervisor or teacher and explain the issues related to activity intolerance. Usually allowances can be made for a part-time or limited work schedule that includes additional rest periods. It is also important to explain the patient's need to get back into a normal social environment as soon as possible because remaining off work or out of school until complete physical recovery is achieved may be detrimental to the patient's psychosocial recovery.

Ongoing nutritional concerns and the need to maximize protein intake are present in the rehabilitative cycle and should be evaluated as an element of activity intolerance. Work by Demling and DeSanti[39] supports a high-calorie, high-protein diet as a means of increasing body weight and muscle function.

SELF-CONCEPT AND DEPRESSION.   During the resuscitative and reparative phases the patient is usually in a state of denial regarding the final outcome of the physical injury. Even during the early stages of rehabilitation, patients may believe that, with scar maturation and reconstructive surgery, the physical deformities will be corrected and their appearance will return to the preinjury state. This early denial may actually be therapeutic in that the patient is motivated to do what is necessary to return to normal. Sometime during rehabilitation, though, patients will begin to deal with the alterations in their physical appearance and physical limitations. As the new physical appearance becomes incorporated, the self-image must change as well. The patient may go through the various stages of grief as the process proceeds. Eventually the patient will develop a revised self-image. How the patient copes with this revised self-image depends on the individual, his or her support system, and the patient's preinjury emotional or psychologic status.[82] Interestingly, the final physical appearance may have little correlation with how the patient copes with this revised self-image.

NONCOMPLIANCE WITH TREATMENT MEASURES.   Noncompliance occurs when patients do not follow a treatment regimen or do not behave in the manner expected by the health care team. The reasons for noncompliance are many, but for the most part they are the result of lack of communication between patients and members of the health care team.[83] This lack of communication on the part of the health care team usually occurs because they are unclear in their instructions, have expectations that are unachievable by patients, or do not listen to what patients are trying to tell them. Lack of communication on the part of patients occurs because they do not understand the instructions, they lack the cognitive ability to understand, they do not have the social or environmental support to comply with the regimen or expectations, or they lack understanding of the consequences of noncompliance.[83] Symptoms of noncompliance may include wound breakdown, exaggerated scarring,[84] decreased range of motion, increased contracture formation, splints that are not worn because they no longer fit properly, increased complaints, and apparent lack of motivation. Noncompliance is a frustrating problem for both patients and members of the health care team and, because of its negative connotation, does not foster solutions to the problem. When the problem is communication breakdown, it can be more readily addressed and corrected. When symptoms of noncompliance appear, the responsibility for the problem lies with the health care worker, not the patient. This approach allows the health care worker to diagnose the problem and deal with it. The first question to ask is, Are the plans and expectations realistic? Next, patient issues must be identified. The key to diagnosing the patient problem is to listen intently to what patients say or do not say concerning the issues. If patients demonstrate the cognitive ability to understand and perform the recommended care, then other avenues of miscommunication should be explored. What in the environment or in the patient's social relationships impinges on the problem? Does the patient have increased pain related to an undiagnosed physical problem such as heterotopic bone formation? Is the patient showing signs of depression? Usually the cause for the communication problem can be

TABLE 31-6 Research Priorities: Effect on Patient Welfare

Rank	Score	Question
1	6.40	What nursing interventions reduce anxiety and pain during dressing changes and other painful procedures?
2	6.33	What is the role of anesthetic agents used in subanesthetic doses for pain control during painful procedures in burned adults and children?
3	6.25	What modalities are effective in controlling postburn itching? Are some of these more effective than others?
4	6.17	What nursing interventions are most effective in the prevention or minimization of contractures (both short and long term)?
4	6.17	What strategies can nurses employ to optimize intake of prescribed nutritional requirements for pediatric and adult patients with burns?
6	6.15	What nursing interventions are most effective in stress reduction in the patient with burns (physiologic and psychologic)?
7	6.13	What is the best method to measure the pain of the patient with burns?
8	6.09	What community-based follow-up would best meet the physical and emotional needs of the patient with burns?
9	6.05	What nursing interventions promote healing of donor sites and skin grafts?
10	6.04	What methods are effective in helping patients with burns (children, adolescents, adults) deal with social reentry?
10	6.04	What is the relationship among type of donor-site dressing, patient pain, mobility, and infection?
12	6.03	What is the relationship between the frequency of performing range-of-motion exercises and maintenance of function?
13	6.02	What nursing interventions are most effective in preventing diarrhea from contaminating the burn wound?
14	5.98	What is the relationship between onset of activity and graft take?
14	5.98	What are the most effective routes and methods of narcotic administration in the adult patient with burns at various times after injury?
16	5.97	What is the most effective wound closing protocol for the patient with burns (e.g., timing, method, temperature regulations)?
16	5.97	What is the effect of early use of elastic wraps or pressure garments on healing of the burn wound?

found and corrected, and the symptoms of noncompliance should resolve.

RESEARCH PRIORITIES IN NURSING MANAGEMENT OF THE BURN PATIENT

A Delphi study to ascertain research priorities in the care of the burn patient was undertaken in 1990.[85] The goal of this study was to delineate those areas in which nursing practice-based research could improve burn care. The research method used, the Delphi technique, consisted of a series of four questionnaires to reach consensus on the priorities. The final questionnaire contained 101 questions distilled from a total of 548 questions submitted in the initial round of the study. Table 31-6 lists the top 20 priorities for research. Although research has been actively conducted on these 20 priorities, conclusive evidence to guide practice has not been formulated. Thus these research priorities remain unaddressed, but answers for consistent and best practice are closer at hand.

SUMMARY

The care of the burn patient is complex. Nursing management over the three phases of care requires the nurse to explore many areas of nursing, continually evaluating signs and symptoms of physical dysfunction and addressing psychosocial impairment associated with the injury. Continued research is needed to improve many aspects of patient care and to ensure optimal rehabilitation.

REFERENCES

1. Christoffel T, Gallagher SS: *Injury prevention and public heath,* Gaithersburg, Md, 1999, Aspen.
2. American Burn Association: *Burn care resources: burn facts,* Chicago, 2000, The Association.
3. Brigham PA, McLoughlin E: Burn incidence and medical care in the United States: estimates, trends, and data sources, *J Burn Care Rehabil* 17(1):95-102, 1996.
4. Wolf SE, Herndon DN: Burns and radiation injuries. In Mattox KL, Feliciano DV, Moore EE, editors: *Trauma,* ed 4, New York, 2000, McGraw-Hill, 1137-1151.
5. Liao CC, Rossignol AM: Landmarks in burn prevention, *Burns* 26(5):422-434, 2000.
6. Rose JK, Herndon DN: Advances in the treatment of burn patients, *Burns* 23(S1):S19-S26, 1997.
7. Arturson G: Pathophysiology of the burn wound and pharmacological treatment, *Burns* 22(4):255-265, 1996.
8. Robson MC, Kucan JO: The burn wound. In Wachtel TL, Kahn V, Frank HA, editors: *Current topics in burn care,* Rockville, Md, 1983, Aspen, 56.
9. Pruitt BA, Goodwin CW, Cioffi WG: Thermal injuries. In Davis JH, Sheldon GF, editors: *Surgery: a problem solving approach,* ed 2, St. Louis, 1995, Mosby.

10. Berkow SG: A method for estimating the extensiveness of lesions (burns and scalds) based on surface area proportions, *Arch Surg* 8:138-142, 1924.

11. Lund CC, Browder NC: Estimation of areas of burns, *Surg Gynecol Obstet* 79:352-357, 1944.

12. LaBorde P, Willis J: Burns. In Sole ML, Lamborn ML, Hartshorn JC, editors: *Introduction to critical care nursing,* ed 3, Philadelphia, 2000, WB Saunders, 612.

13. Greenfield E : Integumentary disorders. In Kinney MR, Dunbar SB, Brooks-Brunn JA et al, editors: *AACN's clinical reference for critical care nursing,* ed 4, St. Louis, 1998, Mosby, 1066.

14. Richard R: Assessment and diagnosis of burn wounds, *Adv Wound Care* 12(9):468-471, 1999.

15. Sparkes BG: Immunological response to thermal injury, *Burns* 23(2):106-111, 1997.

16. Ryan CM, Schoenfeld DA, Thrope WP et al: Objective estimates of the probability of death from burn injuries, *N Engl J Med* 338(6):362-366, 1998.

17. Bert J, Gyege C, Bowen B et al: Fluid resuscitation following a burn injury: implications of a mathematical model of microvascular exchange, *Burns* 23(2):93-101, 1997.

18. Secor VH: The systemic inflammatory response syndrome: role of inflammatory mediators in multiple organ dysfunction syndrome. In Secor VH, editor: *Multiple organ dysfunction and failure,* St. Louis, 1996, Mosby, 46-72.

19. Cuthbertson DP: The disturbance of metabolism produced by bone and nonbony injury with notes on certain abnormal conditions of bone, *Biochem J* 24:1244-1263, 1930.

20. Gottschlich MM, Jenkins ME: Metabolic consequences and nutritional needs. In Carrougher GJ, editors: *Burn care and therapy,* St. Louis, 1998, Mosby, 213-232.

21. Wolfe RR: Metabolic responses to burn injury: nutritional implications. In Herndon DN, editor: *Total burn care,* London, 1996, WB Saunders, 217-222.

22. Bagley SM: Nutritional needs of the acutely ill with acute wounds, *Crit Care Nurs Clin North Am* 8(2):159-168, 1996.

23. Gordon MD, Winfree JH: Fluid resuscitation after a major burn. In Carrougher GJ, editors: *Burn care and therapy,* St. Louis, 1998, Mosby, 107-132.

24. Luterman A: Burns and metabolism, *J Am Coll Surg* 190(2):104-113, 2000.

25. Lund T: Edema generation following thermal injury: an update, *J Burn Care Rehabil* 20(6):445-451, 1999.

26. National Institutes of Health: Consensus conference, *J Trauma* 19(11):S89-S101, 1979.

27. Ahrns KS, Harkins DR: Initial resuscitation after burn injury: therapies, strategies, and controversies, *AACN Clin Issues* 10(1):46-60, 1999.

28. Schoemaker WC, Bishop MH: Clinical algorithms for resuscitation in acute emergency conditions. In Ayers SM, Grenvik A, Holbrook PR et al, editors: *Textbook of critical care,* ed 3, Philadelphia, 1995, WB Saunders, 102-113.

29. Mikhail J: Resuscitation endpoints in trauma, *AACN Clin Issues* 10(1):10-21, 1999.

30. Schiller WR, Bay RC, Garren RL et al: Hyperdynamic resuscitation improves survival in patients with life threatening burns, *J Burn Care Rehabil* 18(1):110-121, 1997.

31. Kao CC, Garner WL: Acute burns, *Plast Reconstr Surg* 101(7):2482-2490, 2000.

32. Schiller WR, Bay RC: Hemodynamic and oxygen transport monitoring in management of burns, *New Horiz* 4(4):475-482, 1996.

33. Bernard F, Gueugniaud PY, Bertin-Maghit M et al: Prognostic significance of early cardiac index measurements in severely burned patients, *Burns* 20(6):529-531, 1994.

34. Barton RG, Saffle JR, Morris SE et al: Resuscitation of thermally injured patients with oxygen transport criteria as goals of therapy, *J Burn Care Rehabil* 18(1):1-9, 1997.

35. Jeng JC, Lee K, Jablonski K et al: Serum lactate and base deficit suggests inadequate resuscitation of patients with burn injuries: application of a point of care laboratory instrument, J Burn Care Rehabil 18(5):402-405, 1997.

36. Shin C, Kinsky MP, Thomas JA et al: Effect of cutaneous burn injury and resuscitation on the cerebral circulation in an ovine model, *Burn* 24(1):39-45, 1998.

37. Ward CG: Burns, *J Am Coll Surg* 186(2):123-126, 1998.

38. Demling RH: Comparison of the anabolic effects and complications of human growth hormone and the testosterone analog, oxandrolone, after severe burn injury, *Burns* 25(3):215-221, 1999.

39. Demling RH, DeSanti L: Increased protein intake during the recovery phase after severe burns increases body weight gain and muscle function, J Burn Care Rehabil 19(2):161-167, 1998.

40. Ramzy PI, Wolf SE, Herndon DN: Current status of anabolic hormone administration in human burn injury, *J Parenter Enteral Nutr* 23(6):S190-S194, 1999.

41. Taber DL, Pollard T: Pathophysiology of inhalation injury. In Herndon DN, editor: *Total burn care,* London, 1996, WB Saunders, 175-183.

42. Ivy ME, Possenti PP, Kepros J et al: Abdominal compartment syndrome in patients with burns, *J Burn Care Rehabil* 20(5):351-353, 1999.

43. Flynn MB: Identifying and treating inhalation injuries in fire victims, *Dimens Crit Care Nurs* 18(4):18-23, 1999.

44. Fitzpatrick JC, Cioffi WG, Ventilatory support following burns and smoke inhalation injury, *Respir Care Clin North Am* 3(1):21-49, 1997.

45. Greenfield E, McManus AT: Infectious complications: prevention and strategies for their control, *Nurs Clin North Am* 32(2):297-309, 1997.

46. Pruitt BA, McManus AT, Kim SH et al: Burn wound infections: current status, *World J Surg* 22(2):135-145, 1998.

47. Rose DD, Jordan EB: Perioperative management of burn patients, *AORN J* 69(6):1211-1221, 1999.

48. Stanley M, Richard R: Management of the acute burn wound: an overview, *Adv Wound Care* 10(2):39-44, 1997.

49. Holder IA, Neely AN: Vacomycin resistant enterococci, *Burns* 24(4):389-391, 1998.

50. Cook N: Methicillin resistant S*taphylococcus aureus* versus the burn patient, *Burns* 24(2):91-96, 1998.

51. Dougherty W, Waxman K: The complexities of managing severe burns with associated trauma, *Surg Clin North Am* 76(4):923-958, 1996.

52. Eldad A: Out of the strong came forth sweetness: on the contribution of military conflicts to the development of burn treatment in Israel, *J Burn Care Rehabil* 19(6):470-478, 1998.

53. Lim JJ, Rehmar SG, Elmore P: Rapid response: care of burn victims, *AAOHN J* 46(4):169-177, 1998.

54. Frye KE, Luterman A: Burns and fractures, *Orthop Nurs* 18(1):30-35, 1999.

55. Shaw JM, Robson MC: Electrical injuries. In Herndon DN, editor: *Total burn care,* London, 1996, WB Saunders, 401-407.

56. Warden GD: Fluid resuscitation and early management. In Herndon DN, editor: *Total burn care,* London, 1996, WB Saunders, 53-62.

57. Chalk L: Wound prevention and healing: everyone's problem, *Surg Serv Manag* 5(11):31-38, 1999.

58. Miller PR, Munn DD, Meredith JW et al: Systemic inflammatory response syndrome in the trauma intensive care unit: who is infected? *J Trauma* 17(6):1004-1008, 1999.

59. Fink R: *Pain assessment guide,* Denver, University of Colorado Health Sciences Center, 1996.

60. Marvin JA: Management of pain and anxiety. In Carrougher GJ, editors: *Burn care and therapy,* St. Louis, 1998, Mosby, 167-184.

61. Davis ST, Sheely-Adolphson P: Psychosocial interventions: pharmacologic and psychologic modalities, *Nurs Clin North Am* 32(2):331-341, 1997.

62. Hildreth M, Gottschlich M: Nutritional support of the burned patient. In Herndon DN, editor: *Total burn care,* London, 1996, WB Saunders, 237-245.

63. Robert R, Blakeney P, Villarreal C et al: Anxiety: current practices in assessment and treatment of anxiety of burn patients, *Burns* 26(6):549-552, 2000.

64. Richard R, Staley M, Miller S et al: To splint or not to splint: past philosophy and present practice, *J Burn Care Rehabil* 17(5):444-450, 1996.

65. Ward RS: Physical rehabilitation. In Carrougher GJ, editors: *Burn care and therapy,* St. Louis, 1998, Mosby, 293-328.

66. Fritsch DE: Hypothermia in the trauma patient, *AACN Clin Issues* 6(2):196-211, 1995.

67. Wiebelhaus P, Hansen S: Burns: handle with care, *RN* 62(11):52-58, 1999.

68. Klasen HJ, A review on the nonoperative removal of necrotic tissue from burn wounds, *Burns* 26(3):207-220, 2000.

69. Boxer AM, Gottesman N, Bernstein H et al: Debridement of dermal ulcers and decubiti with collagenase, *Geriatrics* 24(7):75-86, 1996.

70. Wang HJ, Wan HL, Yang TS et al: Acceleration of skin graft healing by growth factors, *Burns* 22(1):10-14, 1996.

71. Sai P, Babu M: Collagen based dressings: a review, *Burns* 26(1):54-60, 2000.

72. Mertz P, Cazzaniga A, Serralta V et al: *The effect of an antimicrobial gauze dressing impregnated with 0.2% polyhexamethylene biguanide as a barrier to prevent* Pseudomonas aeruginosa *wound invasion,* Mansfield, Mass, Kendall Wound Care Research and Development, 2000.

73. Tredget EE, Shankowsky HA, Groeneveld A et al: A matched paired randomized study evaluating the efficacy and safety of Acticoat silver coated dressings for the treatment of burn wounds, *J Burn Care Rehabil* 19(6):531-537, 1998.

74. Klasen HJ: A historical review of the use of silver in the treatment of burns: renewed interest for silver, *Burns* 26(2):131-138, 2000.

75. Eaglestein WH, Falanga V: Tissue engineering and the development of Apligraf a human skin equivalent, *Adv Wound Care* 11(4):1-9, 1998.

76. Spence RJ, Wong L: The enhancement of wound healing with human skin allograft, *Surg Clin North Am* 77(3):731-744, 1997.

77. Heimbach D, Luterman A, Burke J et al: Artificial dermis for major burns, *Ann Surg* 208(3):313-319, 1988.

78. Sheridan RL, Hegarty M, Tompkins RG et al: Artificial skin in massive burns: results to ten years, *Eur J Plast Surg* 17(1):91-93, 1994.

79. Falanga VJ: Tissue engineering in wound repair, *Skin Wound Care* 13(S2):15-19, 2000.

80. Ratner D: Skin grafting from here to there, *Dermatol Clin* 16(1):75-89, 1998.

81. Rakel BA, Bermel MA, Abbott LI et al: Split thickness skin graft donor site care: a quantitative synthesis of the research, *Appl Nurs Res* 11(4):174-182, 1998.

82. Taal LA, Faber AW: Posttraumatic stress and maladjustment among adult burn survivors 1-2 years post burn, *Burns* 24(4):285-292, 1998.

83. Pessina MA, Ellis SM: Rehabilitation, *Nurs Clin North Am* 32(2):365-374, 1997.

84. Staley MJ, Richard RL: Use of pressure to treat hypertrophic burn scars, *Adv Wound Care* 10(3):44-46, 1997.

85. Marvin JA, Carrougher G, Bayley B et al: Burn nursing Delphi study: setting research priorities, *J Burn Care Rehabil* 12(2):190-197, 1991.

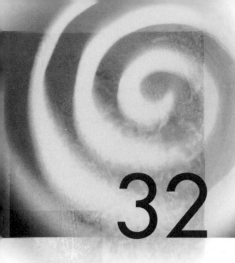

SUBSTANCE ABUSE AND TRAUMA CARE

Janet M. Beebe

32

SUBSTANCE ABUSE AND INJURY EPIDEMIOLOGY

Health problems associated with the use of alcohol, tobacco, and other drugs (ATOD) are currently of epidemic proportions in our society, as documented by recent estimates from the Substance Abuse and Mental Health Services Administration. Approximately 109 million U.S. residents age 12 or older used alcohol in the months before the survey. Of these, 32 million engaged in at least one episode of binge drinking, defined as consumption of five or more drinks on one occasion. Further, 11 million persons were estimated to be heavy drinkers; that is, they have consumed five or more drinks per occasion on 5 or more days in the previous 30 days.[1]

Based on a probability sample interview survey done in 1996, an estimated 13 million Americans age 12 years or older used an illicit drug in the month before the interview. There were an estimated 216,000 heroin users, 1.75 million cocaine users, and 10.1 million marijuana users. Of this latter group, an estimated 6.1 million were frequent marijuana users. "Frequent use" was defined as 51 or more episodes of use in the past year.[1] Additionally, 62 million Americans, 29% of the population, smoke tobacco, making nicotine one of the most widely used psychoactive drugs.[2]

The total economic cost of alcohol and other drug abuse in 1992 was estimated to be $245.7 billion. Of this cost, $97.7 billion was attributed to drugs other than alcohol, making alcohol alone the largest contributor to the total figure. Included in these estimates were costs for substance abuse treatment and prevention efforts; associated health care costs; costs for reduced productivity and lost earnings; and other costs to society, including social welfare and crime. Between 1985 and 1992, the estimated cost of the use of ATOD increased by 50%. The primary factors contributing to this increase were the epidemic of heavy cocaine use, the continuing spread of the human immunodeficiency virus (HIV), an eightfold increase in state and federal incarcerations, and a threefold increase in drug-related crimes. Approximately one third of hospitalizations are linked to alcohol use.[3]

ALCOHOL AND TRAUMA

Recent studies of patients from trauma centers and university hospitals have reported psychoactive drug use rates from 25% to 60%.[4-7] There are well-documented relationships among increasing blood alcohol concentration (BAC) and level of impairment in cognition and motor coordination, likelihood of injury, and severity of injury. Intoxicated patients were shown in one study to have significantly higher Injury Severity Scores (ISSs) than those not intoxicated, and within groups of ISSs, those at the higher end of the range had correspondingly higher BACs.[8] More than 77% of the motor vehicle crashes (MVCs) that led to fatalities in 1997 involved drivers or nonmotorists who were intoxicated.[9] Habitual drunken drivers have demonstrated an increased risk of dying in an alcohol-related crash.[10]

Alcohol abuse has been associated with all types of injuries. Studies evaluating mechanism of injury and alcohol use have reported that 32% to 47% of MVC victims had positive BACs.[5,11,12] Positive BAC rates for injured motorcyclists were comparable at 33% to 39.3%.[11,12] The risks associated with walking under the influence of alcohol are underappreciated. The reported incidence of positive BACs among pedestrians struck is 31% to 49%.[5,13] Alcohol also plays a major role in intentional interpersonal violence. Sixty-one percent of firearm homicide victims in one study were intoxicated[14] and 31% of the intentional injury victims from another[5] had positive BACs. Alcohol has also been linked to 30% of fire fatalities[15] and 48% of drownings.[16] Alcohol is a significant risk factor for sustaining traumatic brain injury and may impair rehabilitation and recovery.[17,18]

A number of researchers have investigated the incidence of alcohol dependence among trauma patients. Trauma patients are at high risk for future trauma but cannot always be identified by their BAC. Rivara et al[13] determined that 75% of acutely intoxicated trauma patients have positive scores on the Short Michigan Alcohol Screening Test and that 25% to 35% of them had biochemical evidence of chronic alcohol use. Soderstrom et al[19] found that 54% of acutely intoxicated trauma patients could be diagnosed as alcohol dependent, along with 11% of trauma patients who had negative BACs.

Alcohol is present in nearly one third of injured adolescents, a population for whom alcohol is an illegal drug. Studies of adolescent trauma patients found that 20% to 30% tested positive for alcohol or other drugs at the time of admission.[20-22]

Research remains inconclusive regarding whether alcohol intoxication results in less favorable outcomes after trauma. Although animal studies have documented alcohol's adverse effects on degree and outcome of injury,[23,24] such results are difficult to duplicate with humans.[25,26] A study of trauma patients from a level I trauma center demonstrated no increased risk of complications from acute intoxication but found a twofold increase in risk of complications in patients with behavioral and biochemical markers of chronic alcohol abuse.[26] Some researchers have suggested that the more severe outcomes seen in BAC-positive patients are the result of correlates of alcohol use such as high speed and not using seat belts.[27] A study of MVC patients from two emergency departments documented more severe crashes among the patients with positive BACs.[28] A study of level I trauma center patients by Cornwell et al failed to find a positive correlation between alcohol use and adverse outcome.[7] Hospitalization costs and length of stay are substantially higher for drinking drivers than for those who had not been drinking. One study documented that mean inpatient hospital and physician charges per collision were $18,258 for drinking drivers compared with $14,181 for nondrinking drivers. Drinking drivers also had longer lengths of stay, even after correction for age, gender, and injury severity.[29] In 1998 the National Safety Council predicted that 3 out of 10 U.S. residents would be involved in alcohol-related MVCs.[9]

OPIATES AND TRAUMA
The incidence of positive opiate tests in patients admitted to urban trauma centers has been reported to be 5% to 16%.[30-32] A prospective study of urban trauma patients conducted 1984 through 1998 documented a 531% increase in the number of patients who tested positive for opiates.[33]

COCAINE AND TRAUMA
Cocaine use may be an underreported cause of trauma. Studies of trauma patients have demonstrated cocaine usage rates from 6% to 22%.[4,34,35] A study of New York City fatalities (persons 15 to 44 years of age) found that 26.7% tested positive for cocaine metabolites and an additional 18.3% tested positive for free cocaine, indicating recent use. Two thirds of the cocaine-positive fatalities were the result of homicides, suicides, traffic collisions, or falls. Based on this study, fatal injury after cocaine use ranks among the top five causes of death for 15- to 44-year-olds in New York City.[36] Soderstrom et al documented a 242% increase in the number of trauma patients who tested positive for cocaine between July 1984 and December 1998.[33]

MARIJUANA AND TRAUMA
A level I trauma center study in Maryland was the first to prospectively document marijuana use among large numbers of trauma patients. The 1023 patients admitted during the study period had an 18.3% positive test rate for marijuana, and an additional 16.5% tested positive for both alcohol and marijuana.[37] One study of orthopedic trauma patients reported a 21% positive test rate and documented that patients who tested positive for marijuana had an additional length of hospital stay that averaged 1.3 days.[4]

CAUSES OF SUBSTANCE ABUSE

The causes of substance abuse are complex phenomena with biologic, psychologic, social, and cultural determinants. Although much research has been done on the various components, there remain many unanswered questions. Hence no single theory or model has yet been developed to comprehensively explain the phenomenon of addiction. Current etiologic theories include genetic influences, behavioral models, neurobiologic models, and environmental stressors. Most clinicians agree, however, that a level of substance use sufficient to cause physical, psychologic, and social impairment for an individual is in itself problematic. Problematic substance abuse is loosely divided into two broad categories—substance abuse (Table 32-1) and substance dependence (Table 32-2)—depending on whether there is evidence of tolerance and physiologic dependence.[38] *Addiction* is the term commonly used synonymously for drug or alcohol dependence. Currently substance use is viewed as a continuum from abstinence to addiction, with several steps along the way. Thus psychoactive substance use disorders are a heterogeneous set of problems perceived in gradations of gray rather than in black and white terms.

TABLE 32-1   Criteria for Substance Abuse

A. A maladaptive pattern of substance use leading to clinically significant impairment or distress, as manifested by one (or more) of the following, occurring within a 12-month period:
   (1) Recurrent substance use resulting in a failure to fulfill major role obligations at work, school, or home (e.g., repeated absences or poor work performance related to substance use; substance-related absences, suspensions, or expulsions from school; neglect of children or household)
   (2) Recurrent substance use in situations in which it is physically hazardous (e.g., driving an automobile or operating a machine when impaired by substance use)
   (3) Recurrent substance-related legal problems (e.g., arrests for substance-related disorderly conduct)
   (4) Continued substance use despite having persistent or recurrent social or interpersonal problems caused or exacerbated by the effects of the substance (e.g., arguments with spouse about consequences of intoxication, physical fights)
B. The symptoms have never met the criteria for substance dependence for this class of substance.

From American Psychiatric Association: *Diagnostic and statistical manual of mental disorders*, ed 4, Washington, DC, 1994, The Association.

TABLE 32-2   Criteria for Substance Dependence

A. A maladaptive pattern of substance use, leading to clinically significant impairment or distress, as manifested by three (or more) of the following, occurring at any time in the same 12-month period:

   (1) Tolerance, as defined by either of the following:
       (a) a need for markedly increased amounts of the substance to achieve intoxication or desired effect
       (b) markedly diminished effect with continued use of the same amount of the substance
   (2) Withdrawal, as manifested by either of the following:
       (a) the characteristic withdrawal syndrome for the substance (refer to criteria A and B of the criteria sets for withdrawal from the specific substances)
       (b) taking the same (or a closely related) substance to relieve or avoid withdrawal symptoms
   (3) The substance is often taken in larger amounts or over a longer period than was intended
   (4) There is a persistent desire or unsuccessful efforts to cut down or control substance use
   (5) A great deal of time is spent in activities necessary to obtain the substance (e.g., visiting multiple doctors or driving long distances), use the substance (e.g., chain-smoking), or recover from its effects
   (6) Important social, occupational, or recreational activities are given up or reduced because of substance use.
   (7) The substance use is continued despite knowledge of having a persistent or recurrent physical or psychological problem that is likely to have been caused or exacerbated by the substance (e.g., current cocaine use despite recognition of cocaine-induced depression, or continued drinking despite recognition that an ulcer was made worse by alcohol consumption)

From American Psychiatric Association: *Diagnostic and statistical manual of mental disorders,* ed 4, Washington, DC, 1994, The Association.

Familial,[39,40] twin,[41-44] and adoption studies[45-47] have all indicated a genetic component of substance abuse. Overall, these studies have supported the observation that alcoholism clusters in families. Children of alcoholic parents have an increased incidence of alcoholism compared with the children of nonalcoholics. These studies have generally found that the incidence of alcoholism among children of alcoholics is much higher than that in the general population. Although rates of alcoholism are lower for women, female children of alcoholics had an overall higher incidence than that found in the general population. One study evaluated subjective reports and physiologic parameters to demonstrate that sons of alcoholics have less intense reactions to ethanol.[48]

Twin studies provide the opportunity to compare human subjects with similar genetic material while assuming a constant environment. Although rates of concordance have varied, the majority of twin studies have indicated that homozygous twins of alcoholics are significantly more likely to be alcoholic themselves than are heterozygous twins of alcoholics.[43,44,49] Cocaine and marijuana dependence have

high concordance rates among identical twins.[50,51] Genetics influences susceptibility to most categories of drugs, with heroin showing the strongest influence.[52] Males appear to be more susceptible to genetic influence than females.[53] Twin studies have indicated an environmental role as well.[52]

Adoption studies have looked at the rates of alcoholism in children born of alcoholic biologic parents but then adopted by nonalcoholics. The aim of these studies was to observe the rates of alcoholism without the effects of growing up in an alcoholic household. Adopted children of biologic alcoholic parents raised in nonalcoholic homes are also significantly more likely to manifest alcoholism.[54,55]

Animal studies have detected physiologic differences between levels of neurotransmitters in alcohol-preferring and non-alcohol-preferring rats.[56] In humans the dopaminergic and serotonergic systems of the brain are implicated in addictions.[57-59] One study of the brain tissue of alcoholic and nonalcoholic men compared variations in gene coding for the D_2 dopamine receptor.[60] One genetic variation of three possible genotypes was found in 76% of the alcoholics but only 24% of the nonalcoholics. This specific genotype resulted in dopamine receptors with significantly lower affinity for dopamine and fewer dopamine-binding sites than either of the other two genotypes. A follow-up study evaluated alcoholism and the presence of this specific receptor type among family members. This study failed to find a strong causative link for the specific genotype, indicating that, although it may play a role in susceptibility to alcoholism, it is not in and of itself sufficient to cause alcoholism.[61]

Various psychologic conditions share a strong associated co-morbidity with substance abuse disorders. These include bipolar disorder,[62] anxiety disorders,[63] depressive disorders,[64] the group B personality disorders,[65,66] and attention deficit hyperactivity disorder.[67]

Environment also plays an important role in substance use. Reactions to psychoactive drugs are determined in part by the user's mental state before use, the set, and the environment or setting in which the use occurs. In an environment with predominantly sexual overtones, the user may experience heightened feelings of arousal. The same individual in a situation perceived as threatening may become aggressive or fearful rather than hypersexual.

Studies comparing alcohol- and non-alcohol-preferring mice have induced alcohol-preferring behavior in the nonalcoholic mice by subjecting them to environmental stressors.[68] In humans, heroin use among Vietnam veterans followed a similar pattern.[69,70] Veterans who began using heroin while overseas usually stopped after they returned to the United States. Most reported complete cessation of heroin use once the extreme environmental stressors were removed. Animal studies seem to suggest that an interaction of environment along with a genetic predisposition is required for the development of addictive behaviors.[68] Ethical concerns have limited such research in humans.

Abusive environments in early childhood may be a substantial risk factor for later drug abuse. A majority of

TABLE 32-3 Psychoactive Drugs

Depressants	Stimulants	Hallucinogenics	
		Minor	Major
Alcohol	Amphetamine (Dexedrine)	Marijuana	Lysergic acid diethylamide (LSD)
Barbiturates	Methamphetamine	Hashish	Mescaline
Short-acting	Nonamphetamines		Psilocybin
Thiopental	Methylphenidate (Ritalin)		Phencyclidine (PCP)
Intermediate-acting	Phendimetrazine (Preludin)		MDMA (Ecstasy)
Secobarbital (Seconal)	Phentermine (Ionamin)		Tetrahydrocannabinol (THC)
Pentobarbital (Nembutal)	Caffeine (coffee, tea, sodas)		Peyote
Tuinal	Nicotine		Dimethyltryptamine (DMT)
Amobarbital (Amytal)	Cocaine		Hash oil
Long-acting	Freon (propellants and		2,5-dimethoxy-4-
Phenobarbital	refrigerants)		methylamphetamine
Barbital			(DOM [STP])
Nonbarbiturates			
Zolpidem (Ambien)			
Glutethimide (Doriden)			
Ethchlorvynol (Placidyl)			
Methaqualone (Quaalude)			
Chloral hydrate			
Meprobamate (Miltown)			
Benzodiazepines			
Diazepam (Valium)			
Chlordiazepoxide (Librium)			
Oxazepam (Serax)			
Flurazepam (Dalmane)			
Triazolam (Halcion)			
Lorazepam (Ativan)			
Midazolam (Versed)			
Volatile solvents (glues, typewriter			
correction fluid)			
Anesthetics			
Nitrous oxide			
Ether			

Opiates

Natural
  Morphine sulfate
  Codeine
Semisynthetic
  Heroin
Synthetic
  Methadone
  Hydromorphone (Dilaudid)
  Meperidine (Demerol)
  Hydrocodone (Vicodin)
  Fentanyl
  Propoxyphene (Darvon)

patients in treatment centers report being victims of childhood physical or sexual abuse.[71] Studies suggest that drug use is a complex interaction between the child, the environment, and level of social support.[72,73] One study of the use of inhalants by adolescents reported a strong correlation between that activity and child abuse.[74] Because not all abused children become drug users, much is still to be determined about the role of childhood abuse in later drug abuse by adults.

PHARMACOLOGIC EFFECTS OF PSYCHOACTIVE DRUGS

Psychoactive drugs (Table 32-3) exert their mood-altering effects by altering levels of neurotransmitters within the brain. Early theories of psychoactive drug action attempted to explain the role of psychoactive drugs by identifying one neurotransmitter affected by a particular drug. As understanding of neurobiochemistry has grown, theories have been amended to incorporate a complex series of interac-

Scientists investigating which brain structures may be involved in the human drug reward system have learned a great deal from studies with rats. Because the chemistries of the human brain and the rat brain are similar, scientists believe that the process of drug addiction may be the same for both. The illustrations shown here use information gathered from animal studies to show what areas may be involved in reward systems in the human brain.

The **cocaine and amphetamine reward system** includes neurons using dopamine found in the ventral tegmental area (VTA). These neurons are connected to the nucleus accumbens and other areas such as the prefrontal cortex.

The **opiate reward system** also includes these structures. In addition, opiates affect structures that use brain chemicals that mimic the action of drugs such as heroin and morphine. This system includes the arcuate nucleus, amygdala, locus coeruleus, and periaqueductal gray area.

The **alcohol reward system** also includes the VTA and nucleus accumbens and affects the structures that use γ-aminobutyric acid (GABA) as a neurotransmitter. GABA is widely distributed in numerous areas of the brain, including the cortex, cerebellum, hippocampus, superior and inferior colliculi, amygdala, and nucleus accumbens.

The VTA and the nucleus accumbens are two structures involved in the reward system for all drugs, including alcohol and tobacco, although other mechanisms might be involved for specific drugs.

COCAINE AND AMPHETAMINES

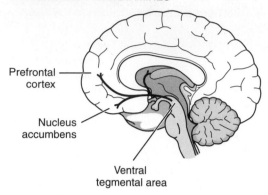

OPIATES

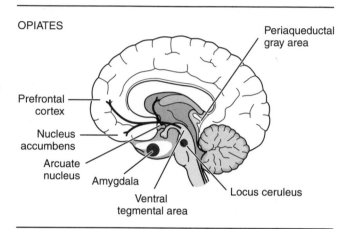

ALCOHOL

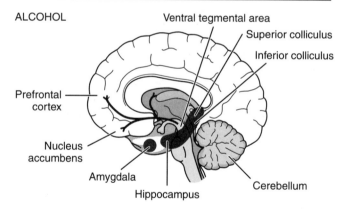

FIGURE 32-1 **The Brain's Reward System.** From: National Institute of Drug Abuse: The brain's drug reward systems, NIDA Notes 11:10, 1996.

tions between various neurotransmitters. The release of one neurotransmitter may result in the release of a second neurotransmitter or direct stimulation of a receptor site, which may enhance or block neurotransmitter function. Either the direct or the secondary action can be responsible for the clinically evident psychoactive effects.[75]

All psychoactive substances exert their effects by binding with receptors located on neurons in the central nervous system (CNS). The presence of such receptors within the body hints at naturally occurring substances to bind with these receptors. Some of these naturally occurring substances, or ligands, have been identified; for other receptor types, no naturally occurring chemical has yet been identified. Thus psychoactive action on the part of a given chemical suggests the existence of an endogenous ligand.

Psychoactive drugs are able to produce their effects by binding with these receptors and either stimulating or suppressing activation of neurons. These actions can prolong the effects of a given neurotransmitter, increase neurotransmitter release, or block receptor response to a neurotransmitter. Thus psychoactive drugs achieve their effects by enhancing or inhibiting the function of the neurons.[75] These actions account for their various analgesic, hallucinogenic, stimulant, anxiolytic, or depressant effects, determined to some degree by the area of the brain containing the affected neural pathways (Figure 32-1).[76]

TOLERANCE AND DEPENDENCE

Tolerance is a common response to the repetitive use of the same drug. It manifests as a reduction in response to a given dose of a drug after repeated administration. A higher dose of the drug is then needed to obtain the same response induced by the original dose. There are several types of tolerance. *Innate tolerance* refers to an individual's resistance or susceptibility to a particular drug. Two individuals drinking alcohol for the first time may have wide variations in their response to the same amount of alcohol. The less impaired person has a higher innate tolerance than does the more impaired person. *Pharmacokinetic and pharmacodynamic tolerance* refers to types of tolerance that occur as the body becomes more efficient at metabolizing a drug or as an organ system becomes habituated to functioning under the influence of a given drug. As these processes take place, ever-increasing doses are required to achieve the desired effects. Pharmacokinetic tolerance occurs when there is a change in the distribution or metabolic pathway of a drug. For example, barbiturates induce the P450 microsomal enzyme system of the liver, resulting in increased metabolism of the barbiturates and any other drugs metabolized by this particular pathway. Thus the system becomes more efficient at processing the chemical. *Pharmacodynamic tolerance* refers to adaptive changes that have taken place in the system as a result of the continued use of the drug. Increases or decreases in the number of neurotransmitter receptors in the CNS as a result of antidepressant use are an example of this type of tolerance. *Learned tolerance* refers to a diminution of drug effect as a result of compensatory mechanisms acquired by the person to counteract the effects of the drug.

Physical and psychologic dependence may also develop with repetitive drug use. Physical dependence is a state of physiologic adaptation to a drug, resulting in a characteristic withdrawal syndrome when the drug is stopped. Adaptation occurs in physiologic systems so that their homeostasis is adjusted to incorporate the additional chemical, resulting in an altered and new homeostasis. Continued administration of the drug then becomes necessary to maintain homeostasis. If the drug is suddenly removed from the system, an imbalance is created.[77] This imbalance is referred to as *withdrawal* or *acute abstinence*. The acute abstinence syndrome for a given drug is typically an exaggerated response that is the opposite of the drug's clinical effects. Generally withdrawal syndromes are characteristic for a given class of drugs. The presence of tolerance and physical dependence do not of themselves satisfy the criteria for addiction.[75] Psychologic dependence or addiction, in contrast to physiologic dependence, is characterized by intense cravings, preoccupation with use of a particular drug, continued use despite adverse consequences, and a tendency to relapse after cessation of drug use. Psychologic dependence includes a constellation of behaviors associated with obtaining and using the drug of choice.

ALCOHOL AND CENTRAL NERVOUS SYSTEM DEPRESSANT PHARMACOLOGY

Ethyl alcohol is the prototypical CNS depressant. It is typically ingested in the form of beer, wine, or liquor. Other CNS depressants include barbiturates, benzodiazepines, chloral hydrate, meprobamate, and methaqualone.

PHARMACOKINETICS. Although small quantities of alcohol can be absorbed directly from the stomach, its primary site of absorption is the proximal portion of the small intestine. Absorption occurs rapidly over a period of 30 to 60 minutes and is generally complete. The rate of absorption is affected by the rate of gastric emptying and, to a lesser extent, by the presence or absence of food in the stomach.[78]

Alcohol is distributed rapidly throughout the body water by way of the circulation. The concentration of alcohol in a particular tissue is dependent on its blood supply. In highly vascular tissue such as the CNS and muscle, ethanol reaches equilibrium with the serum more quickly than it does in relatively avascular tissue such as adipose.[78] A 50-kg person consuming the same amount of ethyl alcohol as a 100-kg person will have a higher BAC because he or she has less total body water to dilute the alcohol. Additionally, a 70-kg woman will achieve a higher BAC than a 70-kg man who consumes the same amount of alcohol. The woman has a higher percentage of body fat, so there will be less body water to dilute the alcohol. Women also have lower levels of gastric alcohol dehydrogenase than men. This results in less alcohol being broken down in the stomach and more alcohol being absorbed by the stomach and reaching the peripheral circulation.[79]

Most of the alcohol consumed is metabolized in the liver by the enzyme alcohol dehydrogenase[80] and to a lesser degree by the microsomal enzyme system.[81] It is converted into acetaldehyde and then rapidly converted into acetyl CoA, which can then be oxidized through the citric acid cycle or used in various anabolic reactions involved in the synthesis of cholesterol, fatty acids, and tissue constituents. This enzymatic step is the rate-limiting portion of the metabolic process. The metabolism of ethanol differs from that of most substances in that the rate of oxidation of ethanol remains relatively constant and is minimally affected by the ethanol concentration.[78] The maximal rate of ethanol clearance is 120 mg/kg or approximately .5 oz/hr. This equates to the amount of alcohol found in a 1-oz shot of 100-proof liquor, a 4- to 5-oz glass of wine, or 12 oz of beer. For the purpose of evaluating alcohol intake, each of these is considered one drink.

Small amounts of alcohol are eliminated via the kidneys and lungs. The kidneys excrete about 2% of alcohol and the lungs excrete about 0.05%. The amount of alcohol in 2100 ml of expired air is approximately the same amount in 100 ml of blood. This direct correlation is the basis for the breathalyzer test.[82]

MECHANISM OF ACTION. γ-Aminobutyric acid (GABA) is the primary inhibitory neurotransmitter in the CNS. Alcohol exerts its depressant effect primarily by binding with the GABA receptors of the brain.[83] Alcohol shares this action with other central nervous system depressants, most notably benzodiazepines and barbiturates. Alcohol and other central nervous system depressants bind to portions of the $GABA_A$ receptors and modulate their primary function of altering chloride influx through the ion channels of the cell.[84] Chloride increases the resting membrane potential, hyperpolarizing the cell and rendering it less reactive, or depressed.[85] At times alcohol seems to act as a CNS stimulant. This paradoxic effect is the result of suppression of areas in the brain responsible for social constraint and judgment.

Alcohol also has a suppressant effect on the glutamate (NMDA) receptors within the CNS.[86] NMDA receptors are excitatory, and suppression of the excitatory function results in further depression of the CNS. The reversal of these effects during acute alcohol withdrawal is thought to be responsible for the clinical manifestations of CNS hyperactivity.[87] Alcohol's action on glutamate receptors is thought to play a role in alcoholic blackouts and acute withdrawal seizures as well.[87,88]

Benzodiazepines and barbiturates have the same GABAergic effects as alcohol, but their effects on other systems of the CNS are more limited.[78] CNS depressants vary with respect to their onset and duration of action. Response to a given dose depends on the resultant blood level, habituation of the user, and, to some extent, his or her expectations of the drug use results. Duration of effects is dependent on the half-life of the drug.

Alcohol also has effects on the endorphin,[89] serotonergic,[90] and dopaminergic[91] systems within the brain, effects that are somewhat different from those of other CNS depressants. The stimulation of the endorphin system accounts for alcohol's weak analgesic effect. Patients sustaining minor injuries may not complain of pain until after their BAC has dropped. Stimulation of the dopaminergic system is thought to be responsible for the euphoric effects of alcohol.[91] Findings also suggest that serotonin may mediate alcohol-seeking behavior in habituated individuals.[59]

POTENTIATION. Alcohol has a synergistic effect when combined with other CNS depressants or opiates.[78] The cumulative effect of the drugs is greater than the anticipated effect of each drug taken alone. Patients with one or more class of drug in their system may be more susceptible to respiratory depression or nervous system suppression when additional drugs are used therapeutically. Intoxicated patients who receive opiates or sedatives in the resuscitation phase of care must be monitored closely for such cumulative effects.

OTHER PHARMACOLOGIC EFFECTS
Central Nervous System.   As previously described, the clinical manifestations of CNS depressant intoxication are directly related to the drug's effects on the CNS. The earliest effect of alcohol ingestion is to alter judgment, causing the drinker to become disinhibited and to behave uncharacteristically (e.g., laugh or talk loudly, become boisterous or argumentative). These manifestations appear with a BAC in the range of 50 to 150 mg/dl. As the blood level of the drug rises, cerebellar and vestibular functions become affected. All individuals with a BAC in the 200 to 300 mg/dl range experience significant motor symptoms, manifesting in slurred speech and an unsteady, ataxic gate. At still higher

levels, individuals develop diplopia. They may then become stuporous and can eventually lose consciousness. At levels higher than 400 to 500 mg/dl, respiration can become impaired and the individual may become comatose. Individuals with this degree of impairment also lose protective gag and cough reflexes. BACs of 500 or more can be fatal.[92] Responses to alcohol intoxication occur in a predictable fashion as BAC rises; however, the level producing stupor in the uninitiated drinker may result in minimal obvious impairment in the alcohol-dependent individual.[93]

Chronic ingestion of alcohol damages the nervous system in multiple ways. Alcohol exerts a direct toxic effect on the peripheral nerves, resulting in peripheral neuropathy. Alcoholic polyneuropathy is one of the most common neurologic complications of alcoholism. It can present as pain, paresthesia, or numbness in a glove-and-stocking distribution over the extremities, most commonly in the feet. On physical examination, deep tendon reflexes are decreased, pain and temperature sensations are reduced, and distal muscle groups may be weakened or atrophied. Patients may also report dysesthesias severe enough to limit ambulation.[94] Documentation of serial physical examinations and a detailed history help distinguish acute changes from preexisting conditions.

Several neurologic disorders result in altered mentation after long-term abuse of alcohol. Delirium tremens associated with alcohol withdrawal is a common cause of altered mentation, but there are several other alcohol-related disorders that may mimic the symptoms of acute brain injury. Thiamine depletion associated with chronic alcohol ingestion results in Wernicke-Korsakoff syndrome. Initially this syndrome was thought to be secondary to malnutrition, but it develops even in adequately nourished alcoholics. A triad of symptoms—ataxia, oculomotor palsies or paralysis, and global confusion—characterizes Wernicke's encephalopathy. Affected patients have gait ataxia with moderately severe limb incoordination. Nystagmus is the most frequent ocular manifestation; patients may also experience bilateral rectus palsies, horizontal conjugate defects, and vertical gaze palsies. Less frequently encountered defects include ptosis, loss of pupillary reflexes, and complete ophthalmoplegia. The associated state of confusion is characterized by inattention to the environment, disorientation, and lethargy. Some patients are agitated, but apathy and indifference are more common findings. Wernicke's encephalopathy should be considered in any alcohol-dependent patient with stupor or coma. Patients who have hypothalamic involvement may also be hypothermic and hypotensive.[94]

A high index of suspicion is prudent because most of the effects of Wernicke's encephalopathy are reversible with proper treatment. Untreated, the syndrome carries a 10% to 20% mortality rate. Persistent gait ataxia, nystagmus, and Korsakoff's psychosis are sequelae of Wernicke's encephalopathy. Korsakoff's psychosis is a chronic amnesic disorder characterized by intact remote memory, retrograde amnesia for recent memories, disorientation to time and place, and a marked inability to learn new information. Immediate recall may remain intact, but new information is lost after several minutes. Patients are often aware of the deficit, so confabulation is common. Patients with Korsakoff's psychosis are generally alert, with other cognitive functions relatively intact.[95]

Other CNS effects of chronic alcohol use include alcoholic cerebellar degeneration, alcoholic dementia, and central pontine myelinolysis. Cerebellar degeneration is characterized by gait ataxia and mild degrees of limb impairment. The lower extremities are more commonly involved than the upper extremities. Cerebellar degeneration does not correlate directly with the amount of alcohol consumed, which may indicate a degree of genetic susceptibility. Cerebellar dysfunction can improve with adequate nutrition and abstinence from alcohol.[94]

Alcoholic dementia is a cluster of cognitive defects attributed to the direct neurotoxic effects of alcohol. It is not clinically different from the other dementias.[94] Imaging studies demonstrate loss of neurons and cortical atrophy, but the tangles and plaques characteristic of other dementias are not usually present.[95] It is characterized by a global degeneration in all cognitive abilities. Individuals may be emotionally labile and irritable and have severe long-term and short-term memory impairment. General problem-solving abilities as well as the ability to use new information are impaired. These individuals may appear disheveled and neglected. Alcohol intoxication at the time of injury also results in greater neuropsychologic impairment after traumatic brain injury than that seen in sober patients.[18]

Central pontine myelinolysis is a rare disorder found most commonly in alcoholics. It is often preceded by hyponatremia, and aggressive reversal of chronic hyponatremia may be responsible for precipitating the syndrome. There is usually bilateral, symmetric, focal destruction of the white matter in the ventral pons although a few patients have destruction of white matter in other areas of the brain. Central pontine myelinolysis evolves over days to weeks, with confusion being a prominent sign. Demyelination of pontine corticobulbar fibers and corticospinal tracts can lead to dysarthria; dysphagia; facial, tongue and neck weakness; and conjugate gaze palsies. Patients can develop paraparesis or quadriparesis as a result of the corticospinal involvement and, in severe cases, may develop a "locked-in" syndrome.[94]

Cardiovascular System.   Alcohol has multiple effects on the cardiovascular system. Acute alcohol intoxication results in mild increases in heart rate.[96] Human and animal studies have demonstrated that, acutely, it results in depressed contractile function.[96-98] Decreases in stroke volume by 20% to 40% along with twofold increases in left ventricular end-diastolic pressure have been documented. Alcohol also decreases the rate of left ventricular pressure development and slows relaxation time.[97] Experimentally, acute alcohol intoxication has been shown to potentiate the physiologic and metabolic derangements accompanying

hemorrhagic shock and may contribute to secondary brain injury as a result.[99]

The resultant decrease in cardiac reserve may have detrimental effects on the trauma patient. During the resuscitation phase, intoxicated patients may require inotropic agents to maintain hemodynamic stability in addition to volume replacement and transfusion therapy. However, acute intoxication decreases myocardial responsiveness to several inotropic agents, including dobutamine, isoproterenol, and phenylephrine.[100] Although acute intoxication may potentiate or produce hypotension in trauma patients, intoxication as a cause of hypotension is rare and diagnosed by excluding other common factors such as blood loss.

Chronic consumption of ethanol results in gross and microscopic changes in the myocardium indistinguishable from those found in patients with idiopathic dilated cardiomyopathy. Changes occurring in the hearts of patients with alcoholic cardiomyopathy include ventricular dilation and wall thickening, endocardial scarring, mild valvular irregularities, reduced left ventricular ejection fraction, and decreased ventricular compliance. These abnormalities are easily detected on echocardiogram. On direct examination the myocardium is dilated, flabby, and pale, with areas of degeneration, fibrosis, and endocardial thickening. Microscopic changes, including integral loss of the sarcolemma and alterations of contractile proteins, are present as well.[97,98]

Clinically patients with alcoholic cardiomyopathy may be asymptomatic or present with severe congestive heart failure. Atrial arrhythmias are a common occurrence in alcoholic cardiomyopathy.[101,102] Asymptomatic patients may experience stroke volume abnormalities only during exercise testing.[96] This would suggest that compensated patients can decompensate acutely with the added cardiovascular stress of traumatic injury.

Respiratory System.   Ethanol taken by itself has minimal respiratory depressant effects, even at levels of 200 mg/dl.[103] Associated respiratory effects include a decreased responsiveness to carbon dioxide and slight reduction in vital capacity and expiratory reserve volume as BAC increases. In nonalcoholic drinkers, respiratory arrest has been associated with BACs of 400 to 500 mg/dl.[93] Studies indicate that alcohol increases pulmonary vascular resistance after soft tissue injury and may increase the risk of posttraumatic acute respiratory distress syndrome (ARDS).[104]

Hematologic System.   Chronic alcohol consumption can result in both folate deficiency and iron deficiency anemia.[80] Alcohol also depresses bone marrow and vacuolizes red blood cell precursors.[78] The alcoholic patient can present a challenge because multiple types of anemia may be present simultaneously.

Alcohol interferes with the production and function of platelets. Chronic alcoholics may have thrombocytopenia from impaired megakaryocyte production. Even brief periods of drinking can alter platelet function. Patients can have normal levels of platelets with impaired platelet function. Alcohol decreases platelet response or activation to several biologic agents that serve as triggers for platelet plug formation in the event of vessel disruption. These agents include collagen, epinephrine, adenosine diphosphate, arachidonate, and platelet-activating factor. Platelet dysfunction and thrombocytopenia may exacerbate coagulopathy associated with acute hemorrhage and impair hemostasis.[105]

Digestive System. Alcohol produces toxic effects on several areas of the digestive tract. Many of these pathologic alterations have implications in the care of the trauma patient.

Esophageal complications of excessive alcohol intake include an increased risk of esophageal malignancy, particularly when associated with smoking.[106] Esophageal irritation from alcohol and regurgitation of acidic gastric contents result in esophagitis. Mallory-Weiss tears may occur from repeated episodes of vomiting, and esophageal varices are associated with alcoholic cirrhosis.[80]

Excessive alcohol ingestion may damage the gastric mucosa, causing chronic gastritis,[80] which can be exacerbated by coexisting *Helicobacter pylori* infection.[107] Chronic gastritis often resolves with appropriate antimicrobial and antacid treatment. Patients are also at risk for acute hemorrhagic gastritis.[81]

Alcohol is inherently hepatotoxic and can injure the liver in the absence of any nutritional deficiencies. Fatty infiltration of the liver is the first manifestation of hepatotoxicity and can begin after a few days of heavy alcohol consumption. This is followed by fibrosis, which sometimes manifests as alcoholic hepatitis.[81] Eventually the fibrosis may progress to necrosis and inflammation, resulting in cirrhosis. The early fatty infiltration is reversible with cessation of drinking, but the latter stages of fibrosis are irreversible.[108]

Microscopically, alcohol directly affects the stellate cells or lipocytes of the liver.[80] Cellular function is altered so that these cells, which normally store lipid, begin to produce collagen in a manner similar to myofibroblasts.[109] Alcohol also alters phospholipid metabolism within liver cells.[80]

Alcohol interferes with the cytochrome P450 enzymatic system in the liver. This system is responsible for the metabolism of a large number of compounds, many of them pharmaceutical agents. Acute alcohol use impairs the function of this system, consequently slowing the metabolism of drugs dependent on the system. This slows the rate of drug elimination, resulting in higher serum levels of agents metabolized via this pathway. In contrast, chronic use of alcohol actually increases the rate of metabolism of the P450 system. Drugs are then more rapidly metabolized, resulting in lower-than-predicted serum concentrations of these medications.[81]

Trauma patients may have hepatic dysfunction significant enough to interfere with hemostasis. In addition to the coagulopathy associated with acute hemorrhagic shock, they can have a chronic coagulopathy from impaired production of vitamin K-dependent clotting factors in the liver. Although serum transaminases are often elevated in liver disease, the prothrombin time is the most sensitive indicator of hepatic dysfunction.[110]

Long-term alcohol use produces a form of chronic pancreatitis associated with irreversible structural and functional alterations in the pancreatic tissue. Episodes of acute pancreatitis can occur as well, with classic symptoms of midepigastric pain, nausea, vomiting, and anorexia, along with associated elevations of serum amylase and lipase.[80] Some alcoholics have pathophysiologic changes associated with chronic pancreatitis even though they remain asymptomatic.[111] Serum enzyme levels are often normal in individuals with subacute forms of pancreatitis. Diarrhea can develop from malabsorption syndromes caused by a loss of pancreatic exocrine secretions.[81]

OPIATE PHARMACOLOGY

Opiate drugs are derivatives of the poppy plant, *Papaver somniferum,* or synthetic compounds that resemble the chemical structure of the naturally occurring substances. Morphine and codeine are naturally occurring opiates found in the resin of the poppy plant seedpod. Heroin is a semisynthetic compound, having undergone processing after being extracted from raw opium gum. Meperidine (Demerol), oxycodone (Percodan), hydromorphone (Dilaudid), and methadone represent synthetic formulations. Naturally occurring opiates are the enkephalins, dynorphins, and endorphins, which are peptide molecules produced in the CNS. Naturally occurring opiates have been found in the brain, spinal cord, and exocrine glands. These peptides are portions of larger precursor protein molecules from which the naturally occurring opiates have been cleaved. After production from the precursor proteins, the peptide molecules are stored in the specific opiate neurons for later use.[112]

PHARMACOKINETICS. Opiate drugs can be ingested, injected subcutaneously (i.e., skin popping) or intravenously, or inhaled either nasally or by smoking. Heroin, the most commonly abused opiate, historically has been injected intravenously. However, the purity of heroin imported into the United States has increased, resulting in greater numbers of intranasal users.[113] Rate of absorption, onset of action, and duration of action are dependent on the route of administration and the half-life of the particular drug used. (Table 32-4).[112]

Absorption of opioid drugs is dependent on how lipophilic a particular compound is. More highly lipophilic drugs are more readily absorbed transdermally and from mucosa. They also better penetrate the blood-brain barrier. The liver metabolizes most opioid drugs. They tend to undergo a large first-pass effect, which accounts for the higher equivalent oral dosages compared with parenteral doses. Drugs with a high first-pass metabolism are absorbed readily by the gastrointestinal tract and then transported to the liver via the portal circulation. During this initial

TABLE 32-4 Opioids

Generic Name	Trade Name	Route	Dose (mg)	Duration of Action (hr)	Half-Life (hr)
Morphine sulfate	Morphine	IM, SC	10	4-5	2
		O	60	4-7	
Diacetylmorphine	Heroin	IM, SC	5	4-5	0.5
		O	60	4-5	
Hydromorphone	Dilaudid	IM, SC	1.3	4-5	2-3
		O	7.5	4-6	
Oxymorphone	Numorphan	IM, SC	1	4-6	2-3
		R	5	4-6	
Levorphanol	Levo-Dromoran	IM, SC	2	4-5	12-16
		O	4	4-7	
Dolophine	Methadone	IM	10	4-5	15-40
		O	20	4-6	
Meperidine	Demerol	IM, SC	75	3-5	3-4
		O	300	4-6	
Fentanyl	Sublimaze	IM	0.1	1-2	3-4
Codeine		O	200	4-6	
		IM	130	4-6	2-4
Hydrocodone	Hycodan	O	5-10	4-5	4
Oxycodone	Roxicodone, Percocet	O	5-10	4-5	
Propoxyphene	Darvon	O	65	4-6	6-12
Buprenorphine	Buprenex	IM	0.4	4-5	5
		SL	0.8	5-6	

Adapted from Reisine T, Pasternak G: Opioid analgesics and antagonists. In Molinoff PB, Ruddon RW, Gilman AG, editors: *Goodman & Gilman's the pharmacological basis of therapeutics,* ed 9, New York, 1996, McGraw-Hill.

IM, Intramuscular; *SC,* subcutaneous; *O,* oral; *R,* rectal; *SL,* sublingual.

circulation through the liver, a large percentage of the drug is metabolized before entering the peripheral circulation, thus resulting in loss of part of the dose. Routes not involving the gastrointestinal tract result in a much larger percentage of the dose entering the peripheral circulation. Some opiates, notably codeine, methadone, and oxycodone, have a higher ratio of oral effectiveness compared with their parenteral form. These drugs experience a lower first-pass effect. Oral bioavailability ranges from 25% for morphine up to 60% for codeine. Unchanged drug and metabolites of opioids are excreted in the urine and, to a lesser degree with some of the drugs, in the feces. Patients with renal or hepatic insufficiency may require lower dosages than unimpaired individuals, but, as with any group of patients, individual tolerance varies widely.[112]

PHARMACOLOGY. Stimulation of opiate receptors, of which three subtypes (μ, δ, and κ) have been identified, results in the familiar analgesic effects of these drugs. The overall effects of opiate neurotransmitters on the CNS include drowsiness, mood alterations, and mental clouding. At doses in excess of that required for analgesia, the drugs can produce euphoria.[112]

There is also a group of synthetic drugs that possess both opiate agonist and antagonist properties. They have analgesic actions similar to opiates when used alone but have antagonistic effects when used in conjunction with opiates.[112] These compounds include pentazocine (Talwin),

buprenorphine (Buprenex), butorphanol (Stadol), and nalbuphine (Nubain). These drugs can precipitate acute withdrawal in the opiate-dependent patient and have little role in providing analgesia to injured patients, particularly those who are opiate dependent.

PSYCHOLOGIC EFFECTS. Psychologic effects of narcotics include decreased awareness of and distress from pain, drowsiness, mood alterations, and, at higher doses, euphoria.[113] The level of euphoria depends to some degree on which agent is used, the dose, and the route of administration.[114]

TOLERANCE AND DEPENDENCE. Tolerance and dependence develop with repeated use of narcotic analgesics. These characteristics are common to all opiate drugs and are not necessarily indicative of abuse. Tolerance can occur with patients who have been on opiates for as few as 7 days. Patients with prolonged hospitalizations may require increased doses of narcotic analgesics because of the development of tolerance. These patients do not necessarily develop the behavioral component of craving associated with addictive behavior. This physical dependence is distinct from addiction with its psychobehavioral component.[112]

TOXICITY. The most serious side effect of opiates is respiratory depression. In overdose, patients can develop respiratory arrest followed by cardiac arrest and hypoxic brain injury. Opiates also suppress the cough reflex, increasing the risk of aspiration.[112] Patients who inject heroin may precipitate acute pulmonary edema.

Miosis, or pupillary constriction, is a common side effect of opiates and occurs even in the tolerant user. Assessment of constricted, poorly reactive pupils may indicate recent narcotic use.[112] Care must be taken to rule out other causes for pupil findings and to determine if any narcotics were administered before the assessment.

Generally opiates have little effect on heart rate and blood pressure in the supine patient although they produce some vasodilation. This vasodilation can result in hypotension in the volume-depleted patient.[112] Adverse blood pressure and heart rate changes noted during administration of narcotics may indicate that the patient requires further volume repletion.

Narcotic analgesics decrease gastric motility and can result in constipation and delayed or impaired gastric emptying. These drugs can cause nausea and vomiting as a result of a direct action on the chemoreceptor trigger zone of the medulla. Urinary retention is another possible adverse effect of opiates. Opiate-dependent patients typically develop tolerance to the respiratory depressant and emetic effects of opiates.[77]

COCAINE AND AMPHETAMINE PHARMACOLOGY

PHARMACOKINETICS. Cocaine hydrochloride is a derivative of the coca plant, *Erythroxylon coca*. There are basically two chemical forms of cocaine—hydrochloride salt and freebase. The hydrochloride salt is a white powder that is water soluble and can be injected intravenously or snorted intranasally in powder form.[115] *Freebase* refers to a compound that has not been neutralized by an acid to make the hydrochloride salt. Freebase cocaine is processed by mixing cocaine hydrochloride with an alkali (e.g., baking soda) and water. This mixture is then heated to remove the hydrochloride, leaving waxy chunks of cocaine. This alkaloidal form of cocaine is volatile at a lower temperature than the hydrochloride form, which allows it to be smoked. The term *crack* refers to the crackling sound made when freebase cocaine is smoked. Regardless of which route is used for administration, cocaine enters the circulation rapidly. Once in the blood, it binds with plasma proteins and is rapidly transported to the CNS.[116] Some of the drug remains unbound or free, this being the active portion of the drug. The onset of action for cocaine is variable, depending on the route of administration. Intravenous (IV) and inhaled administration of cocaine causes an almost immediate increase in blood pressure and heart rate.[117] Peak effects occur 30 minutes after intranasal administration and are generally less intense but more prolonged than with either of the other routes.[116] Cocaine is metabolized primarily in the liver and excreted via the kidneys.[118]

PHARMACOLOGY. Cocaine acts on both the peripheral and central nervous systems. It blocks the reuptake of norepinephrine (NE) in the periphery. In the CNS, cocaine inhibits the reuptake of dopamine.[115] Recent microneurographic evidence has found that cocaine also causes central sympathetic activation.[119] CNS outflow and the resultant increase in circulating norepinephrine are responsible for the signs and symptoms of sympathetic nervous system hyperactivity.[119,120]

PSYCHOLOGIC EFFECTS. Cocaine's psychologic effects are caused by its blockade of dopamine reuptake within the CNS. The heightened sense of mental acuity, euphoria, and decreased fatigue associated with cocaine use are the result of the effect of excessive dopamine on the nucleus accumbens.[75] The cocaine "high" is short lived, lasting 1 to 2 hours with nasal inhalation, 30 to 40 minutes with intravenous administration, and 5 to 10 minutes with smoked cocaine.[116]

TOLERANCE AND DEPENDENCE. Cocaine use results in the rapid development of tolerance to the euphoric effects[117]; however, only partial tolerance develops to the cardiovascular effects.[118] There is some degree of cross-tolerance with other CNS stimulants. Chronic cocaine users have decreased numbers of dopamine receptors in their CNS as a result of the continuous high levels of dopamine. Loss of these receptors is thought to account for the increased anxiety and depression seen during withdrawal from cocaine.[117]

TOXICITY. Cocaine's detrimental physiologic effects occur primarily during periods of active use. Toxic effects of cocaine are most commonly seen in its actions on the cardiovascular system. Excessive norepinephrine leads to generalized vasoconstriction and tachycardia.[120] Increases in heart rate and blood pressure peak early during a binge and return to baseline despite continued increases in the serum cocaine level.[121] Acute elevation of circulating norepinephrine contributes to the development of tachycardias and arrhythmias, mesenteric ischemia,[122] and myocardial infarctions.[123]

Adverse effects of cocaine on the neurologic system include cerebrovascular accidents (CVA), seizures, and altered mental states. Cocaine use has been associated with ischemic and hemorrhagic CVA, often in young persons with no known risk factors for cerebral vascular disease.[124] Research has documented that cocaine use results in altered cerebral perfusion,[125] and some cocaine-induced CVAs can be linked to underlying cerebrovascular abnormalities.[126] Patients with cocaine-induced seizures typically have one generalized seizure after cocaine use via the intravenous route. These patients usually have unremarkable neurologic diagnostic workups after the seizure although further workup to rule out traumatic brain injury is still warranted.[127] The causes of cocaine-induced seizures remain unclear. Mental status changes associated with cocaine use range from anxiety to acute psychosis. "Cocaine psychosis" is typified by paranoid ideation, well-structured delusions, hallucinations, and hypersensitivity to environmental stimuli.[128]

Inhaled or smoked cocaine also has detrimental effects on the bronchial mucosa and ciliary-mucous clearance mechanisms. Alveolar macrophage function is impaired[129] and ciliary clearance mechanisms are effectively paralyzed by the use of crack.[130]

Cocaine and ethanol are often used together. This combination results in greater euphoria and increased perception of well-being relative to cocaine alone. Experimentally, this combination of drugs has resulted in increased cardiac toxicity in selected individuals.[131] Heart rate increases with co-administration of cocaine and alcohol were significantly greater than those with either drug used alone.[132]

METHAMPHETAMINE. Methamphetamine deserves attention here because its use is becoming epidemic in some areas of the country. One study of methamphetamine use in trauma patients documented a doubling of positive results between 1989 and 1994.[34] Methamphetamine is a CNS stimulant with physiologic and psychologic effects much like those seen with cocaine. Its euphoric effects are also the result of increased dopamine in the CNS although this occurs via a slightly different mechanism than with cocaine. It can be ingested orally, snorted, injected intravenously, or smoked. Effects are felt 3 to 5 minutes after inhalation and 15 to 20 minutes after oral ingestion. Unlike cocaine, however, the effects of methamphetamine last from 6 to 8 hours. Psychologic effects include increased attention, euphoria, and decreased fatigue. Adverse psychologic effects include paranoia, hallucinations, and mood disturbances. Hyperthermia and seizures have been associated with acute methamphetamine use.[133]

NICOTINE PHARMACOLOGY
Nicotine is the psychoactive chemical found in the leaves of the tobacco plant, *Nicotiana tabacum*. The dried leaves are typically smoked as cigarettes, as cigars, or in a pipe. Leaves may also be chewed.

PHARMACOKINETICS. Nicotine in tobacco smoke is rapidly absorbed from the lungs after inhalation. Nicotine can also be absorbed through the oral mucosa and skin, the routes employed to deliver "smokeless" tobacco and nicotine replacement therapy. From the lungs, skin, or mucosa it moves rapidly to the blood and is delivered to target organs. The majority of nicotine is metabolized in the liver although some is metabolized by the kidneys and lungs. Nicotine and its metabolites are excreted via the kidney.[77]

PHYSIOLOGIC EFFECTS. Physiologic effects of nicotine include vasoconstriction and tachycardia as a result of catecholamine release from direct action on the adrenal medulla. Stimulation of CNS receptors results in tremor and

nausea or vomiting from actions on the chemoreceptor trigger zone. Parasympathetic stimulation of the gastrointestinal tract by nicotine results in increased gastrointestinal motility. Digestive tract responses to nicotine include nausea, vomiting, and diarrhea, the latter as a result of the effect of nicotine on receptors in the large bowel.[134]

Nicotine has a paralytic effect on the mucociliary transport mechanism of the lungs.[134] In addition, chronic use of tobacco results in a number of histopathologic changes in the tracheobronchial tree.[129] Patients with long histories of smoking are at an increased risk for pulmonary complications after injury.

PSYCHOLOGIC EFFECTS. Nicotine acts directly on nicotinic cholinergic receptors of the CNS. This stimulation in turn causes a release of dopamine within the mesolimbic system of the brain. As with many drugs of abuse, the action of dopamine on the nucleus accumbens of the brain is thought to account for the pleasurable sensations induced by nicotine.[75] Nicotine has both stimulant and depressant activities, which account for its reported paradoxic effects. Smokers report having a cigarette to "get them going" in the morning and smoking at bedtime to help "calm their nerves."[77] Use of nicotine decreases subjective levels of anxiety, alters mood, and subjectively increases concentration.[134]

TOLERANCE AND DEPENDENCE. Nicotine is a highly addictive drug with a short-half life of about 2 hours. Nicotine-dependent patients experience cravings 30 to 60 minutes after their last dose, as the nicotine blood level begins to drop. Tolerance to the drug also develops rapidly. Nicotine withdrawal typically lasts 72 hours although craving persist for several weeks.[135]

MARIJUANA PHARMACOLOGY
Marijuana is the common name for the dried flower buds, stems, and leaves of the *Cannabis sativa* plant. The drug is usually smoked but can be ingested. δ-9-Tetrahydrocannabinol (δ^9-THC) is the major psychoactive ingredient in the plant although more than 400 cannabinoids have been identified. The highest concentration of cannabinoids is in the resin of the plants' flowering tops, where concentrations are 5 to 10 times higher than the amounts found in the leaves.[136] Hash or hashish is the dried resin collected from the plant tops. Selective breeding of plants has increased the level of δ^9-THC in the plants from 1.5% in the 1960s to more recent levels of 3% to 3.5%.[137]

As with other psychoactive drugs, marijuana was assumed to mimic the effects of a naturally occurring physiologic substance. This brought about a search for the substance after the receptor sites for δ^9-THC had been identified. Anandamide, identified in the mid-1990s, is a naturally occurring lipid neurotransmitter that has both peripheral and central receptor sites.[138,139] It binds with the same previously identified cannabinoid receptor sites in the CNS.[140]

PHARMACOKINETICS. When marijuana is inhaled, δ^9-THC is absorbed rapidly into the bloodstream. Initial metabolism takes place in the lungs and liver. The resultant metabolite, 11-hydroxy-THC (11-THC), more readily crosses the blood-brain barrier to affect CNS receptors than does δ^9-THC. Peak 11-THC plasma levels remain lower than the parent compound but stay at a plateau for a prolonged period after smoking has ceased.[136] In one study the plasma δ^9-THC level began to rise after the first inhalation. Peak levels occurred approximately 9 minutes after smoking had started and then decreased to negligible levels after 2 hours; however, some trace of the drug was still present after 12 hours.[141] Although the pathway is similar for that of ingested marijuana, there is a more gradual increase in the δ^9-THC level over a period of 4 to 6 hours. This results in a delay in the onset of psychoactive effects. The peak serum levels of δ^9-THC are higher with ingestion than those resulting from smoking.[140]

Because δ^9-THC is highly lipophilic, it is released slowly from the CNS and other lipid-rich tissues, resulting in a prolonged half-life. Half-life can vary from 18 hours to 4 days. δ^9-THC is converted into inactive metabolites in the liver and is excreted in the urine and feces.[136]

PHYSIOLOGIC EFFECTS. Acute effects of marijuana use include heart rate elevations and increases in diastolic blood pressure. Systolic and mean arterial pressures are not affected significantly. Heart rate remains elevated for up to 3 hours after high-dose exposure in experimental studies but returns to baseline sooner after low-dose exposure. In addition to its effects on heart rate and blood pressure, marijuana causes a significant drop in skin temperature.[141]

Cannabis use impairs gross and fine motor functions and delays reaction time.[142] Despite these effects, no clear link has been established between cannabis use and vehicular crashes or fatalities.[136] One reason is that cannabis users tend to overestimate their degree of impairment and compensate by increasing their attention to driving, whereas drivers under the influence of alcohol tend to underestimate their degree of impairment.[143] Acute marijuana use impairs short-term memory and substantially increases memory intrusions, thus impairing the ability to learn.[142] These effects can persist up to 24 hours after smoking marijuana.[144] Retrieval of previously learned material is largely unaffected. Chronic use of marijuana results in subtle neuropsychologic defects, which persist after periods of abstinence.[145] Effects of long-term cannabis use include impairment of organization and problems integrating complex information involving attention and memory processes.[146,147] It is unknown whether these defects are permanent.

Chronic marijuana use adversely affects the function of alveolar macrophages[129] and alters the tracheobronchial epithelium.[148] Pulmonary alterations from chronic use result in cough and sputum production similar to that observed in cigarette smokers. In trauma patients these effects could conceivably increase the risk for pulmonary complications, particularly pneumonia.

Marijuana can alter ocular examination findings. Conjunctival injection (i.e., red eyes) typically accompanies marijuana use. Marijuana also reduces intraocular pressure and decreases pupillary responsiveness to light, resulting in increased time for light accommodation.[149]

PSYCHOLOGIC EFFECTS. Marijuana induces a state of intoxication characterized by euphoria and relaxation. Psychic manifestations vary depending on user set and setting and can include heightened awareness of the external environment, drowsiness, increased hunger, and depression.[142] At levels producing moderate intoxication, it adversely affects a wide range of behaviors, including simple motor tasks and complex psychomotor and cognitive tasks.[149] Higher levels may induce panic, paranoia, and anxiety. Rarely it may be associated with psychosis, usually in persons with underlying psychiatric disorders characterized by psychotic thought processes.[142]

TOLERANCE AND DEPENDENCE. Marijuana tolerance develops rapidly with regular use, probably as a result of decrease or downregulation of receptor sites in the CNS. An atypical pattern of tolerance has been reported with marijuana, compared with other drugs of abuse. Chronic users report requiring less drug to achieve the customary drug experience. This may reflect increased efficiency in the smoking technique rather than a true reverse tolerance.[136] Although it was originally thought that marijuana use did not result in physiologic dependence, studies of long-term marijuana users refute this. These studies report that sudden abstinence after regular use of cannabinoids causes a withdrawal syndrome.[150]

CLINICAL APPLICATION

Drugs of abuse have numerous physiologic effects that can influence the care of substance-abusing patients. These effects may make assessment, diagnosis, and treatment difficult. Health care providers must consider the effects of psychoactive drugs when caring for trauma patients, given the high incidence of psychoactive substance abuse in this patient population.

RESUSCITATION PHASE

The primary goals of care during the resuscitation phase are (1) identification and treatment of life-threatening conditions and (2) stabilization of the cardiovascular, pulmonary, and neurologic systems. Detailed descriptions of assessment and management strategies for multiple trauma patients are provided elsewhere in this text and are not repeated here. The purpose of the following discussion is to focus on treatment needs unique to the substance-abusing patient.

ASSESSMENT CONSIDERATIONS

Assessment of the substance-abusing trauma patient is complicated by several factors. As with any trauma patient, alterations in neurologic status as the direct effect of injury may obviate obtaining a current or past medical history, including any information about substance abuse. Intoxicated patients may be stuporous and thus unwilling or unable to cooperate with history taking or physical assessment. Further, it may be difficult to determine whether physical findings are the result of trauma or the substance abuse.[151] It is imperative that complete assessment of the trauma patient be accomplished systematically and rapidly. Physical, historical, and laboratory findings consistent with substance abuse should be included in documentation of the physical examination and in the patient database.

IDENTIFYING THE PATIENT WITH A SUBSTANCE ABUSE PROBLEM

Trauma Database. Substance-abusing trauma patients often have a history of previous injuries. Injury can be considered a symptom of substance abuse.[152] Patients should be questioned about previous injuries, including falls, MVCs, assaults, and industrial injuries. This information should be obtained as soon as possible in the trauma cycle, preferably at the time of admission. Pertinent information can be obtained from family members if the patient is unable to provide information; the family can also be used to validate and supplement information received from the patient. Additionally, as much information as possible about the circumstances of the current injury episode should be collected from police officers, first responders, and other eyewitnesses at the scene. Reports of altered behavior or impaired judgment before or immediately after the injury can help identify the substance-abusing patient.[153]

Physical Assessment. Physical assessment of the trauma patient includes a complete head-to-toe examination and frequent monitoring of vital signs and neurologic status. It should also include evaluating the patient for evidence of drug and alcohol use. Drug and alcohol use can affect virtually all the body's systems.

Many of the sequelae of drug and alcohol abuse are manifested as alterations in the integument.[154] Numerous bruises in various stages of healing over the lower extremities can be indicative of repetitive minor trauma caused by bumping into hard, fixed objects. Multiple small burns in various stages of healing are common as a result of dropping ashes while smoking.[155] Abscesses and cellulitis are other common integumentary manifestations seen with intravenous or subcutaneous drug injection. Patients who are using drugs intravenously often have "track marks," lines of multiple injection sites along the course of peripheral veins. Track marks are actually tattooing from impurities in injected drugs. Intravenous drug users may also have signs of phlebitis and sclerosis of veins. Patients occasionally develop venous insufficiency caused by venous scarring, which may be seen in one or both upper extremities rather

than in the lower extremities as would be more common with other venous disorders.[154] Patients may inject drugs subcutaneously ("skin popping"). These needle marks do not necessarily follow veins but are often found in fleshy parts of the body such as the thighs or upper arms. Some patients also inject drugs intraarterially and can develop arteriovenous fistulas or pseudoaneurysms.[156]

Drug use may result in pathologic alterations in the upper and lower respiratory tract. Intranasal inhalation of cocaine often results in damage to the nasal mucosa and destruction of all or part of the nasal septum. This destruction results from to the vasoconstrictive effects of cocaine and subsequent ischemia of the nasal mucosa and septum.[157] Intoxicated patients and those using opiates may vomit and develop aspiration pneumonia and the more severe consequence of ARDS.[158] Alcoholics may develop chronic pneumonia as a result of frequent aspiration. Patients who smoke crack often have a cough productive of copious amounts of soot-stained sputum similar to that found in victims of smoke inhalation. Auscultation of breath sounds and observation of aspirated or expectorated sputum may provide evidence of inhalation drug use, chronic pneumonia, or other pulmonary condition.

Patients who use cocaine are susceptible to mesenteric ischemia or infarction and may have required exploratory laparotomy in the past. A history of abdominal surgery in the cocaine-using patient should be explored carefully.[159] Patients using alcohol or opiates may also have gastrointestinal symptoms, most commonly nausea, vomiting, constipation, and diarrhea. Chronic abdominal pain may result from pancreatitis, and patients may have hepatomegaly from cirrhosis or hepatitis.[81]

Nervous system alterations caused by drug abuse may include a history of seizures, ataxia, peripheral neuropathy, and abnormalities of the deep tendon reflexes. Ocular palsy can result from extensive alcohol use. Cognitive defects often include short-term memory deficits.[94] Other neuropsychiatric manifestations of drug use may include paranoia, hallucinations, agitation, and anxiety.

Patients with recent cocaine use can present with arrhythmias, hypertension, chest pain, cerebral vascular accidents, and electrocardiogram (ECG) changes consistent with myocardial ischemia or infarction.[160] Abuse of other psychoactive drugs may also cause adverse changes in heart rate and rhythm and blood pressure. Alcoholics may have secondary cardiomyopathy, and intravenous drug users frequently develop bacterial endocarditis and subsequent valvular dysfunction.[97,161] Intravenous drug users and alcoholics may present with signs of congestive heart failure.

Substance Abuse History. All trauma patients admitted to the hospital after injury should be questioned about ATOD use. Reassuring patients that such information is needed for comprehensive care often increases their willingness to provide a complete history. Patients should be asked about (1) specific substances they use, (2) date of last use, (3) amount used on a typical day of use, (4) routes of use,

TABLE 32-5	**CAGE Questionnaire**

Giving two or more positive answers is strongly indicative of a substance abuse disorder. Patients are asked if they
(1) have attempted to **cut** down on their alcohol or drug use,
(2) are **annoyed** or **angry** when questioned about their alcohol or drug use,
(3) feel **guilty** about their alcohol or drug use, or
(4) have an **eye-opener** (i.e. drink or drug) upon arising in the morning.

Modified from Ewing JA: Detecting alcoholism: the CAGE questionnaire, *JAMA* 252:1905-1907, 1984.

TABLE 32-6	**TWEAK Test**
T	**Tolerance:** How many drinks can you hold?
W	Have close friends or relatives **worried** or complained about your drinking in the past year?
E	**Eye-opener:** Do you sometimes take a drink in the morning when you first get up?
A	**Amnesia:** Has a friend or family member ever told you about things you said or did while you were drinking that you could not remember?
K(C)	Do you sometimes feel the need to **cut down** on your drinking?

From Russell M, Martier S, Sokel R et al: Screening for pregnancy risk drinking TWEAKing the tests (abstract), *Alcohol Clin Exp Res* 15:368, 1991.

and (5) frequency of use.[153] Additionally, it is crucial to elicit any history of withdrawal symptoms, particularly from patients who use central nervous system depressants. A history of alcohol withdrawal seizures or delirium tremens is the best predictor of subsequent episodes although a negative history does not rule out the possibility of new onset of either phenomenon.[162] Patients should be questioned about past medical illnesses, particularly those known to be highly associated with substance abuse.

Psychosocial Assessment.   Psychosocial assessment includes obtaining information about the patient's social, employment, and legal difficulties and any history of psychiatric illness. This information can be used to assess the progression of the patient's chemical dependency. Impairment in one or more areas may indicate a history of chronic substance abuse if not dependence.

QUESTIONNAIRE SCREENING FOR SUBSTANCE ABUSE. Several instruments are available for detection of and screening for substance abuse. If the patient's condition does not permit use of these tools during the resuscitation phase, they may be administered later during hospitalization. The CAGE[163] and CAGE Adapted for Drugs (CAGE-AID)[164] are the simplest to use (Table 32-5). Both have demonstrated good specificity and validity in screening for alcohol and drug abuse and can be administered rapidly.[165] In a study of level I trauma center patients, the CAGE demonstrated an 84% sensitivity and 90% specificity for alcohol use disorders.[19] Other instruments include the TWEAK test (Table 32-6) and the Alcohol Use Disorder Identification Test (AUDIT) (Table 32-7). The TWEAK test was developed for use in pregnant women. Its five items are weighted, with the first two receiving 2 points and the others 1 point for an affirmative answer.[166] A score of 3 or more is considered positive.[164] The AUDIT test is a 10-item, weighted-score instrument developed by the World Health Organization (WHO).[167,168] Possible scores range from 0 to 40, with a cutoff of 8 considered positive for alcohol abuse. Overall it has demonstrated a sensitivity of 92% and a specificity of 93%. It has the benefit that it can be taken as a pencil-and-paper test, which can be given to patients to complete in privacy.[164] Research on trauma patients has indicated enhanced sensitivity and spec-

ificity for the AUDIT when low-threshold responses for alcohol consumption are used.[169] Screening tools are used in conjunction with laboratory assessment in the evaluation of substance abuse and dependence.

LABORATORY ASSESSMENT

Toxicology Screening.   A model trauma care system plan developed by the U. S. Department of Health and Human Services recommends that all trauma patients be screened for alcohol and other drug use. Serum and urine specimens for toxicologic analysis should be obtained as soon as possible after admission.[170] Despite these recommendations and the strong association between trauma and alcohol use in particular, many trauma patients are still not screened for alcohol and drug use.[171] Practitioners should be familiar with the substances routinely included in the toxicology profiles of their institutions. Many profiles do not include the hallucinogenic compounds because they are unstable and difficult to test for. The usefulness of toxicology screening is limited by the amount of time required to obtain results, which may range from several hours to a few days, depending on what laboratory support is available. Additionally, positive toxicologic testing does not rule out the existence of underlying injury. Research indicates that laboratory tests alone may be insufficient for identifying chemically dependent patients.[172] Rates of detection are enhanced with the use of screening tools in conjunction with laboratory tests.

Tetrahydrocannabinol, cocaine, opiates, and phencyclidine (PCP) are substances most commonly assayed in a urine toxicologic screen. Three methods of urine analysis are currently available: thin-layer chromatography (TLC), enzyme immunoassay, and gas chromatography. TLC is the least expensive technique but also the least sensitive. It can detect methadone, codeine, propoxyphene (Darvon), barbiturates, amphetamine, cocaine, and high levels of morphine. It does not detect marijuana or the hallucinogenic compounds. Because false-positive results are fairly common, positive results from TLC should be verified by another method. Enzyme immunoassay is a more expensive test but also more sensitive than TLC. In addition to the above-mentioned drugs, it can also detect alcohol, benzodiazepines, methaqualone (Quaalude), PCP, and canna-

TABLE 32-7 Alcohol Use Disorder Identification Test (AUDIT)

1. How often do you have a drink containing alcohol?

Never	(0)
Monthly or less	(1)
2 to 4 times a month	(2)
2 to 3 times a week	(3)
4 or more times a week	(4)

2. How many drinks containing alcohol do you have on a typical day when you are drinking?

None	(0)
1 or 2	(1)
3 or 4	(2)
5 or 6	(3)
7 to 9	(4)
10 or more	(5)

3. How often do you have six or more drinks on one occasion?

Never	(0)
Less than monthly	(1)
Monthly	(2)
Weekly	(3)
Daily or almost daily	(4)

4. How often during the last year have you found that you were unable to stop drinking once you had started?

Never	(0)
Less than monthly	(1)
Monthly	(2)
Weekly	(3)
Daily or almost daily	(4)

5. How often during the last year have you failed to do what was normally expected of you because of drinking?

Never	(0)
Less than monthly	(1)
Monthly	(2)
Weekly	(3)
Daily or almost daily	(4)

6. How often during the last year have you needed a first drink in the morning to get yourself going after a heavy drinking session?

Never	(0)
Less than monthly	(1)
Monthly	(2)
Weekly	(3)
Daily or almost daily	(4)

7. How often during the last year have you had a feeling of guilt or remorse after drinking?

Never	(0)
Less than monthly	(1)
Monthly	(2)
Weekly	(3)
Daily or almost daily	(4)

8. How often during the last year have you been unable to remember what happened the night before because you had been drinking?

Never	(0)
Less than monthly	(1)
Monthly	(2)
Weekly	(3)
Daily or almost daily	(4)

9. Have you or someone else been injured as the result of your drinking?

Never	(0)
Less than monthly	(1)
Monthly	(2)
Weekly	(3)
Daily or almost daily	(4)

10. Has a relative, friend, or a doctor or other health worker been concerned about your drinking or suggested you cut down?

Never	(0)
Less than monthly	(1)
Monthly	(2)
Weekly	(3)
Daily or almost daily	(4)

Record the total of the specific items: _____

From Babor TF, Grant M: *Project on Identification and Management of Alcohol-Related Problems. Report on phase II: a randomized clinical trial of brief interventions in primary health care*, Geneva, Switzerland, 1989, World Health Organization.

binoids. Various techniques are available for enzyme immunoassay. Capillary gas-liquid chromatography is the most sensitive test but is also labor intensive and expensive. It should be reserved for cases of obvious poisoning or intoxication in the absence of any known history regarding the nature of the ingested substance. Gas chromatography with mass spectrometry is the most sensitive urine test available. It can be used to verify positive results obtained by the immunoassay method. Chromatography also has the benefit of providing quantitative results that can yield some information about how recently drugs were used. Marijuana in particular can be assigned as recent or old use.[155]

Drugs measured via serum concentrations include ethanol, methanol, acetaminophen, benzodiazepines, barbiturates, and tricyclic antidepressants.[155] Drugs that were administered in the prehospital phase of care or at referring institutions should be noted to prevent misinterpretation of positive toxicology results by subsequent providers.

Saliva, breath, and hair analyses are other laboratory tests available to assess drug use. Breathalyzers and saliva tests are sometimes used in emergency departments, but blood remains the most consistently available means for monitoring BAC.[155]

Other Parameters.   Although serum and urine toxicologic tests are considered the gold standard for documenting acute intoxication, other laboratory tests have been used to assess for chronic alcohol use. These biologic markers include mean corpuscular volume (MCV), the serum transaminases, aspartate aminotransferase (AST), alanine aminotransferase (ALT), and γ-glutamyltransferase (GGT). MCV is commonly elevated in patients with megaloblastic anemias such as that caused by folate deficiency. Folate deficiency anemia is often associated with a history of long-term excessive alcohol use. One study of biologic markers in trauma patients demonstrated only a 27% sensitivity for MCV in predicting excessive alcohol use.[172] AST and ALT have been used in the past as measures of drug-related hepatic involvement but are elevated late in the course of hepatic injury; therefore, they are not particularly sensitive, nor are they specific to alcohol use disorders. GGT is a more sensitive indicator of alcoholic liver disease, with a 51% sensitivity for predicting excessive alcohol use, but it can also be elevated in patients with hepatitis.[173] Caution must be used when interpreting these values because acute liver injury elevates hepatic enzyme levels irrespective of drug or alcohol use. Carbohydrate-deficient transferrin (CDT) is the newest biochemical marker to be used in the assessment of problematic drinking.[174] In medical patients it has a high sensitivity and specificity and correlates well with the amount of alcohol consumed in the previous month.[175] However, in a study of trauma patients it was found to have a sensitivity of only 34% for predicting excessive alcohol use.[176]

MANAGEMENT PRIORITIES

DRUG OVERDOSE IN THE TRAUMA PATIENT.   Management priorities for the trauma patient who has taken a drug

overdose are essentially the same as those for any patient with a drug overdose. Initial resuscitation efforts focus on the timely stabilization of cardiopulmonary function. Additionally, trauma patients may require simultaneous treatment for injuries. Respiratory depression is the most serious effect of CNS depressant and opioid overdoses; hence the first priority is to establish and secure a patent airway. After this, adequate ventilation is ensured, intravenous access obtained, and circulatory function maintained with intravenous fluid and, in some cases, inotropic support. Patients may overdose on a combination of substances and may not fit a clinical profile unique to one category of drugs.

Naloxone Administration.   The classic triad of opioid overdose includes respiratory depression, miotic "pinpoint" pupils, and coma. Reversal of the opioid effects, including their respiratory depressant action, can be achieved with intravenous administration of naloxone. Naloxone should be diluted and administered gradually in 0.4 mg doses while observing for the reversal of respiratory depression and improvement in mental status. Titrated administration with close observation minimizes the risk of precipitating acute opiate withdrawal syndrome. Up to 10 mg of naloxone can be administered, but if no effect is noted at this point, an alternative explanation should be sought. The half-life and duration of action of naloxone is shorter than those of some of the opioid drugs, so patients treated with naloxone need to be monitored closely for a return of respiratory depression from residual opioid after the naloxone dose has been metabolized.[112]

Flumazenil Administration.   Benzodiazepine overdose is rarely fatal unless the benzodiazepine is combined with other drugs, most notably alcohol. Flumazenil is a benzodiazepine antagonist that can be used to reverse the effects of benzodiazepines. It is most commonly used for reversal of drugs administered during anesthesia but is approved for use in overdose. A total of 1 mg given over 1 to 3 minutes usually reverses therapeutic doses of benzodiazepines. In suspected overdose, 1 to 5 mg can be given over 2 to 10 minutes. If no reversal is seen after a 5-mg dose, benzodiazepines are probably not the major cause of sedation.[78]

NEUROLOGIC MANAGEMENT ISSUES.   Serial, comprehensive neurologic assessments are crucial during the resuscitative phase to identify changes caused by acute trauma, particularly to the CNS. Adverse effects of psychoactive drugs may also be detected. When the trauma patient has an altered sensorium or deterioration of other cerebral function, intracranial causes (i.e., brain injury) must be expeditiously ruled out. Acute alterations in neurologic function should never be assumed to be the result of substance abuse alone until other possibilities, such as intracerebral mass effect, shock, hypoxia, and other potential physiologic causes, have been ruled out.[177] One study documented that mild brain injuries were often missed because of the assumption that neurologic alterations were due only to alcohol intoxication.[151] Another study of brain-injured patients with intracranial hematomas noted missed diagnosis and delays in treatment when decreased level of consciousness was attributed solely to intoxication.[178]

Seizures. Seizures are a common neurologic alteration that may occur as a result of substance use, the withdrawal process, or trauma. Seizures may occur after use of alcohol, cocaine,[179] and opiates[112] or present as part of a withdrawal syndrome, typically from alcohol[180] and other CNS depressants.[181] CNS withdrawal is a less likely cause during the resuscitation phase. Other causes of seizures, including intracranial lesions and preexisting seizure disorders, must be ruled out. Seizures can be treated with diazepam (10 mg IV) or lorazepam (4-8 mg IV). Patients who seize should be monitored closely to note the characteristics, duration, and cessation of seizure activity; recurrence of seizure activity; and their condition during the postictal period. Seizure precautions must be initiated to protect the patient from further injury.

Assaultive or Self-Injurious Behavior. Patients who demonstrate aggressive or self-injurious behavior may require the use of chemical or physical restraints to facilitate evaluation and treatment. In some cases, chemical restraint is the only effective alternative for calming the patient. Ideally a concise neurologic exam should be performed before the use of chemical restraints. Other possible causes of combative behavior, including intracranial pathologic conditions and hypoxia, must be ruled out. Care must be taken to document patient responses to chemical restraints, and such measures should be withdrawn as soon as the patient's condition warrants discontinuation. The goals of care are to maintain patient and staff safety while completing the evaluation process. The nurse should remain attuned to the effect that the set and setting can have on the patient's responses to treatment. Keeping sensory stimulation to a minimum is a challenge during the acute assessment phase. Decreasing the number of staff members treating the patient; providing reassurance; offering simple, honest explanations; and maintaining a calm, quiet environment serve to minimize sensory input. Such measures can reduce agitation, gain the patient's trust, elicit cooperation, and lessen the need for restraints.

ALTERATIONS IN RESPIRATORY FUNCTION. Psychoactive drug use can have several adverse effects on pulmonary function, in addition to those resulting from trauma.[148,182] Ongoing, systematic assessments of pulmonary function, including physical examination and monitoring for adequate respiratory gas exchange, are important for early recognition and management of pulmonary complications.[183] Patients with concomitant chest trauma are at an especially high risk for hospital-acquired pneumonias. Patients experiencing respiratory difficulty require prompt, definitive management. Chest radiography or a computed tomography (CT) scan to determine the underlying cause should be performed as soon as possible. Definitive care for

the patient experiencing respiratory distress can include tracheal intubation and mechanical ventilation. In addition to incentive spirometry, deep breathing, and coughing exercises, patients may require chest physiotherapy to mobilize and clear secretions.

CARDIOVASCULAR MANAGEMENT ISSUES
Cardiac. Trauma patients with a history of chronic alcohol use should be evaluated for evidence of impaired myocardial function.[182] Some patients may require the use of a pulmonary artery catheter for serial measurement of cardiac output and other cardiopulmonary parameters. Cardiomegaly on an admission chest film may provide evidence of cardiomyopathy in patients with known alcohol dependency.[97] Patients with a history of intravenous drug use may have valvular dysfunction related to previous episodes of bacterial endocarditis. Evidence of myocardial compromise, or a murmur in the intravenous drug abuser, should prompt further assessment. An echocardiogram provides the most definitive assessment of valvular function and should be undertaken early during hospitalization if there is reason to suspect valvular dysfunction.[184]

Circulation. Drugs of abuse can precipitate several alterations in circulation. The hypertensive effects of acute alcohol use may mask an underlying volume depletion resulting from acute hemorrhage.[185] Acute intoxication blunts compensatory responses to blood loss and has been associated with more profound shock in response to hemorrhage than is seen in nonintoxicated individuals.[186-188] Animal research indicates that use of both cocaine and alcohol may result in more severe alterations of hemodynamic status than would be expected with either drug individually.[132]

Patients who have used opiates recently may have decreased blood pressure and heart rate, which interfere with the normal compensatory mechanisms of acute hemorrhage. These patients are also slower to respond to volume repletion.[112] Patients abusing opiates or intoxicated with CNS depressants may also have decreased pain perception, further complicating the clinical assessment. Health care providers cannot rely solely on reports of patient discomfort to guide clinical assessment. A cause of hemodynamic instability must be sought aggressively before attributing alterations in vital signs to preinjury drug use.

Although cocaine is commonly associated with elevations in vital signs, research on cocaine-intoxicated patients failed to discern any difference in vital signs when compared with nonintoxicated patients. In this group of patients, changes in vital signs are more commonly related to injury type than to the cocaine intoxication.[189,190]

FLUID AND ELECTROLYTE IMBALANCES. Acute and chronic ingestion of alcohol can result in several fluid and electrolyte abnormalities. Alcohol overconsumption has multiple effects on kidney function and on water, electrolyte, and acid-base homeostasis.[191] Accurate measurement and documentation of intake and output and monitoring of electrolyte levels are vital for detection of such imbalances. Critically and acutely ill patients should have electrolyte levels (including calcium, magnesium, and phosphate) monitored closely until levels are consistently stable. Intravenous volume and electrolyte deficits should be corrected to achieve the desired fluid balance, normalized serum electrolyte levels and sufficient urinary output.

Sodium and Water.   Acute ingestion of alcohol induces diuresis because of the suppression of antidiuretic hormone (ADH). As the BAC decreases, the urinary flow rate and sodium excretion normalize in response to the subsequent rise in ADH. Chronic alcohol ingestion results in an overall retention of fluid and salt, with a resultant expansion of plasma volume and extracellular fluid. After withdrawal from alcohol, these abnormalities resolve in 3 to 4 days. Chronic alcoholics tend to be volume overloaded unless they have experienced hemorrhagic blood loss or protracted vomiting.[191] Acutely intoxicated patients typically have elevated serum osmolarities. Estimations of BAC can be made using serum osmolarity; however, this calculation should not be used as a substitute for more definitive toxicologic analysis (Table 32-8).[192]

Calcium.   Severe hypocalcemia is common in chronic alcoholics and may be the result of both increased urinary loss and impaired intestinal absorption. This has ramifications in acute trauma because it may perpetuate acute blood loss secondary to abnormal hemostasis.[193] Symptomatic hypocalcemia causes neuromuscular irritability characterized by tetany, laryngeal spasm, muscle cramps, and positive Chvostek's and Trousseau's signs. Insufficient calcium can also result in hypotension and ineffective myocardial contractility.[194]

Magnesium.   Magnesium loss with and without hypomagnesemia is another common complication of alcoholism. It may be induced by poor nutritional intake, enhanced renal excretion,[195] and diarrhea. Low serum magnesium is associated with muscle weakness, tremors, and other electrolyte disturbances, primarily hypokalemia and hypocalcemia.[180] Alcoholics can have depleted magnesium stores without having abnormally low serum magnesium levels. Serum magnesium levels should be maintained in the high-normal range to facilitate replacement of depleted body stores and correction of hypocalcemia.

Phosphorus.   A study by Ryback et al demonstrated a 30% to 50% incidence of hypophosphatemia in hospitalized alcoholics.[196] Hypophosphatemia results from enhanced urinary loss of phosphate, secondary hyperparathyroidism, enhanced release of calcitonin, and impaired intestinal absorption resulting from vomiting and diarrhea.[191] Severe hypophosphatemia can result in impaired cardiac and skeletal muscle function, blood cell dysfunction, and respiratory impairment. Patients with hypophosphatemia may be unable to wean from mechanical ventilation because of impaired respiratory muscle function.[197]

Glucose.   Alcohol inhibits gluconeogenesis, and the resultant hypoglycemia is a common cause of mental status alterations in the alcoholic. If hypoglycemia is suspected, a finger-stick blood glucose test should be performed. Patients with documented hypoglycemia should be treated with dextrose and concomitant administration of thiamine to prevent the development of Wernicke-Korsakoff syndrome.[198]

PERIOPERATIVE PHASE

ANESTHESIA CONSIDERATIONS

Acute or chronic drug use can alter the patient's response to anesthetic agents used during surgical intervention. The patient may require higher-than-average doses of these drugs to maintain the level of anesthesia. In some cases, drug use may potentiate the effects of anesthetic agents. If a psychoactive drug history is known or suspected, intraoperative care can be planned accordingly. A high tolerance for agents used in induction and maintenance of anesthesia may be the first indication of a substance abuse problem, particularly in patients taken emergently to the operating room. Cocaine use should be considered when the patient develops tachycardia refractory to oxygen, analgesia, and volume repletion during anesthesia induction. Chronic cocaine use renders indirect-acting vasopressors such as ephedrine ineffective, so direct-acting vasopressors should be used.[199,200]

PREVENTING WITHDRAWAL

Patients who are undergoing long operative procedures can be at risk for acute withdrawal during the operation. It is imperative that intraoperative withdrawal be prevented. Patients with known opioid dependence requiring surgery can be given methadone before the procedure to alleviate the risk of intraoperative withdrawal. Those patients at risk for CNS depressant withdrawal should receive a long-acting benzodiazepine such as diazepam or chlordiazepoxide before the initiation of surgery.[201]

TABLE 32-8	**Estimating Blood Alcohol Level From Serum Osmolarity**

To determine the blood alcohol level, subtract the low-normal value of 280 milliosmol/liter (mOsm/L) from the patient's serum osmolarity. Then divide that number by 25 to approximate the blood alcohol level.

For example, given a serum osmolarity of 350mOsmol/l:
1. $350 - 280 = 70$
2. $70 \div 25 = 2.8$
3. $2.8 =$ Approximate blood alcohol level

Modified from Glasser L, Sternglanz PD, Combie ZJ et al: Serum osmolarity and its applicability to drug overdose, *Am J Clin Pharmacol* 60:695-699, 1973.

HEMATOLOGIC CONSIDERATIONS

Management of the chronic alcoholic may be complicated by preexisting coagulopathy caused by impaired production of vitamin K-dependent clotting factors. Patients with extensive cirrhosis may require transfusion or a continuous infusion of fresh frozen plasma to maintain hemostasis. Patients who are thrombocytopenic and show evidence of continued bleeding require platelet transfusion as well. Patients with persistently elevated prothrombin time can be treated with 10 mg of vitamin K administered intravenously, intramuscularly, or subcutaneously daily for 3 days.

CRITICAL CARE PHASE

During the critical care phase the multidisciplinary health care team continues to focus on restoring homeostasis and managing physiologic alterations directly attributable to injury and substance use. Patients in this phase require intensive nursing care because of instability of one or more major organ systems. Acute withdrawal syndromes are some of the most common physiologic alterations encountered during this phase of care.

WITHDRAWAL SYNDROMES

Withdrawal is a psychophysiologic syndrome triggered by the abrupt cessation of a psychoactive drug. Withdrawal syndromes are characteristic for each class of drugs. Onset and duration of withdrawal vary with the half-life of each specific drug. Drugs with short half-lives have a more rapid onset and shorter course of withdrawal than those with longer half-lives. Withdrawal syndromes can vary in severity from mild physical and mental symptoms, such as the headache and fatigue associated with caffeine withdrawal, to life-threatening cardiovascular collapse associated with delirium tremens in alcohol withdrawal. The severity of withdrawal experienced by any one individual also varies in relation to the amount of substance used, the length of exposure, the degree of physiologic dependence, and other co-morbid conditions. Because patients frequently use multiple psychoactive drugs, they may experience more than one type of withdrawal simultaneously.

Every effort should be made to prevent, identify, differentiate, and treat withdrawal syndromes. At the same time, other physiologic causes for the withdrawal symptoms must be ruled out. The trauma patient who exhibits restlessness, agitation, tachycardia, and confusion must be assessed carefully for potential drug withdrawal. Simultaneously hypoxia, brain injury, pain, fluid and electrolyte imbalances, psychiatric disorders, sepsis, sleep deprivation, and medication or transfusion reactions must all be considered and excluded. A major risk, however, when caring for the patient with a history of substance abuse is that the caregivers consider all possible sources of the symptoms except acute withdrawal.

CENTRAL NERVOUS SYSTEM DEPRESSANT WITHDRAWAL
Alcohol Withdrawal. Alcohol withdrawal begins 12 to 24 hours after the cessation of drinking. Patients who are highly alcohol dependent have adapted to functioning with a certain baseline BAC and may begin to experience symptoms of withdrawal before their BAC has reached zero.[180] Because time to withdrawal is variable, vigilant monitoring is required to recognize withdrawal early and prevent or minimize its sequelae.

Alcohol withdrawal is often divided into stages. Severe mental status changes and autonomic hyperactivity generally last 3 to 5 days. A minority of patients develop protracted withdrawal, which can last 2 weeks or more.[202] Anxiety and sleep disturbances commonly last for 2 weeks or more.[180] Patients may pass through all the stages to full-blown delirium tremens or may experience only the relatively mild but unpleasant symptoms of stage I withdrawal. A history of delirium tremens or withdrawal seizures is the best predictor of untoward outcomes, but a negative history does not preclude their development.[162]

Stage I alcohol withdrawal typically begins 4 to 24 hours after the last drink. It is characterized by a reversal of alcohol's sedative and depressant effects. Patients typically experience a dysphoric mood and increased levels of anxiety. Autonomic hyperactivity occurs and is characterized by tachycardia, hypertension, fever, diaphoresis, fine tremor, and possibly mild hyperreflexia. Some patients may also experience nausea, vomiting, or diarrhea. These symptoms are frequently superimposed on the clinical presentation of shock, injury, or evolving infection.[180]

Stage II typically occurs from 24 to 36 hours after cessation of drinking. It is characterized by a worsening of the symptoms seen in stage I withdrawal. Hypertension, tachycardia, and tremor become more pronounced. Patients experience increased levels of anxiety and often are insomnic.[180]

Stage III also occurs from 24 to 36 hours after the last drink. There is further autonomic hyperactivity of a severity at least comparable to stage II. Patients develop further coarsening of their tremors and may experience visual hallucinations or illusions. Visual hallucinations may be subtle, in the form of small, fleeting shadows seen out of the corner of the eye, or they may be more dramatic, with patients reporting the presence of nonexistent persons in their room. Patients in stage III remain oriented relative to their baseline.[180]

Stage IV also occurs 24 to 36 hours after the last drink and includes the development of auditory hallucinations. Patients may report hearing familiar voices and insist a family member is nearby despite a caregiver's assurances to the contrary. Auditory hallucinations can also be unpleasant or accusatory. Some patients experience tactile hallucinations or formication, the experience of feeling nonexistent insects crawling over the skin. Anxiety often reaches the panic level, and patients may attempt to flee the hospital. They become disoriented and often insist they are somewhere other than a hospital. At this stage they are at extremely high risk for falls or self-injury and require constant supervision and possibly physical restraints.[180]

Stage V, delirium tremens (DTs), is one of the most serious complications of alcohol withdrawal. DTs generally appear 72 to 96 hours after the last drink and result in extreme autonomic instability, which can culminate in cardiovascular collapse. Manifestations of DTs include fluctuating level of consciousness, with profound disorientation, delirium, hallucinations, coarse generalized tremor, marked vital sign elevation, severe agitation, nausea, vomiting, and diarrhea. Before the use of benzodiazepines the mortality rate for patients with untreated DTs was 30%; with definitive care, this has decreased to 2% to 4%.[203]

Seizures can occur in the absence of other obvious signs of the withdrawal syndrome. They typically occur within 7 to 48 hours after the cessation of drinking. These are isolated, generalized tonic-clonic seizures, which are usually self-limiting and rarely exceed six episodes over a period of several hours. They can be treated with intravenous lorazepam or diazepam.[180] Alcohol withdrawal seizures usually do not advance to status epilepticus. Patients who develop sequential seizures must be evaluated emergently for other possible causes such as worsening of a head injury or preexisting seizure disorder.

Assessment. Patients who have positive BACs or who are known to be active drinkers should be monitored for signs and symptoms of withdrawal. Parameters to be monitored include heart rate, blood pressure, temperature, orientation, and presence or absence of tremor. Tremor may be noted in the extremities or the protruded tongue.

Treatment. Treatment for alcohol withdrawal should be instituted before or early in the course of the withdrawal syndrome to minimize the risk of DTs or seizures. Patients in withdrawal who are not identified until they develop DTs are at higher risk for complications and require much larger doses of sedatives to control the CNS excitation. Patients with a history of alcohol withdrawal syndrome or a very high admission BAC should be started on a prophylactic regimen of a benzodiazepine.[204]

Benzodiazepines are ideal drugs for prevention and treatment of alcohol withdrawal because they are cross-tolerant with alcohol, do not induce hepatic microsomal enzymes, produce little alteration in coagulation parameters, and have anticonvulsant properties. In patients without liver disease, a long-acting benzodiazepine is most efficacious. Agents such as chlordiazepoxide have active metabolites, which provide a built-in taper of the drug. For patients with severe liver disease, a short-acting benzodiazepine such as lorazepam, without active metabolites, prevents the development of secondary oversedation caused by the buildup of undetoxified metabolites. Table 32-9 presents information about the agents commonly used in the prevention and treatment of alcohol withdrawal.

Various dosing schedules have been used for detoxification. For any of the schedules, dosing must be individualized to adequately relieve the signs and symptoms of withdrawal. Some patients require extremely high doses because of their

TABLE 32-9 Benzodiazepines Commonly Used for Alcohol Withdrawal Management

Drug	Pharmacology
Diazepam (Valium)	Active metabolite
	Long acting
	Incomplete IM absorption; should be given IV or PO
	Total body clearance is inversely proportional to patient's age and directly proportional to liver function
Chlordiazepoxide (Librium)	Active metabolite
	Long acting
	Manufacturer recommends no more than 300 mg/day
	Can be given IV; however, do not use accompanying diluent for IV administration, use sterile normal saline instead; diluent is intended for IM use only
Oxazepam (Serax)	No active metabolite
	Intermediate acting
	Oral route only
	Useful for elderly patients and those with hypoalbuminemia
Lorazepam (Ativan)	No active metabolite
	Short acting
	Useful for patients with hepatic dysfunction
Midazolam (Versed)	Active metabolite
	Ultra short acting
	Most rapidly inactivated benzodiazepine
	May be useful as infusion in critically ill patients

high tolerance for CNS depressants. Three commonly used schedules are tapering, loading, and symptom triggered. Tapering consists of routinely scheduled doses of medication that are tapered gradually over 2 to 3 days. Commonly used drugs are chlordiazepoxide and diazepam. Both drugs are long acting with active metabolites, which provide a natural taper after cessation. If a short-acting agent such as lorazepam is used, the drug must be tapered by decreasing the dose rather than increasing the dosing interval. Increasing the dosing interval of short-acting agents can result in breakthrough of withdrawal symptoms. During tapering, doses are not administered when there is excessive sedation or the patient is sleeping soundly.[162]

Loading is a technique whereby medication is supplied when the withdrawal symptoms are most severe. By using drugs with long half-lives, it is possible to allow a self-taper. Diazepam is often used because it has a half-life of 40 hours. Diazepam (20 mg) is given every 1 to 2 hours to a minimal cumulative dose of 60 mg or until the patient is symptom free. This strategy is often used in outpatient detoxification and may be useful for stable inpatients.[162]

TABLE 32-10 Sullivan Protocol

Symptom	Point Value*	Scale
Tremor	1	Tremor felt by examiner but not visible
	2	Mild, visible tremor
	3	Marked, visible tremor
Tachycardia	1	Pulse rate 80-100 beats/min
	2	Pulse rate 100-130 beats/min
	3	Pulse rate >130 beats/min
Hypertension (valid only in absence of hypertensive history)	1	Systolic 150-175 mm Hg
	2	Systolic 175-200 mm Hg
	3	Systolic >200 mm Hg
Diaphoresis	1	Mild, barely visible
	2	Moderate
	3	Marked; gown/bedding wet
Nausea/vomiting	1	Nausea only
	2	Vomits two or fewer times in 8 hours
	3	Frequent vomiting, dry heaves
Fever	1	38° C or less
	2	38-38.5° C
	3	>38.5° C
Agitation	1	Activity increased
	2	Restless, fidgety
	3	Restless, trashing in bed
Confusion, orientation, contact with reality	1	Detached, decreased sensation, vague orientation
	2	Vague about present illness, disorientation is infrequent
	3	Detached, no staff contact, disoriented
Sleeplessness	1	Awake during night (two or three times)
	2	Awake half the night or more
Hallucinations	1	Auditory only or visual only, not agitated from hallucinations
	2	Unrelated auditory and visual hallucinations
	3	Auditory and visual hallucinations are related
Seizure		Document presence or absence.

From Watling SM, Fleming C, Casey P et al: Nursing-based protocol for treatment of alcohol withdrawal in the intensive care unit, *Am J Crit Care* 4:66-70, 1995.

*If a sign/symptom is not present, score as "0."

Symptom-triggered dosing is the preferred method of withdrawal management. It uses withdrawal signs and symptoms to guide dosing. An inventory of signs and symptoms is used to measure the severity of the withdrawal.[180] Standardized scales such as the Revised Clinical Institute Withdrawal Assessment Scale for Alcohol (CIWA-Ar)[205] provide good validity, interrater reliability, and clinical utility.[180] Doses are given in response to a threshold score obtained from the inventory. Withdrawal scores also offer a means to monitor response to treatment. Research has shown that use of a symptom inventory minimizes the incidence of both oversedation and undertreatment of withdrawal. Use of symptom-triggered dosing ultimately results in lower amounts of drugs used during withdrawal and fewer episodes of excessive sedation.[180]

The Sullivan Protocol (Table 32-10), a modification of the CIWA-Ar, has been adapted for use in critically ill patients. Patients are scored every 2 hours while awake and every 4 while asleep, and they receive a graduated dose depending on their score. Table 32-11 provides examples of graduated dosing using lorazepam and diazepam. The score

TABLE 32-11 Sample Benzodiazepine Dosing Chart

Severity Score	Lorazepam Dose	Diazepam Dose
>12	4 mg	10 mg
10-11	3 mg	7.5 mg
8-9	2 mg	5 mg
6-7	1 mg	2.5 mg
0-5	0 mg	0 mg

From Watling SM, Fleming C, Casey P et al: Nursing-based protocol for treatment of alcohol withdrawal in the intensive care unit, *Am J Crit Care* 4:66-70, 1995.

is reassessed 30 minutes after dosing, and the dose is repeated if the score remains higher than 5 and the respiratory rate is more than 12. Some patients may require higher doses than those shown in the table. When the withdrawal score is consistently greater than 5 after repeated doses of medication, increasing the doses for the patient is indicated.[206]

Haloperidol can be used for hallucinosis and is administered in intravenous or oral doses of 2.5 to 10 mg/hr up to a total dose of 200 mg/day. Haloperidol should not be used as the sole agent for treating alcohol withdrawal because it does not decrease autonomic hyperactivity and can reduce the seizure threshold, thus precipitating or exacerbating withdrawal seizures.[180]

Clonidine is an α-adrenergic blocking agent that mitigates the autonomic hyperactivity seen in alcohol withdrawal syndrome.[162] It is less efficacious in reducing cravings and anxiety. It must be used cautiously in the patient dependent on CNS depressants because it has no anticonvulsant properties.[180] Hypotensive side effects of clonidine may limit its usefulness for withdrawal management. Clonidine dosing starts with a 0.1-mg test dose after measuring baseline heart rate and blood pressure. Vital signs are measured again 30 minutes after the test dose. Depending on the test dose results, patients can be started on 0.1 to 0.2 mg of clonidine four times a day for 2 to 3 days. The clonidine is then tapered over a period of 5 to 10 days. Patients receiving 0.2 mg should have the dose decreased initially and then reduced by discontinuing a dose every 2 to 3 days.[207]

Patients' vital signs and neurologic status should be monitored every 1 to 4 hours for the first 72 hours, depending on the severity of withdrawal and associated injuries. Alterations in vital signs characteristic of withdrawal syndromes may be the first indication that the patient is experiencing acute withdrawal. Other nursing care priorities include monitoring fluid and electrolyte balance and initiating seizures precautions.

Sedative-Hypnotic Withdrawal. Sedative-hypnotic withdrawal symptoms are similar to those of alcohol withdrawal. Onset and duration vary with the half-life of the agent used. Symptoms of sedative-hypnotic withdrawal include tremor, muscle twitching, weakness, nausea, vomiting, anorexia, restlessness, irritability, insomnia, blurred vision, vital sign elevations, mydriasis, and diaphoresis. The clinical picture during withdrawal from moderate use may be dominated by subjective symptoms with few observable signs, as is characteristic with alcohol withdrawal. Seizures and delirium may be seen with abstinence after high-dose use. Sedative-hypnotic withdrawal must be considered in any patient with a history of withdrawal symptoms after cessation of sedative-hypnotics. Patients who have been on a short-acting benzodiazepine for longer than 6 weeks, those taking average daily doses of one and a half to two times the normal dose of longer-acting agents for 45 days, and those who have taken therapeutic doses for a year or more are at risk for withdrawal symptoms after sedative-hypnotic cessation.[208]

Withdrawal management from sedative-hypnotics is most often accomplished with phenobarbital substitution and tapering. Phenobarbital is cross-tolerant with other CNS depressants. Patients are medicated with an initial test dose of 30 mg of phenobarbital or its equivalent. Patients who respond to the test dose should demonstrate a decrease in subjective complaints, reduction in tremor if present, and a decrease in autonomic hyperactivity. The patient is then observed for somnolence, dysarthria, slurred speech, and lack of coordination. If any of these develops, the dose is excessive and should be reduced. After determining the response to the test dose, patients are medicated hourly on an as-needed basis (PRN) with 30 to 60 mg of phenobarbital or its equivalent. The period of PRN dosing is determined by the duration of action of the abused substances. When the patient has received similar 24-hour doses of phenobarbital for 2 consecutive days, the total dose is divided by 2. This stabilizing dose is administered in divided doses over the next 24 hours to determine if adequate stabilization has occurred. The dosage of phenobarbital is then decreased in increments of 30 mg every day for 80% of the dose. The final 20% of the dose should be decreased daily in increments of 15 mg. Tapering too rapidly leads to mental status changes and autonomic hyperactivity.[181]

OPIATE WITHDRAWAL. All the opiates have similar withdrawal signs and symptoms although the time frame and intensity of symptoms vary depending on the drug used. As with other drugs, the time until development of withdrawal depends of the half-life of the drug or drugs used. Short-acting opiates such as heroin, morphine, and meperidine have a brief, intense withdrawal syndrome that typically begins 4 to 6 hours after the last dose and lasts 5 to 10 days.[209] Long-acting agents such as methadone are characterized by a milder withdrawal syndrome that begins 72 to 84 hours after the last dose but may persist for several weeks.

Assessment. Acute withdrawal from heroin peaks in intensity 48 to 72 hours after cessation. Symptoms include yawning, lacrimation, rhinorrhea, diaphoresis, mydriasis, myalgia, tremors, nausea, vomiting, diarrhea, abdominal cramps, fever, chills, tachycardia, hypertension, and piloerection.[209] Many of these symptoms are caused by increased activity of the autonomic nervous system. Patients are anxious and irritable and experience strong drug cravings. Muscle cramping and gastrointestinal hyperactivity are especially distressing. The expression "kick the habit" originated from the observation that heroin users move their legs continuously to relieve the cramping associated with acute withdrawal. Opiate withdrawal is seldom life-threatening in a healthy individual and is often compared to influenza in severity. However, the traumatized patient may be unable to tolerate the added stress of withdrawal.

Treatment. Acute opioid withdrawal can be treated successfully with daily administration of a long-acting opioid such as methadone.[209] The goal of methadone maintenance in the trauma patient is to supplement the patient's previous opioid requirement with methadone in a dose sufficient to prevent signs and symptoms of withdrawal. It is available in oral preparations and a parenteral form. Patients with a known history or objective evidence of opioid abuse, such as positive toxicology results combined with physical signs of intravenous use, can be started on methadone early in their hospital course. If a patient is enrolled in a methadone maintenance program, health care providers can obtain consent and then contact the treatment facility to determine the patient's current dose. Although strict federal guidelines control the use of methadone for detoxification of outpatients, it can be ordered for opioid detoxification for acutely hospitalized inpatients. Initial doses of methadone for detoxification and maintenance range from 60 to 100 mg/day,[210] although 10 to 40 mg is generally sufficient to control symptoms of withdrawal. A patient's initial dose can be determined by assessing the patient's response to 20 mg of methadone. The dose can then be increased if no observable effect is seen.[209] Intravenous doses of methadone, for patients unable to take enteral medication, are typically one half to two thirds of the oral dose.[210] The methadone can be tapered by 5 mg every 2 to 3 days. Patients who require methadone after discharge from the hospital must be referred to methadone maintenance programs.

Clonidine, an α-adrenergic agent, may be used to block much of the sympathetic hyperactivity associated with opioid withdrawal. It has little effect, however, on the drug cravings, mood alterations, and muscle cramps characteristic of this withdrawal syndrome. Clonidine withdrawal from opiates generally takes 5 to 7 days and is similar to the procedure described for alcohol withdrawal. Hypotension is a possible but uncommon side effect of clonidine use for withdrawal.[209]

Buprenorphine, an opioid with both agonist and antagonist properties, may also be used to manage opioid withdrawal in select trauma patients. Although used in many centers for opioid detoxification, it has not been approved for this use by the Food and Drug Administration (FDA). Buprenorphine undergoes a high first-pass metabolism and for this reason is administered sublingually or parenterally. Typical doses for detoxification are 0.3 to 0.6 mg intramuscularly two to four times a day, 8 mg subcutaneously once a day, or 6 to 8 mg sublingually once a day.[112,210] The buprenorphine is then tapered over several days. The once-daily doses can be tapered by 1 or 2 mg/day and, when using the intramuscular route, by decreasing both the dosing interval and dose simultaneously. Buprenorphine should not be used for patients who have required a short-acting opioid in the past 6 hours, those with symptoms of opioid intoxication, or those who have received methadone in the previous 24 hours, because it may precipitate acute withdrawal.[210] Patients who are likely to require surgery or administration of opiates in the near future should also not be considered candidates for buprenorphine use.

Analgesia in Opioid Dependence. Methadone should not be used as the sole analgesic for the treatment of acute pain. Conventional shorter-acting agents such as morphine sulfate or fentanyl should be given in addition to methadone to manage acute pain. Analgesic doses required for pain relief vary widely and must be titrated to the individual patient. Typically, though, patients require doses at the high end of the dosing range and may require more frequent dosing because of the increased metabolism of narcotics. Patient-controlled analgesia (PCA) used in conjunction with methadone can be an effective strategy for the opioid-abusing patient. Use of PCA also prevents power struggles between patients and care providers over administration times. As acute pain decreases, patients can then be switched to oral formulations such as oxycodone or acetaminophen with codeine.[211]

Nonsteroidal antiinflammatory drugs (NSAIDs) are also efficacious in patients addicted to narcotics and can be used in conjunction with narcotic analgesia. Patients should be started on routine scheduled doses of NSAIDs in addition to narcotic analgesics. Ketorolac, an NSAID available in a parenteral form, can be used when patients are unable to take enteral medications.[211]

There are multiple reports documenting the fact that health care providers undermedicate patients for fear of initiating or exacerbating addiction. Studies have demonstrated that, although patients on long-term opioids may become physically dependent, true addiction, with its attendant mental and behavioral components, is rare. When a patient has a known substance abuse disorder, health care providers may be even more vigilant in their attempts to limit the use of opioids to avoid perpetuating the addiction or creating a second addiction.[212] In general, patients with a history of substance dependence have a higher tolerance to narcotics compared with the general population. However, tolerance varies from person to person, just as it does among persons not dependent on chemicals.

Analgesia in Recovering Patients. Health care providers may encounter chemically dependent patients who are in recovery at the time of their injury. These patients and their health care providers share legitimate concerns about reactivating addiction. It is, however, inappropriate to withhold analgesia to prevent relapse. What is warranted is active participation by the patient in identifying pain, communicating adequate pain relief or lack thereof, and describing drug cravings. Health care providers should review daily with the patient the analgesia plan and any drug cravings experienced. Use of nonpharmacologic modalities such as relaxation, heat, and elevation should be used along with nonnarcotic forms of analgesia whenever possible. The patient must also have ready access to support systems. Relapse is not a given when chemically dependent patients are treated for acute pain as long as issues of analgesia, fears about relapse, and coping strategies for drug cravings are addressed.[212]

CENTRAL NERVOUS SYSTEM STIMULANT WITHDRAWAL. Withdrawal of a CNS stimulant, although highly unpleasant for the patient, is not associated with the high morbidity of CNS depressant withdrawal.[209] Because stimulants have relatively short half-lives, they are often used in a binge pattern in which the user continuously readministers the drug in response to declining blood levels. Binges may last for several days. On cessation of this heavy drug use, a person experiences withdrawal, which is usually short term and self-limiting. The period for the development of withdrawal varies with the stimulant used and the route by which it was ingested. Amphetamine withdrawal has a later onset and longer duration than cocaine withdrawal although symptoms of these two abstinence syndromes are similar. As with any withdrawal syndrome, the physiologic and behavioral manifestations tend to be reciprocal of what is seen during acute intoxication.

Stimulant craving begins minutes to hours after the last dose of drug was administered. The initial drug craving is followed by what is often referred to as "the crash," a period of intense dysphoria, depression, anxiety, strong drug cravings, and possible psychomotor agitation.[213] The length of the crash varies from 12 hours to 4 days for cocaine and up to a week for methamphetamine. Some patients experience suicidal ideation during the dysphoric phase. Toward the end of the crash, hypersomnia develops and can last up to 4 days. Although patients are hypersomnic, they may experience sleep cycle alterations. After the crash, sleep cycles begin to normalize, appetite increases, the patient's mood stabilizes, and cravings abate. During the early phase of withdrawal, physiologic parameters, including heart rate, blood pressure, and respiratory rate, return to baseline.[209]

Although stimulant withdrawal is usually mild and self-limiting, a few patients have experienced myocardial ischemia, most during the first week of withdrawal. Stimulant abusers also experience intermittent drug cravings for an indefinite period after cessation. They are particularly susceptible to environmental cues, which serve as triggers for drug use.

Treatment.   Currently there are no specific pharmacologic treatments for acute CNS stimulant withdrawal. Although various drugs have been studied for use during stimulant withdrawal, none is clearly efficacious. Highly anxious patients may benefit from a short-acting benzodiazepine, and those with prolonged dysphoria may benefit from tricyclic antidepressant therapy. Stimulant withdrawal is best treated supportively by permitting the patient to sleep and eat as much as necessary.[213] Ideally treatment should be aimed at promoting return of natural sleep cycles and minimizing anxiety although this may be difficult in the critical care environment. A calm, quiet environment with appropriate lighting and scheduled activities with periods of rest can alleviate some of the distress associated with the withdrawal period. The patient should be encouraged, if possible, to appropriately express any feelings related to the experience, and the health care provider should offer reassurance that these feeling are normal in the setting of cocaine or amphetamine withdrawal.[150] Evidence of suicidal ideation should be reported to the physician immediately.

CANNABIS WITHDRAWAL.   Acute marijuana withdrawal is a mild syndrome associated with abrupt cessation after heavy, regular cannabis use. Withdrawal symptoms include irritability, restlessness, insomnia, anorexia, nausea, diarrhea, weight loss, and muscle twitching. Physiologic alterations include mild increases in heart rate, temperature, and blood pressure. Symptoms of marijuana withdrawal abate without treatment.[213] As with CNS stimulant withdrawal, patients benefit from a calm environment.

NICOTINE WITHDRAWAL.   Because of the short half-life of nicotine, symptoms of nicotine withdrawal begin within 30 minutes after the last nicotine dose and peak in about 24 hours. Full detoxification is reached in about 72 hours although cravings may persist for several weeks. Withdrawal is characterized by intense cravings, irritability, agitation, insomnia, anxiety, dysphoria, difficulty concentrating, decreased heart rate and blood pressure, decreased intestinal motility, and increased appetite with associated weight gain over time.[214] Patients often complain of "needing" a cigarette, and they may attempt to leave the patient care area in an effort to secure one.

Treatment.   Patients can be started on a transdermal nicotine patch at the standard starting dose of 21 mg/day. This provides roughly the equivalent of one pack of cigarettes per day. If the patient has typically smoked more than a pack per day, he or she may experience some symptoms of nicotine withdrawal even at the maximal patch dose; however, the withdrawal severity is decreased. Patients who are hospitalized for a long time may be able to complete the entire series of tapered dosing during that hospital stay. Mitigating the symptoms of nicotine withdrawal can decrease the patient's levels of anxiety, irritability, and insomnia. Severe cardiovascular disease and sensitivity to the patch are the only major contraindications to its use. Patch sites should be rotated daily to avoid local skin irritation, and patches should be applied to relatively hair-free areas to promote maximal absorption.[215]

NURSING MANAGEMENT CONSIDERATIONS

NUTRITIONAL DEFICIENCIES.   Treatment of Wernicke's encephalopathy should be instituted in any patient with a history of alcohol abuse or a positive BAC on admission.[216] Patients should receive 100 mg of thiamine parenterally for a minimum of 3 days. Parenteral administration either as an additive to intravenous fluid or intramuscularly ensures absorption. Patients need thiamine repletion before receiving glucose solutions or feedings because carbohydrates can precipitate or worsen the encephalopathy. Patients should also receive 1 mg/day of folate and a multivitamin supplement either parenterally or enterally.[198] Magnesium levels should be normalized because hypomagnesemia can increase resistance to thiamine.

Consultation with a registered dietitian is invaluable in assessing the dietary needs of substance abusers. Patients with long-standing alcoholism are often deficient in macronutrients, vitamins, and minerals. Alcohol is an energy-dense but nutrient-poor nutritional source. As much as 50% of the chronic alcoholic's caloric intake may be derived from alcohol.[80] Patients with severe hepatic dysfunction may require limited protein to prevent the development of hepatic encephalopathy.[198] Increased protein requirements as a result of injury must be balanced with the risk of encephalopathy. Patients using cocaine may be emaciated because of the appetite suppressant effect of cocaine. In addition, they probably chose to spend their limited financial resources on the drug rather than on food. These patients benefit from small, frequent feedings if they are taking food orally.[162]

The various anemias associated with drug and alcohol abuse can be treated with folic acid or ferrous sulfate. Folic acid is given at 1 mg/day orally or parenterally as an IV fluid additive. Ferrous sulfate (325 mg PO tid) is administered with food to minimize gastric irritation. Ferrous sulfate liquid can be administered to patients receiving liquid enteral feeding.

RISK OF INFECTION.   Research has identified alcohol's adverse effects on the immune system. These adverse effects result in depression of immune function, increasing the person's predisposition for cancer and infectious diseases. Immune system derangements include decreased activity of natural killer cells,[217,218] diminished neutrophil activity, and impaired lymphocyte function.[219] One study of patients with penetrating abdominal trauma found that those with a BAC more than 200 mg/dl at the time of admission experienced a greater than twofold incidence of trauma-related infections.[220] In another study of trauma patients, chronic alcohol use was associated with a twofold increase in infectious complications.[26] Patients who use inhaled drugs are likely to have impaired pulmonary immune response. Tobacco, marijuana, and cocaine smoke all cause dysfunction of alveolar macrophages, one of the primary immune defenses of the pulmonary tree.[129] Patients who abuse alcohol or intravenous drugs have a high incidence of tuberculosis (TB), many with highly resistant strains.

Intravenous drug abusers have a high risk of contracting bloodborne infections and may already have an underlying infection such as hepatitis, human immunodeficiency virus (HIV), or subclinical bacterial endocarditis.[184] Patients with elevated liver enzymes and signs and symptoms consistent with hepatitis infection should be tested for both hepatitis B and C and HIV.[221] Patients who present with or develop opportunistic infections consistent with HIV infection should be tested for that virus.

Bacterial endocarditis (BE) and its sequelae are other common co-morbidities found in intravenous drug abusers. Unlike patients with rheumatic heart disease who develop BE, intravenous drug abusers often have BE in the valves on the right side of the heart.[161] These patients are at risk for pulmonary infarctions from septic emboli. Patients consistently running a temperature of 38.5° C or higher in the absence of other conditions are highly suspect for BE.

Infections should be identified and treated aggressively to minimize complications. Trauma patients who demonstrate clinical evidence of possible infection (e.g., fever, leukocytosis) should be evaluated for sources of infection, including those associated with substance abuse. As with any patient, health care team members should prevent opportunities for nosocomial infections by practicing strict universal precautions and using appropriate sterile technique.

ALTERATIONS IN RESPIRATORY FUNCTION.   Regular pulmonary toilet is a crucial aspect of nursing care for these patients. Those who are able to cooperate with incentive spirometry should have it instituted as soon as possible in their hospital course. Patients who are mechanically ventilated or are unable to cooperate with incentive spirometry as a result of cognitive impairment require chest physiotherapy and either endotracheal or nasotracheal suctioning in order to mobilize secretions. Routine turning and mobilization out of bed to a chair as soon as possible help to mobilize secretions and maintain alveolar patency.

ILLICIT DRUG USE DURING HOSPITALIZATION.   Withdrawal from mood-altering drugs such as alcohol, cocaine, opiates, and nicotine frequently causes strong drug cravings. Hospitalized patients may try to acquire drugs from illicit sources to satisfy themselves. If sudden alterations in mood or behavior suggest that a patient has obtained illicit drugs, a repeat toxicology screen may be required to document the occurrence. Supervised visitation may become necessary under these circumstances.

INTERMEDIATE CARE AND REHABILITATION PHASES

The intermediate care and rehabilitation phases focus on returning patients to their optimal functional status. For the substance-abusing patient, this also includes the need to address the substance abuse as a primary disorder, the outcome of which was traumatic injury. Patient education should focus on the impact of the substance abuse and chemical dependency as a chronic disorder with its own natural history, similar to that of other chronic diseases.

NURSING MANAGEMENT CONSIDERATIONS

FAMILY DYNAMICS.   Alcoholic families are typically unstable and chaotic. Altered communication patterns within these families may include silence, decreased sharing, and active concealment of problems. Individual members are neglected and their needs unmet. Much of the family's energy has been directed at controlling the chemically dependent member and coping with the consequences of substance abuse. High levels of anger and guilt are common. An acute traumatic event exacerbates the level of stress in what is already a stressed system. Family members may be unable to work together for mutual support and problem solving.[222]

In addition to the other fears experienced by all trauma families, families of substance abusers may have the additional burden of wondering if this was another in a series of incidents related to the substance abuse. Family members may inquire about drinking or other drug use before the injury. Toxicology results are confidential and require the patient's written consent before any release of information. Release of information about substance use is governed by strict federal regulations.[153] A family that has secured legal representation for the patient needs to have the patient give written consent for the release of medical records to the attorney.

Roles are often reversed in substance-abusing families. Parents may have abdicated their roles to children, or a spouse may be fulfilling the roles of two people. The legal next of kin might not be able to execute the role of family spokesperson. The nurse may need to identify which person is actually capable of fulfilling the spokesperson role and communicate directly with him or her.[223]

IMPAIRED GASTROINTESTINAL FUNCTION.   Risk for disruption of the gastrointestinal tract after trauma can be exacerbated by preexisting gastritis, gastric ulcerations, and drug-induced liver damage in the substance-abusing patient. All trauma patients who are not receiving or tolerating enteral feedings should be on prophylaxis for stress ulcers. Patients with known cirrhosis or esophageal varices who require gastric intubation should be monitored closely for signs of bleeding because the gastric tube can erode the already friable varices. Esophageal variceal hemorrhage is a medical emergency with high mortality.

SLEEP PATTERN DISRUPTION.   Most patients with a history of substance abuse experience sleep cycle disruption in the acute withdrawal period. Stimulant abusers sleep more during the acute withdrawal period and experience more rapid eye movement (REM) sleep. In contrast, alcoholics experience less total sleep and REM during the acute withdrawal phase.[224] Promoting normalization of sleep cycles by providing uninterrupted rest periods, manipulating room lighting to simulate day and night, and using relaxation techniques is important to prevent sleep deprivation, which can adversely affect respiration and neurologic status.

MOTIVATIONAL CRISIS

An injury episode necessitating hospitalization can serve as a pivotal point in the course of substance abuse. It may provide a window of opportunity with which to confront the substance abuser with the reality of his or her disease process. Although some patients minimize the role of alcohol in causing their injury,[225] hospitalization may diminish some of the psychologic barriers substance abusers maintain to minimize the consequences of their substance use.[226] Studies have indicated that trauma patients are more

willing to change behavior after injury[227] and more amenable to treatment for substance abuse.[228]

INTERVENING IN SUBSTANCE ABUSE

Review of available literature demonstrates that trauma centers have done a fair job of detecting psychoactive drug-abusing and drug-dependent clients and a less adequate job of counseling or referring them for appropriate chemical dependency treatment after acute hospitalization and rehabilitation. There may be a bias on the part of health care providers that there is little they can do to assist these patients.[228] There is evidence, however, that even brief interventions may encourage drug-using patients to alter their behavior.[229-231] Research from a level I trauma center demonstrated a reduction in alcohol consumption and re-injury rates in patients who received brief intervention (BI).[232]

The nurse is usually the person who has greatest amount of patient contact to permit such an intervention. A calm, nonjudgmental approach that helps the patient to examine the consequences of his or her substance use is appropriate. An assessment of the patient's perceptions regarding the need for change and what is necessary to effect the change should be performed in this phase of the trauma cycle. Patients can be referred to a substance abuse clinician if more intensive treatment is warranted.

SUBSTANCE ABUSE TREATMENT.   Patients admitted with positive toxicology screens, those who develop withdrawal syndromes after admission, and patients whose screening tool results indicate substance abuse despite negative toxicology results should be evaluated by a substance abuse clinician. This person may be a physician, advanced practice nurse, or social worker trained in substance abuse assessment, prevention, treatment, and referral. A substance abuse treatment team, if available, should provide consultation for patients and provide referrals for intensive outpatient or inpatient substance abuse treatment after the acute hospitalization. Addiction specialists may also be invaluable for managing patients with protracted withdrawal syndromes or psychiatric co-morbidities.

One study documented a 62% acceptance rate for treatment in a group of trauma patients evaluated by a substance abuse consultation team.[233] The American Society of Addiction Medicine (ASAM) has developed a set of patient placement criteria for determining the appropriate level of treatment. It uses six dimensions for evaluating addiction severity. Levels of treatment range from patient education to long-term residential treatment, depending on the level of dependence.[234] Providers should offer treatment alternatives rather than a single option because research has failed to show consistent outcomes based on type of treatment.[235] If the patient desires treatment, arrangements can be made at this time and incorporated into the discharge planning. Ideally there should be a seamless flow from discharge to entrance into substance abuse treatment.

Many hospitals have no formal chemical dependency counseling available, and nursing staff may be the only link to substance abuse treatment and community support resources. Nurses employed at such facilities can develop a directory of treatment centers and community resources in order to facilitate ongoing care for these patients. At a minimum, content about chemical dependency should be incorporated into the education plan for patients with evidence of drug abuse. This includes information about adverse effects of the substances, the personal and interpersonal impact of substance use, with a focus on traumatic injury as a direct result of substance use, the chronic nature of substance use disorders, and the availability of treatment.

BRIEF INTERVENTION. *Brief intervention* refers to strategic action on the part of a health care provider with the intent of effecting behavioral change.[228] BI is composed of a variety of activities directed at problem drinkers who are not alcohol dependent. These activities are of low intensity and short duration. They usually consist of 3 to 5 sessions, each lasting 5 to 60 minutes. The content is instructional and motivational. It consists of feedback from screening tests and laboratory results, drug education, and practical advice.[236] Although BI was used initially with problem drinkers, it has been applied to other addictive behaviors as well.

BI has been found to be just as effective as more formal interventions. BI performed by primary health care providers has been proven effective for treating socially stable, heavy-drinking medical patients.[237,238] This therapy reduced alcohol consumption by 25% to 35%.[239] BI is not appropriate for highly alcohol-dependent patients. These patients should be referred to an addictionologist or other chemical dependency professional for substance abuse treatment referral.[236] BI has been found efficacious in trauma patients and adolescents seen in emergency departments after alcohol-related incidents. Alcohol consumption and re-injury have been decreased in both groups with the use of BI.[232,240]

Stages of Change. The stages of change model was developed by Prochaska, DiClemente, and Norcross based on their observations of how people change. Much of their research targeted problem behaviors involving alcohol and cigarettes. Their research demonstrated that change is a series of stages, each with distinct characteristics. People move back and forth between the stages, often several times before permanent change occurs. Change is rarely linear.[241]

The six stages of change are precontemplation, contemplation, preparation, action, maintenance, and termination. Each stage has defining behaviors and characteristics. Health care providers can intervene with patients in any of the stages although each stage has different intervention strategies that are most effective. Matching interventions to the patient's current stage is critical because interventions performed at the wrong stage are counterproductive.[241]

Patients in the precontemplation stage do not perceive that a problem exists; thus they do not identify any need to alter their behavior. Although the problem is clear to others, the patient is oblivious. These patients are often said to be in

denial; however, they can be motivated to change with use of the proper tools.[228,241]

Contemplators acknowledge the existence of a problem and contemplate change. They struggle to understand their problem and search for solutions. They frequently tell themselves they need to change but have indefinite plans for change. Generally their intent is to effect change within the next 6 months. Additionally, they are unsure how to change.[228,241]

People in the preparation stage intend to act within the next month. The are committed to action and appear ready but often have unresolved ambivalence. Commonly they are trying to decide which course of action is best.[228,241]

The action stage is characterized by overt modification of behavior and the environment. This stage places the greatest demand on time and energy. It is the most visible to others. Patients receive the most feedback during the action phase, but feedback is critical during all the phases.[228,241]

Maintenance involves the day-to-day struggle to consolidate the changes made during the action phase and avoid relapse. The process of change does not end with action.[228,241]

Termination is the final stage of change. In this phase the former problem is no longer a temptation or threat. No effort is required on the person's part to maintain the change. At this point, change is complete and the cycle of change is exited. Although this is the ultimate goal, many authorities believe that this stage is unattainable for problems like substance dependence. Substance dependence is considered by most to be a chronic problem like diabetes, for which termination is not possible.[228,241]

The FRAMES Model. The FRAMES model of brief alcohol intervention has six components[237]: feedback, responsibility, advice, menu, empathy, and self-efficacy (Table 32-12). Not all components are necessarily used during each counseling session. Some are more relevant than others during the various stages in the change process.[237]

The FRAMES model and other processes are helpful for promoting change in drug use.[226] Consciousness raising and social liberation are effective during precontemplation, when individuals actively resist change. Many are discour-

TABLE 32-12 FRAMES Model

Feedback: respectfully giving specific information that concerns the patient
Responsibility: stressing that the patient is responsible for any change
Advice: respectfully giving advice to the patient
Menu: offering patient a menu of choices
Empathy: listening and forming accurate reflective statements
Self-efficacy: (a) change is possible and (b) change is beneficial

From Bien TH, Miller WR, Tonigan JS: Brief interventions for alcohol problems: a review, *Addiction* 88:315-335, 1993.

aged and unsure if change is possible. Health care providers can explore how patients feel when the behavior is discussed. Defensiveness about the behavior is common at this stage. Consciousness raising presumes that the individual lacks knowledge about the problem. The patient's awareness of the risks and benefits of the behavior and his or her willingness to accept the consequences associated with the behavior should be determined. Consciousness raising includes increasing the level of knowledge about defense mechanisms used to perpetuate the behavior. The patient's defense mechanisms should be explored. Minimizing the problem, acting out, and blaming others are common defense strategies. At this stage it is counterproductive to push for active change. *Social liberation* implies helping patients create more options. They should be helped in identifying available support systems, and their willingness to use the social resources should be assessed.[228] The goal of these interventions is to increase ambivalence, a sign that a patient has moved into the contemplation phase.[241]

Emotional arousal or propaganda is effective during contemplation.[241] The interventionist can review the risks and benefits of continued drug or alcohol use. The goal is to make the risks more prominent in the patient's mind. Videos and photos of injury scenes can be useful at this stage. The patient should be asked to summarize his or her perception of personal risk.[228]

The preparation stage involves assisting the patient in planning how to implement change. Setting a quit date, removing paraphernalia, telling others about the intention to quit, and enlisting social support aid in making the change a priority. Careful planning in the preparation stage can facilitate the transition to the action phase.[228,241]

During the action stage, several interventions promote the change process. Taking purposeful action, identifying and actively avoiding drug use triggers, and engaging in diversional activities all promote successful change. Positive feedback and recognition are crucial in this phase.[228,241]

Maintenance requires sustained long-term effort to continue the lifestyle changes initiated during the action phase. Complacence about maintaining behavioral modifications and overconfidence are pitfalls in this phase. Health care providers can offer ongoing positive feedback while acknowledging any difficulties. They should reinforce the benefits of change. This is a time when external feedback often wanes.[228,241]

During termination, by definition, no further action is required to maintain the change. Recovery from chemical dependency generally does not reach this stage, but with early substance abuse, reaching the termination stage may be possible. Relapse, although not part of the stages of change model, is commonly encountered in the field of addiction medicine. It is a process of reversing the changes made in recovery and ultimately resuming addictive behaviors.[228,242]

SOCIAL NETWORK INTERVENTION. A social network intervention (SNI) or traditional intervention is orchestrated by an interventionist, usually a chemical dependency professional or psychiatrist. An intervention involves several members of the patient's social network. They meet with the interventionist, who provides education about alcoholism or drug addiction and the need for treatment and ascertains how the people have been affected by the substance abuse. The intervention group then meets with the patient. The participants describe the impact and emotional effects of incidents they have witnessed during the individual's substance abuse.[228] This type of intervention is efficacious in trauma patients, but it is time and labor intensive compared with BI.[243]

COMMUNITY REINTEGRATION

OUTPATIENT FOLLOW-UP

After hospital discharge, outpatients should be questioned about ongoing use of psychoactive substances. Any evidence of use should be noted in the patient's chart. Reasons for remaining abstinent previously identified by the patient can be reviewed at this time, and barriers to continued abstinence can be explored.[228] Clinicians can ascertain what patients are doing to promote abstinence and offer feedback to reinforce positive behavioral changes.[244]

COMMUNITY SUPPORT SYSTEMS

Community support resources can be invaluable to the patient with a substance abuse disorder. Alcoholic Anonymous (AA), which is widely available and free, is the most familiar community resource.[245] AA uses a 12-step program of recovery and mutual support to maintain abstinence from alcohol and facilitate spiritual growth. Recent research has identified active participation in AA as a predictor for positive outcome.[246] Health care workers can assist patients by providing them with a local meeting schedule and by being familiar with meetings that address special needs. There are AA meetings for women, for gays and lesbians, and, in some areas, language-specific meetings. Other programs that developed from AA and that may be appropriate for referral are Cocaine Anonymous, Narcotics Anonymous, and Chemically Dependent Anonymous. Patients are encouraged to find meetings where they feel comfortable. Many hospitals have Alcoholics Anonymous or Narcotics Anonymous meetings available, and ambulatory patients should be encouraged to attend.

Although not as widely known or available, there are other self-help groups for substance abusers. These include Rational Recovery, Secular Organization for Sobriety, and Women for Sobriety. Rational Recovery uses a cognitive behavioral approach with no focus on spirituality like that found in the traditional 12-step programs.[245] Women may prefer Women for Sobriety and its focus on enhancing self-esteem.

RECOVERY FROM SUBSTANCE ABUSE

Patients in the earliest phases of alcohol abuse may have some success with controlled drinking. This is not true of those individuals with chemical dependencies. Addictions are chronic, progressive, potentially fatal illnesses of which trauma is a symptom. As such, they require a lifelong program of management, similar in some ways to that required of diabetic or asthmatic patients.[247] This usually necessitates abstinence from the drug of choice and other mood-altering drugs, a structured plan of recovery with emphasis on learning new coping strategies, and personal support from other recovering people. Constant vigilance is required for the continued health and well-being of these patients.

FOLLOW-UP TRAUMA CARE

Recovering substance abusers may require future surgery or hospitalization for continued care related to their injury. Balancing analgesia needs with the potential for relapse requires open communication between patients and their care providers, including the primary physician, anesthesiologist or anesthetist, and nursing staff. Part of the vigilance required includes honesty with health care providers about their chemical dependence. This helps ensure that their anesthesia and analgesia needs can be met in a safe and effective manner, while minimizing the risks of relapse to active chemical use.[245] It also allows other aspects of the patient's substance abuse recovery to be incorporated into the plan of care. This may include liberal visitation from members of the patient's support system or access to a telephone. Nurses can play a large role in advocating for chemically dependent patients in recovery.

FUTURE NEEDS IN SUBSTANCE ABUSE AND TRAUMA

Community prevention should include ongoing public education about the link between all types of trauma and substance abuse. The public has been bombarded with messages about the risks of drinking and driving. They are less well-informed about the links between alcohol and all types of injury. Substance abusers often maintain that they are a threat only to themselves, which is clearly not the case. They present very real and costly hazards to society.[3] Ongoing research should focus on the efficacy of various treatment and trauma prevention programs, with funding provided for those models that effectively bring about results in terms of decreasing injury caused by substance use. Such research needs to identify which patients will best benefit from specific treatment and intervention techniques. For example, clinical trials are currently underway to assess the outcomes of brief intervention in trauma patients. It will be important for clinicians working in the treatment field to document the number of trauma patients and their short and long-term treatment outcomes. It is imperative that long-term successes (e.g., abstinence rates at 1 year) are measured, in addition to short-term outcomes such as the number of patients accepting substance abuse treatment.

Research also needs to focus on determining what period during hospitalization after trauma is the optimal time for successful substance abuse intervention and referral. Such research should also document which health care providers

are most successful in this endeavor. Should this be undertaken by the primary nurse (the provider who has the most patient contact), the physician, or a specialized substance abuse counselor or addictionologist? Other general areas of inquiry include how best to present the information about substance abuse to the patient and how to include family members in the treatment.

SUMMARY

The epidemic of substance abuse in our society is clearly reflected in the trauma population. Substance-abusing trauma patients are challenging not only because of their substance induced co-morbidities but also because of their high risk for subsequent injury. Caring for substance-abusing patients requires knowledgeable and skilled nursing care to develop and implement effective multidisciplinary plans of care throughout each phase of the trauma cycle.

REFERENCES

1. Substance Abuse and Mental Services Health Administration: *Highlights,* www.health.org/pubs/nhsda/96hhs/rtst1006.htm, 1996.
2. National Institute of Drug Abuse: *Tobacco (NIDA Infofax 010),* www.nida.nih.gov/Infofax/tobacco.html, 1998.
3. National Institute of Drug Abuse: *Costs to society (NIDA Infofax 038),* www.nida.nih.gov/Infofax/costs.html, 1998.
4. Levy RS, Hebert CK, Munn BG et al: Drug and alcohol use in orthopedic trauma patients: a prospective study, *J Orthop Trauma* 10:21-27, 1996.
5. Soderstrom CA, Smith GS, Dischinger PC et al: Psychoactive substance use disorders among seriously injured trauma center patients, *JAMA* 277:1769-1774, 1997.
6. Ankney RN, Vizza J, Coil JA et al: Cofactors of alcohol-related trauma at a rural trauma center, *Am J Emerg Med* 16:228-231, 1998.
7. Cornwell EE, Belzberg H, Velmahos G et al: The prevalence and effect of alcohol and drug abuse on cohort-matched critically injured patients, *Am Surg* 64:461-465, 1998.
8. Tulloh BR, Collopy BT: Positive correlation between blood alcohol level and ISS in road trauma, *Injury* 25:538-543, 1994.
9. National Safety Council: *Injury facts,* http://www.org/lrs/statinfo/99ifacts.htm, 1999.
10. Brewer RD, Morris PD, Cole TB et al: The risk of dying in alcohol-related automobile crashes among habitual drunk drivers, *N Engl J Med* 331:513-517, 1994.
11. Soderstrom CA, Dischinger PC, Trifillis AL: Marijuana and other drug use among automobile and motorcycle drivers treated at a trauma center, *Accid Anal Prev* 27:131-135, 1995.
12. Sun SW, Kahn DM, Swan KG: Lowering the legal blood alcohol level for motorcyclists, *Accid Anal Prev* 30:133-136, 1998.
13. Rivara FP, Jurkovich GJ, Gurney JG et al: The magnitude of acute and chronic alcohol abuse in trauma patients, *Arch Surg* 128:907-912, 1993.
14. McGonigal MD, Cole J, Schwa CW et al: Urban firearm deaths: a five-year perspective, *J Trauma* 35:532-536, 1993.
15. Barillo DJ, Goode R: Substance abuse in victims of fire, *J Burn Care Rehabil* 17:71-76, 1996.

16. Wintemute GJ, Kruas JF, Teret SP et al: The epidemiology of drowning in adulthood: implications for prevention. *Am J Prev Med* 4:343-348, 1988.

17. Bombardier CH, Thurber CA: Blood alcohol level and early cognitive status after traumatic brain injury, *Brain Inj* 12: 725-734, 1998.

18. Kelly MP, Johnson CT, Knoller N et al: Substance abuse, traumatic brain injury and neuropsychological outcome, *Brain Inj* 11:391-402, 1997.

19. Soderstrom CA, Smith GS, Kufera JA et al: The accuracy of the CAGE, the Brief Michigan Alcoholism Screening Test, and the Alcohol Use Disorders Identification Test in screening trauma center patients for alcoholism, *J Trauma* 43:962-969, 1997.

20. Davis NB, Hayes JS, Cohen S: Motor vehicle crashes and positive toxicology screens in adolescents and young adults, *J Trauma Nurs* 6:15-18, 1999.

21. Barnett NP, Spirito A, Colby SM et al: Detection of alcohol use in adolescent patients in the emergency department, *Acad Emerg Med* 5:607-612, 1998.

22. Gordon S, Toepper W, Blackman S: Toxicology screening in adolescent trauma, *Pediatric Emerg Care* 12:36-39, 1996.

23. Liedtke AJ, DeMuth WE: Effects of alcohol on cardiovascular performance after experimental nonpenetrating chest trauma, *Am J Cardiol* 35:243-250, 1975.

24. Blomqvist S, Thorne J, Elmer O et al: Early post-traumatic changes in hemodynamics and pulmonary ventilation in alcohol-pretreated pigs, *J Trauma* 27:40-44, 1987.

25. Guohua L, Keyl PM, Smith GS et al: Alcohol and injury severity: reappraisal of the continuing controversy, *J Trauma* 42:562-569, 1997.

26. Jurkovich GJ, Frederick P, Rivara MD et al: The effect of acute alcohol intoxication and chronic alcohol abuse on outcome from trauma, *JAMA* 270:51-56, 1993.

27. Li G, Keyl PM, Smith GS et al: Alcohol and injury severity: reappraisal of the continuing controversy, *J Trauma* 42: 562-569, 1997.

28. Waller PF, Blow FC, Maio RF et al: Crash characteristics and injuries of victims impaired by alcohol versus illicit drugs, *Accid Anal Prev* 29:817-827, 1997.

29. Mueller BA, Kenaston T, Grossman D et al: Hospital charges to injured drinking drivers in Washington State: 1989-1993, *Accid Anal Prev* 30:597-605, 1998.

30. Bailey DN: Drug use in patients admitted to a university trauma center: results of limited toxicology screening, *J Anal Toxicol* 14:22-24, 1990.

31. Clark RF, Harchelroad F: Toxicology screening of the trauma patient: a changing profile, *Ann Emerg Med* 20:151-153, 1991.

32. Hutchinson DT, McClinton MA, Wilgis EF et al: Drug and alcohol use in emergency hand patients, *J Hand Surg* 17A: 576-677, 1992.

33. Soderstrom CA, Tandon M, Dischinger PC et al: Epidemic increases in cocaine and opiate use among 42,981 patients treated at a level I trauma center during a 15-year period [abstract], Poster session presented at the 59th meeting of the American Association for the Surgery of Trauma, Boston, September 1999.

34. Schermer CR, Wisner DH: Methamphetamine use in trauma patients: a population-based study, *J Am Coll Surg* 189: 442-449, 1999.

35. Beech DJ, Mercadel R: Correlation of alcohol intoxication with life-threatening asaults, *J Natl Med Assoc* 90:761-764, 1998.

36. Marzuk PM, Tardiff MD, Leon AC et al: Fatal injuries after cocaine use as a leading cause of death among young adults in New York City, *N Engl J Med* 332:1753-1757, 1995.

37. Soderstrom CA, Trifillis AL, Shandar BS et al: Marijuana and alcohol use among 1023 trauma patients, *Arch Surg* 123: 733-737, 1988.

38. American Psychiatric Association: *Diagnostic and statistical manual of mental disorders,* ed 4, Washington, DC, 1994, The Association.

39. Stabenau JR: Additive independent factors that predict risk for alcoholism, *J Stud Alcohol* 51:164-174, 1990.

40. Hill SY, Yuan H, Locke J: Path analysis of P300 amplitude of individuals from families at high and low risk for developing alcoholism, *Biol Psychiatry* 45:346-359, 1999.

41. Allgulander C, Nowak J, Rice JP: Psychopathology and treatment of 30,344 twins in Sweden. I. The appropriateness of psychoactive drug treatment, *Acta Psychiatr Scand* 82:420-426, 1990.

42. Allgulander C, Nowak J, Rice JP: Psychopathology and treatment of 30,344 twins in Sweden. II. Heritability estimates of psychiatric diagnosis and treatment in 12,884 twin pairs, *Acta Psychiatr Scand* 83:12-15, 1991.

43. Pickens RW, Svikins DS, McGue M et al: Heterogeneity in the inheritance of alcoholism: A study of male and female twins, *Arch Gen Psychiatry* 48:19-28, 1991.

44. McGue M, Pickens RW, Svikis DS: Sex and age effects on the inheritance of alcohol problems: a twin study, *J Abnorm Psychol* 101:3-17, 1992.

45. Goodwin DW, Schulsinger F, Hermansen L et al: Alcohol problems in adoptees raised apart from alcoholic biological parents, *Arch Gen Psychiatry* 28:238-243, 1973.

46. Goodwin DW: Alcoholism and genetics: the sins of the fathers, *Arch Gen Psychiatry* 42:171-174, 1985.

47. Bohman M, Sigvardsson S, Cloninger CR: Maternal inheritance of alcohol abuse: cross-fostering analysis of adopted women, *Arch Gen Psychiatry* 38:965-969, 1991.

48. Schuckit MA: Reactions to alcohol in sons of alcoholics and controls, *Alcohol Clin Exp Res* 12:465-470, 1988.

49. Kendler KS, Heath AC, Neale MC et al: A population-based twin study of alcoholism in women, *JAMA* 268:1877-1882, 1992.

50. Kendler KS, Prescott C: Cannabis use, abuse, and dependence in a population-based sample of female twins, *Am J Psychiatry* 155:1016-1022, 1998.

51. Kendler KS, Prescott C: Cocaine use, abuse, and dependence in a population-based sample of female twins, *Br J Psychiatry* 173:345-350, 1998.

52. Tsuang M, Lyons MJ, Meyer JM et al: Co-occurrence of abuse of different drugs in men, *Arch Gen Psychiatry* 55:967-972, 1998.

53. Van den Bree M, Johnson E, Neale M et al: Genetic and environmental influences on drug use and abuse/dependence in male and female twins, *Drug Alcohol Depend* 52:231-241, 1998.

54. Cadoret RJ, Troughton E, O'Gorman TW et al: An adoption study of genetic and environmental factors in drug abuse, *Arch Gen Psychiatry* 43:1131-1136, 1986.

55. Cutrona CE, Cadoret RJ, Suhr JA et al: Interpersonal variables in the prediction of alcoholism among adoptees: evidence for gene-environment interactions, *Compr Psychiatry* 35:171-179, 1994.

56. McClearn GE, Rogers DA: Differences in alcohol preference among inbred strains of mice, *Q J Stud Alcohol* 20:691-695, 1959.

57. Fadda F, Mosca E, Colombo G et al: Effect of spontaneous ingestion of ethanol on brain dopamine metabolism, *Life Sci* 44:281-287, 1989.

58. McBride WJ, Chernet E, Dyr W et al: Densities of dopamine D2 receptors are reduced in CNS regions of alcohol-preferring P rats, *Alcohol* 10:387-390, 1993.

59. LeMarquand D, Pihl RO, Benkelfat C: Serotonin and alcohol intake, abuse and dependence: clinical evidence, *Biol Psychiatry* 36:326-337, 1994.

60. Noble EP, Blum K, Ritchie T et al: Allelic association of the D2 dopamine receptor gene with receptor-binding characteristics in alcoholism, *Arch Gen Psychiatry* 48:648-654, 1991.

61. Parsian A, Todd RD, Devor EJ et al: Alcoholism and alleles of the human D2 dopamine receptor locus, *Arch Gen Psychiatry* 48:655-663, 1991.

62. Winokur G, Cook B, Liskow B et al: Alcoholism in manic depressive (bipolar) patients, *J Stud Alcohol* 54:574-576, 1993.

63. Kessler RC, McGonagle KA, Zhao S et al: Lifetime and 12-month prevalence of DSM-III-R psychiatric disorders in the United States, *Arch Gen Psychiatry* 51:8-19, 1994.

64. Regier DA, Farmer ME, Rae DS et al: Comorbidity of mental disorders with alcohol and other drug abuse, *JAMA* 264:2511-2518, 1990.

65. Ross HE, Glaser FB, Germanson T: The prevalence of psychiatric disorders in patients with alcohol and other drug problems, *Arch Gen Psychiatry* 45:1023-1031, 1988.

66. Walker R: Substance abuse and B-cluster disorders. I. Understanding the dual diagnosis patient, *J Psychoactive Drugs* 24:223-241, 1992.

67. Gittleman R, Mannuzza S, Shenker R et al: Hyperactive boys almost grown up. I. Psychiatric status, *Arch Gen Psychiatry* 42:937-947, 1985.

68. Piazza PV, LeMoal M: The role of stress in drug self-administration, *Pharmacol Sci* 19:67-74, 1998.

69. Stanton MD: Drugs, Vietnam and the Vietnam veterans: an overview, *Am J Drug Alcohol Abuse* 3:557-570, 1976.

70. Mintz J, O'Brien CP et al: The impact of Vietnam service on heroin-addicted veterans, *Am J Drug Alcohol Abuse* 6:39-52, 1979.

71. Walker GC, Scott PS, Koppersmith G: The impact of child sexual abuse on addiction severity: an analysis of trauma processing, *J Psychosoc Nurs Ment Health Serv* 36:10-18, 1998.

72. Najavits LM, Weiss RD, Shaw SR: The link between substance abuse and posttraumatic stress disorder in women: a research review, *Am J Addictions* 6:273-283, 1997.

73. Najavits LM, Gastfriend, DR, Barber JP et al: Cocaine dependence with and without PTSD among subjects in the National Institute on Drug Abuse Collaborative Cocaine Treatment Study, *Am J Psychiatry* 155: 214-219, 1998.

74. Fendrich M, Mackesy-Amiti ME, Wislar JS et al: Childhood abuse and the use of inhalants: differences by degree of use, *Am J Public Health* 87:765-769, 1997.

75. Stahl S: *Essential psychopharmacology,* New York, 1996, Cambridge University.

76. National Institute of Drug Abuse: The brain's drug reward systems, *NIDA Notes* 11:10, 1996.

77. O'Brien CP: Drug addiction and drug abuse. In Hardman JG, Limbird LE, Molinoff PB et al, editors: *Goodman & Gilman's the pharmacological basis of therapeutics,* ed 9, New York, 1996, McGraw-Hill, 557-578.78.

78. Hobbs WR, Rall TW, Verdoorn TA: Hypnotics and sedatives: ethanol. In Hardman, JG, Limbird, LE, Molinoff PB et al, editors: *Goodman & Gilman's the pharmacological basis of therapeutics,* ed 9, New York, 1996, McGraw-Hill, 361-398.

79. Frezza M, DiPadova D, Pozzato G et al: High blood alcohol levels in women: the role of decreased gastric alcohol dehydrogenase activity and first-pass metabolism, *N Engl J Med* 322:95-99, 1990.

80. Lieber CS: Hepatic and other medical disorders of alcoholism: from pathogenesis to treatment, *J Stud Alcohol* 59:9-25, 1998.

81. Lieber CS: Hepatic disorders. In Grahm W, Schultz TK, editors: *Principles of addiction medicine,* ed 2, Chevy Chase, Md, 1998, American Society of Addiction Medicine, 755-774.

82. Johnson BL, Quander JD: Overview of drug-free workplace programs. In Grahm W, Schultz TK, editors: *Principles of addiction medicine,* ed 2, Chevy Chase, Md, 1998, American Society of Addiction Medicine, 755-774.

83. Schultz TK, editors: *Principles of addiction medicine,* ed 2, Chevy Chase, Md, 1998, American Society of Addiction Medicine, 1241 1254.

84. Ticku MK, Kulkarni SK: Molecular interactions of ethanol with GABAergic systems and potential of RO15-4513 as an ethanol antagonist, *Pharmacol Biochem Behav* 30:501-510, 1988.

85. Treistman SN, Bayley H, Lemos JR: Effects of ethanol on calcium channels, potassium channels & vasopressin release, *Ann N Y Acad Sci* 625:249-263, 1991.

86. Olsen RW, Tobin AJ: Molecular biology of GABA A receptors, *FASEB J* 4:1469-1480, 1990.

87. Weight FF, Lovinger DM, White G et al: Alcohol and anesthetic actions on excitatory amino acid-activated ion channels, *Ann N Y Acad Sci* 625:97-107, 1991.

88. Grant KA, Valverius P, Hudspith M et al: Ethanol withdrawal seizures and the NMDA receptor complex, *Eur J Pharmacol* 176:289-296, 1990.

89. Lovinger DM, White G, Weight FF: Ethanol inhibits NMDA-activated ion current in hippocampal neurons, *Science* 243:1721-1724, 1989.

90. Gianoulakis C: The effect of ethanol on the biosynthesis and regulation of opioid peptides, *Experientia* 45:428-435, 1989.

91. Lovinger DM, White G: Ethanol potentiation of 5-hydroxytryptamine receptor-mediated ion current in neuroblastoma cells & isolated adult mammalian neurons, *Mol Pharmacol* 40:263-270, 1991.

92. Brodie MS, Shefner SA, Dunwiddie TS: Ethanol increases the firing rate of dopamine neurons of the rat ventral tegmental area in vitro, *Brain Res* 508:65-69, 1990.

93. Mayo-Smith MF: Management of alcohol intoxication and withdrawal. In Grahm W, Schultz TK, editors: *Principles of addiction medicine,* ed 2, Chevy Chase, Md, 1998, American Society of Addiction Medicine, 431-440.

94. Urso T, Gavaler JS, VanThiel DH: Blood ethanol levels in sober alcohol users seen in an emergency room, *Life Sci* 28: 1053-1056, 1981. 94. Geller A: Neurological effects. In Grahm W, Schultz TK, editors: *Principles of addiction medicine,* ed 2, Chevy Chase, Md, 1998, American Society of Addiction Medicine, 775-792.

95. Lynch MJG: Brain lesions in chronic alcoholism, *Arch Pathol* 69:342-353, 1960.

96. Thomas AP, Rozanski DJ, Renard DC et al: Effects of ethanol on the contractile function of the heart: a review, *Alcohol Clin Exp Res* 18:121-131, 1994.

97. Waldenstrom A: Alcohol and congestive heart failure, *Alcohol Clin Exp Res* 22:315S-317S, 1998.

98. Constant J: The alcoholic cardiomyopathies-genuine and pseudo, *Cardiology* 91:92-95, 1999.

99. Zink BJU, Sheingerg MA, Wang X et al: Acute ethanol intoxication in a model of traumatic brain injury with hemorrhagic shock: effects of early physiological response, *J Neurosurg* 89:983-990, 1998.

100. Segel LD: Alcoholic cardiomyopathy in rats: inotropic response to phenylephrine, glucagon, ouabain, and dobutamine, *J Mol Cell Cardiol* 19:1061-1072, 1987.

101. Engel TR, Luck JC: Effect of whiskey on atrial vulnerability and "holiday heart," *Am J Coll Cardiol* 1:816-818, 1983.

102. Greenspon AJ, Schaal SF: The "holiday heart": electrophysiologic studies of alcohol effects in alcoholics, *Ann Intern Med* 98:135-139, 1983.

103. Johnston RE, Reier CE: Acute respiratory effects of ethanol in man, *Clin Pharmacol Ther* 14:501-508, 1972.

104. Elmer O, Gustafson I, Gornasson G et al: Acute alcohol intoxication and traumatic shock, *Eur Surg Res* 5:268-275, 1983.

105. Rubin R, Rand ML: Alcohol and platelet function, *Alcohol Clin Exp Res* 18:105-110, 1994.

106. Garro AJ, Lieber CS: Alcohol and cancer, *Ann Rev Pharmacol Toxicol* 30:219-249, 1990.

107. Lieber CS: Gastritis and *Helicobacter pylori*: forty years of antibiotic therapy, *Digestion* 58:203-210, 1997.

108. Lieber CS: Pathogenesis and treatment of liver fibrosis: 1996 update, *Dig Dis* 15:42-66, 1997.

109. Friedman SL: The cellular basis of hepatic fibrosis: mechanisms and treatment strategies, *N Engl J Med* 328:1828-1835, 1993.

110. Parker RI: Etiology and treatment of acquired coagulopathies in the critically ill adult and child, *Crit Care Clin* 13:591-609, 1997.

111. Jaakola M, Frey T, Sillanaukee P et al: Acute pancreatic injury in asymptomatic individuals after heavy drinking over the long-term, *Hepatogastroenterology* 41:477-482, 1994.

112. Reisine T, Pasternak G: Opiod analgesics and antagonists. In Hardman, JG, Limbird, LE, Molinoff PB et al, editors: *Goodman & Gilman's the pharmacological basis of therapeutics*, ed 9, New York, 1996, McGraw-Hill, 521-556.

113. Gold MS: The pharmacology of opioids. In Graham AW, Schultz TK, editors: *Principles of addiction medicine*, ed 2, Chevy Chase, Md, 1998, American Society of Addiction Medicine, 131-136.

114. Cone EJ, Holicky BA, Grant TM et al: Pharmacokinetics and pharmacodynamics of intranasal "snorted" heroin, *J Analyt Toxicol* 17:327-337, 1993.

115. Benowitz NL: Clinical pharmacology and toxicology of cocaine, *Pharmacol Toxicol* 72:3-12, 1993.

116. Cone EJ: Pharmacokinetics and pharmacodynamics of cocaine, *J Anal Toxicol* 19:459-477, 1995.

117. Evans SM, Cone EJ, Henningfield JE: Arterial and venous cocaine plasma concentrations in humans: relationship to route of administration, cardiovascular effects and subjective effects, *J Pharmacol Exp Ther* 279:1345-1356, 1996.

118. Ambre JJ: The urinary excretion of cocaine and metabolite in humans: a kinetic analysis of published data, *J Analyt Toxicol* 9:241-245, 1985.

119. Vongpatanasin W, Mansour Y, Chavoshan B et al: Cocaine stimulates the human cardiovascular system via a central mechanism of action, *Circulation* 100:497-502, 1999.

120. Lange RA, Cigarroa RG, Yancy CW et al: Cocaine-induced coronary artery vasoconstriction, *N Engl J Med* 321:1557-1562, 1989.

121. Foltin RW, Fischman MW, Levin FR: Cardiovascular effects of cocaine in humans: laboratory studies, *Drug Alcohol Depend* 37:193-210, 1995.

122. Martin TJ: Cocaine-induced mesenteric ischemia, *N C Med J* 52:429-430, 1991.

123. Fineschi V, Wetli CV, DiPaolo M et al: Myocardial necrosis and cocaine: a quantitative morphologic study in 26 cocaine-associated deaths, *Int J Legal Med* 110:193-198, 1997.

124. Holland JG, Hume AS, Martin JN: Relation of cocaine use to seizures and epilepsy, *Epilepsia* 37:875-878, 1996.

125. Strickland TL, Miller BL, Kowell A et al: Neurobiology of cocaine-induced organic brain impairment: contributions from functional neuroimaging, *Neuropsychol Rev* 8:1-9, 1998.

126. Sanchez-Ramos JR: Psychostimulants, *Neurol Clin* 11:535-553, 1993.

127. Holland RW, Marx JA, Earnest MP et al: Grand mal seizures temporally related to cocaine use: clinical and diagnostic features, *Ann Emerg Med* 21:772-776, 1992.

128. Gold MS: The pharmacology of cocaine, crack and other stimulants. In Graham AW, Schultz TK, editors: *Principles of addiction medicine*, ed 2, Chevy Chase, Md, 1998, American Society of Addiction Medicine, 137-146.

129. Baldwin GC, Tashkin DP, Buckley DM et al: Marijuana and cocaine impair alveolar macrophage function and cytokine production, *Am J Respir Crit Care Med* 156:1606-1613, 1997.

130. Thadani PV: NIDA conference report on cardiopulmonary complications of "crack" cocaine use, *Chest* 110:1072-1076, 1996.

131. Mueller PJ, Qi G, Knuepfer MM: Ethanol alters hemodynamic responses to cocaine in rats, *Drug Alcohol Depend* 48:17-24, 1997.

132. McCance-Katz EF, Kosten TR, Jatlow P: Concurrent use of cocaine and alcohol is more potent and potentially more toxic than use of either alone—a multiple dose study, *Biol Psychiatry* 44:250-259, 1998.

133. National Institutes of Drug Abuse: *Methemphetamine*, www.nida.nih.gov/researchreports/methamph/ methamph2.html, Research Report Series, 1998.

134. Slade J: The pharmacology of nicotine. In Graham AW, Schultz TK, editors: *Principles of addiction medicine*, ed 2, Chevy Chase, Md, 1998, American Society of Addiction Medicine, 147-152.

135. Rustin TA: Management of nicotine withdrawal. In Graham AW, Schultz TK, editors: *Principles of addiction medicine*, ed 2, Chevy Chase, Md, 1998, American Society of Addiction Medicine, 487-496.

136. Adams IB, Martin BR: Cannabis pharmacology and toxicology in animals and humans, *Addiction* 91:1585-1614, 1996.

137. ElSohly MA, Ross SA: *Quarterly report, NIDA Potency Monitoring Project*, Report No. 50, Rockville, Md, 1994, National Institute on Drug Abuse.

138. Romero J, Garcia L, Fernandez-Ruiz JJ et al: Changes in rat brain cannabinoid binding sites after acute or chronic exposure to their endogenous agonist, anadamide, or to delta 9-tetrahydrocannabinol, *Pharmacol Biochem Behav* 51:731-737, 1995.

139. Axelrod J, Felder CC: Cannabinoid receptors and their endogenous agonist, anadamide, *Neurochem Res* 23:575-581, 1998.

140. Howlett AD: Pharmacology of cannabinoid receptors, *Annu Rev Pharmacol Toxicol* 35:607-634, 1995.

141. Huestis MA, Sampson AH, Holicky BJ et al: Characterization of the absorption phase of marijuana smoking, *Clin Pharmacol Ther* 52:31-41, 1992.

142. Gold MS: The pharmacology of marijuana. In Graham AW, Schultz TK, editors: *Principles of addiction medicine,* ed 2, Chevy Chase, Md, 1998, American Society of Addiction Medicine, 163-172.

143. Robbe HWJ: *Influence of marijuana on driving,* Maastricht, Netherlands, 1994, Institute for Human Psychopharmacology, University of Limberg.

144. Heishman SJ, Huestis MA, Henningfield JE et al: Acute and residual effects of marijuana: profiles of plasma, THC levels, physiological subjective, and performance measures, *Pharmacol Biochem Behav* 37:561-565, 1990.

145. Pope HG, Yurgelun-Todd D: The residual cognitive effects of heavy marijuana use in college students, *JAMA* 275:521-527, 1996.

146. Solowij N: *The long-term effects of cannabis on the central nervous system: I. Brain function and neurotoxicity,* World Health Organization Project on Health Implications of Cannabis Use, Geneva, Switzerland, 1996, WHO.

147. Solowij N: *The long-term effects of cannabis on the central nervous system: II. Cognitive functioning,* World Health Organization Project on Health Implications of Cannabis Use, Geneva, Switzerland, 1996, WHO.

148. Fligiel SE, Roth MD, Kleeny EC et al: Tracheobronchial histopathology in habitual smokers of cocaine, marijuana and/or tobacco, *Chest* 112:319-326, 1997.

149. Fant RV, Heishman SJ, Bunker EB et al: Acute and residual effects of marijuana in humans, *Pharmacol Biochem Behav* 60:777-784, 1998.

150. Haney M, Ward AS, Comer SD et al: Abstinence symptoms following smoked marijuana in humans, *Psychopharmacology* 141:395-404, 1999.

151. Ksiakiewicz B, Bloch-Boguslawska E: Diagnostic difficulties with skull and brain injury complications in alcoholic patients, *Pol Merkuriusz Lek* 3:166-168, 1998.

152. Kaufmann CR, Branas CC, Brawley ML: A population-based study of trauma recidivism, *J Trauma* 45:325-332, 1998.

153. Substance Abuse and Mental Health Services Administration: *TIP: alcohol and other drug screening of hospitalized trauma patients,* 16, Rockville, Md, 1995, SAMHSA.

154. Cherubin CE, Sapira JD: The medical complications of drug addiction and the medical assessment of the intravenous drug user: 25 years later, *Ann Intern Med* 119:1017-1026, 1993.

155. Jaffe-Johnson S: Assessment and diagnosis. In Allen KM, editor: Nursing care of the addicted client, Philadelphia, 1996, JB Lippincott, 117-139.

156. McIlroy MA, Reddy D, Markowitz H et al: Infected false aneurysms of the femoral artery in intravenous drug addicts, *Rev Infect Dis* 11:578-585, 1989.

157. Wartenberg AA: Medical syndromes associated with specific drugs. In Grahm W, Schultz TK, editors: *Principles of addiction medicine,* ed 2, Chevy Chase, Md, 1998, American Society of Addiction Medicine, 731-740.

158. Hojer J, Hulting J: Acute alcohol intoxication: risk of complications, *Nord Med* 107:182-184, 1992.

159. Hoang MP, Lee EL, Anand A: Histologic spectrum of arterial and arteriolar lesions in acute and chronic cocaine-induced mesesteric ischemia: report of three cases and literature review, *Am J Surg Pathol* 22:1404-1010, 1998.

160. Vongpatanasin W, Mansour Y, Chavoshan B et al: Cocaine stimulates the human cardiovascular system via a central mechanism of action, *Circulation* 100:497-502, 1999.

161. Saccente M, Cobbs CG: Clinical approach to infective endocarditis, *Cardiol Clin* 14:351-362, 1996.

162. Haack MR: Treating acute withdrawal from alcohol and other drugs, *Nurs Clin North Am* 33:75-92, 1998.

163. Ewing JA: Detecting alcoholism: the CAGE questionnaire, *JAMA* 252:1905-1907, 1984.

164. Savage C: Screening and detection. In Allen KM, editor: *Nursing care of the addicted client,* Philadelphia, 1996, JB Lippincott, 100-117.

165. Kitchens JM: Does this patient have an alcohol problem? *JAMA* 272:1782-1787, 1994.

166. Russell M, Martier S, Sokel R et al: Screening for pregnancy risk drinking TWEAKing the tests [abstract], *Alcohol Clin Exp Res* 18:1156-1161, 1994.

167. Babor TF, de la Fuente JR, Saunders J et al: *AUDIT: the Alcohol Use Disorders Identification Test: guidelines for use in primary health care,* Geneva, Switzerland, 1992, World Health Organization.

168. Saunders JB, Aasland OG, Babor TF et al: Development of the Alcohol Use Disorders Identification Test (AUDIT). WHO collaborative project on early detection of persons with harmful alcohol consumption, II, *Addiction* 88:791-804, 1993.

169. Soderstrom CA, Dischinger PC, Kerns TJ et al: Screening trauma patients for alcoholism according to the NIAAA guidelines with alcohol use disorders identification test questions, *Alcohol Clin Exp Res* 22:1470-1475, 1998.

170. U. S. Department of Health and Human Services: *Model trauma care system plan,* Rockville, Md, 1992, Health Resources and Services Administration.

171. Buchfuhrer LA, Radecki SE: Alcohol and drug abuse in an urban trauma center: predictors of screening and detection, *J Addict Dis* 15:65-74, 1996.

172. Ryb G, Soderstrom CA, Kufera JA et al: The use of blood alcohol concentration and laboratory tests to detect current alcohol dependence in trauma center patients, *J Trauma* 47:874-880, 1999.

173. Rosman AS, Lieber CS: Biochemical markers of alcohol consumption, *Alcohol Health Res World* 43:210-218, 1990.

174. Gronback M, Henriksen JH, Becker U: Carbohydrate-deficient transferrin: a valid marker of alcoholism in population studies? Results from the Copenhagen City Heart Study, *Alcohol Clin Exp Res* 19:457-461, 1995.

175. Borg S, Beck O, Voltaire A et al: *Clinical characteristics and biochemical markers of alcohol consumption during long-term abstinence in relation to relapses: results from a longitudinal study of alcohol-dependent male patients.* Presented at the 2nd Congress of the European Society for Biomedical Research on Alcoholism, Brussels, 1992.

176. Soderstrom CA, Smith GS, Dischinger PC et al: CDT as a marker of alcoholism in trauma center patients [abstract], *J Addict Dis* 17:165, 1997.

177. Miller TW, Geraci EB: Head injury in the presence of alcohol intoxication, *Int J Trauma Nurs* 3:50-55, 1997.

178. Galbraith S: Misdiagnosis and delayed diagnosis in traumatic intracranial haematoma, *Br Med J* 1:438-1439, 1976.

179. Winbery S, Blaho K, Logan B et al: Multiple cocaine-induced seizures and corresponding cocoaine and metabolite concentrations, *Am J Emerg Med* 16:529-533, 1998.

180. Saitz R, O'Malley SS: Pharmacotherapies for alcohol abuse, *Med Clin North Am* 81:881-907, 1997.

181. Eickelberg SJ, Mayo-Smith MF: Management of sedative-hypnotic intoxication and withdrawal. In Grahm W, Schultz TK, editors: *Principles of addiction medicine,* ed 2, Chevy Chase, Md, 1998, American Society of Addiction Medicine, 441-456.

182. Spies CD, Neuner B, Neumann T et al: Intercurrent complications in chronic alcoholic men admitted to the intensive care unit following trauma, *Intensive Care Med* 22:286-293, 1996.

183. Bellemare JF, Tepas JJ 3rd, Imani ER et al: Complications of trauma care: risk analysis of pneumonia in 10,0001 adult trauma patients, *Am Surg* 62:207-211, 1996.

184. O'Connor PG, Samet JH, Stein MD: Management of hospitalized intravenous drug users: role of the internist, *Am J Med* 96:551-557, 1994.

185. Lip GY, Beevers DG: Alcohol, hyertension, coronary disease and stroke, *Clin Exp Pharmacol Physiol* 22:189-194, 1995,

186. Elmer O, Lim R: Influence of acute intoxication on the outcome of severe non-neurologic trauma, *Acta Chir Scand* 151:305-308, 1985.

187. Desiderio M: The effects of acute, oral ethanol on cardiovascular performance before and after blunt cardiac trauma, *J Trauma* 27:267-277, 1987.

188. Newsome HJ: Ethanol modulation of plasma norepinephrine response to trauma and hemorrhage, *J Trauma* 28:1-9, 1988.

189. Richards CF, Clark RF, Holbrook T et al: The effect of cocaine and amphetamines on vital signs in trauma patients, *J Emerg Med* 13:59-63, 1995.

190. Signs SA, Dickey-White HI, Vanek VW et al: The formation of cocaethylene and clinical presentation of ED patients testing positive for the use of cocaine and ethanol, *Am J Emerg Med* 14:665-670, 1996.

191. Vamvakas S, Teschner M, Bahner U et al: Alcohol abuse: potential role in eletrolyte disturbances and kidney function, *Clin Nephrol* 49:205-213, 1998.

192. Glasser L, Sternglanz PD, Combie ZJ et al: Serum osmolarity and its applicability to drug overdose, *Am J Clin Pharmacol* 60:695-699, 1973.

193. Reynolds HN, Cottingham CA, Sand F et al: Trisodium citrate. In *Continuous renal replacement manual,* ed 2, Baltimore, Md, 1999, University of Maryland Medical System.

194. Marcus R: Agents affecting calcification and bone turnover. In Hardman, JG, Limbird, LE, Molinoff PB et al, editors: *Goodman & Gilman's the pharmacological basis of therapeutics,* ed 9, New York, 1996, McGraw-Hill, 1519-1546.

195. DeMarchi S, Cecchin E, Basile A: Renal tubular dysfunction in chronic alcohol abuse: effects of abstinence, *N Engl J Med* 328:1927-1934, 1993.

196. Ryback RS, Eckardt MJ, Pautier CP: Clinical relationships between serum phosphorus and other blood chemistry values in alcoholics, *Arch Intern Med* 140:673-677, 1980.

197. Newman JH, Neff TA, Ziporin P: Acute respiratory failure associated with hypophosphatemia, *N Engl J Med* 296:1101-1103, 1977.

198. Feinman L, Lieber CS: Nutrition. In Grahm W, Schultz TK, editors: *Principles of addiction medicine,* ed 2, Chevy Chase, Md, 1998, American Society of Addiction Medicine, 741-754.

199. Voight L: Anesthetic management of the cocaine abuse patient, *AANA J* 63:438-443, 1995.

200. Hyatt B, Bensky KP: Illicit drugs and anesthesia, *CRNA* 10:15-23, 1999.

201. Beattie C, Umbricht-Schneiter A, Mark L: Anethesia and analgesia. In Grahm W, Schultz TK, editors: *Principles of addiction medicine,* ed 2, Chevy Chase, Md, 1998, American Society of Addiction Medicine, 877-890.

202. Wolf KM, Shaughnessy AF, Middleton DB: Prolonged delirium tremens requiring massive doses of medication, *J Am Board Fam Pract* 6:502-504, 1993.

203. Worner TM: Propanolol versus diazepam in the management of the alcohol withdrawal syndrome: double-blind controlled trial, *Am J Drug Alcohol Abuse* 22:115-124, 1994.

204. Mayo-Smith MF: Pharmacological management of alcohol withdrawal, *JAMA* 278:144-151, 1997.

205. Sullivan JT, Sykora K, Schneiderman J et al: Assessment of alcohol withdrawal: the revised clinical institute withdrawal assessment for alcohol scale (CIWA-Ar), *Br J Addict* 84:1353-1357, 1987.

206. Watling SM, Fleming C, Casey P et al: Nursing-based protocol for treatment of alcohol withdrawal in the intensive care unit, *Am J Crit Care* 4:66-70, 1995.

207. Novak H, Ward H, Adams M: *Nurses' handbook: for the nursing management of drug and alcohol problems,* Sydney, Australia, 1995, Charles.

208. Hayner G, Galloway G, Wiehl WO: Haight Ashbury free clinics' drug detoxification protocols. Part 3: Benzodiazepines and other sedative-hypnotics, *J Psychoactive Drug* 25:331-335, 1993.

209. Warner EA, Kosten TR, O'Connor PG: Pharmacotherapy for opioid and cocaine abuse, *Med Clin North Am* 81:909-925, 1997.

210. Stine SM, Meandzija B, Kosten TR: Pharmacologic therapies for opioid addiction. In Grahm W, Schultz TK, editors: *Principles of addiction medicine,* ed 2, Chevy Chase, Md, 1998, American Society of Addiction Medicine, 545-556.

211. Stine SM, Kosten TR: *Methadone dose in the treatment of opiate withdrawal,* www.medscape.com/Medscape/MentalHe...97/v02.n11/mh3076.stine.html, 1997.

212. Vourakis C: Substance abuse concerns in the treatment of pain, *Nurs Clin North Am* 33:47-60, 1998.

213. Wilkins JN, Conner BT, Gorelick DA: Management of stimulant, hallucinogen, marijuana and phencyclidine intoxication and withdrawal. In Grahm W, Schultz TK, editors: *Principles of addiction medicine,* ed 2, Chevy Chase, Md, 1998, American Society of Addiction Medicine, 465-486.

214. Rustin TA: Management of nicotine withdrawal. In Grahm W, Schultz TK, editors: *Principles of addiction medicine,* ed 2, Chevy Chase, Md, 1998, American Society of Addiction Medicine, 487-496.

215. Christen AG, Jay SJ, Christen SA: Treating highly dependent smokers with nicotine gum and patches, *Indiana Med* 89:169-174, 1996.

216. Ferguson RK, Soryal IN, Pentland B: Thiamine deficiency in head injury: a missed insult? *Alcohol Alcohol* 32:493-500, 1997.

217. Feng L, Cook TT, Alber C et al: Ethanol and natural killer cells. II. Stimulation of human natural killer activity by ethanol in vitro, *Alcohol Clin Exp Res* 21:981-987, 1997.

218. Cook T, Feng L, Vandersteen D et al: Ethanol and natural killer cells. I. Activity and immunophenotype in alcoholic humans, *Alcohol Clin Exp Res* 21:974-980, 1997.

219. Tamura DY, Moore EE, Partrick DA et al: Clinically relevant concentrations of ethanol attenuate primed neutrophil bactericidal activity, *J Trauma* 44:320-324, 1998.

220. Gentilello LM, Cobean R, Wertz M et al: Acute ethanol intoxication increases the risk of infection after penetrating abdominal trauma, *J Trauma* 34:669-674, 1993.

221. Selwyn PA, O'Connor PG: Diagnosis and treatment of substance users with HIV infection, *Primary Care* 19:119-153, 1992.

222. Rotunda RJ, Scherer DG, Imm PS: Family systems and alcohol misuse: research on the effects of alcoholism on family functioning and effective family interventions, *Prof Psychol Res Pract* 26:95-104, 1995.

223. Brown S, Lewis V: A developmental model of the alcoholic family. In Grahm W, Schultz TK, editors: *Principles of addiction medicine*, ed 2, Chevy Chase, Md, 1998, American Society of Addiction Medicine, 1099-1110.

224. Thompson PM, Gillin JC, Golshan S et al: Polygraphic sleep measures differentiate alcoholics and stimulant abusers during short-term sleep, *Biol Psychiatry* 38:831-836, 1995.

225. Sommers MS, Dyehouse JM, Howe SR et al: Attribution of injury to alcohol involvement in young adults seriously injured in alcohol-related motor vehicle crashes, *Am J Crit Care* 9:28-35, 2000.

226. Dyehouse JM, Sommers MS: Brief intervention after alcohol-related injuries, *Nurs Clin North Am* 33:93-104, 1998.

227. Bombardier CH, Ehde D, Kilmer J: Readiness to change alcohol habits after traumatic brain injury, *Arch Phys Med Rehabil* 78:592-596, 1997.

228. Dunn CW, Donovan DM, Gentilello LM: Practical guidelines for performing alcohol interventions in trauma centers, *J Trauma* 42:299-304, 1997.

229. Gentilello LM, Bonovan DM, Dunn CW et al: Alcohol interventions in trauma centers, *JAMA* 274:1043-1048, 1995.

230. Fleming MF, Barry KL, Manwell LB et al: Brief physician advice for problem alcohol drinkers, *JAMA* 277:1039-1045, 1997.

231. Greber RA, Allen KM, Soeken KL et al: Outcome of trauma patients after brief intervention by a substance abuse consultation service, *Am J Addict* 6:38-47, 1997.

232. Gentilello LM, Rivara FP, Donovan DM et al: Alcohol interventions in a trauma center as a means of reducing the risk of injury recurrence, *Ann Surg* 230:473-483, 1999.

233. Fuller MG, Diamond DL, Jordan ML et al: The role of a substance abuse consultation team in a trauma center, *J Stud Alcohol* 56:267-271, 1995.

234. American Society of Addiction Medicine: *Patient placement criteria for treatment of substance-related disorders*, ed 2, Chevy Chase, Md, 2000, The Society.

235. National Institute of Drug Abuse: Project MATCH secondary a priori hypotheses, *Addiction* 92:1671-1698, 1997.

236. Higgins-Biddle JC, Babor TF, Mullahy J et al: Alcohol screening and brief intervention: where research meets practice, *Conn Med* 61:565-575, 1997.

237. Bien TH, Miller WR, Tonigan JS: Brief interventions for alcohol problems: a review, *Addiction* 88:315-335, 1993.

238. Ockene JK, Wheeler EV, Adams A et al: Provider training for patient-centered alcohol counseling in a primary care setting, *Arch Intern Med* 157:2334-2340, 1997.

239. Anderson P, Scott E: The effect of general practitioners' advice to heavy drinking men, *Br J Addict* 87:891-900, 1992.

240. Monti PM, Colby SM, Barnett NP et al: Brief intervention for harm reduction with alcohol positive older adolescents in a hospital emergency department, *J Consult Clin Psychol* 67:1-6, 1999.

241. Prochaska JO, Norcross JC, DiClemente CC: *Changing for good*, New York, 1994, Avon.

242. Saunders B, Houghton M: Relapse revisited: a critique of current concepts and clinical practice in the management of alcohol problems, *Addict Behav* 21:843-855, 1997.

243. Gentilello LM, Duggan P, Drummond E et al: Major injury as a unique opportunity to initiate treatment in the alcoholic, *Am J Surg* 156:558-561, 1988.

244. Friedman MD, Saitz R, Samet JH et al: Management of adults recovering from alcohol or other drug problems, *JAMA* 279:1227-1231, 1998.

245. Toro IM, Tho DJ, Beam HP et al: Chemically dependent patients in recovery: roles for the family physician, *Am Fam Physician* 53:1667-1673, 1996.

246. Lindeman RW: The efficacy of the twelve steps of alcoholics anonymous in the treatment of alcoholism, *J Psychoactive Drugs* 25:337-340, 1993.

247. Millar JS: A time for everything: changing attitudes and approaches to reducing substance abuse, *Can Med Assoc J* 159:485-487, 1998.

(Modified from The brain's drug reward systems, *NIDA Notes* 11(4):19, 1996.)

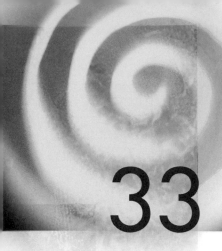

THE ORGAN AND TISSUE DONOR

Cheryl Edwards • Franki Chabalewski

33

This chapter is designed to give the trauma nurse a basic understanding of organ and tissue donation and the significant role that the trauma nurse plays in the donation process. The crisis created by the critical shortage of organs available for transplant will only worsen as the number of people in need of transplantation increases. Trauma nurses, front-line patient advocates and managers, are essential for the early referral of the potential donor.

The process may be confusing because statutes, policies, and parameters vary from state to state, from hospital to hospital, and among organ procurement organizations (OPOs). The OPO staff is the best resource to assist in caring for the donor and the donor's family and to ensure that hospital policies and procedures are current. The trauma team is urged to work collaboratively with the regional OPO to provide the most compassionate approach to potential donor families while preparing their loved one for their final act of generosity: giving an organ to save or enhance another person's life.

DONOR IDENTIFICATION AND REFERRAL

There have been many significant advances in the field of organ transplantation since the first transplant was done in 1956. Thousands of lives that would have otherwise been lost to end-stage organ failure have been saved and thousands of others enjoy an improved quality of life, all as a result of organ transplantation. Improvements in surgical techniques, organ preservation procedures, and immunosuppressive therapies have made it possible for transplant recipients to enjoy a high quality of life. However, there is one factor that severely limits the number of lives affected through transplantation: the shortage of life-saving organs for transplant.

More than 77,330 people are currently waiting for a transplant in the United States.[1] That number grows exponentially each year, whereas the number of organ donors remains unchanged.[2] A new name is added to the waiting list every 10 minutes. Every 2 hours, one of those listed dies because a transplant did not become available in time. Fewer than one third of those patients waiting will receive the transplant they so desperately need (Figure 33-1).

Trauma nurses play an integral role in solving the critical shortage of organs for transplant through the early referral of every potential donor. Referrals to the regional OPO can increase the number of organ donors through a collaborative approach. Coordinated efforts between the organ procurement coordinator (OPC) and the health care team's nurses, physicians, and ancillary personnel can have a dramatic impact on the number of lives saved annually through the "gift of life" as a result of organ donation.

FEDERAL REGULATIONS AND TIMELY REFERRAL OF POTENTIAL ORGAN DONORS

The critical shortage of organs for transplantation has prompted federal initiatives designed to increase professional and public awareness regarding the need for organs and tissues for donation. Research has shown that one third of potential donors are never identified by hospital personnel.[3] In response the Health Care Financing Administration (HCFA) developed the "Medicare Conditions of Participation" regulations. These regulations require all U.S. hospitals to work collaboratively with their regional OPO and tissue recovery agency. Specifically, they charge every hospital with reporting all potential organ donors and inpatient deaths to their OPO. The regulations mandate that hospital staff be required to report every impending death (including the potential for brain death) to the OPO in a timely manner—before life-limiting treatment decisions are made, before termination of life support, and before any discussion regarding organ and tissue donation is initiated with the family. Additionally, according to these regulations, the responsibility for conducting a consent discussion with the family of a potential donor lies with the OPO staff or hospital staff trained by the OPO.[4] These regulations are meant to relieve the hospital staff of the burden of determining donor suitability. They are not designed to exclude hospital staff from the consent discussion but to ensure that the OPC is included in the process.

Early referral to the regional OPO has many benefits to the staff, the patient's family, and the recipients. Staff, who may be uncomfortable with discussing donation or who lack the knowledge to provide the option of donation to a family,

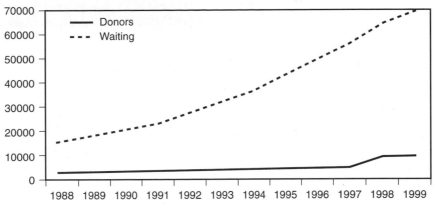

FIGURE 33-1 UNOS Data From Scientific Registry, June 1, 1999.

are now relieved of that burden under the new regulations. Early involvement with the OPC can facilitate a collaborative, sensitive approach to the donation discussion. Potential donor families can be assured that the request for donation occurs at a time that is right for them, with the appropriate options offered based on the individual situation. They need to take time to discuss their options, to have questions answered, and to be assured that their decision will be respected whether or not they choose to donate. The transplant recipients benefits are obvious. Many lives are saved and many people enjoy the benefit of an improved quality of life through organ transplantation. Advances in the field of transplantation have allowed recipients greater survival times than ever before.[1]

Early OPC involvement can assist the staff in caring for the family and prevent well-meaning personnel from offering the option of donation in situations where it is inappropriate (if the deceased person had the human immunodeficiency virus (HIV) or had metastatic disease) and from offering inaccurate information about the options for donation. As donor criteria continue to change, OPO staff is best trained in the most current criteria and possess the information necessary to screen a potential donor. The OPC can spend time with the family answering questions and reinforcing their options. This can be a time-consuming encounter and may require more information than the staff is able to provide.[5] Ideally the trauma staff and OPC will develop a plan and collaboratively decide on the best approach to the family should brain death occur.

DONOR PROFILE

A 16-year-old white male is admitted to the emergency department after a fall from a moving vehicle while "car surfing." He has sustained a severe closed head injury. An emergent computed tomography (CT) scan of his head reveals diffuse cerebral edema and inoperable intraparenchymal hemorrhages. His prognosis for survival is poor. A referral is made to the regional OPO to alert the OPC on call that the patient's condition is deteriorating. The neurosur-

geon places an intracranial pressure monitor and admits the patient to the intensive care unit for aggressive treatment of the increased intracranial pressure.

Six hours after admission it is obvious that all efforts to control this patient's intracranial hypertension have failed and his clinical examination is consistent with herniation syndrome. The OPC on call is again apprised of the situation. A cerebral blood flow study is done to confirm the suspicion of brain death. In accordance with state and hospital policies, the patient is declared brain dead.

Trauma patients, particularly young and otherwise healthy individuals, who have sustained an isolated traumatic brain injury have always constituted and will continue to constitute a significant percentage of the overall organ donor pool. However, factors such as enforced speed limits, seat belt and motorcycle helmet laws, air bags, and more sophisticated prehospital care have changed the potential for organ donation in the trauma population. Many patients who would have been potential donors do not progress to brain death.

Concurrent solid organ injuries in the trauma patient can also preclude donation. Malangoni et al in 1996 showed that trauma patients sustaining isolated, severe head injuries were the most likely to become organ donors (33%). Concurrent injuries decrease that likelihood. Of those patients sustaining trauma to at least one organ system and a traumatic brain injury, only 13% were suitable organ donors. Further, only 1% of those trauma patients with severe organ injury and no head injury were suitable donors.[6]

It is essential for the trauma nurse to realize that trauma patients are not the only potential organ donors. In fact, from 1988 to 1996 the number of persons involved in motor vehicle crashes who become organ donors decreased 29%, whereas the number of patients who became organ donors as a result of a cerebrovascular accident, such as intracerebral hemorrhage or ischemic stroke, rose 57%.[1] Any catastrophic cerebral insult, whether anoxic, hemorrhagic, ischemic, or traumatic, that results in uncontrolled cerebral edema can lead to brain death and the potential for organ donation. Some studies have shown that physicians and staff fail to recognize these patients as potential organ donors and subsequently fail to refer the patient to the OPO.[7] In these cases the opportunity for donation is lost. Not only is the family denied their legal right to be offered the option of donation, but they are deprived of an opportunity to find solace while experiencing the loss of a loved one. Many donor families find comfort in knowing that their loved one's final act of kindness, organ and tissue donation, can help countless others by saving and greatly enhancing the lives of others.

Brain Death

The Uniform Determination of Death Act of 1980, supported by the President's Commission for the Study of Ethical Problems in Medicine and Biomedical and Behavioral Research, confirmed the legality of and set parameters for the declaration of brain death. The act states that any individual sustaining irreversible cessation of circulatory and respiratory function *or* irreversible cessation of *all* cerebral function, including the brainstem, is dead.[8] Technologic advances make it possible to support multiple body systems so that the signs traditionally equated with life, cardiac and respiratory function, can be maintained despite the loss of all cerebral function and control. Therefore the organ donor is traditionally the individual who is brain dead or, more specifically, the patient who has died but remains on mechanical support for purposes of organ donation until organ recovery is completed. The non-heart-beating organ donor, or the donor whose organs are recovered after asystole, is discussed later in this chapter.

Once a primary insult occurs, whether medical or traumatic, the challenge to the health care team is to prevent secondary injury. In the absence of trauma, in older children and adults the cranium is a closed vault. Within this rigid, closed cavity exist three elements: brain matter (80%), cerebrospinal fluid (CSF; 10%), and blood (10%). The Monro-Kellie hypothesis states that when any one of these elements increases in volume, one of the other elements must accommodate that increased volume through a reciprocal reduction in volume.[9] Failure to compensate results in uncontrolled increased intracranial pressure. Irrepressible intracranial hypertension and cerebral edema cause a progressive decrease in cerebral perfusion as intracranial pressure exceeds mean arterial blood pressure. The resultant cerebral ischemia leads to brain death (Table 33-1).

The brain dead individual exhibits no spontaneous respiratory effort, no response to painful stimuli, and absence of all brainstem reflexes (e.g., fixed, dilated pupils; absence of oculocephalic, oculovestibular, cough, gag, and corneal reflexes).

Before declaration of brain death, all medical conditions or metabolic derangements that may affect the neurologic examination should be treated or corrected. Serum chemistries should be within normal limits; body temperature should be at or above 95° F; and there should be no drug levels that would impair neurologic reflexes, such as neuromuscular blockade, sedation, or anesthetics. The patient

TABLE 33-1	**Clinical Criteria for the Declaration of Brain Death**

1. Known cause of death
2. Irreversibility
3. Body temperature >90° F (35° C)
4. Fixed pupils
5. No spontaneous movements in response to external stimuli
6. No reflex activity except that elicited by spinal cord
7. Apnea in the presence of hypercapnia (Pa_{CO_2} >60 mm Hg)

House-Park MA: Nursing care of the potential donor. In Chabalewski FL, editor: *Donation & transplantation: nursing curriculum,* Richmond, Va, 1996, UNOS, 105-130.

should be hemodynamically stable, with a systolic blood pressure equal to or higher than 90 mm Hg.

Apnea Testing

Apnea is an essential component in the determination of brain death. In order to confirm apnea in the course of brain death examination, an apnea test is performed. Before initiating the test, the patient should be normothermic and normotensive with a systolic blood pressure 90 mm Hg or higher and a baseline Pa_{CO_2} between 35 and 45 torr. The patient should not have received any drugs that could potentially suppress respiratory effort.

To perform the apnea test, once these prerequisites are met, the patient is hyperoxygenated with 100% oxygen for at least 10 minutes. The patient is then removed from ventilatory support, and oxygen is fed through the endotracheal tube via cannula at 6 L/min. After cessation of mechanical ventilation, the patient's chest should be clearly visible for the remainder of the test. The patient is then monitored carefully for spontaneous respiratory effort and any change in the baseline vital signs. Any spontaneous effort of breathing or a greater than 10% change in the blood pressure, heart rate, or pulse oximetry is cause to abort the study because spontaneous respiratory effort negates the assumption of brain death.

If an apnea test is aborted because of deterioration in vital signs, in the absence of respiratory effort the supposition of brain death is supported and the patient is returned to ventilatory support at the pretest settings. If the patient remains stable in the absence of respiratory effort for up to 10 minutes an arterial blood gas measurement is repeated and the patient is placed back on ventilatory support at the pretest settings. A Pa_{CO_2} 60 or greater, or at least 2 to 2.5 times the pretest Pa_{CO_2}, supports the diagnosis of brain death.[9]

Confirmatory Testing

Electroencephalography, transcranial Doppler, or cerebral flow studies may be done to confirm the diagnosis of brain death as evidenced by clinical examination (absence of brainstem reflexes). The decision to perform confirmatory studies is based on the judgment of the physician declaring brain death and is done in accordance with state laws and individual hospital policy.[10]

SEQUELAE OF BRAIN DEATH

The inception of brain death presents a challenge to donor stability. Multiple systems are affected once compensatory mechanisms regulated by the central nervous system fail. The sympathetic nervous system accelerates, causing an uncontrolled release of catecholamines. Tachycardia, an increase in systolic blood pressure, and increased cardiac output characterize this "autonomic storm." Once the catecholamine stores are depleted, this phase ends and hemodynamic instability may ensue. Regulatory mechanisms fail; the ability to control blood pressure and heart rate is lost. Hypotension typically ensues because of a lack of autoregulation, causing vasodilation.[11]

Interventions previously employed to control intracranial hypertension (osmotic diuresis, fluid restriction) may result in a dangerously low systolic blood pressure (<80 mm Hg). Left untreated, persistent hypotension may threaten viability of organs for transplant. Vigorous but controlled fluid resuscitation can be successful in treating hypotension. Frequently one or more pressors are infused to maintain a systolic blood pressure of at least 100 mm Hg. Heart rate may vary, and arrhythmias may occur. An initial exaggerated vagal response results in bradycardia but rapidly progresses to tachycardia secondary to catecholamine release and pressor support. As the hypothalamus is destroyed, thermoregulatory mechanisms fail and the patient may develop poikilothermy, whereby body temperature mimics ambient temperature. Infusion of cold blood products may exacerbate hypothermia. To help maintain the patient's body temperature, careful attention of the room temperature, infusion of blood through a warmer, and use of an external hyperthermic unit help to maintain a body temperature above 95° F. Oxygenation is controlled through mechanical ventilation. Aspiration pneumonia, pulmonary contusions, and neurogenic pulmonary edema may impair adequate oxygenation and threaten the viability of the lungs for transplant.

The posterior pituitary gland ceases to compensate for the feedback mechanism and no longer produces antidiuretic hormone (ADH). The subsequent onset of diabetes insipidus can be treated successfully with aqueous pitressin, either subcutaneously or intravenously. Maintaining hemodynamic stability in the brain dead individual presents a tremendous but rewarding challenge to the critical care staff.

THE ORGAN DONATION PROCESS

The steps in the process of organ donation are intricate and interrelated and each is integral to the success of the process. All patients who die or whose death is impending must be referred to the OPC to be evaluated for potential for organ donation. Informed consent cannot be obtained until a patient is declared brain dead, the family is informed of the death, and the family understands the concept of brain death. Donor management is ongoing throughout the organ evaluation process until organ recovery is complete. The steps of the organ donation process are as follows: (1) identification and referral, (2) evaluation, (3) brain death declaration, (4) informed consent, (5) donor management and organ placement, and (6) organ recovery.

The United Network for Organ Sharing (UNOS) developed a critical pathway to assist health care professionals in critical care areas throughout the organ donation process (Table 33-2). The pathway provides an outline for the care of an organ donor from referral through organ recovery. Each step is defined as a phase and is composed of key events, parameters, and diagnostic or clinical values critical to optimal organ function. The donation process is multifaceted and can progress rapidly through each phase, with some events occurring simultaneously. The pathway provides a clear illustration of each phase and identifies the expectations for each. It promotes a collaborative relationship among all disciplines involved in the care of the donor. It is not meant to replace open communication between the OPC and health care team; rather, it keeps all members of the team involved in the process.[12] The pathway is designed to be reviewed, revised, and adapted by each hospital in conjunction with its individual OPOs so that current federal, state, or hospital protocols may be incorporated.

DONOR IDENTIFICATION AND REFERRAL

In accordance with federal regulations, every patient admitted to a hospital with the potential to progress to brain death or who is actually brain dead must be referred to the regional OPO in a timely manner.[4] In some instances it is obvious in the emergency department that the patient meets brain death criteria. In this situation the staff should make the referral before decisions are made regarding withdrawal of care or instituting a do not resuscitate order. An OPC is available on a 24-hour basis to respond to a referral for evaluation. The OPC can work collaboratively with the trauma team to develop a plan regarding potential organ and tissue donation. Figure 33-2 outlines the referral process.

When referring a potential organ donor to the OPO, it is helpful to have the following information: (1) patient name if known, (2) age, (3) gender, and (4) blood type if known. The referral should not be delayed because of a lack of specific information.

Early referral makes the difference in the number of recipients who may benefit from this gift of life. Referral before brain death promotes a collaborative approach between the OPC and the health care team in the development of a plan of care. Early development of a plan can ensure anticipation and early correction of the sequelae commonly seen once brain death occurs, thus preventing organ insult as a result of hemodynamic instability. Any delay in treating hemodynamic instability may threaten the viability of organ function. A timely referral therefore can mean five to seven organs being recovered for transplant as opposed to two or three recovered in cases when the referral is made after the diagnosis of brain death.[5]

EVALUATION OF THE POTENTIAL ORGAN DONOR

Each referral is evaluated by an OPC. The initial referral rarely elicits information that excludes the patient from

TABLE 33-2 Critical Pathway for the Organ Donor©

Patient Name _____ ID Number _____

Collaborative Practice	Phase I Referral	Phase II Declaration of Brain Death and Consent	Phase III Donor Evaluation	Phase IV Donor Management	Phase V Recovery Phase
The following professionals may be involved to enhance the donation process. Check all that apply. ☐ Physician ☐ Critical care RN ☐ Organ Procurement Organization (OPO) ☐ OPO Coordinator (OPC) ☐ Medical Examiner (ME)/Coroner ☐ Respiratory ☐ Laboratory ☐ Radiology ☐ Anesthesiology ☐ OR/Surgery staff ☐ Clergy ☐ Social worker	☐ Notify physician regarding OPO referral ☐ Contact OPO ref: Potential donor with severe brain insult ☐ OPC on site and begins evaluation: Time ___ Date ___ ☐ Ht ___ Wt ___ as documented ☐ ABO as documented ☐ Notify house supervisor/ charge nurse of OPC presence on unit	☐ Brain death documented Time ___ Date ___ ☐ Pt accepted as potential donor ☐ MD notifies family of death ☐ Plan family approach with OPC ☐ Offer support services to family (clergy, etc) ☐ OPC/Hospital staff talks to family about donation ☐ Family accepts donation ☐ OPC obtains signed consent & medical/social history Time ___ Date ___ ☐ ME/Coroner notified ☐ ME/Coroner releases body for donation ☐ **Family/ME/Coroner denies donation–stop pathway– initiate post-mortem protocol–support family.**	☐ Obtain pre/post transfusion blood for serology testing (HIV, Hepatitis, VDRL, CMV) ☐ Obtain lymph nodes and/or blood for tissue typing ☐ Notify OR & anesthesiology of pending case ☐ Notify house supervisor of pending donation ☐ Chest & abdominal circumference ☐ Lung measurements per CXR by OPC ☐ Cardiology consult as requested by OPC ☐ **Organ recovery process discontinued–donor organs unstable for transplantation**	☐ OPC writes new orders ☐ Organ placement ☐ OPC sets tentative OR time ☐ Insert arterial line/ CVP/2 large-bore IVs	☐ Checklist for OR ☐ Supplies given to OR ☐ Prepare patient for transport to OR ☐ IVs ☐ Pumps ☐ O₂ ☐ Ambu ☐ PEEP valve ☐ Transport to OR Date ___ Time ___ ☐ OR nurse reviews consent & brain death documentation & checks patient's ID band
Labs/Diagnostics		☐ Review previous lab results ☐ Review previous hemodynamics	☐ Blood chemistry ☐ CBC + diff ☐ UA ☐ C&S ☐ PT, PTT ☐ ABO ☐ A Subtype ☐ Liver function tests ☐ Blood culture × 2/15 minutes to 1 hour apart ☐ Sputum Gram Stain & C&S ☐ Type & Cross Match ___ # units PRBCs ☐ CXR ☐ ABGs ☐ EKG ☐ Echo ☐ Consider cardiac cath ☐ Consider bronchoscopy	☐ Determine need for additional lab testing ☐ CXR after line placement (if done) ☐ Serum electrolytes ☐ H&H after PRBC Rx ☐ PT, PTT ☐ BUN, serum creatinine after correcting fluid deficit ☐ Notify OPC for ___ PT>14 ___ PTT<28 ___ Urine outout is ___ <1 mL/Kg/hr ___ >3 mL/Kg/hr ___ Hct ↓ 30/Hgb ↓ 10 ___ Na ↑ 150 mEq/L	☐ Labs drawn in OR as per surgeon or OPC request ☐ Communicate with pathology: Bx liver and/or kidneys as indicated

$c i$

Respiratory	☐ Pt on ventilator ☐ Suction q 2 hr ☐ Reposition q 2 hr	☐ Prep for apnea testing: set FiO$_2$ @ 100% and anticipate need to decrease rate if PCO$_2$ ↓ 45 mm Hg	☐ Maximize ventilator settings to achieve SaO$_2$ 98–99% ☐ PEEP = 5cm H$_2$O ☐ Challenge for lung placement FiO$_2$ @ 100%, PEEP @ 5cm H$_2$O × 10 min ☐ ABGs as ordered ☐ VS q 1°	☐ Notify OPC for BP < 90 systolic HR < 70 or > 120 CVP < 4 or > 11 PaO$_2$ < 90 or SaO$_2$ < 95%	☐ Portable O$_2$ @ 100% FiO$_2$ for transport to OR ☐ Ambu bag and PEEP valve ☐ Move to OR
Treatments/ Ongoing care		☐ Use warming/cooling blanket to maintain temperature at 36.5° C–37.5° C ☐ NG to ↓ intermittent suction	☐ Check NG placement & output ☐ Obtain actual Ht ___ & Wt ___ if not previously obtained		☐ Set OR temp as directed by OPC ☐ Post mortem care at conclusion of case
Medications			☐ Medication as requested by OPC	☐ Fluid resuscitation—consider crystolloids, colloids, blood ☐ DC meds except pressors & antibiotics ☐ Broad-spectrum antibiotic if not previously ordered ☐ Vasopressor support to maintain BP>90 mm Hg systolic ☐ Electrolyte imbalance: consider K, Ca, PO$_4$, Mg replacement ☐ Hyperglycemia: consider Insulin drip ☐ Oliguria: consider diuretics ☐ Diabetes insipidus: consider antidiuretics ☐ Paralytic as indicated for spinal reflexes	☐ DC antidiuretics ☐ Diuretics as needed ☐ 350 U heparin/kg or as directed by surgeon
Optimal outcomes	The potential donor is identified & a referral is made to the OPO.	The family is offered the option of donation & their decision is supported.	The donor is evaluated & found to be suitable candidate for donation.	Optimal organ function is maintained.	All potentially suitable, consented organs are recovered for transplant.

ABGs, Arterial blood gases; *BP*, Blood pressure; *Bx*, Biopsy; *BUN*, Blood urea nitrogen; *CBC*, Complete blood count; *CMV*, Cytomegalovirus; *C & S*, Culture and sensitivity; *CXR*, Chest x-ray film; *CVP*, Central venous pressure; *DC*, Discontinue; *ECG*, Electrocardiogram; *FiO$_2$*, Fraction of inspired oxygen; *Hb*, Hemoglobin; *Hct*, Hematocrit; *H & H*, Hemoglobin and hematocrit; *HIV*, Human immunodeficiency virus; *HR*, Heart rate; *OR*, Operating room; *PaO$_2$*, Partial arterial oxygen pressure; *PCO$_2$*, Partial pressure of carbon dioxide; *PEEP*, Positive end-expiratory pressure; *PRBCs*, Packed red blood cells; *Pt*, Patient; *PT*, Prothrombin time; *PTT*, Partial thromboplastin time; *NG*, Nasogastric tube; *Rx*, Prescription; *SaO$_2$*, Arterial oxygen saturation; *UA*, Urinalysis; *VDRL*, Venereal Disease Research Laboratory; *VS*, Vital signs; *Shaded areas*, Organ procurement coordinator activities. Reprinted with permission of the United Network for Organ Sharing, Richmond, Va.

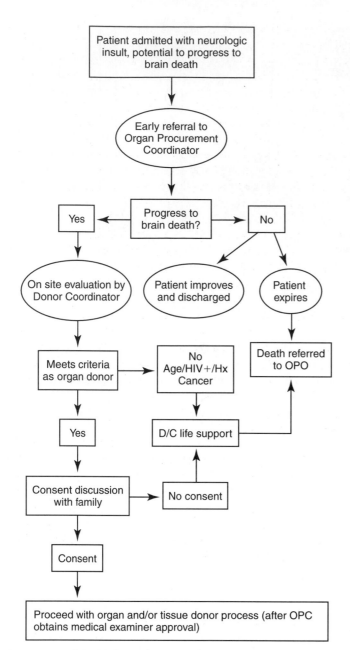

FIGURE 33-2 **Referring a Potential Donor.**

organ donation. Typically this phone consultation is followed by an OPC site visit to review the case. The OPC and staff discuss the family's understanding of the prehospital events, admitting diagnosis, hospital course, and prognosis. Old charts may be requested. The medical history, the description of events leading to this admission, the hospital course since arriving in the emergency department, laboratory data, and any diagnostic tests to determine donor suitability are reviewed.

All organ donors are screened for communicable disease through standard serologic testing. Table 33-3 lists common testing and the implications for organ and tissue donation. Pretransfusion specimens are desirable, a point for the trauma team to remember when drawing specimens for laboratory tests in the emergency department. If there is an

indication that the patient may become an organ donor, obtain two extra blood chemistry specimens to be held in the laboratory if needed.

Hospital staff should never rule out any potential donor without consulting the OPC first. The shortage of precious organs for transplant and advances in the field of transplantation have led to an expansion of donor criteria. Factors that may have ruled out a patient as a potential donor in the past may no longer be applicable.

BRAIN DEATH DECLARATION AND DOCUMENTATION

In accordance with individual state regulations and hospital policy, brain death determination should be documented clearly in the patient record with the time, date, and signature of the physician. Some states require two licensed physicians to declare brain death. Most hospital policies regarding the declaration of brain death prohibit the transplant physicians who may perform the recovery procedure from being involved in the process of declaring a patient brain dead. Some institutions may have separate policies regarding the declaration of brain death in neonates, infants, and children. These policies often dictate a standard waiting period and reexamination to confirm brain death. Hospital policy regarding brain death declaration must be followed. In the brain dead individual the time that brain death is documented is the legal time of death. Whether or not the case progresses to organ recovery, the time that the patient is declared brain dead is the date and time the patient expired, not to be confused with the time of asystole after withdrawal of mechanical support.

INFORMED CONSENT

Much research has been done on the needs of families of the critically ill patient. The family is typically in crisis and needs honest, direct, understandable explanations about their loved one's care and prognosis. They may need to spend time with their loved one and feel supported and accepted by the staff. They need to have hope but to be given the opportunity to discuss the possibility of death. They need to know that the health care team cares about their loved one.[13,14]

Success in obtaining consent depends largely on the family's perception of the hospital experience and the ability to understand the diagnosis of brain death. The family of a potential donor needs to be informed as the patient's condition deteriorates and needs repeated explanations about the patient's potential to progress to brain death. Results of clinical examinations and diagnostic testing should be shared in understandable terms, and questions should be answered honestly. The use of visual aids to explain the injuries may help them to understand. Family members should be allowed to see the CT scan or x-ray films if they will help them to understand the extent of the cerebral damage. Understanding the finality of brain death is difficult for family members when their loved one appears to be "sleeping." The patient may be warm to the touch, have

TABLE 33-3   **Serologic Testing**

Test	Significance of Positive Results	Organ Donation	Tissue Donation
HIV I, HIV II			
Human immunodeficiency viruses I, II	Indicates antibodies to HIV I and II	NO	NO
HTLV I, HTLV II			
Human lymphocyte viruses I, II	Indicates presence of antibodies to HTLV I and II	NO	NO
HCV			
Hepatitis C antibody	Indicates presence of antibodies to hepatitis C	YES	NO
HBsAg			
Hepatitis B surface antigen	Indicates a current hepatitis B infection	YES*	NO
HBc			
Hepatitis B core antibody	Indicates exposure to hepatitis B virus	YES	NO
AUSab			
Australian antibody	Indicates immunity to hepatitis B virus through	YES	YES
Hepatitis B surface antibody	previous infection or immunization		
VDRL or RPR			
Rapid plasma reagin	Indicates exposure to *Treponema pallidum* spirochete, which causes syphilis	YES	NO
CMV			
Cytomegalovirus	Indicates presence of antibodies to CMV	YES	YES

*Life-saving organs only—heart, lungs, and liver.

good color and a visible heart rate, and appear to be breathing, albeit with mechanical means.[15] This scenario lends itself more to the perception that the patient is sleeping or in a coma rather than the reality that that person has died. Timing is of paramount importance when discussing the option of organ donation. This discussion should not take place until the family understands and accepts the death of their loved one. The introduction of the subject of organ donation too early in the hospital course, or before the family accepts the death, can cause unnecessary anguish and ensure that that family will not be willing to discuss the option of donation if and when brain death occurs.[5] The explanation of brain death and the discussion about organ donation should be separated to give the family time to accept that their loved one has died before they make a decision regarding organ or tissue donation.

Staff may be reluctant to refer a potential donor to the OPO because the family is upset over the news of their loved one's death. Fear that a discussion about organ donation will further traumatize the family is a common misperception. In reality the knowledge that a loved one's final act of kindness saved other lives may be very comforting. Early involvement of the OPC ensures the proper timing of such a conversation and relieves staff from the responsibility of discussing donation with a family.

The manner in which the option of organ donation is presented to the family and their personal feelings regarding donation play integral roles in the family's decision to donate. It is important to provide the family with a quiet, private setting when offering the option of donation. The OPC discusses the benefits of donation, answers their questions honestly, explains the process, and addresses common concerns associated with organ and tissue dona-

TABLE 33-4   **Transplantable Organs and Tissues**

Organs	Tissues
Heart	Bone
Kidneys	Bone marrow
Lungs (segment)	Corneas
Liver (segment)	Dura
Pancreas	Heart valves
Small bowel	Skin
Stomach	Tendons
	Vessels

tion. The option for the family to donate organs includes heart, lungs, liver, kidneys, pancreas, and small bowel. Tissue donation can include the cornea and eye, heart valves, bone, skin, vessels, tendons, and, in some states, bladder. The consent form lists each option for donation, and only those organs and tissues indicated for donation by the family are removed. Families need to know that an open-casket viewing is possible without detection of the donation. They should also be aware that there is no cost to them for any expense related to organ or tissue donation.

The family is offered the option of organ and tissue donation for both transplant and research, and they may decline any or all of these options. Consent is given for each individual organ and tissue to be transplanted. Table 33-4 lists all organs and tissues that may be used for transplant. The family is assured that their decision is confidential. The choice is theirs, and whether or not they wish to pursue organ donation, they will be supported in their decision.

The operating room staff and anesthesia personnel are notified soon after consent is obtained, in anticipation of the organ recovery that will take place several hours later.

SPECIFIC ORGAN EVALUATION

Once a patient is declared brain dead and informed consent is obtained, organ evaluation commences. Age, medical history, existing laboratory values, and the specific organs designated on the consent form determine which organs are evaluated for transplantation. Figure 33-3 outlines an overview of the evaluation process. Pertinent laboratory studies are ordered at the onset of this evaluation process and compared with previous values. Laboratory studies may be ordered on a regular basis throughout the organ placement process and just before the recovery procedure.

DONOR MANAGEMENT

The goal of donor management is to maximize the viability of each organ system for transplant. With the onset of brain death, all compensatory mechanisms are impaired or fail altogether. Donor management is directed at maintenance of optimal oxygenation and organ perfusion, while maintaining fluid, electrolyte, and acid-base balance.[16] In the adult organ donor the rule of 100s is a guideline: urine output 100 ml/hr or more, Pao_2 100 torr or more on the least Fio_2 possible, and systolic blood pressure 100 mm Hg or greater.

Donor management begins with a review of the patient's status. The OPC, nurse, and physician discuss the patient's clinical status and the goals for management of the donor. A collaborative relationship and open communication facilitate the best outcome possible for organ recovery. Again, a

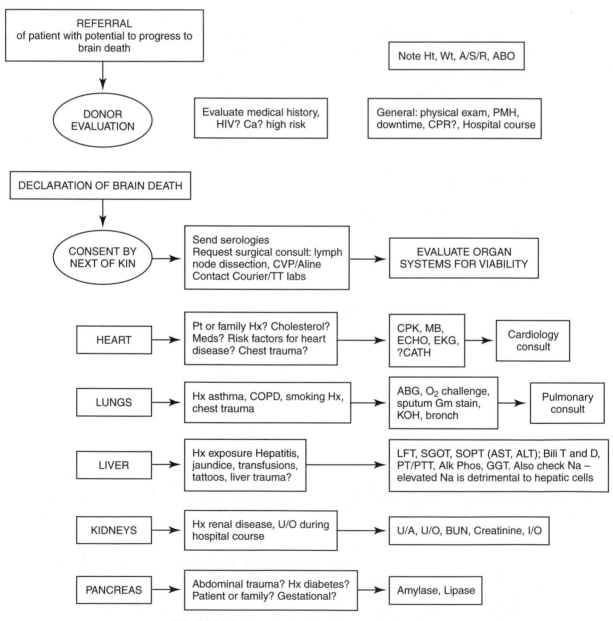

FIGURE 33-3 Organ Evaluation Process: An Overview.

good tool to guide the care of the organ donor is the critical pathway for the organ donor (see Table 33-2).[12] It provides an outline for the plan of care and defines parameters that the nurse should be aware of when caring for the donor. It can be used by the novice nurse to learn the donor process or as a guide for the experienced nurse.

Even for the most experienced staff, maintaining hemodynamic stability after brain death is a challenge. Hypotension is a result of osmotic diuresis and fluid restriction induced to prevent or treat cerebral edema before brain death. Hemorrhage caused by concurrent injury or coagulopathies caused by open head trauma or hypothermia may threaten hemodynamic stability. Unless fluid deficits are treated aggressively and appropriately with colloid, crystalloid, and blood, prolonged hypotension may threaten the viability of organs for transplant. Table 33-5 outlines a formula to calculate the fluid deficit in these individuals.

Further insult ensues with the relative hypovolemia resulting from systemic vasodilation after brain death. Vasopressors can be infused to replace lost catecholamine stores. Thyroid hormone replacement may be used to replace levels of triiodothyronine, thyroxin, insulin, and cortisol in an effort to restore hemodynamic stability. Ideally a systolic blood pressure of at least 100 mm Hg should be achieved and maintained.

The potential donor requires support for other functions lost to brain death as well. Because the hypothalamus is not functioning, the body cannot regulate body temperature; care needs to be taken to maintain a temperature at 95° F or above. Temperatures below 95° F may induce coagulopathies that cannot be reversed with transfusion of blood products. Hyperthermia units and warmed blood products and intravenous fluids can help maintain the body temperature above 95° F. Diabetes insipidus may result from depletion of antidiuretic hormone, a result of absent pituitary function. Continuous infusion of aqueous pitressin can control polyuria and prevent dehydration and provides the best control of hourly urine output. It is common to see a mild vasopressor effect with the continuous infusion of pitressin.

Fluid and electrolyte imbalances are common and can be related to aggressive fluid resuscitation or dehydration. An elevated serum sodium level can indicate a need for aggressive fluid replacement. Potassium, magnesium, phosphates, and calcium repletion may be indicated.

TABLE 33-5 Fluid Deficit Calculation

1. $0.6 \times$ (kg in body weight) = Total body H_2O
2. Current serum sodium $\times$ (total body H_2O) $\div$ 140 (normal Na) = X
3. X – (total body H_2O) = Amount of deficit in liters
   Replace with 0.45 normal saline over 8-24 hours

Modified from North American Transplant Coordinators Organization: *An introductory course for the transplant coordinator,* Lenexa, Kan, 1998, North American Transplant Coordinators Organization.

Hyperglycemia is not unusual, even in the absence of a history of diabetes. Infusion of dextrose solutions, response to stress, and the β-adrenergic effects of infused catecholamines may elevate glucose levels. Hyperglycemia should be treated aggressively to prevent further derangement of electrolytes and polyuria. Although not common, it is reasonable to consider an insulin infusion to control serum glucose levels.

Ideally arterial and central venous lines are placed early to facilitate repeated blood sampling. Meticulous attention to strict aseptic technique must be observed. Aseptic technique should be practiced when drawing blood, performing invasive procedures, and performing dressing changes. The organ donor is just as susceptible to nosocomial infection as any other patient. When the donor develops an infection, it compromises the many recipients who will require immunosuppressive therapy after transplant. Each donor should be monitored closely for the sequelae of brain death. Many problems associated with the loss of all cerebral function can be anticipated and treated early. The OPC guides the management of the donor. In most states the OPC assumes care of the donor after brain death declaration, once informed consent is obtained. The OPC writes all orders and directs the care of the donor.

PLACEMENT OF ORGANS

After each organ system is evaluated, the OPC attempts to place each organ that is suitable for transplant within the constraints of the consent. Data are provided to UNOS, specifically the donor's height, weight, age, gender, and race. Donor-specific lists are generated for each organ.

The transplant surgeon for each potential recipient is contacted and given the appropriate data. Then a decision is made based on the evaluation of each organ. Once all the organs deemed suitable are placed with a primary and backup recipient, arrangements are made for each transplant team to be brought to the hospital. The operating room staff is contacted and a time for the recovery is scheduled.

ORGAN RECOVERY PROCESS

The procedure for the recovery of organs begins after the intended recipients are identified and the transplant teams arrive at the donor hospital. The transplant teams can vary from two to twelve people, depending on the number of organs to be recovered.

A midline incision is made from the top of the sternum to the symphysis pubis. The sternum is opened with a sternal saw or Lebsche knife. All organs are removed through this single incision. The organs to be recovered are dissected free from all but their vasculature. This generally takes 30 minutes to 3 hours, depending on the organs to be recovered. Unusual findings are documented, and the surgeon may perform a biopsy of an organ. Once the dissection is complete, preparation is made to cross-clamp the aorta. After the cross-clamping, the organs are removed sequentially in the following order: heart, lungs, liver, kidneys, and pancreas.

Once removed, each organ is inspected and then preserved for transportation to the transplant center. A member of the recovery team closes the incision. The entire procedure, depending on the number of organs recovered, can take 45 minutes (kidneys only) to 6 hours (multiorgan donor). The OPC assists the staff with postmortem care and transporting the body to the morgue.

Ischemic time, or the amount of time from cessation of blood flow to an organ until reperfusion, is always kept to the minimal time to optimize organ function after transplantation. The heart and lungs are limited to 4 hours or less of ischemic time although some programs have reported successful transplantation after 6 hours for the heart only. Pancreas and liver transplants are done within 24 hours, whereas kidneys are transplanted within 24 hours but can be transplanted up to 48 hours. All efforts are made to transplant the organs as soon after recovery as possible.

FOLLOW-UP AFTER DONATION

After each case, the hospital staff from the emergency department, intensive care unit, and surgical services are told about the outcome of the donor family's decision to donate. Information about each of the recipients, such as age, gender, disease process, and progress since the transplant, is shared with all those involved in the process. Written follow-up may also be sent to all staff involved in the care of the donor, from the trauma nurse to ancillary staff.

Unless otherwise requested by the donor family, the OPC contacts them after organ recovery to inform them which organs could be recovered for transplantation. Emotional support continues through this time, and referral to the appropriate support groups can be made. Information may be provided regarding the National Kidney Foundation's Donor Family Council and other avenues of support to the family of an organ or tissue donor. Written correspondence is mailed after the phone contact. Information such as age, gender, and marital status of each recipient is shared with the donor family. Written communication between the donor family and recipients can be an option if both parties agree and the OPO can facilitate such communication. Occasionally both parties wish to meet, which can also be facilitated by the OPO staff. There is much controversy over issues surrounding the direct contact between donor families and recipients. A majority of the literature supports such contact if both parties wish to pursue it.[17,18]

ROLE OF UNOS IN ORGAN ALLOCATION

ABOUT UNOS

The National Organ Transplant Act (NOTA; Public Law 98-507), passed in 1984, established the national Organ Procurement and Transplantation Network (OPTN) and the Scientific Registry for Transplant Recipients (SR). In 1986 UNOS was awarded two federal contracts with the U.S. Department of Health and Human Services, Health Resources and Services Administration, Division of Transplan-

tation, to administer the OPTN and the SR. In 1999 the University Renal Research and Education Association was awarded the contract to administer the SR. Under the OPTN, UNOS maintains the national waiting list for all patients in need of a solid organ for transplant, conducts educational activities, and coordinates the communication network necessary to attain its organizational directive. The SR collects data on all transplant recipients and provides a national database for basic and clinical research on organ transplantation.

UNOS is a private, nonprofit corporation organized to improve the effectiveness of organ transplantation in the United States. UNOS promotes, facilitates, and scientifically advances organ procurement and transplantation on a national level. UNOS does more than coordinate the matching and placement of donor organs with the potential recipients on the national waiting list; policy development and education are also important functions of UNOS.

ORGAN ALLOCATION

Policies governing the transplantation system are based on medical and scientific criteria and do not permit favoritism based on political influence or discrimination on the basis of race, gender, or financial status. The policies are also in a continuous state of evaluation and modification in order to meet the rapidly changing technology.[19]

The allocation of organs uses a complex computer matching system. Information about each cadaveric organ donor is entered into the UNOS computer and compared with the list of potential recipients waiting nationally to determine priority for organ allocation. Based on UNOS policies, a different algorithm is applied for each organ system to initially eliminate incompatible potential recipients. The computer system then assigns a point score to every compatible waiting recipient based on factors such as medical urgency, time waiting, blood group compatibility, and tissue type similarity (for kidney and pancreas).

For kidney allocation, the computer identifies all potential recipients who have an identical tissue type match with the donor. Policy requires that all perfectly matched (six-antigen match) patients be offered a kidney first. The computer algorithm for kidney allocation gives some priority to children under the age of 10 and to highly sensitized patients who are waiting for transplant.[2]

UNOS, through the Organ Center, is available to all OPOs 24 hours a day every day of the year to help place organs in an equitable and efficient manner. Current information and statistics about transplantation can be accessed through the Web site at www.UNOS.org.

NON–HEART-BEATING DONORS

The limited number of brain dead organ donors has resulted in the search for and identification of other appropriate organ donor sources. Traditionally the organ donor is an individual who has been declared brain dead but is maintained on mechanical support until the organ donation process is complete. Oxygenation and perfusion are maintained for optimal organ function. However, the non-heart-beating donor (NHBD) has suffered cardiopulmonary death within a very limited period of time before organ recovery. Kidneys are more tolerant of ischemic time (the time from cross-clamping until reperfusion in the recipient) and therefore are most commonly recovered. Less common is the recovery of liver and pancreas. Recovery of heart and lungs in this situation is rare.

In contrast to the heart-beating or brain dead donor, the NHBD has also suffered a devastating neurologic insult but has not progressed to brain death. These potential donors are asystolic and pronounced dead, thus making donation possible in accordance with the family's wishes.

Each case is evaluated carefully. Criteria tend to be stricter for the NHBD because anoxic damage is expected. Protocols for the NHBD vary from OPO to OPO and hospital to hospital. Procedures and withdrawal of support can be performed in the intensive care unit, operating room, or Post Anesthesia Care Unit (PACU). In contrast to the family of a heart-beating donor, the family of an NHBD usually has made the decision to withdraw support before a discussion about donation.

NHBDs offer another option in dealing with the shortage of organs for transplantation. They currently constitute approximately 1% of all organ donors, but the number can be expected to increase in response to the ever-growing numbers of persons listed for a transplant. As NHBD programs become a more accepted practice, more families for whom organ donation would not be an option will have the opportunity to choose donation.[20,21]

TISSUE DONATION

In accordance with federal regulations, every hospital must report all inpatient deaths to their regional OPO. The OPO coordinator, or hospital staff trained by the OPO, review the following information: patient's name, age, gender, race, date and time of admission and death, admitting diagnosis, cause of death, and known medical history. If the patient is a potential tissue donor, the identity of the next of kin, their relationship to the patient, and their phone number are also requested. The coordinator confirms that the family has been notified of the patient's death.

Tissues that can be donated include eyes and corneas, bone, skin, heart valves, pericardium, bladder, vessels, and ligaments. As with the organ donor, tissue donation is undetectable with an open-casket viewing. In contrast to the organ donation discussion, the discussion about the family's options for tissue donation can occur after they arrive home and have had time to accept the death of their loved one. In most cases, tissue recovery can take place up to 24 hours after death, except for eyes, which are optimally recovered within 6 to 10 hours. As with organ donation, it is the coordinator's responsibility to obtain permission from the

medical examiner before proceeding with tissue recovery. The family receives written follow-up regarding the recipients of their generosity. Less common, but possible, is communication between the donor family and the recipients.

MEDICAL EXAMINER CASES

The primary responsibility of the medical examiner or coroner is the determination of the cause and manner of death. Collection and documentation of all available evidence are necessary to arrive at and support such determinations. Cases that are reportable to the medical examiner include, but are not limited to, deaths resulting from trauma, homicide or suicide, and occupational injury; deaths within 24 hours of admission to the hospital; intraoperative deaths; deaths occurring under suspicious circumstances; and deaths resulting from poisoning or electrocution. In those states where the OPO and the medical examiners have a cooperative relationship and enjoy open communication, organ donation can and does happen without impeding the investigation of the cause of death.

Clear and concise documentation of injuries before organ recovery is essential. In some cases the medical examiner is present during the organ recovery surgery to determine if bruising of the chest or abdominal wall occurred before or as a result of the recovery procedure. Pictures may be taken to document injuries. The National Association of Medical Examiners (NAME) supports a working relationship between the medical examiners and the local OPO, and some states have developed written protocols to facilitate such cooperative relationships. The key is for the OPO to develop and maintain a collaborative relationship with the medical examiners to save lives through organ donation while avoiding loss of evidence, which may result in the inability to prosecute a criminal case.[22]

TRANSPLANT RECIPIENTS AS TRAUMA PATIENTS

The transplant recipient admitted to the emergency department after sustaining trauma can present many challenges. As with any trauma situation, the priorities are the primary survey followed by the secondary survey. Adequate oxygenation and hemodynamic stability are of paramount importance because the transplanted organ may be less tolerant of sustained hypotension. Trauma resuscitation protocols should be followed as with any victim, but the health care team should maintain an awareness of special considerations (e.g., a donated kidney or pancreas is implanted in the anterior abdominal cavity). The index of suspicion for donor organ damage should be high in patients with blunt or penetrating abdominal trauma.

Immunosuppressive therapy can also present a challenge in treating injured organ recipients. Those who are taking drugs such as cyclosporine should avoid certain concurrent drug regimens; for example, the use of neuromuscular blockade in the chronically immunosuppressed recipient can result in a prolongation of the effects of those drugs. Certain antibiotics, H_2 antagonists, and even steroids may promote hepatic or renal toxicity.

The complex implications of caring for a transplant recipient who has suffered trauma are best handled through a multidisciplinary approach, including the transplant team involved with the recipient's surgery. They can best guide the care to avoid tragic complications that could result in loss of donor organ function.

SUMMARY

The critical shortage of organs for transplant challenges all members of the health care community to maintain an awareness regarding their essential role in donor awareness. The option of organ and tissue donation is often one of the few choices the family is allowed when their loved one suffers a sudden and traumatic injury. It is well documented that choosing donation can provide the family with solace and peace of mind. When modern technology can no longer sustain their loved one's life, the nurse can still facilitate a positive outcome for the family during this crisis. This can be realized best when a timely referral is made, involving the OPC early in the process. A collaborative effort with the OPC to promote the best outcome possible affirms the integral part each nurse plays in saving lives through organ transplantation. It is only through these efforts that the recipient's hope for a life-saving transplant is transformed into reality.

REFERENCES

1. United Network for Organ Sharing (UNOS): www.unos.org, June 1, 1999.
2. *1998 Annual report of the U.S. Scientific Registry of Transplant Recipients and the Organ Procurement and Transplantation Network, transplant date 1988-1997,* Richmond, Va, 1999, UNOS.
3. Gortmaker SL, Beasley CL, Brigham LE et al: Organ donor potential and performance: size and nature of the organ donor shortfall, *Crit Care Med* 24(3):432-439, 1996.
4. Department of Health and Human Services, Health Care Financing Administration: Medicare and Medicaid programs; hospital conditions of participation; provider agreements and supplier approval. Final rule, *Fed Reg* 63:119, 1998.
5. Ehrle RN, Shafer TJ, Nelson KR: Referral, request and consent for organ donation: best practice: a blueprint for success, *Crit Care Nurse* 19(2):21-33, 1999.
6. Malangoni MA, Mancuso C, Jacobs DG et al: Analysis of deaths within 24 hours of injury: cost benefit implications for organ and tissue donation, *J Trauma* 40:632-635, 1996.
7. McNamara P, Franz HG, Fowler RA et al: Medical record review as a measure of the effectiveness of organ procurement practices in the hospital, *Jt Comm J Qual Improv* 23:321-333, 1997.
8. Guidelines for the determination of death: report of the medical consultants on the diagnosis of death to the President's Commission for the Study of Ethical Problems in Medicine and Biomedical and Behavioral Research, *JAMA* 246: 2184-2186, 1981.
9. Hickey JV: Intracranial pressure: theory and management of increased intracranial pressure. In *The clinical practice of neurologic and neurosurgical nursing,* ed 4, Philadelphia, 1997, JB Lippincott, 256-257.
10. House-Park MA: Nursing care of the potential donor. In Chabalewski FL, editor: *Donation & transplantation: nursing curriculum,* Richmond, Va, 1996, UNOS, 105-130.
11. Sullivan J, Seem DL, Chabalewski F: Determining brain death, *Crit Care Nurse* 19(2):37-46, 1999.
12. Holmquist, M, Chabalewski F, Blount T et al: A critical pathway: guiding care for organ donors, *Crit Care Nurse* 19(2):84-100, 1999.
13. Riley LP, Coolican MB: Families of organ donors: facing death and life, *Crit Care Nurse* 19(2):53-59, 1999.
14. Titler MG, Bombei C, Schutte DL: Developing family focused care, *Crit Care Nurs Clin North Am* 7(2):375-386, 1995.
15. Bartucci M: Organ donation: a study of the donor family's perspective, *J Neurosci Nurs* 19:305-309, 1987.
16. Boyd GL, Phillips MG, Henry ML: Cadaver donor management. In *UNOS: organ procurement, preservation and distribution in transplantation,* ed 2, Richmond, Va, 1996, UNOS.
17. Albert P: Direct contact between donor families and recipients: crisis or consolation? *J Transplant Coordination* 8(3):139-144, 1998.
18. Coolican MB, Politoski BA: Donor family programs, *Crit Care Clin North Am* 6(3):613-623, 1994.
19. Lewis DD, Valeruis W: Non-heart-beating organ donation: an answer to the organ shortage, *Crit Care Nurse* 19(2):70-74, 1999.
20. Heffernan L: Legal, economic and religious issues. In Chabalewski FL, editor: *Donation & transplantation: nursing curriculum,* Richmond, Va, 1996, UNOS.
21. Potts JT Jr: *Non-heart-beating organ transplantation: medical and ethical issues in procurement,* Washington, DC, 1997, National Academy.
22. Sheridan FP: A medical examiner's review of organ and tissue donation. In *UNOS: organ procurement, preservation and distribution in transplantation,* ed 2, Richmond, Va, 1996, UNOS.

INDEX

Page numbers followed by f indicate figures; t, tables.